Textbook of Cardiovascular Intervention

Craig A. Thompson
Editor

Textbook of Cardiovascular Intervention

Springer

Editor
Craig A. Thompson, MD, MMSc
Cardiovascular Catheterization and Intervention
Yale New Haven Hospital
New Haven, CT
USA

Cardiology Section, Department of Medicine
Invasive Cardiology and Vascular Medicine
Yale University School of Medicine
New Haven, CT
USA

ISBN 978-1-4471-4527-1 ISBN 978-1-4471-4528-8 (eBook)
DOI 10.1007/978-1-4471-4528-8
Springer London Heidelberg New York Dordrecht

Library of Congress Control Number: 2013953237

Printed on acid-free paper

Springer is part of Springer Science+Business Media (www.springer.com)

My wife, Christi Moore, and daughter, Ainsley Thompson,
who make it all possible and worthwhile…

Preface

We currently live in an extraordinary time in the management of cardiovascular diseases. Catheter-based interventions have evolved to address a variety of needs through innovation and clinical evidence. Interventional cardiovascular medicine continues to be likely the most rapidly evolving and best-studied field in all of the medical and surgical disciplines. Less than four decades have passed since the first coronary balloon angioplasty by Andreas Grüntzig. In this time, the field has grown to a mature specialty where many appropriate patients with coronary disease can have definitive improvements in lifestyle with PCI compared with stand-alone medical therapy, and many patients with complex disease can have competitive results and outcomes with bypass surgery. The evolution of current PCI techniques, drug-eluting stent support, and success in negotiating even the most complex chronic total occlusions can extend therapy to a lost generation of patients who have historically had poor to no options with any of the aforementioned strategies. It is a testament to the tireless work and dedication of clinicians, medical staff, scientists, and industry that this model for technology and technique development has extended to a variety of other comorbidities that affect our patients' lives on a daily basis. Peripheral vascular disease, a major marker for poor cardiovascular and cerebrovascular outcomes, can be effectively managed with simple percutaneous techniques. These patients can have improved quality of life and, importantly, an opportunity for better cardiovascular health with well-selected and executed interventional methods. Patients with significant stroke risk can have that likelihood reduced in many settings with endovascular techniques. The patient with critical aortic stenosis and clearly impaired longevity and heart failure with high or extreme risk for standard surgical valve replacement now has an option and a potential "lease on life" with transcatheter aortic valve replacement. The list is extensive, but the point is consistent and robust. Surgical and interventional fields continue to blend in gray scale with significant synergy and overlap, and medical therapy and understanding of disease are as good as ever.

Given the vast expansion of technologies, techniques, and the clinical evidence base in the information age, it can be challenging for the practicing clinician, fellow-in-training, or technology developer to maintain general knowledge of the interventional cardiovascular space. With this dilemma in mind, I was delighted to collaborate with Springer to develop a textbook of interventional cardiology. Our goal is to provide a practical, information dense, compact textbook with enhanced graphics and broad exposure to the current interventional field that can be digested by the reader as well as a reference tool. We have given a strengthened voice to noncoronary interventional medicine to recognize the current importance and need for total patient management. We will provide the message in a classic text format but also in a variety of digital formats to provide optimal access to information. For readers requiring additional detail on given topics, our chapters are well referenced and linkage to the sources, simple.

The greatest asset of this text is the perspectives of the best-in-class author-contributors. It has been my honor and deep pleasure to work with the world's greatest minds on chapters in their specialty areas. This editorial process has been an educational and enlightening experience for me. While there are far too many individuals to acknowledge in this preface, I would like to thank the efforts for all who contributed chapters; to Margaret Burns, who was fantastic with the logistics of project development; to Vicky John, the associate editor from Springer; and to the entire team (editorial, illustrations) at Springer. Finally, I would like to acknowledge Grant Weston from Springer, who championed the need for this type of educational platform in its early inception and is in many ways responsible for this being a reality today.

The contributors, to a person, have my deepest gratitude for helping with this project.

New Haven, CT, USA Craig A. Thompson, MD, MMSc

Contents

1 **Invasive Hemodynamics** 1
Robert R. Attaran and Michael W. Cleman

2 **Optimal Angiographic Technique and Quantitative Analysis** 9
Alexandra J. Lansky, Cody Pietras, Kamran Haleem, and Vivian Ng

3 **Quantitative, Qualitative, and Diagnostic Intravascular Ultrasound** 23
Ning Guo and Gary S. Mintz

4 **Patient Selection for Coronary Intervention** 41
N.S. Rajendra and A.H. Gershlick

5 **Contrast Nephropathy and Kidney Injury** 53
Jeremiah R. Brown and Peter A. McCullough

6 **Vascular Access, Closure, and Management** 65
Matthew W. Sherwood and Sunil V. Rao

7 **Guide Catheter Selection, Manipulation, and Support Augmentation for PCI** 79
Jean-Michel Paradis and Stéphane Rinfret

8 **Guidewires and Angioplasty Balloons: The Primer** 91
Vijay S. Ramanath and Craig A. Thompson

9 **Coronary Atherectomy (Rotational, Laser, Directional) and Thrombus Extraction** 99
Bruce D. Hettleman and Jason R. Foerst

10 **Stents: Safety and Efficacy** 115
Marvin H. Eng and David E. Kandzari

11 **Adjunctive Pharmacology for Coronary Intervention** 143
John K. Forrest and Osman Faheem

12 **Robotic-Assisted Coronary Intervention** 157
Jorge C. Magallon and Giora Weisz

13 **The Transradial Approach for Coronary Angiography and Intervention** 167
Michael Mok, Philippe Généreux, and Stéphane Rinfret

14 **Percutaneous Cell Therapy for Acute and Chronic Cardiac Disease** 173
Abdul M. Mozid, S. Arnous, and Anthony Mathur

15 **Physiologic Evaluation of Patients with Ischemic Heart Disease** 193
William F. Fearon

16 **Interventional Management of Acute Myocardial Infarction** 207
Nur Jamal, Ron Reiter, and M. Nicholas Burke

17 **Hemodynamic Support in PCI:** ***From Chronic Heart Failure to Cardiogenic Shock*** 221
Jooby John and Kirk N. Garratt

18 **PCI Considerations in Women: Gender-Specific Outcomes and Challenges** 227
Christopher J. Varughese, Rebecca Pinnelas, Jennifer Yu, and Roxana Mehran

19 **Percutaneous Coronary Interventions in the Elderly** 243
Emmanouil S. Brilakis and Subhash Banerjee

20 **Left Main PCI: Patient Selection and Technique** 253
Seung-Jung Park and Duk-Woo Park

21 **Multivessel Disease** 265
Vishal Kapur, Ajay J. Kirtane, and Jeffrey W. Moses

22 **Coronary Bifurcation Lesions** 277
James T. DeVries and Aaron V. Kaplan

23 **Chronic Total Occlusion Angioplasty: Indications, Appropriateness, and Strategy** 289
J. Aaron Grantham and Craig A. Thompson

24 **The Retrograde Approach to Chronic Total Occlusion PCI** 299
David V. Daniels and William L. Lombardi

25 **Intravascular Ultrasound Applications for Chronic Total Occlusion Percutaneous Intervention** 311
Satoru Sumitsuji

26 **Percutaneous Mitral and Aortic Balloon Valvuloplasty** 317
Igor F. Palacios, Sammy Elmariah, and Dabit Arzamendi

27 **Transcatheter Aortic Valve Therapy** 341
Anita Asgar and Raoul Bonan

28 **Percutaneous Management of Mitral Regurgitation** 351
Jason H. Rogers and John M. Lasala

29 **Upper Extremity Interventions** 371
Tracy Huynh and Carlos Mena-Hurtado

30 **Percutaneous Management of Lower Extremity Arterial Disease: Patient Selection, Techniques, and Technologies** 381
Subhash Banerjee and Kimberly Brayton

31 **Application of Advanced Technologies for the Treatment of Lower Extremity Arterial Disease** 395
Faisal Hasan

32 **Percutaneous Management of Renovascular Diseases** 405
R. Kevin Rogers and Joseph M. Garasic

33 **Endovascular Therapy for Mesenteric Disease** 429
R. Kevin Rogers and Joseph M. Garasic

34 **Endovascular Management of Aortic Aneurysmal and Stenotic Disease** 445
Giovanni Teruzzi and Antonio L. Bartorelli

35 Percutaneous Management of Carotid and Vertebral Artery Disease 481
Zehra Jaffery and Christopher J. White

36 Acute Stroke Intervention 499
James T. DeVries

37 Venous Thromboembolic Disease 511
Ido Weinberg and Michael R. Jaff

Index 531

Contributors

S. Arnous, BSc, MRCP Department of Cardiology, London Chest Hospital, London, UK

Dabit Arzamendi, MD, MSc Interventional Cardiology & Structural Heart Disease, Cardiology Division, Massachusetts General Hospital, Boston, MA, USA

Anita Asgar, MD, FRCPC Transcatheter Valve Therapy Clinic, Institut de Cardiologie de Montreal, Montreal, QC, Canada

Robert R. Attaran, FACC, FASE, FSCAI Miami International Cardiology Consultants, Miami, FL, USA

Subhash Banerjee, MD Division of Cardiology, VA North Texas Healthcare System, Dallas, TX, USA

UT Southwestern Medical School, Dallas, TX, USA

Antonio L. Bartorelli, MD Cardiovascular Section, Department of Clinical Sciences and Community Health, Centro Cardiologico Monzino, University of Milan, Milan, Italy

Raoul Bonan, MD, FACC Department of Medicine, Montreal Heart Institute, Montreal, QC, Canada

Kimberly Brayton, MD Division of Cardiology, VA North Texas Health Care System, Dallas, TX, USA

UT Southwestern Medical School, Dallas, TX, USA

Emmanouil S. Brilakis, MD, PhD UT Southwestern Medical School, Dallas, TX, USA

Cardiac Catheterization Laboratories, VA North Texas Healthcare, Dallas, TX, USA

Jeremiah R. Brown, PhD, MS The Dartmouth Institute for Health Policy and Clinical Practice and Section of Cardiology, Department of Medicine, Community and Family Medicine, Audrey and Theodore Geisel School of Medicine at Dartmouth, Lebanon, NH, USA

M. Nicholas Burke, MD Department of Cardiology, Minneapolis Heart Institute Foundation, Minneapolis, MN, USA

Michael W. Cleman, MD Cardiac Catheterization Laboratory, Heart and Vascular Center, Yale-New Haven Hospital, New Haven, CT, USA

David V. Daniels, MD Palo Alto Medical Foundation, Palo Alto, CA, USA

James T. DeVries, MD, FACC, FSCAI Department of Medicine, Dartmouth Medical School, Lebanon, NH, USA

Division of Cardiology, Dartmouth-Hitchcock Medical Center, Lebanon, NH, USA

Sammy Elmariah, MD, MPH Division of Cardiology, Department of Medicine, Massachusetts General Hospital, Boston, MA, USA

Marvin H. Eng, MD Division of Cardiology, Department of Medicine, University of Texas Health Science Center-San Antonio, San Antonio, TX, USA

Osman Faheem, MD Division of Cardiology, Department of Internal Medicine, Yale University School of Medicine, New Haven, CT, USA

William F. Fearon, MD Division of Cardiovascular Medicine, Stanford University Medical Center, Stanford, CA, USA

Jason R. Foerst, MD Virginia Tech-Carilion School of Medicine and Research Institute, Roanoke, VA, USA

John K. Forrest, MD Yale Transcatheter Valve Program, Section of Cardiology, Cardiac Catheterization Laboratory, Yale Vascular Center and Yale New Haven Hospital, New Haven, CT, USA

Joseph M. Garasic, MD Division of Cardiology, Massachusetts General Hospital, Boston, MA, USA

Kirk N. Garratt, MSc, MD Interventional Cardiology, Lenox Hill Hospital, New York, NY, USA

Philippe Généreux, MD Angiographic Core Laboratory, Cardiovascular Research Foundation, New York, NY, USA

A.H. Gershlick, MB, BS, BSc, FRCP Department of Cardiology, University Hospitals of Leicester, Leicester, UK

J. Aaron Grantham, MD, FACC Department of Medicine, University of Missouri School of Medicine, Columbia, MO, USA

St. Luke's Mid America Heart Institute, Kansas City, MO, USA

Ning Guo, MD, PhD Department of Cardiology, First Affiliated Hospital of Medical College of Xi'an Jiaotong University, Xi'an, China

Faisal Hasan, MD, FACC Section of Cardiovascular Medicine, Yale New Haven Hospital, New Haven, CT, USA

Bruce D. Hettleman, MD, FACC, SCAI Section of Cardiology, Department of Medicine, Dartmouth-Hitchcock Medical Center, Lebanon, NH, USA

Tracy Huynh, MD Interventional Cardiology, Yale-New Haven Hospital, New Haven, CT, USA

Michael R. Jaff, DO Section of Vascular Medicine, Department of Medicine, Massachusetts General Hospital, Boston, MA, USA

Zehra Jaffery, MD John Ochsner Heart and Vascular Institute, Department of Cardiovascular Diseases, Ochsner Clinic Foundation, New Orleans, LA, USA

Nur Jamal, MD Department of Cardiology, Minneapolis Heart Institute Foundation, Minneapolis, MN, USA

Jooby John, MD, MPH Interventional Cardiology, Lenox Hill Hospital, New York, NY, USA

Kamran Haleem, MD Department of Cardiovascular Medicine, Yale New Haven Hospital, New Haven, CT, USA

David E. Kandzari, MD Piedmont Heart Institute, Atlanta, GA, USA

Piedmont Hospital, Atlanta, GA, USA

Aaron V. Kaplan, MD Device Development and Research, Geisel School of Medicine at Dartmouth, Dartmouth Hitchcock Medical Center, Lebanon, NH, USA

Vishal Kapur, MD Division of Cardiology, Department of Medicine, Columbia University Medical Center, New York-Presbyterian Hospital, New York, NY, USA

Ajay J. Kirtane, MD, SM Division of Cardiology, Department of Medicine, Columbia University Medical Center, New York-Presbyterian Hospital, New York, NY, USA

Alexandra J. Lansky, MD Yale Cardiovascular Research, Valve Program, Yale University School of Medicine, New Haven, CT, USA

John M. Lasala, MD, PhD Interventional Cardiology, Cardiac Catheterization Laboratory, Washington University School of Medicine, One Barnes-Jewish Hospital, St. Louis, MO, USA

William L. Lombardi, MD North Cascade Cardiology and St. Joseph Hospital, Bellingham, WA, USA

Jorge C. Magallon, MD Division of Cardiology, Department of Medicine, New York Presbyterian Hospital-Columbia University Medical Center, New York, NY, USA

Anthony Mathur, PhD, FRCP NIHR Biomedical Research Unit, Department of Cardiology, London Chest Hospital, London, UK

Peter A. McCullough, MD, MPH St. John Providence Health System, Providence Park Hospital, Cardiovascular Institute, Warren, MI, USA

Roxana Mehran, MD, FACC, FACP Department of Cardiology, Mount Sinai Medical Center, New York, NY, USA

Carlos Mena-Hurtado, MD Coronary and Peripheral Interventions, Department of Medicine, Yale New Haven Hospital/Yale University, New Haven, CT, USA

Gary S. Mintz, MD Cardiovascular Research Foundation, New York, NY, USA

Michael Mok, MBBS, FRACP Quebec Heart & Lung Institute, Laval University, Quebec City, QC, Canada

Jeffrey W. Moses, MD Division of Cardiology, Department of Medicine, Columbia University Medical Center, New York-Presbyterian Hospital, New York, NY, USA

Abdul M. Mozid, BMedSci, MRCP NIHR Biomedical Research Unit, Department of Cardiology, London Chest Hospital, London, UK

Vivian Ng, MD Department of Internal Medicine, Cardiology Section, Yale University School of Medicine, New Haven, CT, USA

Igor F. Palacios, MD Department of Medicine, Division of Cardiology, Interventional Cardiology, Massachusetts General Hospital, Boston, MA, USA

Harvard Medical School, Boston, MA, USA

Jean-Michel Paradis, MD Multidisciplinary Department of Cardiology, Quebec Heart & Lung Institute, Laval University, Quebec City, QC, Canada

Duk-Woo Park, MD, PhD Division of Cardiology, Department of Medicine, University of Ulsan College of Medicine, Asan Medical Center, Songpa-gu, Seoul, South Korea

Seung-Jung Park, MD, PhD Division of Cardiology, Department of Medicine, University of Ulsan College of Medicine, Asan Medical Center, Songpa-gu, Seoul, South Korea

Cody Pietras, BA Department of Internal Medicine (Division of Cardiology) and the Yale Cardiovascular Research Group, Yale University School of Medicine, New Haven, CT, USA

Rebecca Pinnelas, BS Office of Interventional Cardiology Research, Mount Sinai Medical Center, New York, NY, USA

N.S. Rajendra, MBBS, MRCP, MD Department of Cardiology, Glenfield Hospital, Leicester and Queen's Hospital, Burton, Leicester, UK

Vijay S. Ramanath, MD, FACC Department of Medicine, Texas A & M Health Science Center, College of Medicine, Bryan, TX, USA

Sunil V. Rao, MD Department of Medicine, Duke University Medical Center, Durham, NC, USA

Cardiac Catheterization Laboratories, Durham VA Medical Center, Durham, NC, USA

Ron Reiter, MD Department of Cardiology, Minneapolis Heart Institute Foundation, Minneapolis, MN, USA

Stéphane Rinfret, MD, SM, FRCPC Multidisciplinary Department of Cardiology, Quebec Heart & Lung Institute, Laval University, Quebec City, QC, Canada

Jason H. Rogers, MD Division of Cardiovascular Medicine, UC Davis Medical Center, Sacramento, CA, USA

R. Kevin Rogers, MD, MSc Division of Cardiology, Massachusetts General Hospital, Boston, MA, USA

Matthew Sherwood, MD Department of Cardiovascular Medicine, Duke University Medical Center, Durham, NC, USA

Saturo Sumitsuji, MD Advanced Cardiovascular Therapeutics, Osaka University, Suita, Osaka, Japan

Giovanni Teruzzi, MD Cardiovascular Section, Department of Clinical Sciences and Community Health, Centro Cardiologico Monzino, University of Milan, Milan, Italy

Craig A. Thompson, MD, MMSc Director, Cardiovascular Catheterization and Intervention, Yale New Haven Hospital, New Haven, CT, USA

Cardiology Section, Department of Medicine, Director, Invasive Cardiology and Vascular Medicine, Yale University School of Medicine, New Haven, CT, USA

Christopher J. Varughese, MD Department of Cardiology, The Mount Sinai Hospital, New York, NY, USA

Ido Weinberg, MD, MSc Department of Cardiology, Massachusetts General Hospital, Boston, MA, USA

Giora Weisz, MD Columbia University, New York, NY, USA

Center for Interventional Vascular Therapy, New-York Presbyterian Hospital – Columbia University Medical Center, New York, NY, USA

Christopher J. White, MD Department of Cardiovascular Diseases, Ochsner Clinic Foundation, New Orleans, LA, USA

Jennifer Yu, MBBS, FRACP Department of Cardiology, Mount Sinai Medical Center, New York, NY, USA

Invasive Hemodynamics

1

Robert R. Attaran and Michael W. Cleman

The first cardiac catheterization for scientific enquiry was arguably performed in the 1700s by English pastor and veterinarian, Stephen Hales. In 1727, Hales recorded the first blood pressure by inserting pipes into the arteries of animals. He also inserted tubes, including gun barrels, into cardiac chambers in order to measure stroke volume.

It is the aim of invasive hemodynamics to determine, as accurately as possible, heart and circulatory system pressure, flow, and resistance. Pressure is typically measured by connecting a fluid (saline)-filled catheter to a pressure transducer that is usually an electrical strain gauge. After transduction of pressure changes into electricity using the Wheatstone bridge principle, the obtained signal is demonstrated as a continuous pressure tracing. Before pressure measurements are taken, the transducer setup is "zeroed" at the same elevation as the atria by momentarily directing its connection to atmospheric air.

Right Atrium

The normal right atrial pressure waveform (mean 0–8 mmHg) has three positive components, *a*-, *c*-, and v-waves, as well as x and y descents (Fig. 1.1, Tables 1.1 and 1.2). During examination of neck pulsations, the x descent coincides with systole and therefore the carotid upstroke. Typically the a-wave follows the P wave on the ECG and is greater in amplitude than the v-wave. The mean RA pressure falls with natural inspiration and rises with expiration. The a-wave can be preceded by a small peak called the "h-wave," which is typically absent unless there is bradycardia or elevated venous pressures.

Left Atrium

Mean pressures (5–10 mmHg) tend to be higher than in the right atrium with v-waves being more prominent than a-waves. Left atrial pressures can reflect left ventricular preload as well as compliance. They can be estimated invasively by obtaining the pulmonary artery wedge pressure (PAWP). In the setting of mitral stenosis, there will be a pressure gradient between the left atrium and left ventricle. Throughout diastole, the PAWP will be higher than the LV pressure *and* will remain higher at end-diastole. The area under the curve of the pressure gradient can be utilized to calculate mitral valve area (discussed later).

Right and Left Ventricle

The ventricular waveform includes a brisk early systolic rise and a brisk fall in early diastole (typical values 25/5 mmHg in the right, 120/10 mmHg in the left). There can be an end-diastolic peak corresponding to atrial contraction, sometimes referred to as the "post-a-wave" left ventricular end-diastolic pressure. Elevated LVEDP (greater than 12 mmHg) can be associated with abnormal left ventricular filling or compliance. A thorough evaluation should mention both pre- and post-a-wave values for LVEDP.

Aortic and Pulmonic Artery Pressures

In the aorta and pulmonary artery, there is a pronounced systolic upstroke, followed by a downstroke with a brief positive deflection due to aortic valve closure (dicrotic notch)

R.R. Attaran, FACC, FASE, FSCAI
Miami International Cardiology Consultants,
3801 Biscayne, Blvd, Miami, FL, USA

M.W. Cleman, MD (✉)
Cardiac Catheterization Laboratory. Heart and Vascular Center,
Yale-New Haven Hospital, New Haven, CT, USA
e-mail: michael.cleman@yale.edu

C.A. Thompson (ed.), *Textbook of Cardiovascular Intervention*,
DOI 10.1007/978-1-4471-4528-8_1, © Springer-Verlag London 2014

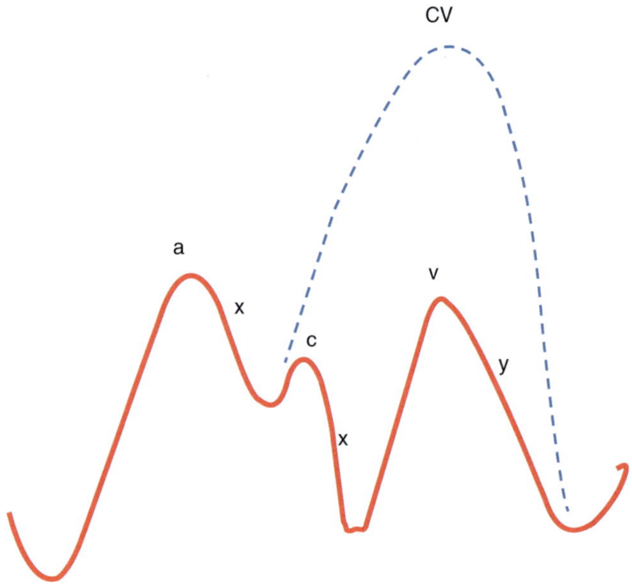

Fig. 1.1 Atrial pressure waveforms. The *dotted line* represents the "c-v"-wave seen in the right atrium from severe tricuspid regurgitation

Table 1.1 Atrial waveforms and their etiology

a	Atrial contraction
x	Right atrial rela(x)ation
c	Early ventricular contraction resulting in upward tricuspid valve movement
v	Atrial filling
y	Right atrial empt(y)ing

Table 1.2 Right atrial pressure in specific scenarios

Atrial septal defect (large)	Equalization of a and v amplitudes
Severe tricuspid regurgitation	Large "c-v"-waves
Atrial fibrillation or flutter	Absence of a-waves
AV dissociation or dyssynchrony (e.g., complete AV block)	Cannon a-waves
Pericardial tamponade	Loss of y (and possibly x) descent; equalization of right and left atrial (wedge) pressure
Constriction	Rapid y descent – more pronounced with inspiration
Restriction	Rapid x and y descent

(Fig. 1.2). The mean aortic pressure is somewhat lower distally than proximally, although there may be a slight rise in the systolic pressure. In the setting of significant aortic regurgitation, there can be end-diastolic pressure equalization between the LV and aorta (Fig. 1.3).

Mean pulmonary artery pressures less than 21 mmHg are considered normal. Mean values above 25 mmHg suggest pulmonary hypertension.

Pulmonary *arterial* hypertension is a more specific diagnosis and carries four criteria:

1. Resting mean pulmonary artery pressure >25 mmHg
2. Pulmonary vascular resistance >3 Wood units
3. Pulmonary artery wedge pressure <15 mmHg
4. Absence of other causes of pulmonary hypertension

Echocardiography has largely replaced right heart catheterization as the modality of choice for evaluating pulmonary artery pressures. In certain circumstances, both modalities are used. For instance, heart transplant recipient candidates are typically referred for both procedures. While some studies show a good correlation between pulmonary pressures as estimated by both modalities, results from the clinical arena show both poor correlation and modest agreement, due to a number of factors including patient hydration and sedation status during invasive studies as well as echocardiographic technique.

Pulmonary Artery Wedge Pressure (PAWP)

The PAWP estimates left atrial pressure (normal range 8–12 mmHg). The careful advancement of a pulmonary artery catheter, with its balloon tip inflated, will normally "wedge" the balloon such that arterial flow is interrupted beyond that point and the pressure tracing changes. In case of uncertainty, an arterial sample obtained from this position should yield an oxygen saturation very similar to aortic values.

Wedge pressure waveforms follow those of the left atrium, with an a-wave corresponding to atrial contraction followed by an x descent due to atrial rela(x)ation, a v-wave corresponding to atrial filling, followed by a y descent due to atrial empt(y)ing. The x descent corresponds with the QRS complex on ECG. The v-wave has a larger amplitude than the a-wave, reflecting left atrial pressure characteristics.

PAWP, as with the PA pressure, should typically be measured at the end of expiration, just before the inspiratory decline. With mechanically ventilated patients, PAWP is measured just before the inspiratory rise in pressure. While the PAWP reflects left atrial pressure, it can be higher in the presence of mitral stenosis or pulmonary venous hypertension, for example (Fig. 1.4). If suspected, a simultaneous LVEDP should be measured.

Cardiac Output

Indicator dilution and Fick equation are the principal invasive means in present use to estimate cardiac output. Indicator dilution is based on the principle that if a known quantity of a tracer is introduced into the circulation, its concentration over time can be used to estimate circulating volume. One

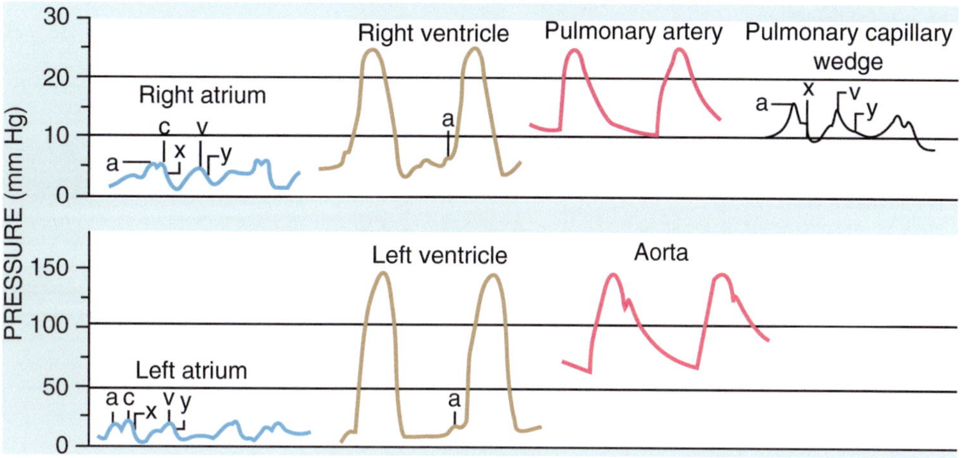

Fig. 1.2 Classic atrial, ventricular, and pulmonary artery pressure tracings

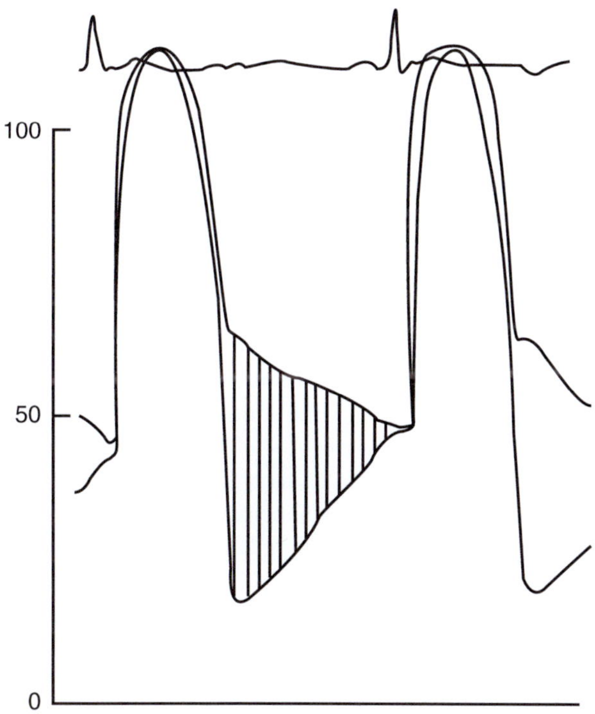

Fig. 1.3 Left ventricular and aortic pressure tracings in severe aortic regurgitation. Note the wide aortic pulse pressure and the end-diastolic equalization of pressures

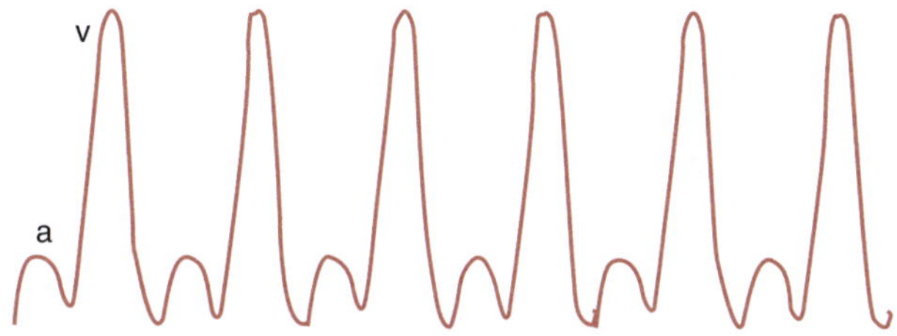

Fig. 1.4 Pulmonary artery wedge pressure waveform with "giant v-waves" that can be seen in severe mitral regurgitation, ventricular septal defect, as well as mitral stenosis and with a stiffened left ventricle

example of this principle, thermodilution, measures iced or room temperature saline, injected from a more proximal port within the RA and measured by a thermistor in the PA. The area under curve provides an estimate of cardiac output. Usually 3–5 separate measurements are made and outlier values eliminated. This technique can be less reliable in the setting of severe tricuspid and pulmonic regurgitation, as well as intracardiac shunting.

German physiologist and inventor of the contact lens, Adolf Fick (1829–1901) determined that regional uptake of a substance by an organ, in this case oxygen by the lungs, is the product of blood flow to the lungs and the arteriovenous oxygen concentration difference across the lungs. To determine intravascular oxygen content, oxygen saturation samples obtained from the pulmonary artery and aorta are essential for this calculation. In clinical practice the femoral artery sheath is often used to draw an aortic blood sample surrogate. The utilization of pulmonary and aortic blood to estimate pulmonary oxygen uptake assumes that there is no R-to-L shunting at the intracardiac level. The Fick equation also requires estimation of lung oxygen uptake. While some labs measure this directly, for example, using a Douglas bag or polarography, another approach is to estimate it. The normal oxygen consumption rate is approximately 125 ml/m^2 of body surface area, or 3 ml O_2/min/kg, but this value differs with age and sex:

$$\text{Cardiac Output} = O_2 \text{ consumption} \left(\text{ml}/\text{min}\right) / \text{arteriovenous } O_2 \text{ difference} \times [\text{Hb}] \times 10 \left(\text{Normal cardiac output } 4-8\ \text{L}/\text{min, normal cardiac index } 2.5-4\ \text{L}/\text{min}/\text{m}^2\right)$$

[Hb] = serum hemoglobin concentration

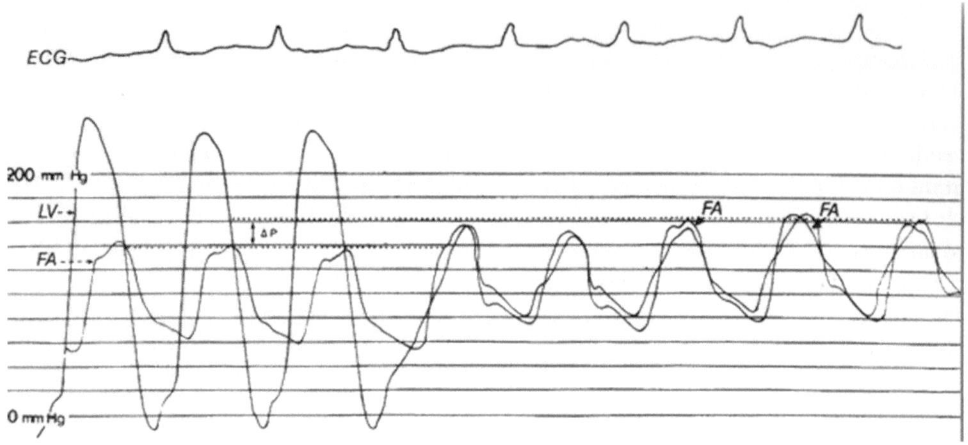

Fig. 1.5 Simultaneous ventricular and aortic pressure recordings during a "pullback" through a severely stenosed aortic valve. Note the slight rise in aortic systolic pressures once the catheter has been pulled out, a phenomenon described by Carabello, seen to occur in aortic valve areas ≤0.6 cm²

Vascular Resistance

Derived from Ohm's law ($R = \Delta P/Q$), vascular resistance is calculated by dividing the pressure gradient across a vascular bed by the flow through it:

$$\text{Pulmonary vascular resistance} = \left(\frac{\text{mPAP} - \text{mPAWP}}{\text{cardiac output}}\right)$$

$$\text{Systemic vascular resistance} = \left(\frac{\text{mSBP} - \text{mRAP}}{\text{cardiac output}}\right)$$

mPAP = mean pulmonary artery pressure, mPAWP = mean pulmonary artery wedge pressure, mSBP = mean systolic blood pressure, mRAP = mean right atrial pressure

Resistance is measured in hybrid reference units or Wood units (mmHg/L/min). By multiplying by 80, the value is converted into dynes.s.cm^{-5}. Pulmonary vascular resistance (PVR) is normally less than 1.7 Wood units, about one tenth that of systemic vascular resistance (SVR). PVR is increased by various factors including blood viscosity, hypoxia, and acidosis. Pulmonary hypertension is said to be reversible with vasodilators if mean PAP falls by ≥10 mmHg to below 40 mmHg, or PVR must fall below 5 Wood units, without loss of cardiac output.

Calculations of Valvular Area

An ideal valve should provide little or no resistance to forward flow of blood. Valvular stenosis or obstruction results in a pressure gradient, the extent of which can be influenced by not only the severity and length of the stenosis but also cardiac output, chamber compliance, and afterload, among others. A normal aortic valve area is in the 3–4 cm² range. Values less than 1 cm² are consistent with severe stenosis (Fig. 1.5). Valvular area is typically calculated by simultaneous measurement of pressure waveforms before and after the valve of interest using catheters such as the pigtail and measuring cardiac output by right heart catheterization.

Gorlin's formula measures valve area as follows:

$$\text{Valve area} = \text{CO} / \text{HR} \times (\text{DFP or SEP})\ K \times C \times \sqrt{\ }\text{mean}\Delta P$$

CO = cardiac output. HR = heart rate; K is 44.3, a constant derived by Gorlin. C is 1 for the aortic and pulmonic valves, and 0.85 for the mitral valve. DFP = diastolic filling period. SFP = systolic filling period

In order to apply the Gorlin formula, for instance, to the aortic valve area, simultaneous left ventricular and aortic pressure tracings should be recorded and any difference should be measured by planimetry, incorporating systolic ejection period. Catheterization lab software will readily make such calculations.

An easier formula to apply is the Hakki:

$$\text{Valve area} = \text{CO} / \sqrt{\ }\text{peak}\Delta P$$

CO = cardiac output; $\sqrt{\ }$ peakΔP = square root of peak-to-peak pressure gradient

As cardiac output is within the numerator of both the Gorlin and Hakki formulae, a low cardiac output state can overestimate the severity of aortic stenosis.

Most operators will incorporate pullback of a pigtail catheter into their left heart catheterization. While this method is not relied upon as the sole means of evaluating aortic stenosis, it can help screen for a significant peak-to-peak gradient across the aortic valve. Furthermore, a slow pullback can help identify a significant subaortic gradient, such as that seen with a subaortic membrane.

A commonly used technique for the measurement of aortic stenosis severity is the simultaneous recording of pressures within the left ventricle and the femoral artery, where the arterial access has been made. Error can be introduced into this technique due to downstream augmentation of pressures as well as time delays between pressure waveforms, although some lab software can offer correction for the latter. The authors prefer to use the double-lumen pigtail catheter (Langston, Vascular Solutions) for continuous recording. This double-lumen design allows for simultaneous measurement of pressures on either side of the aortic valve. These techniques can all be confounded by the Carabello sign. In aortic valve areas ≤0.6 cm², the catheter can be significantly occlusive and aortic pressure rises when the catheter is backed out of the aorta (Fig. 1.5).

When comparing estimates of aortic valvular stenosis obtained by cardiac catheterization to echocardiography, discrepancies can be noted. The severity of aortic stenosis can be exaggerated by echocardiography. One explanation is the presence of pressure recovery. Pressure recovery is the increase in pressure downstream from a stenotic segment. Echo estimates of pressure are derived from velocity of flow, as applied to the continuity equation. Hydrodynamic theory suggests that a flow "field" will taper just proximal to a stenotic orifice, converges even more within the stenosis, and reaches its smallest just beyond the stenotic segment (vena contracta). As the blood field diverges and loses momentum beyond the stenotic valve, its pressure rises. Therefore, pressure is lower immediately upon entering the aortic root, after which the pressure rises ("recovers"). Doppler echocardiography estimates valvular stenosis by comparing the velocity within the left ventricular outflow tract to that within the vena contracta.

Post-Premature Ventricular Contraction Pulse Pressure in Hypertrophic Obstructive Cardiomyopathy (HOCM) Versus Aortic Stenosis

In aortic stenosis, pulse pressure classically increases post-PVC, whereas in HOCM it decreases. Post-PVC, due to Starling's law, the compensatory pause will result in a greater force of ventricular contraction. In aortic stenosis, the obstruction is fixed; therefore, the powerful post-PVC ventricular contraction will lead to a higher systolic aortic pressure (and therefore higher pulse pressure). With HOCM, the obstruction is dynamic. Post-PVC, though the ventricular contraction is more forceful, the severity of the stenosis increases dramatically; therefore, the peak aortic pressure falls, as does the pulse pressure. This post-PVC drop in pulse pressure in HOCM is known as the Brockenbrough–Braunwald–Morrow sign.

A frequently used technique to provoke a PVC is to gently probe the left ventricular endocardial surface with a multipurpose catheter while observing pressure tracings from the femoral artery sheath.

Shunt Calculations

Cardiac output, as a singular concept, becomes inaccurate in the presence of shunts, where it is often more accurate to state systemic and pulmonic flow separately and to consider the extent and direction of shunting. Effective flow is the theoretical flow of blood through a system if no shunt was present. Recirculated systemic and pulmonary flow is calculated by subtracting effective flow from systemic and pulmonic flow, respectively. Recirculated pulmonic flow is the amount of L-to-R shunting (of oxygenated blood), and recirculated systemic flow represents R-to-L shunting (of deoxygenated blood).

In the absence of a shunt, effective flow, systemic flow, and pulmonic flow are all equal:

$$\text{Oxygen content}\ (\text{ml}/\text{L}) = 1.36 \times 10 \times [\text{Hb}] \times \text{oxygen saturation}$$

$$\text{Mixed venous oxygen saturation} = (3\text{SVC O}_2 + \text{IVC O}_2)/4$$

$$\text{Systemic flow}\ (Q_s) = \text{VO}_2 / \left[\begin{array}{l} (\text{FAO}_2 - \text{MVO}_2) \\ \times 1.36 \times [\text{Hb}] \times 10 \end{array} \right]$$

$$\text{Pulmonic flow}\ (Q_p) = \text{VO}_2 / \left[\begin{array}{l} (\text{PVO}_2 - \text{PAO}_2) \\ \times 1.36 \times [\text{Hb}] \times 10 \end{array} \right]$$

$$\text{Effective flow}\ (Q_e) = \text{VO}_2 / \left[\begin{array}{l} (\text{PVO}_2 - \text{MVO}_2) \\ \times 1.36 \times [\text{Hb}] \times 10 \end{array} \right]$$

$$Q_p / Q_s = (\text{FAO}_2 - \text{MVO}_2)/(\text{PVO}_2 - \text{PAO}_2)$$

or in practice FAO_2 or sometimes the value 95 % is substituted for PVO_2, assuming no shunt

$$\text{Recirculated pulmonary flow} = \text{pulmonic flow} - \text{effective flow}$$

$$\text{Recirculated systemic flow} = \text{systemic flow} - \text{effective flow}$$

VO_2 = oxygen uptake rate, FAO_2 = femoral artery oxygen saturation, PVO_2 = pulmonary vein oxygen saturation, MVO_2 = mixed venous oxygen saturation, PAO_2 = pulmonary artery oxygen saturation, SVC O_2 = superior vena cava oxygen saturation, IVC O_2 = inferior vena cava oxygen saturation

The location of a shunt is determined by measuring oxygen saturation within the great vessels and cardiac chambers, wherever accessible by catheters. For instance, an increase in oxygen saturations above that expected for the right-sided

Table 1.3 Significant oxygen saturation step-up percentage values suggesting a shunt

Right atrium/SVC/IVC	7 %
Ventricular/great vessels	5 %

Table 1.4 Hemodynamic changes with pericardial tamponade

Tachycardia, hypotension, and reduced cardiac output
Elevated filling pressures in all cardiac chambers
Diastolic equalization of cardiac chamber pressures
Inspiratory decline in peak aortic pressure >10–12 mmHg (pulsus paradoxus)

chambers implies L-to-R shunting of oxygenated blood (Table 1.3). Smaller shunts, however, e.g., less than 20 % of pulmonary blood flow, may be undetectable by saturation measurements alone.

Special Case Scenarios

Pericardial Tamponade

The rapid recognition of this emergency is vital in order to institute rapid treatment. While echocardiography is now the gold standard means of evaluating a patient with tamponade, understanding the invasive hemodynamics remains important (Table 1.4).

Pericardial tamponade is not an all-or-none phenomenon, but rather a continuum. It begins with rising pericardial pressures that lead to elevated atrial and ventricular filling pressures, eventually resulting in a fall in cardiac output and death. Pulsus paradoxus, the inspiratory fall with systolic blood pressure, becomes greater as tamponade progresses. In tamponade, the y descent, which represents atrial emptying, is absent or attenuated. This is because right atrial and RV diastolic pressures are equalized; thus, little or no flow occurs in early ventricular diastole.

Constriction Versus Restriction

Despite their differing pathophysiologies, differentiation of constriction from restriction remains a challenge due to some overlap in hemodynamic features. Simply put, pericardial constraint occurs due to scarring and stiffening of the pericardial sac. This results in impaired ventricular filling in the later phases of diastole as the stiff pericardial sac is stretched to its limits. As a result, ventricular filling is brisk in early diastole. The limited space created by this inelastic pericardium results in ventricular interdependence. Constriction also results in isolation of intracardiac chambers from transmission of respiratory intrathoracic pressure changes. Restriction occurs due to a rigid, non-dilated ventricular myocardium with resultant severe diastolic dysfunction and restrictive filling.

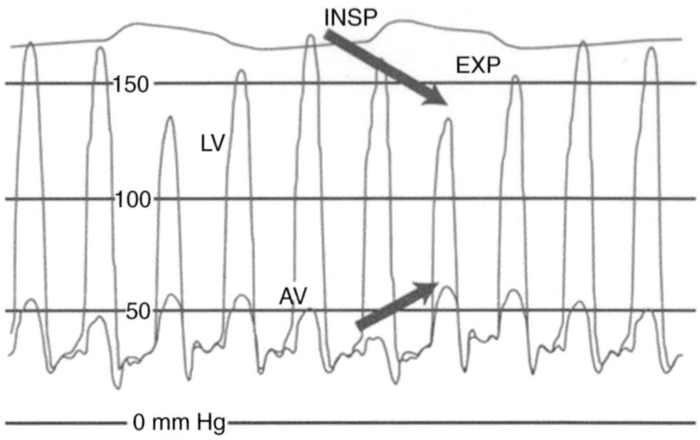

Fig. 1.6 Discordance of right and left ventricular pressure with respiration in pericardial constriction

The pericardium covers all cardiac chambers with the exception of the left atrium that is only partially covered. With a normal pericardium, inspiration transmits a decreased intrathoracic pressure uniformly to the pulmonary veins, pericardial space, and all four cardiac chambers. In constriction, the inelastic and thickened pericardium can isolate the right atrium, right ventricle, and left ventricle from intrathoracic pressure changes. Therefore, inspiratory declines in intrathoracic pressure are transmitted to the pulmonary veins and left atrium (PAWP), but not to the other cardiac chambers ("dissociation"). During inspiration, the left atrial pressure falls whereas the LV diastolic pressure does not. This results in a lower transmitral diastolic flow, less LV filling, and therefore a lower LV stroke volume. The presence of an inelastic pericardium will result in ventricular interdependence. Reduced LV filling will allow space for proportionately more RV filling; thus, RV stroke volume will be higher.

The opposite will occur during expiration where left atrial pressures will rise compared to LV diastolic pressure, resulting in greater transmitral flow, greater LV filling and stroke volume, and concomitant reduced RV filling due to interdependence. Greater LV stroke volumes translate to higher LV pressures and these will be noted during continuous pressure recordings. In restriction, the pericardium remains compliant, and if anything, it is the interventricular septum that may be noncompliant. Therefore, in constriction there is significant respiratory variation in LV/RV filling, but not in restriction. A very useful technique to distinguish constriction from restriction, therefore, is the simultaneous recording of pressures within the LV and RV. Respiratory ventricular pressure discordance will support diagnosis of constriction (Fig. 1.6). Pressure concordance will suggest restriction (Fig. 1.7).

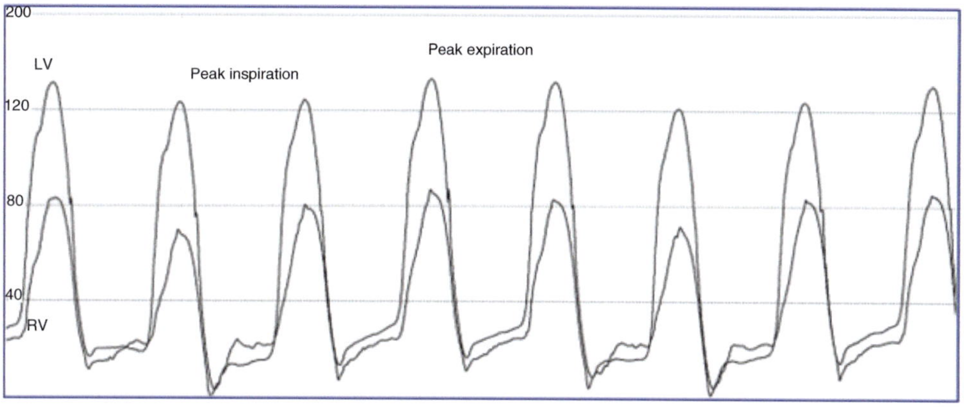

Fig. 1.7 Concordance of right and left ventricular pressure changes with respiration in restrictive cardiomyopathy

Table 1.5 Traditional and novel criteria used to differentiate constriction from restriction

Hemodynamic criteria	Constriction	Restriction
LVEDP–RVEDP (mmHg)	≤5	>5
PASP (mmHg)	≤50	>50
RVEDP/RVSP	>1/3	<1/3
Inspiratory decrease in RAP (mmHg)	<5	>5
Systolic area index	>1.1	<1.1

In both constriction and restriction, atrial pressures should be classically elevated, unless the patient has been diuresed. The authors, if encountering a patient with RAP less than 15 mmHg, referred for evaluation of possible constriction or restriction, will often bolus a liter of normal saline.

In constriction, the inspiratory fall in right atrial pressure is blunted or absent, for reasons given above. However, the y descent may be more pronounced. The so-called dip and plateau effect is controversial and has been described in both constriction and restriction and cannot help distinguish between the two.

The first four criteria cited in Table 1.5 for the diagnosis of constriction lack specificity. Systolic area index is a measure of ventricular discordance and follows concepts described above. Using high-fidelity manometry, ventricular pressure tracings obtained from the LV and RV were obtained during exaggerated respiration and areas under curve compared. The systolic area index was defined as the ratio of the RV area (mm Hg × s) to the LV area (mm Hg × s) in inspiration versus expiration. Values greater than 1.1 were 97 % sensitive and 100 % specific for constriction [12].

References

1. Attaran R, Sorrell VL, Movahed MR. Poor correlation of pulmonary systolic pressure using echocardiography versus right heart catheterization in patients awaiting heart transplantation. Transplant Proc. 2009;41:3827–30.
2. Brown L, Kahl F, Link K, et al. Anatomic landmarks for use when measuring intracardiac pressure with fluid-filled catheters. Am J Cardiol. 2000;86:121–4.
3. Campbell P, Drazner MH, Kato M. Mismatch of right- and left-sided filling pressures in chronic heart failure. J Card Fail. 2011;17:561–8.
4. Carabello BA, Barry WH, Grossman W. Changes in arterial pressure during left heart pullback in patients with aortic stenosis: a sign of severe aortic stenosis. Am J Cardiol. 1979;44:424–7.
5. Fuchs RM, Heuser RR, Yin FC, et al. Limitations of pulmonary wedge V waves in diagnosing mitral regurgitation. Am J Cardiol. 1982;49:849–54.
6. Gorlin R, Gorlin SG. Hydraulic formula for calculation of stenotic mitral valve, other cardiac valves, and central circulatory shunts. Am Heart J. 1951;41:1–29.
7. Gössl M, Rihal CS. Cardiac shunt calculations made easy: a case-based approach. Catheter Cardiovasc Interv. 2010;76:137–42.
8. Hakki AH, Iskandrian AS, Bemis CE, et al. A simplified valve formula for the calculation of stenotic aortic valve areas. Circulation. 1981;63:1050–5.
9. Hillis LD, Firth BG, Winniford MD. Analysis of factors affecting the variability of Fick versus indicator dilution measurements of cardiac output. Am J Cardiol. 1985;56:764–8.
10. Kendrick AH, West J, Papouchado M, et al. Direct Fick cardiac output: are assumed values of oxygen consumption acceptable? Eur Heart J. 1988;9:337–42.
11. Sorajja P. Invasive hemodynamics of constrictive pericarditis, restrictive cardiomyopathy, and cardiac tamponade. Cardiol Clin. 2011;29:191–9.
12. Talreja DR, Nishimura RA, Oh JK, et al. Constrictive pericarditis in the modern era: novel criteria for diagnosis in the cardiac catheterization laboratory. JACC. 2008;51:315–19.

Optimal Angiographic Technique and Quantitative Analysis

2

Alexandra J. Lansky, Cody Pietras, Kamran Haleem, and Vivian Ng

The rapid rise of new percutaneous coronary intervention (PCI) techniques and devices has necessitated standardized methods of evaluating coronary artery disease (CAD) severity and the effect of treatments on the natural history of the disease. Coronary angiography is the gold standard for evaluating coronary artery disease (CAD), but subjective evaluation of angiographically apparent CAD is limited by high levels of intra- and inter-observer variability [1–3]. Thus, methods and algorithms for quantitative coronary angiography (QCA) have been developed in order to objectively quantify the extent of CAD. This chapter will discuss proper techniques for angiographic image acquisition, the current tools and practice of quantitative angiographic analysis, and common angiographic measurement parameters.

Angiographic Image Acquisition

Basic Anatomic Projections and Vessel Orientation

Optimal coronary angiography is dependent on a thorough knowledge of coronary anatomy and its variations and a systematic imaging sequence protocol that enables visualization of all coronary segments, particularly areas of vessel overlap, bifurcations, or tortuous anatomy.

A basic map of the coronary anatomy is delineated in Fig. 2.1 and the optimal views for imaging each coronary segment are summarized in Table 2.1. The right and left coronary systems including the left main, left anterior descending coronary artery (LAD), and left circumflex (LCx) with their respective branch vessels are best visualized by a series of imaging views that include the anterior-posterior (AP) (Fig. 2.2), the left anterior oblique (LAO) (Fig. 2.3), the right anterior oblique (RAO) (Fig. 2.4), and the left lateral (Fig. 2.5) views with varying degrees of cranial or caudal angulation. While standard views are generally consistent from one patient to the next, the precise angulations tend to vary based on variations in anatomical orientation. The Coronary Artery

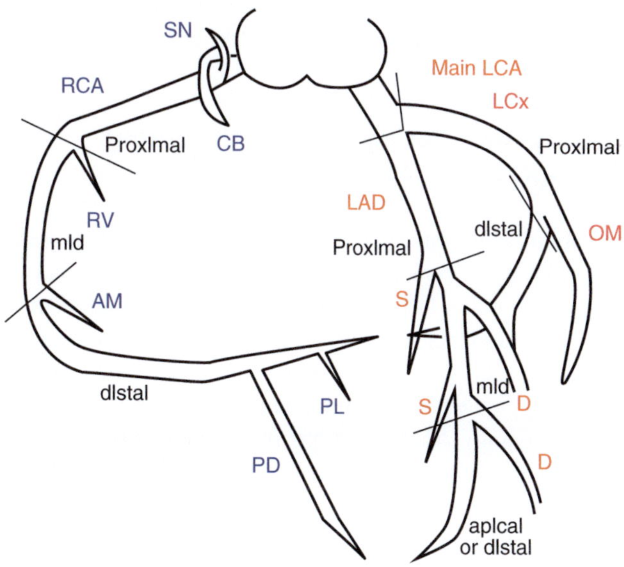

Fig. 2.1 Schematic diagram of the coronary anatomy. *RCA* right coronary artery, *SN* sinus nodal artery, *CB* conus branch, *RV* right ventricular artery, *AM* acute marginal artery, *PD* posterior descending artery, *PL* posterior lateral artery, *LCA* left coronary artery, *LAD* left anterior descending artery, *S* septal branch, *D* diagonal branch, *LCx* left circumflex, *OM* obtuse marginal artery

A.J. Lansky, MD (✉)
Yale Cardiovascular Research Group, Valve Program, Yale University School of Medicine, One Church Street, Suite 330, New Haven, CT, 06510, USA
e-mail: alexandra.lansky@yale.edu

C. Pietras, BA
Department of Internal Medicine (Division of Cardiology) and the Yale Cardiovascular Research Group, Yale University School of Medicine, New Haven, CT, USA

K. Haleem, MD
Department of Cardiovascular Medicine, Yale New Haven Hospital, 333 Cedar St., New Haven, CT 06520, USA

V. Ng, MD
Department of Internal Medicine, Cardiology Section, Yale University School of Medicine, 333 Cedar St., New Haven, CT 06520, USA

C.A. Thompson (ed.), *Textbook of Cardiovascular Intervention*,
DOI 10.1007/978-1-4471-4528-8_2, © Springer-Verlag London 2014

Table 2.1 Views for optimal visualization of the coronary anatomy

	AP	LAO	RAO	Left lateral
Left main	Optimal view for LM	*LAO/caudal:* bifurcation of LAD, LCx, and Ramus		
LAD	AP/cranial	*LAO/cranial:* prox LAD, diagonals, septals *Straight LAO:* mid and distal LAD	*RAO cranial or caudal:* mid, distal LAD, diagonals	Mid and distal LAD
LCX		*Steep LAO/cranial:* prox LCx	*RAO/caudal:* proximal, mid LCx, and OMs	
RCA		*Steep LAO:* ostial, proximal RCA *LAO/cranial:* distal RCA, PDA, crux and PLSA	*Straight RAO:* mid RCA *RAO/cranial:* PDA and PLSA	Mid and distal RCA, PDA

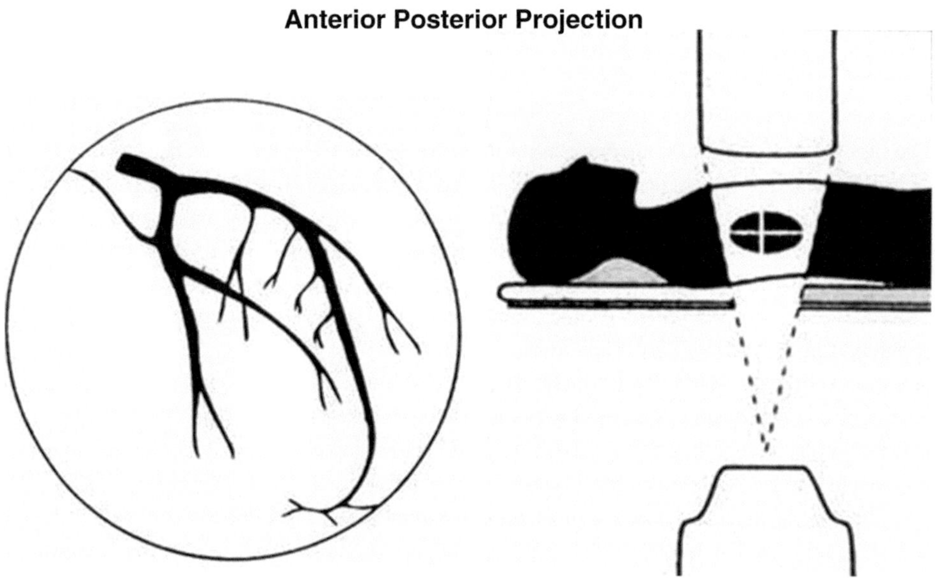

Fig. 2.2 Anterior-posterior (*AP*) view of the left coronary artery. Ideal view to visualize the left main coronary segment

Surgery Study (CASS) numbering system is the most commonly used coronary segment numbering system and has gained wide acceptance in interventional clinical trials [4].

Factors Contributing to Variability during Angiographic Image Acquisition

Variability in the angiographic assessment of vessel diameter and other measurements can be introduced by a number of factors, including biologic differences among lumen diameters (e.g., reference vessel size, vasomotor tone, thrombus) and inconsistencies in radiographic image acquisition parameters (e.g., quantum mottling, out-of-plane magnification, foreshortening). Acquisition parameters should be carefully controlled in order to optimize the overall diagnostic accuracy of quantitative angiography. Common sources of error during angiographic image acquisition and potential corrections are summarized in Table 2.2.

Biologic Variability

Studies that include a wide range of vessel sizes have more biologic variability in vessel diameters (as reflected in the standard deviation of the measurements) than those with more restrictive inclusion criteria. Vasomotor tone may also affect the reference vessel size, resulting in distal vasoconstriction and vasospasm that dynamically affect the arterial diameter in paired measurements. Transient maximum coronary vasodilation may be achieved with intracoronary (50–200 μ(micro)g), intravenous (>10 μ(micro)g/min), or sublingual (0.4–0.8 mg) nitroglycerin, or intracoronary (3 mg) isosorbide dinitrate.

Acquisition Variability

Variable acquisition factors include cardiac and respiratory motion artifact, vessel foreshortening, inadequate filling of the coronary artery ("streaming"), overfilling of the aortic cusp with contrast, and failure to separate overlapping branch vessels from the stenosis. These factors may lead to either overestimation or underestimation of lesion severity. Out-of-plane magnification and pincushion distortion may also contribute to small errors in angiographic imaging. For sequential studies, using the identical angiographic imaging laboratory allows replication of the X-ray generator, tube, and image intensifier parameters.

Data Compression Variability

One limitation of the cineless catheterization laboratory is the vast volume of digital data required for storage and real time retrieval. On average a single interventional case requires a 7.5 MB per second transfer rate. Data compression and subsequent decompression may minimize archiving space and data transfer time but can also introduce variability if not

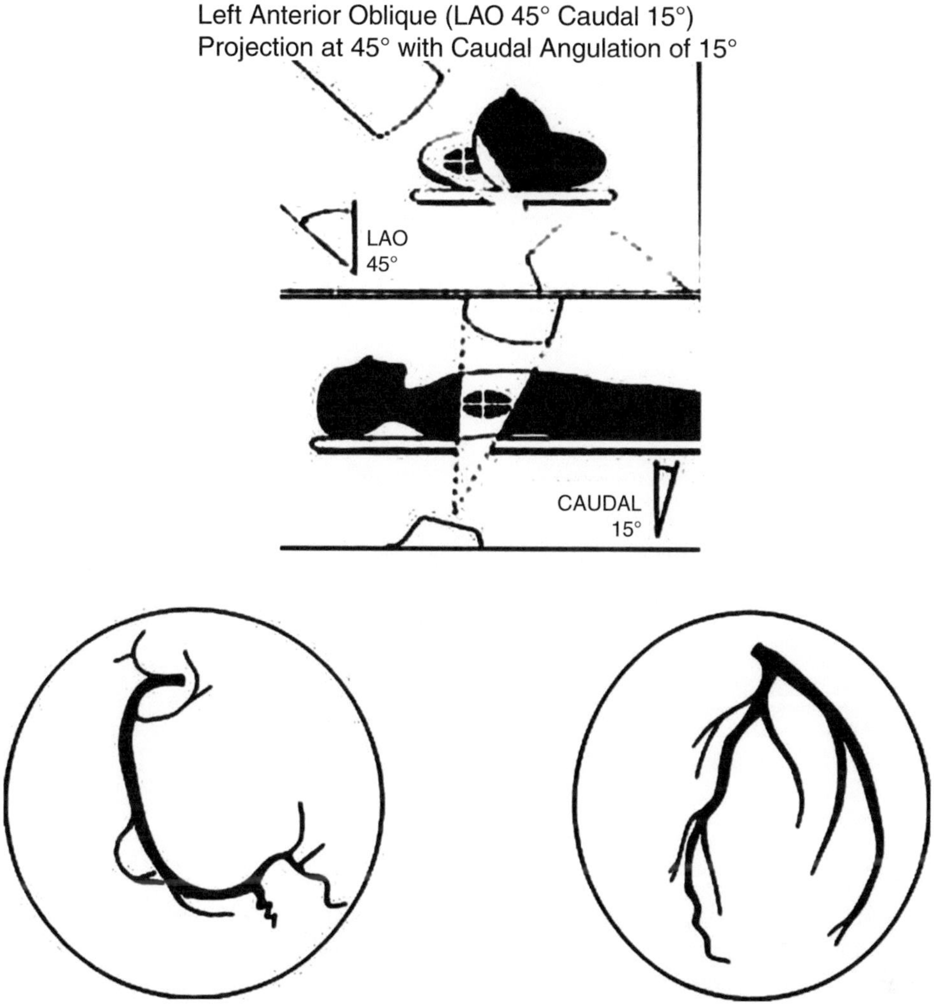

Fig. 2.3 Left anterior oblique (*LAO*) view of the left and right coronary arteries. Ideal view to visualize the mid and distal left anterior descending and right coronary

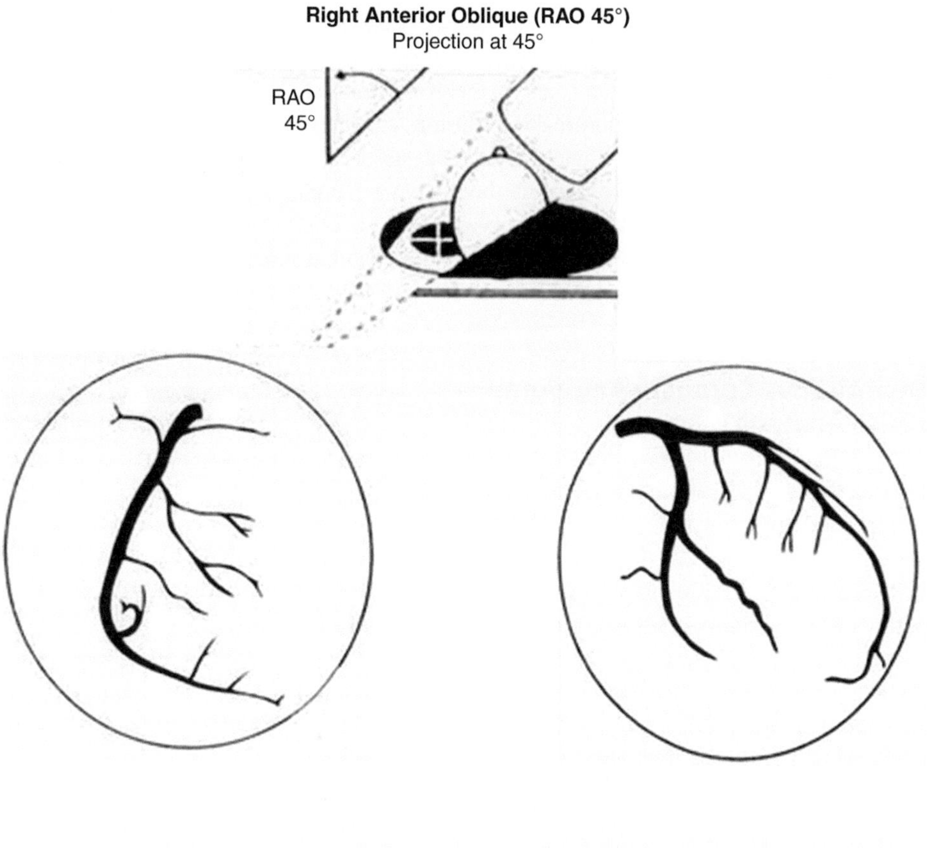

Fig. 2.4 Right anterior oblique (*RAO*) view of the left and right coronary arteries. Ideal view to visualize the left circumflex and mid right coronary artery

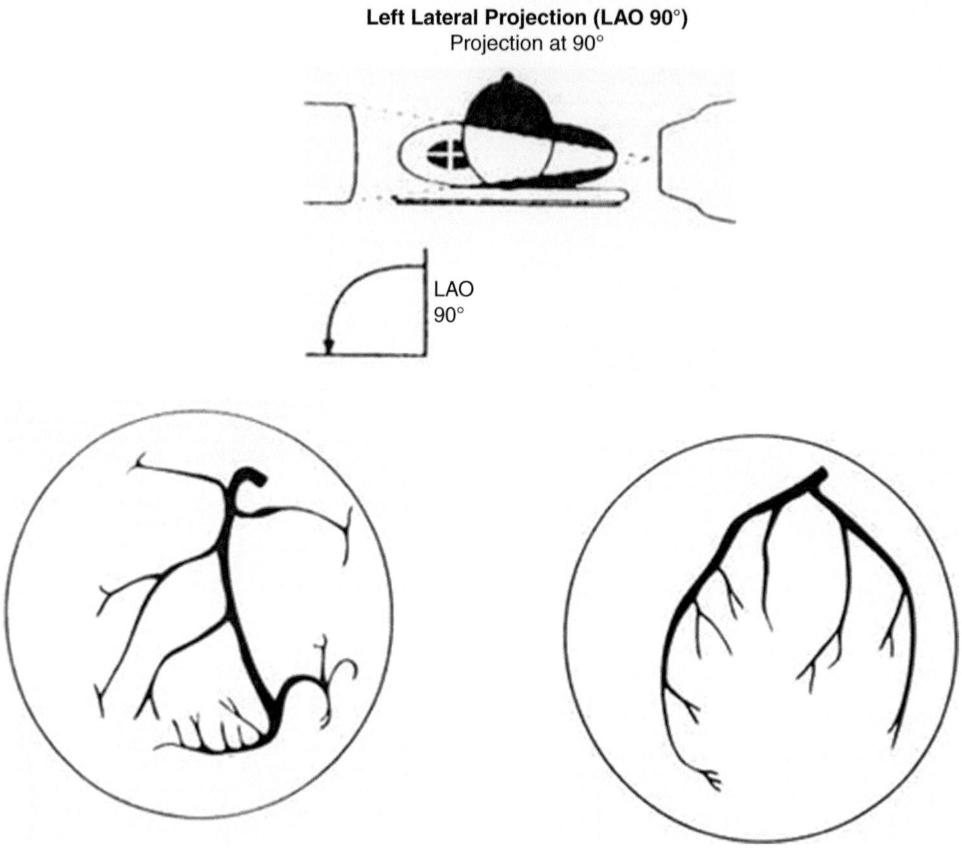

Fig. 2.5 Left lateral (*LLat*) view of the left and right coronary arteries. Ideal view to visualize the mid and distal segment of the left anterior descending and right coronary arteries

properly implemented. Compression can be achieved using the Joint Photographic Experts Group (JPEG) standard, where lossless compression of up to 3-fold can be completely recovered upon retrieval of the image and where lossy compression results in irretrievable loss of data. In clinical practice, JPEG lossy compression up to 15:1 has been shown to have no effect on identification of dissections, thrombus, or the presence of intracoronary stents and is therefore deemed acceptable for clinical decision-making during coronary interventions [4]. Quantitative angiographic analysis of 5:1, 8:1, and 12:1 lossy JPEG compression has been shown in one study to result in higher intra-observer variability (0.23–0.31 mm) compared to original images (<0.13 mm) and is therefore not recommended for QCA in clinical trials [5].

Quantitative Coronary Angiography (QCA) Analysis

Limitations of Qualitative Estimates of Lesion Severity

In clinical practice, estimation of coronary artery lesions is performed by visually assessing 2-dimensional angiograms taken in multiple projections. While this method provides acceptable estimates of luminal narrowing for basic clinical decision-making, multiple studies have demonstrated that it is prone to significant inter- and intra-observer variability [1–3] and frequently causes either overestimation or underestimation of lesion severity [2, 6–8]. A blinded review of angiograms by experienced cardiologists reported an average diameter stenosis of 85 % before PCI and 30 % post-procedurally, with a bimodal distribution. QCA revealed average pre- and post-procedural stenosis of 68 % and 49 %, respectively, with a Gaussian distribution. These differences corresponded to a 200 % error in the estimation of percent diameter stenosis [6]. In addition, visual estimates of stenosis severity frequently result in values which are physiologically incompatible with anterograde flow (e.g., 90–99 % diameter stenosis). Handheld and digital calipers were later developed to provide absolute vessel diameters and improve reproducibility of measurements; however, this method continued to over- and underestimate stenosis [9]. The limited utility of visual estimates of lesion severity in clinical trials led to the development of computer-assisted QCA, which improves accuracy and reproducibility and provides a wide variety of measurements useful in both research and clinical settings.

Computer-Assisted Quantitative Coronary Angiography (QCA)

Several generations of QCA systems have been developed based on edge-detection algorithms to improve measurement accuracy. First-generation algorithms improved the reliability of coronary measurements; [10–12] however, these

Table 2.2 Correctable sources of imaging error during angiographic acquisition

Source of error	Potential corrections
Biologic variation in lumen diameter	
Vasomotor tone	Nitroglycerin, 200 μmUg intracoronary every 10 min
Variations in image acquisition	
Single studies	
Vessel motion	
Cardiac	End-diastolic/end-systolic frame
Respiration	Breath holding
Vessel foreshortening	Obtain multiple angiographic projections
Insufficient contrast injection	Use 7 or 8 French large, high-flow catheters
Branch vessel overlap	Obtain multiple angiographic projections
Pincushion distortion	Image objects in center of image
Sequential studies	
X-ray generator (pulse width/dose/beam quality)	Repeat study in same imaging laboratory
X-ray tube (focal spot/shape/tube current)	As above
Image intensifier (magnification/resolution)	As above
Differences in angles and gantry height	Record gantry height/angle/skew on worksheet
Image calibration	Use measured catheter diameter
Errors in image analysis	
Electronic noise	Recursive digitization and frame averaging
Quantum noise	Spatial filtering of digital image data
Automated edge-detection algorithm	Minimize observer interaction
Selection of reference positions	Interpolated or averaged normal segment
Identification of lesion length	Use of side branches, other landmarks
Frame selection	End-diastolic frame showing "worst" view

systems tended to overestimate the diameters of small vessels [13]. Second-generation systems corrected for overestimation of small vessel sizes (diameter approximation <1.2 mm) and produced more reliable results in small vessels [14]. Further improvements were made in third-generation systems to take advantage of images from new digital flat-panel detectors instead of the conventional image intensifier systems. These systems are better able to determine smaller-diameter vessels [15] and analyze complex lesion morphology with irregular borders [16].

2-Dimensional Quantitative Coronary Angiography

The process of QCA can be subdivided into several distinct steps: digitization, image calibration, and arterial contour detection. Advances have been made to each of these steps over the last several decades. The process of digitization from cine film using cine-video converter is obsolete and was replaced by digital systems with direct digital input to a video camera. The analog video output signal is modified electronically and results in a greater contrast differences in areas with high X-ray absorption and lower contrast differences in areas with low X-ray absorption, significantly improving image quality. Conventional vacuum tubes have largely been replaced by flat-panel detectors which do not affect the quality of QCA but reduce geometric distortions. Image calibration is often done with contrast-filled injection catheters and can be problematic due to variable image quality and out-of-plane magnification. This can be overcome by using biplane calibration, but this is rarely used in routine QCA. The contour-detection procedure determines the vessel edge based on the weighted sum of the first- and second-derivative functions of the brightness values of scan lines perpendicular to the center line which in turn undergoes a minimal cost analysis that determines the optimal contour path along the segment (Fig. 2.6). Systems also take into account the image resolution and vessel diameter. Vessel contour editing can be performed manually but should be minimized. The two most commonly used angiographic analysis systems are the Cardiovascular Angiography Analysis System (CAAS, Pie Medical B.V., Maastricht, the Netherlands) and the Coronary Measurement System (CMS, Medis system, Leiden, the Netherlands) (Fig. 2.7).

3-Dimensional Quantitative Coronary Angiography

Currently, 2-dimensional (2D) QCA is the most commonly used and validated form of QCA. However, 2D angiography technology has limitations because of vessel overlap and vessel foreshortening during image acquisition. This is especially problematic in more complex lesions such as bifurcations. A 3D angiography utilizes standard 2D angiographic images obtained at least 30° apart and with minimal vessel overlap and reconstructs 3D images. Several 3D QCA programs are now available: CardiOp-B (Paieon Medical Ltd., Park Afek, Israel) and CAAS 5 (Pie Medical Imaging, Maastricht, the Netherlands, and Medis, Leiden, the Netherlands). In these systems, the user defines the area of interest by defining the proximal end, distal end, and area of stenosis. Their calibration methods differ, however: CardiOp-B requires the operator to input the size of the catheter in the image into the program, whereas the Medis and CAAS 5 system automatically calibrates the images using Digital Imaging and Communications in Medicine (DICOM) information embedded in the images [17, 18]. After image creation, operators can rotate or zoom the image to find an optimal visualization angle [19, 20]. 3D QCA programs have been validated [21, 22] and can provide information on vessel size, percent diameter stenosis, minimal lumen diameter,

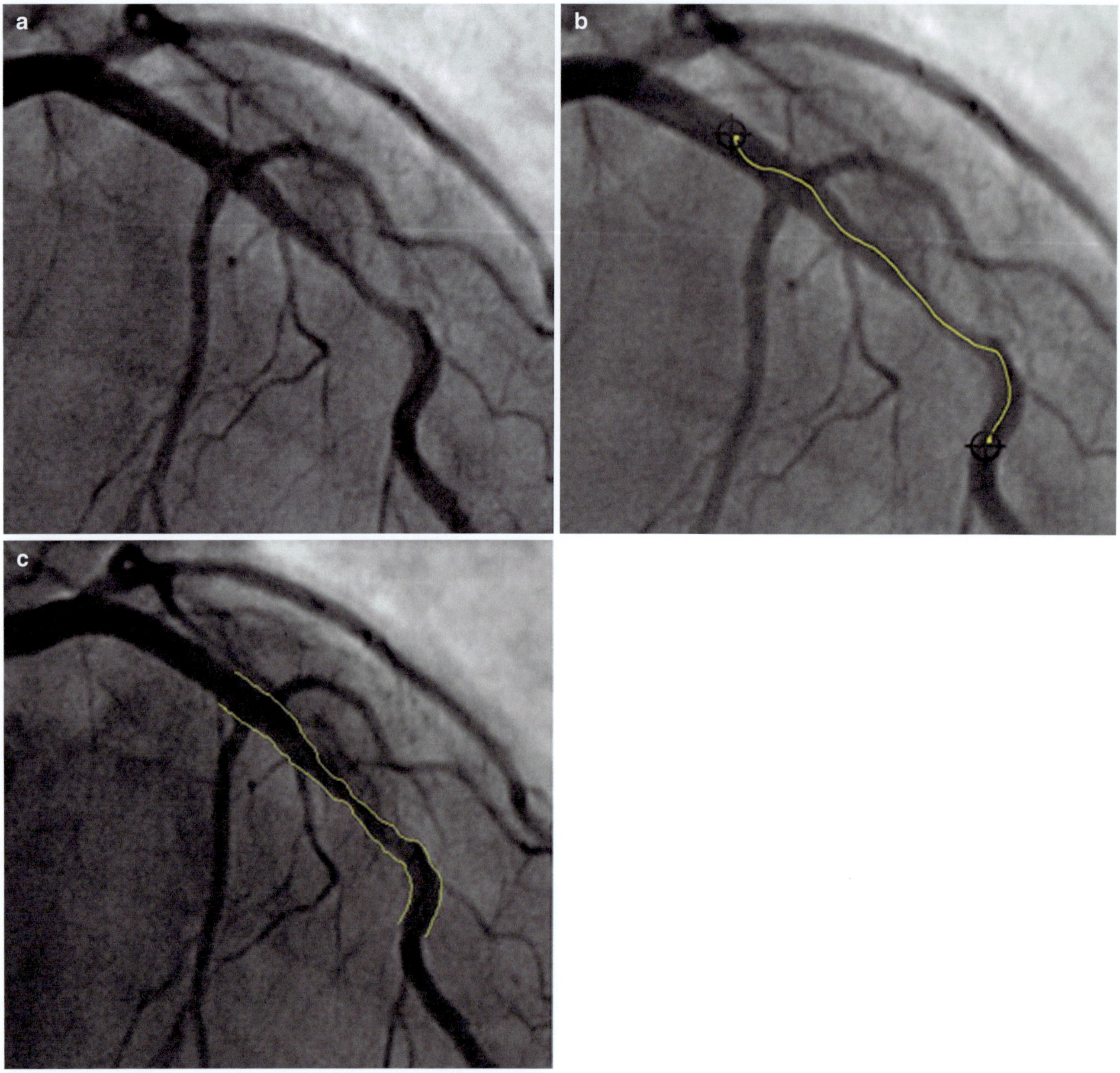

Fig. 2.6 Quantitative coronary angiogram segment analysis. (**a**) Preprocedural angiogram of lesion. (**b**) Manual selection of lesion segment. (**c**) Result of automatic contour-detection algorithm

bifurcation angle, and other QCA values. It was thought that 3D QCA would improve accuracy by resolving problems with vessel foreshortening and out-of-plane magnification, but thus far, comparisons to conventional 2D QCA programs have reported mixed results [18, 19, 22–25].

Inherent Limitations of Angiography in Detecting Coronary Artery Disease

Coronary atherosclerosis is a dynamic cycle of progression, regression, healing, and development of new atherosclerotic lesions. A complicating factor in the angiographic evaluation of the severity and degree of coronary atherosclerosis is the occurrence of compensatory mechanisms, characterized by enlargement of the atherosclerotic coronary artery that occurs in the early stages of plaque formation [26, 27]. This compensatory enlargement preserves a near-normal lumen cross-sectional area (and angiographic appearance), so that the early atherosclerotic plaque will have minimal hemodynamic effects. As the maximal stretching capacities of the vessel is reached, the expansion of the vessel will stop and further plaque deposition will begin to impinge on the lumen. Only once the lumen of the vessel becomes impaired does it become visible on arteriography, which visualizes only the 2-dimensional contrast-filled lumen. Because X-ray arteri-

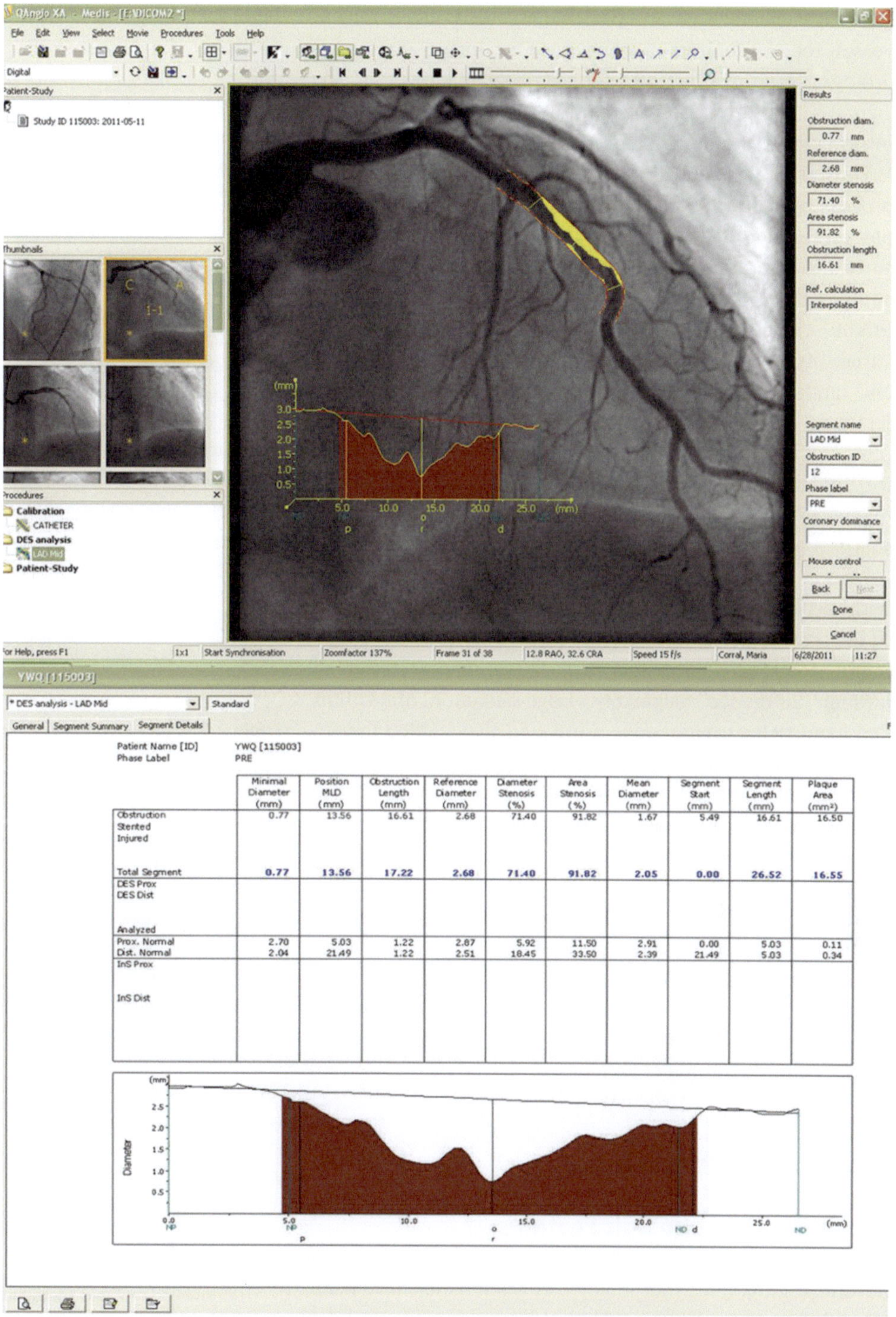

Fig. 2.7 The results of the minimal cost analysis using the Medis QAngio XA software (Version 7.2.34.0). The images include the reconstructed original vessel contours, plaque area (*shaded*), and the diameter function. The absolute and relative QCA parameters are presented in the lower analysis box

ography only depicts the coronary lumen, it underestimates the presence of diffuse atherosclerosis. Cross-sectional imaging of the coronary arteries is better assessed in these early stages by intravascular ultrasound (IVUS), which provides high-resolution cross sections of the arterial wall and demonstrates the presence or absence of plaque deposition and compensatory arterial enlargement. For intermediate lesions, precise physiologic measurements of stenosis severity, such as fractional flow reserve or coronary Doppler measurements, are better suited for clinical decision-making.

Measurement Factors Contributing to QCA Variability

In addition to biologic differences among lumen diameters and inconsistencies in radiographic image acquisition parameters (discussed previously), angiographic measurements can also introduce variability into the assessment of vessel diameters. Analysis of two or more orthogonal projections permits a more accurate assessment of the physiologic significance of lesion severity, although a second, technically suitable projection is not available in many cases due to vessel foreshortening, overlap, or poor image quality. If orthogonal projections are not available, analyses of the "worst-view" projection may provide sufficiently accurate information for clinical studies. Herrington and colleagues [13] used a components-of-variance model to show that the process of acquiring and performing quantitative angiography on selected frames accounted for 57 % of the total measurement variability, whereas patient, procedure, and equipment variations accounted for 30 % of total variability. Frame selection accounted for the remaining 13 % of total variability. When direct digital angiography is performed and random errors associated with noise in the cine-video pathway are eliminated, frame selection may be a much more important contributor to overall measurement variability. Frame selection has been associated with substantial inter-observer variability, and the frame demonstrating the sharpest and tightest view of the stenosis should be used.

Automated quantitative angiographic systems also differ with respect to the preferred method of calibration, location of the arterial border and construction of its contour, use of minimal cost or "smoothing" algorithms, and selection of normal "reference" segments. Edge-detection algorithms that identify the arterial edge using a 50 % weighted threshold of the first- and second-derivative extrema may have systematically larger reference and obstruction diameters than those using a 75 % weight (weighted toward the first-derivative extremum) or the first-derivative extremum. These systematic differences may also affect the accuracy and reproducibility of the absolute and relative angiographic measurements. Accordingly, each Angiographic Core Laboratory should independently determine its own variability during the performance of quantitative angiographic studies, potentially allowing standardization of techniques among different Core Laboratories.

Table 2.3 ACC-AHA characteristics of Type A, B and C coronary lesions

Type A lesions (high success [> 85 %]; low risk)	
Discrete (<10 mm)	Little or no calcium
Concentric	Less than totally occlusive
Readily accessible	Not ostial in location
Nonangulated segment (<45°)	No major side branch involvement
Smooth contour	Absence of thrombus
Type B lesions (moderate success [60–85 %]; moderate risk)	
Tubular (10–20 mm length)	Moderate to heavy calcification
Eccentric	Total occlusions <3 months old
Moderate tortuosity of proximal segment	Ostial in location
Moderately angulated (45–90°)	Bifurcation lesion requiring double guidewire
Irregular contour	Some thrombus present
Type C lesions (low success [< 60 %]; high risk)	
Diffuse (>20 mm length)	Total occlusion >3 months old
Excessive tortuosity of proximal segment	Inability to protect major side branches
Extremely angulated segment (> 90°)	Degenerated vein grafts with friable lesions

Modified from Ryan et al. [4], with permission

Table 2.4 SCAI lesion classification system: Class I–IV lesions

Type I lesion (highest success expected; lowest risk)
(1) Does not meet criteria for C lesion
(2) Patent
Type II lesions
(1) Meets any of these criteria for ACC/AHA C lesion
Diffuse (greater than 2 cm length)
Excessive tortuosity of proximal segment
Extremely angulated segments greater than 90°
Inability to protect major side branches
Degenerated vein grafts with friable lesions
(2) Patent
Type III lesions
(1) Does not meet criteria for C Lesion
(2) Occluded
Type IV lesions
(1) Meets any of these criteria for ACC/AHA C lesion
Diffuse (greater than 2 cm length)
Excessive tortuosity of proximal segment
Extremely angulated segments greater than 90°
Inability to protect major side branches
Degenerated vein grafts with friable lesions
(2) Occluded

Modified from Krone et al. [28], with permission

Angiographic Parameters

Qualitative Morphologic Features

Several angiographic morphologic characteristics have been identified that have short- and long-term prognostic implications after coronary intervention with balloon angioplasty and new device angioplasty. The joint task force of the American College of Cardiology (ACC) and American Heart Association (AHA) established criteria in 1988 to estimate procedural success and complication rates after balloon angioplasty based on the presence or absence of specific high-risk lesion characteristics (Table 2.3). These were validated with good correlation with procedural success among patients undergoing multivessel PCI. The Society for Cardiac Angiography and Interventions (SCAI) more recently developed and validated a simplified score based on four groups: non-Type C-patent, Type C-patent, non-Type C-occluded, and Type C-occluded (Table 2.4) [28]. This classification provided better discrimination for procedure success or complications (c statistic of 0.75) compared to the original ACC/AHA classification (c statistic of 0.69) or to the modified ACC/AHA system (c statistic of 0.71) [28]. The Mayo Clinic Risk Score, developed and validated in a database of 5,064 contemporary PCI patients, was based on the presence or absence of eight morphologic variables [29]. Compared to the ACC/AHA lesion classification, the Mayo Clinic risk score better predicts cardiovascular complications but is a less accurate determinant of angiographic success.

In addition to composite scores based on lesion complexity and other risk score systems, estimation of procedural risk based on the presence of one or more specific adverse morphologic features may be useful.

Lesion Angulation

Vessel curvature at the site of maximum stenosis should be measured in the most unforeshortened projection using a length of curvature that approximates the balloon length used for coronary dilation. Balloon angioplasty of highly angulated lesions is associated with an increased risk of coronary dissection, whereas stenting of angulated lesions may prohibit delivery of the stent or impose stent strain with arterial contour straightening and predispose to stent fracture.

Lesion Calcification

Coronary calcification reduces the compliance of the vessel, may predispose to dissections after balloon angioplasty, can reduce the ability to cross chronic total occlusions, and can impede stent strut expansion. Calcification within saphenous vein grafts (SVGs) is generally within the reference vessel wall rather than within the lesion and is associated with older graft age, diabetes, and smoking.

Degenerated Saphenous Vein Grafts (SVGs)

SVGs develop progressive degeneration over time with 25 % occluding within the first year and 50 % within 10 years. Extensive SVG degeneration and plaque volume are both independent predictors of 30-day major adverse cardiac events after PCI of SVG.

Thrombus

Angiography has a low sensitivity but high specificity in detecting coronary thrombus, defined by the appearance of discrete, intraluminal filling defects within the arterial lumen. The presence of thrombus is associated with a higher risk of ischemic complications after PCI, and the associated incidence of distal embolization and thrombotic occlusion are variable (ranging from 6 to 73 %) and related to the size of the coronary thrombus.

Ostial Lesions

Ostial lesions are those within 3 mm of the origin of the coronary artery and are classified as aorto-ostial and non-aorto-ostial. Stenting has become the default therapy for most aorto-ostial lesions, although there are unique challenges of stent placement in the aorto-ostial location. Isolated non-aorto-ostial stenoses of the left circumflex and left anterior descending arteries and ostial side branch bifurcation lesions also pose unique challenges with vessel wall geometry, adequate ostial branch coverage (particularly those with a narrow angle with the adjacent branch), and plaque shifting causing compromise of the parent or adjacent branch vessels.

Lesion Length

Lesion length may be estimated quantitatively as the "shoulder-to-shoulder" extent of atherosclerotic narrowing greater than 20 %, although many clinicians estimate the lesion length based on the identification of a "normal to normal" segment, which is generally longer than the length obtained with quantitative methods. While stents improve late outcomes in long lesions compared with balloon angioplasty, long stented segments and lesion length remain the most important predictors of restenosis in the stent era [30].

Bifurcation Lesions

The Medina bifurcation classification is broadly accepted as an equivalent but simpler alternative to the Duke classification (Fig. 2.8) [31–33]. The risk of side branch occlusion in bifurcation lesions relates to the extent of atherosclerotic

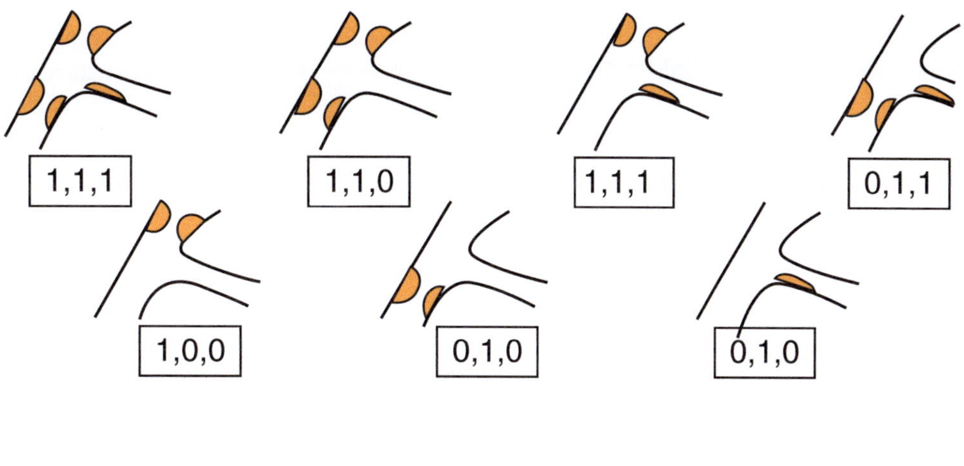

Fig. 2.8 Schematic Medina and Duke classification systems for bifurcation stenoses

involvement of the side branch and ranges from 14 to 27 % in side branches with ostial involvement. Recurrence at the origin of the side branch is the most common location of failure after bifurcation stenting.

Total Occlusions

Total coronary occlusion is identified as an abrupt termination of the epicardial vessel; anterograde and retrograde collaterals may be present and are helpful in quantifying the length of the totally occluded segment. Coronary occlusions are common findings and often lead to the decision to perform coronary bypass surgery rather than PCI in the setting of multivessel disease. The success rate for recanalization of occlusions depends on the occlusion duration and on certain lesion morphologic features, such as bridging collaterals, occlusion length greater than 15 mm, a blunt- rather than funnel-shaped occlusion, and side branch at the side of occlusion, which all increase difficulty of guide-wire advancement. Although newer technologies and techniques have been used to recanalize refractory occlusions, better guidewires and wire techniques have accounted for much of the improvement in crossing success over recent years. Simultaneous dual coronary injections are useful for identifying the length and anatomy of the total occlusion.

Collateral Assessment

A key component of total occlusion assessment is grading of collateral blood flow to the jeopardized myocardium [34]. Collateralization can be assessed by degree of distal filling according to the Rentrop classification and by the size of the collateral connection—Group 0 (no continuous connection between the donor and recipient artery), Group 1 (continuous threadlike connection ≤0.3 mm), and Group 2 (continuous small side-branch-like sized collateral through its course ≥0.4 mm). Other less well-validated parameters include collateral size, collateral frame count (measured by the number of frames from opacification of the guiding catheter to the filling of the collaterals), and collateral density (measured as the number of collaterals >1 mm in size in a region of interest).

Measures of Myocardial Perfusion

Angiographic measures of coronary perfusion are the predominant determinant of survival among patients with ST-segment elevation myocardial infarction (STEMI) after thrombolytic and primary PCI. The Thrombolysis In Myocardial Infarction (TIMI) flow grade classification scheme characterizes the extent of coronary flow in patients with STEMI treated with systemic thrombolytic agents and in patients presenting with non-ST-segment elevation myocardial infarction and unstable angina. The TIMI frame count [35] and the TIMI myocardial perfusion grade were developed to further quantify anterograde flow and assess distal microvascular perfusion.

TIMI Flow Grade Classification

The TIMI flow grade system is a valuable tool for assessing the efficacy of reperfusion strategies in patients with STEMI and for identifying patients at higher risk for an adverse outcome with acute coronary syndromes undergoing PCI.

Patients reperfused with primary angioplasty within 2 h of symptom onset have lower mortality and greater myocardial salvage after primary PTCA than those with delayed reperfusion. The importance of early reperfusion is underscored in patients spontaneously achieving TIMI-3 flow prior to primary PTCA, as demonstrated in approximately 10–20 % of patients at the time of initial angiography. In the Primary Angioplasty in Myocardial Infarction (PAMI) trials, spontaneous reperfusion or TIMI-3 flow occurred in 16 % of patients and was a powerful and independent predictor of in-hospital and late survival in patients undergoing mechanical reperfusion. The survival benefit of spontaneous reperfusion persisted even when corrected for post-procedural TIMI-3 flow. Other studies have demonstrated that patients achieving early TIMI-3 flow (whether spontaneously or pharmacologically mediated) have improved myocardial salvage, which has spurred interest in investigating other pharmacologic combinations upstream of mechanical reperfusion.

There are a number of limitations of the TIMI classification system. Substantial observer variability exists with the TIMI flow grade, when comparing angiographic core laboratory and clinical center assessment, with best agreement occurring when the artery is closed (TIMI-0 or TIMI-1 flow: kappa value = 0.84), moderate agreement for TIMI grade 3 flow (kappa value = 0.55), and poor agreement with TIMI grade 2 flow (kappa value = 0.38); similar findings have been shown between experienced angiographic core laboratories. Another limitation of the TIMI flow grade is that it provides ordinal values rather than continuous ones, limiting its statistical power in clinical trials. Furthermore, although TIMI flow grade has classically compared flow in the infarct-related vessel to flow in the "normal" non-culprit artery, flow in the non-infarct-related artery in patients with STEMI is not truly normal compared with flow in patients without STEMI. Difficulties in reproducibly assessing myocardial flow relative to other vessels (e.g., the right coronary artery or in the setting of total occlusions of the contralateral vessel) led some investigators to modify the definition of "TIMI grade 3 flow" as opacification of the distal coronary artery within three cardiac cycles [36]. The "three cardiac cycle" definition of "TIMI-3" flow results in an absolute rate increase of approximately 10 % compared with the original definition of TIMI grade 3 flow.

TIMI Frame Count (TFC)

A quantitative assessment of the number of frames required for epicardial contrast to reach standardized distal landmarks may provide a more objective method of estimating coronary blood flow than the TIMI flow grade [35]. TFC is measured from the first frame in which a column of dye touches both borders of the coronary artery and moves forward to a final frame in which the dye begins to enter a standard distal landmark in the artery. The TFC is corrected for the longer length of the LAD to arrive at a corrected TIMI frame count (CTFC; TFC divided by 1.7). Advantages of CTFC over TIMI flow grades include that it is quantitative, objective, continuous, and subject to less inter-observer variability. CTFC is predictive of clinical outcomes in the setting of elective PCI and STEMI.

TIMI Myocardial Perfusion Grade (TMPG)

Epicardial flow does not necessarily imply tissue-level or microvascular perfusion, a finding that prompted development of the TMPG and the myocardial blush grade (MBG). These measures are independent predictors of mortality in acute myocardial infarction after thrombolytic therapy and after mechanical reperfusion [37, 38]. The TMPG permits risk stratification even within grades of epicardial flow: patients with TIMI grade 3 flow after reperfusion therapy have an elevated mortality rate if diminished microvascular perfusion (TMPG 0 or 1) is present. Accordingly, the TIMI flow grades and the TMPGs can be combined to identify a group of patients at "very low" and "very high" risk for mortality after STEMI.

Angiographic Complications after PCI

Angiographic complications occur in 5–10 % of PCIs as a result of atherosclerotic plaque disruption, embolization, thrombus formation, or vasoactive mediators.

Coronary Dissection

The National Heart, Lung, and Blood Institute (NHLBI) coronary dissection classification categorizes the severity of coronary dissection following PCI. Prognosis depends on dissection severity, length, contrast staining, and impact on coronary perfusion. Coronary dissections resulting in lumen compromise and reduce flow are uncommon (<3 % of cases).

No Reflow

No reflow is a reduction in flow despite a patent lumen at the site of PCI. As a strong predictor of mortality after PCI, no reflow occurs in 1–5 % of PCIs (as many as 15 % of primary angioplasties for STEMI). Other predictors of no reflow include higher plaque burden, thrombus, lipid pools by IVUS, higher lesion elastic membrane cross-sectional area, pre-infarction angina, and initial TIMI-0 flow.

Distal Embolization

Distal embolization is the migration of a filling defect or thrombus to distally occlude the target vessel or one of its branches. It occurs in approximately 10 % of PCIs for AMI and is also common during PCI of SVG lesions.

Coronary Perforation

Coronary perforation is a rare complication associated with a high rate of major adverse outcomes [39–43], occurring in 0.1 % of patients undergoing balloon angioplasty but more commonly during atheroablative therapy (1.3 %; $P<0.001$). Perforations can be graded based on the angiographic appearance of the perforation as Type I (extraluminal crater without blood extravasation), Type II (pericardial or myocardial blushing), or Type III (>1 mm perforation with contrast streaming and cavity spilling) [44]. Rates of emergent bypass surgery and a composite of death, myocardial infarction, and pericardial tamponade increase by perforation grade. These outcomes have significantly improved with the use of coronary stent grafts [45].

Coronary Spasm

Coronary spasm is a transient reduction of more than 50 % diameter in an arterial segment that otherwise has insignificant (<25 %) narrowing. Coronary spasm occurs in approximately 5 % of cases, but its frequency has been reduced with the routine use of coronary vasodilators.

Abrupt Closure

Abrupt closure is an abrupt cessation of coronary flow to TIMI-0 or TIMI-1. Occurring in 3–5 % of balloon angioplasty procedures, its incidence has been markedly reduced in the stent era. Abrupt closure may be due to coronary dissection, embolization, or thrombus formation within the vessel.

Late Aneurysm Formation

A coronary aneurysm is a focal or fusiform expansion (>50 % of maximum reference diameter) of the vessel lumen late following PCI. Coronary artery aneurysms are actually pseudoaneurysms and occur rarely after balloon angioplasty, atheroablation, or stent implantation (<1 %). They typically develop from tears or dissection and incomplete healing that compromises the vessel wall integrity and result in vessel wall expansion. Under rare circumstances, coronary artery aneurysms can become infected requiring surgical intervention.

Angiographic Indices of Procedural Results

Early and late angiographic results after PCI have been described using a number of quantitative angiographic criteria. Common angiographic indices, which allow objective evaluation of procedural results, include the following:

Angiographic Success

Angiographic success after stent implantation is usually defined as attainment of a <20 % residual diameter stenosis within the stent or a <30 % residual diameter stenosis within the segment (allowing for higher "inflow" or "outflow" diameter stenosis at the stent margins) [5]. Relative diameter stenosis changes are provided by the relationship: Percent diameter stenosis = (1 − (MLD/Reference Diameter)) × 100.

Binary Angiographic Restenosis

Binary angiographic restenosis is best defined as a ≥50 % diameter stenosis at follow-up, although a number of other criteria have been used. Binary restenosis after drug-eluting stent placement may occur within the stent ("in-stent" restenosis"), within the 5 mm margins of the stent ("edge" restenosis) or within the segment between the proximal and distal reference segments ("in-segment" or in-lesion" restenosis). In defining ischemia-driven target lesion revascularization, a 70 % diameter stenosis is the follow-up angiographic threshold used in the absence of clinical symptoms.

Late Lumen Loss

Serial quantitative angiographic studies have shown there is an approximate 0.50 mm reduction in lumen diameter that develops within three to six months after balloon angioplasty, although angiography cannot differentiate whether this reduction is due to intimal hyperplasia or arterial remodeling. Because there is little or no arterial remodeling after bare-metal stent placement, late lumen loss is primarily due to intimal hyperplasia and follows a near-Gaussian distribution. In contrast, the distribution of late lumen loss after drug-eluting stent placement suggests a near "all-or-nothing" response. Late lumen loss and target lesion revascularization have a monotonic and curvilinear relationship, with the likelihood of TLR not exceeding 5 % until the late loss is >0.5 mm for the analysis segment and not exceeding 10 % until late loss is >0.65 mm [46]. A surrogacy meta-analysis found that late loss and percent diameter stenosis strongly predicted the risk of TLR, with in-segment percent diameter stenosis being the most highly predictive (c statistic approximately 0.95) [47]. However, the usefulness of late lumen loss in drug-eluting stent comparative trials remains controversial [48].

Applications of Coronary Angiography

Quantitative coronary angiography measurements are often used in clinical trials as surrogate end points for clinical outcomes because of the low frequency of clinical events associated with the advancement of percutaneous interventions. For example, in-stent and in-segment late loss and percent diameter stenosis at angiographic follow-up have been extensively validated as surrogates for target lesion revascularization rates [49]. Furthermore, certain angiographic characteristics such as lesion length, lesion location, presence of bifurcation lesions, and multivessel disease are associated with increased mortality after PCI [50–52].

In addition to the high-risk lesion characteristics and scores discussed previously, validation of specific QCA measurements associated with clinical outcomes has led to their incorporation into various scoring systems (Table 2.5), several of which also include clinical information. These systems can provide valuable insights into prognosis and optimal management, improving patient outcomes.

Table 2.5 Risk scoring systems incorporating angiographic characteristics

Scoring system (Study)	Clinical characteristics included?	Description
Duke Jeopardy Score Califf et al. [53]	No	Weighted score depending on significant stenoses locations of significant stenosis. More proximal lesions are weighed more heavily
Myocardial Jeopardy Index Alderman et al. [54]	No	Weighted score based on the size of the arteries with significant stenoses. Size of arteries is surrogate for amount of myocardium supplied
APPROACH Score Graham et al. [57]	No	Weighted score based on amount of myocardium supplied by arteries with significant stenoses
SYNTAX score Sianos et al. [60]	No	Complex scoring system which takes into account lesion complexity in addition to the amount of myocardium supplied by a stenosed artery
ACUITY risk model Lansky et al. [59]	Yes	Combination of clinical risk factors and angiographic describing severity of coronary disease to risk stratify ACS patients undergoing early intervention
BC-PCI Risk Score Hamburger et al. [58]	Yes	Uses age, gender, severity of symptoms, renal function, 3v-disease and left main disease to predict 30-mortality risk
Clinical SYNTAX score Garg et al. [56]	Yes	Combines angiographic SYNTAX score with clinical characteristics (age, ejection fraction, creatinine clearance) to predict long-term mortality in patients receiving PCI
NERS Score Chen et al. [55]	Yes	Contains 17 clinical, 4 procedural and 33 angiographic characteristics to predict 6 month ischemic outcomes in patients with unprotected left main disease

Conclusion

Iterative improvements in QCA equipment and measurements have provided increasingly accurate descriptions of the coronary vascular tree. The value of QCA is predicated on a thorough knowledge of the principles, limitations, and challenges of data acquisition and the use of standardized, validated analysis methods, and carefully defined surrogate end points. With these fundamentals in mind, QCA will continue to be an invaluable tool for clinical decision-making and clinical research evaluating new and evolving therapies for coronary artery disease.

References

1. DeRouen TA, Murray JA, Owen W. Variability in the analysis of coronary arteriograms. Circulation. 1977;55(2):324–8.
2. Katritsis D, Lythall DA, Cooper IC, Crowther A, Webb-Peploe MM. Assessment of coronary angioplasty: comparison of visual assessment, hand-held caliper measurement and automated digital quantitation. Cathet Cardiovasc Diagn. 1988;15(4):237–42.
3. Fisher LD, Judkins MP, Lesperance J, et al. Reproducibility of coronary arteriographic reading in the coronary artery surgery study (CASS). Cathet Cardiovasc Diagn. 1982;8(6):565–75.
4. Ryan TJ, Faxon DP, Gunnar RM, et al. Guidelines for percutaneous transluminal coronary angioplasty. A report of the American College of Cardiology/American Heart Association Task Force on Assessment of Diagnostic and Therapeutic Cardiovascular Procedures (Subcommittee on Percutaneous Transluminal Coronary Angioplasty). Circulation. 1988;78(2):486–502.
5. Smith S, Feldman T, Hirshfeld J, et al. ACC/AHA/SCAI 2005 guideline update for percutaneous coronary intervention–summary article: a report of the American College of Cardiology/American Heart Association Task Force on Practice Guidelines (ACC/AHA/SCAI Writing Committee to Update the 2001 Guidelines for Percutaneous Coronary Intervention). Circulation. 2006;113(1):156–75.
6. Fleming RM, Kirkeeide RL, Smalling RW, Gould KL. Patterns in visual interpretation of coronary arteriograms as detected by quantitative coronary arteriography. J Am Coll Cardiol. 1991;18(4):945–51.
7. Bertrand ME, Lablanche JM, Bauters C, Leroy F, Mac Fadden E. Discordant results of visual and quantitative estimates of stenosis severity before and after coronary angioplasty. Cathet Cardiovasc Diagn. 1993;28(1):1–6.
8. Desmet W, Willems J, Van Lierde J, Piessens J. Discrepancy between visual estimation and computer-assisted measurement of lesion severity before and after coronary angioplasty. Cathet Cardiovasc Diagn. 1994;31(3):192–8.
9. Kalbfleisch SJ, McGillem MJ, Pinto IM, Kavanaugh KM, DeBoe SF, Mancini GB. Comparison of automated quantitative coronary angiography with caliper measurements of percent diameter stenosis. Am J Cardiol. 1990;65(18):1181–4.
10. Reiber JH, Serruys PW, Kooijman CJ, et al. Assessment of short-, medium-, and long-term variations in arterial dimensions from computer-assisted quantitation of coronary cineangiograms. Circulation. 1985;71(2):280–8.
11. Mancini GB, Simon SB, McGillem MJ, LeFree MT, Friedman HZ, Vogel RA. Automated quantitative coronary arteriography: morphologic and physiologic validation in vivo of a rapid digital angiographic method. Circulation. 1987;75(2):452–60.
12. Spears JR, Sandor T, Als AV, et al. Computerized image analysis for quantitative measurement of vessel diameter from cineangiograms. Circulation. 1983;68(2):453–61.
13. Herrington DM, Siebes M, Walford GD. Sources of error in quantitative coronary angiography. Cathet Cardiovasc Diagn. 1993;29(4):314–21.
14. Hausleiter J, Jost S, Nolte CW, et al. Comparative in-vitro validation of eight first- and second-generation quantitative coronary angiography systems. Coron Artery Dis. 1997;8(2):83–90.
15. Van Herck PL, Gavit L, Gorissen P, et al. Quantitative coronary arteriography on digital flat-panel system. Catheter Cardiovasc Interv. 2004;63(2):192–200.
16. van der Zwet PM, Reiber JH. A new approach for the quantification of complex lesion morphology: the gradient field transform; basic principles and validation results. J Am Coll Cardiol. 1994;24(1):216–24.
17. Gradaus R, Mathies K, Breithardt G, Bocker D. Clinical assessment of a new real time 3D quantitative coronary angiography system: evaluation in stented vessel segments. Catheter Cardiovasc Interv. 2006;68(1):44–9.
18. Ramcharitar S, Daeman J, Patterson M, et al. First direct in vivo comparison of two commercially available three-dimensional quantitative coronary angiography systems. Catheter Cardiovasc Interv. 2008;71(1):44–50.
19. Dvir D, Marom H, Guetta V, Kornowski R. Three-dimensional coronary reconstruction from routine single-plane coronary angiograms: in vivo quantitative validation. Int J Cardiovasc Intervent. 2005;7(3):141–5.
20. Agostoni P, Biondi-Zoccai G, Van Langenhove G, et al. Comparison of assessment of native coronary arteries by standard versus three-dimensional coronary angiography. Am J Cardiol. 2008;102(3):272–9.
21. Schuurbiers JC, Lopez NG, Ligthart J, et al. In vivo validation of CAAS QCA-3D coronary reconstruction using fusion of angiography and intravascular ultrasound (ANGUS). Catheter Cardiovasc Interv. 2009;73(5):620–6.
22. Tsuchida K, van der Giessen WJ, Patterson M, et al. In vivo validation of a novel three-dimensional quantitative coronary angiography system (CardiOp-B): comparison with a conventional two-dimensional system (CAAS II) and with special reference to optical coherence tomography. EuroIntervention. 2007;3(1):100–8.
23. Meerkin D, Marom H, Cohen-Biton O, Einav S. Three-dimensional vessel analyses provide more accurate length estimations than the gold standard QCA. J Interv Cardiol. 2010;23(2):152–9.
24. Wellnhofer E, Wahle A, Mugaragu I, Gross J, Oswald H, Fleck E. Validation of an accurate method for three-dimensional reconstruction and quantitative assessment of volumes, lengths and diameters of coronary vascular branches and segments from biplane angiographic projections. Int J Card Imaging. 1999;15(5):339–53. discussion 355–336.
25. Tu S, Koning G, Jukema W, Reiber JH. Assessment of obstruction length and optimal viewing angle from biplane X-ray angiograms. Int J Cardiovasc Imaging. 2010;26(1):5–17.
26. Glagov S, Weisenberg E, Zarins CK, Stankunavicius R, Kolettis GJ. Compensatory enlargement of human atherosclerotic coronary arteries. N Engl J Med. 1987;316(22):1371–5.
27. Stiel GM, Stiel LS, Schofer J, Donath K, Mathey DG. Impact of compensatory enlargement of atherosclerotic coronary arteries on angiographic assessment of coronary artery disease. Circulation. 1989;80(6):1603–9.
28. Krone R, Shaw R, Klein L, et al. Evaluation of the American College of Cardiology/American Heart Association and the Society for Coronary Angiography and Interventions lesion classification system in the current "stent era" of coronary interventions (from the ACC-National Cardiovascular Data Registry). Am J Cardiol. 2003;92(4):389–94.

29. Singh M, Rihal CS, Lennon RJ, Garratt KN, Holmes DR. Comparison of Mayo Clinic risk score and American College of Cardiology/American Heart Association lesion classification in the prediction of adverse cardiovascular outcome following percutaneous coronary interventions. J Am Coll Cardiol. 2004;44:357–61.
30. Popma JJ, Leon MB, Moses JW, et al. Quantitative assessment of angiographic restenosis after sirolimus-eluting stent implantation in native coronary arteries. Circulation. 2004;110:3773–80.
31. Gobeil F, Lefevre T, Guyon P, et al. Stenting of bifurcation lesions using the Bestent: a prospective dual-center study. Catheter Cardiovasc Interv. 2002;55:427–33.
32. Medina A, de Lezo J. A new classification of coronary bifurcation lesions. Rev Esp Cardiol. 2006;59(2):183–4.
33. Lefevre T, Louvard Y, Morice MC, et al. Stenting of bifurcation lesions: classification, treatments, and results. Catheter Cardiovasc Interv. 2000;49:274–83.
34. Seiler C. The human coronary collateral circulation. Heart (England). 2003;89:1352–7.
35. Gibson CM, Cannon CP, Daley WL, et al. TIMI frame count: a quantitative method of assessing coronary artery flow. Circulation. 1996;93(5):879–88.
36. Stone GW, Brodie BR, Griffin JJ, et al. Prospective, multicenter study of the safety and feasibility of primary stenting in acute myocardial infarction: in-hospital and 30-day results of the PAMI stent pilot trial. Primary Angioplasty in Myocardial Infarction Stent Pilot Trial Investigators. J Am Coll Cardiol. 1998;31(1):23–30.
37. van 't Hof AW, Liem A, Suryapranata H, Hoorntje JC, de Boer MJ, Zijlstra F. Angiographic assessment of myocardial reperfusion in patients treated with primary angioplasty for acute myocardial infarction: myocardial blush grade. Zwolle Myocardial Infarction Study Group. Circulation. 1998;97(23)):2302–6.
38. Stone GW, Peterson MA, Lansky AJ, Dangas G, Mehran R, Leon MB. Impact of normalized myocardial perfusion after successful angioplasty in acute myocardial infarction. J Am Coll Cardiol. 2002;39(4):591–7.
39. Fasseas P, Orford JL, Panetta CJ, et al. Incidence, correlates, management, and clinical outcome of coronary perforation: analysis of 16,298 procedures. Am Heart J. 2004;147:140–5.
40. Dippel EJ, Kereiakes DJ, Tramuta DA, et al. Coronary perforation during percutaneous coronary intervention in the era of abciximab platelet glycoprotein IIb/IIIa blockade: an algorithm for percutaneous management. Catheter Cardiovasc Interv. 2001;52:279–86.
41. Javaid A, Buch AN, Satler LF, et al. Management and outcomes of coronary artery perforation during percutaneous coronary intervention. Am J Cardiol. 2006;98:911–14.
42. Klein LW. Coronary artery perforation during interventional procedures. Catheter Cardiovasc Interv. 2006;68:713–17.
43. Stankovic G, Orlic D, Corvaja N, et al. Incidence, predictors, in-hospital, and late outcomes of coronary artery perforations. Am J Cardiol. 2004;93:213–16.
44. Ellis SG, Ajluni S, Arnold AZ, et al. Increased coronary perforation in the new device era. Incidence, classification, management, and outcome. Circulation. 1994;90(6):p2725–30.
45. Lansky AJ, Yang YM, Khan Y, et al. Treatment of coronary artery perforations complicating percutaneous coronary intervention with a polytetrafluoroethylene-covered stent graft. Am J Cardiol. 2006;98:370–4.
46. Ellis SG, Popma JJ, Lasala JM, et al. Relationship between angiographic late loss and target lesion revascularization after coronary stent implantation: analysis from the TAXUS-IV trial. J Am Coll Cardiol. 2005;45:1193–200.
47. Pocock SJ, Lansky AJ, Mehran R, et al. Angiographic surrogate end points in drug-eluting stent trials: a systematic evaluation based on individual patient data from 11 randomized, controlled trials. J Am Coll Cardiol. 2008;51(1):23–32. doi:10.1016/j.jacc.2007.07.084
48. Mauri L, Orav EJ, Candia SC, Cutlip DE, Kuntz RE. Robustness of late lumen loss in discriminating drug-eluting stents across variable observational and randomized trials. Circulation. 2005;112: 2833–9.
49. Pocock SJ, Lansky AJ, Mehran R, et al. Angiographic surrogate end points in drug-eluting stent trials: a systematic evaluation based on individual patient data from 11 randomized, controlled trials. J Am Coll Cardiol. 2008;51(1):23–32.
50. Mercado N, Boersma E, Wijns W, et al. Clinical and quantitative coronary angiographic predictors of coronary restenosis: a comparative analysis from the balloon-to-stent era. J Am Coll Cardiol. 2001;38(3):645–52.
51. Dauerman HL, Higgins PJ, Sparano AM, et al. Mechanical debulking versus balloon angioplasty for the treatment of true bifurcation lesions. J Am Coll Cardiol. 1998;32(7):1845–52.
52. Kandzari DE, Tcheng JE, Gersh BJ, et al. Relationship between infarct artery location, epicardial flow, and myocardial perfusion after primary percutaneous revascularization in acute myocardial infarction. Am Heart J. 2006;151(6):1288–95.
53. Califf RM, Phillips 3rd HR, Hindman MC, Mark DB, Lee KL, Behar VS, Johnson RA, Pryor DB, Rosati RA, Wagner GS, et al. Prognostic value of a coronary artery jeopardy score. J Am Coll Cardiol. 1985;5:1055–63.
54. Alderman EL, Stadius M. The angiographic definitions of the Bypass Angioplasty Revascularization Investigation. Coron Artery Dis. 1992;3:1189–207.
55. Chen SL, Chen JP, Mintz G, Xu B, Kan J, Ye F, Zhang J, Sun X, Xu Y, Jiang Q, Zhang A, Stone GW. Comparison between the ners (new risk stratification) score and the syntax (synergy between percutaneous coronary intervention with taxus and cardiac surgery) score in outcome prediction for unprotected left main stenting. JACC Cardiovasc Interv. 2010;3:632–41.
56. Garg S, Sarno G, Garcia-Garcia HM, Girasis C, Wykrzykowska J, Dawkins KD, Serruys PW. A new tool for the risk stratification of patients with complex coronary artery disease: the clinical syntax score. Circ Cardiovasc Interv. 2010;3:317–26.
57. Graham MM, Faris PD, Ghali WA, Galbraith PD, Norris CM, Badry JT, Mitchell LB, Curtis MJ, Knudtson ML. Validation of three myocardial jeopardy scores in a population-based cardiac catheterization cohort. Am Heart J. 2001;142:254–61.
58. Hamburger JN, Walsh SJ, Khurana R, Ding L, Gao M, Humphries KH, Carere R, Fung AY, Mildenberger RR, Simkus GJ, Webb JG, Buller CE. Percutaneous coronary intervention and 30-day mortality: the British Columbia PCI risk score. Catheter Cardiovasc Interv. 2009;74:377–85.
59. Lansky AJ, Goto K, Cristea E, Fahy M, Parise H, Feit F, Ohman EM, White HD, Alexander KP, Bertrand ME, Desmet W, Hamon M, Mehran R, Moses J, Leon M, Stone GW. Clinical and angiographic predictors of short- and long-term ischemic events in acute coronary syndromes: results from the acute catheterization and urgent intervention triage strategy (acuity) trial. Circ Cardiovasc Interv. 2010;3:308–16.
60. Sianos G, Morel MA, Kappetein AP, Morice MC, Colombo A, Dawkins K, van den Brand M, Van Dyck N, Russell ME, Mohr FW, Serruys PW. The syntax score: an angiographic tool grading the complexity of coronary artery disease. EuroIntervention. 2005;1: 219–27.

Quantitative, Qualitative, and Diagnostic Intravascular Ultrasound

3

Ning Guo and Gary S. Mintz

Angiography is a shadowgraph technique that visualizes the lumen in multiple projected longitudinal "silhouettes"; it assesses coronary artery disease by comparing stenotic to supposedly "normal" segments. However, atherosclerosis is a diffuse process involving the entire arterial wall; and coronary arteries are complex three-dimensional structures with branch points, tortuous segments, and bends. Intravascular ultrasound (IVUS) provides tomographic imaging to provide a more accurate quantitative and qualitative assessment of the disease process and coronary artery anatomy.

An important publication is "Standards for the Acquisition, Measurement, and Reporting of Intravascular Ultrasound studies: A Report of the American College of Cardiology Task Force on Clinical Expert Consensus Documents" [1]. While 11+ years old, this consensus document continues to be the gold standard for IVUS imaging. It contains the preferred nomenclature for describing an IVUS image both qualitatively and quantitatively.

The pre-intervention diagnostic uses of IVUS are (1) to assess the severity of a coronary artery stenosis (lumen dimensions and plaque burden); (2) to assess lesion morphology including composition, distribution, morphometry, and unusual features; and (3) to measure reference vessel size and lesion length prior to performing percutaneous coronary intervention (PCI).

The following are the basic steps in performing a pre-intervention or diagnostic IVUS study:

- Make sure that the patient is adequately anticoagulated.
- Administer intracoronary nitroglycerin to avoid coronary spasm.
- Position the guidewire in the distal vessel.
- Advance the IVUS catheter over the guidewire to a position distal to the target site.
- Begin imaging and verify that the image is acceptable or, if necessary, tweak the overall gain to compensate for a weak catheter and adjust the zoom (depth) for large vessels.
- If imaging an aorto-ostial lesion, retract the guiding catheter back into the aorta and verify that the path of the IVUS transducer will still be coaxial to the ostium of the vessel.
- Begin recording.
- Using uninterrupted pullback, withdraw the transducer or catheter to a point proximal to the target site, but ideally back to the aorta especially when imaging the left anterior descending or left circumflex in order to assess left main disease. (While both manual and motorized transducer pullbacks are acceptable for cross-sectional vessel assessment, length measurements require the use of a motorized pullback device.)
- The transducer can be seen fluoroscopically and its position relative to angiographic anatomy checked using small amounts of contrast injection.
- Remove the catheter and review the recorded study to make the necessary measurements and decisions.

The following are the sequence of structures that are viewed (when imaging from distal to proximal) and the basic decisions that must be made:

- Assessment of distal reference vessel: (1) amount of disease, (2) selection of the distal reference site, and (3) measurement of the distal reference site lumen and/or medial and midwall dimensions.
- Assessment of the target lesion: (1) measurement of lumen compromise and (2) qualitative analysis of morphology, morphometry, etc.
- Assessment of the proximal reference vessel: (1) amount of disease, (2) selection of the proximal reference site, and (3) measurement of the proximal reference site lumen and/or medial and midwall dimensions.

N. Guo, MD, PhD
Department of Cardiology,
First Affiliated Hospital of Medical College
of Xi'an Jiaotong University, Xi'an, China

G.S. Mintz, MD (✉)
Cardiovascular Research Foundation,
111 East 59th St, New York 10022, NY, USA
e-mail: gsm18439@aol.com

C.A. Thompson (ed.), *Textbook of Cardiovascular Intervention*,
DOI 10.1007/978-1-4471-4528-8_3, © Springer-Verlag London 2014

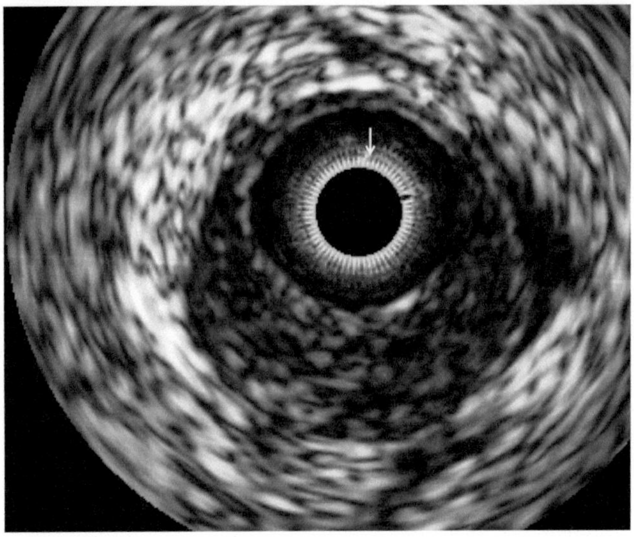

Fig. 3.1 *Ring-down*. Ring-down artifacts (*arrow*) are usually observed as bright halos of variable thickness surrounding the catheter and create a zone of uncertainty adjacent to the transducer surface

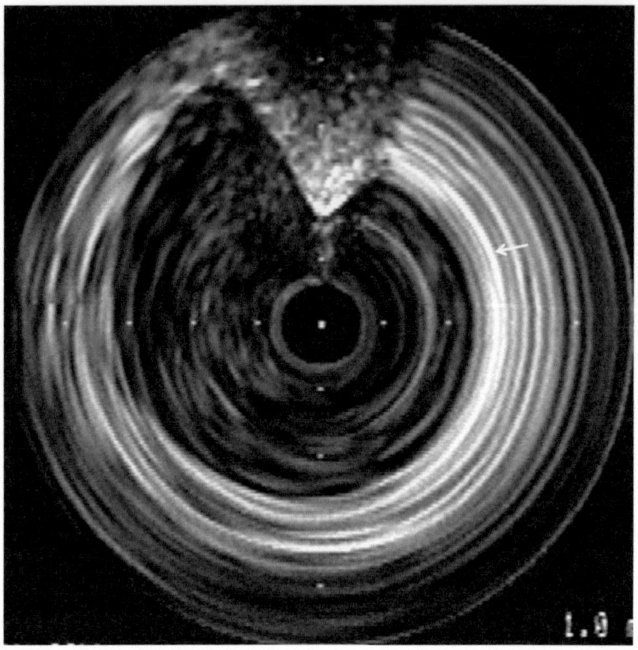

Fig. 3.2 *Non-uniform rotational distortion* (*NURD*). Non-uniform rotational distortion (*NURD*), indicated by *white arrow*, causes a smeared appearance to the image. The arc of vessel wall is alternatively expanded or compressed. Area measurements are no longer reliable. This is an artifact unique to rotating transducers

- Visualization of the rest of the proximal vessel checking for occult stenoses and proximal vessel calcification and, especially if imaging a left coronary artery, assessment of left main disease.
- Measure lesion length – the distance between distal and proximal reference sites.

In the stent era, qualitative morphology assessment is less important than quantitative measurements for proper stent sizing (diameter and length).

Quantitative Analyses

IVUS measurements should be performed at the leading edge of each interface, never the trailing edge. Measurements should be avoided if artifacts are present or if the IVUS catheter is positioned obliquely. It is important for each laboratory to establish standards and have an acceptable inter- and intra-observer variability. This is true for both quantitative and qualitative analyses.

IVUS artifacts can lead to the misinterpretation of IVUS image, including ring-down, non-uniform rotational distortion (NURD), side-lobes, reverberations, blood speckle, air bubbles, etc. Ring-down artifacts are usually observed as bright halos of variable thickness surrounding the catheter and are present in all medical ultrasound devices (Fig. 3.1). Excessive ring-down suppression can reduce signals from true targets. NURD is unique to mechanical catheter systems and results in geometric distortion or smearing of the image when the mechanical binding of the drive cable rotates the transducer nonuniformly (Fig. 3.2); this can occur for a number of reasons, including the presence of acute bends in the artery, tortuous guiding catheter shapes, variance in manufacturing of the hub or driveshaft, excessive tightening of a hemostatic valve, kinking of the imaging sheath, or a small guiding catheter lumen.

During clinical IVUS imaging of non-stented lesions, there are only two distinct boundaries that have consistent histologic correlates: the lumen-intima (or lumen-plaque) interface and the media-adventitia interface. Thus, in non-stented vessels, there are only two cross-sectional area (CSA) measurements that can be reproducibly performed: external elastic membrane (EEM) CSA (a reproducible measure of the area within the media-adventitia interface) and lumen CSA (a reproducible measure of the area within the intima).

Lumen Borders

The first "structure" that the IVUS beam sees is the blood-filled lumen. Saline (or contrast) injection through the guiding catheter is useful in differentiating blood speckle from tissue and defining true lumen borders, especially when blood speckle is intense as when a tight stenosis becomes more occlusive (and blood flow more static) with the IVUS catheter across the lesion. Lumen measurements are performed at the leading edge of the intima relative to the center of mass of the lumen. Measurements include lumen CSA, minimum lumen diameter (the shortest diameter through the center point of the lumen), and maximum lumen diameter (the longest diameter through the center point of the lumen) (Fig. 3.3).

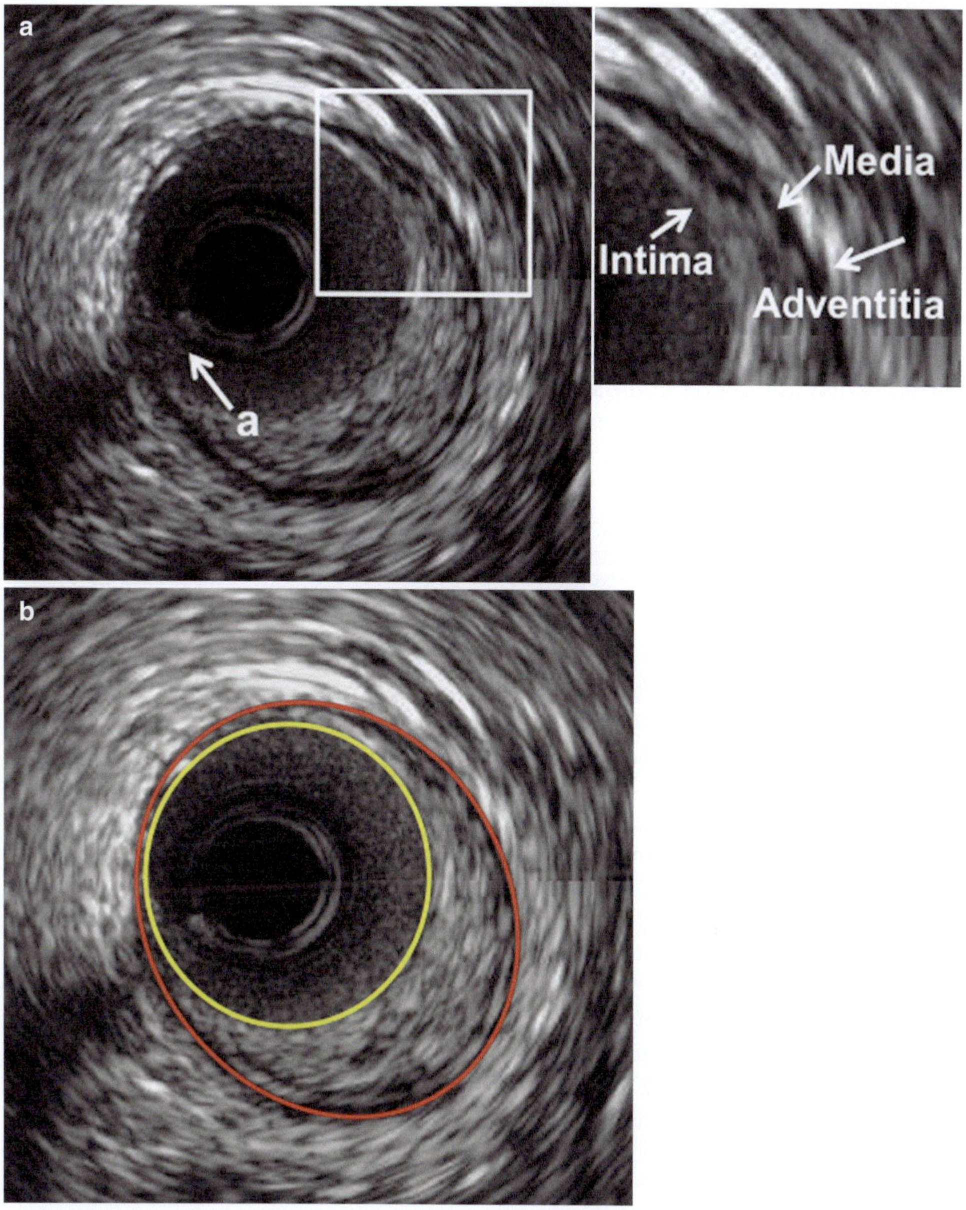

Fig. 3.3 *Cross-sectional appearance and measurements*. This is an example of a diseased coronary artery with eccentric plaque. *Panel A* shows intima, media, and adventitia. Note the guidewire artifact with *shadowing* (**a**). Measurements are shown in *Panel B*. The *yellow line* highlights lumen. The *red line* indicates the external elastic membrane (*EEM*). Measurements should be performed at the leading edge of the intima or the border between the media and the adventitia, respectively. Plaque&media CSA is calculated as EEM minus lumen CSA

Media

Truly normal coronary arteries are rare in the practice of interventional cardiology; only 160 μm of intimal thickening are needed to consistently produce an intimal layer using current imaging frequencies [2]. In normal arteries the material that most strongly reflects ultrasound is collagen. The adventitia of coronary arteries has high collagen content and is, therefore, echoreflective. Conversely, the media of coronary arteries has low collagen content and is typically echolucent (Fig. 3.3).

The internal elastic membrane separates the intima from the media. Although the internal elastic membrane is composed of strong echogenic elastic tissue, fibrous changes in the inner third of the media decrease the difference in acoustic impedance (reflectivity) between these adjacent layers blurring the distinction between the internal elastic membrane and the inner border of the media [3]. With increasing atherosclerosis, the intima/plaque layer increases in thickness and tends to merge with the internal elastic lamina. All of these changes preclude reliable measurement or even estimation of media thickness [4].

External Elastic Membrane (EEM)

The adventitia is 300–500 μm thick and is composed of loose collagen and elastic tissue that merges with the surrounding peri-adventitia. A discrete interface exists at the border between the media and the adventitia; it is almost invariably present on an IVUS image and corresponds closely to the location of the EEM. Measurements should be made at the leading edge of the border between the media and the adventitia (Fig. 3.3).

EEM circumference and CSA cannot be measured reliably at sites where large side branches originate or in the setting of extensive calcific acoustic shadowing. If acoustic shadowing involves a relatively small arc (<90°), planimetry of the EEM circumference can be performed by extrapolation from the closest identifiable EEM borders although measurement accuracy and reproducibility will be reduced. In addition, some stent designs may obscure the EEM. Finally, longitudinal image reconstruction can identify the media-adventitia border just proximal or distal to calcium or stent metal and, therefore, aid in interpolation. Because arteries decrease in size from immediately proximal to a large side branch to immediately distal to that branch, interpolation should not be used to "reconstruct" an EEM interrupted by a branch.

Plaque and Media

Because the media cannot be quantified accurately, IVUS measurements cannot determine true histological plaque area (the area bounded by the internal elastic membrane). Instead, IVUS studies use EEM and lumen measurements to create a surrogate for true plaque (or atheroma) – the plaque plus media – and the cross-sectional measurement of atherosclerotic plaque is reported as plaque and media CSA that is calculated as EEM minus lumen CSA and abbreviated as P&M CSA (Fig. 3.3). In practice, the inclusion of the media into the atheroma area does not constitute a major limitation because the media represents only a very small fraction of the P&M CSA. In addition, the percentage of media represented in the P&M complex does not change measurably during serial studies.

Plaque typically appears eccentric by IVUS in that there is usually more on one side of the lesion than the other. IVUS can assess the degree of eccentricity of plaque distribution. However, there is no consensus as to the exact IVUS definition of an eccentric plaque. One qualitative, indicative measure of eccentricity is the ratio of maximum P&M thickness to minimum P&M thickness and qualitatively as eccentric plaque as maximum/minimum P&M thickness ≥2 [5]. It also can be quantified as the difference between maximum and minimum P&M thickness divided by maximum P&M thickness [1].

Qualitative Analyses

Atherosclerotic lesions are heterogeneous and include varying amounts of calcium, dense fibrous tissue, lipid, smooth muscle cells, thrombus, etc. While grayscale IVUS cannot provide histologically accurate information regarding plaque composition, IVUS imaging has been used grossly to separate lesions into subtypes according to echodensity of different plaque components and presence or absence of shadowing and reverberations. However, it should be noted that plaques frequently contain more than one acoustical subtype. In fact, atherosclerotic plaques are rarely homogeneous and should be described as mixed, "fibrocalcific," "fibrofatty," etc. Furthermore, with the exception of calcification, plaque composition assessment using grayscale IVUS should be performed with caution. With improved pharmacology, the assessment of atheroma burden and plaque morphology has become important. Several technologies have been developed to improve on the limitations of grayscale IVUS to assess plaque composition, including virtual histology (VH)-IVUS, iMAP-IVUS, and integrated backscatter (IB)-IVUS. Of these technologies, VH-IVUS in combination with grayscale IVUS data has been used most frequently in serial trials [6].

Calcified Plaques

Calcium is a powerful reflector of ultrasound; little of the beam penetrates through or even into the calcium. Thus, calcium casts a shadow over deeper arterial structures, only the leading edge of the calcific deposit can be seen, and even calcium thickness cannot be measured. In practice the grayscale IVUS signature of calcium is hyperechoic plaque (brighter than the reference adventitia) that shadows. Occasionally, calcium will produce reverberations: one or more equidistantly spaced rings at intervals that are a multiple of the distance from the transducer to the leading edge of the calcium. Reverberations are more specific for calcium than mere shadowing and are more common after calcium is treated with rotational atherectomy (Fig. 3.4).

Detection of lesion-associated calcium by IVUS also depends on the histologic pattern. Small calcific deposits within a necrotic lipid core appear different from larger calcific elements, and microcalcifications can be missed entirely. With the exception of microcalcifications, IVUS is sensitive and specific for detecting calcium within a plaque.

Using IVUS, calcium can be localized to the lesion versus the reference segment, characterized as superficial (closer to the tissue-lumen interface) versus deep (closer to the media-adventitia junction), and quantified according to its arc and length. IVUS routinely detects target lesion calcification – even severe calcium – that is angiographically "silent." Both pathologic and IVUS studies have shown that arterial calcification is a marker for and an index of the overall arterial atherosclerotic plaque burden.

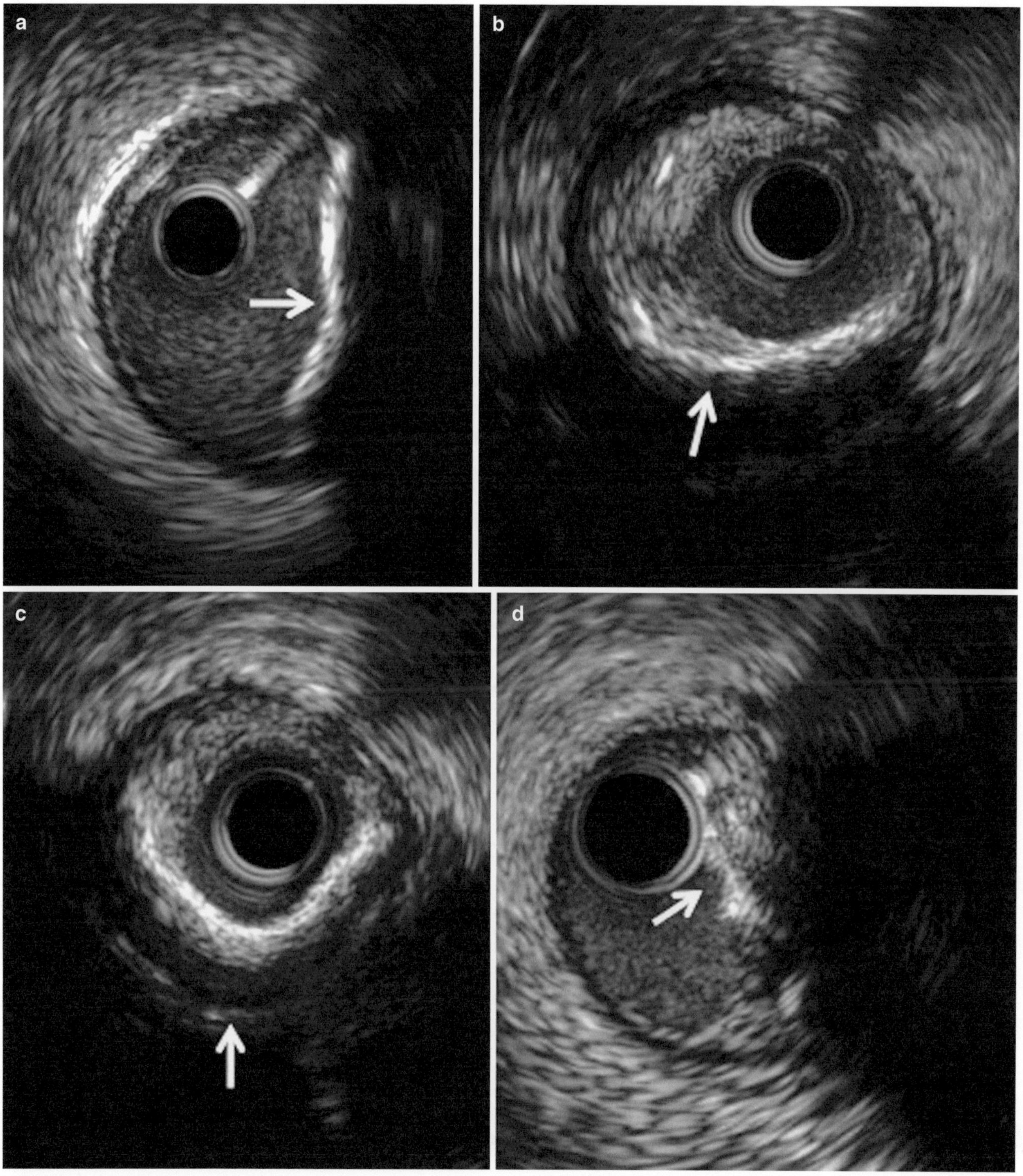

Fig. 3.4 *Calcified plaques*. Hyperechoic plaque (plaque that is brighter than the reference adventitia and shadows deeper wall structures) can be superficial (**a**: closer to the tissue-lumen interface) or deep (**b**: closer to the media-adventitia junction). (**c**) is an example of reverberation (*arrow*); reverberation is more specific for calcium while shadowing is more sensitive. A calcific nodule is presented in (**d**)

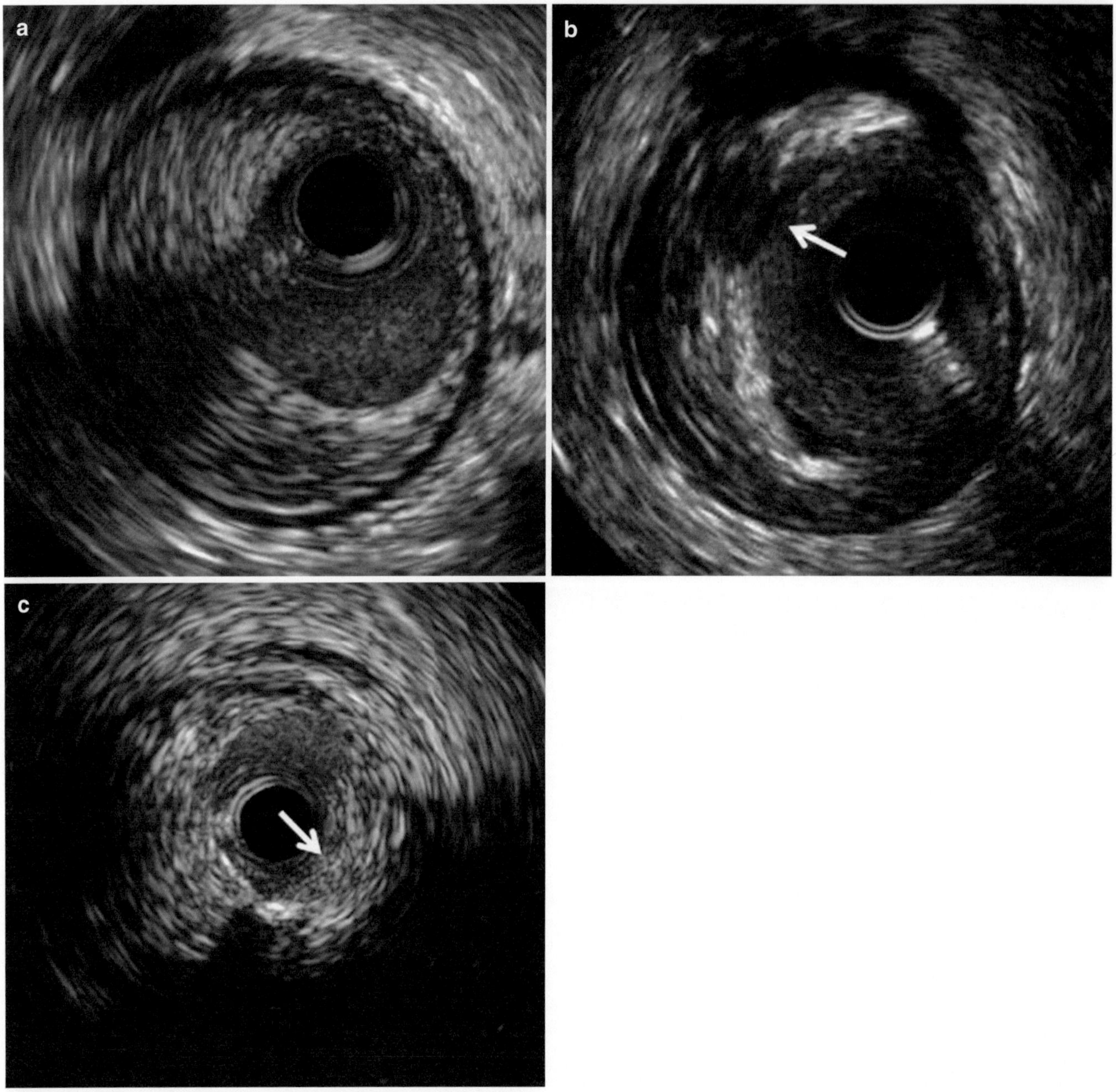

Fig. 3.5 *Fibrous plaque, echolucent plaque, and attenuated plaque.* A fibrous plaque is shown in (**a**) – plaque that is as bright as the adventitia, but without shadowing. (**b**) presents an echolucent plaque that is characterized by a hypoechoic zone within the plaque (*arrow*). An attenuated plaque (hypoechoic or isoechoic, but without penetration to the adventitia) is shown in (**c**) (*arrow*)

Fibrous Plaques

Fibrous plaques represent the majority of atherosclerotic lesions. In general, the greater the fibrous tissue content, the greater the echogenicity of the tissue. Both calcified and fibrotic plaques are hyperechoic, and very dense fibrous plaques may produce sufficient attenuation to be misclassified as calcification with acoustic shadowing (Fig. 3.5).

Echolucent Plaques

Echolucent plaques are less bright compared to the reference adventitia. Alternative terms are hypoechoic and "soft." Echolucent plaques contain varying amounts of fibrous and fatty tissue. Pure fat is much more echolucent than muscle. A lipid pool, therefore, should appear as a dark or echolucent zone within a lesion (Fig. 3.5); however, in practice, the in

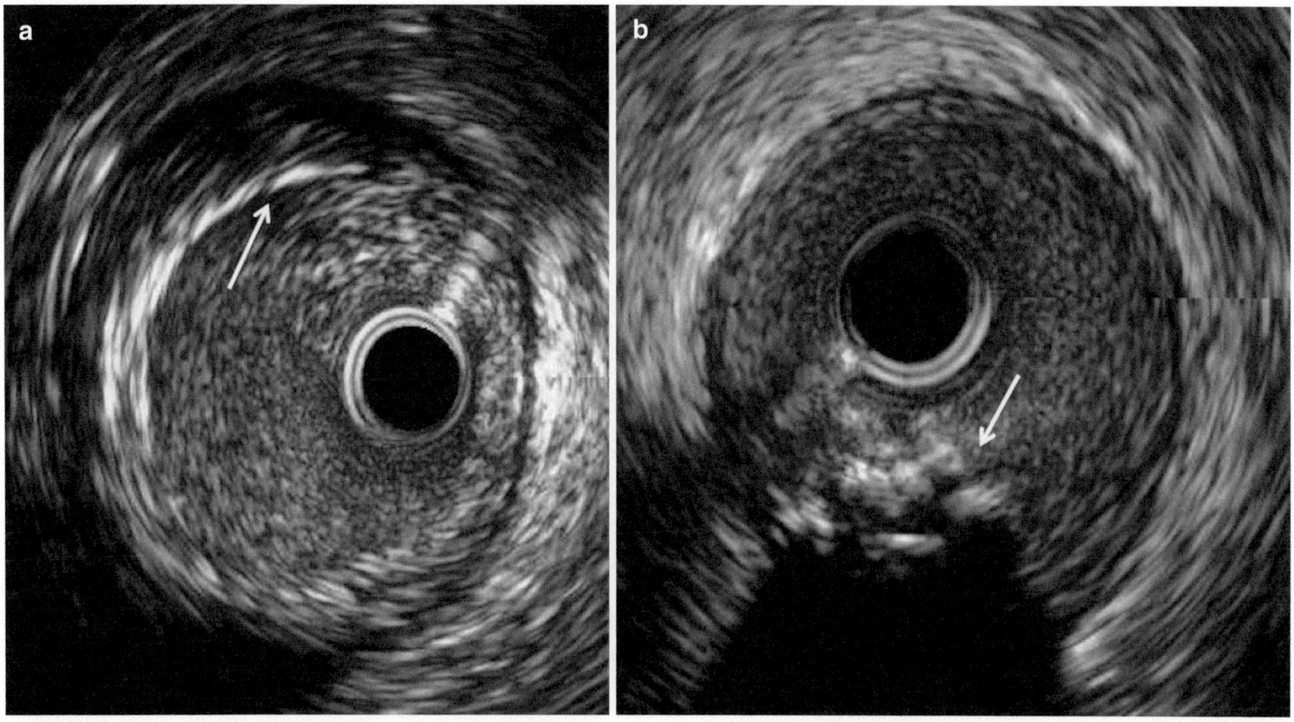

Fig. 3.6 *Thrombus*. Thrombus is a discrete and mobile intraluminal mass with a distinct interface with the underlying vessel wall (**a**) or as a lobulated mass projecting into the lumen with sparkling "scintillating" appearance (**b**), in this case superimposed on a calcified nodule

vivo identification of lipid pools (as well as of rupture-prone plaques or thin-capped atheromas) is not possible with the current grayscale IVUS technology. Most echolucent plaques contain minimal collagen and elastin. The term "soft" should be avoided since it implies "sponginess", and even fatty plaques are hard to the touch.

Attenuated Plaques

Attenuated plaque is hypoechoic plaque with deeper ultrasound attenuation that is not due to calcification or very dense fibrous plaque (Fig. 3.5). Several histopathologic analyses of attenuated plaques have shown microcalcifications, thrombi, or cholesterol crystals [7, 8]. Histologically, attenuated plaques contains more fibrofatty tissue and necrotic core compared to fibrous plaque without attenuation [9]. Comparison with VH-IVUS has suggested that these contain large necrotic cores. 10].

Thrombus

The identification of thrombus is one of the most difficult aspects of IVUS imaging. Clues to the presence of thrombus include the following: (1) a sparkling "scintillating" appearance, (2) a lobulated mass projecting into the lumen, (3) a distinct interface between the suspected thrombus and underlying plaque, (4) identification of blood speckle within the thrombus indicating microchannels through the thrombus, and (5) mobility (Fig. 3.6). While the combination of these features is, in general, specific, it is not sensitive; and the IVUS diagnosis of thrombus should be considered presumptive. However, there are no recent studies assessing the accuracy of the IVUS diagnosis of thrombus. Furthermore, it is important to emphasize that while the routine IVUS diagnosis of thrombus in native coronary arteries is difficult, the diagnosis of thrombus in saphenous vein grafts (where degenerated tissue can have all of these same features) is, frankly, totally unreliable. Furthermore, the IVUS signature of thrombus changes with the age and composition of the clot.

Lesion and Reference Segment Assessment

Within a segment, there will always be a worst stenosis, but there can be multiple secondary stenoses. In the case of multiple lesions within a single coronary segment, distinct stenoses (or other important morphologies such as the site of plaque rupture) require at least 5 mm of reference segment between them.

The worst stenosis should be the slice with the smallest lumen CSA. This may or may not represent the site with the largest plaque burden. However, if there are multiple image slices with the same minimum lumen area, the one with the largest P&M area should be selected for quantitative analysis. In some cases quantitative analysis of a single slice may describe the lesion adequately. In other cases, proper description may require analysis of an entire segment with quantitative analysis and measurement of a number of image slices. Lesion morphology can vary from slice to slice within a segment.

Plaque Burden Versus Stenosis

The P&M CSA is often divided by EEM CSA to generate a measurement called the plaque burden or atheroma burden. This is distinct from the luminal area stenosis. The former represents the area within the EEM occupied by atheroma regardless of lumen compromise, and a large plaque burden can occur in the absence of any obstruction in the presence of sufficient positive remodeling. Thus, it is a measure of plaque accumulation, not of luminal compromise. Conversely, lumen area stenosis (or diameter stenosis) is a measure of luminal compromise in which the lesion site lumen CSA is compared to the reference lumen CSA; this is analogous to the calculation of the angiographic diameter stenosis.

Reference Segments

The proximal image slice is the site with the largest lumen proximal to a stenosis, but within the same segment (usually within 10 mm of the stenosis with no major intervening branches). This may not be the site with the least plaque. However, among slices with the same largest lumen area, the one with the least plaque should be selected. Ostial lesions and lesions immediately distal to a large side branch will not have a proximal reference.

Similarly, the distal reference is the site with the largest lumen distal to a stenosis, but within the same segment (usually within 10 mm of the stenosis with no intervening branches). Again, this may not be the site with the least plaque; however, among slices with the same largest lumen area, the one with the least plaque should be selected. It should be noted that the distal reference may be underperfused, especially during pre-intervention imaging, and may "grow" during an intervention as the stenosis is relieved. Once the reference segments are selected, quantitative and qualitative assessment should be similar to the stenosis.

There are discrepancies between IVUS and coronary angiography assessment of reference segments. IVUS reference segment measurements are usually larger than angiography; however, in individual patients this difference is very variable, and some IVUS reference measurements are actually smaller than angiography. IVUS routinely shows significant atherosclerosis in angiographically "normal" reference segments in patients with significant stenoses undergoing intervention. In a study of 884 patients, only 6.8 % of the angiographically "normal" reference segments were truly normal; the average plaque burden of the most normal-looking reference segment was 51 ± 13 % [11]. Importantly, a greater stent edge plaque burden and residual reference segment stenosis are associated stent edge restenosis and stent thrombosis [12, 13].

Remodeling

Vascular remodeling, originally described by Glagov et al. from necropsy specimens, refers to the increase or decrease in EEM area that occurs during the development of atherosclerosis [14]. EEM CSA increase is termed "positive remodeling." Conversely, EEM CSA decrease has been termed "negative remodeling."

The ideal natural history study of atherosclerosis and remodeling requires serial observations, perhaps multiple studies over a span of years. The slope of the line relating the change in EEM CSA to the change in P&M CSA would indicate the direction and magnitude of remodeling [1].

- A slope >1.0 would indicate positive remodeling with overcompensation (resulting in net lumen increase).
- A slope = 1.0 would indicate perfect positive remodeling where the increase in plaque was exactly balanced by the increase in EEM CSA leading to no lumen change.
- A slope <1.0 would indicate inadequate positive remodeling (incomplete compensation).
- A slope <0 (or reduction in EEM CSA) would indicate negative remodeling.

Most IVUS reports of remodeling have been based on IVUS studies performed at a single point in time. Here are two sets of definitions among the many that have been published. Lesion remodeling may be studied by calculating a remodeling index (RI = lesion EEM CSA/reference EEM CSA). In one paradigm, RI >1.05 is termed positive remodeling, RI between 0.95 and 1.05 is termed intermediate remodeling, and RI <0.95 is termed negative remodeling. In another paradigm, lesion EEM CSA > proximal reference is termed positive remodeling, lesion EEM CSA between the proximal and distal reference is termed intermediate remodeling, and lesion EEM CSA < distal reference is termed negative remodeling [1, 15].

As shown in a number of IVUS studies, positive remodeling is seen in the stetting of acute coronary syndromes, plaque vulnerability, and late acquired stent malapposition [15–21]. Thus, the cumulative evidence indicates that positively remodeled lesions are more biologically active than intermediate or negatively remodeled lesions.

Lengths and Volumes

Longitudinal representation of IVUS images is useful for length measurements, for interpolation of shadowed deep arterial structures, and for quickly identifying the minimal lumen area and the proximal and distal reference image slices. However, area, diameter, and thickness measurements must be performed on the appropriate cross-sectional image slices.

Motorized transducer pullback (ideally at 0.5 mm/s) yields accurate length measurements especially with mechanical systems because the transducer is pulled through a stationary imaging sheath (length = number of seconds × pullback speed). This approach can be used to determine the length of a lesion, stenosis, calcium, or any other longitudinal feature. Lengths should not be measured with manual transducer pullback.

Angiography measures lesion length from shoulder-to-shoulder in the least foreshortened projection. However, it is not always possible to eliminate foreshortening; and a single projection cannot deal with vessel tortuosity or bend points. IVUS measures lesion length by tracking the transducer through the coronary artery regardless of bend points or tortuosity; and, of course, foreshortening is not an issue. In addition lesion length determination requires identification of the ends of the lesion – a process that can be difficult because these ends are rarely disease free.

Volumetric Analysis

Motorized transducer pullback can also permit volumetric IVUS calculations using either Simpson's rule (in which multiple image slices acquired at a fixed interval are added) or multiple longitudinal views. A typical set of volumetric measurements will include EEM volume, lumen volume, stent volume, intimal hyperplasia (IH) volume, %IH volume (IH volume divided by stent volume), P&M volume, and volumetric plaque (or atheroma) burden (P&M volume divided by EEM volume). Volumes should not be measured when using manual transducer pullback.

Longer imaged segments, lesions, and stents will have larger volumes compared to shorter segments. Therefore, mean planar analysis (in which measured volumes are normalized for lesion length) should be reported along with actual volumes when comparing segments of unequal length. A typical set of mean planar (or cross-sectional area) measurements will include mean EEM CSA, mean lumen CSA, mean stent CSA, mean IH CSA, %IH (mean IH CSA divided by mean stent CSA), mean P&M CSA, and mean plaque burden (mean P&M CSA divided by mean EEM CSA).

Monitoring changes in the extent of coronary atherosclerosis with IVUS has been increasingly used in clinical trials to assess progression and regression of atherosclerosis. Nearly all IVUS studies of progression/regression employ volumetric IVUS methodology. A recent clinical expert consensus document issued the standards for acquisition, measurement, and reporting of IVUS progression/regression studies [6].

Diagnostic Imaging

The use of IVUS to assess stenosis severity has come under justifiable criticism. Similarly, in the stent era – especially, the drug-eluting stent era – assessment of lesion morphology is less important than previously since stent implantation tends to minimize the impact of lesion morphology on the acute and chronic results of percutaneous intervention.

Stenosis Severity

Studies performed more than 10 years ago suggested that an IVUS minimum lumen area (MLA) >4 mm^2 was a valid criteria *to defer an intervention* based on both comparisons to physiologic measures and from follow-up data. In these studies a pre-intervention MLA ≥4.0 mm^2 had a diagnostic accuracy of 92 % in predicting a coronary flow reserve ≥2.0 [22] and a diagnostic accuracy of 93 % versus stress myocardial perfusion imaging [23]. Takagi found similar results when the IVUS MLA was compared to fractional flow reserve measured by the pressure wire [24]. In support of these studies, PCI was deferred based on IVUS findings in 300 patients. Events occurred in 24 patients. There was an important difference between lesions with MLA above and below 4.0 mm^2. In 248 lesions with a MLA ≥4.0 mm^2, the event rate was only 4.4 %; and the revascularization rate was only 2.8 % [25]. However, this cutoff only applied to major epicardial vessels excluding the left main coronary artery (LMCA) and excluding saphenous vein grafts, and it was necessary to interrogate the lesion carefully to identify and measure the image slice with the smallest lumen, especially in very focal stenoses. Recently this cutoff has come under criticism for a number of reasons including the size of the vessels (studies were done mostly in 3.5 mm vessels), the average MLA of the intermediate lesions studied (4 mm^2), and the fact that these studies have been misinterpreted incorrectly to suggest that lesions with an IVUS MLA <4 mm^2 justified stent implantation. For example, Lee et al. found that an MLA ≤2.0 mm^2, plaque burden of ≥80 %, and lesion length of ≥20 mm predicted a fractional flow reserve (FFR) of <0.75 with good sensitivity and specificity in reference vessels <3 mm [26]. Kang et al. reported that an MLA ≥2.4 mm^2 may be useful to exclude FFR <0.80, but its 63 % specificity limited the value or an MLA <2.4 mm^2 for predicting an FFR <0.80. Thus, it is recommended that for major epicardial vessels excluding the LMCA, physiologic lesion assessment (using an intracoronary pressure wire and

Table 3.1 Comparisons of angiography, IVUS, and physiologic methodology to assess lesion severity

	Abizaid [22]	Nishioka [23]	Takagi [24]	Briguori [27]	Takayama [28]	Lee [26]	Kang [29]	Ahn [30]	Ben-Dor [31]	Koo [32]
Physiologic methodology	CFR	SPECT	FFR	FFR	FFR	FFR	FFR	SPECT	FFR	FFR
Patient number	112	70	51	53	14	94	236	170	92	267
Abnormal percentage	40 %	65 %	49 %	23 %	50 %	40 %	21 %	26 %	26 %	33 %
IVUS parameters										
Reference lumen CSA, mm^2	8.3 7.4	11.9 10.6	9.3	7.8	10.3	5.9 5.5	7.6			7.8 6.7
MLA, mm^2	4.4	4.3	3.9	3.9	3.5	2.3	2.6	2.1		3.0
MLA cutoff, mm^2	4.0	4.0	3.0	4.0	n/a	2.0	2.4	2.1	3.2	2.75
Other determinants	LL				MLA/LL	LL PB	PB LAD	PB	Vessel size	Proximal-mid LAD Vessel size
QCA parameters										
Length, mm			14	8.5	17.9	15.1		21.2		16.5
QCA reference, mm			3.0	3.1	2.9	2.7		3.3		3.1
DS, %			46	52	53			55		50

IVUS intravascular ultrasound, *CFR* coronary flow reserve, *SPECT* single-photon emission computed tomography, *FFR* fractional flow reserve, *CSA* cross-sectional area, *MLA* minimal lumen area, *LL* lesion length, *PB* plaque burden, *LAD* left anterior descending coronary artery, *QCA* quantitative coronary angiography, *DS* diameter stenosis

maximum hyperemia with intravenous adenosine to measure FFR) should be the preferred approach to assess lesion severity. A summary of the published comparisons are shown in Table 3.1. While the most common MLA associated with ischemia in these studies is 3.0 mm^2, in the current era the best technique for assessing lesion severity in non-left main coronary artery (LMCA) lesions is FFR and not IVUS.

Assessment of LMCA disease has emerged as an important indication for IVUS imaging. An IVUS left main minimum lumen diameter (MLD) of 2.8 mm had a sensitivity of 93 % and a specificity of 98 %, and an IVUS MLA of 5.9 mm^2 had a sensitivity of 93 % and a specificity of 95 % compared to a FFR of 0.75 [33]; and studies have shown that the FFR cutoff 0.75–0.8 is useful for triaging patients with left main disease [34, 35]. LITRO was a large-scale, multicenter prospective registry to evaluate the long-term results of the prospective application of 6 mm^2 as an MLA IVUS criterion for assessment of intermediate lesions of LMCA. In a 2-year follow-up period, cardiac death-free survival was 97.7 % in the group with an MLA >6 mm^2 versus 94.5 % in the revascularized group ($p=0.5$), and event-free survival was 87.3 % versus 80.6 % ($p=0.3$). In the 2-year period only 8 (4.4 %) patients in the group with an MLA >6 mm^2 required subsequent LMCA revascularization, none with an infarction. However, patients with an MLA <6 mm^2 in whom revascularization was deferred had a significantly worse event-free survival (68 %) and survival free of cardiac death, MI, and revascularization was 62.5 % [36].

Unstable Lesion Morphology

In the stent era, especially the drug-eluting stent era, assessment of lesion morphology is less important than previously since stent implantation tends to minimize the impact of lesion morphology on the acute and chronic results of percutaneous intervention. Nevertheless, several aspects of morphologic assessments are important, especially for some unusual images that coronary angiogram cannot access accurately.

The most common type of vulnerable plaque is a thin-capped fibroatheroma (TCFA) that first ruptures and then thromboses. It is estimated that approximately 60 % of acute coronary events are the result of TCFA rupture and thrombosis. Histopathologic characteristics of a TCFA include positive remodeling, fibrous cap thickness <100 μ and perhaps <65 μ, macrophage infiltration of the fibrous cap, and lipid/necrotic core >10 % of total plaque area often with intraplaque hemorrhage or rich vasa vasorum. The majority of TCFAs are found within the proximal segments of the left anterior descending (LAD) and left circumflex (LCX) arteries and within the right coronary artery (RCA) from its ostium to its distal bifurcation. Grayscale IVUS can assess remodeling, but cannot identify other features indicative of a TFCA. In a retrospective three-vessel grayscale IVUS study, Kim et al. defined vulnerable plaques as plaques with rupture, hypoechoic core, dissection, or thrombus [37]. On multivariate cox regression analysis, the multiplicity of vulnerable plaques in nontarget vessels was the only independent predictor of long-term (mean follow-up was

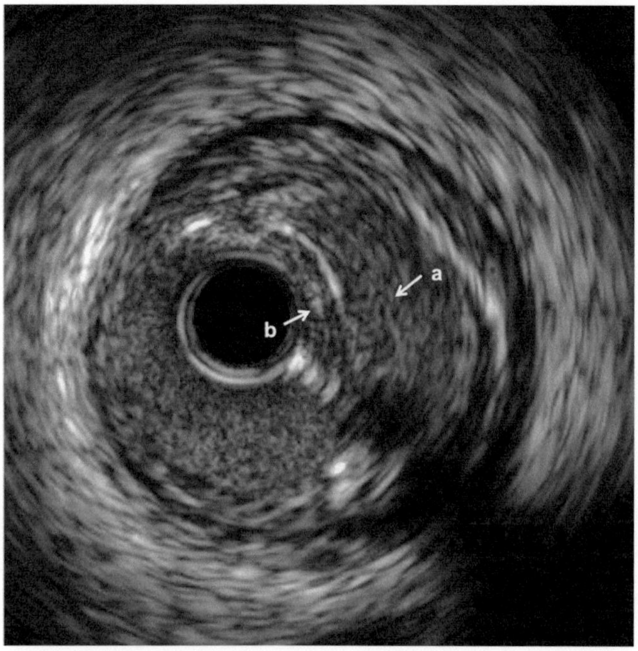

Fig. 3.7 *Ruptured plaque*. This IVUS image shows a plaque containing a cavity (*arrow* "a") that communicates with the lumen with an overlying residual fibrous cap fragment (*arrow* "b") that typically appears to be incomplete relative to the mouth of the ruptured plaque cavity in its circumferential extent

50 months) critical events, while ACS and diabetes mellitus were independent predictors of multiple vulnerable plaques.

The IVUS features of a ruptured plaque are consistent with the reported histology – a cavity that communicated with the lumen with an overlying residual fibrous cap fragment [16, 38]. The fibrous cap remnant typically appears to be incomplete relative to the mouth of the ruptured plaque cavity in either its circumferential or axial extent (Fig. 3.7). Most rupture plaques are associated with acute coronary syndromes and cause angiographically complex plaques. However, not all ruptured plaques are associated with acute events. A minority will be clinically and angiographically silent [39]. Maehara et al. demonstrated the occurrence of plaque rupture in patients with stable symptom or asymptomatic ischemia [38]. Almost all (90 %) angiographic complex lesions – either ulceration, intimal flap, lumen irregularity, thrombus, and aneurysm – were associated with IVUS ruptured plaques validating the commonly used Ambrose angiographic identification of ACS lesions. However, angiography missed plaque ruptures especially multiple discrete plaque ruptures in the same artery. Three-vessel IVUS imaging showed that plaque ruptures occurred mainly in proximal segments of the LAD (83 % of LAD plaque rupture), the proximal and distal segments of the RCA (48 and 32 % of RCA plaque ruptures, respectively), and the entire LCX [40]. Recognizing that some ruptured plaques can be asymptomatic or only associated with stable coronary artery disease, Fujii et al. compared the morphology of ruptured plaques that were culprit ACS lesions with "incidental" ruptured plaques [41]. Multivariate analysis identified smaller minimum lumen area and presence of thrombus as independent predictors of ACS culprit plaque ruptures. This suggests that plaque rupture, itself, did not lead to symptoms. Instead, it was the association of plaque rupture with a smaller lumen area and/or thrombus formation causing lumen compromise that led to symptoms. Thus, vulnerable plaques can also rupture silently and heal or contribute to disease progression [42].

Conversely, an identifiable plaque rupture in the setting of an acute myocardial infarction (MI) has a worse outcome compared to an MI without plaque rupture that is presumably caused by plaque erosion and thrombosis, and multiple plaque ruptures have a worse prognosis than a single plaque rupture [43–45]. However, the prevalence of multiple plaque ruptures in the setting of an acute myocardial infarction has been the subject of debate with the frequencies ranging from approximately 80 % down to approximately 20 % [46].

Not all vulnerable plaques are TCFAs. Erosions are the next most common type of vulnerable plaques that lead to thrombosis and acute event. Eroded plaques are rich in smooth muscle cells and proteoglycan and are less calcified compare to ruptured plaques. They are more common in women, younger individuals, and diabetics; are associated with smoking and an absence of positive remodeling; and have less luminal stenosis compared to rupture plaques. The surface features of erosions are below the resolution of grayscale IVUS.

Calcific nodules are the least common type of vulnerable plaques. Calcific nodules are often confused with intracoronary thrombi when seen angiographically in patients presenting with an ACS. They are seen more often in the right coronary and in older patients. No data have been published yet concerning the population at risk for this type of vulnerable plaque.

Attenuated plaques are more common in patients with ACS than in patients with stable angina and are also more common in patients with ST-elevation myocardial infarction (STEMI) than in patients with non-STEMI. Attenuated plaques are usually associated with a high level of C-reactive protein, positive remodeling, and distal embolization or slow or no-reflow before and especially after PCI [47, 48]. However, ASTEROID (A Study to Evaluate the Effect of Rosuvastatin on Intravascular Ultrasound-Derived Coronary Atheroma Burden) trail showed that attenuated plaque is present in a significant number of nonculprit segments and remains stable during follow-up [5]. These findings challenge the assumption that attenuated plaque is a finding limited to culprit lesions associated with acute clinical presentation.

Angiographic Aneurysms

Maehara published an IVUS classification of angiographic coronary artery aneurysms [49]. In this study of 77 angiographic

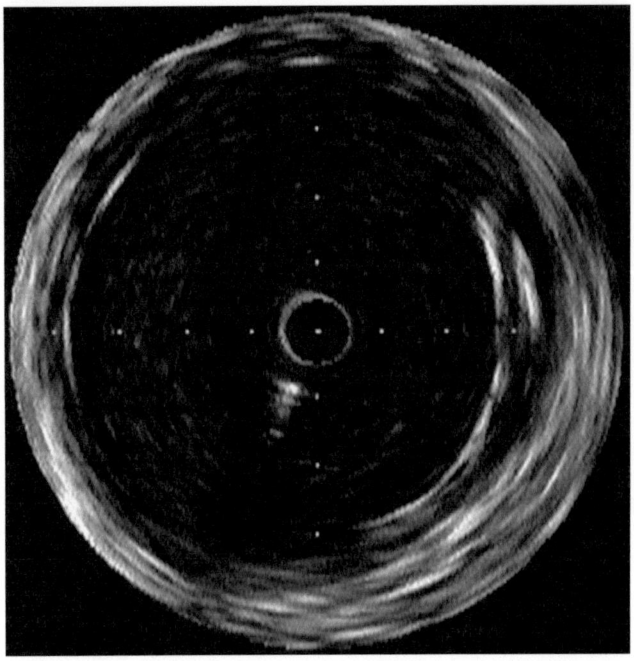

Fig. 3.8 *True aneurysm*. This IVUS image shows a true aneurysm caused by Kawasaki's disease with intact intimal, medial, and adventitial layers. The *dots* are 1 mm apart

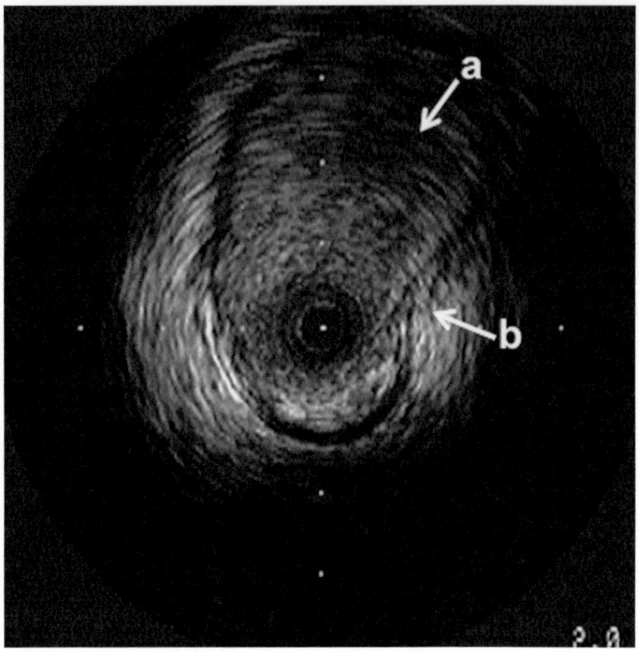

Fig. 3.9 *Pseudoaneurysm*. This is a follow-up IVUS image with previously directional coronary atherectomy illustrating a pseudoaneurysm (*arrow* "a") and discontinuous adventitia at the point of the transition from the vessel to the aneurysm (*arrow* "b"). The *dots* are 2 mm apart

"aneurysmal" lesions, 21 (27 %) were classified as true aneurysms (Fig. 3.8), 3 (4 %) were classified as pseudoaneurysms (all having previous intervention) (Fig. 3.9), and 12 (16 %) were lesions with ruptured or disrupted plaques or spontaneous or unhealed dissections. A true aneurysm was defined as both an EEM and lumen area 50 % larger than the proximal reference with an intact vessel wall – typically with one or more adjacent severe stenoses. A pseudoaneurysm (or false aneurysm – ruptures of the vessel wall that are sealed by an overlying hematoma that organizes into thin-walled fibrous tissue that bridges the break in vessel wall integrity) was defined as a maximum lumen area 50 % larger than the proximal reference with loss of vessel wall integrity. For all practical purposes, pseudoaneurysms were only seen in the setting of a prior intervention although post-intervention aneurysms can be either true aneurysms or pseudoaneurysms. However, the most common finding – seen in 41 patients (53 %) – was a normal arterial segment adjacent to one or more stenoses that had the angiographic appearance of an aneurysm.

Myocardial Bridges

Normally, EEM and lumen CSA are largest in midsystole and smallest in late diastole. In a muscle bridge (MB), the artery (most often the left anterior descending artery) runs under a band of epicardial muscle causing systolic compression of the artery. IVUS studies have clarified why ischemia can occur in such patients when the angiogram shows just systolic compression, and coronary flow is minimal during systole. IVUS shows both phasic systolic compression and – importantly – the fact that compression persists into mid-to-late diastole when most coronary flow occurs. Ge has described a specific "half moon" phenomenon surrounding myocardial bridges; this is only present over the intramyocardial length of the artery [50] (Fig. 3.10). Visualization of the typical systolic compression depends on the severity of the abnormality, although it can be provoked or exaggerated by nitroglycerin. Although angiography detected a MB in only 3 % of patients, IVUS-detectable MBs were observed in approximately 1/4 of patients undergoing LAD imaging [51]. Moreover, in-stent restenosis was more common in the stented MB segments versus without [52, 53].

Spontaneous Dissections

Spontaneous coronary artery dissection is a rare cause of ACS and sudden death. It has traditionally been described in three groups of patients: patients with coronary artery disease; women during the peripartum period; and a heterogeneous group of patients with idiopathic disease, comprising individuals without cardiovascular risk factors, those with

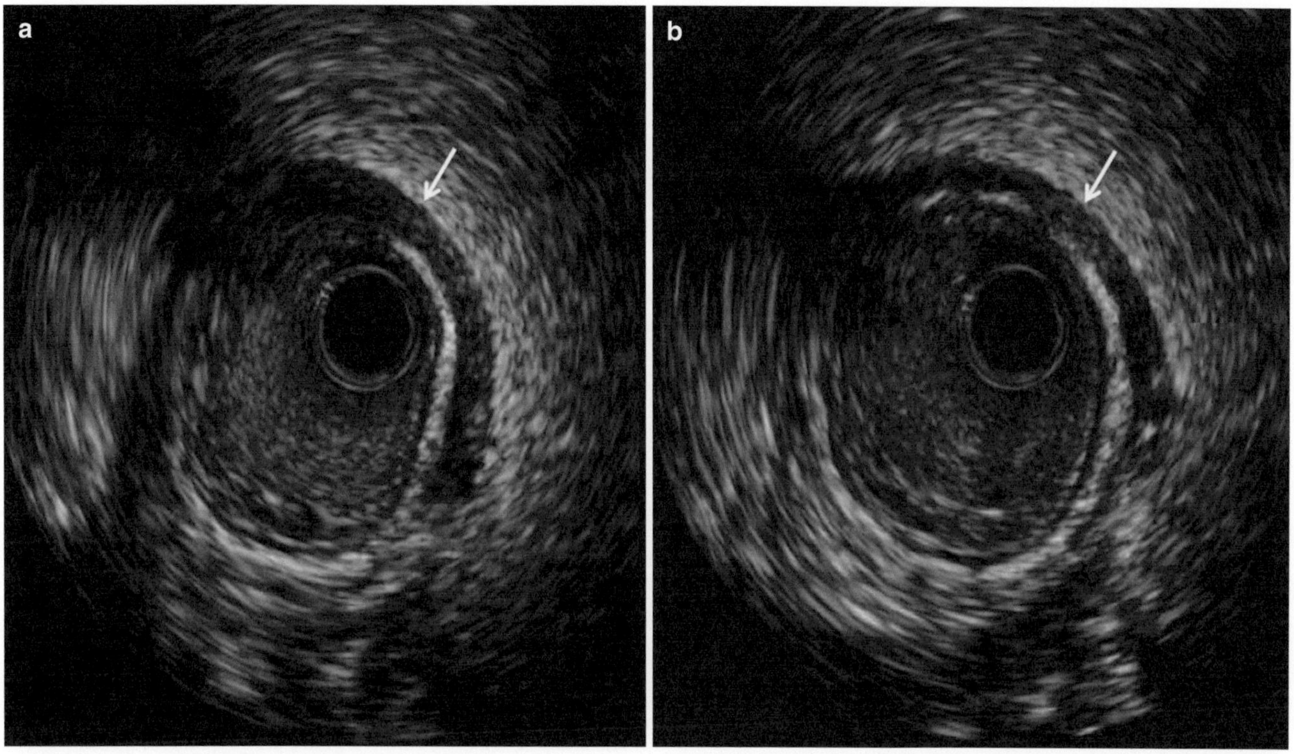

Fig. 3.10 *Myocardial bridge*. The "half moon" appearance (*arrows* in both *Panel A* and *B*) is characteristic of a myocardial bridge that causes typical systolic compression of the vessel (*Panel A* in systole vs. *Panel B* in diastole)

connective tissue disorders, and cases of intoxication. Spontaneous dissections occur in the absence of any history of an intervention: 80 % of the cases are in women and 25 % occur either postpartum or with oral contraceptive use. The most commonly affected artery in women is the left anterior descending, whereas in men the right coronary artery is more often affected [54]. Cases of left main coronary artery dissection have also been described [55]. The common angiographic finding is the presence of flow in two lumens separated by a radiolucent flap. However, the angiogram may be unimpressive or show diffuse disease [56]. On IVUS, these are medial dissections that are often circumferential with an intramural hematoma occupying part of the dissected false lumen. Intimal tears are rare, and there is usually no communication between the true and false lumens (Fig. 3.11).

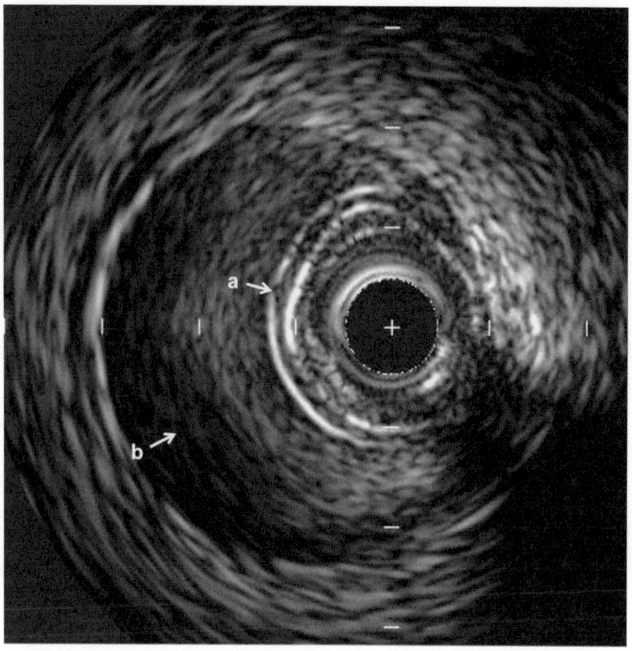

Fig. 3.11 *Spontaneous dissection*. This is an example of spontaneous dissection showing a circumferential medial dissection (*arrow* "a") with an intramural hematoma (*arrow* "b"). There is no evidence of atherosclerosis

Angiographic Hazy Lesions

Angiographic hazy lesions can represent the full spectrum of pre-intervention anatomic morphologies including calcium, spontaneous dissections, thrombus, and a large plaque burden with positive remodeling.

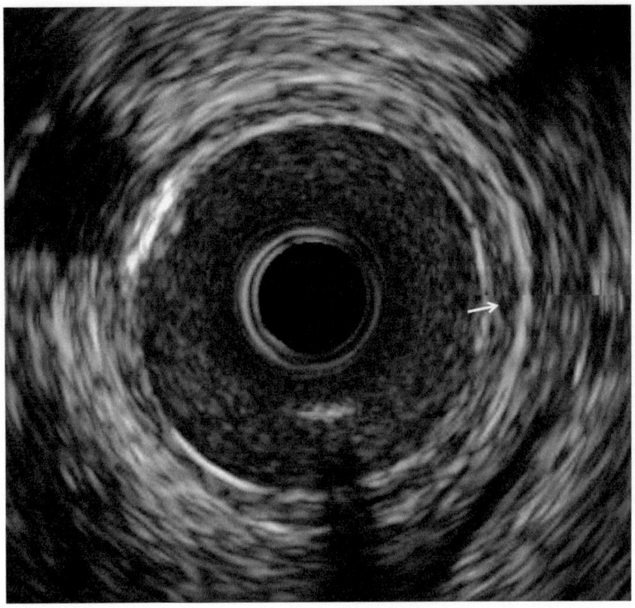

Fig. 3.12 *Saphenous vein graft* (*SVG*). A normal, recently explanted saphenous vein appears to be a monolayer. This is an example of an arterialized saphenous vein with intimal fibrous thickening (*arrow*)

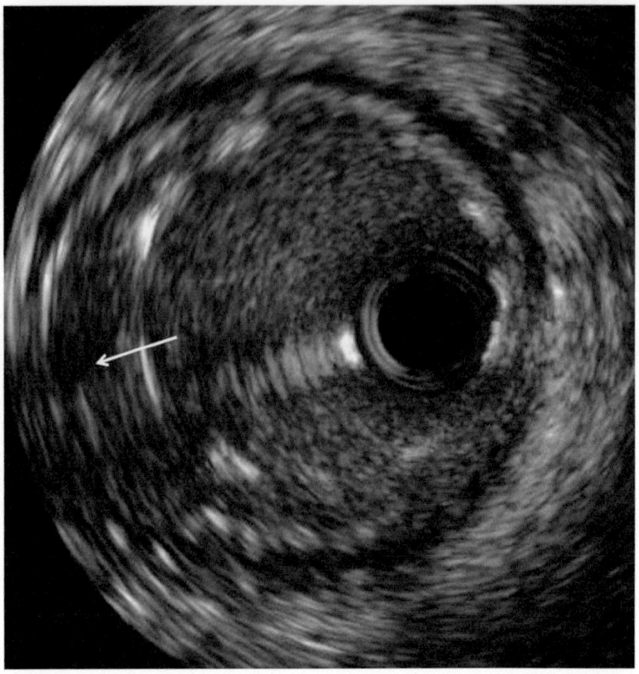

Fig. 3.13 *Stent malapposition*. The space and blood speckle between the stent struts and vessel wall (*arrow*) indicates the stent malapposition

Saphenous Vein Grafts

In vein grafts, wall morphology and plaque characteristics are different from those in native coronary arteries. The vein graft wall is free from the surrounding tissue and has no side branches (Fig. 3.12). In situ veins do not have an EEM. However, saphenous vein grafts typically undergo "arterialization" with morphologic changes that include intimal fibrous thickening, medial hypertrophy, and lipid deposition to create an echolucent zone [57]. The "EEM" area – which is actually the vein graft CSA – is measured by tracing the outer border of this echolucent zone. All other measurements including "P&M" CSA and plaque burden are calculated similar to native coronary disease.

Saphenous vein grafts that fail early are more likely to (1) be ostial or proximal; (2) have smaller reference vein graft and plaque CSAs, but a larger plaque burden; and (3) have less calcium and mobile plaque elements compared to vein grafts that fail late [58]. Negatively remodeled vein graft lesions typically are echodense, contain little plaque, and can have very thick walls without an echolucent zone; they may represent intrinsic vein graft wall or perigraft fibrosis or occur at anastomotic sites. Degenerated vein grafts contain exceptionally large plaque burdens.

Previously Stented Lesions

Endovascular stents are intensely echoreflective. The metallic prosthesis creates a third IVUS boundary besides the lumen and the EEM: lumen CSA, stent CSA, and EEM CSA. When tracing the stent, it is important not to mistake the guidewire for a stent strut; both are metallic reflectors. Post-intervention – in the absence of tissue protrusion or stent malapposition – the stent CSA will be equivalent to the lumen CSA. Measurements include stent CSA, minimum stent diameter, maximum stent diameter, stent symmetry (ratio of minimum to maximum stent diameter), and stent expansion (the minimum stent CSA compared with a predefined reference which can be the proximal, distal, largest, or average reference lumen CSA or, even, the lesion or reference EEM CSA). Expansion is different from apposition, and the two terms should not be used interchangeably. Serial IVUS studies have identified that stent underexpansion contributes to both DES restenosis and thrombosis [12, 59]. Stent underexpansion may be associated with longer stent length and is an important preventable mechanism of ISR [59, 60]. Strut apposition refers to the proximity of stent struts to the arterial wall. Good apposition is defined as sufficiently close contact to preclude blood flow between any strut and the underlying wall. Stent malapposition, synonymous with incomplete stent apposition, was blood speckle behind stent struts not overlying a side branch (Fig. 3.13). Stent malapposition could be acute (occurring at the time of stent implantation) or late (detected at follow-up) [20, 61]. There is an increased frequency of late stent malapposition after DES implantation that may lead to late stent thrombosis and other adverse clinical outcomes [62, 63]. At follow-up, the lumen CSA is typically smaller than the stent CSA because of IH accumulation within the stent. Unless IVUS was performed at stent implantation, it is not possible to differentiate intimal hyperplasia from acute tissue protrusion.

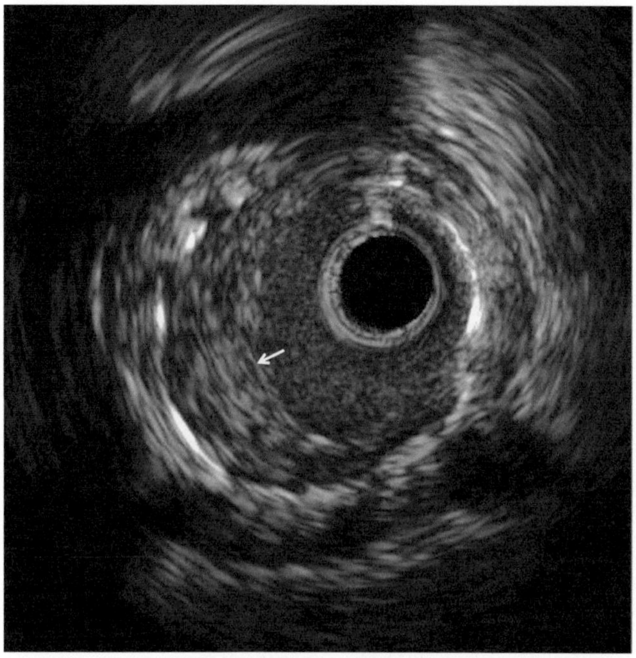

Fig. 3.14 *Neointimal hyperplasia*. The proliferation of new tissue inside of the stent (*arrow*) following implantation indicates neointimal hyperplasia and compromises the vessel lumen

The neointimal hyperplasia that is characteristic of early in-stent restenosis often appears to have low echogenicity, even at times less echogenic than blood speckle (Fig. 3.14). Appropriate system settings are critical to avoid suppressing this relatively non-echogenic material. The intimal hyperplasia of late in-stent restenosis may appear more echogenic. Finally, in some patients with brachytherapy failure or drug-eluting stent restenosis, in-stent restenosis tissue can be truly echolucent – the so-called black hole or black wall phenomenon. However, a VH-IVUS analysis showed that in-stent necrotic core and dense calcium increased over time, suggesting that the development of in-stent neoatherosclerosis may be another mechanism of ISR besides intimal hyperplasia [64]. A study of very late stent thrombosis found that disease progression with neointimal rupture was seen in two third of very late stent thrombosis [65]. A recent publication of using optical coherence tomography (OCT) also suggested that in-stent neoatherosclerosis may be an important mechanism of ISR, especially late after implantation [66].

References

1. Mintz GS, Nissen SE, Anderson WD, et al. Standards for the acquisition, measurement, and reporting of intravascular ultrasound studies: a report of the American College of Cardiology Task Force on Clinical Expert Consensus Documents. J Am Coll Cardiol. 2001;37:1478–92.
2. Fitzgerald PJ, St. Goar FG, Connolly AJ, et al. Intravascular ultrasound imaging of coronary arteries. Is three layers the norm? Circulation. 1992;86:154–8.
3. Isner JM, Donaldson RF, Fortin AH, et al. Attenuation of the media of coronary arteries in advanced atherosclerosis. Am J Cardiol. 1986;58:937–9.
4. Mallery JA, Tobis JM, Griffith J, et al. Assessment of normal and atherosclerotic arterial wall thickness with an intravascular ultrasound imaging catheter. Am Heart J. 1990;119:1392–400.
5. Bayturan O, Tuzcu EM, Nicholls SJ, et al. Attenuated plaque at nonculprit lesions in patients enrolled in intravascular ultrasound atherosclerosis progression trials. JACC Cardiovasc Interv. 2009;2:672–8.
6. Mintz GS, Garcia-Garcia HM, Nicholls SJ, et al. Clinical expert consensus document on standards for acquisition, measurement and reporting of intravascular ultrasound regression/progression studies. EuroIntervention. 2011;6:1123–30.
7. Hara H, Tsunoda T, Moroi M, et al. Ultrasound attenuation behind coronary atheroma without calcification: mechanism revealed by autopsy. Acute Card Care. 2006;8:110–12.
8. Ito S, Saio M, Suzuki T. Advanced atherosclerotic plaque as potential cause of no-reflow in elective percutaneous coronary intervention: intravascular ultrasound and histological findings. J Invasive Cardiol. 2004;16:669–72.
9. Yamada R, Okura H, Kume T, et al. Histological characteristics of plaque with ultrasonic attenuation: a comparison between intravascular ultrasound and histology. J Cardiol. 2007;50:223–8.
10. Wu X, Maehara A, Mintz GS, et al. Virtual histology intravascular ultrasound analysis of non-culprit attenuated plaques detected by grayscale intravascular ultrasound in patients with acute coronary syndromes. Am J Cardiol. 2010;105:48–53.
11. Mintz GS, Painter JA, Pichard AD, et al. Atherosclerosis in angiographically "normal" coronary artery reference segments: an intravascular ultrasound study with clinical correlations. J Am Coll Cardiol. 1995;25:1479–85.
12. Fujii K, Carlier SG, Mintz GS, et al. Stent underexpansion and residual reference segment stenosis are related to stent thrombosis after sirolimus-eluting stent implantation. J Am Coll Cardiol. 2005;45:995–8.
13. Liu J, Maehara A, Mintz GS, et al. An integrated TAXUS IV, V, and VI intravascular ultrasound analysis of the predictors of edge restenosis after bare metal or paclitaxel-eluting stents. Am J Cardiol. 2009;15:501–6.
14. Glagov S, Weisenberg E, Zarins CK, et al. Compensatory enlargement of human atherosclerotic coronary arteries. N Engl J Med. 1987;316:1371–5.
15. Schoenhagen P, Ziada KM, Kapadia SR, et al. Extent and direction of arterial remodeling in stable versus unstable coronary syndromes: an intravascular ultrasound study. Circulation. 2000;101:598–603.
16. von Birgelen C, Klinkhart W, Mintz GS, et al. Plaque distribution and vascular remodeling of ruptured and nonruptured coronary plaques in the same vessel: an intravascular ultrasound study in vivo. J Am Coll Cardiol. 2001;37:1864–70.
17. Nakamura M, Nishikawa H, Mukai S, et al. Impact of coronary artery remodeling on clinical presentation of coronary artery disease: an intravascular ultrasound study. J Am Coll Cardiol. 2001;37:63–9.
18. Higashikuni Y, Tanabe K, Yamamoto H, et al. Relationship between coronary artery remodeling and plaque composition in culprit lesions: an intravascular ultrasound radiofrequency analysis. Circ J. 2007;71:654–60.
19. Takeuchi H, Morino Y, Matsukage T, et al. Impact of vascular remodeling on the coronary plaque compositions: an investigation with in vivo tissue characterization using integrated backscatter-intravascular ultrasound. Atherosclerosis. 2009;202:476–82.
20. Guo N, Maehara A, Mintz GS, et al. Incidence, mechanisms, predictors, and clinical impact of acute and late stent malapposition after primary intervention in patients with acute myocardial infarction: an intravascular ultrasound substudy of the Harmonizing Outcomes with Revascularization and Stents in Acute Myocardial Infarction (HORIZONS-AMI) trial. Circulation. 2010;122:1077–84.

21. Kang SJ, Mintz GS, Park DW, et al. Late and very late drug-eluting stent malapposition: serial 2-year quantitative IVUS analysis. Circ Cardiovasc Interv. 2010;3:335–40.
22. Abizaid A, Mintz GS, Pichard AD, et al. Clinical, intravascular ultrasound, and quantitative angiographic determinants of the coronary flow reserve before and after percutaneous transluminal coronary angioplasty. Am J Cardiol. 1998;82:423–8.
23. Nishioka T, Amanullah AM, Luo H, et al. Clinical validation of intravascular ultrasound imaging for assessment of coronary stenosis severity: comparison with stress myocardial perfusion imaging. J Am Coll Cardiol. 1999;33:1870–8.
24. Takagi A, Tsurumi Y, Ishii Y, et al. Clinical potential of intravascular ultrasound for physiological assessment of coronary stenosis: relationship between quantitative ultrasound tomography and pressure-derived fractional flow reserve. Circulation. 1999;100: 250–5.
25. Abizaid AS, Mintz GS, Mehran R, et al. One year follow-up after percutaneous transluminal angioplasty was not performed based on intravascular ultrasound findings. Importance of lumen dimensions. Circulation. 1999;100:256–61.
26. Lee CH, Tai BC, Soon CY, et al. New set of intravascular ultrasound-derived anatomic criteria for defining functionally significant stenoses in small coronary arteries (results from Intravascular Ultrasound Diagnostic Evaluation of Atherosclerosis in Singapore [IDEAS] study). Am J Cardiol. 2010;105:1378–84.
27. Briguori C, Anzuini A, Airoldi F, et al. Intravascular ultrasound criteria for the assessment of the functional significance of intermediate coronary artery stenoses and comparison with fractional flow reserve. Am J Cardiol. 2001;87:136–41.
28. Takayama T, Hodgson JM. Prediction of the physiologic severity of coronary lesions using 3D IVUS: validation by direct coronary pressure measurements. Catheter Cardiovasc Interv. 2001;53: 48–55.
29. Kang SJ, Lee JY, Ahn JM, et al. Validation of intravascular ultrasound-derived parameters with fractional flow reserve for assessment of coronary stenosis severity. Circ Cardiovasc Interv. 2011;4:65–71.
30. Ahn JM, Kang SJ, Mintz GS, et al. Validation of minimal luminal area measured by intravascular ultrasound for assessment of functionally significant coronary stenosis comparison with myocardial perfusion imaging. JACC Cardiovasc Interv. 2011;4:665–71.
31. Ben-Dor I, Torguson R, Gaglia Jr MA, et al. Correlation between fractional flow reserve and intravascular ultrasound lumen area in intermediate coronary artery stenosis. EuroIntervention. 2011;7: 225–33.
32. Koo BK, Yang HM, Doh JH, et al. Optimal intravascular ultrasound criteria and their accuracy for defining the functional significance of intermediate coronary stenoses of different locations. JACC Cardiovasc Interv. 2011;4:803–11.
33. Jasti V, Ivan E, Yalamanchili V, et al. Correlations between fractional flow reserve and intravascular ultrasound in patients with an ambiguous left main coronary artery stenosis. Circulation. 2001;110: 2831–6.
34. Bech GJ, Droste H, Pijls NH, et al. Value of fractional flow reserve in making decisions about bypass surgery for equivocal left main coronary artery disease. Heart. 2001;86:547–52.
35. Hamilos M, Muller O, Cuisset T, et al. Long-term clinical outcome after fractional flow reserve-guided treatment in patients with angiographically equivocal left main coronary artery stenosis. Circulation. 2009;120:1505–12.
36. de la Torre Hernandez JM, Hernández Hernandez F, Alfonso F, et al. Prospective application of pre-defined intravascular ultrasound criteria for assessment of intermediate left main coronary artery lesions results from the multicenter LITRO study. J Am Coll Cardiol. 2011;58:351–8.
37. Kim SH, Hong MK, Park DW, et al. Impact of plaque characteristics analyzed by intravascular ultrasound on long-term clinical outcomes. Am J Cardiol. 2009;103:1221–6.
38. Maehara A, Mintz GS, Bui AB, et al. Morphologic and angiographic features of coronary plaque rupture detected by intravascular ultrasound. J Am Coll Cardiol. 2002;40:904–10.
39. Hong MK, Mintz GS, Lee CW, et al. Comparison of coronary plaque rupture between stable angina and acute myocardial infarction: a three-vessel intravascular ultrasound study in 235 patients. Circulation. 2004;110:928–33.
40. Hong MK, Mintz GS, Lee CW, et al. The site of plaque rupture in native coronary arteries: a three-vessel intravascular ultrasound analysis. J Am Coll Cardiol. 2005;19:261–5.
41. Fujii K, Kobayashi Y, Mintz GS, et al. Intravascular ultrasound assessment of ulcerated ruptured plaques: a comparison of culprit and non-culprit lesions of patients with acute coronary syndromes and lesions in patients without acute coronary syndromes. Circulation. 2003;108:2473–8.
42. Burke AP, Kolodgie FD, Farb A, et al. Healed plaque ruptures and sudden coronary death: evidence that subclinical rupture has a role in plaque progression. Circulation. 2001;103:934–40.
43. Tanaka A, Shimada K, Namba M, et al. Ruptured plaque is associated with larger infarct size following successful percutaneous coronary intervention in ST segment elevation acute myocardial infarction. Coron Artery Dis. 2009;20:260–6.
44. Kusama I, Hibi K, Kosuge M, et al. Impact of plaque rupture on infarct size in ST-segment elevation anterior acute myocardial infarction. J Am Coll Cardiol. 2007;50:1230–7.
45. Okura H, Kobayashi Y, Sumitsuji S, et al. Effect of culprit-lesion remodeling versus plaque rupture on three-year outcome in patients with acute coronary syndrome. Am J Cardiol. 2009;103:791–5.
46. Rioufol G, Finet G, Ginon I, et al. Multiple atherosclerotic plaque rupture in acute coronary syndrome: a three-vessel intravascular ultrasound study. Circulation. 2002;106:804–8.
47. Lee SY, Mintz GS, Kim SY, et al. Attenuated plaque detected by intravascular ultrasound: clinical, angiographic, and morphologic features and post-percutaneous coronary intervention complications in patients with acute coronary syndromes. JACC Cardiovasc Interv. 2009;2:65–72.
48. Wu X, Mintz GS, Xu K, et al. The relationship between attenuated plaque identified by intravascular ultrasound and no-reflow after stenting in acute myocardial infarction: the HORIZONS-AMI (Harmonizing Outcomes With Revascularization and Stents in Acute Myocardial Infarction) trial. JACC Cardiovasc Interv. 2011; 4:495–502.
49. Maehara A, Mintz GS, Ahmed JM, et al. An intravascular ultrasound classification of angiographic coronary artery aneurysms. Am J Cardiol. 2001;88:365–70.
50. Ge J, Jeremias A, Rupp A, et al. New signs characteristic of myocardial bridging demonstrated by intracoronary ultrasound and Doppler. Eur Heart J. 1999;20:1707–16.
51. Tsujita K, Maehara A, Mintz GS, et al. Comparison of angiographic and intravascular ultrasonic detection of myocardial bridging of the left anterior descending coronary artery. Am J Cardiol. 2008;102: 1608–13.
52. Tsujita K, Maehara A, Mintz GS, et al. Impact of myocardial bridge on clinical outcome after coronary stent placement. Am J Cardiol. 2009;103:1344–8.
53. Tsujita K, Maehara A, Mintz GS, et al. Serial intravascular ultrasound analysis of the impact of myocardial bridge on neointimal proliferation after coronary stenting in patients with acute myocardial infarction. J Interv Cardiol. 2010;23:114–22.
54. Micha M, Peter A, Walter A, et al. Idiopathic spontaneous coronary artery dissection: incident, diagnosis and treatment. Int J Cardiol. 2005;101:363–9.

55. Klein AJ, Hudson PA, Kim MS, et al. Spontaneous left main coronary artery dissection and the role of intravascular ultrasonography. J Ultrasound Med. 2010;29:981–8.
56. Maehara A, Mintz GS, Castagna MT, et al. Intravascular ultrasound assessment of spontaneous coronary artery dissection. Am J Cardiol. 2002;89:466–8.
57. Spray TL, Roberts WC. Changes in saphenous veins used as aortocoronary bypass grafts. Am Heart J. 1977;94(4):500–16.
58. Castagna MT, Mintz GS, Weissman NJ, et al. Calcification in saphenous vein grafts: clinical correlated and intravascular ultrasound findings. J Am Coll Cardiol. 2002;39:36A.
59. Liu X, Doi H, Maehara A, et al. A volumetric intravascular ultrasound comparison of early drug-eluting stent thrombosis versus restenosis. JACC Cardiovasc Interv. 2009;2:428–34.
60. Kang SJ, Mintz GS, Park DW, et al. Mechanisms of in-stent restenosis after drug-eluting stent implantation: intravascular ultrasound analysis. Circ Cardiovasc Interv. 2011;4:9–14.
61. Mintz GS. What to do about late incomplete stent apposition? Circulation. 2007;115:2379–81.
62. Hassan AK, Bergheanu SC, Stijnen T, et al. Late stent malapposition risk is higher after drug-eluting stent compared with bare-metal stent implantation and associates with late stent thrombosis. Eur Heart J. 2010;31:1172–80.
63. Cook S, Wenaweser P, Togni M, et al. Incomplete stent apposition and very late stent thrombosis after drug-eluting stent implantation. Circulation. 2007;115:2426–34.
64. Kang SJ, Mintz GS, Park DW, et al. Tissue characterization of in-stent neointima using intravascular ultrasound radiofrequency data analysis. Am J Cardiol. 2010;106:1561–5.
65. Lee CW, Kang SJ, Park DW, et al. Intravascular ultrasound findings in patients with very late stent thrombosis after either drug-eluting or bare-metal stent implantation. J Am Coll Cardiol. 2010;55:1936–42.
66. Kang SJ, Mintz GS, Akasaka T, et al. Optical coherence tomographic analysis of in-stent neoatherosclerosis after drug-eluting stent implantation. Circulation. 2011;123:2954–63.

Patient Selection for Coronary Intervention

4

N.S. Rajendra and A.H. Gershlick

Since its inception in the late 1970s, use of percutaneous coronary intervention (PCI) for revascularization has grown inexorably, with more than three million procedures undertaken worldwide. Both the range of presenting clinical indication of patients and anatomical subsets regarded as suitable for the procedure have increased for a number of reasons. Predominant are evidence-based developments and standardization in device technology, but also increase in operator skills and improved understanding of the need for adjunctive pharmacotherapy have played important roles. There is no doubt that the development of stents and subsequently drug-eluting stents were pivotal developments in the adoption of PCI. Subsequently, since the 1990s, PCI has become the dominant revascularization strategy compared with coronary artery bypass surgery (CABG). Current ratios of PCI: CABG range in different parts of Europe from 4:1 to 10:1. With such a meteoric rise in PCI adoption, there have been, despite and somewhat because of the wealth of evidence base, issues and controversies surrounding PCI, including whether patients are appropriately selected, whether there is too much so-called "inappropriate" PCI/stenting, and whether it is always in the patients' best interest to undergo this procedure rather than alternative strategies of CABG or stand-alone best medical therapy, especially since it appeals to patients as a less invasive, and quicker to recover from, procedure. This chapter will set out to address some of these issues.

N.S. Rajendra, MBBS, MRCP, MD (✉)
Department of Cardiology, Glenfield Hospital,
Leicester and Queen's Hospital, Burton,
Groby Road, Leicester LE3 9QP, UK
e-mail: drrajendra_ns@rediffmail.com

A.H. Gershlick, MB, BS, BSc, FRCP
Department of Cardiology,
University Hospitals of Leicester,
Groby Road, Leicester LE3 9QP, UK
e-mail: agershlick@aol.com

Stable Coronary Artery Disease

Chronic stable angina (CSA) is characterized by stable coronary plaque disease with patients experiencing exertional angina. Gruntzig first described angioplasty in 1978 [1] and proposed it as a potential treatment strategy for CSA. Over the subsequent three decades, important technological advancements have been made progressing from the balloon angioplasty era to the bare-metal stent era and to the current drug-eluting stent era, with progressive improvements in clinical outcomes. It is interesting to note that the quoted 10-year survival rate for subjects with stable coronary artery disease has improved from 58 % [2] to 84 % [3] over a period of just two decades. However, there have been significant advances in medical therapy during the same period, with trials of ACE inhibitors, statins, and beta blockers demonstrating significant benefit. The importance of such agents as constituents of optimal medical therapy (OMT) for CSA is fully accepted.

Initial Work-Up of CSA

In keeping with abovementioned issues, initial work-up prior to cardiac catheterization should involve certainty that it is CSA and that intervention is needed: taking a good history, performing a full physical examination, ensuring that the patient is on optimal medical therapy (that they can tolerate), and, importantly, testing for inducible ischemia using exercise tolerance test, dobutamine stress echo, myocardial perfusion scan, or cardiac stress MRI.

In the UK, the current NICE (National Institute for Health and Clinical Excellence) guideline for recent onset stable chest pain [4] recommends stratifying patients on the basis of estimated likelihood of CAD into categories of low (10–29 % estimated likelihood), intermediate (30–60 % estimated likelihood), and high (61–90 % estimated likelihood) risk groups. The guideline recommends CT calcium scoring for the low-risk group; noninvasive functional testing in the form of MPS, stress echo, or cardiac MRI for the intermediate group; and

C.A. Thompson (ed.), *Textbook of Cardiovascular Intervention*,
DOI 10.1007/978-1-4471-4528-8_4, © Springer-Verlag London 2014

offering coronary angiography if appropriate and if revascularization is being considered for the high-risk group. The guideline discourages the use of exercise tolerance test to diagnose or exclude stable angina in patients with known CAD. We (the authors) personally disagree however and believe that the exercise test still has an important screening role.

The exercise tolerance test, although limited by low sensitivity and specificity (68 % and 77 % respectively), has an important role when there is an intermediate probability of CAD and is recognized by the ACC/AHA Task Force on practice guidelines as an important diagnostic/screening tool in such patients for clinical decision making [5]. However, an abnormal resting ECG (e.g., LBBB) and the presence of patient comorbidities such as peripheral vascular disease, prior stroke, arthritis, lung disease, neurological disorders, and/or deconditioning in the aged population may preclude exercise testing.

In such circumstances, stress imaging in the form of dobutamine stress echocardiography or myocardial perfusion imaging (dobutamine, dipyridamole, or adenosine) can be considered. A large evidence base exists to support the use of such noninvasive screening, which also have certain limitations. Patients with suboptimal echo windows remain a challenge for DSE. Adenosine can cause flushing, dyspnea, chest pain, and bradyarrhythmias and cannot be used in a patient with sick sinus syndrome or high-grade AV block. Dipyridamole may cause bronchospasm and is not used in asthmatics. MPS carry a radiation load. With these techniques however, reversible areas of ischemia may be quantified and localized to specific areas of the myocardium and may be correlated with coronary artery territory. Importantly, ischemic burden can stratify patients who may potentially receive prognostic benefit above and beyond symptomatic and cardiac performance improvement expected with PCI.

Cardiac MRI with stress (dobutamine/adenosine) and delayed enhancement is a recent addition to the batch of noninvasive investigations for angina and has higher spatial resolution, better sensitivity/specificity, and ability to quantify valvular lesions and delineate viable myocardium as its advantages. Availability and general contraindications to MRI may limit the use of this investigation.

Evidence of more than minor ischemia on noninvasive testing against a background of tolerated optimal medical therapy is generally considered necessary before coronary angiography is indicated – but individual patient-based and informed decisions are also acceptable (recurrent admissions with chest pain despite no evidence of significant myocardial ischemia).

Diagnostic coronary angiography remains the gold standard for demonstrating the actual presence of coronary disease, but its utilization differs vastly. A recent study [6] reflecting American practice reported on the low yield of demonstrable obstructive coronary artery disease and advocated better strategies for risk stratification to increase the diagnostic yield, whereas on the other hand, in some parts of the world, only those with significant and truly limiting symptoms, enforced OMT and high ischemic burden, are allowed access to this useful test.

Importance must be given to the presenting history, existing risk factors for ischemic heart disease, coexisting noncardiac conditions like anemia, chronic kidney disease, and peptic ulcer disease, and also drug compliance as these will play an important role if there arises a need for coronary intervention and, for example, need for subsequent dual antiplatelet therapy.

Once a decision has been made to proceed to cardiac catheterization, it is important that the patient is given all the necessary information regarding the procedure, preprocedure checks, and the risks and benefits of the procedure. This is all done best in a preadmission clinic. It is important for the physician to emphasize that in the stable angina group, intervention is mainly to limit angina symptoms, which to many patients is very important.

Fractional Flow Reserve as an Aid to Intervention

Measurement of fractional flow reserve (FFR), in recent years, has assumed a valuable role in selecting patients and coronary lesions for intervention. In fact, FFR-guided PCI for detection of ischemia-related lesion(s) in the absence of vessel-related ischemia has been assigned a class I indication with level of evidence A in the latest ESC guidelines on myocardial revascularization [7]. FFR is an index of the physiological significance of a coronary stenosis and is defined as the ratio of maximal blood flow in a stenotic artery to normal maximal flow. It is easily measured during coronary angiography by calculating the ratio of distal coronary pressure (Pd) measured with a coronary pressure guidewire to aortic pressure (Pa) measured simultaneously with the guiding catheter. FFR in a normal coronary artery (Pd/Pa) equals 1.0. An FFR value of 0.80 or less identifies ischemia-causing coronary stenoses with an accuracy of more than 90 % [8, 9].

The information provided by FFR is similar to that obtained with noninvasive myocardial perfusion studies, but it is more specific and has a better spatial resolution, because every artery or segment is analyzed separately, and masking of one ischemic area by another, more severely ischemic, zone is avoided. It is particularly helpful when there is doubt on the table regarding lesion importance.

In multivessel disease, Berger et al. [10] reported that PCI of hemodynamically nonsignificant stenoses (FFR > 0.75) can often be safely deferred, even if initially planned on the basis of the angiogram. In a separate study, patients scheduled for PCI were subjected to FFR and patients whose FFR was ≥0.75 were randomly assigned to deferral or performance of PCI. PCI was performed as planned if FFR <0.75. The authors report that the 5-year outcome of deferral of PCI of an intermediate coronary stenosis based on FFR ≥0.75 is excellent. The risk of cardiac death or myocardial infarction related to this stenosis is <1 % per year and not decreased by intervening by stenting.

In the FAME (Fractional Flow Reserve Versus Angiography for Multivessel Evaluation) study, 1,005 subjects with multivessel disease undergoing PCI with drug-eluting stents (96 %) were randomly assigned to either angiography-guided PCI or FFR-guided PCI (FFR<080). In the FFR-guided PCI group, a significantly less number of stents were used. At 1 year follow-up, the primary end point (composite of death, myocardial infarction, and repeat revascularization) was significantly lower in the FFR-guided group compared to angiography-guided PCI group (13.2 vs. 18.7 $p=0.02$) [11] which was sustained at 2 years follow-up [25]. The authors also report a significant economic advantage with the mean overall costs at 1 year being significantly less in the FFR-guided arm ($14,315 vs. $16,700; $p<0.001$) [12]. The recently reported FAME II trial [13] extended the evidence base supporting the association with ischemic burden and poor outcomes in patients with coronary disease. The primary end point was a composite of death, myocardial infarction, or urgent revascularization. Results recruitment was halted prematurely after enrollment of 1,220 patients (888 who underwent randomization and 332 enrolled in the registry) because of a significant between-group difference in the percentage of patients who had a primary end-point event: 4.3 % in the PCI group and 12.7 % in the medical therapy group (hazard ratio with PCI, 0.32; 95 % confidence interval [CI], 0.19–0.53; $P<0.001$). The difference was driven by a lower rate of urgent revascularization in the PCI group than in the medical therapy group (1.6 % vs. 11.1 %; hazard ratio, 0.13; 95 % CI, 0.06–0.30; $P<0.001$). The authors concluded, "FFR-guided PCI plus the best available medical therapy, as compared with the best available medical therapy alone, decreased the need for urgent revascularization. In patients without ischemia, the outcome appeared to be favorable with the best available medical therapy alone."

PCI Versus Optimal Medical Therapy and PCI Versus CABG

COURAGE Study

Part of the backlash against PCI involves the contention that it is undertaken too early, without too much thought and against a background of inadequate medical therapy. The COURAGE trial sought to address this issue and has become one of the most contentious trials published. The Clinical Outcomes Utilizing Revascularization and Aggressive Drug Evaluation (COURAGE) [14] study reported that PCI did not reduce the risk of death, myocardial infarction, or major cardiovascular events when added to OMT in patients with stable CAD. The study randomized 2,287 patients to OMT+PCI or OMT. There was no significant difference between the groups with respect to composite of death, myocardial infarction, and stroke over a median follow-up period of 4.6 years (20 % PCI group vs. 19.5 % OMT group, OR 1.05, $p=0.62$). There was however a significant improvement in angina scores and quality of life in the PCI+OMT group which was sustained until 3 years after randomization [15].

A nuclear substudy of COURAGE reports that adding PCI to OMT resulted in a greater ischemia reduction as assessed by serial myocardial perfusion scans [16], with the anti-ischemic benefit of PCI being greatest for patients with more severe ischemia at baseline (>20 % ischemic burden). Revascularization in the presence of moderate to severe ischemia (defined as ≥10 % ischemic burden on MPS) is deemed to provide survival benefit according to observational studies [16].

The COURAGE study has generated intense debate with regard to patient selection for intervention in the stable CAD group. It is very important to note that COURAGE was an angiographic triage trial and not a study primarily of medical therapy versus PCI for stable coronary disease. Many patients with angiographically critical disease were revascularized and not enrolled, therefore providing a cohort with low adverse events for randomization and analysis. Other limitations of the study have been highlighted by various authors [17–19] and include:

1. The predominant usage of bare-metal stents for PCI.
2. Patient selection – over 35,000 patients were screened and ultimately <10 % recruited, therefore limiting broad extrapolation of results.
3. ~30 % crossover to PCI in OMT group during follow-up. There was a highly significant difference in the rate of revascularization performed during follow-up: 21 % in PCI group (bare-metal stents) versus 32 % in OMT group ($P<0.001$).
4. >85 % of patients were male and Caucasian.

PCI Versus CABG in Higher-Risk Groups

SYNTAX (Synergy Between Percutaneous Coronary Intervention with TAXus and Cardiac Surgery)

SYNTAX was a 5-year "all comers" study that randomized 1,800 patients with multivessel CAD and is to date the largest randomized study in this cohort. 1,077 patients have been entered into a CABG registry (those who were deemed not suitable for PCI) and 198 patients in PCI registry (those who were deemed at excessive surgical risk). In the randomized study, the primary end point of MACCE included death from any cause, myocardial infarction, stroke, and repeat revascularization. At 1 year, the rates of major adverse cardiac or cerebrovascular events were significantly higher in the PCI group (17.8 %, vs. 12.4 % for CABG; $P=0.002$), as a result of an increased rate of repeat revascularization (13.5 % vs. 5.9 %, $P<0.001$). Stroke rate was significantly higher with

2.2 % compared to PCI at 0.6 % [20]. These results were maintained to 3 years. The SYNTAX score was predictive of outcomes in the PCI group, and when SYNTAX score was divided into terciles, MACCE rates were 13.0 % versus 7.7 % ($P=0.19$), 15.5 % versus 12.6 % ($P=0.54$), and 12.9 % versus 25.3 % ($P=0.08$) for CABG versus PCI in the lower (0–22), intermediate (23–32), and high (≥33) terciles, respectively. Current consensus is to recommend surgery in patients with SYNTAX score >32, while PCI is undertaken if SYNTAX score is <22 and intervention should be best tailored to suit the needs of the individual patient in those who score between 22 and 32. However, it is unclear at this point from the published and presented data if a CABG-specific advantage exists for this subset or if this is reflective of incomplete revascularization or inadequate management of chronic total occlusions and bifurcations in this subset.

Currently, an ongoing study, EXCEL, aims to evaluate the second-generation everolimus-eluting stents XIENCE PRIME ™ or XIENCE V ® (ABBOTT Vascular) versus CABG for left main stem revascularization (2,500 patients) [21]. The primary end point for this study is a composite of all-cause mortality, myocardial infarction, or stroke. Repeat revascularization is a secondary end point of the study which is currently randomizing subjects, and the results are likely to impact future guidelines and practice.

In the recently reported BARI2D (Bypass Angioplasty Revascularization Investigation 2 Diabetes Mellitus) in subjects with stable angina and type 2 diabetes, 1,173 patients were randomly assigned to optimal medical treatment with an option of subsequent revascularization and 1,173 to revascularization (796-PCI, 377-CABG). At 5 year follow-up, there was no significant difference in the rates of death and myocardial infarction between patients undergoing revascularization and those undergoing medical therapy [22]. However, compared to medical treatment, revascularization strategy reduced the occurrence of worsening angina (13 % vs. 8 %, $p<0.001$), new angina (51 % vs. 37 %, $p=0.001$), and subsequent coronary revascularizations (33 % vs. 18 %, $p<0.001$) [22].

In keeping with the available evidence base, the ESC and AHA guidelines [7, 23–25] for chronic stable angina recommend:

1. Optimal medical therapy constitutes antiplatelet agent, ACE inhibitor/ARB, beta blocker, statin, and antianginal medications (e.g., nitrates). ACE inhibitors, beta blockers, and statins are called vasculoprotective agents because of their effect on endothelial function. While their use has increased enormously, it is not uncommon to find side effects of these medications that either preclude the up titration of doses or necessitate cessation of medication and/or substitution. OMT should therefore be considered in this context and not forced to the nth degree.
2. Coronary revascularization on symptomatic grounds (despite OMT) and prognostic grounds based on ischemic burden or particular anatomy (left main stem/proximal LAD).

Acute Coronary Syndrome

Pathogenesis

Unlike CSA, the majority of patients with an acute coronary syndrome suffer sudden reduction of coronary blood flow due to a discrete plaque event: rupture, erosion, or hemorrhage in association with a vulnerable plaque [26]. This disruption of the plaque exposes platelets to underlying collagen, initiating platelet adhesion and aggregation, while tissue factor in plaque induces coagulation and thrombus formation ensues with variable degrees of arterial occlusion. Vulnerable plaques may not be visualized during coronary angiography. Subclinical microembolism, smooth muscle hyperreactivity, and endothelial dysfunction may also contribute to progression of the syndrome. Many fatal intra-arterial occlusions arising from plaque rupture do not occur at highly stenotic areas in coronary arteries. As prognosis after myocardial infarction is significantly determined by the amount of muscle destroyed during ischemia/reperfusion [27], ensuring vessel patency and limiting injury to preserve myocardium are the overriding concerns.

The concept of vulnerable patient is as important as the concept of vulnerable plaque as this high-risk group subjects will need aggressive secondary prevention following revascularization strategies.

Risk Stratification in ACS

GRACE Risk Score

The GRACE (Global Registry of Acute Coronary Events) score is a well-validated risk assessment tool that takes into consideration factors like age, heart rate, systolic blood pressure, serum creatinine level, Killip class at admission, presence of ST depression, and elevated cardiac biomarkers as well as cardiac arrest. Computer or PDA software of a simplified nomogram is freely available at http://www.outcomes.org/grace.

The latest ESC guidelines recommend using the GRACE risk score as the preferred classification to apply on admission and at discharge in routine clinical practice.

TIMI Score

The TIMI risk score [28], although deemed less accurate in predicting outcomes, is simpler to use and is widely accepted and incorporates age (>65 years), three or more risk factors for CAD, known coronary stenosis of 50 % or more, aspirin use in the past 7 days, severe angina defined as 2 or more episodes in 24 h, presence of ST changes (0.5 mv or more), and biomarkers as the variables. Event rates of 4.7 % for a score of 0/1, 8.3 % for 2, 13.2 % for 3, 19.9 % for 4, 26.2 % for 5, and 40.9 % for 6/7 at 14 days were observed in the TIMI 11B cohort.

There are other risk scoring systems that are less widely used. They include the FRISC and the PURSUIT risk scores which are based on the FRISC 2 and PURSUIT studies, respectively [29, 30]. The importance of the risk scoring is that it allows evidence-based selection of patients for angiography and PCI if indicated which it generally is. The currently available risk assessment tools are elaborated in Table 4.1 [31–35].

Ideal Timing for Intervention

Timing of intervention for NSTE-ACS continues to be a hotly debated topic. As mentioned earlier, vulnerable plaque results in variable degrees of coronary arterial occlusion and is responsible for the varied presentation from mild chest pain (usually at rest) to severe ongoing chest pain with ST-segment depression, rather than ST elevation (unlike STEMI). It can be argued that patients who do not have ongoing pain, hemodynamic compromise, or dynamic ECG changes do not need to be rushed to the cath lab on presentation. Recent data and meta-analyses have helped the development of protocols and guidelines. The timing of intervention in randomized studies has varied from as early as 12 h and the major randomized studies are depicted in Table 4.2.

A collaborative meta-analysis of seven randomized controlled trials of routine versus selective intervention strategy by Mehta et al. [36] that included over 9,000 patients found that at 17 months follow-up, the routine invasive strategy was associated with a reduction in MI, severe angina, and rehospitalizations compared to selective intervention strategy. However, they also found that routine intervention was associated with a higher early mortality (1.8 % during initial hospitalization compared to 1.1 % in selective intervention group). This highlighted the importance of risk stratification as patients in the higher-risk groups derived greater absolute benefit from a routine invasive strategy.

A meta-analysis of individual subjects of three randomized studies (RITA 3, FRISCII, and ICTUS) at 5 years follow-up [37] reports a significant reduction in the composite of death and myocardial infarction with routine invasive treatment (14.7 % vs. 17.9 % with selective intervention) driven primarily by reduction in MI. The absolute reduction in cardiovascular death or MI was 2.0 % in the low-risk, 3.8 % in the intermediate-risk, and 11.1 % in the high-risk groups emphasizing again that high-risk groups have the most to gain with a routine intervention strategy.

A recent meta-analysis by Katritsis et al. [38] which included 4,013 patients from the ABOARD, ELISA, ISAR-COOL, and TIMACS study concludes that although early intervention did not reduce the risk of death or myocardial infarction, there was a significant reduction in the risk of recurrent ischemia and the duration of hospital stay.

The ESC guidelines [7] therefore recommend an early intervention strategy within 24 h of admission for high-risk groups (GRACE score >140) and angiography and revascularization in the same admission (preferably within 72 h) for the low-risk groups. The NICE guidelines [39] recommend 96 h as the timeframe to perform angiography and revascularization on the basis that data from randomized trials reflect time from randomization to intervention rather than from presentation.

STEMI

Reperfusion therapy has been recognized as highly beneficial for patients with STEMI (Fig. 4.1). It is indicated in all patients with history of chest pain/discomfort of <12 h and with persistent ST-segment elevation or (presumed) new left bundle branch block. Guidelines recommend reperfusion in patients with ST elevation even after 12 h of symptom onset if there is ongoing ischemia (clinical or ECG).

Table 4.1 Tools available for risk assessment of patients with ACS

Risk assessment tools	
Clinical presentation and history	Risk factors, nature of chest pain
Physical examination	Anemia, blood pressure, heart failure, arrhythmias
Chest X ray	Cardiomegaly, left ventricular failure
ECG	12 lead, dynamic monitoring, exercise ECG
Echo	Bedside echo, stress echo, and contrast echo
Biomarkers	Creatinine kinase, creatinine kinase-myoglobin, troponin (I and T), BNP, NT-proBNP, hsCRP
Assessment of coronary anatomy	Coronary CT angiography, invasive coronary angiography

Table 4.2 Major randomized studies with early and delayed interventional strategies in ACS

Study	*N*	Arms	Outcomes	Result
FRISC II [31]	2,457	Invasive (<10 days) vs. conservative	Death/MI at 12 months	10.4 % vs. 14.1 % $P=0.005$
TACTICS TIMI [32]	2,220	Early invasive (median 25 h) vs. selective invasive (median 93 h) for PCI	Death/MI/readmission at 6 months	9.4 % vs. 15.9 % $P=0.025$
RITA 3 [33]	1,890	Early invasive (median 3 days to PCI) vs. conservative	Death/MI/refractory angina at 12 months	9.6 % vs. 14.5 $p=0.001$
ICTUS [34]	1,200	Early invasive (median 23 h) vs. selective invasive (median 283 h)	Death/MI/readmission with ACS at 12 months	22.7 % vs. 21.2 % $P=0.35$
TIMACS [35]	3,031	Early invasive (median time 16 h to PCI) vs. delayed invasive (median time 52 h to PCI)	Death/MI/stroke at 6 months	9.6 % vs. 11.3 % $p=0.15$

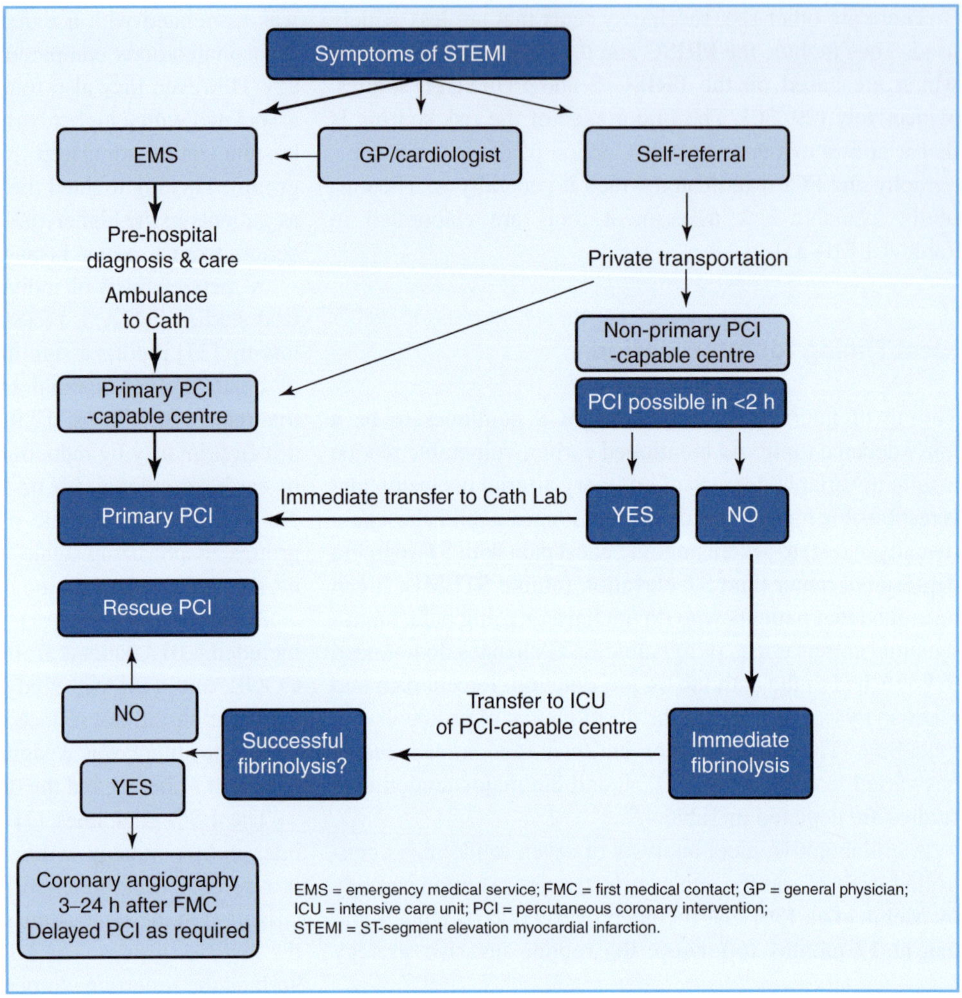

Fig. 4.1 Reperfusion strategies (From Wijns et al. [7], with permission)

PCI of a totally occluded artery >24 h after symptom onset in a stable patient is however not recommended. Fibrinolysis studies have consistently demonstrated mortality and morbidity benefits, and it has been well recognized that "time is muscle."

Primary PCI (PPCI) has emerged as the gold standard treatment in recent years, and both the ESC and the American guidelines recommend PPCI where feasible and when the PPCI can be undertaken within the relatively tight guideline mandated times. PPCI can also be performed in patients in whom fibrinolysis is contraindicated due to any of the causes mentioned in Table 4.3, although mortality and morbidity is higher in this cohort [40].

Selecting Patients for PCI When They Have Been Given Fibrinolysis

Reperfusion therapy initiated prior to planned PCI for STEMI in order to bridge the time gap is defined as facilitated PCI. A variety of agents have been used like full-dose or half-dose

Table 4.3 Contraindications to fibrinolysis

Absolute contraindications
Hemorrhagic stroke or stroke of unknown origin at any time
Ischemic stroke in preceding 6 months
Central nervous system trauma or neoplasms
Recent major trauma/surgery/head injury (within preceding 3 weeks)
Gastrointestinal bleeding within the last month
Known bleeding disorder
Aortic dissection
Noncompressible punctures (e.g., liver biopsy, lumbar puncture)
Relative contraindications
Transient ischemic attack in preceding 6 months
Oral anticoagulant therapy
Pregnancy or within 1 week postpartum
Refractory hypertension (systolic blood pressure 180 mmHg and/or diastolic blood pressure 110 mmHg)
Advanced liver disease
Infective endocarditis
Active peptic ulcer
Refractory resuscitation

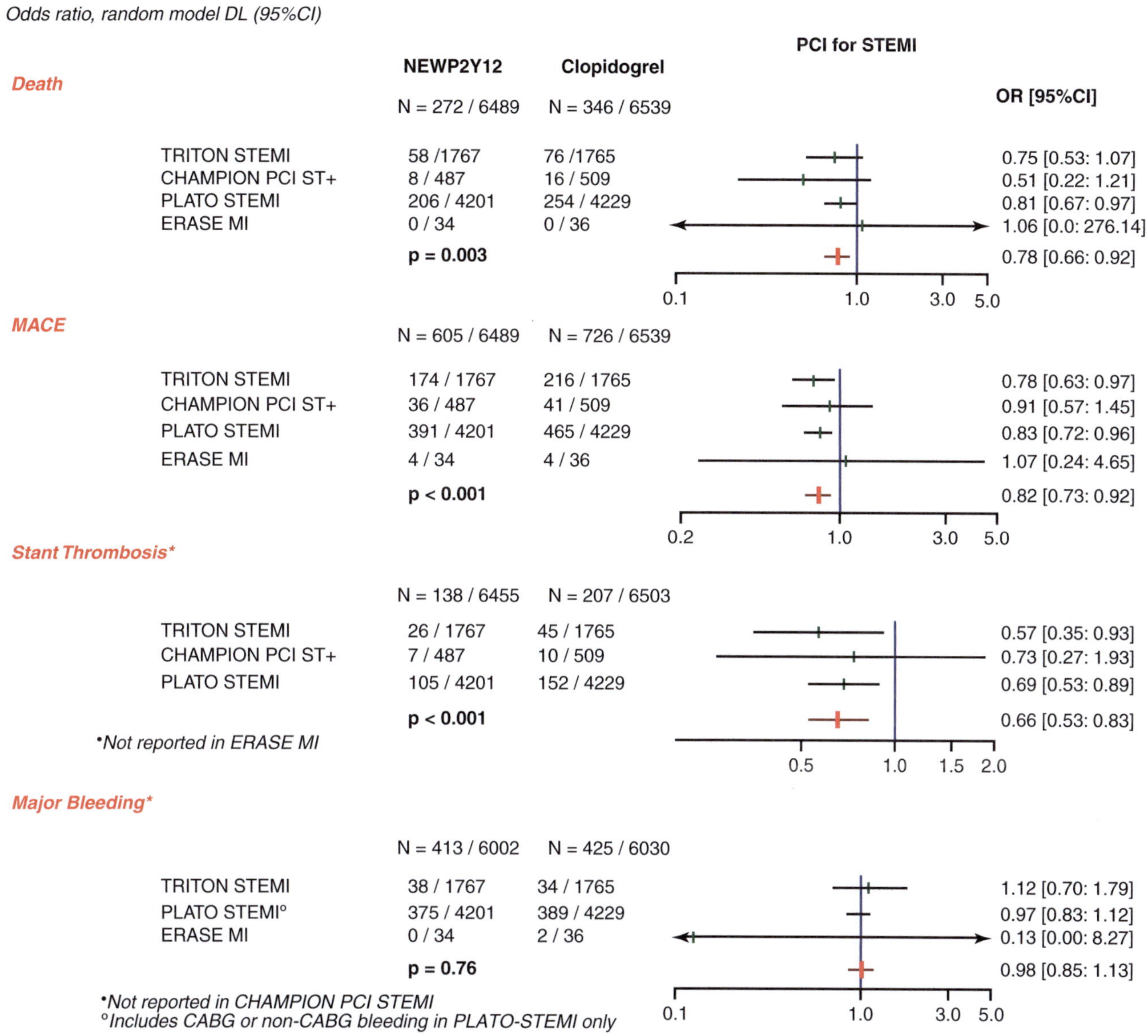

Fig. 4.2 Effect of New P2Y$_{12}$ in PCI for STEMI (From Bellemain-Appaix et al. [55], with permission)

fibrinolytics and GPIIb/IIIa inhibitors, and results were not consistent [41, 42], and facilitated PCI is not recommended by the 2008 ESC guidelines (class III) since it is not better and may be worse than PPCI (Fig. 4.2).

Pharmacoinvasive strategy on the other hand is defined as pharmacological reperfusion with an invasive strategy backup where patients are transferred to a PCI-capable hospital after being administered fibrinolytic therapy, following which they undergo rescue PCI if they have failed to reperfuse or routine angiography during inpatient stay.

The TRANSFER AMI [43] study published in 2009 randomized 1,059 patients with STEMI treated with fibrinolysis to standard treatment or immediate transfer and PCI (median 2.8 h). There was a significant reduction in the composite of death, reinfarction, recurrent ischemia, new or worsening congestive heart failure, or cardiogenic shock at 30 days (OR 0.64, $p=0.0004$) in the group who were treated with fibrinolysis and transferred for PCI within 6 h with no significant difference in major bleeding between the two groups. In keeping with new evidence, pharmacoinvasive therapy in high-risk patients with low-bleeding risk has a class IIB recommendation in the 2009 ACC/AHA/SCAI focused update for STEMI [44].

Achieving timely PCI still presents a considerable challenge. The ongoing The Strategic Reperfusion Early After Myocardial Infarction (STREAM) study [45] is a prospective, randomized, parallel, comparative, international multicenter trial which is randomizing patients with STEMI to fibrinolysis combined with enoxaparin, clopidogrel, and aspirin, and cardiac catheterization within 6–24 h or rescue coronary intervention if reperfusion fails within 90 min of fibrinolysis versus PCI performed according to local guidelines. The outcome of this study which includes efficacy and safety end points should provide useful additional information to optimize therapeutic decisions. 1,500 of 2,000 patients have been randomized.

Rescue PCI

Failure of restoration of vessel patency after thrombolysis is not uncommon, manifesting as persistent ST elevation, and PCI in this situation is termed rescue PCI. Rescue PCI should be considered in this context up to 12 h after symptom onset. The REACT study was a multicenter randomized study in 427 patients which showed that rescue PCI was associated with a significantly higher event-free survival at 6 months when compared to repeat thrombolysis or conservative management [46]. A meta-analysis of randomized studies including REACT [47] also concludes that rescue PCI is associated with improved clinical outcomes.

Adjunctive Pharmacotherapy to PCI

Aspirin is recommended in the dose of 150–325 mg orally as part of dual antiplatelet agent strategy prior to PPCI. Clopidogrel is used in the dose of 300–600 mg for loading followed by 75 mg/day. A recent large Swedish observational study reports that upstream clopidogrel prior to arrival at the cath lab in patients undergoing PPCI was associated with a significant reduction in death/MI as well as death alone at 12 months follow-up. The dose of 300 mg for loading was found to be as effective as that of 600 mg in the Korean acute myocardial infarction registry [48]; however, other studies report that 600 mg loading dose is associated with better outcomes [49, 50]. The 2010 ESC guidelines on myocardial revascularization recommend 600 mg of clopidogrel as the loading dose [7].

Two new antiplatelet agents that have been approved recently are prasugrel and ticagrelor, and both have class I recommendation in the 2010 ESC guidelines for STEMI.

In the TRITON-TIMI 38 study [51], prasugrel, a thienopyridine that is more potent, more rapid in onset, and more consistent in inhibition of platelets than clopidogrel, was compared to clopidogrel in 13,608 patients with ACS scheduled for PCI. Prasugrel was associated with a significant reduction in the primary efficacy end point of cardiovascular death, nonfatal MI, and nonfatal stroke (hazard ratio 0.81). Prasugrel was also associated with a significant increase in major and life-threatening bleeding in certain high-risk subgroups. In the predefined STEMI group, 3,534 patients were randomized to receive either prasugrel (loading dose 60 mg, regular dose 10 mg/day) or clopidogrel (loading dose 300 mg, regular dose 75 mg)[52]. Treatment with prasugrel resulted in significant reductions in 30-day rates of cardiovascular death, nonfatal MI, or nonfatal stroke, a benefit that persisted out to 15 months with no difference in fatal or non-CABG-related bleeding.

Ticagrelor is an oral, reversible, direct-acting inhibitor of the adenosine diphosphate receptor P2Y12 that has a more rapid onset and more pronounced platelet inhibition than clopidogrel [53–55]. Of the 18,624 patients randomized to receive ticagrelor or clopidogrel in the PLATO study [53], 7,026 had STEMI. Ticagrelor (loading dose 180 mg, regular dose 90 mg BD) was associated with a significant reduction in the rate of death from vascular causes, myocardial infarction, or stroke without an increase in the rate of overall major bleeding but with an increase in the rate of non-procedure-related bleeding. The recommended duration of dual antiplatelet therapy after PPCI for STEMI is 12 months irrespective of the type of stent but should be tailored to individual patient.

The ACC/AHA/SCAI 2009 focused update for the management of ST-elevation myocardial infarction [44] advocates starting GPIIb/IIIa inhibitors during PPCI (class IIa) in selected patients and a class IIb recommendation for initiating GP GPIIb/IIIa inhibitors prior to PPCI. Following the HORIZONS AMI study [55], bivalirudin has class I recommendation for use in STEMI with or without prior treatment with unfractionated heparin and class IIa recommendation in patients with STEMI undergoing PCI who are at high risk of bleeding. The recent NICE guidance on the use of bivalirudin in STEMI concludes that there was sufficient evidence to demonstrate that bivalirudin was more clinically effective than glycoprotein IIb/IIIa inhibitor plus heparin, leading to lower rates of major bleeds and mortality [56] and cost dominant. Despite the improved clinical outcomes in HORIZIONS AMI for patients receiving bivalirudin, there was a statistically significant increase in the number of patients experiencing acute stent thrombosis (< 24 h) when compared to those in the unfractionated heparin arm. This difference disappeared after 24 h and did not affect overall clinical outcomes and a loading dose of 600 mg clopidogrel is recommended. Newer antiplatelets like prasugrel or ticagrelor could also potentially reduce the incidence of stent thrombosis and currently a trial comparing prasugrel plus bivalirudin with clopidogrel plus heparin is underway (BRAVE-4 NCT00976092).

Manual thrombus aspiration has class IIa recommendation in both AHA [44] and ESC [7]. Thrombectomy is recommended in STEMI patients with short ischemic times and large thrombus burden, while its use in STEMI patients with long ischemic times, side branches with small infarct territories, and low thrombus burden remains questionable. The ongoing TOTAL (ThrOmbectomy vs. PCI Alone for STEMI) study – a multicenter randomized trial which aims to recruit 4,000 subjects with STEMI randomizing them to either manual aspiration thrombectomy or PCI and evaluating for cardiovascular death, recurrent MI, cardiogenic shock, or new or worsening class IV heart failure at 180 days – promises to contribute considerably to existing evidence base in this regard.

The question about the type of stent (bare-metal stent or drug-eluting stent) to be used in STEMI is an interesting one also. Current evidence suggests that DES use is not associated with any increase in mortality, MI or stent thrombosis compared to BMS. At the same time DES use is associated with reduced target vessel revascularization rates [57–60]. This potential advantage has to be balanced against the need for prolonged dual antiplatelet therapy and could be challenging when dealing with an emergency situation such as STEMI.

Summary and Conclusion

PCI use continues to expand and is a viable robust and preferred alternative to CABG in most patients. In order to obtain the maximum benefit of PCI, appropriate selection of patients is therefore of paramount importance. We have discussed the different presentations of CAD and the issues pertaining to PCI in these populations. Patient selection for any procedure must always be based on what is best for that patient with rigorous reflection on the applicability of any evidence base/guideline recommendations as applied to that patient. It should also be kept in mind that the backlash against PCI evident among some groups (who may support unwaveringly the "COURAGE perspective") may indeed also not be in the patients' best interest.

A patient needing to stop and look in a shop window that they are not interested in because they have poorly controlled angina or suffering the oft un-asked about side effects from blunderbuss medication, when a low-risk cost-effective PCI could change their quality of life, are infrequently aired aspects of the discussion. That said, there are routine recognized steps that need to be gone through to ensure any patient "needs" (i.e., will benefit from PC I). Advances have also occurred in coronary artery bypass grafting and medical therapy. Therefore, very careful consideration is to be given when selecting patients for revascularization in order to optimize patient outcomes. When selecting patients for intervention, it is important to consider the following factors:

1. The clinical presentation (stable angina/acute coronary syndrome)
2. Severity of angina (asymptomatic, Canadian Cardiovascular Society [CCS] class I, II, III, or IV)
3. The age and ethnicity of the patients (elderly patients and some ethnic groups do not present with classical anginal symptoms)
4. Extent of ischemia on noninvasive testing and the presence or absence of other prognostic factors, such as congestive heart failure (CHF), depressed left ventricular function, chronic kidney disease, or diabetes
5. Concomitant of medical therapy
6. Anatomic disease (1-, 2-, or 3-vessel disease, with or without proximal LAD/left main coronary disease, SYNTAX score)

References

1. Gruntzig A. Transluminal dilatation of coronary-artery stenosis. Lancet. 1978;1:263.
2. Roberts R. Stable angina as a manifestation of ischemic heart disease: medical management. Circulation. 1985;72(6 Pt 2):V145–54.
3. Braunwald E, Domanski MJ, Fowler SE, et al. Angiotensin-converting-enzyme inhibition in stable coronary artery disease. N Engl J Med. 2004;351(20):2058–68.
4. www.nice.org.uk/guidance/CG95
5. Gibbons RJ, Abrams J, Chatterjee K. ACC/AHA 2002 guideline update for the management of patients with chronic stable angina–summary article: a report of the American College of Cardiology/American Heart Association Task Force on practice guidelines (Committee on the Management of Patients with Chronic Stable Angina). J Am Coll Cardiol. 2003;41(1):159–68.
6. Patel MR, Peterson ED, Dai D, et al. Low diagnostic yield of elective coronary angiography. N Engl J Med. 2010;362(10):886–95.
7. Wijns W, Kohl P, Danchin N, et al. Guidelines on myocardial revascularisation ESC/EACTS. Eur Heart J. 2010;31(20):2501–55.
8. Pijls N, De Bruyne B, Peels K, et al. Measurement of fractional flow reserve to assess the functional severity of coronary-artery stenoses. N Engl J Med. 1996;334:1703–8.
9. Pijls N, Van Gelder B, Van der Voort P, et al. Fractional flow reserve. A useful index to evaluate the influence of an epicardial coronary stenosis on myocardial blood flow. Circulation. 1995;92:3183–93.
10. Berger A, Botman KJ, McCarthy P, et al. Long-term clinical outcome after fractional flow reserve-guided percutaneous coronary intervention in patients with multivessel disease. J Am Coll Cardiol. 2005;46(3):438–42.
11. Torino PA, Be Bruyne B, Pijls NH, et al. Fractional flow reserve versus angiography for guiding percutaneous coronary intervention. N Engl J Med. 2009;360(3):213–24.
12. Fearon WF, Bornschein B, Torino PA, et al. Economic evaluation of fractional flow reserve-guided percutaneous coronary intervention in patients with multivessel disease. Circulation. 2010;122(24):2545–50.
13. De Bruyne B, Pijls NH, Kalesan B, Barbato E, Tonino PA, Piroth Z, Jagic N, Mobius-Winckler S, Rioufol G, Witt N, Kala P, Maccarthy P, Engstrom T, Oldroyd KG, Mavromatis K, Manoharan G, Verlee P, Frobert O, Curzen N, Johnson JB, Juni P, Fearon WF. Fractional flow reserve-guided pci versus medical therapy in stable coronary disease. N Engl J Med. 2012;367:991–1001.
14. Boden WE, Teo KK, et al. Optimal medical therapy with or without PCI for stable coronary disease. N Engl J Med. 2007;356(15):1503–16.
15. Weintraub WS, Spertus JA, Kolm P, et al. Effect of PCI on quality of life in patients with stable coronary disease. N Engl J Med. 2008;359(7):677–87.
16. Shaw LJ, Berman DS, Maron DJ, et al. Optimal medical therapy with or without percutaneous coronary intervention to reduce

ischemic burden: results from the Clinical Outcomes Utilizing Revascularization and Aggressive Drug Evaluation (COURAGE) trial nuclear substudy. Circulation. 2008;117:1283–91.
17. Hachamovich R, Hayes SW, Friedman JD, et al. Comparison of the short-term survival benefit associated with revascularization compared with medical therapy in patients with no prior coronary artery disease undergoing stress myocardial perfusion single photon emission computed tomography. Circulation. 2003;107:2900–7.
18. Prasad A, Rihal C, Holmes Jr DR. The COURAGE trial in perspective. Catheter Cardiovasc Interv. 2008;72:54–9.
19. Curzen N. Is there evidence for prognostic benefit following PCI in stable patients? COURAGE and its implications: an interventionalist's view. Heart. 2010;96(2):103–5.
20. Borden WB, Redberg RF, Mushlin AI, et al. Patterns and intensity of medical therapy in patients undergoing percutaneous coronary intervention. JAMA. 2011;305(18):1882–9.
21. Serruys PW, Morice MC, Kappetein AP, et al. Percutaneous coronary intervention versus coronary-artery bypass grafting for severe coronary artery disease. N Engl J Med. 2009;360(10):961–72.
22. http://clinicaltrials.gov/ct2/show/NCT01205776
23. Frye RL, August P, Brooks MM, et al. A randomized trial of therapies for type 2 diabetes and coronary artery disease. N Engl J Med. 2009;360(24):2503–15.
24. Dagenais GR, Lu J, Faxon DP, Kent K, et al. Effects of optimal medical treatment with or without coronary revascularization on angina and subsequent revascularizations in patients with type 2 diabetes mellitus and stable ischemic heart disease. Circulation. 2011;123(14):1492–500.
25. Kim YH, Park DW, Lee JY, et al. Impact of angiographic complete revascularization after drug-eluting stent implantation or coronary artery bypass graft surgery for multivessel coronary artery disease. Circulation. 2011;123:2373–81.
26. Fraker Jr TD, Fihn SD, et al. 2007 chronic angina focused update of ACC/AHA 2002 guidelines. Eur Heart J. 2010;31(20):2501–55.
27. Libby P, Theroux P. Pathophysiology of coronary artery disease. Circulation. 2005;111(25):3481–8.
28. Pfeffer M, Braunwald E. Ventricular remodeling after myocardial infarction: experimental observations and clinical implications. Circulation. 1990;81:1161–72.
29. Antman EM, Cohen M, Bernink PJ, et al. The TIMI risk score for unstable angina/non-ST elevation MI: a method for prognostication and therapeutic decision making. JAMA. 2000;284(7):835–42.
30. Brilakis ES, Wright RS, Kopecky SL. Association of the PURSUIT risk score with predischarge ejection fraction, angiographic severity of coronary artery disease, and mortality in a nonselected, community-based population with non-ST-elevation acute myocardial infarction. Am Heart J. 2003;146(5):811–18.
31. Lagerqvist B, Diderholm E, Lindahl B, et al. FRISC score for selection of patients for an early invasive treatment strategy in unstable coronary artery disease. Heart. 2005;91(8):1047–52.
32. Wallentin L, Lagerqvist B, Husted S, et al. Outcome at 1 year after an invasive compared with a non-invasive strategy in unstable coronary-artery disease: the FRISC II invasive randomised trial. FRISC II investigators. Fast revascularisation during instability in coronary artery disease. Lancet. 2000;356(9223):9–16.
33. Cannon CP, Weintraub WS, Demopoulus LA, et al. Comparison of early invasive and conservative strategies in patients with unstable coronary syndromes treated with the glycoprotein IIb/IIIa inhibitor tirofiban. N Engl J Med. 2001;344(25):1879–87.
34. Fox KA, Poole-Wilson PA, Henderson RA, et al. Interventional versus conservative treatment for patients with unstable angina or non-ST-elevation myocardial infarction: the British Heart Foundation RITA 3 randomised trial. Randomized intervention trial of unstable angina. Lancet. 2002;360(9335):743–51.
35. De Winter RJ, Windhausen F, Cornel JH, et al. Early invasive versus selectively invasive management for acute coronary syndromes. N Engl J Med. 2005;353:1095–104.
36. Mehta SR, Granger CB, Boden WE, et al. Early versus delayed invasive intervention in acute coronary syndromes. N Engl J Med. 2009;360(21):2165–75.
37. Mehta SR, Cannon CP, Fox KA, et al. Routine vs selective invasive strategies in patients with acute coronary syndromes: a collaborative meta-analysis of randomized trials. JAMA. 2005;293(23): 2908–17.
38. Fox KA, Clayton TC, Damman P, et al. Long-term outcome of a routine versus selective invasive strategy in patients with non-ST-segment elevation acute coronary syndrome a meta-analysis of individual patient data. J Am Coll Cardiol. 2010;55(22):2435–45.
39. Katritsis DG, Siontis GC, Kastrati A, et al. Optimal timing of coronary angiography and potential intervention in non-ST-elevation acute coronary syndromes. Eur Heart J. 2011;32(1):32–40.
40. www.nice.org.uk/CG94
41. Kastrati A, Mehilli J, Nekolla S, et al. A randomized trial comparing myocardial salvage achieved by coronary stenting versus balloon angioplasty in patients with acute myocardial infarction considered ineligible for reperfusion therapy. J Am Coll Cardiol. 2004;43(5):734–41.
42. Di Mario C, Dudek D, Piscione F, et al. Immediate angioplasty versus standard therapy with #rescue angioplasty after thrombolysis in the Combined Abciximab REteplase Stent Study in Acute Myocardial Infarction (CARESS-in-AMI): an open, prospective, randomised, multicentre trial. Lancet. 2008;371(9612):559–68.
43. Ellis SG, Tendera M, de Belder MA, et al. Facilitated PCI in patients with ST-elevation myocardial infarction. N Engl J Med. 2008;358(21):2205–17.
44. Cantor WJ, Fitchett D, Borgundvaag B, et al. Routine early angioplasty after fibrinolysis for acute myocardial infarction. N Engl J Med. 2009;360(26):2705–18.
45. Kushner FG, Hand M, Smith Jr SC, et al. 2009 focused updates: ACC/AHA guidelines for the management of patients with ST-elevation myocardial infarction (updating the 2004 guideline and 2007 focused update) and ACC/AHA/SCAI guidelines on percutaneous coronary intervention (updating the 2005 guideline and 2007 focused update) a report of the American College of Cardiology Foundation/American Heart Association Task Force on practice guidelines. J Am Coll Cardiol. 2009;54:2205–41.
46. Armstrong PW, Gershlick A, Goldstein P. The Strategic Reperfusion Early After Myocardial Infarction (STREAM) study. Am Heart J. 2010;160(1):30–5.
47. Gershlick AH, Stephens-Lloyd A, Hughes S, et al. Rescue angioplasty after failed thrombolytic therapy for acute myocardial infarction. N Engl J Med. 2005;353(26):2758–68.
48. Wijeysundera HC, Vijayaraghavan R, Nallamothu BK, et al. Rescue angioplasty or repeat fibrinolysis after failed fibrinolytic therapy for ST-segment myocardial infarction: a meta-analysis of randomized trials. Am Coll Cardiol. 2007;49(4):422–30.
49. Choi CU, Rha SW, Oh DJ, et al. Standard versus high loading doses of clopidogrel in Asian ST-segment elevation myocardial infarction patients undergoing percutaneous coronary intervention: insights from the Korea Acute Myocardial Infarction Registry. Am Heart J. 2011;161(2):373–382.e1-3.
50. Larson DM, Duval S, Sharkey SS, et al. Clopidogrel pretreatment in ST-elevation myocardial infarction patients transferred for percutaneous coronary intervention. Am Heart J. 2010;160(1):202–7.
51. Dangas G, Mehran R, Guagliumi G, et al. Role of clopidogrel loading dose in patients with ST-segment elevation myocardial infarction undergoing primary angioplasty: results from the HORIZONS-AMI (harmonizing outcomes with revascularization

and stents in acute myocardial infarction) trial. J Am Coll Cardiol. 2009;54(15):1438–46.

52. Wiviott SD, Braunwald E, McCabe CH, et al. Prasugrel versus clopidogrel in patients with acute coronary syndromes. N Engl J Med. 2007;357(20):2001–15.
53. Montalescot G, Wiviott SD, Braunwald E, et al. Prasugrel compared with clopidogrel in patients undergoing percutaneous coronary intervention for ST-elevation myocardial infarction (TRITON-TIMI 38): double-blind, randomised controlled trial. Lancet. 2009;373(9665):723–31.
54. Wallentin L, Becker RC, Budaj A, et al. Ticagrelor versus clopidogrel in patients with acute coronary syndromes. N Engl J Med. 2009;361(11):1045–57.
55. Bellemain-Appaix A, Brieger D, Beygui F, et al. New P2Y12 inhibitors versus clopidogrel in percutaneous coronary intervention: a meta-analysis. J Am Coll Cardiol. 2010;56(19):1542–51.
56. Mehran R, Lansky AJ, Witzenbichler B, et al. Bivalirudin in patients undergoing primary angioplasty for acute myocardial infarction (HORIZONS-AMI): 1-year results of a randomised controlled trial. Lancet. 2009;374(9696):1149–59.
57. www.nice.org.uk/guidance/TA230
58. Di Lorenzo E, Sauro R, Varricchio A, et al. Long-term outcome of drug-eluting stents compared with bare metal stents in ST-segment elevation myocardial infarction: results of the paclitaxel- or sirolimus-eluting stent versus bare metal stent in Primary Angioplasty (PASEO) Randomized Trial. Circulation. 2009;120(11):964–72.
59. Iijima R, Byrne RA, Dibra A, et al. Drug-eluting stents versus bare-metal stents in diabetic patients with ST-segment elevation acute myocardial infarction: a pooled analysis of individual patient data from seven randomized trials. Rev Esp Cardiol. 2009;62(4):354–64.
60. Piscione F, Piccolo R, Cassese S, et al. Clinical impact of sirolimus-eluting stent in ST-segment elevation myocardial infarction: a meta-analysis of randomized clinical trials. Catheter Cardiovasc Interv. 2009;74(2):323–32.

Contrast Nephropathy and Kidney Injury

5

Jeremiah R. Brown and Peter A. McCullough

National Statistics and Prevalence

Contrast-induced acute kidney injury (CI-AKI), also referred to as contrast-induced nephropathy, is a major complication following cardiac catheterizations and other procedures using intravascular, iodinated radio-contrast for imaging. CI-AKI occurs in approximately 10 % or more of patients undergoing cardiac catheterization. Variation in reported rate of CI-AKI exists because of a variety of definitions and variability in the timing and frequency of measurement after contrast exposure. In the United States, approximately 1.2 million cardiac catheterization are performed [1, 2], which translates into approximately 120,000 annual cases of CI-AKI. Patients developing CI-AKI have an increased risk of short- and long-term mortality, new onset of dialysis-dependent renal failure, and increased length of stay and utilization of healthcare resources [3, 4]. According to a systematic review and meta-analysis of clinical trials, CI-AKI is associated with a threefold increased risk of death (RR: 2.89; 95 % CI: 2.32–3.61) [5]. With the rate of overall AKI-related hospitalizations on the rise (Fig. 5.1) [6], AKI is anticipated to be a source of rapidly increasing healthcare costs. Therefore, every effort should be taken to anticipate and minimize this complication. In this chapter, we will summarize the pathophysiology, diagnosis, and prevention of CI-AKI for your clinical practice.

J.R. Brown, PhD, MS (✉)
The Dartmouth Institute for Health Policy and Clinical Practice and Section of Cardiology, Department of Medicine, Community and Family Medicine,
Audrey and Theodore Geisel School of Medicine at Dartmouth, HB 7505 DHMC One Medical Center Drive, Lebanon, NH, USA
e-mail: jbrown@dartmouth.edu

P.A. McCullough, MD, MPH
St. John Providence Health System, Providence Park Hospital, Cardiovascular Institute, Warren, MI, USA

Pathophysiology: CI-AKI and Acute Tubular Necrosis

CI-AKI occurs when there is chronic kidney disease (CKD) with reduced nephron capacity as a result of hypertension, diabetes, and other determinants of kidney disease. As contrast travels in the bloodstream, it triggers a transient release of nitric oxide, which induces endothelium-dependent vasodilation. Within the renal vascular arcades, this results in transient renovascular dilation and increased renal blood flow, which lasts for a few minutes. When the water-soluble contrast passes into the glomerulus through the fenestrated endothelium, it enters the Bowman's capsule and the urinary space with rapid exposure to the tubular epithelial cells. The contrast material is then taken up by these cells and permeates gap junctions and the basal side of the tubule with entry into the peritubular space. In response, there is tubuloglomerular feedback through adenosine release from the macula densa, endothelin release, prostaglandin dysregulation, and subsequent decreased nitric oxide synthesis. These mechanisms combine to cause sustained intrarenal vasoconstriction lasting for approximately 2 h. During this time, there is a substantial reduction in renal blood flow and accumulation of contrast in the in the renal medulla, causing further vasoconstriction, prolonged contrast exposure

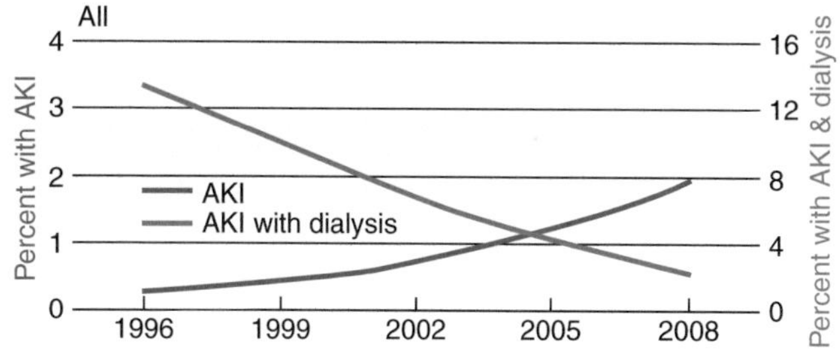

Fig. 5.1 Statistics from the United States Renal Database System (USRDS), graphing the increase in percent of hospitalizations with acute kidney injury (*AKI*, *Blue*) and percent of hospitalizations with AKI and dialysis (*red*) (From USRDS 2010 report: http://www.usrds.org/2010/pdf/V1_08.pdf)

C.A. Thompson (ed.), *Textbook of Cardiovascular Intervention*,
DOI 10.1007/978-1-4471-4528-8_5, © Springer-Verlag London 2014

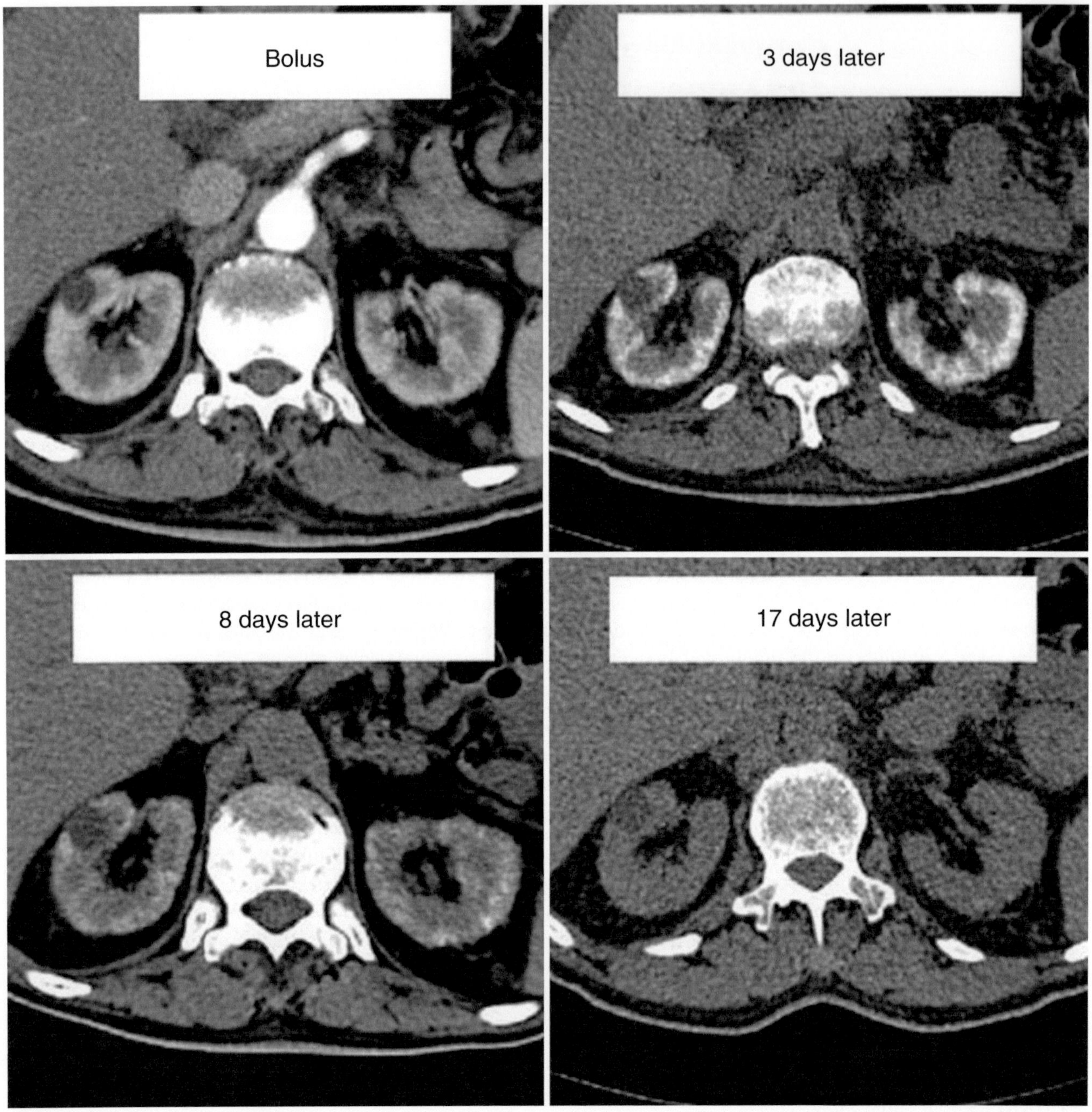

Fig. 5.2 (**a**) CT image of a patient exposed to intravenous iodixanol contrast (0.5 g I/kg). (**b–d**) Serial CT scans (unenhanced) on day 3 (**b**), day 8 (**c**), and day 17 (**d**) after exposure to iodixanol (From Koneth et al. [7], with permission)

to the renal tubular cells, and direct chemotoxic cellular injury. This phenomenon has been illustrated in numerous case reports of persistent nephrograms, where contrast has been shown to be trapped in the medulla for days and weeks (Fig. 5.2) [7]. During this time, the prolonged contrast exposure to renal tubules propagates direct cellular injury inducing tubular apoptosis and cell death (Fig. 5.3). A critical biochemical component to renal tubular cell damage appears to be the liberation of labile or poorly liganded iron from cellular organelles. Catalytic iron in the cytosol and pericellular space allows the Fenton and Haber-Weiss equations to rapidly produce reactive oxygen species including the destructive hydroxyl radical. By this process, adjacent cells then injured, propagating tissue damage after the initial waves of ischemic and chemotoxic attack have occurred. Following renal tubule dysfunction and cell death, there is dissolution of the basement membrane and sloughing of tubular epithelial cells into the u-ring. A rise in the serum creatinine and decreased urine output signal this process has occurred over the preceding 48 h [8]. As a normal

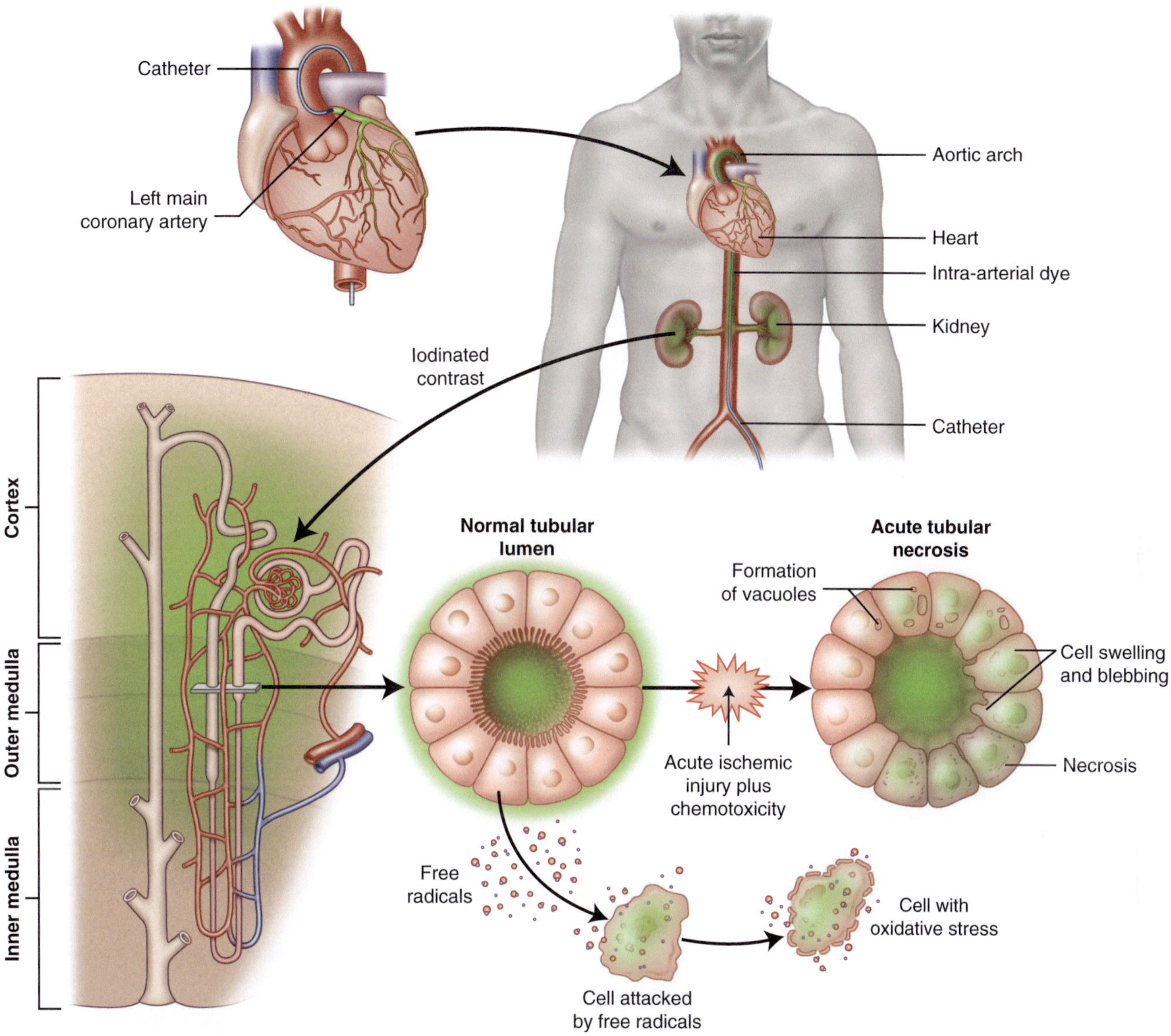

Fig. 5.3 Pathophysiology of contrast-induced acute kidney injury (*CI-AKI*) and acute tubular necrosis

response to injury, renal tubular cells regenerate from bone stem cells; however this process takes time and can be compromised by preexisting disease (e.g., diabetes) or reexposure to contrast. Over 90 % of patients exhibit considerable recovery with no evidence of worsened CKD at follow-up. However, other patients progress more quickly to worsened chronic kidney disease or kidney failure requiring persistent dialysis or transplantation (Fig. 5.4) [6].

How to Diagnose CI-AKI: Definitions

CI-AKI is diagnosed by a sudden increase in SCr, normally occurring within 48 h after contrast exposure. The consensus definition for CI-AKI was previously a 25 % or 0.5 (mg/dL) increase from baseline to the peak SCr within 48 h [9]. Other definitions after reevaluation of AKI occurring in the hospital setting include the Acute Kidney Injury Network of ≥0.3 (mg/dL) or ≥50 % increase in the highest SCr within 48 h [10]. The measurement of peak SCr after cardiac catheterizations is often difficult to do on a routine basis because outpatient cardiac catheterizations and same-day percutaneous coronary interventions (PCI), where patients remain in the hospital for brief periods of time do not allow for repeat measurement. However, SCr is known to reach its peak after contrast administration between 48 and 96 h – a time when most patients have returned home. In high-risk patients, discharge planning should include a 72–96-h follow-up from the time of catheterization to determine presence of CI-AKI.

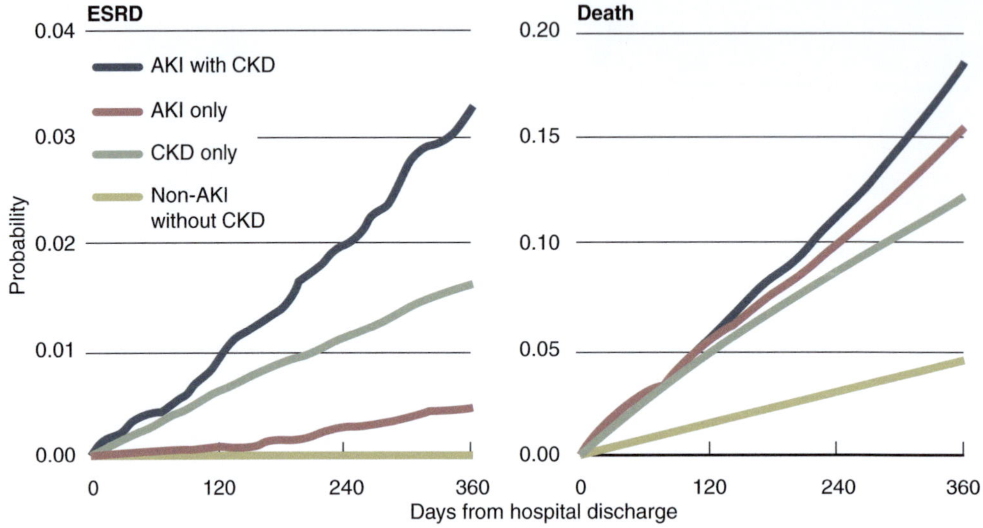

Fig. 5.4 Probability of progressing to end-stage renal disease (*left*) or death with acute kidney injury (*AKI*) with or without chronic kidney disease (*CDK*) (From the United States Renal Database System (USRDS) 2010 report: http://www.usrds.org/2010/pdf/V1_08.pdf)

What Does a Serum Creatinine Elevation Mean?

When a positive SCr signal is detected that diagnoses the patient with CI-AKI, care should be taken to discontinue any drugs that could be considered nephrotoxic. Most patients experience a transient elevation in SCr and return to their baseline and resume normal renal function with 2 weeks [11, 12]. However, 30–48 % of patients have a persistent elevation of SCr for up to 90 days [13, 14]. Among patients with persistent elevations, 36 % have been reported to require dialysis [14]. Most importantly, it has been reported that regardless of transient or persistent CI-AKI diagnoses, both groups of patients have significant increased risks of death and morbidity (Fig. 5.5) [3].

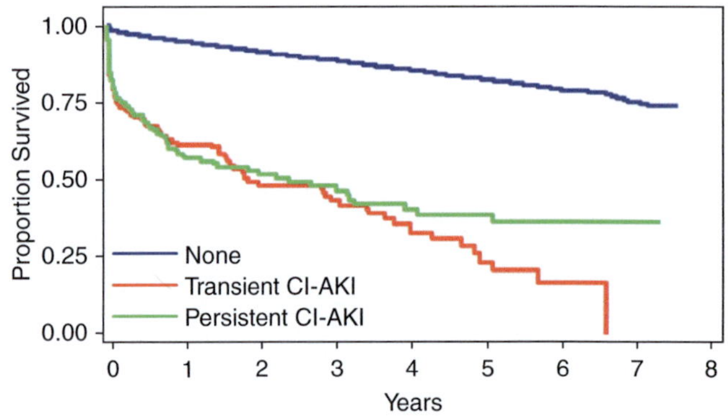

Fig. 5.5 Kaplan-Meier survival curves for contrast-induced acute kidney injury (*CI-AKI*). *Blue*: no CI-AKI (<0.5 mg/dL increase in creatinine from baseline). *Red*: transient CI-AKI (≥0.5 mg/dL increase in creatinine from baseline and creatinine returned to normal within 2 weeks). *Green*: persistent CI-AKI (≥0.5 mg/dL increase in creatinine from baseline and creatinine remained elevated within 2 weeks) (Courtesy of Jeremiah R. Brown, Ph.D., Lebanon, NH)

Novel Biomarkers for Early Detection

Due to the latency period to detect a rise in SCr, which takes up to 48 h after contrast exposure or kidney injury, there is considerable interest in the development of urinary and/or serum biomarkers for CI-AKI that could accurately identify the problem before the rise in SCr. There are several blood biomarkers that have been identified as possible candidates: cystatin C, neutrophil gelatinase-associated lipocalin (NGAL), IL-18, and kidney injury molecule-1 (KIM-1). A recent meta-analysis demonstrated NGAL had strong predictive ability for AKI in critical illness and after cardiac surgery in both children and adults [15]. A single investigation of serum cystatin-C, which is a renal filtration marker, suggested that a 10 % elevation in cystatin C at 24 h was predictive of CI-AKI with a negative predictive value of 100 % but only a positive predictive value of 39.1 % [16]. Additional investigations have been conducted on hospital-acquired AKI on panels of urinary markers; however much of this work has not been extended into investigating patients exposed to contrast [17]. While progress is being made in the field of developing urinary and serum biomarkers for early detection of CI-AKI, much work remains to be done. The ideal biomarker would show detection of acute tubular necrosis on arrival to the ICU after cardiac catheterization or within 4 h of contrast exposure to flag patients prior to discharge. Additional research will be required to validate these biomarkers in the clinical setting and evaluate their clinical utility in routine patient care.

Risk Score for Predicting CI-AKI

Decreased baseline renal function measured by the estimated glomerular filtration (eGFR) rate is the leading risk factor for developing CI-AKI. eGFR is commonly reported by

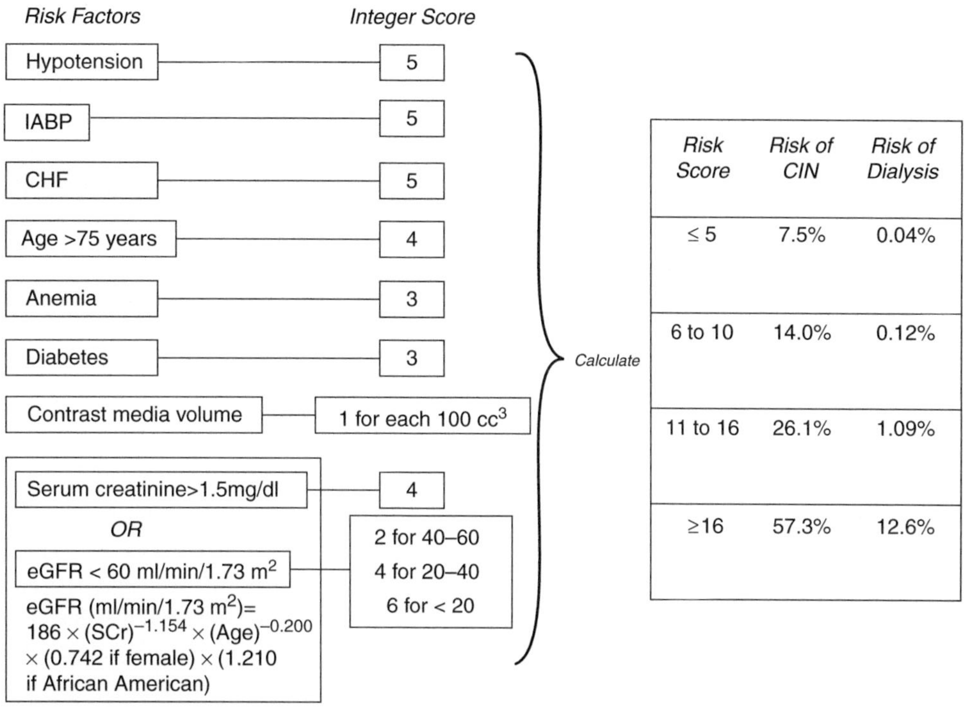

Fig. 5.6 Clinical risk prediction tool for contrast-induced acute kidney injury (*CI-AKI*). As defined by Mehran and colleagues: *Anemia* = baseline hematocrit value <39 % for men and <36 % for women; *CHF* = congestive heart failure class III/IV by New York Heart Association classification and/or history of pulmonary edema; *eGFR* = estimated glomerular filtration rate; *hypotension* = systolic blood pressure <80 mmHg for at least 1 h requiring inotropic support with medications or intra-aortic balloon pump (*IABP*) within 24 h peri-procedurally (From Mehran et al. R, Aymong ED, Nikolsky E, et al. [23], with permission)

clinical laboratories along with the patient's serum creatinine (SCr) and calculated using the Modification of Diet in Renal Disease (MDRD) equation (mL/min/1.73 m^2) where eGFR$_{MDRD}$ = 186 × (serum creatinine mg/dL)$^{-1.154}$ × (age)$^{-0.203}$ × (0.742 for women) [18–20]. Patients with an eGFR < 60 are considered to have chronic kidney disease stage 3 or worse. The new CKD-EPI equation has been introduced to the clinical setting and can be calculated as: CKD-EPI equation: eGFR$_{CKD\text{-}EPI}$ = 141 × (minimum of standardized serum creatinine [mg/dL]/κ or 1)α × (maximum of standardized serum creatinine [mg/dL]/κ or 1)$^{-1.209}$ × 0.993^{age} × (1.018 if female) or (1.159 if black), where κ is 0.7 if female and 0.9 if male and α is 0.329 if female and 0.411 if male [21, 22]. The CKD-EPI equation appears to be better calibrated for patients with eGFR ≥ 60 and middle-aged patients and will likely replace the 4-variable MDRD equations in laboratory reporting of the eGFR.

Risk scores have been developed to more accurately identify the patients at highest risk of CI-AKI. The most widely used risk score for CI-AKI was developed by Dr. Mehran and colleagues in 2004 (Fig. 5.6) [23]. The model included known risk factors including age greater than 75 years, diabetes, anemia, congestive heart failure, hypotension, intra-aortic balloon pump use, eGFR or baseline SCr, and contrast volume. Brown and colleagues developed a similar model focusing on pre-procedural risk and included baseline SCr, congestive heart failure, and diabetes mellitus provide approximately three-quarters of the predicted of risk, while the other factors included age 80 years or older, female gender, urgent or emergent priority of the procedure, and pre-procedural intra-aortic balloon pump use [24]. Predicting the risk of CI-AKI is critical to providing informed consent for the patient and family, planning peri-procedure prophylaxis, and ordering follow-up assessments.

CI-AKI Prevention

A critical component to preventing CI-AKI is the avoidance of dehydration. Volume depletion reduces renal blood flow and accentuates the degree of vasoconstriction that occurs with contrast. In addition, reducing urine flow allows greater penetration of contrast into the renal tubular epithelium. Patients can do at-home prevention by hydrating with water before and after the procedure. This has been shown to be modestly effective and safe. While in the hospital, intravenous hydration with normal saline or sodium bicarbonate has been evaluated as a strategy to reduce the incidence of CI-AKI in patients undergoing cardiac catheterizations [25, 26].

Traditionally, NPO orders have been used in clinical practice restricting patients to no food or drink after midnight, thus, increasing the risk of dehydration. Patients can be educated at the time the procedure is scheduled and reminded in a letter and by phone to drink 1–2 L of water before going to bed the night before the procedure and 1–2 L in the morning. To meet anesthesia requirement for partial sedation, orders should be rewritten for NPO 2 h prior to the procedure. When the patient arrives for the procedure, an IV infusion of saline at 1.5 mL/kgmL/h can be started and continued through the procedure for up to 6 h afterwards. For patients with eGFR<60 begin NaCL or sodium bicarbonate 1–3 h before the procedure at 3 mL/kg/h and 1,200 mg *N*-acetylcysteine (PO 12 h×4) can be given.

Hydration, Sodium Bicarbonate, and *N*-Acetylcysteine

Numerous clinical trials and meta-analyses have evaluated the effectiveness of normal saline compared with sodium bicarbonate. Several meta-analyses have shown sodium bicarbonate to be more effective than hydration with normal saline with pooled relative risk estimates at 0.52–0.62 [27–29]. Based on a 48 % reduction in CI-AKI, it was determined that treating only 16 patients with sodium bicarbonate were needed to prevent one case of CI-AKI. Total cost to treat 16 patients with sodium bicarbonate is $50 [27]. Approximate cost in additional hospital expenses for each case of CI-AKI is $7,500 [4]. However, two large trials that have evaluated NaCl and sodium bicarbonate have shown similar rates of CI-AKI, and thus the early positive findings for sodium bicarbonate are believe to be the result of alpha error or random chance [30, 31].

N-acetylcysteine, a mild antioxidant, has shown to have a dose–response effect on preventing CI-AKI. A meta-analysis of randomized trials reported that when 1,200 mg of *N*-acetylcysteine was used in comparison to 600 mg, CI-AKI was reduced by 54 % [32, 33]. The use of *N*-acetylcysteine for high-risk patients can be considered with a 1,200 mg dose given PO twice before the procedure and twice after (PO 1,200 mg 12 h×4). However, a recent trial from Brazil consisting of 2,308 patients reported no difference in the use of high-dose *N*-acetylcysteine (RR 1.00, 95 % CI: 0.81–1.25), causing clinicians to reconsider the effectiveness of *N*-acetylcysteine among patients with normal renal function or patients with CKD stage 3 (eGFR 30–59) [34].

Limited trials have evaluated the combination of both *N*-acetylcysteine and sodium bicarbonate in comparison to normal saline alone. A meta-analysis summarizing this combination effect yielded mixed results, but demonstrated a trend towards a 35 % reduced incidence of CI-AKI (Fig. 5.7) [35]. Based on this evidence, it appears that using multiple pharmacological agents to prevent CI-AKI may reach the highest degree of prevention.

CI-AKI Prevention: Contrast Agent and Volume

Contrast Agents

The choice of nonionic contrast agent has been an issue of uncertainty and mostly driven by operator preference and institutional contracts. Multiple industry-sponsored and investigator-initiated *t*-randomized controlled trials and meta-analyses have been conducted to determine the efficacy and safety of the available contrast agents used in percutaneous procedures. Higher osmolality contrast agents have been shown to result in more CI-AKI in the past. The main question has focused on the relative renal safety of iso-osmolar or low-osmolar contrast. Iso-osmolar contrast (iodixanol) has been shown in some trials to reduce the risk of CI-AKI [36], mainly in intra-arterial studies [37]. However, other trials and a meta-analysis have demonstrated no difference between the iso-osmolar agent and low-osmolar agents with a summary relative risk of 0.79 (95 % CI: 0.56–1.19) [38–42]. A long-term follow-up of the CARE trial recently revealed that patients receiving iopamidol were less likely to develop CI-AKI and other long-term events than patients receiving iodixanol [43]. The evidence for choice of contrast for the overall population with eGFR<60 remains at equipoise. However, based on the best evidence to date, those with both eGFR<60 and diabetes mellitus, iodixanol appears to result in less CI-AKI. New contrast-manufacturing technology has introduced contrast reformulated with cyclodextrin; this technology may provide improved solubility and stability while improving retention of the contrast dye in the blood and urine and minimizing penetration to cells and tissues [44].

Contrast Volume

While there exists uncertainly around the right contrast agent, the volume of contrast is one of the most important factors in preventing CI-AKI. Over 20 years ago, Cigarroa developed an equation in 1989 called the maximum acceptable contrast dose or MACD. The equation takes into account the body weight (Kg) and baseline renal function (SCr): MACD=(5 mL contrast volume × body weight, Kg/baseline serum creatinine, md/dL) [45]. This equation has been incorporated into progressive catheterization laboratories as a measure of safe dosing of contrast tailored to the individual patient's size and renal function. The MACD has been evaluated in several clinical trials and confirmed that patients who received contrast volumes in excess of the MACD were more likely to develop CI-AKI [46]. Another clinical trial confirmed these results and demonstrated a dose–response effect between exceeding the MACD and risk of CI-AKI (Fig. 5.8) [47, 48]. Each 50 % increment above the MACD increased the risk of CI-AKI by 7 % [47, 48]. It is important to realize that the lower the eGFR at baseline, the smaller the volume of contrast needed to induce CI-AKI. Thus, there is no "safe" contrast limit and the policy of "as low as reasonably possible" for each patient should be followed.

Device Solutions

A cost-effective way to reduce the amount of contrast given to the patient while reducing the overall contrast use could

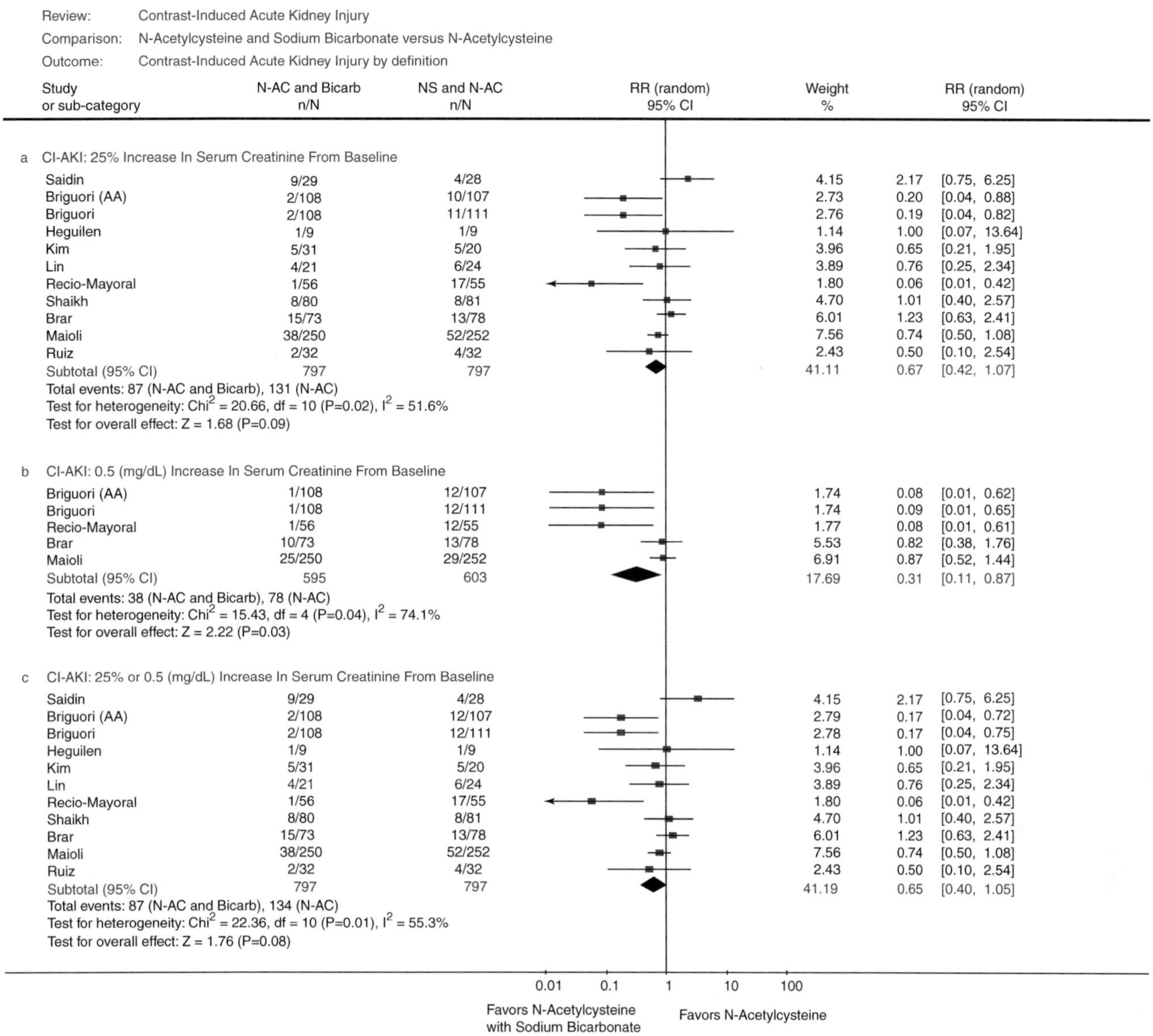

Fig. 5.7 Meta-analysis of individual randomized controlled trials is listed in order by year of publication. Outcome is contrast-induced AKI. (**a**): contrast-induced AKI (25 % relative increase in serum creatinine from baseline). (**b**): contrast-induced AKI (≥0.5 mg/dL increase in serum creatinine from baseline). (**c**): contrast-induced AKI (≥25 % or ≥0.5 mg/dL increase in serum creatinine from baseline). CI: 95% confidence interval. The size of each *square* denotes the weight of each trial's relative risk in calculating the combined relative risk. The *diamond* represents the combined relative risk at the center; opposing points of the *diamond* represent the 95 % confidence intervals. Treatment: *N*-acetylcysteine plus sodium bicarbonate. AA: *N*-acetylcysteine plus ascorbic acid (From Brown et al. [35], with permission)

be obtained by converting from a manual injection system to an automated contrast injector. Automated contrast injectors have been an effective tool to reduce the volume and cost of contrast [49]. Clinical trials have demonstrated that contrast can be reduced by 39–50 % [49, 50]. In addition to the benefits in safety for the patient, institutions have seen a dramatic fall in the cost of contrast and utilization after converting to automated contrast injectors.

Other technologies have been developed for reducing CI-AKI including the Benephit catheter system, Reitan Pump, and Renal Guard. The Benephit catheter system (AngioDynamics Inc.) uses a miniaturized catheter system to engage both renal arteries and facilitate targeted renal pharmacotherapy [51]. Early results demonstrate that renal blood flow is improved during a case from adjunctive infusion of human recombinant B-type natriuretic peptide (BNP), fenoldopam, and other agents using the catheter system [52–54]. The Reitan pump allows for hemodynamic augmentation for high-risk patients undergoing PCI [55]. Early results suggest that the Reitan pump can improve renal function by improving renal hemodynamics [55]. Renal Guard is another new technology that incorporates furosemide-induced

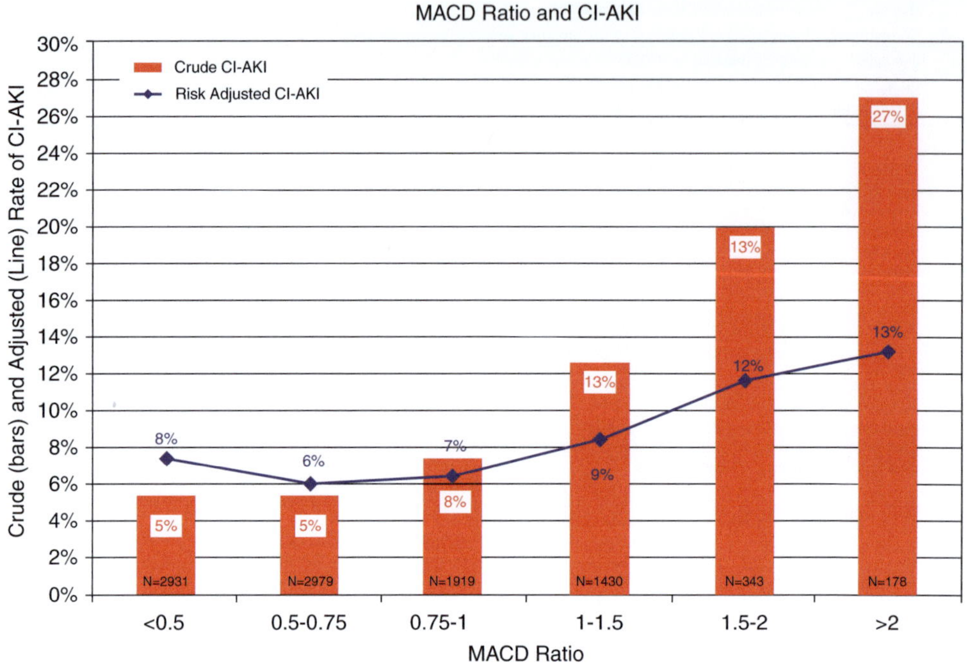

Fig. 5.8 Calculated ratios of contrast volume to the predicted maximum acceptable contrast dose (*MACD*) are plotted by the crude (*grey bars*) and risk-adjusted (*black diamonds*) rates of contrast-induced acute kidney injury (*CI-AKI*) [48] (From Brown et al. [48], with permission)

diuresis with matched hydration. Patients receive a 30-min bolus of 250 mL of normal saline and an IV bolus of furosemide (0.5 mg/kg) with continued intravenous volume infusion until the procedure (90 min). Each mL of urine is replaced with 1 mL of normal saline. Matched hydration is continued for 4 h after the procedure. This method can increase the urine flow rate in patients with significant CKD up to 800 mL/min in the peri-procedural period allowing for more rapid contrast transit through the tubules into the collecting ducts and ureters. Preliminary results from the Mythos Trial reduced CI-AKI from 17 % with regular IV hydration to 6 % with Renal Guard ($P=0.06$) [56].

Novel Solutions

There are novel solutions being investigated to tackle the issue of CI-AKI at the molecular level through labile iron chelation with deferiprone. As discussed above, is thought that local release of catalytic iron may contribute to CI-AKI through its catalysis of oxidative injury [57]. Iron chelators have begun to be investigated to evaluate the mitigation of iron and subsequent reduction myoglobinuric renal injury and myohemoglobinuric injury [58–60]. New clinical trials in humans are recruiting patients to further investigate the utility of iron chelators for the prevention of CI-AKI.

Iloprost, a prostacyclin analog, was investigated among patients with renal dysfunction undergoing cardiac catheterization or PCI. The investigators of a 208-patient trial reported that 1 (ng/kg/min) of intravenous Iloprost injection from 30 to 90 min prior to the case and continuing until 4 h after the case significantly reduced the incidence of CI-AKI with and odds ratio of 0.29 (0.12–0.69) [61].

The pleiotropic effects of statin have begun to be investigated as a beneficial treatment for reducing CI-AKI. Recently, two trials investigated the peri-procedural use of statin and CI-AKI. One study demonstrated 80 mg of atorvastatin before and after contrast injection had no effect on CI-AKI with RR 0.97 (95 % CI: 0.67–1.38) [62]. However, a head-to-head trial comparing 20–80 mg of simvastatin among PCI patients, demonstrated a significant reduction in CI-AKI with the 80 mg simvastatin with RR 0.63 (95 % CI: 0.48–0.83) [63].

Cardiac Catheterization and Cardiac Surgery

Kidney injuring resulting from contrast exposure prior to cardiac surgery can increase the risk for cardiac surgery-associated AKI. Ranucci and colleagues reported cardiac surgery-associated AKI was highest among patients that underwent a cardiac catheterization on the same day of cardiac surgery (11.2 %) compared to patients receiving catheterizations on 1–5 days prior to surgery (4.2 %) [64]. Medalion and colleagues confirmed these findings by demonstrating a significant trend in AKI rates following cardiac surgery depending on timing between the cardiac catheterization: ≤1 day (20 % AKI), 1–5 days (12 %), and ≥5 days (8 %) [65]. Hennessy and colleagues reported a similar effect in valve patients, where patients with a diagnostic cardiac catheterization within 24 h of valve surgery had a fivefold increased risk of developing AKI (OR: 5.3; 95 % CI: 1.9–15.2) [66]. Kramer and colleagues reported that patients having a diagnostic cardiac catheterization during the same admission as cardiac surgery compared to patients that were discharged and returned to the hospital for surgery had a 54 % increased risk of developing AKI after surgery: adjusted OR 1.54, 95 % CI 1.11–2.13); this report highlighted the need to stabilize patients after catheterization procedures – targeting elective and urgent procedures – and readmit the patient for cardiac surgery after the kidneys have had a chance to filter out the contrast dye [67]. These reports demonstrate a need to change practice to prevent patients from receiving a double hit to the kidneys back to back by building in recovery times for patients to reduce additional post-cardiac surgery end organ injury.

Discharge Planning and Follow-Up

Patients should be educated at the time of discharge about the risks associated with receiving intravascular iodinated contrast and the risk of kidney injury or failure. Patients should be encouraged to drink four to eight glasses of water after leaving the hospital over the next 6 h to assist the augmentation of urine output and contrast exit from the urinary system.

SCr should be measured at 24 h if inpatient and before discharge. If there has been a 25 % of 0.5 increase in SCr, the patient should be evaluated for CI-AKI. The presence of CI-AKI prior to discharge should trigger a 2–3-day follow-up SCr to determine if the renal function is worsening or recovering. Both transient and persistent forms of CI-AKI have been shown to be associated with higher rates of rehospitalization and poor long-term mortality (Fig. 5.5).

Patients with a higher risk of CI-AKI should be flagged for a 72-h postcatheterization follow-up by the cardiologist or nurse practitioner to determine presence or absence of CI-AKI. If present, the patient should be evaluated 1 week later to determine if the kidney injury persists or not; if the SCr elevation (or reduced eGFR) persists at 1 week, a nephrology consult is recommended until normal renal function can be obtained with routine follow-up.

Quality Improvement Monitoring and Action Plans

Efforts should be undertaken to monitor risk factors for CI-AKI on a regular basis. We have found it helpful to develop dashboards for patient safety issues such as CI-AKI. On a weekly, monthly, or quarterly basis, one can plot the use contrast volume, type of contrast agent, and proportion of patients with CKD Stage 3, 4, and 5. It is important to track the hydration status since it is one of the key system factors associated with CI-AKI. For institutions with good electronic medical records, the pre-cath, intra-cath, and postcath hydration volume (NaCl or $NaHCO_3$) can be recorded. For institutions without comprehensive EMRs, conducting system audits on the amount of fluids ordered and given pre-cath, intra-cath, and postcath are very informative tools for evaluating the system of care. Occasionally, it may be necessary to follow several patients through the process to identify areas of improvement to maximize IV hydration and CI-AKI prophylaxis. When CI-AKI is made a QI item of interest, greater attention is paid to detail and in general the safety and quality of care improve with respect to this complication [68].

Conclusions

CI-AKI is a serious complication for patients undergoing iodinated contrast procedures. CI-AKI has been associated with poor survival, worse morbidity, and increased healthcare resource utilization and cost. There are effective tools to risk-assess patients prior to and following contrast procedures. These tools can be used to identify patients at high risk of developing CI-AKI or renal failure. In order to prevent CI-AKI, the following should be incorporated into standard of care: aggressive hydration protocols including patient education and at-home hydration, IV normal saline and/or sodium bicarbonate protocols, and consider high-dose *N*-acetylcysteine (1,200 mg) before and after the procedure. Patients should be educated about the risks of contrast on kidney function and the importance of complying with at-home hydration protocols, post-discharge SCr measurement, and follow-up with cardiology and their primary care physician. These strategies are inexpensive and help to maximize patient safety while reducing overall healthcare expenditures.

References

1. Health, United States, 2009: with special feature on medical technology. Hyattsville, MD: National Center for Health Statistics; 2010.
2. DeFrances CJ, Hall MJ. National Hospital discharge survey. Adv Data. 2005;385:1–19.
3. Brown JR, Malenka DJ, DeVries JT, et al. Transient and persistent renal dysfunction are predictors of survival after percutaneous coronary intervention: insights from the Dartmouth Dynamic Registry. Catheter Cardiovasc Interv. 2008;72(3):347–54.
4. Chertow GM, Burdick E, Honour M, Bonventre JV, Bates DW. Acute kidney injury, mortality, length of stay, and costs in hospitalized patients. J Am Soc Nephrol. 2005;16(11):3365–70.
5. Coca SG, Yusuf B, Shlipak MG, Garg AX, Parikh CR. Long-term risk of mortality and other adverse outcomes after acute kidney injury: a systematic review and meta-analysis. Am J Kidney Dis. 2009;53(6):961–73.
6. USRDS 2010 annual data report: atlas of chronic kidney disease and end-stage renal disease in the United States. U.S. Renal Data System, National Institutes of Health, National Institute of Diabetes and Digestive and Kidney Diseases, Bethesda; 2010.

7. Koneth I, Weishaupt D, Bachli EB. Persistent nephrogram after administration of an isoosmolar contrast medium. Nephrol Dial Transplant. 2004;19(6):1654–5.
8. McCullough PA. Contrast-induced acute kidney injury. J Am Coll Cardiol. 2008;51(15):1419–28.
9. McCullough PA, Adam A, Becker CR, et al. Epidemiology and prognostic implications of contrast-induced nephropathy. Am J Cardiol. 2006;98(6A):5K–13.
10. Mehta RL, Kellum JA, Shah SV, et al. Acute Kidney Injury Network: report of an initiative to improve outcomes in acute kidney injury. Crit Care. 2007;11(2):R31.
11. Mathew R, Haque K, Woothipoom W. Acute renal failure induced by contrast medium: steps towards prevention. BMJ. 2006;333(7567):539–40.
12. Rocha-Singh KJ, Ahuja RK, Sung CH, Rutherford J. Long-term renal function preservation after renal artery stenting in patients with progressive ischemic nephropathy. Catheter Cardiovasc Interv. 2002;57(2):135–41.
13. Madyoon H, Croushore L, Weaver D, Mathur V. Use of fenoldopam to prevent radiocontrast nephropathy in high-risk patients. Catheter Cardiovasc Interv. 2001;53(3):341–5.
14. Xu H, Chen LM, Li XW. Risk factors and prognosis of contrast-induced nephropathy with renal dysfunction. Zhongguo Yi Xue Ke Xue Yuan Xue Bao. 2005;27(2):232–6.
15. Haase M, Bellomo R, Devarajan P, Schlattmann P, Haase-Fielitz A. Accuracy of neutrophil gelatinase-associated lipocalin (NGAL) in diagnosis and prognosis in acute kidney injury: a systematic review and meta-analysis. Am J Kidney Dis. 2009;54(6):1012–24.
16. Briguori C, Visconti G, Rivera NV, et al. Cystatin C and contrast-induced acute kidney injury. Circulation. 2010;121(19):2117–22.
17. Vaidya VS, Waikar SS, Ferguson MA, et al. Urinary biomarkers for sensitive and specific detection of acute kidney injury in humans. Clin Transl Sci. 2008;1(3):200–8.
18. Anonymous. Executive summary-K/DOQI clinical practice guidelines. Am J Kidney Dis. 2002;39 Suppl 1:S17–31.
19. Levy EM, Viscoli CM, Horwitz RI. The effect of acute renal failure on mortality. A cohort analysis. JAMA. 1996; 275(19):1489–94.
20. Best PJ, Reddan DN, Berger PB, Szczech LA, McCullough PA, Califf RM. Cardiovascular disease and chronic kidney disease: insights and an update. Am Heart J. 2004;148(2):230–42.
21. Levey AS, Stevens LA, Schmid CH, et al. A new equation to estimate glomerular filtration rate. Ann Intern Med. 2009;150(9):604–12.
22. Matsushita K, Selvin E, Bash LD, Astor BC, Coresh J. Risk implications of the new CKD Epidemiology Collaboration (CKD-EPI) equation compared with the MDRD Study equation for estimated GFR: the Atherosclerosis Risk in Communities (ARIC) Study. Am J Kidney Dis. 2010;55(4):648–59.
23. Mehran R, Aymong ED, Nikolsky E, et al. A simple risk score for prediction of contrast-induced nephropathy after percutaneous coronary intervention: development and initial validation. J Am Coll Cardiol. 2004;44(7):1393–9.
24. Brown JR, DeVries JT, Robb JF, et al. Serious renal dysfunction after percutaneous coronary intervention can be predicted. Am Heart J. 2008;155(2):260–6.
25. Merten GJ, Burgess WP, Gray LV, et al. Prevention of contrast-induced nephropathy with sodium bicarbonate: a randomized controlled trial. JAMA. 2004;291(19):2328–34.
26. Solomon R, Werner C, Mann D, D'Elia J, Silva P. Effects of saline, mannitol, and furosemide to prevent acute decreases in renal function induced by radiocontrast agents. N Engl J Med. 1994;331(21):1416–20.
27. Kanbay M, Covic A, Coca SG, Turgut F, Akcay A, Parikh CR. Sodium bicarbonate for the prevention of contrast-induced nephropathy: a meta-analysis of 17 randomized trials. Int Urol Nephrol. 2009;41(3):617–27.
28. Meier P, Ko DT, Tamura A, Tamhane U, Gurm HS. Sodium bicarbonate-based hydration prevents contrast-induced nephropathy: a meta-analysis. BMC Med. 2009;7:23.
29. Zoungas S, Ninomiya T, Huxley R, et al. Systematic review: sodium bicarbonate treatment regimens for the prevention of contrast-induced nephropathy. Ann Intern Med. 2009;151(9):631–8.
30. Maioli M, Toso A, Leoncini M, et al. Sodium bicarbonate versus saline for the prevention of contrast-induced nephropathy in patients with renal dysfunction undergoing coronary angiography or intervention. J Am Coll Cardiol. 2008;52(8):599–604.
31. Kim YH. Preventive strategies of REnal insufficiency in patients with diabetes undergoing interVENTion or arteriography: the PREVENT trial. Paper presented at: American College of Cardiology 59th Annual Scientific Sessions; March 15, 2010, Atlanta, GA.
32. Marenzi G, Assanelli E, Marana I, et al. N-acetylcysteine and contrast-induced nephropathy in primary angioplasty. N Engl J Med. 2006;354(26):2773–82.
33. Trivedi H, Daram S, Szabo A, Bartorelli AL, Marenzi G. High-dose N-acetylcysteine for the prevention of contrast-induced nephropathy. Am J Med. 2009;122(9):874 e879–e815.
34. Acetylcysteine for prevention of renal outcomes in patients undergoing coronary and peripheral vascular angiography: Main results from the randomized acetylcysteine for contrast-induced nephropathy trial (ACT). Circulation. 2011;124(11):1250–9.
35. Brown JR, Block CA, Malenka DJ, O'Connor GT, Schoolwerth AC, Thompson CA. Sodium bicarbonate plus N-acetylcysteine prophylaxis: a meta-analysis. JACC Cardiovasc Interv. 2009; 2(11):1116–24.
36. Hernandez F, Mora L, Garcia-Tejada J, et al. Comparison of iodixanol and ioversol for the prevention of contrast-induced nephropathy in diabetic patients after coronary angiography or angioplasty. Rev Esp Cardiol. 2009;62(12):1373–80.
37. McCullough PA, Brown JR, Weisbord S. The effects of iso-osmolar contrast media on contrast-induced acute kidney injury: a meta-analysis. Cath Cardiovasc Interv. 2010;75(6):S78, B-034.
38. Reed M, Meier P, Tamhane UU, Welch KB, Moscucci M, Gurm HS. The relative renal safety of iodixanol compared with low-osmolar contrast media: a meta-analysis of randomized controlled trials. JACC Cardiovasc Interv. 2009;2(7):645–54.
39. Wessely R, Koppara T, Bradaric C, et al. Choice of contrast medium in patients with impaired renal function undergoing percutaneous coronary intervention. Circ Cardiovasc Interv. 2009;2(5):430–7.
40. Alexopoulos E, Spargias K, Kyrzopoulos S, et al. Contrast-induced acute kidney injury in patients with renal dysfunction undergoing a coronary procedure and receiving non-ionic low-osmolar versus iso-osmolar contrast media. Am J Med Sci. Jan 2010;339(1):25–30.
41. Laskey W, Aspelin P, Davidson C, et al. Nephrotoxicity of iodixanol versus iopamidol in patients with chronic kidney disease and diabetes mellitus undergoing coronary angiographic procedures. Am Heart J. 2009;158(5):822–828 e823.
42. Mehran R, Nikolsky E, Kirtane AJ, et al. Ionic low-osmolar versus nonionic iso-osmolar contrast media to obviate worsening nephropathy after angioplasty in chronic renal failure patients: the ICON (Ionic versus non-ionic Contrast to Obviate worsening Nephropathy after angioplasty in chronic renal failure patients) study. JACC Cardiovasc Interv. 2009;2(5):415–21.
43. Solomon R. Nephrotoxicity of iodixanol versus iopamidol inpatients with chronic kidney disease and diabetes mellitus undergoing coronary angiographic procedures. Am Heart J. 2010;159(2):e7. author reply e9.
44. Biswas S, Rowe ES, Mosher G, Tejada L, Ozias MK, Rowe VD. Nephroprotective effects of substituted cyclodextrins. Paper presented at: 15th international cyclodextrin symposium, May 10, 2010, Vienna, Austria.

45. Cigarroa RG, Lange RA, Williams RH, Hillis LD. Dosing of contrast material to prevent contrast nephropathy in patients with renal disease. Am J Med. 1989;86(6 Pt 1):649–52.
46. Marenzi G, Assanelli E, Campodonico J, et al. Contrast volume during primary percutaneous coronary intervention and subsequent contrast-induced nephropathy and mortality. Ann Intern Med. 2009;150(3):170–7.
47. Brown JR, Robb JF, Malenka DJ. Does "safe" dosing of iodinated contrast prevent contrast-induced acute kidney injury? Circulation. 2009;120(18):S435.
48. Brown JR, Robb JF, Block CA, et al. Does safe dosing of iodinated contrast prevent contrast-induced acute kidney injury? Circ Cardiovasc Interv. 2010;3(4):346–50.
49. Anne G, Gruberg L, Huber A, et al. Traditional versus automated injection contrast system in diagnostic and percutaneous coronary interventional procedures: comparison of the contrast volume delivered. J Invasive Cardiol. 2004;16(7):360–2.
50. Brosh D, Assali A, Vaknin-Assa H, et al. The ACIST power injection system reduces the amount of contrast media delivered to the patient, as well as fluoroscopy time, during diagnostic and interventional cardiac procedures. Int J Cardiovasc Intervent. 2005;7(4):183–7.
51. Weisz G, Filby SJ, Cohen MG, et al. Safety and performance of targeted renal therapy: the Be-RITe! Registry. J Endovasc Ther. 2009;16(1):1–12.
52. Chen HH, Cataliotti A, Schirger JA, Martin FL, Harstad LK, Burnett Jr JC. Local renal delivery of a natriuretic peptide a renal-enhancing strategy for B-type natriuretic peptide in overt experimental heart failure. J Am Coll Cardiol. 2009;53(15):1302–8.
53. Teirstein PS, Price MJ, Mathur VS, Madyoon H, Sawhney N, Baim DS. Differential effects between intravenous and targeted renal delivery of fenoldopam on renal function and blood pressure in patients undergoing cardiac catheterization. Am J Cardiol. 2006;97(7):1076–81.
54. Grube E, Baim D, Burkhoff D, Mueller R, Buellesfeld L, Teirstein P. Local intra-renal fenoldopam infusion causes greater increases in renal artery flow velocity than systemic intravenous fenoldopam infusion: a pilot study. EuroIntervention. 2005;1(3):305–8.
55. Smith EJ, Reitan O, Keeble T, Dixon K, Rothman MT. A first-in-man study of the Reitan catheter pump for circulatory support in patients undergoing high-risk percutaneous coronary intervention. Catheter Cardiovasc Interv. 2009;73(7):859–65.
56. Marenzi G, Assanelli E, Ferrari C, et al. (2010) Furosemide-induced diuresis with matched hydration compared to standard hydration for prevention of contrast-induced nephropathy. The MYTHOS trial. Eur Heart J Suppl 12(F):F88–F88.
57. Tumlin J, Stacul F, Adam A, et al. Pathophysiology of contrast-induced nephropathy. Am J Cardiol. 2006;98(6A):14K–20.
58. Zager RA, Burkhart KM, Conrad DS, Gmur DJ. Iron, heme oxygenase, and glutathione: effects on myohemoglobinuric proximal tubular injury. Kidney Int. 1995;48(5):1624–34.
59. Zager RA. Combined mannitol and deferoxamine therapy for myohemoglobinuric renal injury and oxidant tubular stress. Mechanistic and therapeutic implications. J Clin Invest. 1992;90(3):711–19.
60. Paller MS. Hemoglobin- and myoglobin-induced acute renal failure in rats: role of iron in nephrotoxicity. Am J Physiol. 1988;255(3 Pt 2):F539–44.
61. Spargias K, Adreanides E, Demerouti E, et al. Iloprost prevents contrast-induced nephropathy in patients with renal dysfunction undergoing coronary angiography or intervention. Circulation. 2009;120(18):1793–9.
62. Toso A, Maioli M, Leoncini M, et al. Usefulness of atorvastatin (80 mg) in prevention of contrast-induced nephropathy in patients with chronic renal disease. Am J Cardiol. 2010;105(3):288–92.
63. Xinwei J, Xianghua F, Jing Z, et al. Comparison of usefulness of simvastatin 20 mg versus 80 mg in preventing contrast-induced nephropathy in patients with acute coronary syndrome undergoing percutaneous coronary intervention. Am J Cardiol. 2009;104(4):519–24.
64. Ranucci M, Ballotta A, Kunkl A, et al. Influence of the timing of cardiac catheterization and the amount of contrast media on acute renal failure after cardiac surgery. Am J Cardiol. 2008;101(8):1112–18.
65. Medalion B, Cohen H, Assali A, et al. The effect of cardiac angiography timing, contrast media dose, and preoperative renal function on acute renal failure after coronary artery bypass grafting. J Thorac Cardiovasc Surg. 2010;139(6):1539–44.
66. Hennessy SA, LaPar DJ, Stukenborg GJ, et al. Cardiac catheterization within 24 hours of valve surgery is significantly associated with acute renal failure. J Thorac Cardiovasc Surg. 2010;140(5):1011–17.
67. Kramer RS, Quinn RD, Groom RC, et al. Same admission cardiac catheterization and cardiac surgery: is there an increased incidence of acute kidney injury? Ann Thorac Surg. 2010;90(5):1418–23. discussion 1423–4.
68. Moscucci M, Rogers EK, Montoye C, et al. Association of a continuous quality improvement initiative with practice and outcome variations of contemporary percutaneous coronary interventions. Circulation. 2006;113(6):814–22.

Vascular Access, Closure, and Management

6

Matthew W. Sherwood and Sunil V. Rao

Vascular access is a critical part of each cardiac catheterization, and success is built upon knowledge of anatomy, individual patient characteristics, and basic procedural skill. While the incidence of periprocedural major bleeding has declined to approximately 2 % in 2010, vascular access site complications continue to be the most common type of complication arising from cardiac catheterization [1]. Catheterization procedures can be performed from the femoral, brachial, or radial arteries, and while there is some debate about the optimal site for access, a competent operator should be proficient at performing procedures from all three access sites. Basic manual compression techniques are most often used to obtain hemostasis from femoral and brachial access sites, although there are several mechanical compression devices as well as vascular closure devices that, if properly used, can aid in achieving and maintaining access site hemostasis. This chapter will review the risks and benefits of femoral, brachial, and radial access, as well as provide guidance on obtaining safe arterial access. In addition, access site management techniques including vascular closure devices are reviewed.

Anatomy

Knowledge of arterial anatomy, useful landmarks, and appropriate points of access will improve the odds of safe arterial access.

M.W. Sherwood, MD (✉)
Department of Cardiovascular Medicine,
Duke University Medical Center, Durham, NC, USA
e-mail: matthew.sherwood@duke.edu

S.V. Rao, MD
Department of Medicine,
Duke University Medical Center, Durham, NC, USA

Cardiac Catheterization Laboratories,
Durham VA Medical Center, Durham, NC, USA

Femoral Anatomy

The femoral artery is a direct continuation of the external iliac artery and begins immediately beneath the inguinal ligament, which is located between the anterior superior iliac spine and the symphysis pubis. The inferior epigastric artery branches off of the external iliac artery just proximal to the inguinal ligament. It courses through the femoral sheath, which is created by the meeting of the transversalis and iliac fascia, with the femoral vein and femoral nerve (Fig. 6.1). The femoral artery lies between these structures, bordered on its lateral aspect by the femoral nerve and on its medial aspect by the femoral vein. As the artery passes under the inguinal ligament, it then provides branches to superficial structures via the superficial epigastric artery and the superficial circumflex iliac artery. Further along its course it also gives off the superficial and deep external pudic artery. It passes just medial to the head of the femur and finally bifurcates to the deep femoral artery (profunda femoris) and continues as the superficial femoral artery down the medial aspect of the thigh.

As detailed below, optimal femoral arterial access is in the common femoral artery (CFA) between the inferior epigastric artery superiorly and the bifurcation of the CFA inferiorly (the so-called safe zone) (Fig. 6.2).

Brachial Anatomy

The brachial artery begins at the inferior border of the teres major muscle tendon as a continuation of the axillary artery. It continues its course down the medial aspect of the upper arm and lies in a superficial plane, covered only by the integument and superficial and deep fascia. It initially gives off the deep brachial artery (profunda) and then the superficial ulnar and deep ulnar collateral arteries. It terminates at the bifurcation to the radial and ulnar arteries just distal to the articulation of the elbow (Fig. 6.3).

C.A. Thompson (ed.), *Textbook of Cardiovascular Intervention*,
DOI 10.1007/978-1-4471-4528-8_6, © Springer-Verlag London 2014

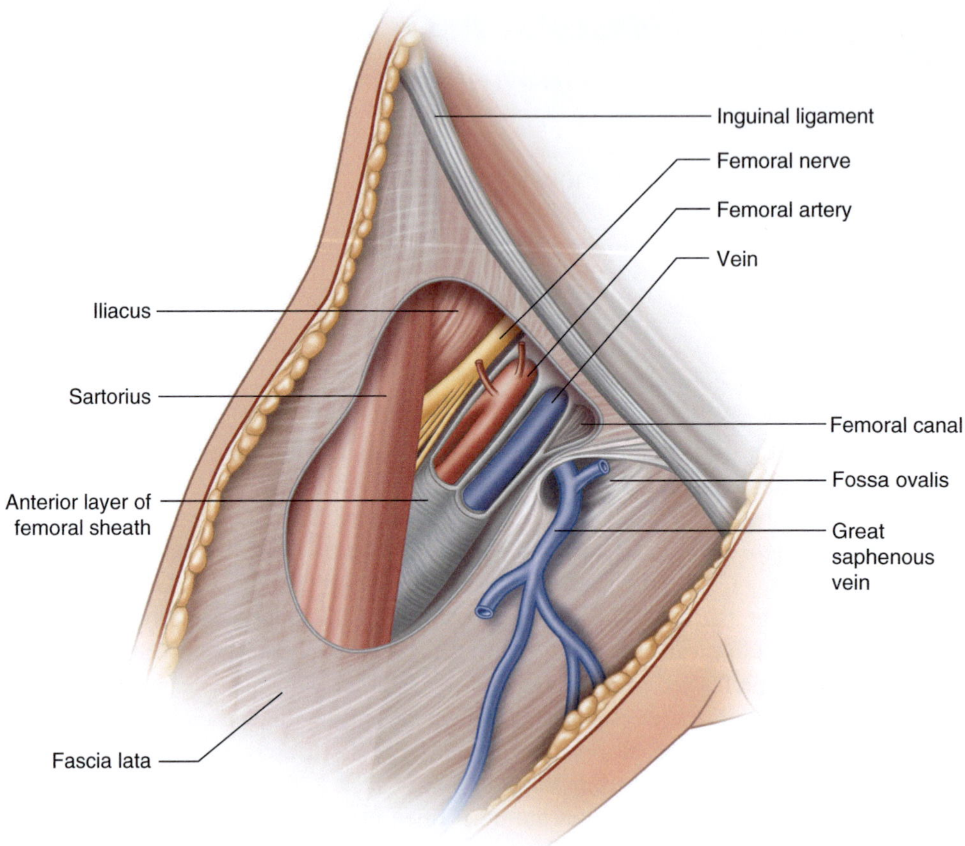

Fig. 6.1 Femoral artery within the femoral sheath. The femoral artery courses under the inguinal ligament within the femoral sheath, bordered on its lateral aspect by the femoral nerve and on its medial aspect by the femoral vein

Radial Anatomy

The radial artery begins as the continuation of the brachial artery just distal to the articulation of the elbow. The brachial artery bifurcates into the ulnar artery, which is larger but runs deeper within the tissue, and radial artery, which remains fairly superficial. For anatomic purposes the radial artery and its branches are separated into three distinct regions, the forearm, the wrist, and the hand. At the forearm the radial artery gives off three branches, proximally the radial recurrent artery, then the muscular artery, and at the distal forearm, the volar radial carpal artery and the superficial volar artery. At the wrist the radial artery provides the dorsal carpal branch and then the first dorsal metacarpal artery. The radial dorsal carpal branch forms an anastomosis with the ulnar dorsal carpal branch and the volar and dorsal interosseous arteries to form the dorsal carpal network. Finally in the hand the radial artery gives off five branches: the princeps pollicis, volaris indicis radialis, volar metacarpal, the perforating branches, and the recurrent branches (Fig. 6.4).

Vascular Access

Femoral

The femoral artery remains the most commonly utilized access site in cardiac catheterization laboratories. As mentioned above, the optimal entry point for femoral arteriotomy is the CFA, superior to the bifurcation to the superficial and profunda branches, but inferior to the superficial epigastric branch. Operators often use the inguinal skin crease as a landmark for skin access, but it is important to note that this can be misleading because the inguinal crease rarely coincides with the location of the CFA. Instead, using either ultrasound or fluoroscopy guidance significantly increases the likelihood of puncture in the safe zone. Because the safe zone typically coincides with the inferior half of the femoral head, femoral head fluoroscopy prior to arterial puncture is a useful technique (see below). Another technique is to palpate the symphysis pubis and the anterior superior iliac spine to denote the location of the inguinal ligament. Femoral arteriotomy should be inferior to the inguinal ligament, but given

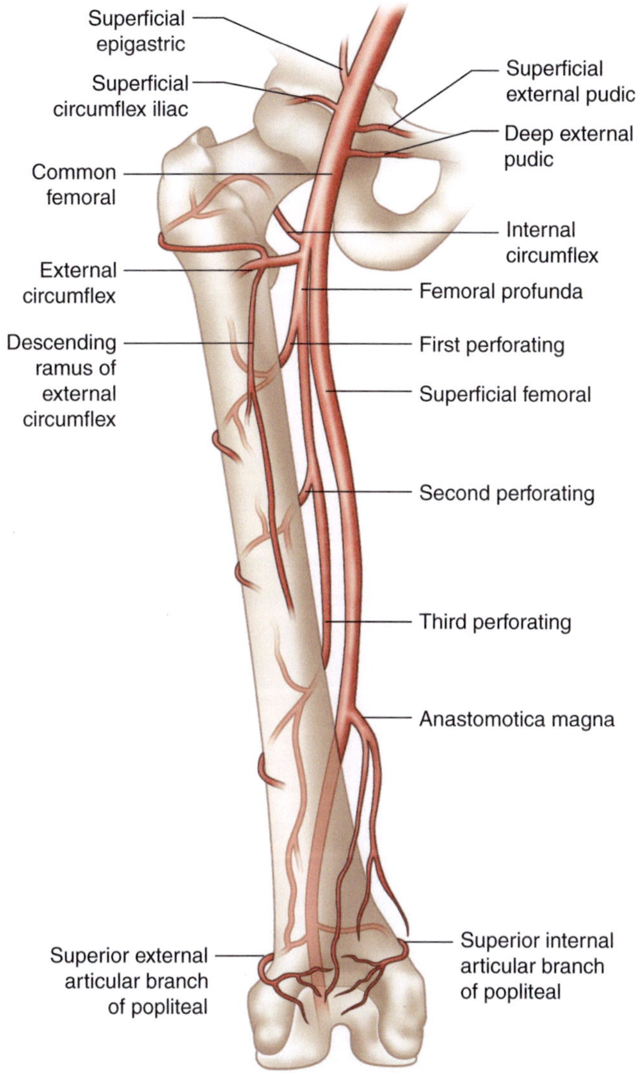

Fig. 6.2 Femoral arterial anatomy. The optimal entry point for femoral arteriotomy is the common femoral artery, superior to the bifurcation to the superficial and profunda branches, but inferior to the superficial epigastric branch

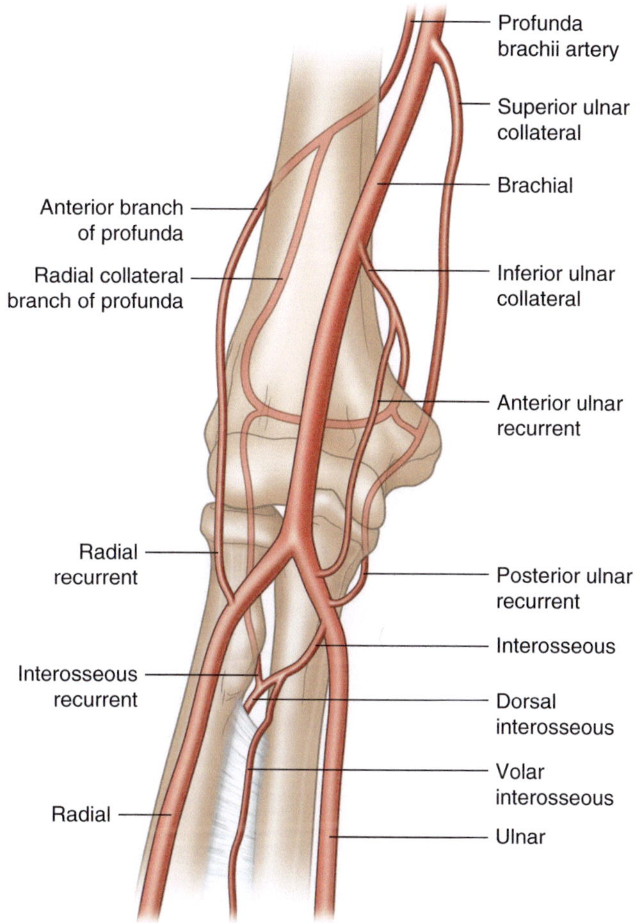

Fig. 6.3 Brachial artery anatomy. The brachial artery begins at the inferior border of the teres major muscle tendon and continues down the medical aspect of the arm terminating at the bifurcation to the radial and ulnar arteries just distal to the articulation of the elbow

the variation in patient anthropometric measurements, fluoroscopy or ultrasound is preferred. Puncture of the femoral artery in the safe zone allows for compression of the access site against the femoral head after arterial sheath removal, thus facilitating hemostasis.

The optimal skin entry site is approximately 3 cm below the inguinal ligament directly over the femoral arterial pulsation. A needle is positioned at this point and advanced through the skin at a 30–45° angle. Often the operator can feel the pulsation of the artery transmitted from the needle tip to the hub, and the needle can be placed through the front wall of the artery at which time pulsating arterial blood flow should come through the needle indicating proper position. A J-tipped guidewire can then be advanced, the needle withdrawn, and finally the arterial sheath inserted over the guidewire with a twisting motion to aid entry through the soft tissue into the artery. Improper placement of the vascular sheath can cause vascular complications during and after the case. Needle and sheath insertion above the inguinal ligament can often lead to retroperitoneal bleeding after the case, occasionally severe enough to require transfusion [2]. Insertion below the optimal point of the CFA may cause the formation of an arteriovenous fistula, can lead to vascular injury to the bifurcation site, insertion into the profunda, or cause the formation of a pseudoaneurysm [3, 4]. Thus, appropriate placement of the needle and vascular sheath into the CFA cannot be overemphasized.

Femoral Head Fluoroscopy

Several methods have been used to aid in proper cannulation of the CFA. Traditional anatomic landmarks such as the

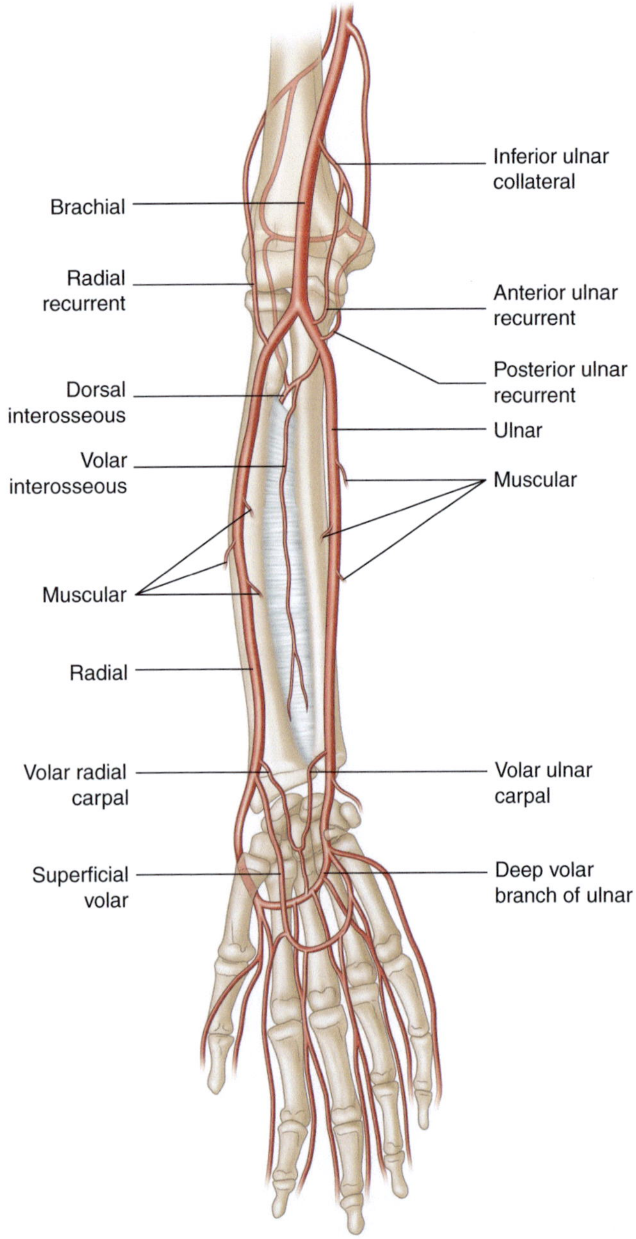

Fig. 6.4 Radial artery anatomy. The radial artery begins just distal to the articulation of the elbow bifurcating into the ulnar artery and radial artery which each contributes to the palmar arches and the anastomoses around the hand

inguinal crease, maximal femoral pulse, and bony prominences help guide the operator, but can be misleading, especially in obese patients. There is a consistent radiographic relationship between the inferior and middle third of the femoral head and the CFA as shown by small radiologic studies [5, 6]. Indeed, in a descriptive femoral artery angiography study performed in ~150 patients, the bifurcation of the CFA was below the center of the femoral head in 99 % of patients. Observational analyses have suggested that fluoroscopic guidance, using the femoral head, can aid in proper placement of the vascular sheath in the safe zone [6–8].

There have been very few randomized controlled clinical trials to evaluate fluoroscopic guidance, and the results are mixed. A very small, single-center randomized trial of ~200 patients showed that palpation with fluoroscopic guidance compared with traditional palpation of anatomic landmarks alone resulted in a small but statistically nonsignificant increase in the successful cannulation of the CFA (90 % vs. 85 %, respectively, $p=0.49$), while increasing the number of attempts and time to access [9]. This study was relatively small, and the authors suggested that a larger study may have found benefit to fluoroscopic guidance. A larger single-center randomized trial performed in 986 patients evaluated the use of fluoroscopic guidance vs. traditional landmarks in achieving CFA access for cardiac catheterization [10]. The authors found that fluoroscopy significantly decreased the incidence of low arteriotomies (defined as below the femoral head) without increasing the number of high arteriotomies (defined as above the femoral head), time to access, and number of needle passes or arterial punctures. A standard technique was used, locating the inferior border of the femoral head on an anterior-posterior fluoroscopic projection, and then utilizing this location as the skin entry site for the needle. While very little data are available for review, it seems femoral head fluoroscopy is a simple and effective way to decrease the number of low arteriotomies, which can reduce vascular bifurcation injuries and pseudoaneurysms, with the caveat that it may increase the time required for access.

Femoral Ultrasound

The utility of ultrasound (US) in gaining central venous access has been proven in multiple clinical trials to reduce time to access and complications, and thus its use has become widespread. Very little research has been performed to evaluate the utility of US in femoral arterial access, though it would seem there could be benefit, especially in obese patients and in those with difficult anatomy. The first randomized study in 2004 was a very small trial of 112 patients undergoing cardiac catheterization [11]. Patients were randomized to either traditional landmark/palpation-guided access vs. US-guided access of the femoral artery (Fig. 6.5). The authors found that US guidance was only beneficial in patients with weak arterial pulses and those with a leg circumference of 60 cm or greater, significantly decreasing the number of attempts needed as well as the time for successful arterial puncture. There was no benefit in patients with normal pulses, and there was no difference in vascular complications. A larger, multicenter, randomized controlled trial was performed in 1,004 patients to evaluate a US-guided technique vs. fluoroscopy-guided technique in obtaining CFA access

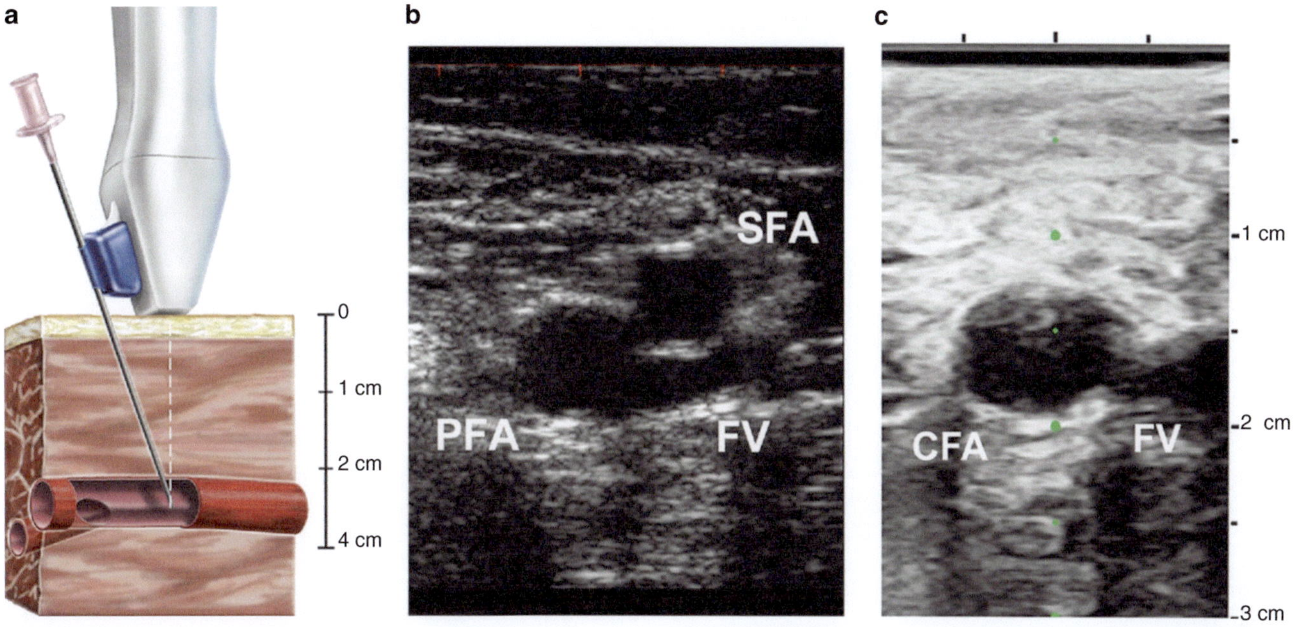

Fig. 6.5 Ultrasound guidance technique for femoral artery access. Femoral artery access with ultrasound guidance can be achieved with a needle attached to the ultrasound probe (**a**). The femoral artery bifurcation to the profunda femoris (*PFA*) and superficial femoral artery (*SFA*) is located (**b**), and then the probe is advanced towards the head until the common femoral artery is visualized (**c**). The femoral vein (*FV*) can be distinguished from the common femoral artery (*CFA*) by location, pulsation, and compression (From Seto et al. [12], with permission)

[12]. There was no significant difference in successful CFA cannulation between US and fluoroscopy techniques (86 % vs. 83 % $p=0.17$), though US did show benefit in the small subgroup of patients with the CFA bifurcation occurring above the inferior border of the femoral head. US guidance did, however, decrease the mean number of attempts (1.3 vs. 3.0 $p<0.000001$), rate of venipuncture (2.4 % vs. 15.8 % $p<0.000001$), and mean time to access (185 s vs. 213 s $p=0.016$) as compared with fluoroscopic guidance. The US guidance technique also significantly decreased the number of access site hematomas (0.6 % vs. 2.2 % $p=0.03$), but had no effect on rates of pseudoaneurysm, dissection, or bleeding requiring transfusion compared with fluoroscopic guidance. Based on the limited data, US guidance appears to be most useful in obese patients or those with weak arterial pulses and may decrease time to access, although its effect on reducing vascular complications is unclear.

Brachial

The brachial artery is a potential access site for cardiac catheterization, but is often used in cases where neither the femoral nor the radial arteries are possible sites of access. In the early years of cardiac catheterization, brachial artery catheterization was performed through the cut-down (Sones) approach. However, if entry through the brachial artery is necessary, the percutaneous approach has been adopted and is similar to modern femoral artery cannulation. The brachial pulse is identified just medial to the biceps brachii tendon 1–2 cm above the articulation of the elbow. The site is prepared and anesthetized and can be accessed with either a micropuncture or standard femoral access needle inserted through the skin and soft tissue at a 30–45° angle. Because of the loose soft tissue in this area, palpation and stabilization of the artery with index and middle fingers distal and proximal to the needle entry site may aid in successful cannulation of the brachial artery. The needle is slowly advanced until pulsatile flow is seen, and then either a 0.018″ guidewire (used with a micropuncture needle) or a short 0.035″ guidewire (used with a standard femoral access needle) is introduced into the brachial artery. The needle is then removed, and the sheath is passed over the wire into the artery.

Radial

The transradial approach to cardiac catheterization is gaining in popularity based on evidence showing its association with a lower rate of vascular complications. Most operators verify that there is collateral flow in the hand by checking either the Allen's or the Barbeau test [13] (Fig. 6.6), although it should be noted that there are no strong data showing an association between radial access and adverse vascular outcomes in patients with abnormal Allen's or Barbeau tests.

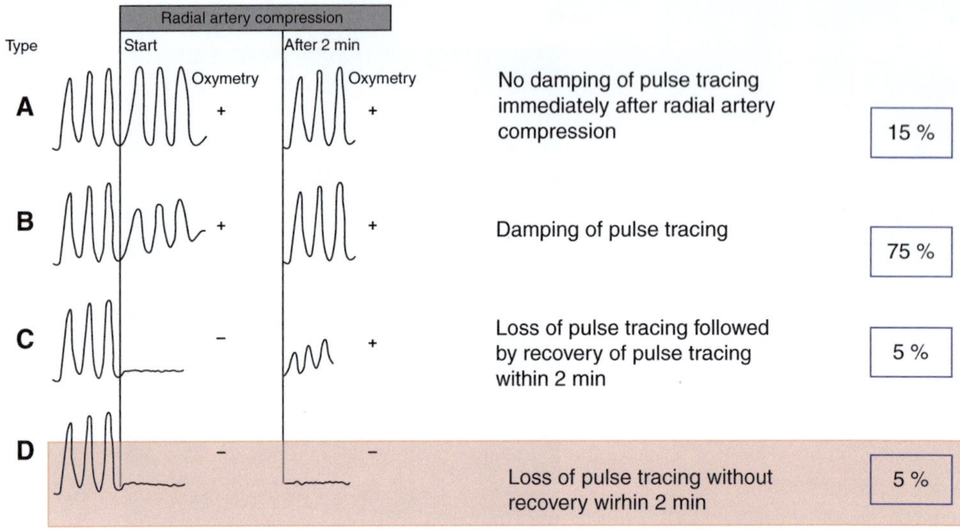

Fig. 6.6 The Barbeau test. The Barbeau test consists of a combination of plethysmography and pulse oximetry before and after manually occluding the radial artery. Transradial cardiac catheterization can be performed safely with *patterns A*, *B*, or *C* but should be avoided with *pattern D* (From Barbeau et al. [13], with permission.)

There are two generally accepted approaches to radial artery access. Both start with palpation of the radial pulse at the wrist and then identifying the bony prominence of the radial styloid process. Optimal radial artery entry site is just proximal to the radial styloid or approximately 2 cm proximal to the wrist. The anterior wall approach is, in essence, much like the traditional femoral artery front wall access. The access needle is inserted through the skin at the aforementioned site at a 30–45° angle and slowly advanced until blood pulsates out of the needle. Then a guidewire is introduced with a twirling motion ensuring it passes freely into the radial artery. The needle is then removed, and the sheath is passed over the wire into the artery. A micropuncture needle with compatible low-profile guidewire is commonly used. A small skin nick may be necessary to advance the sheath through the skin.

The counterpuncture (through and through) approach starts with the same skin and radial artery entry site. In this approach a 20-gauge Teflon cannula is inserted through the soft tissue and advanced through the radial artery. Often a blood flash is seen in the hollow chamber within the cannula, which marks initial entry to the artery. The cannula is advanced further through the posterior wall of the artery in a counterpuncture, or through and through, technique, and then the needle is removed. The hollow cannula is then slowly retracted until pulsatile flow is seen. A low-profile guidewire is then introduced with a twirling motion into the radial artery, and the cannula is removed. The sheath is then passed over the wire into the artery. Advantages of this technique include the presence of pulsatile arterial flow through the cannula (the caliber of micropuncture needles does not allow for pulsatile flow when the anterior wall puncture technique is used) and avoiding losing access to the artery with the micropuncture needle.

Vascular Closure

Femoral Closure Methods

Manual Compression

Manual compression remains the gold standard for achieving hemostasis after diagnostic cardiac catheterization and percutaneous coronary intervention through the femoral artery. For either procedure, the arterial sheath is removed once the activated clotting time is <170 s. Manual pressure is applied with three fingers, 2–3 cm proximal to the skin entry site, directly over the arterial entry site. Initially, heavy pressure is applied to control bleeding and nearly obliterate pedal pulses. Pressure is gradually lessened to allow arterial flow to the distal limb. Pressure is maintained in this area for 10–20 min or longer, depending on sheath size, until hemostasis is achieved. If anticoagulation and antiplatelet medications are used, mostly in the setting of interventional cases, then manual compression times will be longer. After hemostasis is achieved, a sterile, clear, waterproof dressing is applied to the site, and the site is observed for signs of hematoma or oozing. Pedal pulses are also monitored during recovery to ensure adequate distal limb perfusion. The patient is instructed to lay flat under strict bed rest for 2–6 h (depending on type of procedure, size of sheath, and adjunctive antithrombotic therapy) after hemostasis is achieved to promote proper healing of the arteriotomy site.

Assisted Compression (FemoStop, Safeguard, Boomerang Device)

Assisted compression devices mimic manual compression (to a degree) and are meant to decrease operator fatigue when a longer period of compression is necessary for hemostasis. Modern-assisted compression devices include the FemoStop

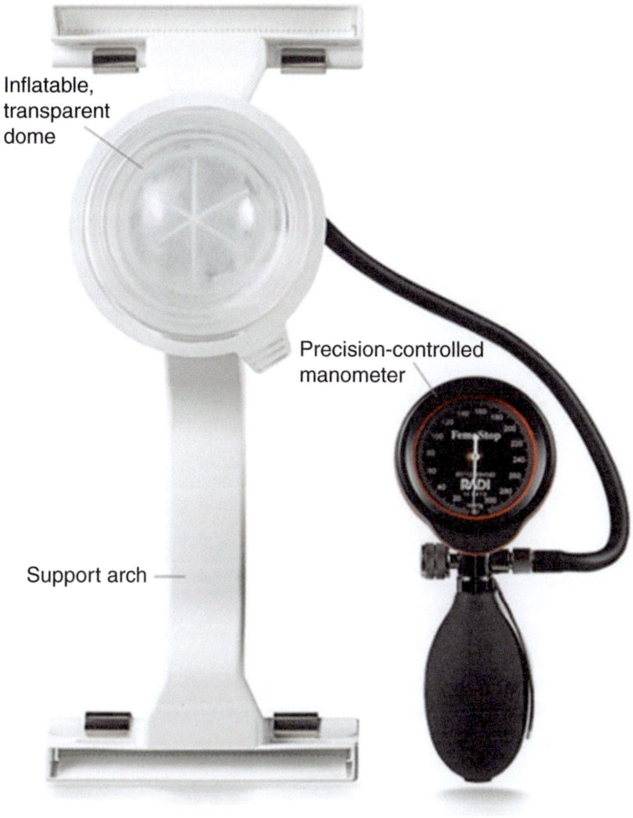

Fig. 6.7 The FemoStop device. The FemoStop device consists of a pneumatic bubble mounted to a support arch that is attached to the patient by a band around the hips. The bubble is then inflated by the precision control manometer to apply pressure to the arteriotomy site

(Radi Medical System/St. Jude Medical System, Reading, MA), Safeguard (Maquet Cardiovascular/Datascope Corporation, Fairfield, NJ), and the Cardiva Catalyst (Boomerang device, Cardiva Medical Inc., Sunnyvale, CA), which is a hybrid closure device.

The FemoStop II Plus device is a pneumatic bubble mounted on a plastic frame that is fastened to the patient by a belt/strap system around the hips (Fig. 6.7). The bubble is positioned 1–2 cm above the skin nick, directly at the arteriotomy site, and then initially inflated to 70 mmHg with the attached sphygmomanometer. The bubble is then inflated to a maximum of 20 mmHg above systolic blood pressure for 1–3 min, then deflated and maintained at just below systolic blood pressure for 15 min. The pressure is then decreased 20 mmHg every 2 min until the pneumatic pressure in the bulb is 30 mmHg. The device is kept in place for 1–2 h at this pressure and then carefully removed. Time may vary depending on anticoagulant status and sheath size. The success rate for application of the device has been reported to be nearly 100 %, and reported complication rates are very low [14, 15]. The FemoStop device, however, does not shorten time to hemostasis, ambulation, or discharge as compared to manual compression [14].

The Safeguard device is a 24-cm adhesive bandage with a clear, plastic, pneumatic bubble in the center. It is applied directly to the skin and is designed to aid in manual compression of femoral arteriotomy sites. It can be used in a pre-hemostasis technique or a post-hemostasis technique strategy. For the pre-hemostasis technique, the Safeguard device is applied directly over the site of arteriotomy with the femoral sheath having been withdrawn ~3 cm so that the sheath hub does not interfere with appropriate device placement. The pneumatic bubble is then inflated with up to 40 cm^3 of air from the Luer lock syringe port. Manual pressure is then applied to the bubble, and the femoral sheath is withdrawn. Manual compression is held until femoral vessel hemostasis is achieved. The device can then be deflated every 2 h to assess for oozing or hematoma formation, and re-inflated as necessary, or promptly removed. In the post-hemostasis technique, the Safeguard device is applied directly to the clean, dry skin site directly over the femoral arteriotomy, and the pneumatic bubble is inflated with up to 40 cm^3 of air. The site is checked frequently for oozing or hematoma formation and again is deflated every 2 h to assess the site. It can then be removed at the clinician's discretion. As with previous devices, the Safeguard is successfully applied near 100 % of the time with very low complication rates. In a subset of the RACE trial, application of the Safeguard device was associated with a decreased time of active compression to achieve hemostasis when compared with historical controls [16]. It did not, however, decrease the time to ambulation or discharge in this study.

The Boomerang device is a hybrid closure device that is placed immediately after diagnostic or interventional procedures and, upon removal, leaves no foreign material in the artery. The device is a flexible mesh 6.5 mm disc coated with protamine sulfate and is deployed through the existing arterial sheath (up to 7 French). It expands like an umbrella at the intraluminal arteriotomy site and is held in place by a tension clip (Fig. 6.8). It remains at the site for a short period of time (~20 min. for Diagnostic cases; 120 min for Interventional cases) and is then removed with the sheath. It does require an additional 5 min. of manual compression to achieve hemostasis after removal. In a small study of 96 patients undergoing diagnostic catheterization [17], the Boomerang device was successful in achieving hemostasis in 99 % of patients with a very low complication rate (minor bleeding in 5 % of patients). No major adverse events were observed. In this small study, the device was successfully utilized in 6 patients with significant vascular disease and even in 19 patients with arterial access at the bifurcation of the femoral artery or in the profunda femoris.

Vascular Closure Devices (StarClose, Perclose/ProGlide, Angio-Seal)

Over time, more advanced methods of active closure have been developed with the goals of reducing time to ambulation

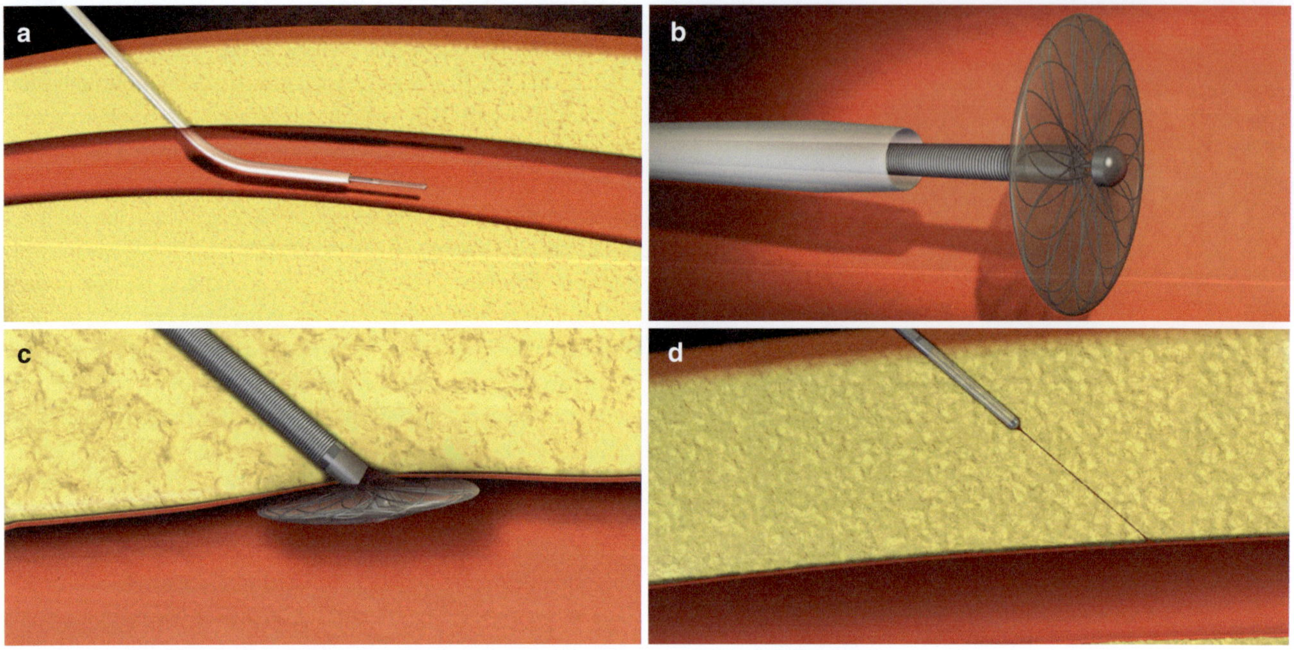

Fig. 6.8 Deployment of the Boomerang device. The Boomerang device is inserted in the artery (**a**) and expands once deployed from the sheath (**b**). It is secured to the anterior wall of the artery with traction (**c**) and then completely withdrawn (**d**) after a short "dwell time" (From Doyle et al. [17], with permission.)

after catheterizations, decreasing patient discomfort, and reducing major bleeding complications. While these newer devices deliver on some of these goals, their use may come at increased cost, a significant learning curve to ensure proper deployment, and the risk of device-related vascular complications [18]. A recent meta-analysis of active closure devices (including the Angio-Seal, Vasoseal, and Perclose devices) showed that there was no decrease in groin bleeding, groin hematomas, arteriovenous fistulas, or pseudoaneurysm formation with closure devices when compared with manual compression [19]. In this analysis, closure devices did significantly decrease the time to hemostasis (mean – 17 min), duration of bed rest (mean – 10 h), and time to discharge (mean – 0.6 days), though the authors noted significant statistical heterogeneity in the studies analyzed.

The safety of closure devices has been brought into question by several analyses that evaluated complications after device deployment. An observational analysis of >5,000 consecutive patients at a single center undergoing cardiac catheterization showed that vascular closure devices (specifically the Angio-Seal, Vasoseal, Duett, Techstar) were more often associated with hematoma, significant hematocrit drop (>15 %), and need for surgical closure of access site, when compared to manual compression. Conversely, Applegate et al. [20]. performed an observational analysis of 4,525 patients undergoing percutaneous coronary intervention (receiving abciximab) who received either manual compression, Angio-Seal, or Perclose device post-procedure. They found no difference in minor or major vascular complication rates between treatments. Finally, the Perclose, Angio-Seal, and Vasoseal devices were studied in a meta-analysis comparing each of these devices to manual compression for the rates of bleeding and vascular injury. The Perclose and Angio-Seal devices were found to have similarly low rates of complication when compared to manual compression, while the Vasoseal device was found to have higher rates of local vascular complications [21].

Angio-Seal

The Angio-Seal device (St. Jude Medical Inc., Minn.) contains a small absorbable collagen plug attached to a suture, which is deployed within the vasculature to aid in hemostasis (Fig. 6.9). To operate the Angio-Seal, the existing arterial sheath is exchanged for an Angio-Seal-designed sheath that aids in deployment of the plug through an arteriotomy locator. Once position with the artery is confirmed via aspiration, the guidewire and arteriotomy locator are removed, and the Angio-Seal device is inserted with an audible click. The

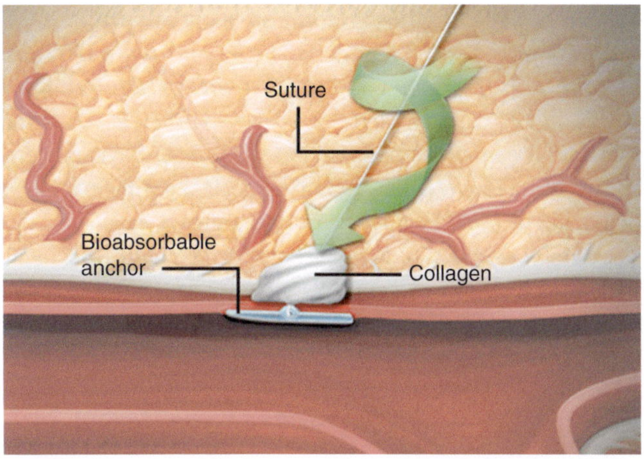

Fig. 6.9 The Angio-Seal device mechanism. The Angio-Seal device is a collagen plug deployed at the arteriotomy site and held in place by an absorbable anchor

Angio-Seal anchor is then released, and traction is applied to position it against the anterior wall of the artery. Further gentle traction is applied to expose the collagen material to the exterior of the artery wall, while the anchor holds it in place at the arteriotomy site. The remainder of the device is then removed through the tissue tract, and the suture is cut just above the skin.

The Angio-Seal device can be used to close the arteriotomy sites of up to 8 French in size and has a high rate of successful deployment (97 %) [20]. It has also been shown to improve patient comfort after cardiac catheterization when directly compared to manual compression or assisted compression with the FemoStop device [14, 22]. In two large meta-analyses of both the Angio-Seal and Perclose devices vs. manual compression, there was no difference found in groin bleeding or other vascular complications [19, 21].

Perclose/ProGlide

The Perclose ProGlide device (Abbott Vascular) is a suture-mediated closure device designed for use in 5–8 French arteriotomy closures. The existing sheath is removed, and the Perclose ProGlide is inserted over a guidewire into the artery. A continuous drip of blood indicates the device is in proper position within the artery lumen, and then the device is initially deployed by lifting the lever. This deploys the device "foot" which is then slowly pulled back to position it against the anterior wall of the artery. Once properly positioned, the plunger is depressed which automatically deploys the needles and suture. The plunger is then pulled back, and the needles are withdrawn with the device leaving two suture ends in place coming out of the skin tract. A surgical knot is then tied and pushed down into the wound to complete closure of the arteriotomy site.

Successful deployment of the Perclose ProGlide device has been reported to be as high as 90–94 % [20, 22]. The aforementioned meta-analyses of both the Perclose and Angio-Seal devices found no difference found in groin bleeding or other vascular complications when compared with manual compression [19, 21]. However, both devices may decrease time to hemostasis, ambulation, and length of stay compared with manual compression [19].

StarClose

The StarClose device is a clip-mediated closure device designed for 5–6 French arteriotomies. First the existing sheath is removed over a guidewire, and the StarClose exchange sheath is inserted. The StarClose device is then advanced through the sheath, and the locator wings are positioned with the depression of a plunger. The device is then slowly withdrawn until resistance is felt indicating the wings are positioned on the anterior wall of the artery. A 4-mm nitinol clip is then deployed approximating the edges of the arteriotomy site and facilitating closure. The device is removed, and adjunctive manual compression may be applied to ensure complete hemostasis.

Successful deployment of the StarClose device has been reported to be as high as 87–92 % in both diagnostic and interventional procedures [23, 24]. While the StarClose device has not been studied as extensively as other active closure devices, there was a prospective randomized trial of 456 patients undergoing cardiac catheterization, who were randomized in a 1:1:1 fashion to the StarClose device, the Angio-Seal device, or standard manual compression [25]. Neither the StarClose nor the Angio-Seal device significantly lowered the rates of hematoma or vascular complications (14 % vs. 11 % vs. 9 %, $p=\text{NS}$) compared with manual compression. The StarClose device was associated with persistent oozing at the closure site significantly more often than the Angio-Seal device (38 % vs. 25 %, $P=0.002$). However, both closure devices were rated as less painful than manual compression by patients in the study. Safety reports of the StarClose device show it has a low complication rate with ~1 % of patients experiencing a device complication (arterial occlusion or high-grade stenosis) requiring surgical repair [23, 24].

Brachial Closure Methods

Percutaneous brachial artery cardiac catheterization is performed far less often than femoral and radial procedures, and manual compression remains the preferred method for closure of the brachial arteriotomy. The patient's arm is held against an arm board, and pressure is applied to the arteriotomy site just proximal to the skin puncture site, while the sheath is removed. Pressure is held to control bleeding, while the radial pulse is palpated to assess distal perfusion. Pressure is maintained in the area for 15–20 min until hemostasis is achieved. Afterward, the radial pulse and arm circumference are monitored to ensure adequate distal perfusion and to detect the presence of a hematoma. Given the amount of loose soft tissue at the cannulation site, there is a significant risk for large hematomas to go unnoticed. Hematoma in the arm may cause compression of soft tissue and nerves, leading to compartment syndrome. The patient is maintained on bed rest with the arm held straight for 4–6 h, though they may sit up in bed for comfort. Using an arm board during the recovery process may aid in reminding the patient not to bend their elbow.

Radial Closure Methods

Following cardiac catheterization through the radial artery, hemostasis can be achieved through the use of manual compression, gauze pads and tape, or dedicated radial artery compression devices. Manual compression is the least practical since most radial cases, including diagnostic angiography, are performed with anticoagulation. The use of dedicated radial compression devices facilitates hemostasis with minimal operator effort. The device or band is placed on the wrist directly over the radial artery puncture site, and occlusive pressure is applied. Time may vary depending on procedure and medications administered, but in general, pressure is maintained for 90 min after diagnostic procedures and 180 min after interventional procedures. In either case, pressure is then gradually withdrawn until hemostasis is achieved. Examples of available devices include, but are not limited to, the TR Band (Terumo), the Hemoband (Terumo), the RadiStop (St. Jude), the RadAR device (MedPoint Technologies), and the RADstat device (Merit Medical). There are limited data comparing the safety and efficacy of these devices. Two small clinical trials have evaluated the TR Band vs. the Hemoband and subsequently vs. the RadiStop.

The first trial enrolled 500 consecutive patients undergoing transradial cardiac catheterization with the first 250 patients enrolled receiving the Hemoband device and the next 250 consecutive patients receiving the TR Band [26]. Both devices achieved and maintained hemostasis in nearly 100 % of patients; however, the TR Band showed significantly lower rates of radial artery occlusion at early (11.2 % vs. 4.4 % $p<0.001$ at 24 h) and late (7.2 % vs. 3.2 % $p<0.001$ at 30 days) follow-up. The authors also reported that patients reported discomfort less frequently with the TR Band compared to the Hemoband (2 % vs. 7 % $p<0.05$). A more recent trial evaluated the TR Band vs. the RadiStop device in 790 patients randomized 1:1 to either device after transradial cardiac catheterization [27]. Both devices were similarly effective in achieving hemostasis with low rates of oozing or local hematoma in either group. However, the TR Band was found to be more comfortable and associated with no discomfort in a significantly larger part of the study patients. The TR Band was also associated with a longer time to achieve hemostasis.

Patent Hemostasis

As will be described in detail later in the chapter, radial artery occlusion (RAO) is one limitation of transradial cardiac catheterization. While most reports suggest that it is almost always clinically silent, it does limit repeat arterial access through the same site. Complete obliteration of antegrade radial artery flow during the hemostasis process is a significant contributor to RAO. "Patent hemostasis" [28, 29] is the technique of maintaining hemostasis while also allowing antegrade radial artery flow. Two studies have demonstrated significant reductions in RAO both early and late after PCI. The PROPHET study [28] randomly assigned 436 consecutive patients who underwent transradial cardiac catheterization to either a conventional strategy of hemostasis or the "patent hemostasis" procedure (Table 6.1). Compared with traditional occlusive hemostasis, patent hemostasis resulted in a significant decrease in radial artery occlusion at 24 h (4 % vs. 12 %, $p<0.05$) and at 30 days (6 % vs. 2 %, $p<0.05$). Approximately 3.6 % of patients required manual compression in the patent hemostasis arm. As mentioned above, the TR Band when studied against the Hemoband also promotes radial artery patency likely due to the titratability of the pressure applied to the radial arteriotomy site, which facilitates "patent hemostasis."

Table 6.1 Patent hemostasis technique

1. Apply hemostasis device (e.g., Hemoband, RADstat, TR Band) to wrist
2. Place pulse oximeter on ipsilateral index finger or thumb
3. Tighten hemostasis device and remove sheath
4. Occlude ipsilateral ulnar artery
5. Loosen hemostasis device until plethysmographic signal returns or bleeding occurs
If bleeding occurs, use manual compression
If hemostasis is maintained in the presence of the plethysmographic signal, then leave hemostasis device in place for 2 h
6. Monitor each hour

Adapted from Pancholy et al. [28], with permission

Management

Femoral Access

Cardiac catheterization through the femoral artery is the default approach for the vast majority of operators. The femoral access site is utilized by many operators due to its ease of use, familiarity, and speed to access. Because of the large diameter of the femoral artery, the large-bore catheters often used in complex procedures can easily traverse the femoral artery. These include, but are not limited to, larger atherectomy burrs, closure devices for patent foramen ovale or atrial septal defects, valvular clips, and transcatheter aortic valves. In addition, given the larger size of the femoral artery, the risk of occlusion post-procedure is very low.

Risks

There are major risks associated with femoral artery access mostly involving hemorrhagic complications or vascular injury. Retroperitoneal hematoma (RPH) is a rare but significant complication of femoral access and is associated with increased mortality and prolonged hospital stay. Many patients do not exhibit the classic signs and symptoms of flank pain and bruising; therefore, RPH should be suspected in any patient who develops hypotension, tachycardia, or acute anemia shortly after a transfemoral procedure. RPH is a significant risk of high arterial punctures (above inguinal ligament) in women and in smaller patients [30]. Diagnosis is often made by CT scan, and treatment is mostly supportive, though patients may require transfusion or active management with endovascular covered stent graft repair. Arterial pseudoaneurysm is another vascular complication of femoral access, which presents as a painful, pulsatile mass at the femoral access site, often with an audible bruit. The incidence is reported as 0.1–0.2 % in diagnostic procedures and between 3 and 5 % in interventional procedures [31]. Independent risk factors for pseudoaneurysm formation include low arterial puncture (below the femoral head), larger sheath sizes, and use of anticoagulants [3, 31]. Treatment depends on the size of the pseudoaneurysm; those <2 cm are often spontaneously close, while those >2 cm can be treated by ultrasound-guided thrombin injection or compression. Rarely, pseudoaneurysms require surgical repair if persistent.

Arteriovenous (AV) fistula is another complication of femoral cardiac catheterization with a reported incidence of 0.3–1 % [32]. AV fistula is frequently asymptomatic and is found on exam as an audible bruit and occasionally a palpable thrill. Female gender and high arterial pressure are independent risk factors for AV fistula, as well as procedural factors such as very low arterial puncture (inferior to femoral head) or puncture of the left femoral artery from the right side of the table. In a large prospective study of >10,000 patients, nearly 38 % of AV fistulas closed within 1 year, and very few patients experienced high-output heart failure or limb ischemia from their AV fistulas [32]. Therefore, conservative medical management in asymptomatic patients seems reasonable for 1 year, then, if the AV fistula is persistent, surgical repair can be considered.

Femoral bleeding, including local hematoma formation, is the most common complication of femoral access. It can be seen either early or late after cardiac catheterization and can present as overt bleeding or as a hematoma. While small hematomas are typically self-limited and reabsorbed with little effect on the patient, large hematomas can cause vascular and neural compression and occasionally require transfusion. Major bleeding, defined as fatal bleeding, intracranial hemorrhage, or bleeding associated with ≥3 g/dL hemoglobin drop or requiring transfusion or surgery, is associated with morbidity and mortality in patients with ACS undergoing PCI [33, 34]. A recent large meta-analysis estimated rates of major bleeding at 2.3 % among patients undergoing femoral, diagnostic, or interventional cardiac catheterization [35].

Brachial

Risks

As mentioned above, the brachial artery site is rarely used for cardiac catheterization. It is a medium-sized caliber vessel and can support larger sheaths (up to 8 French) when larger devices are necessary. However, there is potential for both hemorrhagic and significant thrombotic complications. Thrombosis at the arteriotomy site or embolism to the radial artery can cause limb ischemia and may result in limb loss if not rapidly recognized and treated. Incidence of thrombotic complications was estimated at 1 % in an observational study of over 12,000 patients undergoing catheterization through the brachial artery [36]. Bleeding and hematoma formation are more common and can also result in neurovascular compromise due to the closed compartment of the forearm. Thus the brachial artery route is generally considered the least desirable option for arterial access.

Radial

Benefits

Transradial cardiac catheterization offers several potential advantages. Foremost is the decreased risk of vascular complications and access site bleeding. Two large meta-analyses of radial vs. femoral access trials have shown that the transradial approach is associated with a significantly decreased rate of major bleeding [35, 37]. The most recent, large-scale, international randomized trial of radial vs. femoral access for cardiac catheterization in ACS showed that though non-CABG major bleeding was similar among the

Table 6.2 Transradial approach to cardiac catheterization

Benefits	Risks
Reduced bleeding risk	Limits guide catheter size
Early ambulation	Possible greater radiation exposure to operator
Improved patient comfort	Long-term consequences to radial artery (e.g., for reaccess or for use as bypass graft) unknown
Reduced length of stay and costs	
Same-day discharge possible	

Table 6.3 EASY trial hematoma scale

Type	Description
I	≤5 cm diameter
II	≤10 cm diameter
III	>10 cm but not above the elbow
IV	Extending above the elbow
V	Anywhere with ischemic threat of the hand

Adapted from Bertrand et al. [40], with permission

two groups, major vascular complications were significantly reduced in the transradial group [38]. Outcomes such as death, MI, and stroke were similar between radial and femoral groups, but radial approach was superior in the subgroup of patients with ST segment elevation myocardial infarction. Patients in this trial were more likely to prefer the radial approach for subsequent cardiac catheterization procedures. Other nonclinical advantages of transradial catheterization include reduced hospital length of stay and decreased healthcare utilization [39] (Table 6.2).

Risks

Risks of radial artery access include bleeding (with the potential for compartment syndrome), RAO, radial/brachial/axillary/subclavian artery dissection, radial artery perforation, and the exceedingly rare "cardiovocal syndrome" (injury to the right or left recurrent laryngeal nerve from damage to the subclavian arteries). All of these complications are relatively rare with sporadic reports in the literature. The most common are hemorrhagic complications such as large forearm hematomas causing compartment syndrome. These events are still rare with the incidence of major bleeding events estimated at 0.05 % [37]. Grading of hematomas related to radial access can be accomplished using the EASY Trial hematoma scale [40] (Table 6.3).

Summary

Vascular access is the most common source of complications from cardiac catheterization. Appropriate technique, knowledge of anatomy, and awareness of possible pitfalls are critical to success. There are several important methods for managing the access site after cardiac catheterization. Knowledge of the risks and benefits of manual compression, passive closure devices, as well as active vascular closure devices can aid in avoiding bleeding complications. Finally the ability to perform cardiac catheterization from multiple access sites will help the operator handle the challenges present in the modern-day cardiac catheterization lab and facilitates patient outcomes and comfort with cardiac catheterization.

References

1. Marso SP, Amin AP, House JA, et al. Association between use of bleeding avoidance strategies and risk of periprocedural bleeding among patients undergoing percutaneous coronary intervention. JAMA. 2010;303(21):2156–64.
2. Tiroch KA, Arora N, Matheny ME, Liu C, Lee TC, Resnic FS. Risk predictors of retroperitoneal hemorrhage following percutaneous coronary intervention. Am J Cardiol. 2008;102(11):1473–6.
3. Altin RS, Flicker S, Naidech HJ. Pseudoaneurysm and arteriovenous fistula after femoral artery catheterization: association with low femoral punctures. AJR Am J Roentgenol. 1989; 152(3):629–31.
4. Kim D, Orron DE, Skillman JJ, et al. Role of superficial femoral artery puncture in the development of pseudoaneurysm and arteriovenous fistula complicating percutaneous transfemoral cardiac catheterization. Cathet Cardiovasc Diagn. 1992;25(2):91–7.
5. Spijkerboer AM, Scholten FG, Mali WP, van Schaik JP. Antegrade puncture of the femoral artery: morphologic study. Radiology. 1990;176(1):57–60.
6. Grier D, Hartnell G. Percutaneous femoral artery puncture: practice and anatomy. Br J Radiol. 1990;63(752):602–4.
7. Dotter CT, Rosch J, Robinson M. Fluoroscopic guidance in femoral artery puncture. Radiology. 1978;127(1):266–7.
8. Spector KS, Lawson WE. Optimizing safe femoral access during cardiac catheterization. Catheter Cardiovasc Interv. 2001; 53(2):209–12.
9. Huggins CE, Gillespie MJ, Tan WA, et al. A prospective randomized clinical trial of the use of fluoroscopy in obtaining femoral arterial access. J Invasive Cardiol. 2009;21(3):105–9.
10. Abu-Fadel MS, Sparling JM, Zacharias SJ, et al. Fluoroscopy vs. traditional guided femoral arterial access and the use of closure devices: a randomized controlled trial. Catheter Cardiovasc Interv. 2009;74(4):533–9.
11. Dudeck O, Teichgraeber U, Podrabsky P, Lopez Haenninen E, Soerensen R, Ricke J. A randomized trial assessing the value of ultrasound-guided puncture of the femoral artery for interventional investigations. Int J Cardiovasc Imaging. 2004;20(5):363–8.
12. Seto AH, Abu-Fadel MS, Sparling JM, et al. Real-time ultrasound guidance facilitates femoral arterial access and reduces vascular complications: FAUST (Femoral Arterial Access With Ultrasound Trial). JACC Cardiovasc Interv. 2010;3(7):751–8.
13. Barbeau GR, Arsenault F, Dugas L, Simard S, Lariviere MM. Evaluation of the ulnopalmar arterial arches with pulse oximetry and plethysmography: comparison with the Allen's test in 1010 patients. Am Heart J. 2004;147(3):489–93.
14. Amin FR, Yousufuddin M, Stables R, et al. Femoral haemostasis after transcatheter therapeutic intervention: a prospective randomised study of the angio-seal device vs. the femostop device. Int J Cardiol. 2000;76(2–3):235–40.
15. Pracyk JB, Wall TC, Longabaugh JP, et al. A randomized trial of vascular hemostasis techniques to reduce femoral vascular complications after coronary intervention. Am J Cardiol. 1998; 81(8):970–6.

16. Sanborn TA, Ogilby JD, Ritter JM, et al. Reduced vascular complications after percutaneous coronary interventions with a nonmechanical suture device: results from the randomized RACE study. Catheter Cardiovasc Interv. 2004;61(3):327–32.
17. Doyle BJ, Godfrey MJ, Lennon RJ, et al. Initial experience with the Cardiva Boomerang vascular closure device in diagnostic catheterization. Catheter Cardiovasc Interv. 2007;69(2):203–8.
18. Dauerman HL, Applegate RJ, Cohen DJ. Vascular closure devices: the second decade. J Am Coll Cardiol. 2007;50(17):1617–26.
19. Koreny M, Riedmuller E, Nikfardjam M, Siostrzonek P, Mullner M. Arterial puncture closing devices compared with standard manual compression after cardiac catheterization: systematic review and meta-analysis. JAMA. 2004;291(3):350–7.
20. Applegate RJ, Grabarczyk MA, Little WC, et al. Vascular closure devices in patients treated with anticoagulation and IIb/IIIa receptor inhibitors during percutaneous revascularization. J Am Coll Cardiol. 2002;40(1):78–83.
21. Nikolsky E, Mehran R, Halkin A, et al. Vascular complications associated with arteriotomy closure devices in patients undergoing percutaneous coronary procedures: a meta-analysis. J Am Coll Cardiol. 2004;44(6):1200–9.
22. Martin JL, Pratsos A, Magargee E, et al. A randomized trial comparing compression, Perclose Proglide and Angio-Seal VIP for arterial closure following percutaneous coronary intervention: the CAP trial. Catheter Cardiovasc Interv. 2008;71(1):1–5.
23. Hermiller J, Simonton C, Hinohara T, et al. Clinical experience with a circumferential clip-based vascular closure device in diagnostic catheterization. J Invasive Cardiol. 2005;17(10):504–10.
24. Hermiller JB, Simonton C, Hinohara T, et al. The StarClose Vascular Closure System: interventional results from the CLIP study. Catheter Cardiovasc Interv. 2006;68(5):677–83.
25. Deuling JH, Vermeulen RP, Anthonio RA, et al. Closure of the femoral artery after cardiac catheterization: a comparison of Angio-Seal, StarClose, and manual compression. Catheter Cardiovasc Interv. 2008;71(4):518–23.
26. Pancholy SB. Impact of two different hemostatic devices on radial artery outcomes after transradial catheterization. J Invasive Cardiol. 2009;21(3):101–4.
27. Rathore S, Stables RH, Pauriah M, et al. A randomized comparison of TR band and radistop hemostatic compression devices after transradial coronary intervention. Catheter Cardiovasc Interv. 2010;76(5):660–7.
28. Pancholy S, Coppola J, Patel T, Roke-Thomas M. Prevention of radial artery occlusion-patent hemostasis evaluation trial (PROPHET study): a randomized comparison of traditional versus patency documented hemostasis after transradial catheterization. Catheter Cardiovasc Interv. 2008;72(3):335–40.
29. Cubero JM, Lombardo J, Pedrosa C, et al. Radial compression guided by mean artery pressure versus standard compression with a pneumatic device (RACOMAP). Catheter Cardiovasc Interv. 2009;73(4):467–72.
30. Farouque HM, Tremmel JA, Raissi Shabari F, et al. Risk factors for the development of retroperitoneal hematoma after percutaneous coronary intervention in the era of glycoprotein IIb/IIIa inhibitors and vascular closure devices. J Am Coll Cardiol. 2005;45(3):363–8.
31. Kronzon I. Diagnosis and treatment of iatrogenic femoral artery pseudoaneurysm: a review. J Am Soc Echocardiogr. 1997;10(3):236–45.
32. Kelm M, Perings SM, Jax T, et al. Incidence and clinical outcome of iatrogenic femoral arteriovenous fistulas: implications for risk stratification and treatment. J Am Coll Cardiol. 2002;40(2):291–7.
33. Rao SV, O'Grady K, Pieper KS, et al. Impact of bleeding severity on clinical outcomes among patients with acute coronary syndromes. Am J Cardiol. 2005;96(9):1200–6.
34. Eikelboom JW, Mehta SR, Anand SS, Xie C, Fox KA, Yusuf S. Adverse impact of bleeding on prognosis in patients with acute coronary syndromes. Circulation. 2006;114(8):774–82.
35. Jolly SS, Amlani S, Hamon M, Yusuf S, Mehta SR. Radial versus femoral access for coronary angiography or intervention and the impact on major bleeding and ischemic events: a systematic review and meta-analysis of randomized trials. Am Heart J. 2009;157(1):132–40.
36. McCollum CH, Mavor E. Brachial artery injury after cardiac catheterization. J Vasc Surg. 1986;4(4):355–9.
37. Agostoni P, Biondi-Zoccai GG, de Benedictis ML, et al. Radial versus femoral approach for percutaneous coronary diagnostic and interventional procedures; systematic overview and meta-analysis of randomized trials. J Am Coll Cardiol. 2004;44(2):349–56.
38. Jolly SS, Yusuf S, Cairns J, et al. Radial versus femoral access for coronary angiography and intervention in patients with acute coronary syndromes (RIVAL): a randomised, parallel group, multicentre trial. Lancet. 2011;377(9775):1409–20.
39. Rao SV, Cohen MG, Kandzari DE, Bertrand OF, Gilchrist IC. The transradial approach to percutaneous coronary intervention: historical perspective, current concepts, and future directions. J Am Coll Cardiol. 2010;55(20):2187–95.
40. Bertrand OF, De Larochelliere R, Rodes-Cabau J, et al. A randomized study comparing same-day home discharge and abciximab bolus only to overnight hospitalization and abciximab bolus and infusion after transradial coronary stent implantation. Circulation. 2006;114(24):2636–43.

Guide Catheter Selection, Manipulation, and Support Augmentation for PCI

7

Jean-Michel Paradis and Stéphane Rinfret

Functions of Guiding Catheters

Selection of guiding or guide catheter is a critical component in performance of percutaneous coronary interventions. It can make the difference between a failure and a successful procedure. There are three main roles of a guiding catheter during PCI [1]:

1. *Balloon-stent catheter delivery*. The guiding catheter serves as the delivery tool of the balloon catheter to the coronary artery.
2. *Contrast injection*. The guiding catheter allows visualization of the vessel by contrast injection with or without the balloon catheter in place.
3. *Pressure monitoring*. The guiding catheter monitors aortic pressure for evaluation of the trans-stenotic pressure gradient for physiologic lesion assessment, ostial lesions, and hypotension during extended ischemia.

A guiding catheter must offer adequate backup support. It also has to be atraumatic, with proper alignment and correct engagement in the coronary ostium. Guiding catheters are available in multiple shapes. Each has a unique design and construction. To chose the most appropriate guiding catheter, it is very important to analyze the diagnostic angiogram with multiple views to take into consideration the size of the aortic root, the coronary ostial origin (high, anterior), the ostial orientation (superior, horizontal, inferior), the length of the left main, the takeoff of the target artery, and the location of the lesion. The next step is to plan the coronary intervention technique, to study the required devices, and to anticipate circumstances during the procedure. All of this will influence the size of the guiding catheter, the inner lumen, and backup support required. For example, for rotational atherectomy, 6 Fr allows the use of 1.5-mm burr, a 7-Fr catheter is mandatory to employ a 1.75-mm burr, while an 8-Fr catheter is needed for burrs ≥2 mm. The improvement of balloon and stent technology, together with evolution in fluoroscopic image quality, affords a progressive shift toward the use of lower profile, smaller equipment for PCI. In the early 1980s, 9-Fr guiding catheters were most often used while 8-Fr catheters took over in the late 1990s. Today, most procedures can be performed with 5- or 6-Fr guide catheters introduced through the same sheath used for the diagnostic coronary angiography. In an exhaustive economic analysis, Talley et al. [2] proved a cost-saving effect of coronary interventions performed with 6-Fr guiding catheters because of smaller arteriotomy accompanying sheath insertion and lower rate of clinically significant coronary and peripheral vascular complications (Table 7.1).

Passive vs. Active Support

In this chapter, we distinguish two types of support. *Passive* support is typically needed when deep active engagement of the coronary is not possible. Examples include the presence of a moderate left main lesion, aorto-ostial disease, or a severe proximal RCA lesion. In such situations, selection of a guide catheter curve and size that provides the best support despite few active manipulations will be desired. An additional situation would be for chronic total occlusion (CTO) PCI, when deep engagement is often not possible. Typically, larger bore catheters are stronger than smaller catheters and provide more passive support. For such reason, it is often possible, through 8-Fr guide catheters, to perform complex PCI in a calcified LAD lesion even with JL 4 curves. However, 6-Fr JL 4 guides will only provide poor support for such a purpose. Smaller guides are more easily manipulated for the *active* support maneuvers. They typically

J.-M. Paradis, MD • S. Rinfret, MD, SM, FRCPC (✉)
Multidisciplinary Department of Cardiology,
Quebec Heart & Lung Institute,
Laval University, Quebec City,
QC, Canada
e-mail: stephane.rinfret@criucpq.ulaval.ca

C.A. Thompson (ed.), *Textbook of Cardiovascular Intervention*,
DOI 10.1007/978-1-4471-4528-8_7, © Springer-Verlag London 2014

Table 7.1 Advantages and disadvantages associated with the size of the guiding catheter

	≤5 Fr	6 Fr	≥7 Fr
Advantages	Smaller puncture	Smaller puncture	Increased support
	Small vessel access	Small vessel access	Improved visualization
	Radial access	Radial access	Increased torque
	Deeper engagement possible for active support	Deeper engagement	Facilitate the use of 2 balloons (kissing)
	Smaller quantity of contrast		Allows the use of any covered stent
	Improved patient comfort		
Disadvantages	↓ passive support	↓ support	Larger puncture site/recovery time
	↓ visualization	↓ visualization	Less radial access possible
	↓ torque	↓ torque	Pressure dampening
	Device limiting (no thrombectomy, no simultaneous balloon inflation (kissing) technique possible, no Rotablator)	Device limiting	Increased contrast usage
			Increased risk of ostial dissection

involve deeper engagement of the catheter, with push or rotation, to allow for delivery of the equipment. 5- or 6-Fr JR 4 guides can be actively rotated clockwise to engage the mid-RCA segment to allow for better support in case a distal lesion cannot be crossed with balloons or stents. However, some curves, even when used in 6 Fr, never allow for active engagement of the coronary and are typically used for passive support. This is the case of AL or AR catheters. Therefore, proper selection curve of the catheter, for passive or active support, will be crucial, especially when using 5- or 6-Fr guide catheters from the transradial approach.

Table 7.2 Internal diameters of standard, large, and giant lumen guiding catheters

French	Standard (in.)	Large (in.)	Giant (in.)
6	≤0.061	0.062–0.065	≥0.066
7	≤0.071	0.072–0.075	≥0.076
8	≤0.079	0.080–0.085	≥0.086
9	≤0.089	0.090–0.096	≥0.096
10	≤0.099	0.100–0.107	≥0.108

Ref: Safian and Freed [3]

Construction

Guide catheter construction differs between manufacturers and usually are very different from their diagnostic counterparts. A stiffer shaft, thinner walls, larger internal lumen diameter, a shorter and more angulated tip (110° vs. 90°), and a reinforced construction (3 vs. 2 layers) are some of the characteristics that differentiate guide catheters from diagnostic catheters. In fact, to allow passage of interventional devices, guiding catheters must have very thin walls (<0.12 mm or 0.005 in.) to achieve a lumen diameter at least twice that of a typical diagnostic catheter (2 mm or 0.076 in. vs. 1 mm or 0.038 in.) while maintaining good rotational response and avoiding kinking issues (Table 7.2).

Guiding catheters are generally composed of three layers. The outer layer is a soft nylon elastomer jacket composed of either polyurethane or polyethylene for overall stiffness. The smooth outer coating must also resist thrombus formation. The middle layer is a stainless-steel braid (wire matrix) for increased strength and torque generation. The lubricious PTFE inner coating is conceived for smooth passage of guidewires and balloon catheters. Additionally, to reduce the risk of vessel trauma or dissection during coronary cannulation of the non-tapered tip, most guiding catheters now also incorporate a very soft material in the most distal 2 mm of the catheter (Figs. 7.1 and 7.2).

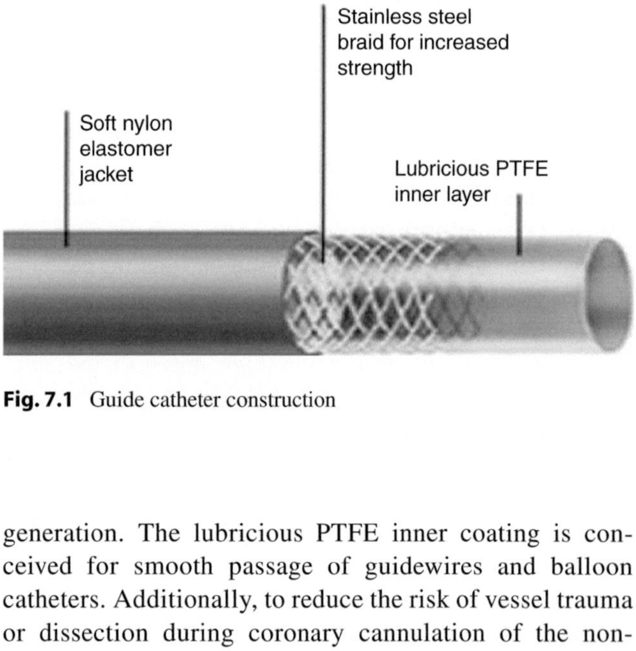

Fig. 7.1 Guide catheter construction

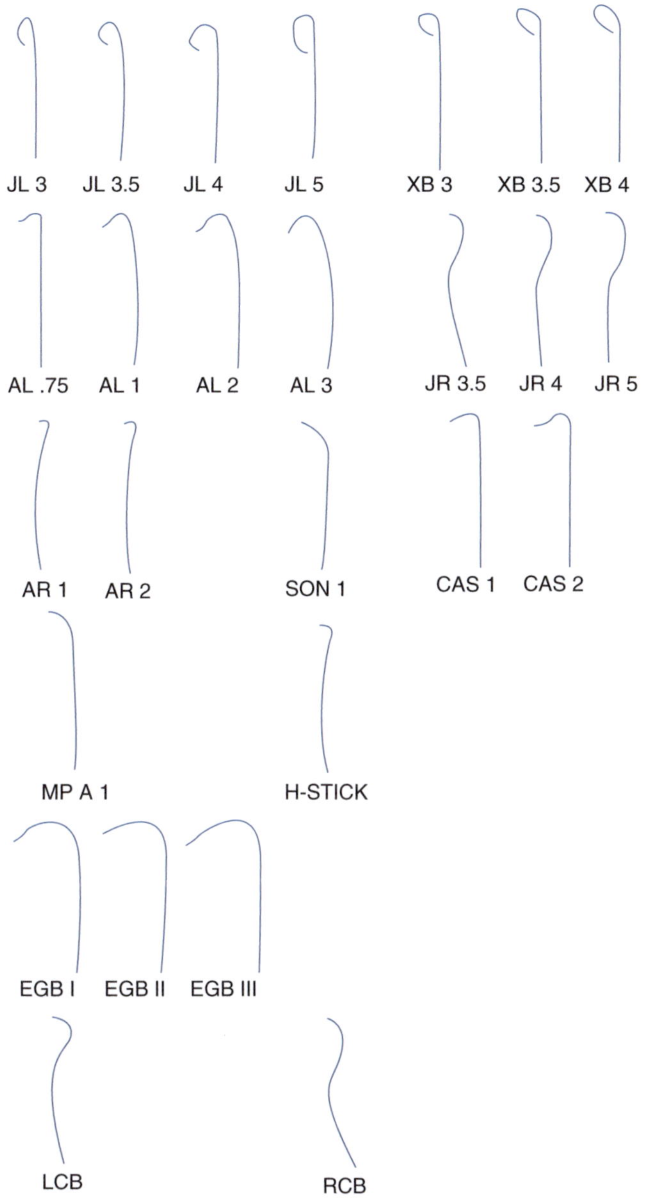

Fig. 7.2 Shapes of some of the most popular guiding catheters

Side Holes

Guiding catheter with side holes might be useful to secure pressure monitoring despite intubation of a diseased vessel (e.g., CTO PCI interventions) or when it is crucial to monitor the pressure throughout a risky procedure (like in left main interventions or while performing interventions on a unique surviving index artery). Side holes are mainly valuable to avoid catheter damping, to allow supplementary blood flow out of the tip to perfuse the coronary artery, and to help avoid dissection of the coronary ostium when the catheter is not perfectly coaxial or if it is engaged into a plaque, by allowing contrast to flow in the side hole and reduce risk of hydraulic antegrade dissection. On the other hand, the presence of side holes may give a false sense of security because the aortic pressure is monitored and not the coronary pressure. Therefore, the catheter can still occlude the coronary flow and induce ischemia but reduce recognition because the pressure curve on the monitor could remain normal. Other drawbacks of using side-hole catheters include increased contrast utilization, and suboptimal opacification of the index artery.

Also, measurement of coronary flow reserve (CRF) is dependent on the presence of side holes on the guiding catheter and on the vasodilator dose. In a small animal study published by Abizaid et al. [4], when CFR measurement was done with an 8-Fr guiding catheter without side holes, a maximum vasodilatory response was obtained using intracoronary adenosine dose of 12 μg. To the contrary, with side hole and 8- or 9-Fr guiding catheters, an approximate doubling of the adenosine dose was required to provoke a maximal vasodilatory response. Consequently, larger doses of adenosine should be given to assess coronary flow parameters when guiding catheter with side holes is used.

Transfemoral Interventions

From the femoral approach, in the presence of a normal aorta and a normal length of the left main, engaging the left coronary ostium is usually feasible with an Extra Backup (XB or EBU depending on the vendor), 4 in males and 3.5 in females, or Judkins left (JL) 4. Judkins *diagnostic* catheter is useful because its fixed primary curve permits to intubate only a little segment of the ostium of either the left main coronary artery or right coronary artery. Therefore, there is less risk of trauma to these vessels. On the contrary, when performing PCI, this fixed primary curve might cause a limitation because the Judkins catheter may not be oriented coaxially with the index artery. Moreover, the secondary curve of JL guiding catheters usually makes a 90° angle at the point of contact on the ascending aorta and has limited back wall support. Therefore, it may be difficult to deliver interventional devices through all the curves, and angles. Unless 7 or 8 Fr is used to increase passive support, the inability to effectively and coaxially engage a 5- or 6-Fr JL catheter make it unsuitable for complex LCX or LAD intervention, one exception being ostial left main intervention, where support is often less necessary and deep engagement is not preferred.

In the presence of a large aorta, it is preferable to upsize to an EBU 4.5 or JL 5 or to an Amplatz left (AL) 2–3 if a better support is needed. The AL guiding catheter is also valuable for the posterior and anterior left main takeoff and for interventions on a circumflex artery with a sharp angulation or abrupt downward origin from the left main. Amplatz catheters can be very valuable in providing Extra Backup passive support when proximal vessel tortuosity, chronic total occlusion, or a distal target lesion is present. Although ensuring a deep engagement with the coaxial alignment and a strong backup support for complex lesions, the AL catheter is a more aggressive and potentially traumatic catheter and must be manipulated cautiously to avoid vessel dissection, especially using 8-Fr size, where passive support will become maximized. In fact, just a simple withdrawal can advance the tip of the AL catheter even further into the coronary artery. Therefore, to disengage an AL catheter properly, one should advance the catheter slightly and then rotate it out of the ostium. If the ostium of the left main is high or the aortic root is small, a JL catheter may be selected, acknowledging the loss of passive support. Therefore, larger catheter could be favored to counteract this. If the left main is short, a short-tip guide may provide a better coaxial alignment, which can be verified in a left anterior oblique view.

The right coronary artery is usually more difficult to cannulate than the left coronary artery. The Judkins right (JR) 4 is usually a good guiding catheter for percutaneous interventions in the right coronary artery (RCA), in the presence of a normal aorta with a regular 90° origin of the RCA. With JR catheters, there is no point of contact with the aorta. Thus, this catheter customarily provides less passive support for right coronary interventions. When a stronger passive support is required, the AL 0.75 or 1 is a good alternative. With a large aorta, the Amplatz right (AR) 2–3 or the Hockey stick (HS) may be chosen by the operator. For a RCA superior takeoff, which means that the RCA points upward from the sinus, AL, AR, or HS catheters are decent choices. JR, JR short tip, Multipurpose, and the bypass right catheter are best for the inferior takeoff.

Shepherd's Crook configuration (severe superior angulation and tortuosity) of right coronary artery represents a challenge for the interventional cardiologist. Effectively, studies have demonstrated that angioplasty of a RCA with a sharp upturn with a near-180° switchback turn is associated with a lower primary success rate, essentially because there is less support provided by the guiding catheter [5]. While JR catheter is particularly inadequate for this type of RCA anatomy, AL 1 or AL 0.75, SCR, Hockey stick, internal mammary, El Gamal, Voda right, or Multipurpose are best suited for this anatomy.

It may be demanding to easily cannulate the left internal mammary (LIMA) when using a femoral approach. This situation may occur because of proximal tortuosity of subclavian artery or acute angle between the subclavian artery and the LIMA. Moreover, because LIMA may be tortuous and extremely redundant, it can be very difficult to reach the culprit lesion with interventional devices. Interventions in arterial mammary grafts are usually performed with 90 cm internal mammary catheter, which offers contralateral wall support from the subclavian artery and is expressly designed to sit coaxially in the ostium of the internal mammary artery and allow for an extra 10 cm to the balloons and stents to reach the lesion. Since there is a high risk of dissection and spasm, forceful engagement of internal mammary artery should be avoided. Pretreatment with nitroglycerin or verapamil and frequent boluses of nitroglycerin may be used to minimize spasm. Finally, after balloon dilation, it is essential to assure that withdrawal of balloon catheter does not intubate the guiding catheter more deeply into the internal mammary artery, inducing a traumatic dissection.

Saphenous vein bypass grafts are often challenging to engage, particularly grafts to the obtuse marginal, which are usually located above and lateral to RCA grafts and may have superior angulation. Left coronary bypass (LCB) catheter, with a 90° primary bend and a 70° secondary bend, is specially designed for left coronary bypass grafts but often provides limited passive support. AL 1–2 offers a good backup force in such cases. The Multipurpose curve, the HS, or the right coronary bypass (RCB) catheter, which has a 120° tip and secondary bend, are nice options for grafts to RCA, which typically arise from the anterior wall of the aorta several centimeters above the aortic root and have horizontal to downward takeoff and direction. Multipurpose catheters may deeply engage a right graft; therefore, large 8-Fr catheters must be manipulated carefully. For grafts with abnormal takeoffs from aorta, especially inferior orientations, the Multipurpose guiding catheter might be useful.

Long Soft Tips Guide Catheters

Some catheters come in two versions: regular tip or longer soft tip. In our experience, the longer soft tip is associated with some compromise in terms of support. It allows to more easily engage the coronary, as its tip will bend before penetrating the ostium. Therefore, an operator can use such catheters placed in non-diseased proximal segments of the LAD or the LCX in the case of a short left main, to increase passive and active support, especially when using smaller equipment. However, if the selected catheter curve is too short, its soft tip will sit at the ostium of the left main or the RCA and will reduce passive support (Table 7.3).

Table 7.3 Choice of guiding catheters – transfemoral procedures

Target ostium	Guiding catheter (in order of preference)
Left coronary artery	
Normal aorta	EBU or XB 4, XB 3.5, JL 4, AL 2 (especially for LCX),
Dilated aorta	XB ≥4, JL 5, AL ≥2,
Narrow aorta	XB or EBU 3.0 or 3.5 (especially long soft tip), AL 1, JL 3.5
Superior/high takeoff	AL 2, AL 3, AL 4, JL 3.5, XB, EBU
Inferior/low takeoff	XB 4, XB 3.5, Multipurpose, JL 4 MOD, AL 1.5
Posterior	AL 2
Anomalous circumflex	Multipurpose, AL 1
Right coronary artery	
Normal aorta	JR 4, AR 2, AL 0.75 or 1, IMA, HS,
Dilated aorta	JR ≥5, AL ≥2, AR ≥2
Narrow aorta	JR 3, AR 1, AL 0.75
Superior takeoff	AL 0.75 or 1, IMA, AR 2, HS
Anterior origin	AL 1, Multipurpose, HS
Posterior origin	AL 1, AR 2
Shepherd's Crook	AL 0.75 or 1, HS,
Saphenous vein graft	
LCA graft	JR, LCB, AL 1, HS, Multipurpose,
RCA graft	Multipurpose, RCB,
Internal mammary artery	IMA, JR 4

Table 7.4 Choice of guiding catheters – transradial procedures

Target artery – vessel	Guiding catheter (in order of preference)
Left coronary artery	XB (or EBU) 3.5 in most, XB 4 in large aortas, XB 3 in small females, AL 1 or 2 (especially for LCX intervention)
	Rarely used: Fajadet left, Kimny radial, Ikari left, Multipurpose, El Gamal
Right coronary artery	JR 4, AL 0.75 or 1, Barbeau, AR 2,
	Rarely used: Fajadet right, Kimny radial, Ikari right, Multipurpose, El Gamal
Both left and right coronary arteries	Kimny radial, Multipurpose, El Gamal, AL
Saphenous bypass graft	AL, Multipurpose, Bypass graft catheter (LCB, RCB), Barbeau, JR
	Rarely used: Kimny radial, , El Gamal,
Internal mammary artery	IMA, modified IMA

Transradial or Brachial Interventions

Transradial interventions [6] are more technically demanding. However, they are becoming more widely used by interventional cardiologists who wish to reduce bleeding complications and increase patient comfort while decreasing staff workload compared to transfemoral interventions [7]. Ability of the patient to resume ambulation immediately after the intervention is greatly appreciated. However, the radial artery is one of the most spasm-prone in the human body. Mechanical stimuli can precipitate radial spasm. Consequently, reducing catheter manipulations will diminish the risk of radial spasm and thereby will cause less pain and will increase procedural success. Other drawbacks associated with transradial procedures are the inability to cannulate the radial artery, found in approximately 3–4 % of patients [8]; inability to cannulate the coronaries, which ranges in from 1 to 7 % [9]; and potential lack of guide support for coronary interventions [10]. Saito et al. [11] have measured by ultrasound a mean radial diameter of 3.10 ± 0.60 mm and 2.80 ± 0.60 mm in Japanese male and females, respectively. Consequently, 5-Fr introducer can be utilized in approximately 93 % of patients, 6-Fr in 85 % of men and 72 % of women, 7-Fr in 71 % of male and 40 % of female, and 8-Fr in 45 % and 24 %, respectively, if the objective is not to overstretch the vessel. However, currently, most transradial operators use 6-Fr catheters even in small radials.

Some of the characteristic features the guiding catheter should have when a transradial coronary intervention is performed include an optimal stiffness for optimal support, sufficient flexibility of the primary curve, contact with the aortic root, and a coaxial alignment with the target coronary artery. Guiding catheter manipulation differs between radial and femoral approaches. Some maneuvers facilitate guide positioning. The operator may ask the patient to take a deep breath to facilitate catheter movement and positioning of the wire into the ascending aorta. It is also valuable to use an exchange-length wire to avoid the need to recross the great vessels. Alternatively, some operators will leave the short 0.035' J guidewire against the aortic valve during the exchange, with the use of a syringe with flush. The next catheter is then advanced without proximal guidewire control, until the back end of the wire exits the guide catheter with further advancement. Finally, when cannulating the left main, most cannulation of the left main involves pushing and counterclockwise rotation of the catheter, especially with XB or AL catheters.

When the procedure is performed from a radial or brachial access, the EBU or XB, JL, or Voda catheters are good options for the left coronary artery. However, when approaching from the right radial artery, it is helpful to use a curve 0.5 cm shorter than that employed in the femoral route with a comparable aortic root (i.e., EBU 3.5 or JL 3.5). For RCA interventions from the right radial artery, the JR catheter offers good engagement. On the contrary, procedures from the left radial artery can be achieved with conventional "transfemoral" curves. The AR catheter may also be used for RCA procedures, although the passive support of such catheter is limited. Therefore, we prefer the use of JR or Barbeau catheter for active support, especially when there is minimal proximal disease. However, when maximal passive support is warranted, AL curves are preferred. The AL 0.75 offers the advantage of good backup support while limiting deep seating of the catheter, which may become problematic with proximal RCA disease. AL catheters may also be advantageous for LCX interventions (Tables 7.4 and 7.5).

Table 7.5 Guiding catheter designs and functions

Catheter	Description	Function – use
JL	Judkins left	Left coronary artery interventions
JR	Judkins right	Right coronary artery and SVG interventions; may not provide coaxial alignment for vein grafts to the RCA
AL	Amplatz left	Useful for difficult anatomy of the left coronary artery (especially left circumflex), SVG, Shepherd's Crook or high anterior RCA
AR	Amplatz right	RCA interventions or SVG to RCA with inferior origin
ALR 1–2	Amplatz left-right (modified)	Longer reach than AR and shorter reach than AL
XB or EBU	Extra Backup	Useful for difficult anatomy in LCA; offers backup support from opposite wall of aorta
K	Kimny	Useful in transradial procedures for bath LCA and RCA. Support may be limited
FL	Fajadet left	LCA interventions from a radial approach
FR	Fajadet right	RCA interventions from a radial approach
IL	Ikari left	LCA interventions; offers good backup support
IR	Ikari right	RCA interventions; offers good backup support
VL	Voda left	Useful for difficult anatomy in LCA; offers backup support from opposite wall of aorta
VR	Voda right	Useful for difficult anatomy in RCA, Shepherd's Crook RCA, or SVG to LCA with vertical upward origin
MP	Multipurpose	Useful for RCA or SVG to RCA or LCA with inferior origin
SON	Sones	Useful for RCA or SVG to RCA or LCA with inferior origin
HS	Hockey stick	Useful for RCA with horizontal or slightly superior origin or SVG to LCA
Barbeau	Barbeau	Useful for transradial RCA interventions, especially in the RCA. Limited support in the left coronary
ELG	El Gamal	LCA and RCA interventions from a radial route
LCB	Left coronary bypass	Useful for SVG to LCA with horizontal or slightly superior origin
RCB	Right coronary bypass	Useful for SVG to RCA
IMA	Internal mammary	LIMA, RIMA, or native vessel beyond anastomosis lesions. Sometimes fits well for RCA interventions
CAS	Castillo	Intended use from brachial approach, configuration similar to an Amplatz catheter

Adapted from the Safian and Freed [3]

Backup

A primary function of guiding catheter is support of devices such as balloon, stents, and guidewires. Four major characteristics determine guiding catheter support: (1) physical characteristics of the catheter material, (2) geometry and surface characteristics of the catheter's supportive points, (3) catheter bends, and (4) catheter intubation into the vessel [12]. In a study published by Ikari et al. [13], it was demonstrated that when measured in an in vitro arterial tree model, backup force was significantly greater with progressively larger French size (Fig. 7.3).

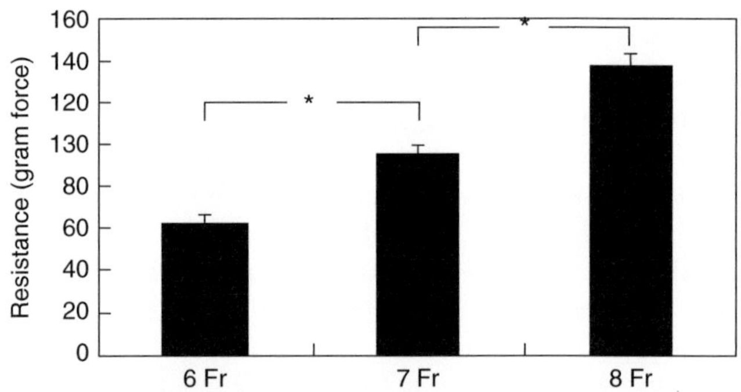

Fig. 7.3 Relation between catheter size and backup force. "*" represents $p<0.001$ (Figure from Ikari et al. [13])

However, in a retrospective analysis of consecutive patients undergoing ad hoc PCI, when compared with 6-Fr guides, 5-Fr guiding catheters were associated with a higher technical success rate (99 % vs. 95 %), less fluoroscopy time (16 ± 9 min vs. 19 ± 12 min), less contrast medium usage (274 ± 101 ml vs. 313 ± 124 ml), and no difference in MACE and in serious vascular complications [14]. Therefore, some operators use the 5-Fr approach in their routine interventional practice, acknowledging several limitations, such as the incompatibility of 5-Fr catheters with thrombectomy device, kissing balloon technique, and other advanced PCI techniques.

Moreover, the same in vitro modeling by Ikari showed that the backup force is associated with the angle (θ (phi)) of the catheter on the reverse side of the aorta (Fig. 7.4). As the angle increases, the backup force is greater. In the model, because the angle (θ (phi)) was greater via the transfemoral route, the backup force with a Judkins left guiding catheter was 60 % greater in transfemoral interventions than in transradial interventions (Fig. 7.5).

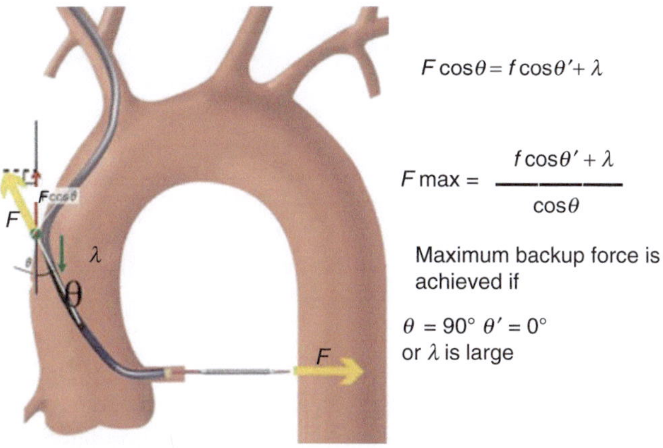

Fig. 7.4 Relation between backup force and the angle of the catheter on the reverse side of the aorta (formula explaining the backup force) (Ikari et al. [13])

Another factor associated with the backup force is the contact area on the aorta. The measured backup force is greater in catheters with longer length of contact with the aorta. However, beyond a certain limit, if the flat portion of the catheter is too long, there was no further increase in the backup force in Ikari's study. The friction of the catheter at the supportive point on the aortic wall is one more feature defining catheter backup force. One of the properties that establishes catheter friction is the character of the catheter's surface. A surface that possesses high friction offers better stability and support for the catheter.

An additional determinant of catheter support is the alignment. Coaxial alignment of the catheter with the vessel is superior for support than non-coaxial alignment. When forces are transmitted in a straight line, minimal force is lost. Conversely, when forces are applied with an angle, the greater the angle, the more force is lost. At 90°, there is a complete loss of force transmission. Changes in forces can be calculated from the following formula: $F_2 = F_1 \times \cos \alpha$ (alpha) (Fig. 7.6).

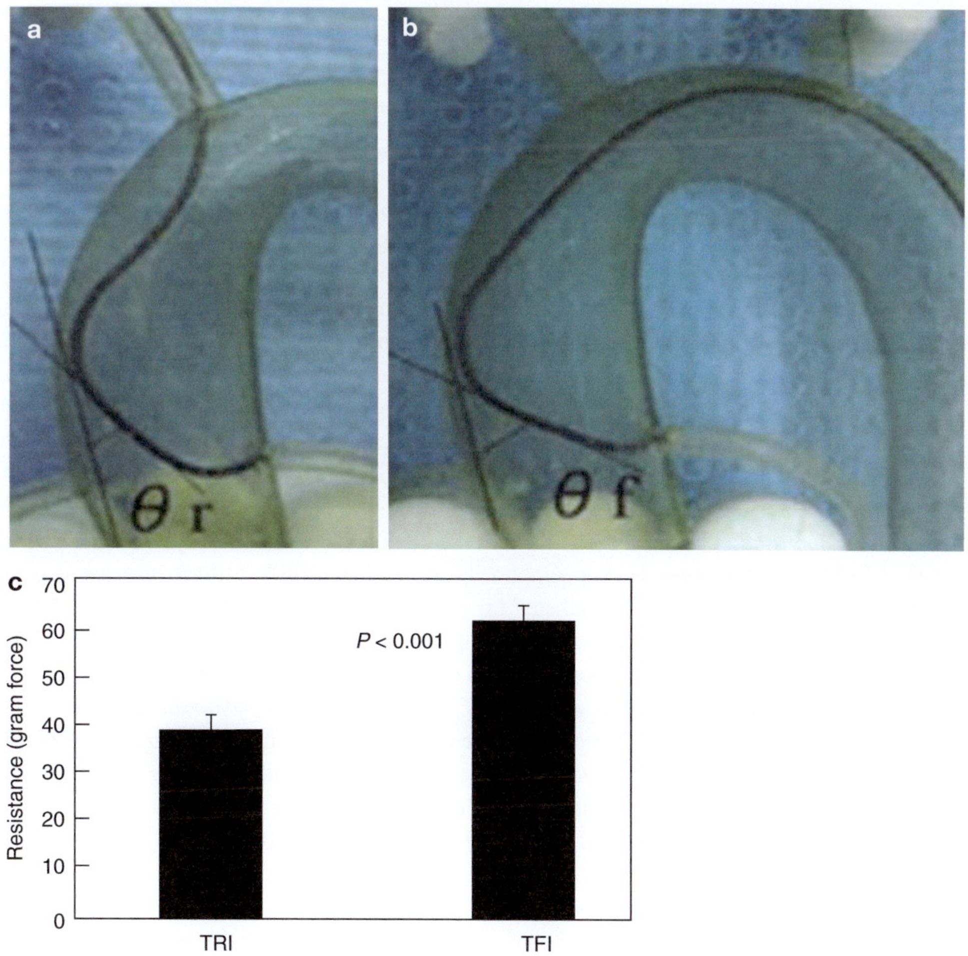

Fig. 7.5 Difference in backup force between transfemoral (*TFI*) and transradial (*TRI*) interventions. (**a**) Angle of the catheter on the opposite side of the aorta in TRI. (**b**) Angle of the catheter on the opposite side of the aorta in TFI. (**c**) In vitro modeling showing greater backup force in TFI

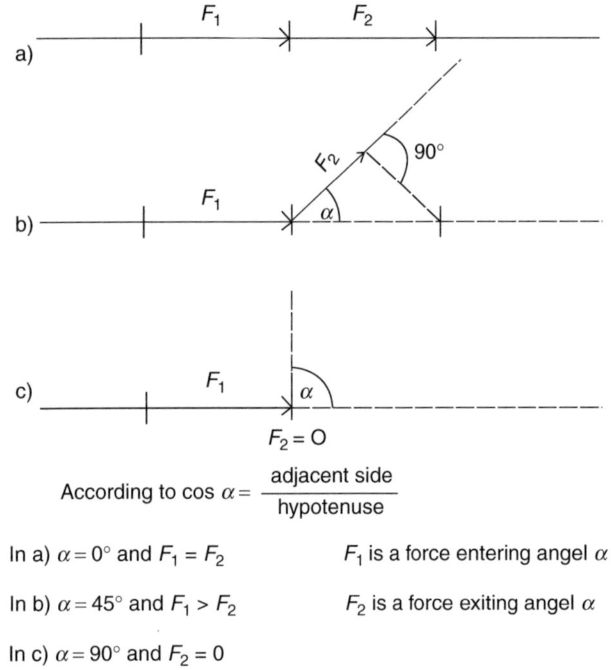

Fig. 7.6 Relation between alignment and backup force [12]

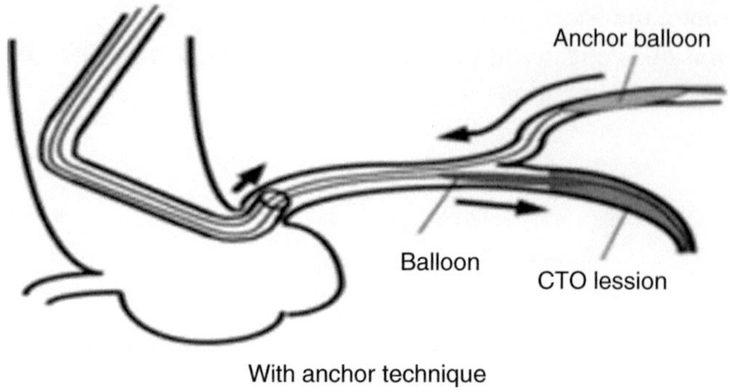

Fig. 7.7 Anchor technique. Enhanced guiding catheter support can be obtained by pulling an anchor balloon inflated in the side branch while advancing another balloon through a lesion [18]

Methods to Increase Backup Force

Changing a guiding catheter to a larger size or to one with a special design that gives stronger support (e.g., Amplatz or Voda guiding catheter) can provide improved backup force, although such decision needs to be considered before significant commitment to the PCI work. Indeed, exchange of guiding catheter while keeping PCI guidewires in place is technically challenging and often risky to lose position.

In transradial or transfemoral interventions with the JL catheter, experienced operators use a deep engagement technique [15] which increases the angle on the reverse side of the aorta (θ (phi)) and the friction between the guide and the coronary artery, therefore creating more backup support. Deep seating can be defined as positioning the catheter tip greater than 20 mm into the target vessel. Deep engagement of right coronary artery or left circumflex can be accomplished by applying clockwise (for RCA) or counterclockwise (for LCX) rotation and gently advancing the guiding catheter over the guide wire. For left anterior descending artery, clockwise rotation of the catheter is required. To minimize the risk of dissection and distal artery embolization associated with deep seating, it is preferable to use a smaller size catheter (5 or 6 Fr) and a soft-tip guide catheter and to reduce the period of time during which the catheter remains deeply engaged. Some authors recommend to deeply intubate only for a brief moment when maximal support is required. The prolonged profound intubation probably enhances the risk of the coronary intervention [12].

The buddy wire strategy has also been developed to solve the problem of lack of support, especially in transradial coronary stenting of complex, calcified lesions [16]. When delivery of balloon or stent is difficult due to instability of the guiding catheter, it is useful to use another guidewire placed in parallel with the previous wire. In circumstances such as RCA and SVG intervention, a third wire (the buddy's buddy) can offer further incremental stability and support. By reducing tortuosity and friction of coronary artery and maintaining coaxial alignment, the balloon or stent can be more easily delivered to the lesion site.

For greater guide catheter support, it is also possible to inflate a balloon in a nontarget vessel and hold its shaft with backward force while advancing another balloon to cross the target lesion. This method is called the "anchor technique," which can be helpful in CTO interventions [17], in side-branch PCI following stent jail, or when it is hard to pass a balloon or a stent across a lesion [18] (Fig. 7.7). The anchor technique is generally a more productive and powerful method to enhance device delivery compared with buddy wire strategies.

Another method to optimize backup force provided by guide catheter system is the mother-in-child technique or the five-in-six system [19, 20]. It involves a 110-cm-long 5-Fr guide (child) inserted in a regular 100-cm-long 6- or 7-Fr guide catheter (mother) [21]. The longer the insertion of the 5-Fr catheter into the artery, the stronger is the backup force generated by this system. In fact, this technique may offer up to 70 % more backup force and may generate a better backup support compared to a 6- or even a 7-Fr guiding catheter alone. However, trauma to the coronary resulting in dissection and air embolism occurring during the intubation of child catheter are complications sometimes encountered with this method.

A safer method of mother-in-child technique involves the use of the newly developed GuideLiner catheter (Vascular Solutions, Inc, Minneapolis, Minnesota) (Fig. 7.8). An other alternative is the Boston Guidezilla catheter, built on the same principles compared to the GuideLiner. The Guideliner

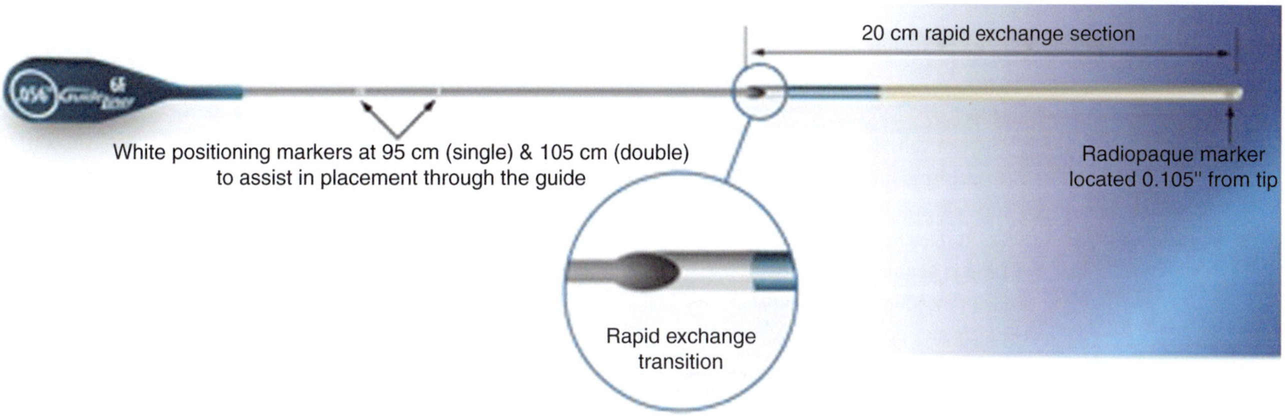

Fig. 7.8 Guideliner catheter

is a catheter guiding extension delivered on a monorail through a standard guiding catheter. It includes a flexible 20-cm straight extension connected to a stainless-steel push tube. The extension is made of an inner polytetrafluoroethylene (PTFE, Teflon) lining, surrounded by a stainless-steel coil, and an outer layer of Pebax polymer, which imparts lubricity. Available in three sizes (5-in-6-Fr, 6-in-7-Fr, 7-in-8-Fr), the Guideliner enables very deep intubation of the target vessel, thus providing very strong backup support. Delivery of the extension into the coronary is facilitated by a radiopaque marker located 2.7 mm from the tip. Delivering the Guideliner over an inflated or uninflated balloon or on a microcatheter can enhance optimal positioning and minimize proximal vessel trauma.

Catheter Complications

Procedural complications have been linked to many institutional [22], operator [23], and patient [24] variables. Between January 2001 and December 2006, in 21 institutions, 103,070 consecutive patients who underwent PCI with 6-, 7-, or 8-Fr guiding catheters were included in a registry evaluating the association between guiding catheter size and complications of PCI [25]. Femoral access was employed in 98.9 % of patients, radial access in 0.6 %, and brachial access in 0.5 %. 62.4 % of procedures were done with 6-Fr guides, 31.7 % with 7-Fr guides, and 5.9 % with 8-Fr guides. After multivariate analysis, when compared with PCI performed with 6-Fr guide catheters, the use of 7- or 8-Fr guides was associated with a higher risk of vascular complications (pseudoaneurysm, arteriovenous fistula, femoral neuropathy, retroperitoneal hematoma, hematoma requiring transfusion), contrast-induced nephropathy, decline in hemoglobin >3 g/dl, and post-procedural blood transfusions. Moreover, 8-Fr guiding catheters were associated with a significantly higher risk of major adverse cardiac events and in-hospital mortality. Therefore, currently, use of smaller size catheters when possible is likely warranted. Furthermore, the use of the transradial approach is associated with further reduction in bleeding and vascular events. (Table 7.6)

New Developments for Transradial PCI

The introduction of arterial catheters through a sheath is the standard technique to facilitate catheter manipulation while maintaining access during catheter exchange. However, the artery diameter-to-sheath size ratio is an independent predictor of post-procedural radial thrombosis [11]. The use of smaller sheaths could help prevent this complication. The effective outer diameter of the introducer sheaths is about 1.5 Fr larger than the labeled (internal diameter) size (Fig. 7.9).

Therefore, omitting the sheath provides a smaller arterial access, may facilitate hemostasis, and may avoid costly use of vascular closure devices. In a study by Bayard et al. [27], it was demonstrated that 5-Fr transfemoral PCI without sheath could be performed safely in daily practice, with comparable, if not lower, vascular access bleeding complication rates than conventional 6-Fr interventions with or without closure devices. This approach also allows substantial savings due to less equipment used. Another article demonstrated that sheathless transradial PCI using standard large-bore (7- or 8-Fr) guiding catheters is a safe and effective technique for the treatment of complex lesions [26]. A new sheathless catheter has been developed by Asahi Intecc. The Sheathless Eaucath possesses approximately the same outer diameter as a 6-Fr sheath introducer but has an internal diameter of a 7.5-Fr guide catheter. Techniques such as simultaneous kissing stents can thus be easily performed through this new device, although accepting that this system may increase the risk of radial artery spasm and silent occlusion due to its longer length [28]. However, whether the sheathless guides offer similar support remains controversial.

Table 7.6 Unadjusted outcomes for patients with 6-, 7-, and 8-F guide catheter size

In-hospital outcomes	Aggregate (n = 103,070)	6-F (n = 64,335)	7-F (n = 32,676)	8-F (n = 6,059)	p Value[a]
CIN[b]	3.83	3.39	4.38	6.21	<0.0001
NRD	0.24	0.22	0.22	0.51	<0.0001
Vascular complication	2.50	2.35	2.69	3.85	<0.0001
Vascular complication with VCD	2.37	2.41	2.06	3.6	0.04
Vascular complication without VCD	2.62	2.33	2.79	3.89	<0.0001
Gastrointestinal bleeding	1.19	1.12	1.27	1.93	<0.0001
Drop in hemoglobin >3 (g/dl)[c]	9.20	8.55	10.23	14.01	<0.0001
Post-procedure transfusion	5.15	4.72	5.26	9.23	<0.0001
Emergency coronary artery bypass graft surgery (CABG)	0.39	0.37	0.35	0.81	<0.0001
Any CABG[d]	1.08	0.99	1.08	1.86	<0.0001
Revascularization (same site)	0.59	0.48	0.67	0.53	0.0007
Myocardial infarction (MI)	1.66	1.56	1.74	2.67	<0.0001
Stroke	0.37	0.33	0.42	0.63	0.0005
Death	1.13	0.97	1.20	2.38	<0.0001
MACE[e]	4.29	3.84	4.54	7.21	<0.0001

Values are %

CIN contrast-induced nephropathy, *MACE* major adverse cardiac event, *NRD* nephropathy requiring dialysis, *VCD* vascular closure device

[a]The p value for comparison of 6-, 7-, and 8-F categories

[b][Peak creatinine -baseline creatinine] ≥0.5 (mg/dl). Patients with a history of dialysis excluded

[c][Baseline hemoglobin – nadir hemoglobin] >3 g/dl

[d]Any CABG includes emergency and nonemergency CABG

[e]Major adverse cardiac events are a composite of stroke, MI, post-PCI CABG or repeat PCI (same site), or death

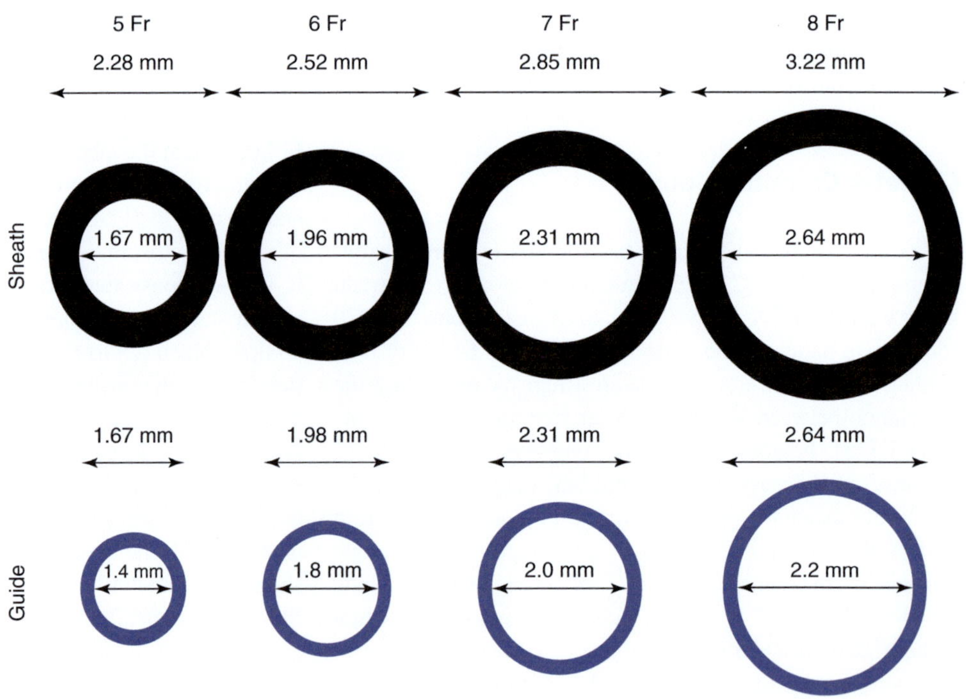

Fig. 7.9 Sheath to guide catheter diameter comparison [26]

The miniaturization of interventional devices continues. Tanaka et al. [29] have developed the "slender" virtual 2-Fr system. This system uses a 4-Fr guiding catheter without a sheath introducer. The outer diameter of the guiding catheter is 1.43 mm, which is equal to a French size of two (2 Fr). This smaller new technology may contribute to reduce vascular access complications, decrease patient morbidity, and improve patient comfort as well. However, because of the limited internal diameter (1.27 mm), this system does not accommodate simultaneous coronary guidewires, balloons, large coronary stents, intravascular ultrasound catheter, and certainly not rotational atherectomy. This system is therefore not recommended for bifurcation lesions. Finally, catheter manipulation is more difficult and more prone to kinking, and backup force is weaker with this smaller shaft system.

Takeshita et al. have developed a novel coronary "accessor" (KIWAMI, Heartrail II, TERUMO, Tokyo, Japan) [30, 31]. The shape of the 4-Fr accessor resembles that of conventional guiding catheters (Judkins, Amplatz, Extra Backup) with an outer diameter of 1.43 mm. Intended to achieve easier coronary cannulation but not to provide Extra Backup force, this 4-Fr accessor system may have a positive impact on contrast dye usage and on vascular access complications. On the other hand, deep intubation technique seems essential to accomplish PCI with the Kiwami system. Again, the small inner diameter (1.27 mm) of this coronary accessory limits the use of several angioplasty devices (rotational atherectomy, intravascular ultrasound, some microcatheters such as Tornus, and some of the coronary stents). Such devices are currently only available in Asia.

Summary

A variety of guide catheter shapes and sizes exist for coronary intervention. The interventional cardiologist become familiar with them to appropriately select the guide system that is optimal for a given procedure and balances effectiveness and safety. Additional maneuvers such as mother-in-child technique, anchor balloons, deep seating, and active guide management extend the interventionalists' ability to manage complex coronary disease.

References

1. Kern MJ. The cardiac catheterization handbook. 4th ed. Philadelphia: Mosby; 2003.
2. Talley JD, Mauldin PD, Becker ER. A prospective randomized trial comparing the benefits and limitations of 6Fr and 8Fr guiding catheters in elective coronary angioplasty: clinical, procedural, angiographic, and economic end points. J Interv Cardiol. 1995;8(4): 345–53.
3. Safian RD, Freed MS. The manual of interventional cardiology. Royal Oak: Physicians' Press; 2002.
4. Abizaid A, Kornowski R, Mintz GS, et al. Influence of guiding catheter selection on the measurement of coronary flow reserve. Am J Cardiol. 1997;79(5):703–4.
5. Tuzcu EM, Simpfendorfer C, Gossman D, Badwhar K. Long-term follow-up of PTCA of the right coronary artery with shepherd's crook morphology. Cleve Clin J Med. 1989;56(6):577–9.
6. Kiemeneij F, Laarman GJ, Odekerken D, Slagboom T, van der Wieken R. A randomized comparison of percutaneous transluminal coronary angioplasty by the radial, brachial and femoral approaches: the access study. J Am Coll Cardiol. 1997;29(6):1269–75.
7. Brueck M, Bandorski D, Kramer W, Wieczorek M, Holtgen R, Tillmanns H. A randomized comparison of transradial versus transfemoral approach for coronary angiography and angioplasty. JACC Cardiovasc Interv. 2009;2(11):1047–54.
8. Mann 3rd JT, Arrowood M, Cubeddu G. PTCA using the right radial artery access site. J Invasive Cardiol. 1995;7(5):142–7.
9. Kiemeneij F, Laarman GJ, de Melker E. Transradial artery coronary angioplasty. Am Heart J. 1995;129(1):1–7.
10. Kiemeneij F, Laarman GJ. Transradial artery Palmaz-Schatz coronary stent implantation: results of a single-center feasibility study. Am Heart J. 1995;130(1):14–21.
11. Saito S, Ikei H, Hosokawa G, Tanaka S. Influence of the ratio between radial artery inner diameter and sheath outer diameter on radial artery flow after transradial coronary intervention. Catheter Cardiovasc Interv. 1999;46(2):173–8.
12. Voda J. Long-tip guiding catheter: successful and safe for left coronary artery angioplasty. Cathet Cardiovasc Diagn. 1992;27(3):234–42.
13. Ikari Y, Nagaoka M, Kim JY, Morino Y, Tanabe T. The physics of guiding catheters for the left coronary artery in transfemoral and transradial interventions. J Invasive Cardiol. 2005;17(12): 636–41.
14. Rakhit RD, Matter C, Windecker S, Garachemani AR, Seiler C, Eberli FR. Five French versus 6 French PCI: a case control study of efficacy, safety and outcome. J Invasive Cardiol. 2002;14(11):670–4.
15. Von Sohsten R, Oz R, Marone G, McCormick DJ. Deep intubation of 6 French guiding catheters for transradial coronary interventions. J Invasive Cardiol. 1998;10(4):198–202.
16. Rigattieri S, Hamon M, Grollier G. The buddy wire technique is useful in transradial coronary stenting of complex, calcified lesions: report of three cases. J Invasive Cardiol. 2005;17(7):376–7.
17. Hirokami M, Saito S, Muto H. Anchoring technique to improve guiding catheter support in coronary angioplasty of chronic total occlusions. Catheter Cardiovasc Interv. 2006;67(3):366–71.
18. Fujita S, Tamai H, Kyo E, et al. New technique for superior guiding catheter support during advancement of a balloon in coronary angioplasty: the anchor technique. Catheter Cardiovasc Interv. 2003;59(4):482–8.
19. Takahashi S, Saito S, Tanaka S, et al. New method to increase a backup support of a 6 French guiding coronary catheter. Catheter Cardiovasc Interv. 2004;63(4):452–6.
20. Hayashida K, Louvard Y, Lefevre T. Transradial complex coronary interventions using a five-in-six system. Catheter Cardiovasc Interv. 2011;77(1):63–8.
21. Ohlow MA, von Korn H, Lauer B. Mother-and-baby technique for catheterization of the left coronary artery in a patient with a huge aneurysm of the ascending aorta. Clin Res Cardiol. 2007;96(7):524–5.
22. Ho V. Certificate of need, volume, and percutaneous transluminal coronary angioplasty outcomes. Am Heart J. 2004;147(3): 442–8.

23. Harjai KJ, Berman AD, Grines CL, et al. Impact of interventionalist volume, experience, and board certification on coronary angioplasty outcomes in the era of stenting. Am J Cardiol. 2004;94(4):421–6.
24. Cheng CI, Yeh KH, Chang HW, et al. Comparison of baseline characteristics, clinical features, angiographic results, and early outcomes in men vs women with acute myocardial infarction undergoing primary coronary intervention. Chest. 2004;126(1):47–53.
25. Grossman PM, Gurm HS, McNamara R, et al. Percutaneous coronary intervention complications and guide catheter size: bigger is not better. JACC Cardiovasc Interv. 2009;2(7):636–44.
26. From AM, Gulati R, Prasad A, Rihal CS. Sheathless transradial intervention using standard guide catheters. Catheter Cardiovasc Interv. 2010;76(7):911–6.
27. Bayard YL, Jakob D, Meier B. All comers 5 French transfemoral percutaneous coronary intervention without sheath. Catheter Cardiovasc Interv. 2011;78(1):47–51.
28. Liang M, Puri A, Linder R. Transradial simultaneous kissing stenting (SKS) with SheathLess access. Catheter Cardiovasc Interv. 2010;75(2):222–4.
29. Tanaka A, Saito S. Percutaneous coronary intervention with a virtual 2-Fr system. Catheter Cardiovasc Interv. 2010;76(5):684–6.
30. Takeshita S, Shiono T, Takagi A, Ito T, Saito S. Percutaneous coronary intervention using a novel 4-French coronary accessor. Catheter Cardiovasc Interv. 2008;72(2):222–7.
31. Takeshita S, Tanaka S, Saito S. Coronary intervention with 4-French catheters. Catheter Cardiovasc Interv. 2010;75(5):735–9.

Guidewires and Angioplasty Balloons: The Primer

8

Vijay S. Ramanath and Craig A. Thompson

Introduction and Historical Perspective

The year 1963 marked one of the greatest achievements in cardiovascular medicine when Dr. Charles Dotter recanalized an occluded right common iliac artery percutaneously by crossing the catheter across the artery in a retrograde fashion [1]. Quickly realizing the therapeutic potential of this technique, he constructed balloon-mounted dilating catheters to restore flow to occluded or stenotic vessels in the peripheral circulation [2]. This was followed by the first successfully performed percutaneous transluminal coronary angioplasty (PTCA) in man by Dr. Andreas Gruentzig in 1977. In this procedure, no coronary guidewires or balloons were used. Rather, a preshaped guiding catheter was placed at the ostium of the coronary artery through which a dilatation catheter was advanced across the stenotic lesion and subsequently inflated (Fig. 8.1) [3]. It was not until 1982 when the first coronary angioplasty wire was developed by Simpson et al. [4]. From this time forward, coronary guidewires and balloons have rapidly developed into highly sophisticated devices with continual advancements in the technology being made each year. This chapter will discuss the basic construction of angioplasty guidewires and balloons to provide the reader a fundamental understanding of how and why these devices are designed.

V.S. Ramanath, MD, FACC
Department of Medicine, Texas A & M Health Science Center, College of Medicine, Bryan, TX, USA

C.A. Thompson, MD, MMSc (✉)
Cardiovascular Catheterization and Intervention, Yale New Haven Hospital, New Haven, CT, USA

Cardiology Section, Department of Medicine, Invasive Cardiology and Vascular Medicine, Yale University School of Medicine, 789 Howard Avenue, Dana 305, New Haven, CT 06520, USA
e-mail: craig.a.thompson99@icloud.com

C.A. Thompson (ed.), *Textbook of Cardiovascular Intervention*, DOI 10.1007/978-1-4471-4528-8_8, © Springer-Verlag London 2014

Guidewires

Basic Construction

Guidewire technology has rapidly evolved since the early 1980s to meet the demands of complex coronary anatomy and pathology. As the severity and complexity of CAD increase, the need for more sophisticated devices also rises in concert. When designing guidewires, the following performance characteristics are vital:

(a) Flexibility: the ability of the wire to bend when direct pressure is applied to the wire tip.
(b) Trackability: the ability of the wire to be advanced around tortuous segments of a vessel and provide adequate support to deliver equipment around bends.
(c) Torque transmission: a wire must be able to follow the course of the vessel. Torque transmission is the ability of the wire to transmit rotational forces to the distal tip of the wire in a 1:1 ratio to direct the wire into the desired vessel and maneuver around plaque or tortuous segment(s).
(d) Support: the ability of the wire to deliver equipment (balloons, stents, atherectomy devices, intravascular ultrasound probe, etc.) particularly around vessel bends without the wire buckling. This characteristic is dependent on the core diameter and core material (discussed below).
(e) Stiffness, including wire tip stiffness, is dependent primarily on the core material (steel vs. nitinol) and wire diameter.

Guidewires are made up of four components: (i) core, (ii) outer coating, (iii) the presence or absence of a polymer jacket or cover, and (iv) wire tip (Fig. 8.2).

(i) Core: The core of a coronary guidewire determines many of its performance characteristics. Core material is predominantly either stainless steel or nitinol or, more recently, a combination of the two. Stainless steel is a stiff material providing excellent support and has an enhanced ability to transmit push force and torque.

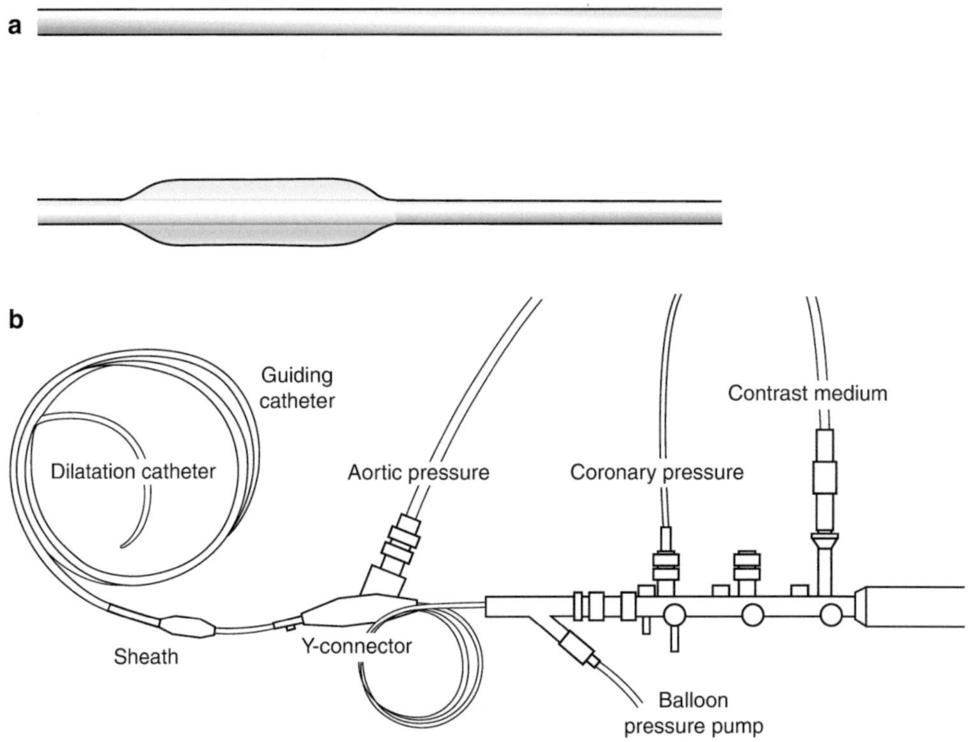

Fig. 8.1 Gruentzig's original coronary balloon angioplasty catheter. (**a**) First in man balloon made of polyvinyl chloride; (**b**) Double-lumen balloon catheter

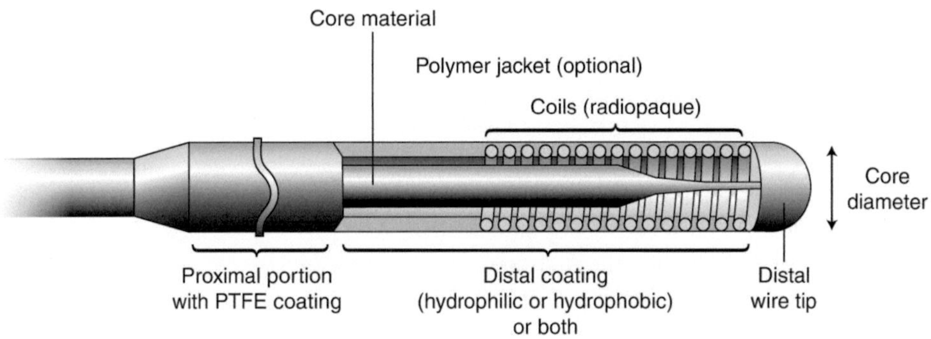

Fig. 8.2 Guidewire components. The proximal portion of most wires manufactured today are coated with polytetrafluoroethylene (*PTFE*), a hydrophobic material that provides a smooth, relatively frictionless surface across which balloons and stents can be passed with ease. The portion of the wire proximal to the PTFE-coated segment is composed of stainless steel

Thus, historically, stainless steel wires have been used to deliver stents in more difficult-to-reach areas (i.e., calcified, tortuous segments). When employed in the wire tip, it allows easy shaping, though, stainless steel tends to unshape ("poor shape memory"). Nitinol (a nickel titanium metal alloy) was discovered in 1962 and became a core material of coronary guidewires in 1996. Nitinol possesses many favorable features as a core material. It has considerable flexibility, durability, and has excellent "shape memory" which is particularly important in the wire tip. Furthermore, it has the ability to resist both kinking and deformation. These characteristics make nitinol more difficult to form; however, once the desired shape has been achieved, its durability allows the wire to more likely maintain its shape for the duration of the procedure. Table 8.1 summarizes the key features of stainless steel versus nitinol. Since both materials have characteristics that are desirable in a guidewire, attempts have been made to design "hybrid" guidewires (e.g., Balanced Middleweight [BMW] family of wires, Abbot Vascular, Runthrough™ NS, Terumo Corporation), which provide the support of stainless steel and the flexibility and shape memory of nitinol. In such a construction, the wire core is composed of stainless steel "jointed" to a segment of nitinol using either an adhesive or is welded together. The BMW wire core, for example, is stainless steel proximally with the distal portion consisting of nitinol. The Runthrough™ NS wire has a nitinol core proximal end with the tip overlayed

Table 8.1 Key features of nitinol and stainless steel as the core material

	Nitinol	Stainless steel
Rigidity/stiffness	Decreased	Increased
Shape memory	Increased	Decreased
Flexibility	Increased	Decreased
Susceptibility to kinking	Decreased	Increased

with platinum and stainless steel coils. An additional advantage to this hybrid construction is that such wires may be more reliably be used on more than 1 vessel in a single procedure due to its ability to maintain its shape and its ability to maintain a new shape if needed. Further developments in these two types of core material have resulted in variations within stainless steel and nitinol. As in any angioplasty guidewire, the core material possesses a certain degree of mechanical strength, which is best measured using a stress-strain curve (Fig. 8.3). With this in mind, developments have been made to improve the core material's ability to withstand stress and resist deformation. For example, newer stainless steel wires often are "spring tempered," which makes these wires more elastic, allowing them to withstand greater amounts of stress while still maintaining their original dimension. In other words, they are more resistant to damage during use. Likewise, certain nitinol wires possess super elastic properties that provide further resistance to kinking than conventional nitinol wires. Regardless of the material used, the wire core tapers towards the distal tip end (Fig. 8.2). If the guidewire core starts tapering more distally towards the tip, the coronary guidewire as a whole becomes more rigid providing increased support, steerability, and better torque transmission. However, with this design, there is a higher chance for wire prolapse. The opposite occurs when the core tapers more proximally allowing for a longer and more flexible tip (Fig. 8.4). An advantage of a more proximal taper is improved trackability of the wire. All coronary guidewires come in a range of overall diameters (0.010″–0.018″), the most common diameter being 0.014″.

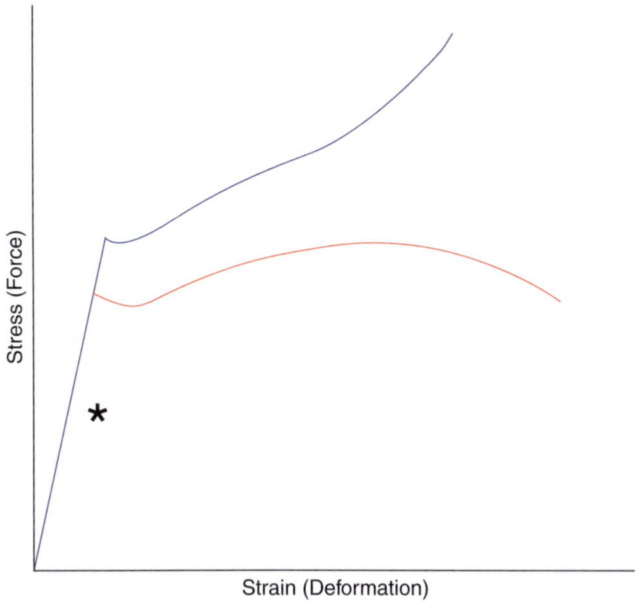

Fig. 8.3 Stress-strain curve of a guidewire. * denotes the elastic portion of the wire's core material in which the material will return to its original dimension when the stress is relieved. The part of the curve beyond the linear portion denotes permanent deformation in which the material does not return to its original dimension even if the stress is relieved. The *red curve* is an example of a wire with non-spring-tempered stainless steel; the *blue curve* exemplifies a wire with spring-tempered stainless steel and demonstrates the increased elasticity seen with spring-tempered stainless steel

(ii) Hydrophobic and hydrophilic coating: Guidewires are equipped with either a hydrophobic or hydrophilic

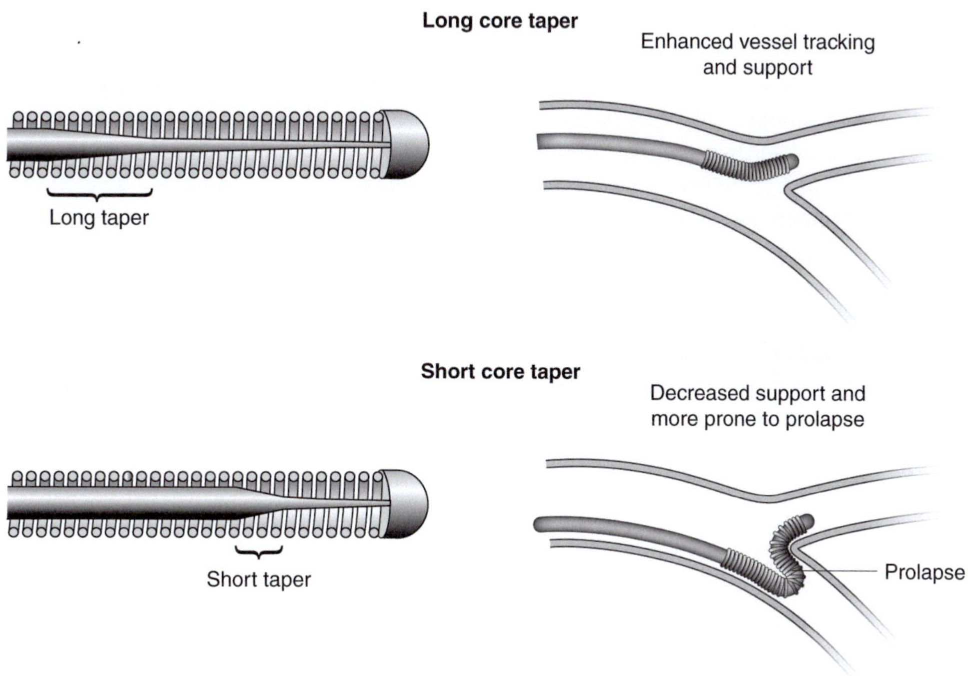

Fig. 8.4 Core taper lengths (long taper vs. short taper)

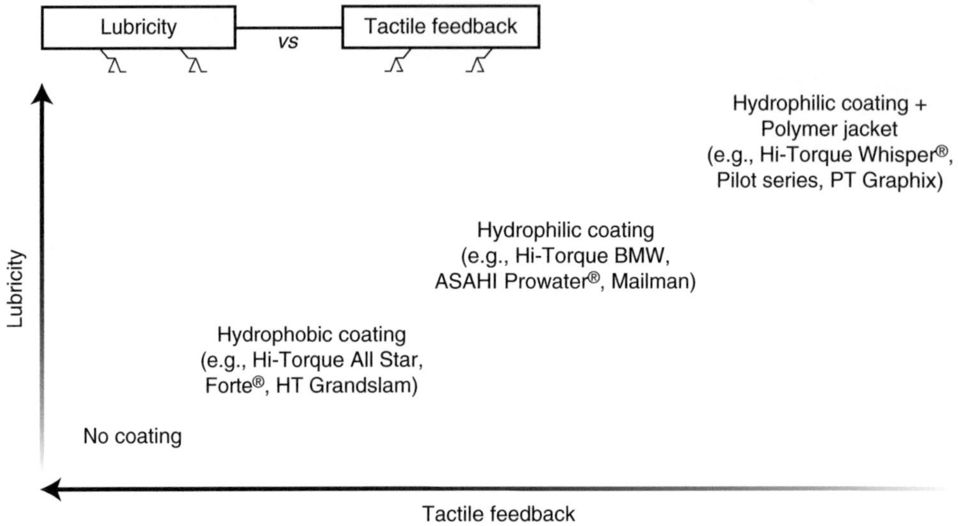

Fig. 8.5 Lubricity vs. tactile feedback

coating for the majority of their length. Typically, guidewires have a hydrophobic polytetrafluoroethylene (PTFE, Teflon®) coat proximally and either a hydrophobic or hydrophilic coating in the distal 30 cm of the wire to provide lubricity and aide in the delivery of equipment. As one would expect, hydrophilic coats provide greater lubricity than hydrophobic coatings. Hydrophilic coatings typically consist of two compounds: polyethylene oxide (PEO) and polyvinylpyrrolidone (PVP). These hydrophilic compounds are used because of their biocompatibility and ability to reduce friction between wire and vessel wall in order to maneuver through areas of tortuosity and stenoses. However, the more hydrophilic a wire is, the less tactile feedback the wire provides the operator and the more likely the wire can enter the subintimal space. This is important when confronted with complex lesions where the operator may require better tactile cues. In contrast, hydrophobic coatings are silicone-based and are less lubricious than hydrophilic coatings. They provide improved tactile feedback and are more likely to stay in the true lumen and thus less likely to cause vessel perforations. Thus, there is a "tug-of-war" between lubricity and tactile feedback, wherein a wire may be more lubricious due to a hydrophilic coating ± polymer cover but will have less tactile feedback, compared to a wire with a hydrophobic coating (Fig. 8.5). There are, however, variations on the distal coating: some wires such as the Asahi Miracle Bros wires possess a hydrophilic coat distally with a hydrophobic coating at the most distal 1–2 cm of the wire. The rationale for this construction is to provide the lubricity of a hydrophilic coat while the most distal 1–2 cm of hydrophobic coating provides enhanced tactile feedback. In contrast, some wires do not have any coating on the distal tip, which theoretically provides additional tactile feedback. An example of this is the Balanced Middleweight (Abbott Vascular, CA), ACS Hi-Torque Floppy (Boston Scientific, MA), and Choice PT (Boston Scientific, MA). Finally, some wires contain a combination of hydrophilic and hydrophobic coat (examples include the Asahi Prowater and Confianza Pro 9 and Pro 12 [Abbott Vascular, CA]).

(iii) Wire tip: The construction of the wire tip consists of coils and the core material. Coils allow the tip to be formed while maintaining a certain degree of rigidity for torque control in addition to providing friction for tactile feedback. Wire tips either consist of stainless steel in its entirety or can consist of steel bonded to nitinol approximately 3 cm from the wire tip. Wire tip construction can either be of the type in which the core material extends in its entirety all the way to the very distal tip without interruption (so-called core-to-tip) or be of the type in which a length of flattened stainless steel is soldered onto the end of the core to bridge the gap (so-called shaping ribbon). The shaping ribbon design was developed after nitinol began to be used as core material to allow the tip to retain its curve during shaping, as a tip made purely of nitinol (particularly super elastic nitinol) will spring back to a straight position upon shaping. One theoretical advantage to a core-to-tip style over the shaping ribbon is that it may provide a slight improvement in torque transmission, as the soldered joint of the shaping ribbon may not transmit torque as efficiently. Guidewires contain wire tips with varying degrees of resistance to wire buckling ("tip load"). The higher the tip load, the more the wire is able to withstand and pierce the lesion without buckling. Table 8.2 provides examples of coronary guidewires with their corresponding tip loads. Wire tips range from 0.009″ to 0.014″ and are manufactured either with a preformed J-tip or straight in which case the operator forms the tip to his/her needs.

(iv) Polymer jackets/covers: A number of wires manufactured today possess a polymer coating either over the entire wire including the coiled tip or excluding the distal coils (Fig. 8.1). This flexible polymer is commonly made of polyurethane with tungsten fillers, which allows the wire to be radio-opaque. The purpose of the polymer jacket is to provide a smooth surface and additional lubricity for enhanced maneuverability.

Table 8.2 Tip loads of some commonly used guidewires

Guidewire	Tip load[a] (g)
Forte Moderate Support	0.6
Forte Extra Support	0.6
Hi-Torque Balance Middleweight	0.7
Asahi Grand Slam	0.8
Mailman	0.8
Kinetix	0.8
Hi-Torque Whisper MS	1
Hi-Torque Iron Man	1
Asahi Prowater	1.1
Hi-Torque Whisper Extra Support	1.2
Hi-Torque Advance	1.3
Hi-Torque Pilot 50	1.3
PT Graphix	1.7
Choice PT	2.1
Asahi Miracle Bros 3	3.9
Asahi Miracle Bros 6	8.8
Asahi Confianza Pro	9.3
Asahi Confianza Pro 12	12.4
Asahi Miracle Bros 12	13
Luge	0.9
Kinetix Plus	1.3

[a]Tip load is a measurement of tip resistance to buckling. For example, the Asahi Miracle Bros 12 has a 13× more resistant tip to buckling than the Hi-Torque Whisper MS wire

Specialty Guidewires

As angioplasty guidewires become more sophisticated, the demand for performing successful percutaneous interventions also rises, which include percutaneous interventions on complex lesions such as chronic total occlusions (CTOs). In order to meet this challenge, a variety of specialty guidewires have been developed which include extra-support wires. Such wires possess an extra thick core material (stainless steel or nitinol). Examples of such wires include the Hi-Torque Balance Heavyweight (Abbott Vascular, CA), Hi-Torque All Star (Abbott Vascular, CA), Hi-Torque Iron Man (Abbott Vascular, CA), and the Asahi Grand Slam wire (Abbott Vascular, CA). Other extra-support wires, particularly used in CTOs, occasionally include the Asahi Miracle Bros series (3, 4.5, 6, 12 g [Abbott Vascular, CA]), Asahi Confianza (including the tapered tip Confianza Pro 12 [Abbott Vascular, CA]), and Hi-Torque Pilot series wires (50, 150, 200 [Abbott Vascular, CA]). These wires will be discussed in more detail in the chapter regarding complex interventions.

With the fundamental characteristics and construction discussed above, Table 8.3 summarizes the features of some commonly used coronary guidewires.

Table 8.3 Characteristics of some commonly used guidewires

Guidewire	Core material	Coating	Wire tip	Polymer jacket	Tip stiffness (g)
Workhorse wires					
HT Balance Middleweight	Nitinol	Hydrophilic	Shaping Ribbon	Absent	0.7
Asahi Prowater	Stainless steel	Hybrid	Core-to-tip	Absent	1.1
PT Graphix	Stainless steel	Hydrophilic	Core-to-tip	Present	1.7
PT2	Nitinol	Hydrophilic	Shaping Ribbon	Present	2.9
Forte	Stainless steel	Hydrophobic	Core-to-tip	Absent	0.6
Luge	Stainless steel	Hybrid	Core-to-tip	Present	0.9
Runthrough NS	Hybrid	Hydrophilic	Core-to-tip	Absent	1
Kinetix, Kinetix Plus	Nitinol	Hydrophilic	Shaping ribbon	Absent	0.8, 1.3
HT Whisper MS	Stainless steel	Hydrophilic	Core-to-tip	Present	1
HT Pilot 50	Stainless steel	Hydrophilic	Core-to-tip	Present	1.5
Choice PT floppy	Stainless steel	Hydrophilic	Core-to-tip	Present	2.1
Asahi Fielder FC	Stainless steel	Hydrophilic	Core-to-tip	Present	1.6
Extra support wires					
Mailman	Stainless steel	Hydrophilic	Core-to-tip	Absent	0.8
HT Balance Heavyweight	Nitinol	Hydrophilic	Shaping ribbon	Absent	0.7
HT Grand Slam	Stainless steel	Hydrophobic	Core-to-tip	Absent	0.8
Choice Extra Support	Stainless steel	Hydrophilic	Core-to-tip	Present	0.9
HT Iron Man	Stainless steel	Hydrophobic	Core-to-tip	Absent	1
Specialty wires					
HT Pilot 150, 200	Stainless steel	Hydrophilic	Core-to-tip	Present	2.7, 4.1
Asahi Fielder XT	Stainless steel	Hydrophilic	Core-to-tip	Present	1.2
Asahi Miracle Bros (3, 4.5, 6, 12)	Stainless steel	Hydrophobic	Core-to-tip	Absent	3.9, 4.4, 8.8, 13.0
Asahi Confianza Pro (9, 12)	Stainless steel	Hybrid	Core-to-tip	Absent	9.3, 12.4

Angioplasty Balloons

General Construction

The basic components of angioplasty balloon catheters include the balloon tip, wire port, mid-shaft, and manifold (Fig. 8.6). The distal tip typically measures 0.017–0.019″ in diameter and is typically designed with a tapered tip to aide in crossing lesions, maneuver around vessel bends, or to avoid getting hung up on plaque, calcified areas, or stent struts (during post-stent deployment dilatation). The shaft of the balloon similar to the balloon itself is composed of nylon or nylon along with a copolymer (discussed below).

Evolution of Angioplasty Balloons

Angioplasty balloons, like guidewires (discussed above), have evolved significantly since its initial prototype in 1970. The earliest angioplasty balloons in the 1980s were made of low-density polyethylene (LDPE), a flexible material with a low-pressure range, large profile (i.e., thicker, bulkier), and thus were more difficult to deliver to the distal vessel and more likely to rupture. In order to improve on this limitation, the next generation of balloons was constructed out of polyethylene terephthalate (PET), a stiff material with a higher pressure range and smaller profile, which increased their deliverability and threshold to rupture upon inflation. The current era angioplasty balloons are most commonly made of nylon or the low-density copolymer polyether block amide (PEBA or PEBAX®). Nylon is a very stiff and noncompliant material while PEBA is extremely compliant, thin, and flexible. Thus, the material of currently manufactured balloons optimizes a balloon's flexibility and profile and allows for a wide range of pressure inflations with a resultant high threshold to rupture. Because PEBA is a very thin yet durable material, it allows the ability for balloons to be designed with multiple layers to increase the durability of the balloon and increase the balloon's puncture resistance from calcified or fibrotic lesions. For example, a 2.5 or 3 mm semi-compliant balloon typically has a thickness of<1/1,000″. For this reason, the majority of coronary angioplasty balloons today are made of PEBA, while most peripheral angioplasty balloons are made of the bulkier nylon material. Balloon material in combination with its manufacturing process (e.g., stretching the material at high temperatures to change its compliance) determines the performance of the balloon, such as its compliance and rated burst pressure.

There are a number of grades of stiffness within PEBA. In balloons with multilayers of PEBA, the outer surface of the balloon may consist of a more rigid grade of PEBA while the inner layer may be made of the softer grade (e.g., NC Trek, Abbott Vascular, CA), though this may vary depending on the balloon's manufacturer. Other manufacturers of NC balloons consist of single layer of a stiff grade of PEBAX (e.g., Quantum Apex, Boston Scientific, MA).

Characteristics of Angioplasty Balloons

The primary characteristic of an angioplasty balloon is its degree of compliance or noncompliance. Compliance refers to the ability of a balloon to expand in diameter for a given amount of applied internal pressure. Most angioplasty balloons used today are either of the semi-compliant or noncompliant type. Semi-compliant balloons are those that grow as the atmospheres of internal hydraulic pressure increase. The more compliant the balloon, the more limited

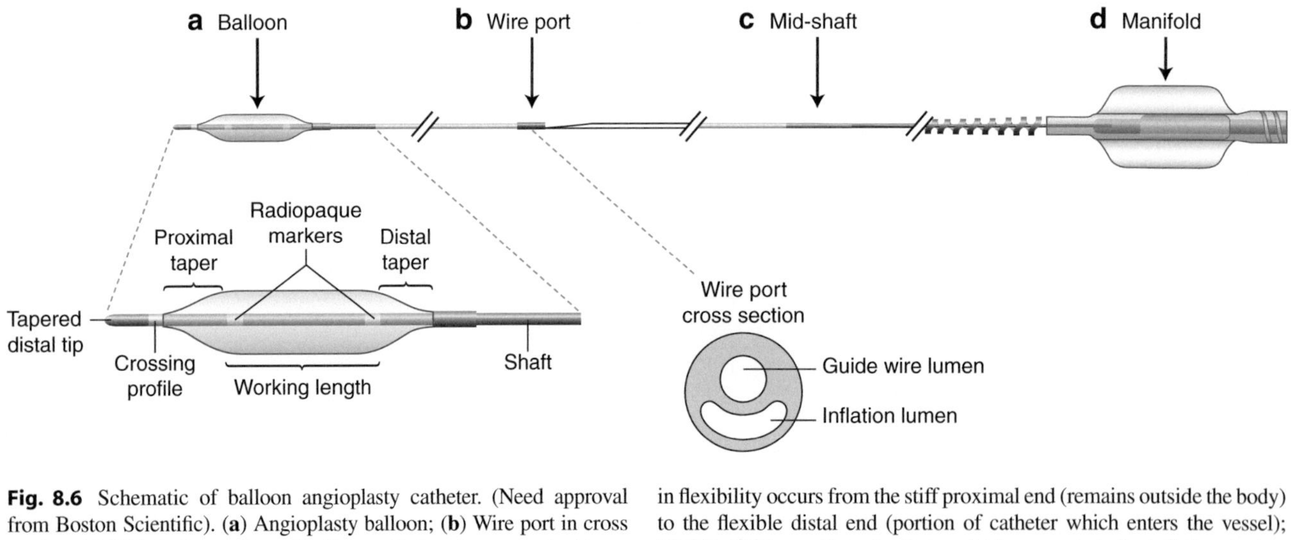

Fig. 8.6 Schematic of balloon angioplasty catheter. (Need approval from Boston Scientific). (**a**) Angioplasty balloon; (**b**) Wire port in cross section; (**c**) Mid-shaft – portion of balloon catheter where a gradual taper in flexibility occurs from the stiff proximal end (remains outside the body) to the flexible distal end (portion of catheter which enters the vessel); (**d**) Manifold – portion of catheter which connects to the inflation device

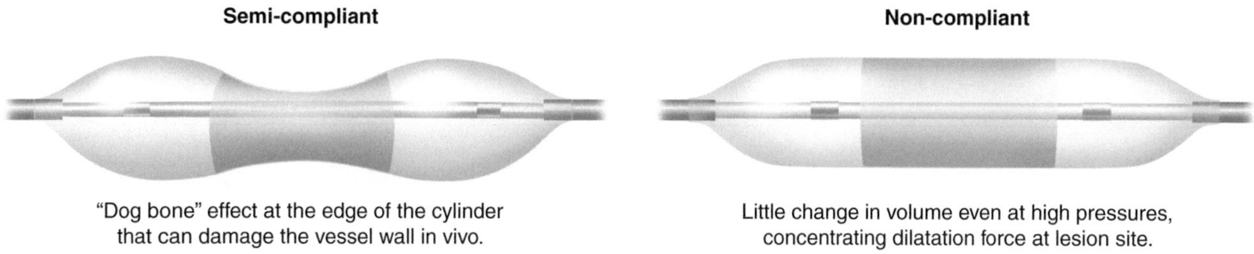

Fig. 8.7 (*Left*) "Dog bone" effect at the edge of the cylinder that can damage the vessel wall in vivo. (*Right*) Little change in volume even at high pressures, concentrating dilatation force at the lesion site

Fig. 8.8 Schematic of cutting balloon® (Boston Scientific, MA)

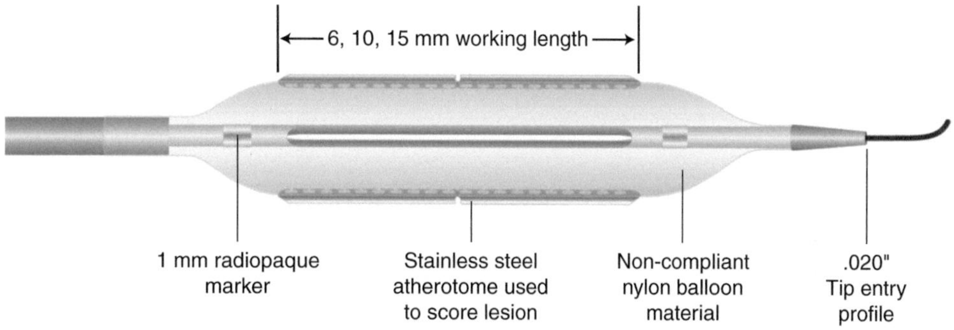

the pressure range in which it can expand without rupturing. In contrast, noncompliant balloons are those whose growth is limited despite increasing atmospheres of internal hydraulic pressure. The more noncompliant a balloon, the more limited its diameter will increase as the internal pressure increases. Compared to compliant or semi-compliant balloons, noncompliant balloons are thick walled, bulkier, and consist of stiffer grade of PEBA or have multiple layers of PEBA with a stiffer grade of PEBA on the outer surface and a softer grade of PEBA on the inner surface. This stiffer grade of PEBA that is used along with techniques during manufacturing allows this class of balloons to have higher burst pressures than their semi-compliant counterparts. The goal of noncompliant balloons is to apply dilatory force to an area of interest while limiting the growth at its edges. In doing so, it avoids stretching outside the lesion or stent margins, a concept often referred to as "dog-boning" (Fig. 8.7). As such, it is ideal for dilating stented segments of a vessel or unyielding calcified lesions. Other important characteristics of a balloon include its nominal pressure (the pressure at which the balloon reaches its stated diameter) and rated burst pressure (the pressure below which 99.9 % of balloons will not rupture as determined during bench testing).

Finally, a more recent classification of angioplasty balloons were designed in the late 1990s with "blades" or wires mounted on them in order to cut or score lesions upon inflation. Cutting balloons (e.g., Flextome, Boston Scientific, MA) are nylon-based noncompliant balloons with stainless steel atherotomes ("blades") that are mounted longitudinally on the balloon surface (Fig. 8.8). These devices are particularly useful in in-stent restenotic lesions or lesions with heavy calcification or fibrosis that are unyielding with conventional semi-compliant balloons or even with noncompliant balloons. Scoring balloons such as AngioSculpt (AngioScore, Fremont, CA) work with a similar premise in that the wire braid on the external surface of the balloon improves stability during inflation and provides superior preparation with controlled dissection and expansion.

Choice of Angioplasty Balloon

There are a number of important considerations when choosing the appropriate balloon. When doing so, the operator must take into account the size of the vessel, the morphology of the lesion (calcified, thrombus, etc.), and other factors such as the presence of proximally located diseased segments through which the balloon will need to pass through to reach the index lesion. In addition to the features mentioned above, currently available balloons are frequently designed to reach ~1/4 mm larger than the stated size. This reduces the degree of precision when deciding on a balloon based on vessel or lesion diameter. In addition, current balloons are designed as either over-the-wire (OTW) or monorail. Historically, the original balloons were of the OTW design. However, this design made the balloons more difficult to manage outside the body, particularly during single operator procedures. Thus, angioplasty balloons were later designed as monorail or rapid exchange which is far easier to manage for a single operator and as a result can reduce procedure times.

Summary

Both angioplasty guidewires and balloons have evolved into very sophisticated devices since the time of Drs. Dotter and Gruentzig to successfully maneuver around complex lesions and anatomy. These devices continue to evolve rapidly as the technology develops and play an enormous role as angioplasty becomes the very forefront in the management of coronary and peripheral atherosclerosis.

References

1. Dotter CT. Presentation at the 1963 Czechoslovak Radiological Congress, Prague, 1963 June 10.
2. Dotter CT. Transluminal angioplasty: a long view. Radiology. 1980;135:561–4.
3. Gruentzig A. Transluminal dilatation of coronary-artery stenosis. Lancet. 1978;1(8058):263.
4. Simpson JB, Baim DS, Robert EW, Harrison DC. A new catheter system for coronary angioplasty. Am J Cardiol. 1982;49:1216–22.

Coronary Atherectomy (Rotational, Laser, Directional) and Thrombus Extraction

9

Bruce D. Hettleman and Jason R. Foerst

When compared to balloon angioplasty with or without coronary stenting, ablative devices including coronary atherectomy (both directional and rotational), laser angioplasty, or cutting balloon angioplasty failed to show improved mortality, restenosis rates, repeat revascularization rates, or cumulative adverse cardiac event rates up to 1 year after treatment (Fig. 9.1) [1, 2]. In fact, periprocedural myocardial infarction and major adverse cardiac events were increased. Drug-eluting stents have eclipsed prior results providing markedly reduced angiographic restenosis and target vessel revascularization with low procedural complication. Balloon angioplasty followed by drug-eluting stent placement provides improved long-term outcome with less procedural complexity, time, radiation exposure, and cost. Thus, trials and common practice do not support routine plaque modification with these tissue ablative devices prior to stent placement [3]. In fact, directional coronary atherectomy is no longer supported in the United States as the only available device; the FlexiCut catheter (Abbott Vascular) is no longer available and there are no plans for replacement. Laser coronary angioplasty did not fulfill initial expectations of photochemical effects with vascular sparing. Despite these problems, rotational atherectomy remains a valuable tool facilitating durable success when stents cannot otherwise be delivered or expanded [4–6].

Heavily calcified, dilation-resistant fibrotic coronary lesions continue to represent a significant challenge for the coronary interventionalist. These lesions typically reside in vessels with advanced disease sometimes in association with proximal vessel curvature or scattered moderate fibrocalcific disease. Balloon dilation-resistant lesions may also occur unexpectedly in relatively focal disease but with significant superficial calcification. These situations provide technical challenges of two types: dilating severe lesions and delivering stents to those lesions. These lesions typically dilate poorly even with modern noncompliant high-pressure balloons and dissections and perforations may occur. Even if the lesions yield at high pressure, stent delivery may be problematic and refractory to advanced delivery techniques including supportive guides, "buddy" wires, and anchoring methods. Inadequate results occur if a stent is unable to be delivered or well expanded with increased risks of stent thrombosis (Fig. 9.2). Importantly, the excessive vessel manipulation required to treat these lesions may result in vessel dissection and occlusion with poor bailout options. If a target vessel is clearly heavily calcified by either fluoroscopy or IVUS or if there is difficulty advancing a balloon to or through the target lesion or balloon expansion is poor, then it is reasonable to assume that the standard balloon and stent approach will fail.

Rotational Atherectomy

Rotational atherectomy is currently a reliable, well-tested technique to achieve successful and durable percutaneous revascularization in these circumstances. This method bears little resemblance to the standard techniques commonly used by the coronary interventionalist and thus a different skill set needs to be acquired. Common experience has shown that rotational atherectomy needs to be performed early in the procedure prior to causing significant vessel dissection, which may limit the advisability of rotational atherectomy.

The only available high-speed rotational atherectomy system approved for coronary vessels is the Rotablator (Boston Scientific, Natick, MA) approved by the FDA in 1993. This device employs a diamond chip-coated brass burr able to rotate at high speeds (Fig. 9.3). The burr is attached to a drive shaft able to accommodate a steerable 0.009-in. stainless steel guidewire over which the device is advanced. The distal portion of the burr is embedded with diamond crystals having 5 μm extruding from a nickel coating. The burr has a smooth

B.D. Hettleman, MD, FACC, SCAI (✉)
Section of Cardiology, Department of Medicine,
Dartmouth-Hitchcock Medical Center,
Geisel School of Medicine, Lebanon, NH, USA
e-mail: bruce.d.hettleman@hitchcock.org

J.R. Foerst
Virginia Tech-Carilion School of Medicine and Research Institute,
Roanoke, VA, USA

C.A. Thompson (ed.), *Textbook of Cardiovascular Intervention*,
DOI 10.1007/978-1-4471-4528-8_9, © Springer-Verlag London 2014

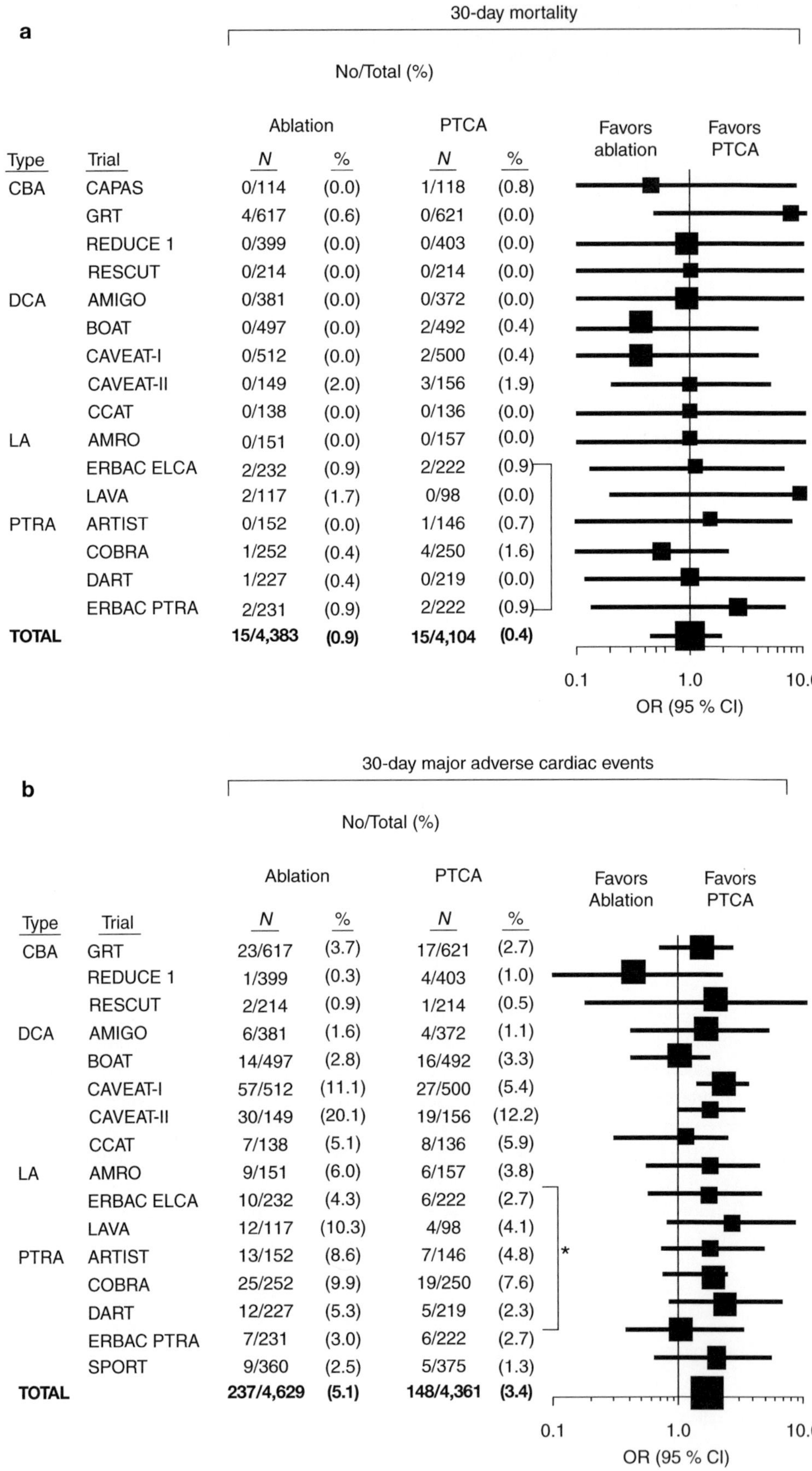

a 30-day mortality

Type	Trial	Ablation *N*	Ablation %	PTCA *N*	PTCA %
CBA	CAPAS	0/114	(0.0)	1/118	(0.8)
	GRT	4/617	(0.6)	0/621	(0.0)
	REDUCE 1	0/399	(0.0)	0/403	(0.0)
	RESCUT	0/214	(0.0)	0/214	(0.0)
DCA	AMIGO	0/381	(0.0)	0/372	(0.0)
	BOAT	0/497	(0.0)	2/492	(0.4)
	CAVEAT-I	0/512	(0.0)	2/500	(0.4)
	CAVEAT-II	0/149	(2.0)	3/156	(1.9)
	CCAT	0/138	(0.0)	0/136	(0.0)
LA	AMRO	0/151	(0.0)	0/157	(0.0)
	ERBAC ELCA	2/232	(0.9)	2/222	(0.9)
	LAVA	2/117	(1.7)	0/98	(0.0)
PTRA	ARTIST	0/152	(0.0)	1/146	(0.7)
	COBRA	1/252	(0.4)	4/250	(1.6)
	DART	1/227	(0.4)	0/219	(0.0)
	ERBAC PTRA	2/231	(0.9)	2/222	(0.9)
TOTAL		**15/4,383**	**(0.9)**	**15/4,104**	**(0.4)**

b 30-day major adverse cardiac events

Type	Trial	Ablation *N*	Ablation %	PTCA *N*	PTCA %
CBA	GRT	23/617	(3.7)	17/621	(2.7)
	REDUCE 1	1/399	(0.3)	4/403	(1.0)
	RESCUT	2/214	(0.9)	1/214	(0.5)
DCA	AMIGO	6/381	(1.6)	4/372	(1.1)
	BOAT	14/497	(2.8)	16/492	(3.3)
	CAVEAT-I	57/512	(11.1)	27/500	(5.4)
	CAVEAT-II	30/149	(20.1)	19/156	(12.2)
	CCAT	7/138	(5.1)	8/136	(5.9)
LA	AMRO	9/151	(6.0)	6/157	(3.8)
	ERBAC ELCA	10/232	(4.3)	6/222	(2.7)
	LAVA	12/117	(10.3)	4/98	(4.1)
PTRA	ARTIST	13/152	(8.6)	7/146	(4.8)
	COBRA	25/252	(9.9)	19/250	(7.6)
	DART	12/227	(5.3)	5/219	(2.3)
	ERBAC PTRA	7/231	(3.0)	6/222	(2.7)
	SPORT	9/360	(2.5)	5/375	(1.3)
TOTAL		**237/4,629**	**(5.1)**	**148/4,361**	**(3.4)**

Fig. 9.1 Meta-analysis of randomized trials of percutaneous transluminal coronary angioplasty versus atherectomy, cutting balloon atherotomy, or laser angioplasty. (**a**) Mortality by treatment assignment up to 30 days. (**b**) Major adverse cardiac events up to 30 days. (**c**) Major adverse cardiac event rates up to 360 days. *CBA* coronary balloon atherotomy, *CI* confidence interval, *DCA* directional coronary atherectomy, *LA* (excimer or holmium) laser angioplasty, *OR* odds ratio, *PTRA* percutaneous transluminal rotational atherectomy, *PTCA* percutaneous transluminal coronary angioplasty (*The ERBAC control groups are identical) (From Bittl et al. [1], with permission.)

Fig. 9.1 (continued)

c

Cumulative major adverse cardiac events up to 360 days

No/Total (%)

Type	Trial	Ablation *N*	Ablation %	PTCA *N*	PTCA %
CBA	CAPAS	31/144	(27.2)	46/118	(39.0)
	GRT	84/617	(13.6)	94/621	(15.1)
	REDUCE 1	92/399	(23.1)	84/403	(20.8)
	RESCUT	35/214	(16.4)	33/214	(15.4)
DCA	BOAT	115/497	(23.1)	153/492	(31.1)
	CAVEAT-I	216/512	(42.4)	193/500	(38.7)
	CAVEAT-II	60/149	(40.3)	69/156	(44.3)
	CCAT	40/138	(29.0)	39/136	(28.7)
LA	AMRO	50/151	(33.1)	47/157	(29.9)
	ERBAC ELCA	10/211	(47.9)	70/191	(36.6)
	LAVA	41/117	(35.0)	33/98	(33.7)
PTRA	ARTIST	31/152	(20.4)	13/146	(8.9) *
	COBRA	72/210	(35.7)	75/213	(35.2)
	DART	59/227	(26.0)	54/219	(24.7)
	ERBAC PTRA	94/205	(45.9)	70/191	(36.6)
	SPORT	63/360	(17.5)	51/375	(13.6)
TOTAL		**1187/4,273**	**(27.8)**	**1054/4,039**	**(26.1)**

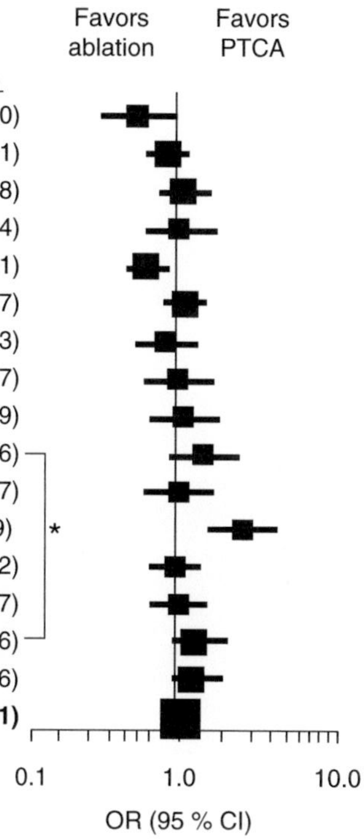

proximal surface not coated with diamond crystals. The driveshaft is covered by a 4.3F (0.058 in.) Teflon sheath that protects tissue from the spinning driveshaft and allows flush solutions to lubricate the driveshaft and burr and provides vasodilators during use. Typical flush solutions (rotaflush) contain 20 cm^3 of Rotaglide Lubricant (emulsion of olive oil and egg yolks), 4 mg of nitroglycerin, 5,000–10,000 units of heparin, and some add 4 mg of verapamil per liter of normal saline. The RotaWire guidewire is a specialized product 330 cm long constructed of stainless steel. Having a 0.014-in. diameter 2.2 cm spring tip, the wire then transitions from 0.005 in. diameter to 0.009 in. on its proximal end. The RotaWire Floppy is used in nearly all cases due to its ability to follow vessel contours with reduced guidewire bias compared to the RotaWire Extra Support (Fig. 9.4). This reduces the possibility of ablation of healthy tissue due to a more asymmetric course taken by the stiffer, extra support wire resulting in greater engagement of the lumen wall by the burr. The stiffer wire was designed to reach distal lesions. The Rotalink burr catheter is available in 1.25–2.5 mm sizes. The Rotalink system allows the burr size to be changed without replacing the entire drive unit. The catheter's driveshaft is connected to a turbine driven by compressed nitrogen. The burr is activated by a foot pedal, and the rotational speed is measured by a fiber optic cable and controlled by a dial on the device's monitor.

Mechanism

Rotational atherectomy works by mechanical plaque abrasion and pulverization applying the principle of differential cutting and orthogonal displacement of friction. Orthogonal displacement of friction allows the spinning burr to negotiate tortuous segments allowing access to more distal lesions that might impede a stent or even at times a balloon-dilating catheter. Differential cutting spares normal elastic tissue while destroying inelastic fibrocalcific plaques. Inelastic calcified elements are pulverized by the advancing burr while elastic elements are deflected and spared. IVUS studies have shown that fibrocalcific material is removed without arterial expansion [7–9]. In addition, angiographic follow-up studies have shown that adjacent segments are not adversely affected and do not show accelerated atherosclerosis (Fig. 9.5). Plaque pulverization ideally produces particulate debris small enough to pass through the myocardial capillary bed. Some studies have shown that uncomplicated rotational atherectomy can be performed without significant impact on myocardial perfusion. Rotational atherectomy and adjunctive PTCA significantly improved basal and hyperemic blood flow velocity and diastolic predominance of coronary blood flow with some improvement in coronary flow reserve [10]. However, the physiologic effects of rotational atherectomy

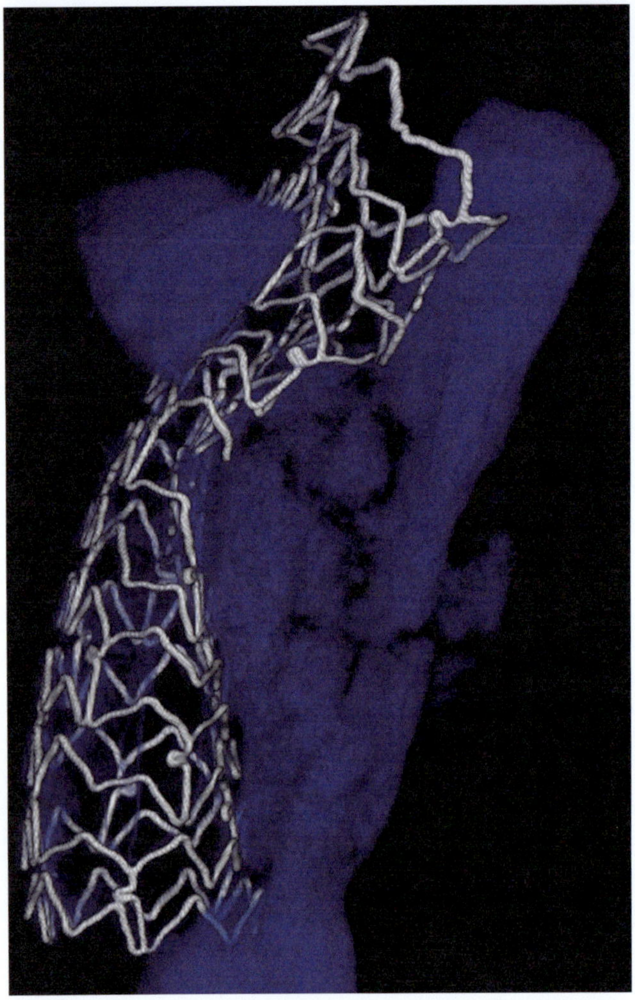

Fig. 9.2 MicroCT of incomplete stent expansion. A 72-year-old man presented with an anterior STEMI and underwent primary PCI of a calcified, proximal LAD lesion but ultimately died of cardiogenic shock. Postmortem microcomputed tomography image of the proximal LAD stent revealed poor stent expansion despite high-pressure balloon inflations with a noncompliant balloon (calcium shown in *blue*)

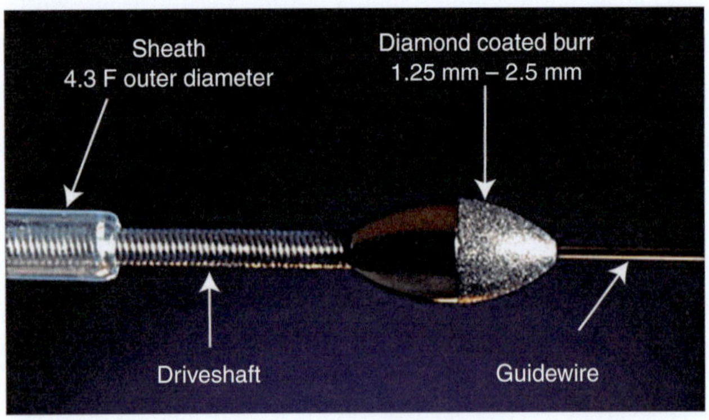

Fig. 9.3 Rotalink burr catheter (Courtesy of Boston Scientific)

can result in slow or no reflow in approximately 7–10 % of patients with associated myocardial injury and infarction including persistent ST elevation, CK release, and new Q waves in even higher percentages of treated patients. The mechanism for this is likely multifactorial and includes plaque debris, platelet aggregation, microcavitation, and vascular spasm, with capillary plugging and tissue edema. Using nuclear imaging, Koch et al. found that 87 % of patients having rotational atherectomy had transient perfusion defects which was decreased to 33 % in patients who received abciximab during the procedure [11–13].

Procedure

Rotational atherectomy is initiated with conventional angioplasty equipment. A 6F guide is able to accommodate the 1.25 and 1.5 mm burrs. Larger burrs up to 2.15 mm require an 8F guide (Table 9.1). A guide that is coaxial with the vessel and sits easily in the ostium should be chosen. Patients should be well hydrated and not hypotensive prior to initiating rotablation. If the target lesion is in the right coronary artery or dominant circumflex, then a temporary pacing wire should be placed in the right ventricle as significant transient bradycardia is unpredictable and common. Many operators use IIb/IIIa agents which have been shown to reduce burr-induced platelet activation and CK release [12, 14–16]. The presence of a IIb/IIIa agent substantially worsens the prognosis of perforation should that occur. The rotablator guidewire does not steer well and is prone to kinking. Although some operators favor steering this wire directly past the target lesion, it is generally best delivered distal to the target lesion via a transport catheter previously advanced over a "workhorse" 0.014-in. guidewire. The rotablator guidewire is placed distal to the lesion but not in the distal narrow vasculature. This allows the burr to remain centered when activated. The activated burr should not come into contact with the 0.014-in. spring tip. The rotablator guidewire is then back loaded through the rotalink burr catheter and brought through the rotalink advancer unit. A specialized clip torquer is then attached to keep the wire from spinning when the burr is activated. The device's compressed gas connector, fiber optic cable, and pressurized rotaflush saline solution infusion port are connected, and the burr is advanced over the wire to within a few cm of the guide catheter. Flowing pressurized saline solution is essential to cool and lubricate the spinning parts of the system. With the pressurized saline solution running, the system is activated and tested prior to advancing the burr into the guide catheter. The burr speed is adjusted to 150,000–160,000 rpm; saline flush solution is ensured and the advancer knob and wire brake are tested. Prior to inserting the burr into the guide catheter, the advancer knob is moved forward approximately 2–3 cm and locked in position. With the guide catheter well seated in the vessel ostium, the static burr is then advanced over the wire to a widely patent position in the target vessel at least 1–2 cm proximal to the lesion. The advancer knob is then retracted fully to relieve any tension on the driveshaft. This can be verified

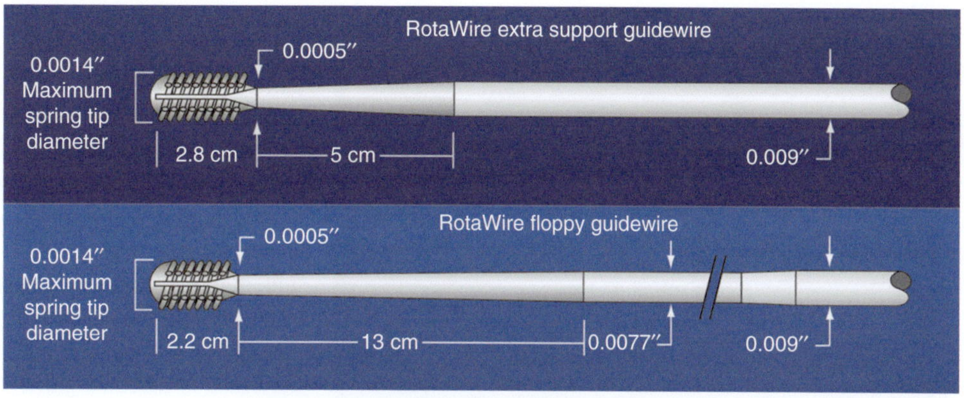

Fig. 9.4 RotaWire specifications

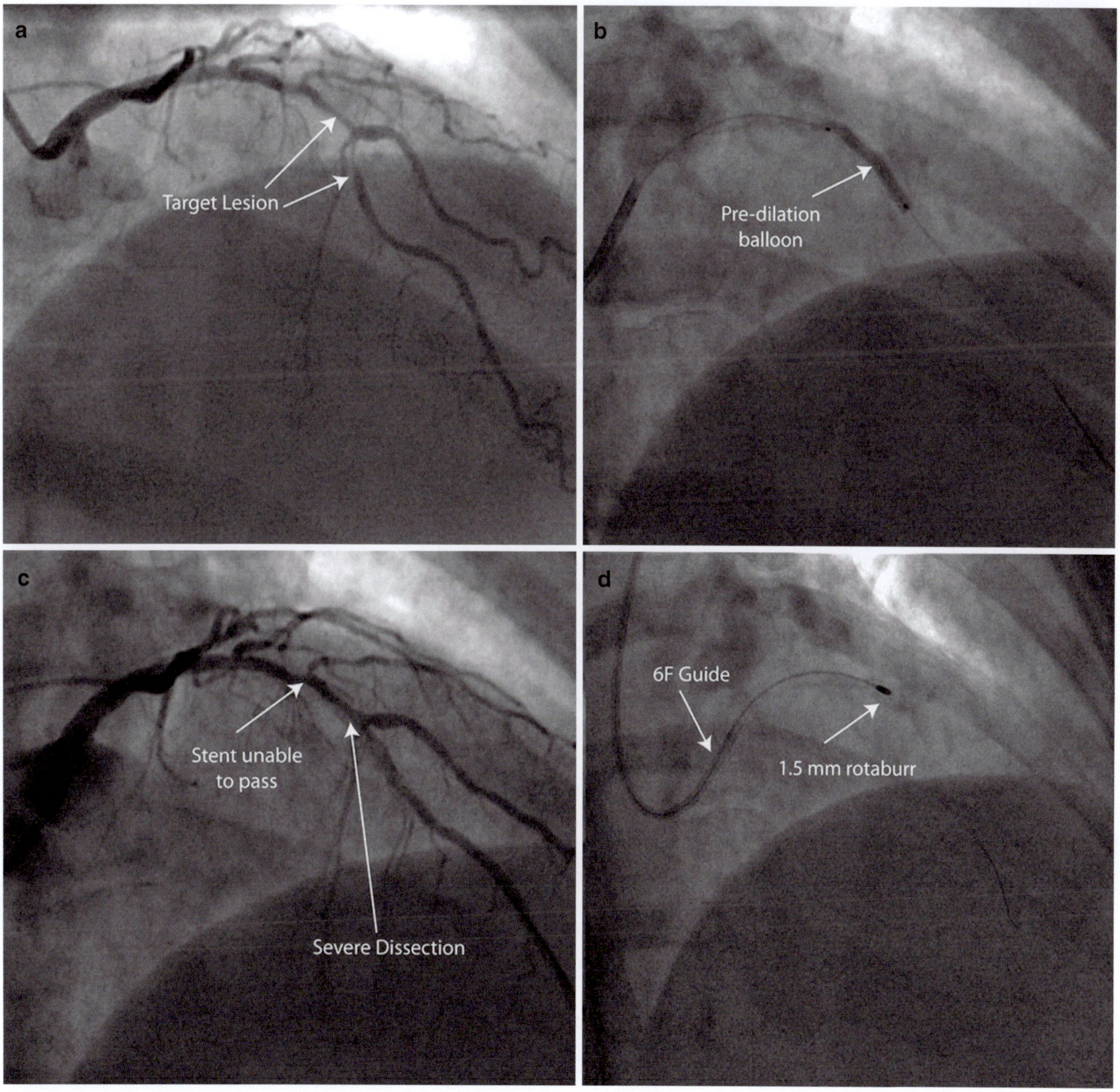

Fig. 9.5 Rota rescue case. (**a**) A 61-year-old woman presented with unstable angina and (**b**) developed severe dissection following pre-dilation of the mid LAD lesion. (**c**) Stents were unable to pass through an undilatable proximal segment until (**d**) rotational atherectomy was performed (**e**) allowing successful stent delivery

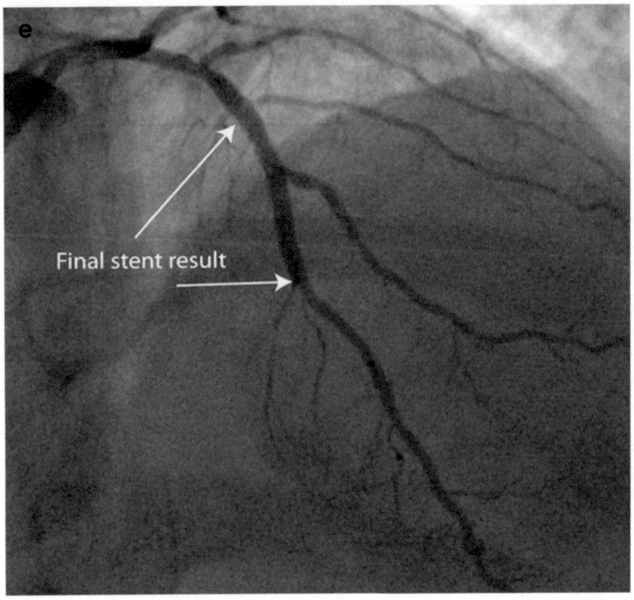

Fig. 9.5 (continued)

Table 9.1 Rotalink burr catheter and guide selection

Burr (mm)	Diameter (in.)	Recommended guide catheter (French)[a]	Minimum recommended guide catheter internal diameter (in.)
1.25	0.049	6.0	0.060[b]
1.50	0.059	6.0	0.063
1.75	0.069	7.0	0.073
2.00	0.079	8.0	0.083
2.15	0.085	8.0	0.089
2.25	0.089	9.0	0.093
2.38	0.094	9.0	0.098
2.50	0.098	9.0	0.102

[a]Guide sizes are based on larger lumen guide catheters
[b]The sheath size is the determinant of the minimum ID on the 1.25 mm burr

fluoroscopically by watching the burr retract slightly. Relieving drive shaft tension keeps the burr from jumping forward into the stenosis when the system is activated. The burr's rotational speed in the free lumen is checked again and adjusted prior to negotiating the lesion (platforming). The burr is then activated and gently advanced into the lesion with a tapping motion by advancing the controlling knob under fluoroscopic guidance. Intermittently pulling back on the advancer knob will allow improved blood flow during the rotablator run. Care should be taken not to allow decelerations of greater than 5,000 RPM to occur as this is associated with slow or no reflow and myocardial injury. The operator listens to the sound of the turbine, is aware of the RPM display on the monitor, and advances and withdraws the burr under fluoroscopic guidance deciding how firmly the burr can be safely advanced. After a 30-s run, the burr is then promptly withdrawn more proximally in the vessel free of the lesion and immediately deactivated. The patient is assessed both hemodynamically and with a small contrast injection to verify preserved flow and no perforation and to allow the patient time to recover. Small doses of intravenous phenylephrine may be required to treat transient hypotension. In addition, intracoronary calcium blockers such as nicardipine are commonly administered to treat abnormal flow. Once the hemodynamics and coronary flow have recovered, this sequence is repeated. The goal is to be able to pass the burr with minimal resistance and no decrease in the RPM measurement through the length of the lesion. Once this is accomplished, the foot pedal is used to switch to the dynaglide mode, the brake is defeated either manually or with the aid of the wire clip torquer, and the burr is removed maintaining distal wire position. A transport catheter is used to exchange the rotawire for a "workhorse" 0.014-in. wire, and adjunctive balloon angioplasty is typically performed prior to stent placement. Most operators no longer use a stepped burr approach and use only a single burr to facilitate lesion modification and PTCA/stent placement with a burr/artery of 0.5–0.6. In the unusual event the initial burr will not pass at 160,000 RPM, success may be achieved by downsizing to a 1.25 mm burr.

Early Studies

Rotablator was approved and used before modern stents were in widespread use. Much of the early experience is of historical significance, as rotational atherectomy is no longer performed without stent placement. The early trials defined acute outcomes and complications, restenosis rates, target vessel revascularization rates, and compared these parameters to other devices available at the time [1]. Early experience with rotational atherectomy was difficult with significant complication rates and no clear advantage over other modalities. Vessel perforation did occur. Adjunctive balloon angioplasty was essential to improve acute success rate [17, 18]. The angiographic restenosis rate ranged from 39 to 62 % which has been eclipsed by drug-eluting stents [19, 20]. The Stratas and Carat trials found no advantage to aggressive debulking with larger burrs (>0.7 burr/artery) and longer ablation times compared to more conservative debulking strategies [21, 22]. Aggressive debulking was associated with more serious angiographic complications and higher angiographic restenosis and target lesion revascularization. The incidence of reduced flow and myocardial injury resulting from rotational atherectomy is technique dependent [21–24]. Kini reported improvement in the incidence of slow flow from 9 to 2 % [24]. With optimized technique the incidence of slow flow and non-Q wave MI can be reduced to a few percent [25]. Several risk factors for the myocardial injury have been identified. These include long burr runs (greater than 30 s), decelerations (greater than 5,000 RPM for 5 s), aggressive burr sizing, and long lesions with presumed greater burden of pulverized debris.

Perforation

The incidence of coronary perforation with rotational atherectomy is 0.7–1 % in highly calcified coronary disease [5, 24, 26]. Al-Lamee et al. reported a 0.23 % incidence of grade III coronary perforations in a study of 24,445 patients undergoing interventions from 1993 to 2009 [27, 28]. Multivariate regression showed the odds ratio for grade III perforation was 5.36 for IVUS-guided procedures, 3.75 for type B2/C lesions, 3.47 if rotational atherectomy was performed, and 1.91 for total occlusions. A similar rate of grade III perforations (0.2 %) was found in another large cohort when no rotablation was performed [29]. Other large series reporting the incidence of coronary perforation list rotational atherectomy as a cause; however, perforation is also found with balloon angioplasty, stent placement, or due to manipulation of hydrophilic guidewires [30, 31]. While the incidence of perforation is higher with rotational atherectomy compared to balloon angioplasty, the high pressures required to expand these calcific lesions is also associated with an increased risk of balloon-induced vessel perforation. If perforation does occur, the presence of IIb/IIIa inhibitors is clearly an issue as more patients require placement of a covered stent or emergency surgery [15]. For this reason, some operators avoid IIb/IIIa inhibitors with rotational atherectomy.

Special Lesion Sets for Rotablator Use

Other than its use to facilitate stent delivery, rotablator has been reported to be useful in treating other lesion sets. Jailed side branches in previously stented vessels may be treated once the stent cell overlying the branch has been successfully balloon dilated but with a significant restenosis rate [32]. Calcified ostial RCA lesions are well treated with rotational atherectomy with durable results [33]. Ostial saphenous vein graft lesions may be treated with rotational atherectomy as well as lesions in internal mammary grafts [34, 35]. There is increasing use of rotational atherectomy in treatment of chronic total occlusion. While this is an evolving application, there is increasing experience and success within the lesion segment and even the subintimal space.

Rotational atherectomy should be avoided in lesions found in the body of saphenous vein grafts, situations with thrombus that cannot be removed, and in the acute MI setting because of the risk of distal embolization from thrombus or soft particulate matter. It is tempting to consider rotational atherectomy for diffuse in-stent restenosis as it does remove intimal hyperplasia compared to balloon dilation which works via tissue extrusion and further stent expansion. Compared to balloon angioplasty in the Artist trial, however, there was no significant benefit to rotational atherectomy for this indication [36]. Rotablator should be avoided in low ejection fraction situations or last vessel situations in which slow or no reflow would be catastrophic. Data from the Protect II trial showed less clinical benefit for patients undergoing high-risk percutaneous revascularization when rotational atherectomy was used in the group with Impella support. This may be related to the more vigorous use of rotational atherectomy in the impella 2.5 arm [37]. Other situations to avoid include eccentric lesions on a severe bend where wire bias is significant and the burr would be deflected away from the lesion toward normal vessel wall. Stand-alone rotablator or rotablator followed by adjunctive balloon angioplasty is not recommended due to unacceptably high restenosis rates.

Rotational Atherectomy in the Drug-Eluting Stent Era

Today, rotablator is used as an adjunct to balloon angioplasty to facilitate successful stent placement (Fig. 9.5). Intravascular ultrasound can be used to define which lesions will require rotablator to allow adequate stent expansion [9, 38, 39]. Superficial calcium deposits of over 180° are best treated with rotational atherectomy prior to stent placement. If vessels appear heavily calcified or if there is significant difficulty passing a balloon to or through a lesion or if a lesion will not yield at moderate pressures, rotational atherectomy is likely to facilitate successful revascularization. In the drug-eluting stent era, best practice parameters have established an excellent safety and outcome profile for rotational atherectomy in heavily calcified arteries [4, 5]. When used favoring a single conservatively sized burr approach followed by adjunctive balloon angioplasty and stent placement, Clavijo et al. found that lesions requiring rotational atherectomy prior to drug-eluting stent placement had similar acute and chronic outcomes to drug-eluting stent placement that did not require rotablator for successful implantation [4]. The primary success rate was 98 % with a low rate of in-hospital ischemic events. The target vessel revascularization rate was less than 5 % in both groups. Rotational atherectomy may be performed without harm in these circumstances as was found in a large multicenter registry of 1,537 stented patients with moderate to severe calcification in whom 7.5 % received rotational atherectomy prior to stent placement [40]. There was no difference in the efficacy and safety outcomes regardless of the use of rotational atherectomy in this study. Rathore et al. found that in a series of patients with heavily calcified coronary disease, rotational atherectomy followed by balloon angioplasty and stenting provided excellent primary success rates (97 %) using a single burr strategy 81 % of the time. In addition, the use of drug-eluting stents resulted in a 50 % reduction in angiographic binary restenosis compared to bare metal stents after rotational atherectomy (11 % vs. 28 %) [5]. Independent predictors of restenosis after rotational atherectomy were the use of bare metal stents, ostial location, chronic total occlusion, and dialysis-dependent chronic renal failure. But, lesion length, minimal lumen diameter, and final lumen area and diameter failed as independent predictors. Restenosis rates with bare metal stents after rotational atherectomy have been reported to be 22–28 % range [5, 41]. Although data are limited, available data favors drug-eluting stents over bare metal stents after rotational atherectomy with significantly less restenosis. The ROTAXUS study randomized 240 patients with complex calcified coronary lesions to either routine rotablation or balloon angioplasty prior to paclitaxel-eluting stent placement. A higher initial success rate was found in the routine rotablation group (92.5 % versus 83.3 %) with a crossover rate of 12.5 % in the balloon angioplasty arm. Routine rotational atherectomy before pacitaxel-eluting stent placement, however, was not superior to balloon agioplasty before stent placement with no difference in 9 month endpoints of binary restenosis (11 %), target lesion revascularization, stent thrombosis or MACE. Ballon angioplasty with only provisional rotational atherectomy is a reasonable default strategy for drug-eluting stent placement in complex calcified coronary lesions [42].

Laser Atherectomy

Excimer laser (XeCl) angioplasty catheters are available and are approved for use in the coronary vasculature (Spectranetics Corporation, Colorado Springs, Colorado) for the treatment of chronic total occlusions that are crossable with a guidewire, saphenous vein graft lesions, ostial lesions, long lesions, moderately calcified lesions, in-stent restenosis prior to the administration of intravascular brachytherapy, and balloon angioplasty dilatation failures. This excimer laser system is a pulsed-wave device operating at a wavelength of 308 nm in the ultraviolet spectrum and delivering pulses of 125 ns duration at a repetitive rate of up to 40 Hz. Laser energy is transmitted as a standing wave of intense monochromatic, coherent light which travels down optical fibers in the laser catheter appropriately positioned in a coronary artery or saphenous vein graft. The biologic effects of laser light depend on the tissue and its surrounding medium's ability to absorb the laser's wavelength and the mode of laser operation (pulsed or continuous) including the energy density (fluence). Radiation in the ultraviolet spectrum is absorbed by the atherosclerotic plaque and also has significant interaction with water. Pulsed systems were designed to reduce heating of surrounding tissue. Rather than photochemical effects, which provide enough energy to break molecular bonds with direct breakdown of molecules potentially providing vascular sparing, the excimer laser energy works predominantly through photothermal and photoacoustic effects [43–45]. Each excimer laser pulse generates a rapidly expanding and imploding vapor bubble. Powerful acoustic waves result which can cause tissue injury and dissection.

Excimer laser angioplasty can be performed with conventional guiding catheters. Coaxial guiding catheter alignment is important for successful device delivery. A catheter with a diameter at least 1 mm smaller than the reference vessel diameter is chosen. The Spectranetics Rx excimer laser catheters are available in sizes from 0.9 to 2.0 mm diameter and are 0.014 in. guidewire compatible. The 0.9 mm Rx and OTW catheters (Spectranetics Corporation) are 6F guide compatible and are used to treat lesions that cannot be crossed with a balloon-dilating catheter as long as local dissection has not occurred. With the laser catheter placed at the proximal end of the target lesion, the guide catheter and vessel are flushed with at least 30 ml of saline to eliminate the interaction of laser energy with contrast medium which may result in vessel dissection. Very slow catheter advancement is important. Once the process is complete, adjunctive balloon angioplasty and stenting are performed.

The initial expectation was that laser angioplasty would provide improved outcomes compared to balloon angioplasty. This was not the case based on published data and trials from the 1990s when the perforation rates were 1–2 % [1, 20, 46–48]. In addition, the experience with excimer laser angioplasty for calcified lesions was disappointing in comparison to rotational atherectomy in the ERBAC trial [20], and rotational atherectomy is preferred for advanced calcification. Improvements in the catheter design and technique with slow advancement and saline infusions may have reduced the risk of dissection and perforations [49–51]. The currently available excimer laser device is used to debulk plaque prior to stent placement in niche applications at experienced centers.

Directional Coronary Atherectomy

The only available device to perform directional coronary atherectomy (FlexiCut catheter, Abbott Vascular, Chicago, IL) has been withdrawn without plans for replacement, and thus this review of DCA is from an historical perspective. This original device (AtheroCath) consisted of a metallic housing with a balloon fixed to one side and a nosecone chamber to collect the cuttings provided by a cup-shaped cutter attached to a drive shaft activated by a battery-operated drive unit. The device could be rotated and oriented by the interventionalist to achieve debulking via directional atheroma excision. Some of the lumen gain achieved by the device was attributed to an angioplasty mechanism related to vessel dilation during atheroma excision. The device received its original FDA approval in 1990 and was quite bulky requiring large guiding catheters (10F) with specialized shapes and smooth curves. The AtheroCath was revised, and five generations of improvements were made to the design. The FlexiCut was 8F compatible but gave up some of the performance benefits of the larger catheters. Multiple trials comparing directional coronary atherectomy to balloon angioplasty with and without coronary stenting were performed [52–58]. These trials generated significant controversy in the interventional

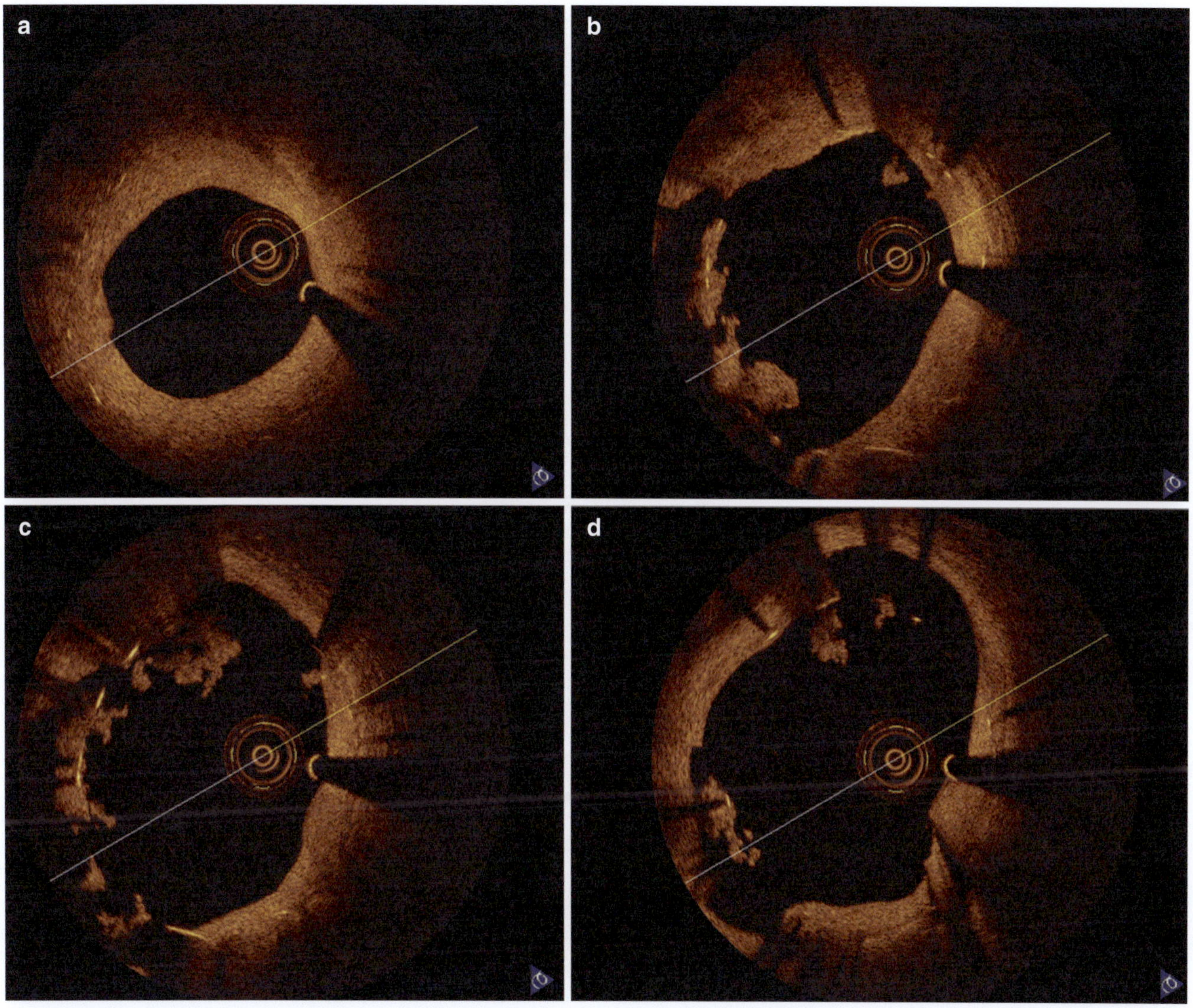

Fig. 9.6 Late stent thrombosis OCT image. A 67-year-old man with bare metal stent implanted in his proximal RCA 6 months prior developed chest pain 5 days after discontinuation of clopidogrel in anticipation of vascular surgery. OCT images demonstrate the bare metal stent with intimal hyperplasia distally (**a**) and poorly apposed struts with adherent thrombus as the imaging catheter is withdrawn proximally into an area of ectasia (**b–d**)

community about the relative merits of two techniques. After further analysis, routine directional coronary atherectomy was not found to have significant benefit over balloon angioplasty [1]. Acute complications were higher with directional coronary atherectomy including a 1 % risk of perforation. Due to its more technically demanding requirements, many interventionalists did not gain sufficient experience with DCA. In addition, once the benefits of routine stent placement were defined, use of DCA decreased.

Thrombus Extraction

Acute coronary syndromes develop as a result of plaque rupture or erosion with a common pathophysiologic pathway of thrombosis within the coronary artery [59]. The presence of intracoronary thrombus is associated with an increased risk of adverse outcomes after coronary angioplasty [60]. Furthermore, ballooning and stenting these thrombotic lesions can result in embolization of atherothrombotic debris. Significant residual thrombus at the time of stent deployment may result in incomplete late stent apposition and possible increased incidence of stent thrombosis (Fig. 9.6).

Silvain et al. used electron microscopy to analyze the contents of serial manual aspirations from ST elevation MI patients and better defined thrombus composition [61]. Platelet, fibrin, and red blood cell components were found in variable concentrations depending on the ischemic time frame. As the ischemic time increased, the thrombus was primarily a fibrin mesh; however, earlier presentations had a much more platelet dense thrombus (Fig. 9.7).

Despite primary PCI, only 35 % of ST elevation MI patients have optimal myocardial reperfusion based on TIMI 3 flow, myocardial blush grades 2 or 3, and greater than 70 %

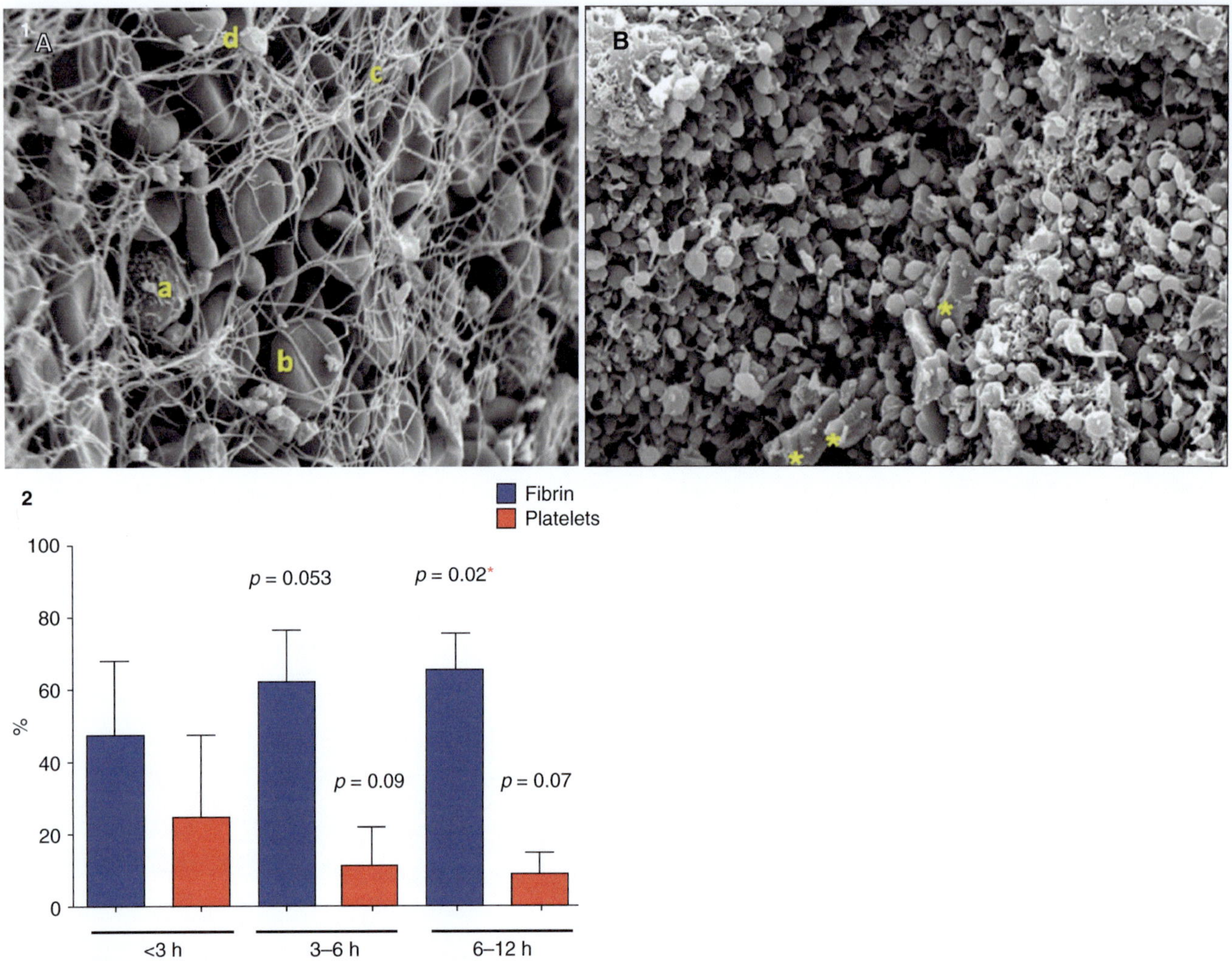

Fig. 9.7 Thrombectomy aspirate composition by ischemic time frame. (*1*) Scanning Electron Micrograph at 3,000× Magnification. (**A**) This portion is mainly composed of erythrocytes (*b*) trapped in a fibrin mesh (*c*) with few platelet aggregates (*d*) and rare white cells (*a*). (**B**) This portion is mainly composed of platelet aggregates with a few cholesterol crystals (*yellow asterisks*) (Adapted from Silvain et al. [61], with permission.) (*2*) Description of the impact of time on thrombus composition demonstrating that the earlier the ischemic time frame, the more platelet rich the extracted thrombus while longer ischemic time frames are associated with more fibrin rich thrombus. The p values are given for comparison with the group <3 h as a reference with multiple Student t test. $*p<0.05$. Multiple comparisons were done with the Dunnett's test, resulting in a $p=0.044$ for fibrin and nonsignificant for platelet content

ST segment elevation resolution [62]. The lack of reperfusion of the microvasculature despite appropriate treatment and reperfusion of the epicardial artery is termed slow or no reflow. This phenomenon has a negative impact on short- and long-term outcomes including higher levels of creatinine kinase release, worsened left ventricular function, and worsened 6-month mortality (12.5 % vs. 4.3 % of patients undergoing primary PCI without no reflow) [63]. One of the most important mechanisms and predictors for this microvascular obstruction is thrombus at the site of the plaque rupture with atherothrombotic embolization. Angiographic predictors of no reflow include thrombus with the greatest linear dimension more than 3 times the reference lumen diameter, an abrupt cutoff without taper at the site of occlusion, greater than 5 mm accumulated thrombus proximal to the occlusion, floating thrombus proximal to the occlusion, persistent contrast distal to the obstruction, and large reference lumen diameters of the infarct artery [64].

These concepts have led to the development of numerous devices aimed at reducing thrombus burden and minimizing the embolic consequences which occur with coronary intervention in the treatment of acute ischemic syndromes.

Distal Protection

One of the early concepts of preventing slow or no reflow after stent placement in the native coronary vasculature was to utilize distal protection devices similar to those shown to be successful in saphenous vein graft interventions. Saphenous vein grafts are prone to slow or no reflow due to embolization of particulate matter. Several products have been shown to

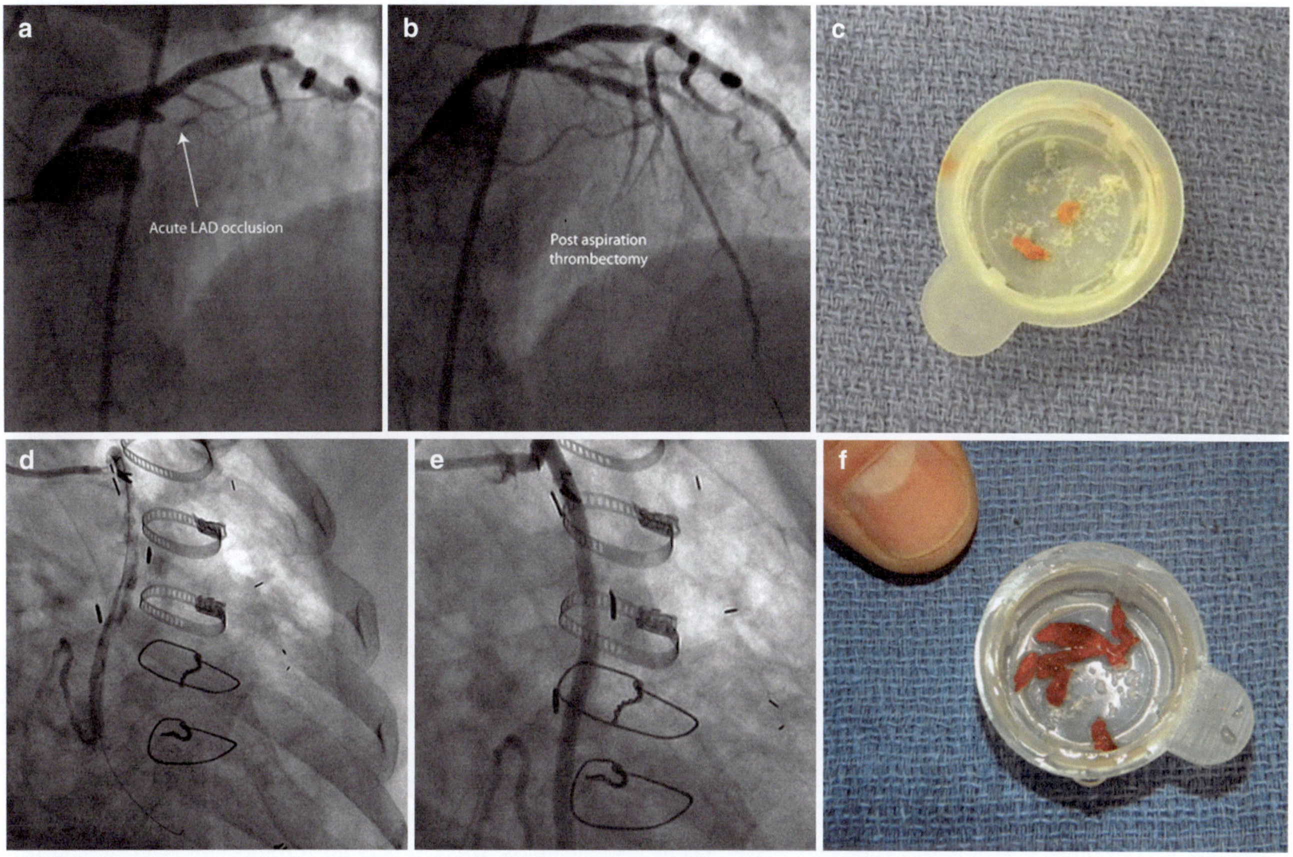

Fig. 9.8 Thrombus cases. A 50-year-old man presented with an anterior STEMI and was recanalized with primary aspiration thrombectomy (**a**–**b**) yielding moderate thrombus (**c**). In contrast, aspiration thrombectomy performed in a saphenous vein graft (**d**–**e**) yielded copious large, red thrombus (**f**)

significantly reduce the incidence of slow or no reflow in saphenous vein graft interventions by capturing released debris resulting in reduction in 30-day MACE driven primarily by reduction in myocardial infarctions [65–68].

This approach in native coronary thrombotic lesions has been unsuccessful as demonstrated in the large, multicenter EMERALD trial which compared use of the PercuSurge GuardWire Plus (Medtronic Corp, Santa Rosa, CA) distal protection device vs. no distal protection in ST elevation MI patients undergoing primary PCI [68]. The PercuSurge GuardWire Plus balloon was advanced just beyond the lesion and inflated to prevent subsequent debris from travelling to the distal coronary bed. PCI was then performed with the distal protection balloon inflated. Following stenting a 5F Export aspiration catheter was passed to aspirate residual debris prior to deflation of the PercuSurge balloon. Despite a high rate of technical success and visible thrombotic debris in the aspirates, there was no benefit in microvascular flow, reperfusion success, infarct size, or event-free survival. Several years later, distal protection was revisited in the DEDICATION trial from Denmark comparing use of the FilterWire-EZ (Boston Scientific, Santa Clara, CA) or SpiderX (eV3, Minneapolis, Minnesota) filter wire versus no distal protection during primary PCI of ST elevation MI patients [69]. Again, this trial showed no benefit in microvascular perfusion, infarct size, or reduction of MACCE.

Trials of direct thrombus extraction devices that do not provide distal protection have shown more promise in improving microvascular perfusion and potentially improving long-term clinical outcomes. Modern thrombectomy devices can be classified broadly as aspiration catheters, mechanical disruption plus extraction, and thrombus dissolution devices.

Manual Aspiration Catheters

Manual aspiration catheters are the simplest of all the devices used in treatment of coronary thrombus. These are dual lumen devices that are composed of a guidewire lumen and a thrombus extraction lumen. With a guidewire placed distal to the lesion and thrombus, the aspiration catheter is advanced just proximal to the thrombotic portion of the coronary artery. Negative suction pressure is applied via a syringe as the catheter is advanced and withdrawn over the thrombotic area. Once the vacuum syringe is full and 25–50 cm^3 of blood are removed, the aspiration catheter is withdrawn over the wire, and the guide catheter is then back bled to minimize the possibility of any residual thrombus remains in the catheter. The aspirate is typically injected into a filter to examine for successful thrombectomy. Figures 9.7 and 9.8 document two cases of successful thrombectomy achieved with aspira-

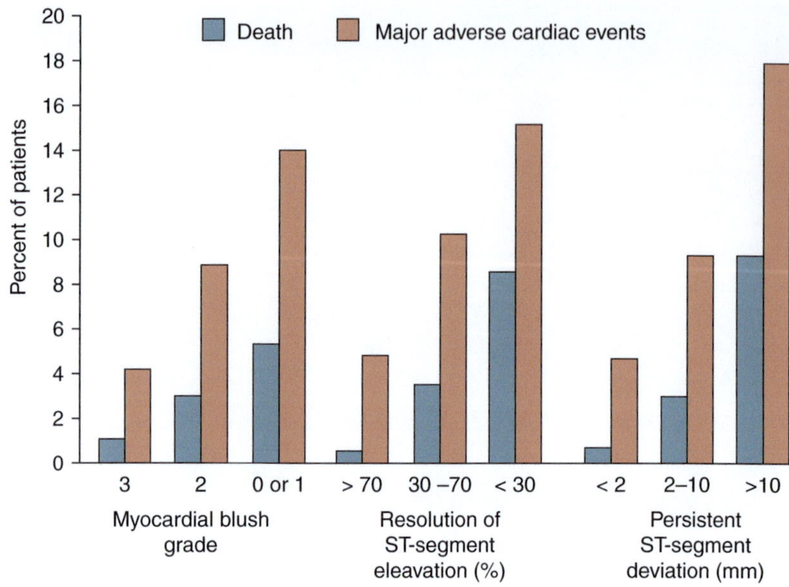

Rate of death (%)	1.0	2.9	5.2	0.7	3.6	8.6	0.6	3.0	9.3
Rate of major adverse cardiac events (%)	4.2	8.8	14.1	4.8	10.3	15.2	4.7	9.2	18.0

Fig. 9.9 Rates of death and major adverse cardiac events, according to myocardial blush grade and ST-segment variable. Rates are shown for 968 patients for whom the data were available. $P = 0.003$ for the association between myocardial blush grade and death. $P < 0.001$ for all other associations: that between myocardial blush grade and major adverse cardiac events, between ST-segment resolution and death, between ST-segment resolution and major adverse cardiac events, between persistent ST-segment deviation and death, and between persistent ST-segment and major adverse cardiac events

tion catheters and contrast the difference between native coronary artery and vein graft thrombus.

Numerous thrombus aspiration catheters have been approved and are available for use in the coronary vasculature. Aspiration is directly related to the suction pressure and lumen radius to the fourth power. Aspiration is indirectly related to blood viscosity and the length of the catheter:

Q= Δ (delta) pressure*Pi*radius4 / 8*viscosity*length

The most important variable for aspiration potential is the minimal lumen diameter of the extraction lumen; however, there are other considerations. A larger catheter may be able to aspirate more material but will require a larger guide catheter. Bulkier devices are challenging when navigating a tortuous coronary vessel or crossing a high-grade lesion. Engineers have developed a variety of strategies to overcome these trackability issues including variable tip designs, hydrophilic coatings, and differences in shaft stiffness to minimize kinking.

Most of the aspiration catheters have a distal monorail guidewire lumen and a more proximal extraction lumen varying distances from the tip and tapered at variable angles. There are no large head-to-head comparisons between these devices, and in vitro aspiration tests of saline do not necessarily correlate with in vivo thrombus extraction.

Numerous small trials comparing aspiration catheters versus no aspiration catheters in primary PCI for ST elevation MI patients have demonstrated short-term benefits including lower creatine kinase release, lower rates of no reflow, and improved ST segment resolution and myocardial blush grades [70, 71]. More definitive data was obtained from the TAPAS trial which enrolled 1071 ST elevation MI patients treated with primary PCI and randomized to thrombus aspiration with the 6-French Export Catheter (Medtronic, Minneapolis, MN) versus no thrombectomy [72]. The primary end point of myocardial blush grade 0 or 1 occurred in 17.1 % in the thrombectomy group versus 26.3 % in the conventional PCI group. The 30-day mortality for patients with a blush grade 0 or 1, 2, and 3 was 5.2 %, 2.9 %, and 1.0 %, respectively. While not a primary end point, the trial concluded that since thrombectomy improved blush grade and better blush grade correlated with better survival, thrombectomy can be presumed to improve survival (Fig. 9.9). The secondary endpoint of cardiac death or nonfatal myocardial infarction at one year occurred significantly less often in the thrombus aspiration group (5.6 % versus 9.9 %). The strategy of thrombus aspiration prior to stenting in acute MI resulted in a lower cardiac mortality at one year compared to conventional treatment without thrombus aspiration (3.6% versus 6.7 %) [73]. Similarly, the EXPIRA trial demonstrated improved primary end points of myocardial blush grade greater than or equal to 2 (88 % with aspiration vs. 60 % without aspiration) and 90-min ST segment elevation resolution >70 % (64 % with aspiration vs. 39 % without aspiration) [74]. Other secondary clinical end points included smaller infarct size by MRI and lower 9-month mortality with aspiration thrombectomy.

Based on the success of the TAPAS and EXPIRA trials of aspiration catheters, the ACC/AHA revised the 2009 STEMI Guidelines to make aspiration thrombectomy a Class IIa, level of evidence B recommendation prior to PTCA or stenting the culprit artery [75].

Mechanical Disruption and Extraction

While the manual aspiration catheters are quite simple and easy to use, several more complex devices for thrombus extraction have been developed in an effort to better prevent atherothrombotic embolization. The Angiojet (Medrad Interventional/Possis, Minneapolis, MN) rheolytic thrombectomy device employs the Venturi effect via three high pressure saline jets directed from distal to proximal within the shaft of the catheter. A powerful suction effect is generated as each jet passes a narrow aperture that draws the thrombus into the catheter shaft where it is disrupted by the water jets and extracted. The system consists of a drive unit that generates the jet pressure, the Spiroflex coronary catheter, and a pump that connects the drive unit to the catheter. This device was FDA approved in the USA in 1999 following the favorable results of the VEGAS-2 trial that demonstrated that rheolytic thrombectomy with the Angiojet was more effective than local infusion of urokinase for treatment of angiographically evident thrombus in saphenous vein grafts and native coronary arteries [76]. Subsequently, the multicentered AIMI trial randomized 480 ST elevation MI patients from 2001 to 2004 to either primary PCI or rheolytic thrombectomy plus PCI [77]. The primary end point of reducing sestamibi imaging infarct size at 14–28 days was not met. Though the study was not powered to look at differences in clinical events, it was also concerning that the secondary end points of 30-day MACE and mortality were higher in the Angiojet arm. A repeat evaluation of the Angiojet in ST elevation MI patients was performed after revisions to the catheter design and protocol modifications. The newer protocol required proximal device activation and antegrade advancement through the thrombus rather than activation once the catheter was through the thrombus as was done in the AIMI trial. This was studied in the JETSTENT trial which randomized ST elevation MI patients to rheolytic thrombectomy with primary PCI versus primary PCI alone [78]. This trial only included patients with high thrombus burden (grade 3–5) and reference vessels at least 2.5 mm in diameter. The co-primary end points of ST segment resolution and sestamibi-measured infarct size were not met, and none of the secondary surrogate end points were met including improvement in myocardial blush grade or TIMI flow. The secondary end points of 30-day, 6-month, and 12-month MACE were better with rheolytic thrombectomy. Early versions of the device were complicated by higher rates of bradycardia possibly related to distal embolization of particulate matter. The JETSTENT trial was associated with <1 % of any need for temporary pacemakers [78]. More data is warranted before use of rheolytic thrombectomy can be recommended for treatment of ST elevation MI patients.

X-SIZER (ev3 Inc., Plymouth, MN) is CE marked for use in the coronaries and FDA approved for removing thrombi from synthetic dialysis grafts. While more complex than manual aspiration catheters, the setup does not require a large external console. The X-SIZER is an aspiration catheter that contains a helical, Archimedes screw cutter that disrupts the thrombus as it is pulled into the catheter. A 9-V battery-powered control unit is used to operate the cutter, and a vacuum bottle is used to generate suction for thrombus aspiration. This device was studied in several small trials of ST elevation MI patients and found to improve ST segment resolution when randomized to no thrombectomy [79–81]. A retrospective review of 200 consecutive patients at a single center found that the device was associated with a 24 % failure rate defined as the occurrence of 1 or more of the following conditions: failure of the X-SIZER to reach the target segment, failure to achieve final TIMI 3 flow, slow flow or no

Table 9.2 Summary of meta-analysis of the major thrombectomy trials comparing aspiration catheters, mechanical thrombectomy devices and embolic protection devices. Simple aspiration catheters have the clearest safety profile with the most likely benefit in clinical outcomes

Group	Mortality	MI	TVR	Stroke	MACE	TIMI blush 3	St-resolution
Catheter aspiration devices							
Overall	**0.63 (0.43–0.93)**	0.65 (0.37–1.12)	0.83 (0.64–1.08)	3.43 (0.85–13.9)	**0.76 (0.62–0.95)**	**1.69 (1.26–2.28)**[a]	**1.41 (1.21–1.64)**[a]
Published	**0.60 (0.39–0.95)**	0.59 (0.32–1.09)	0.89 (0.64–1.22)	2.30 (0.34–15.4)	0.83 (0.65–1.05)	**1.54 (1.36–1.74)**	**1.34 (1.21–1.48)**
Abstract	0.71 (0.34–1.47)	1.01 (0.26–3.92)	0.72 (0.45–1.14)	5.15 (0.61–43.7)	**0.60 (0.38–0.94)**	**1.75 (1.04–2.95)**[a]	**1.46 (1.06–2.03)**[a]
Mechanical thrombectomy devices							
Overall	**1.93 (1.00–3.72)**	0.67 (0.19–233)	1.14 (0.43–3.01)	2.67 (0.71–100)	1.64 (0.60–4.44)[a]	1.16 (0.71–1.90)[a]	1.25 (0.99–1.58)[a]
Published	**1.93 (1.00–3.72)**	0.67 (0.19–233)	1.14 (0.43–3.01)	2.67 (0.71–100)	1.64 (0.60–4.44)[a]	1.16 (0.71–1.90)[a]	1.25 (0.99–158)[a]
Abstract	NA	NA	NA	NA	NA	NA	NA
Ernbolic protection devices							
Overall	0.92 (0.60–1.40)	0.82 (0.44–1.51)	1.04 (0.74–1.47)	0.99 (0.34–2.92)	0.95 (0.69–1.30)	**1.18 (1.02–1.38)**[a]	1.07 (0.98–1.16)
Published	0.92 (0.55–1.54)	0.85 (0.45–1.60)	1.07 (0.71–1.62)	0.99 (0.34–2.92)	0.94 (0.61–1.44)	1.09 (0.95–1.26)[a]	1.06 (0.97–1.15)
Abstract	0.91 (0.42–1.96)	0.33 (0.014–8.10)	1.06 (0.55–2.02)	NA	0.95 (0.60–1.52)	**1.55 (1.16–2.07)**	1.23 (0.80–1.88)

All values are RR (95 % CI) Bold values indicate statistical significance

CI confidence internal, *MACE* major adverse cardiovascular events, *M* myocardial infarction, *TIM* Thrombolysis in Myocardial Infarction, *TVR* target vessel revascularization, *RR* risk ratio

[a]DerSimon and Laird random effects model

reflow, distal embolization, or coronary perforation. Ostial lesions were an independent predictor of device failure, and the device was independently associated with 30-day adverse events [82].

Meta-analyses of adjunctive thrombectomy and embolic protection device trials used in acute myocardial infarction demonstrate that manual catheter thrombus aspiration during acute myocardial infarction is beneficial in reducing mortality compared with PCI alone. Mechanical thrombectomy appeared neutral with a trend toward a higher incidence of stroke and cannot be recommended for routine use while embolic protection had a neutral effect, (Table 9.2) [83, 84].

References

1. Bittl JA, Chew DP, Topol EJ, Kong DF, Califf RM. Meta-analysis of randomized trials of percutaneous transluminal coronary angioplasty versus atherectomy, cutting balloon atherotomy, or laser angioplasty. J Am Coll Cardiol. 2004;43(6):936–42.
2. King 3rd SB, Yeh W, Holubkov R, et al. Balloon angioplasty versus new device intervention: clinical outcomes. A comparison of the NHLBI PTCA and NACI registries. J Am Coll Cardiol. 1998;31(3):558–66.
3. King 3rd SB, Smith Jr SC, Hirshfeld Jr JW, et al. 2007 Focused Update of the ACC/AHA/SCAI 2005 Guideline Update for Percutaneous Coronary Intervention: a report of the American College of Cardiology/American Heart Association Task Force on Practice Guidelines: 2007 Writing Group to Review New Evidence and Update the ACC/AHA/SCAI 2005 Guideline Update for Percutaneous Coronary Intervention, Writing on Behalf of the 2005 Writing Committee. [Erratum appears in Circulation. 2008;117(6):e161]. Circulation. 2008;117(2):261–95.
4. Clavijo LC, Steinberg DH, Torguson R, et al. Sirolimus-eluting stents and calcified coronary lesions: clinical outcomes of patients treated with and without rotational atherectomy. Catheter Cardiovasc Interv. 2006;68(6):873–8.
5. Rathore S, Matsuo H, Terashima M, et al. Rotational atherectomy for fibro-calcific coronary artery disease in drug eluting stent era: procedural outcomes and angiographic follow-up results. Catheter Cardiovasc Interv. 2010;75(6):919–27.
6. Tran T, Brown M, Lasala J. An evidence-based approach to the use of rotational and directional coronary atherectomy in the era of drug-eluting stents: when does it make sense? Catheter Cardiovasc Interv. 2008;72(5):650–62.
7. Kovach JA, Mintz GS, Pichard AD, et al. Sequential intravascular ultrasound characterization of the mechanisms of rotational atherectomy and adjunct balloon angioplasty. J Am Coll Cardiol. 1993; 22(4):1024–32.
8. Dussaillant GR, Mintz GS, Pichard AD, et al. Effect of rotational atherectomy in noncalcified atherosclerotic plaque: a volumetric intravascular ultrasound study. J Am Coll Cardiol. 1996;28(4):856–60.
9. Mintz GS, Potkin BN, Keren G, et al. Intravascular ultrasound evaluation of the effect of rotational atherectomy in obstructive atherosclerotic coronary artery disease. Circulation. 1992;86(5):1383–93.
10. Bowers TR, Stewart RE, O'Neill WW, Reddy VM, Safian RD. Effect of Rotablator atherectomy and adjunctive balloon angioplasty on coronary blood flow. Circulation. 1997;95(5):1157–64.
11. Koch KC, Kleinhans E, Klues HG, et al. Quantitative assessment of transient regional ischemia during rotational atherectomy. J Nucl Med. 1998;39(3):402–8.
12. Koch KC, vom Dahl J, Kleinhans E, et al. Influence of a platelet GPIIb/IIIa receptor antagonist on myocardial hypoperfusion during rotational atherectomy as assessed by myocardial Tc-99m sestamibi scintigraphy. J Am Coll Cardiol. 1999;33(4):998–1004.
13. Koch K-C, Radke PW, Kleinhans E, et al. Mechanisms of myocardial hypoperfusion during rotational atherectomy of de novo coronary artery lesions and stenosed coronary stents: insights from serial myocardial scintigraphy. J Nucl Cardiol. 2002;9(3):304–11.
14. Braden GA, Applegate RJ, Young TM, Love WW, Sane DC. Abciximab decreases both the incidence and magnitude of creatine kinase elevation during rotational atherectomy. J Am Coll Cardiol. 1997;29(2 Suppl. A):499A.
15. Fasseas P, Orford JL, Panetta CJ, et al. Incidence, correlates, management, and clinical outcome of coronary perforation: analysis of 16,298 procedures. Am Heart J. 2004;147(1):140–5.
16. Williams MS, Coller BS, Vaananen HJ, Scudder LE, Sharma SK, Marmur JD. Activation of platelets in platelet-rich plasma by rotablation is speed-dependent and can be inhibited by abciximab (c7E3 Fab; ReoPro). Circulation. 1998;98(8):742–8.
17. Zimarino M, Corcos T, Favereau X, et al. Rotational coronary atherectomy with adjunctive balloon angioplasty for the treatment of ostial lesions. Cathet Cardiovasc Diagn. 1994;33(1):22–7.
18. Zimarino M, Corcos T, Favereau X, et al. Rotational coronary atherectomy with adjunctive balloon angioplasty: evaluation of lumen enlargement by quantitative angiographic analysis. Am Heart J. 1997;133(2):203–9.
19. Safian RD, Niazi KA, Strzelecki M, et al. Detailed angiographic analysis of high-speed mechanical rotational atherectomy in human coronary arteries. Circulation. 1993;88(3):961–8.
20. Reifart N, Vandormael M, Krajcar M, et al. Randomized comparison of angioplasty of complex coronary lesions at a single center. Excimer Laser, Rotational Atherectomy, and Balloon Angioplasty Comparison (ERBAC) study. Circulation. 1997;96(1):91–8.
21. Safian RD, Feldman T, Muller DW, et al. Coronary angioplasty and Rotablator atherectomy trial (CARAT): immediate and late results of a prospective multicenter randomized trial. Catheter Cardiovasc Interv. 2001;53(2):213–20.
22. Whitlow PL, Bass TA, Kipperman RM, et al. Results of the study to determine rotablator and transluminal angioplasty strategy (STRATAS). Am J Cardiol. 2001;87(6):699–705.
23. Sharma SK, Dangas G, Mehran R, et al. Risk factors for the development of slow flow during rotational coronary atherectomy. Am J Cardiol. 1997;80(2):219–22.
24. Kini A, Marmur JD, Duvvuri S, Dangas G, Choudhary S, Sharma SK. Rotational atherectomy: improved procedural outcome with evolution of technique and equipment. Single-center results of first 1,000 patients. Catheter Cardiovasc Interv. 1999;46(3):305–11.
25. Matsuo H, Watanabe S, Watanabe T, et al. Prevention of no-reflow/slow-flow phenomenon during rotational atherectomy–a prospective randomized study comparing intracoronary continuous infusion of verapamil and nicorandil. Am Heart J. 2007;154(5):994 e991–996.
26. Cohen BM, Weber VJ, Relsman M, Casale A, Dorros G. Coronary perforation complicating rotational ablation: the U.S. multicenter experience. Cathet Cardiovasc Diagn. 1996;Suppl 3:55–9.
27. Al-Lamee R, Ielasi A, Latib A, et al. Incidence, predictors, management, immediate and long-term outcomes following grade III coronary perforation. JACC Cardiovasc Interv. 2011;4(1):87–95.
28. Ellis SG, Ajluni S, Arnold AZ, et al. Increased coronary perforation in the new device era. Incidence, classification, management, and outcome. Circulation. 1994;90(6):2725–30.

29. Shimony A, Zahger D, Van Straten M, et al. Incidence, risk factors, management and outcomes of coronary artery perforation during percutaneous coronary intervention. Am J Cardiol. 2009;104(12):1674–7.
30. Javaid A, Buch AN, Satler LF, et al. Management and outcomes of coronary artery perforation during percutaneous coronary intervention. Am J Cardiol. 2006;98(7):911–4.
31. Kiernan TJ, Yan BP, Ruggiero N, et al. Coronary artery perforations in the contemporary interventional era. J Interv Cardiol. 2009; 22(4):350–3.
32. Sperling RT, Ho K, James D, Laham R, Gibson M, Carrozza J. Treatment of stent-jailed side branch stenoses with rotational atherectomy. J Invasive Cardiol. 2006;18(8):354–8.
33. Motwani JG, Raymond RE, Franco I, Ellis SG, Whitlow PL. Effectiveness of rotational atherectomy of right coronary artery ostial stenosis. Am J Cardiol. 2000;85(5):563–7.
34. Thomas WJ, Cowley MJ, Vetrovec GW, Malloy W, Goudreau E. Effectiveness of rotational atherectomy in aortocoronary saphenous vein grafts. Am J Cardiol. 2000;86(1):88–91.
35. Thomas WJ, Cowley MJ, Vetrovec GW, Malloy W, Goudreau E. Effectiveness of rotational atherectomy in narrowed left internal mammary artery grafts to the left anterior descending coronary artery. Am J Cardiol. 2000;86(1):86–8.
36. vom Dahl J, Dietz U, Haager PK, et al. Rotational atherectomy does not reduce recurrent in-stent restenosis: results of the angioplasty versus rotational atherectomy for treatment of diffuse in-stent restenosis trial (ARTIST). Circulation. 2002;105(5):583–8.
37. O'Neill WW, Kleiman NS, Moses J, et al. A prospective, randomized clinical trial of hemodynamic support with impella 2.5 versus intra-aortic balloon pump in patients undergoing high risk percutaneous coronary intervention. Circ 2012;126:1717–1727.
38. Mintz GS, Pichard AD, Kovach JA, et al. Impact of preintervention intravascular ultrasound imaging on transcatheter treatment strategies in coronary artery disease. Am J Cardiol. 1994;73(7):423–30.
39. Henneke KH, Regar E, Konig A, et al. Impact of target lesion calcification on coronary stent expansion after rotational atherectomy. Am Heart J. 1999;137(1):93–9.
40. Bangalore S, Vlachos HA, Selzer F, et al. Percutaneous coronary intervention of moderate to severe calcified coronary lesions: insights from the National Heart, Lung, and Blood Institute Dynamic Registry. Catheter Cardiovasc Interv. 2011;77(1):22–8.
41. Moussa I, Di Mario C, Moses J, et al. Coronary stenting after rotational atherectomy in calcified and complex lesions. Angiographic and clinical follow-up results. Circulation. 1997;96(1):128–36.
42. Abdel-Wahab M, Richardt G, Joachim Buttner H, et al. High speed rotational atherectomy before paclitaxel-eluting stent implantation in complex calcified coronary lesions: the randomized ROTAXUS trial. JACC Cardiovasc Interv 2013;6:10.
43. Clarke RH, Isner JM, Donaldson RF, Jones 2nd G. Gas chromatographic-light microscopic correlative analysis of excimer laser photoablation of cardiovascular tissues: evidence for a thermal mechanism. Circ Res. 1987;60(3):429–37.
44. van Leeuwen TG, van Erven L, Meertens JH, Motamedi M, Post MJ, Borst C. Origin of arterial wall dissections induced by pulsed excimer and mid-infrared laser ablation in the pig. J Am Coll Cardiol. 1992; 19(7):1610–8.
45. van Leeuwen TG, Meertens JH, Velema E, Post MJ, Borst C. Intraluminal vapor bubble induced by excimer laser pulse causes microsecond arterial dilation and invagination leading to extensive wall damage in the rabbit. Circulation. 1993;87(4):1258–63.
46. Appelman YE, Piek JJ, Strikwerda S, et al. Randomised trial of excimer laser angioplasty versus balloon angioplasty for treatment of obstructive coronary artery disease. Lancet. 1996;347(8994):79–84.
47. Holmes Jr DR, Reeder GS, Ghazzal ZM, et al. Coronary perforation after excimer laser coronary angioplasty: the Excimer Laser Coronary Angioplasty Registry experience. J Am Coll Cardiol. 1994;23(2):330–5.
48. Baumbach A, Bittl JA, Fleck E, et al. Acute complications of excimer laser coronary angioplasty: a detailed analysis of multicenter results. Coinvestigators of the U.S. and European Percutaneous Excimer Laser Coronary Angioplasty (PELCA) Registries. J Am Coll Cardiol. 1994;23(6):1305–13.
49. Tcheng JE, Wells LD, Phillips HR, Deckelbaum LI, Golobic RA. Development of a new technique for reducing pressure pulse generation during 308-nm excimer laser coronary angioplasty. Cathet Cardiovasc Diagn. 1995;34(1):15–22.
50. Deckelbaum LI, Natarajan MK, Bittl JA, et al. Effect of intracoronary saline infusion on dissection during excimer laser coronary angioplasty: a randomized trial. The Percutaneous Excimer Laser Coronary Angioplasty (PELCA) Investigators. J Am Coll Cardiol. 1995;26(5):1264–9.
51. Bilodeau L, Fretz EB, Taeymans Y, Koolen J, Taylor K, Hilton DJ. Novel use of a high-energy excimer laser catheter for calcified and complex coronary artery lesions. Catheter Cardiovasc Interv. 2004;62(2):155–61.
52. Simonton CA, Leon MB, Baim DS, et al. 'Optimal' directional coronary atherectomy: final results of the Optimal Atherectomy Restenosis Study (OARS). Circulation. 1998;97(4):332–9.
53. Holmes Jr DR, Garratt KN, Isner JM, et al. Effect of subintimal resection on initial outcome and restenosis for native coronary lesions and saphenous vein graft disease treated by directional coronary atherectomy. A report from the CAVEAT I and II investigators. Coronary Angioplasty Versus Excisional Atherectomy Trial. J Am Coll Cardiol. 1996;28(3):645–51.
54. Baim DS, Cutlip DE, Sharma SK, et al. Final results of the Balloon vs Optimal Atherectomy Trial (BOAT). Circulation. 1998;97(4): 322–31.
55. Stankovic G, Colombo A, Bersin R, et al. Comparison of directional coronary atherectomy and stenting versus stenting alone for the treatment of de novo and restenotic coronary artery narrowing. [Erratum appears in Am J Cardiol. 2004;94(1):150]. Am J Cardiol. 2004;93(8):953–8.
56. Holmes Jr DR, Topol EJ, Califf RM, et al. A multicenter, randomized trial of coronary angioplasty versus directional atherectomy for patients with saphenous vein bypass graft lesions. CAVEAT-II investigators. Circulation. 1995;91(7):1966–74.
57. Elliott JM, Berdan LG, Holmes DR, et al. One-year follow-up in the Coronary Angioplasty Versus Excisional Atherectomy Trial (CAVEAT I). Circulation. 1995;91(8):2158–66.
58. Adelman AG, Cohen EA, Kimball BP, et al. A comparison of directional atherectomy with balloon angioplasty for lesions of the left anterior descending coronary artery. N Engl J Med. 1993;329(4):228–33.
59. Fuster V, Badimon L, Cohen M, Ambrose JA, Badimon JJ, Chesebro J. Insights into the pathogenesis of acute ischemic syndromes. Circulation. 1988;77(6):1213–20.
60. White CJ, Ramee SR, Collins TJ, et al. Coronary thrombi increase PTCA risk. Angioscopy as a clinical tool. Circulation. 1996;93(2):253–8.
61. Silvain J, Collet JP, Nagaswami C, et al. Composition of coronary thrombus in acute myocardial infarction. J Am Coll Cardiol. 2011;57(12):1359–67.
62. Niccoli G, Burzotta F, Galiuto L, Crea F. Myocardial no-reflow in humans. J Am Coll Cardiol. 2009;54(4):281–92.
63. Brosh D, Assali AR, Mager A, et al. Effect of no-reflow during primary percutaneous coronary intervention for acute myocardial infarction on six-month mortality. Am J Cardiol. 2007;99(4):442–5.
64. Yip HK, Chen MC, Chang HW, et al. Angiographic morphologic features of infarct-related arteries and timely reperfusion in acute myocardial infarction: predictors of slow-flow and no-reflow phenomenon. Chest. 2002;122(4):1322–32.

65. Stone GW, Rogers C, Hermiller J, et al. Randomized comparison of distal protection with a filter-based catheter and a balloon occlusion and aspiration system during percutaneous intervention of diseased saphenous vein aorto-coronary bypass grafts. Circulation. 2003;108(5):548–53.
66. Baim DS, Wahr D, George B, et al. Randomized trial of a distal embolic protection device during percutaneous intervention of saphenous vein aorto-coronary bypass grafts. Circulation. 2002; 105(11):1285–90.
67. Mauri L, Cox D, Hermiller J, et al. The PROXIMAL trial: proximal protection during saphenous vein graft intervention using the Proxis Embolic Protection System: a randomized, prospective, multicenter clinical trial. J Am Coll Cardiol. 2007;50(15):1442–9.
68. Stone GW, Webb J, Cox DA, et al. Distal microcirculatory protection during percutaneous coronary intervention in acute ST-segment elevation myocardial infarction: a randomized controlled trial. JAMA. 2005;293(9):1063–72.
69. Kelbaek H, Terkelsen CJ, Helqvist S, et al. Randomized comparison of distal protection versus conventional treatment in primary percutaneous coronary intervention: the drug elution and distal protection in ST-elevation myocardial infarction (DEDICATION) trial. J Am Coll Cardiol. 2008;51(9):899–905.
70. Silva-Orrego P, Colombo P, Bigi R, et al. Thrombus aspiration before primary angioplasty improves myocardial reperfusion in acute myocardial infarction: the DEAR-MI (Dethrombosis to Enhance Acute Reperfusion in Myocardial Infarction) study. J Am Coll Cardiol. 2006;48(8):1552–9.
71. Burzotta F, Trani C, Romagnoli E, et al. Manual thrombus-aspiration improves myocardial reperfusion: the randomized evaluation of the effect of mechanical reduction of distal embolization by thrombus-aspiration in primary and rescue angioplasty (REMEDIA) trial. J Am Coll Cardiol. 2005;46(2):371–6.
72. Svilaas T, Vlaar PJ, van der Horst IC, et al. Thrombus aspiration during primary percutaneous coronary intervention. N Engl J Med. 2008;358(6):557–67.
73. Vlarr PJ, Svilaas T, van der Horst IC, et al. Cardiac death and reinfarction after one year in the thrombus aspiration during percutaneous coronary intervention in acute myocardial infarction study (TAPAS): a one year follow-up study. Lancet 2008;371:1915.
74. Sardella G, Mancone M, Bucciarelli-Ducci C, et al. Thrombus aspiration during primary percutaneous coronary intervention improves myocardial reperfusion and reduces infarct size: the EXPIRA (thrombectomy with export catheter in infarct-related artery during primary percutaneous coronary intervention) prospective, randomized trial. J Am Coll Cardiol. 2009;53(4):309–15.
75. Kushner FG, Hand M, Smith Jr SC, et al. 2009 focused updates: ACC/AHA guidelines for the management of patients with ST-elevation myocardial infarction (updating the 2004 guideline and 2007 focused update) and ACC/AHA/SCAI guidelines on percutaneous coronary intervention (updating the 2005 guideline and 2007 focused update): a report of the American College of Cardiology Foundation/American Heart Association Task Force on Practice Guidelines. Circulation. 2009;120(22): 2271–306.
76. Kuntz RE, Baim DS, Cohen DJ, et al. A trial comparing rheolytic thrombectomy with intracoronary urokinase for coronary and vein graft thrombus (the Vein Graft AngioJet Study [VeGAS 2]). Am J Cardiol. 2002;89(3):326–30.
77. Ali A, Cox D, Dib N, et al. Rheolytic thrombectomy with percutaneous coronary intervention for infarct size reduction in acute myocardial infarction: 30-day results from a multicenter randomized study. J Am Coll Cardiol. 2006;48(2):244–52.
78. Migliorini A, Stabile A, Rodriguez AE, et al. Comparison of AngioJet rheolytic thrombectomy before direct infarct artery stenting with direct stenting alone in patients with acute myocardial infarction. The JETSTENT trial. J Am Coll Cardiol. 2010;56(16): 1298–306.
79. Beran G, Lang I, Schreiber W, et al. Intracoronary thrombectomy with the X-sizer catheter system improves epicardial flow and accelerates ST-segment resolution in patients with acute coronary syndrome: a prospective, randomized, controlled study. Circulation. 2002;105(20):2355–60.
80. Stone GW, Cox DA, Low R, et al. Safety and efficacy of a novel device for treatment of thrombotic and atherosclerotic lesions in native coronary arteries and saphenous vein grafts: results from the multicenter X-Sizer for treatment of thrombus and atherosclerosis in coronary applications trial (X-TRACT) study. Catheter Cardiovasc Interv. 2003;58(4):419–27.
81. Lefevre T, Garcia E, Reimers B, et al. X-sizer for thrombectomy in acute myocardial infarction improves ST-segment resolution: results of the X-sizer in AMI for negligible embolization and optimal ST resolution (X AMINE ST) trial. J Am Coll Cardiol. 2005;46(2): 246–52.
82. Lee CH, Tan HC, Wong HB, et al. Incidence, predictors, and outcomes of device failure of X-sizer thrombectomy: real-world experience of 200 cases in 5 years. Am Heart J. 2007;153(1):14 e13–19.
83. Bavry AA, Kumbhani DJ, Bhatt DL. Role of adjunctive thrombectomy and embolic protection devices in acute myocardial infarction: a comprehensive meta-analysis of randomized trials. Eur Heart J. 2008;29(24):2989–3001.
84. Kumbhani DJ, Bavry AA, Desai MY, et al. Role of aspiration and mechanical thrombectomy in patients with acute myocardial infarction undergoing primary angioplasty: An updated meta-analysis of randomized trials. J Am Coll Cardiol. 2013;62: 1409–18. doi:10.1016/j.jacc.2013.04.025.

Stents: Safety and Efficacy

10

Marvin H. Eng and David E. Kandzari

Historical Perspective

In 1964, Charles Dotter and Melvin Judkins conceptualized angioplasty laying the groundwork for Andreas Grüntzig to pioneer the first coronary angioplasty in 1977 (Fig. 10.1) [1, 2]. Hampered by high rates of restenosis and abrupt closure rates approaching more than 50 and 8 %, respectively, coronary angioplasty was performed with some trepidation [3]. Julio Palmaz devised the first balloon-expandable slotted stent for the peripheral vasculature in 1985, and Richard Schatz successfully modified it for implantation in the coronary vessels [4, 5]. Sigwart et al. were the first to implant a self-expanding covered mesh graft to treat coronary dissections and abrupt closure; however, the balloon-expandable Palmaz-Schatz stent was the first to prove superiority to balloon angioplasty and become commercially available leading to an evolution of safety in percutaneous coronary intervention [4, 6]. Although commercially successful, the initial generation of coronary stents remained limited due to device embolization, stent thrombosis, and poor deliverability. Through dual-antiplatelet therapy and recognition of stent underexpansion, cardiologists were able to mitigate thrombotic complications [7]. With the introduction of stents and optimization of anticoagulation to include glycoprotein IIb/IIIa inhibitors, successive decreases in abrupt closure and referrals for emergent CABG were seen [3]. While safety of PCI continued to improve, in-stent restenosis (ISR) remained a major liability of stents. In 2002, the first drug-eluting stent (DES), a sirolimus-eluting stenting (SES), Cypher® (Cordis Corp., Bridgewater, NJ), was released and subsequently, three major DES types are now commercially available in the United States and additional geographies: paclitaxel-eluting stents (PES), zotarolimus-eluting stents (ZES), and everolimus-eluting stents (EES). At present, these constitute the majority of intracoronary devices utilized globally. This chapter serves to delineate the key components of stent design as well as examine safety and efficacy of the current generation of stents.

Stent Design

Integral components to the current and newest generation of stents include stent platform, polymer coating, and antiproliferative drugs.

Stent Platform

Metallurgy

Stents were initially constructed of 316 L stainless steel, composed of iron, chromium, cobalt, and molybdenum, the latter three which are resistant to corrosion. The L indicates the low (<0.03 % m/m) carbon content to prevent formation of chromium carbide, a promoter of corrosion. The backbone for first-generation DES, 316 L stent platforms were not very deliverable due their inflexible nature and high crossing profiles.

Newer generation stents are composed of cobalt, nickel, chromium, and molybdenum that offer increased radial strength and radiopacity [8, 9]. This enabled construction of stents with lower crossing profiles, increasingly thinner struts, flexibility, and hence improved deliverability compared to its stainless steel counterparts. Evidence for these improvements in deliverability was in part reflected in the higher procedural success of thin cobalt chromium to 316 L stainless steel platform DES in the ENDEAVOR III trial

M.H. Eng, MD (✉)
Division of Cardiology, Department of Medicine,
University of Texas Health Science Center-San Antonio,
7703 Floyd Curl Dr., MC 7872,
San Antonio, TX 78229-3901, USA
e-mail: marvin-eng@yahoo.com

D.E. Kandzari, MD
Piedmont Heart Institute, 275 Collier Road North West Suite 300,
Atlanta, GA 30309, USA

Piedmont Hospital, Atlanta, GA, USA
e-mail: david.kandzari@piedmont.org

C.A. Thompson (ed.), *Textbook of Cardiovascular Intervention*,
DOI 10.1007/978-1-4471-4528-8_10, © Springer-Verlag London 2014

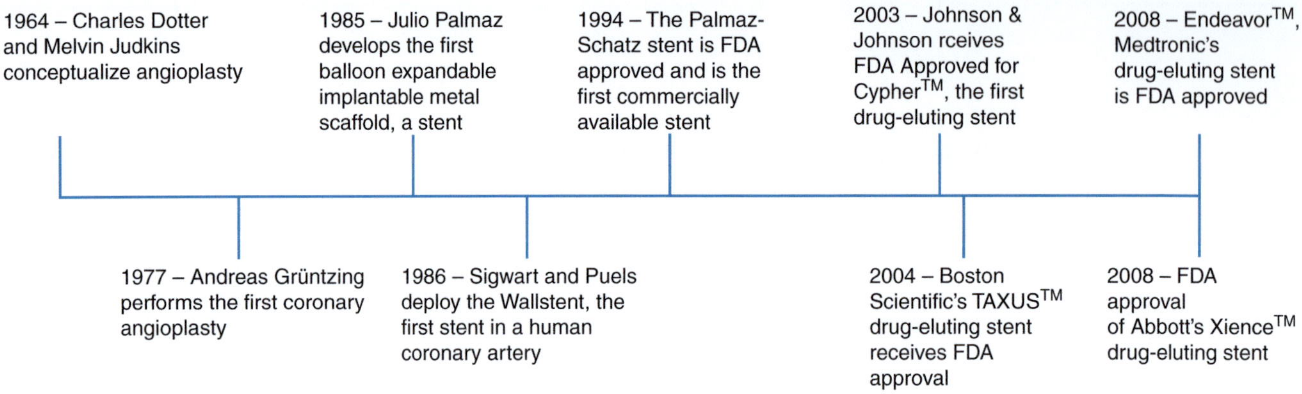

Fig. 10.1 Abbreviated timeline of percutaneous coronary intervention and stent development (Courtesy of Richard Schatz, MD)

(procedure success Endeavor 98.8 % vs. Cypher 94.7 % $p=0.02$) [10]. Aside from improved deliverability, thinner struts have reproducibly decreased restenosis rates when compared to thicker bare-metal comparators as demonstrated in the ISAR-STERO studies [11, 12].

Stent Architecture

Current stent architecture is primarily based on the initial slotted tube design by Julio Palmaz [5]. Importance of stent architecture was evident when neointimal hyperplasia and mural thrombus were significantly decreased when stent geometry was matched to the circular vessel lumen instead of distorting it into nonnative geometry [13]. A prospective study randomizing various bare-metal stents showed differences in freedom from myocardial infarction and follow-up angiographic percent diameter stenosis and late loss between different stent designs, reinforcing the concept of optimal stent architecture [14]. The current design of cellular stents is generalized as either open- or closed-cell design (Figs. 10.2 and 10.3). Computer modeling suggests that there is less tissue prolapse with open-cell design and direct comparisons of bare-metal open-cell to closed-cell stents show that the restenosis rates favor open-cell designs [14, 16]. In theory, open-cell designs should allow greater access to side branches and possibly improve patency of covered side branches. Open-cell DES may have advantages with respect to decreasing myocardial infarction (MI) and target lesion revascularization (TLR) when jailing side branches as reported in a post hoc analysis of SPIRIT III [17]. Closed-cell design may enable even distribution of drugs across the endovascular surface, although there is no prospective data indicating this significantly impacts restenosis rates.

Polymer

Most biological agents require a coating matrix for drug retention and controlling drug-release kinetics. Drugs are released either by particle dissolution or diffusion when polymer breakdown is incorporated (absorbed) into a biodegradable substance. The material should be biologically inert but be able to retain physiochemical composition after sterilization and stent expansion. First-generation DES utilized polymers, long-chained molecules in several small repeating units (Table 10.1) [18]. Although successful in retaining and delivering drug, first-generation polymers have been suspected in causing inflammation implicated in late restenosis and stent thrombosis [19]. An alternate strategy is to improve biocompatibility by using biomimetic compounds. Phosphorylcholine is a naturally occurring zwitterionic compound that emulates a phospholipid membrane that may bind drugs but has a shortened drug elution capacity [20]. Similarly, in an effort to synthetically mimic the phospholipid bilayer structure, the next generation of biocompatible copolymers is Biolinx® (Medtronic, Santa Rosa, CA), a proprietary bled of three polymers: hydrophilic c-19 copolymer, water-soluble polyvinyl pyrrolidinone, and hydrophobic c-10 copolymer [21]. Further details of polymer coatings of individual stents will be discussed further in subsequent sections ascribed to each individual stent.

Drug

Restenosis remains the chief liability of percutaneous interventions and was the impetus for the development of DES. The pathophysiology of restenosis consists of elastic recoil and negative arterial remodeling, followed by neointimal hyperplasia [22]. Inflammation from the endothelial injury and proliferation of smooth muscle cells are largely responsible for the neointimal hyperplasia; therefore, delivery of antiproliferative agents has been the dominant theme of restenosis therapy. Thus far, the armamentarium of drugs to decrease the proliferative response post-endothelial injury have been derived from chemotherapeutic agents and immunomodulators.

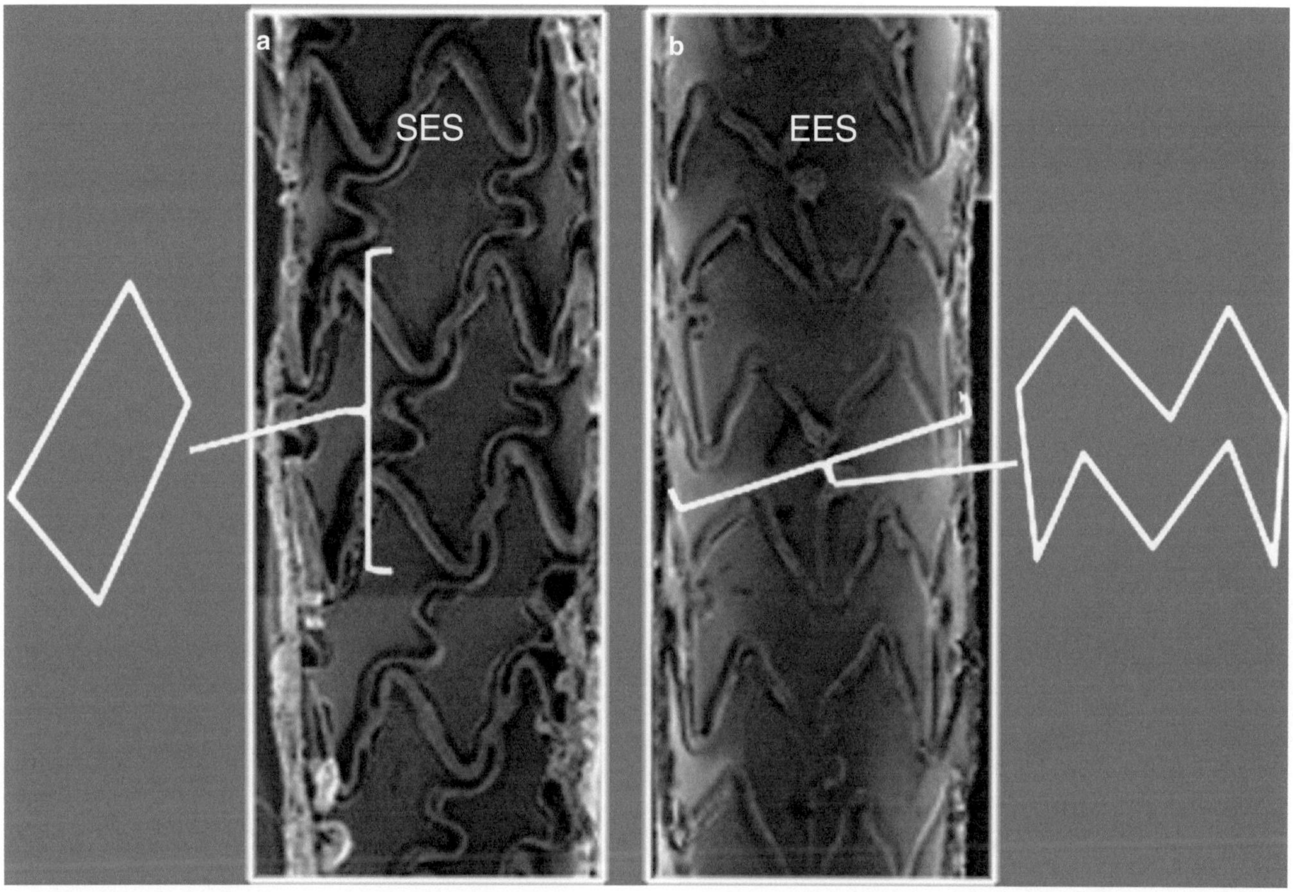

Fig. 10.2 Closed- and open-cell stent design. (**a**) Closed-cell design of the sirolimus-eluting stent (*SES*). The cell is enclosed within a simple geometric shape and retains the area regardless of how stretched the stent becomes. (**b**) Open-cell design of the everolimus-eluting stents (*EES*). The area enclosed by the cell is more complex in shape with convex and concave inflection points throughout the shape. The cell area is capable of increasing greatly with stent expansion (Adapted from Joner et al. [15], with permission)

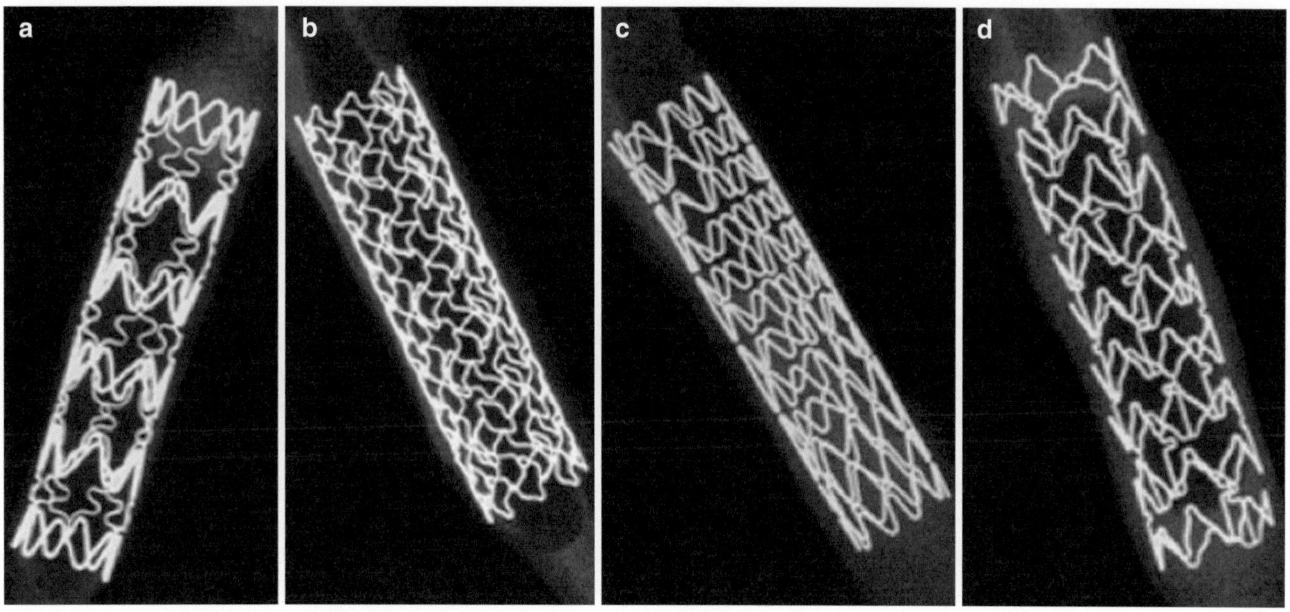

Fig. 10.3 High-resolution radiographs of each drug-eluting stent platform. (**a**) Cypher platform, BX Velocity (Cordis Corp., Johnson & Johnson, Miami, Florida). (**b**) TAXUS platform, Liberté (Boston Scientific, Natick, Massachusetts). (**c**) Endeavor platform, Driver (Medtronic Vascular, Santa Rosa, California). (**d**) XIENCE platform, Multilink Vision (Abbott Vascular, Santa Clara, California) (Adapted from Joner et al. [15], with permission)

Table 10.1 Characteristics of drug-eluting stents commercially available in the United States

	Cypher	TAXUS	Endeavor	Xience
Platform	Bx Velocity	Express/Liberte	Driver	Multilink Vision
Architecture	Closed cell	Open/open cell	Modular, open cell	Open cell
Alloy	316 L	316 L	Cobalt chromium	Cobalt chromium
Strut thickness	140 μm	132 μm/97 μm	91 μm	81 μm
Drug	Sirolimus	Paclitaxel	Zotarolimus	Everolimus
Polymer	PEVA/PMBA	SIBS (Translute®)	Phosphorylcholine	VDF-HFP
Drug elution kinetics	80 % eluted within 30 days	Slow release 10.2 % released in 10 days	98 % eluted within 14 days	80 % eluted within 30 days
Total elution time	168 days	Unknown	21–22 days	120 days

PEVA/PMBA polyethylene-co-vinyl acetate/poly-n-butyl methacrylate, *SIBS* styrene-isobutylene-styrene, *VDF-HFP* vinylidene fluoride and hexafluoropropylene

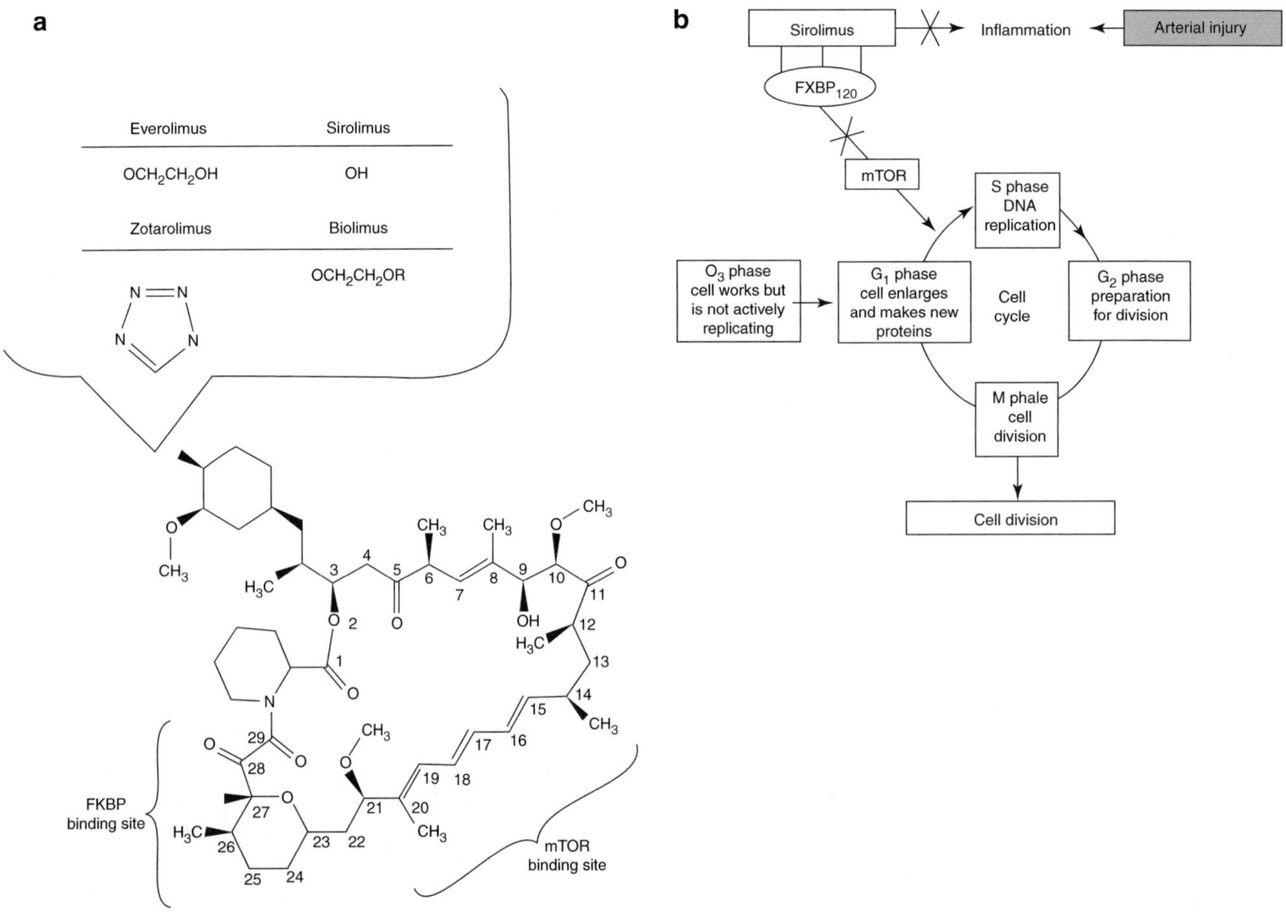

Fig. 10.4 Structure and molecular mechanism of sirolimus and its analogues. (**a**) Chemical structure of sirolimus showing the FKBP12 and mTOR binding sites. Position 42 is a hydroxyl group in sirolimus but is substituted with various side groups as shown below in other analogues. (**b–c**) Sirolimus binds to FK-binding protein 12 (FKBP12) and is then enabled to bind to mammalian target of rapamycin (mTOR). mTOR inhibits downregulation of p27[kip1], halting the cell cycle between the G1 and S1 phases (Adapted from Garg and Serrys [23], with permission)

Sirolimus and Limus Analogues

Sirolimus is a macrolide antibiotic derived from cultured *Streptomyces hygroscopicus* and clinically utilized to prevent transplantation rejection. A potent antifungal, immunosuppressive, and antimitotic agent, sirolimus binds to specific cytosolic proteins instrumental to cell cycle progression (Fig. 10.4). Sirolimus binds to FK506 (FKBP12), and this complex inhibits the activation of mammalian target of rapamycin (mTOR). Binding of mTOR in turn prevents the downregulation of p27, increasing intracellular levels resulting in cyclin-dependent kinase (CDK)-clin complexes. Ultimately arrest of the G1-S phase of the cell cycle halts smooth muscle cell proliferation. Formerly used as an immunosuppressant to treat organ transplant rejection, application towards vascular restenosis was recognized and applied in the Cypher stent [18].

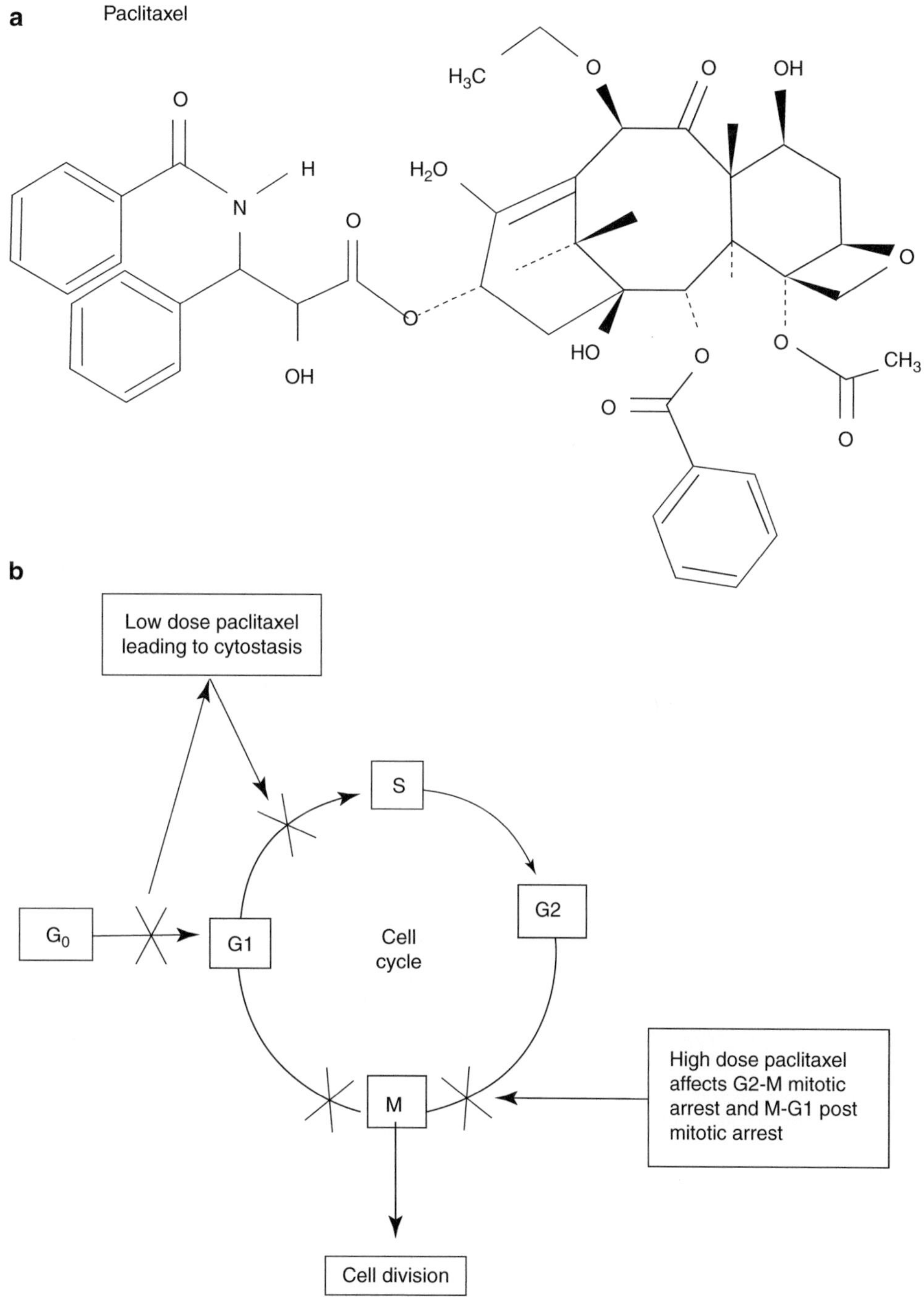

Fig. 10.5 (**a**) Chemical structure and function (**b**) of paclitaxel. Paclitaxel stabilizes microtubules resulting in arrest at the mitotic spindle checkpoint of cell division (Adapted from Garg and Serrrys [23], with permission)

Zotarolimus

Zotarolimus is a proprietary analogue created by substituting a tetrazole ring for the hydroxyl group at position 42 in sirolimus as this site was the most tolerant to modification without altering biological activity (Fig. 10.4). The most hydrophilic of DES drugs, the poor water solubility prevents rapid release into the circulation and favors crossing cell membranes to reach its molecular target [20].

Everolimus

Another analogue of sirolimus, the mechanism of action is identical but its immunosuppressive activity is two to threefold lower than sirolimus in vitro. Nevertheless, in vivo animal data has shown a potent anti-restenotic effect when delivered orally or via DES [18].

Biolimus

Another sirolimus analogue, biolimus has an alkoxy-alkyl group replacing the hydrogen at position 42-o (Fig. 10.4) [24].

Paclitaxel

Isolated from the bark of the Western yew tree, paclitaxel has a complex 8-member ring in its center that stabilizes microtubule formation (Fig. 10.5). Binding to the β-tubulin subunit of microtubules, it antagonizes disassembly and the cell arrests in the middle of mitosis (G2/M phase). Due to its stabilization of microtubules, paclitaxel impacts cell mobility, notably inhibition of smooth muscle cell migration in vitro and in vivo [25].

Drug-Eluting Stents

Bare-metal restenosis rates of at least 20–25 % in randomized clinical trials prompted the development of strategies to improve the efficacy of stenting [26]. While the mechanical optimization of stenting approached its limits, initial attempts at localized delivery of anti-restenotic medications were unsuccessful due to washout [18]. Stents were appealing as a vehicle for local drug delivery as scaffolding evenly distributed drug to the underlying tissue and served as a reservoir for drug with the possibility of controlling the release kinetics. Harmonizing biocompatibility, drug dose, release kinetics, and drug coating elasticity to yield adequate safety and efficacy proved challenging but at last produced the first clinically efficacious drug-eluting stent, the sirolimus-eluting stent [27].

Sirolimus-Eluting Stents

The Cypher® (Cordis Corporation, Bridgewater, NJ) sirolimus-eluting stent (SES) was the first commercially available DES in the United States in 2003. A 316 L stainless steel platform, the Bx Velocity has relatively thick struts (140 μm) and is a closed-cell stent configuration (Table 10.1). A base coat of PEVA/PMBA (polyethylene-co-vinyl acetate/poly-n-butyl methacrylate) is combined with sirolimus as a base layer while a topcoat is applied to serve as a drug diffusion barrier. Approximately 80 % of sirolimus is released in the first 30 days and becomes undetectable at 168 days [28].

First-in-man experience of SES confirmed durable suppression of neointimal proliferation verified by serial angiographic and intravascular ultrasound over the duration of 12 months laying the foundation for prospective clinical evaluation of SES to treat coronary artery disease [28]. Initial randomized trials RAVEL and SIRIUS proceeded to report consistent decreases in target lesion and vessel revascularization without an increased signal of harm (RAVEL SES TLR 0.0 % vs. BMS 26.6 % $P<0.05$) (Table 10.2) [27]. Continued benefit of SES compared to BMS was reproducible across various studies (Table 10.2) in broader patient subgroups including acute myocardial infarction (MI) and more complex coronary artery disease such as long lesions, chronic total occlusions, and diabetes. Analysis of 14 SES vs. BMS trials revealed that SES decreased the risk for the combined endpoint of death, MI, and revascularization (HR 0.43 CI 0.34 to 0.54 $P<0.0001$) compared to BMS largely driven by target vessel revascularization [29]. Analysis of stent thrombosis found no significant difference between SES and BMS; however, there was very low rate but trend towards increased late stent thrombosis in patients receiving SES (SES 0.8 % vs. BMS 0.3 % $P=0.16$) [29].

Paclitaxel-Eluting Stents

The TAXUS family of DES has gone through several iterative advances involving the stent platform and polymer/drug formulation. The first-generation commercially available TAXUS Express utilized a 316 L stainless steel platform and

Table 10.2 Major clinical trial and pooled analysis results of patients receiving sirolimus-eluting stents (SES) in different clinical settings

Study	Patient population	Follow-up	N	Cardiac death	MI	TLR/TVR	MACE	ST[a]
Kastrati A et al. analysis of 14 trials[b] [29]	Pooled analysis	6–58 months	14 trials	HR 1.03	HR 0.93	HR 0.43	NA	0.8 %
Spaulding C et al. pooled analysis [30]	Pooled analysis	1,440 days	878	3.5 %	6.4 %	NA	NA	3.6 %
SIRIUS[c] [31]	Stable CAD, on-label	5 year	533	8.4 %	6.2 %	9.4 %	20.3 %	3.9 %
TYPHOON[c] [32]	Acute MI, off-label	4 year	294	2.4 %	5.2 %	7.6 %	NA	5.2 %
ARTS II [33]	Unrestricted, multivessel disease	5 year	607	5.4 %	4.4 %	14.5 %	27.2 %	9.0 %
RAVEL[c] [34]	Stable CAD, on-label	5 year	120	12.1 %	7.3 %	7.4 %	25.8 %	3.3 %
SCANDSTENT [35]	Unrestricted	3 year	163	2.5 %	3.7 %	4.9 %	12.3 %	3.1 %
J-Cypher [36]	Unrestricted, ACS	3 year	2,308	7.2 %	3.3 %	12.1 %	NA	2.2 %
RESEARCH [37]	Unrestricted	6 year	508	16.3 %	NA	13.6 %	29.7 %	3.1 %
SESAMI[c] [38]	Acute MI, off-label	3 year	157	3.2 %	2.5 %	7.0 %	12.7 %	5.1 %
ENDEAVOR III[c] [39]	Stable CAD, on-label	3 year	113	7.2 %	4.5 %	12.2 %	18.7 %	1.7 %

CAD coronary artery disease, *MI* myocardial infarction, *ACS* acute coronary syndrome
[a]All ARC defined stent thrombosis including definite, possible, and probable
[b]HR calculated against bare-metal controls in randomized trials
[c]Study protocol mandated angiographic follow-up

Table 10.3 Clinical results of patients receiving paclitaxel-eluting stents (PES) for different indications from major studies

Study	Patient population	Follow-up	*N*	Cardiac death	MI	TLR/TVR	MACE	ST[a]
TAXUS II[b] [42]	Stable CAD, on-label	5 year	131	2.4 %	4.7 %	10.3 %	20.4 %	2.7 %
TAXUS IV[b] [43]	Stable CAD, on-label	5 year	643	4.4 %	7.2 %	9.1 %	24 %	2.2 %[c]
WDHR [44]	Unrestricted, off-label	2 year	1,991	3.2 %	5.3 %	32 % RR[d]	NA	3.3 %
PASSION [45]	Acute MI, off-label	5 year	310	8.9 %	6.8 %	7.7 %	18.6 %	4.2 %
HORIZONS[b] [46]	Acute MI, off-label	3 year	2,257	3.2 %	7.0 %	9.4 %	20.0 %	4.8 %[c]
SPIRIT III[b] [47]	Stable CAD, on-label	3 year	332	1.9 %	6.6 %	12.8 %	16.4 %	1.7 %[c]
ENDEAVOR IV[b] [48]	Stable CAD, on-label	3 year	775	2.4 %	4.9 %	6.1 %	13.6 %	3.0 %
T-SEARCH [37]	Unrestricted, off-label	6 year	576	16.0 %[e]	NA	12.5 %	29.9 %	2.8 %

[a]All ARC defined stent thrombosis including definite, possible, and probable
[b]Study protocol mandated angiographic follow-up
[c]Reported only definite and probable stent thrombosis
[d]Relative reduction of TLR compared to bare-metal stents
[e]All-cause mortality

was coated with a hydrophobic, elastomeric triblock copolymer (styrene-isobutylene-styrene) commercially known as Translute™ (Boston Scientific, Natick, MA) [40]. Three formulations were developed with increasing drug to polymer ratio from 8.8 to 35 % weight in weight (w/w) at a constant dose density to yield a slow-, moderate-, and fast-release stent coating. The slow-release (TAXUS-SR) drug-polymer combination is commercially available on both the TAXUS Express and TAXUS Liberté stents, while the moderate-release (TAXUS-MR) version of TAXUS was clinically tested in prospective trials, but not made commercially available [41].

TAXUS clinical trial development mirrored that of the Cypher stent. Initial studies determined efficacy of PES in patients with CAD and simple complexity lesions (Table 10.3). TAXUS I showed that PES was indeed superior to BMS with respect to repeat revascularization [49]. TAXUS II compared efficacy of slow-release to moderate-release PES, and while moderate-release PES was found to have lower rates of TLR, it was not commercially developed (5-year TLR TAXUS-SR 10.3 % vs. TAXUS-MR 64.5 %) [42]. The pivotal trial for FDA approval of PES was TAXUS IV, a prospective randomized study comparing TAXUS Express to its identical bare-metal counterpart in treating simple coronary lesions. In short-term and 5-year follow-up, durable efficacy relative to bare-metal stents with respect to TLR was maintained with comparable rates of stent thrombosis between each group (5-year ST BMS 2.1 % vs. TAXUS-SR 2.2 % P=NS) [43].

In order to enhance procedural performance, paclitaxel and Translute were affixed to a different stainless steel platform, the Liberté™ (Natick, MA, Boston Scientific) stent. The Liberté is a 316 L stainless steel platform with significantly thinner struts (Express 132 μm vs. Liberté 97 μm) and a more uniform strut pattern to improve distribution of drug. Subsequently, TAXUS Liberté was clinically tested in the TAXUS ATLAS prospective trial, comparing patients receiving TAXUS Liberté to historical controls pooled from TAXUS IV and V trials [50]. Overall, the TAXUS Liberté platform met its endpoints for non-inferiority compared to the TAXUS Express stent at 9-month follow-up; however, in a prespecified subgroup analysis, TAXUS Liberté treatment of small vessels was superior to TAXUS EXPRESS in reducing 9-month TLR in small vessels (16.9 % vs. 6.1 % $P<0.05$) [51].

Expansion of PES utilization in the setting of acute MI showed consistent results in decreased TLR rates compared to bare-metal counterparts (PES 4.5 % vs. BMS 7.5 % $P=0.002$) in HORIZONS-AMI, a multicenter trial with a 2×2 factorial design randomizing against bivalirudin and heparin/glycoprotein IIb/IIIa inhibitors and PES vs. BMS [52, 53]. Notably, stent thrombosis for both BMS and PES remained relatively high for each cohort (ST PES 3.2 % vs. BMS 3.4 % $P=0.77$) at 1 year [54].

Sirolimus-Eluting Stents vs. Paclitaxel-Eluting Stents

After the release of both first-generation DES, head to head comparisons were drawn as both stents had contrasting drug mechanisms, elution kinetics, and polymers. Direct comparisons in patients with stable CAD in real-world context were performed in the SIRTAX trial comparing SES and PES [55]. Angiographic follow-up showed increased late lumen loss and binary restenosis translating into increased TLR for the PES group (Table 10.4). Increased late loss and binary restenosis were again observed in a trial with simpler lesion subsets, the REALITY trial, signaling that PES intrinsically may carry greater risks of in-stent restenosis [61]. Despite higher rates of binary restenosis, no significant clinical impact was observed as similar rates of TLR occurred in both SES and PES cohorts (TLR SES 6.0 % vs. PES 6.1 % $P>0.99$) [61]. Based on the less favorable angiographic restenosis seen in studies with angiographic follow-up, expectation for greater separation in TLR events between SES and PES would have

Table 10.4 Results of major studies comparing the performance of sirolimus-eluting stents (SES) and paclitaxel-eluting stents (PES) against the background of different clinical indications

				MACE		MI		TLR/TVR		Death		ST	
Study	Stent	Follow-up	*N*	%	*P*	%	P	%	*P*	%	*P*	%	*P*
SORT OUT II [56]	SES	546 d	1,065	10	0.21	4.2	0.32	4.5	0.14	1.7	0.8	2.6	0.7
	PES		1,033	11.6		5.1		5.9		1.5		2.8	
SIRTAX [55]	SES	9 mo	503	6.2	0.009	2.8	0.49	4.8	0.03	0.6	0.15	2.0	0.62
	PES		509	10.8		3.5		8.3		1.6		1.6	
Diabetes [57]	SES	2 year	200	3.5	0.001	0.5	0.999	3.5	0.004	0	0.248	1.0	0.499
	PES		200	12.5		1.0		11.0		1.5		0	
ISAR DIABETES [58]	SES	9 mo	125	NA	NA	4.0	0.72	6.4	0.13	3.2	0.52	NA	NA
	PES		125	NA		2.4		12.0		4.8		NA	
ISAR DESIRE [59]	SES	1 year	100	NA	NA	1.0	NS	8.0	0.02	2.0	NS	NA	NA
	PES		100	NA		2.0		19.0		1.0		NA	
ISAR DESIRE 2 [60]	SES	1 year	225	20.4	0.71	2.7	0.53	16.6	0.52	3.4	0.60	0.4	0.67
	PES		225	19.6		1.8		14.6		4.5		0.4	
RESEARCH [37]	SES	6 year	508	29.7	HR 1.01	NA	NA	13.6	HR 1.06	16.3	HR 1.0	3.1	0.9
	PES		576	29.9	(0.9–1.14)	NA		12.5	(0.89–1.26)	16.0	(0.86–1.17)	2.8	
REALITY [61]	SES	1 year	684	10.7	0.73	5.1	0.55	6.0	0.99	1.5	0.63	NA	NA
	PES		669	11.4		6.0		6.1		1.0			
Meta-analysis [62]	SES						HR 0.84		HR 0.74		HR 0.92		HR 0.66
	PES						(0.69–1.03)		(0.63–0.87)		(0.74–1.13)		(0.46–0.94)

D days, *HR* hazard ratio, *mo* months, *NA* not applicable

been expected in diabetic populations. While PES was found to have more in-stent restenosis (ISR) in the DIABETES trial (TLR SES 2.0 % vs. PES 7.5 % $P=0.017$) [63], equivalent performance with respect to major adverse cardiac events (MACE) and target lesion revascularization/target vessel revascularization (TLR/TVR) was seen in subsequent head to head SES/PES trials for different lesion subsets including randomized comparison for treating bare-metal or SES restenosis (Table 10.4) [59, 64]. A nonrandomized comparison of SES and PES in a real-world context was published from the Rotterdam DES registries also showing no significant difference in terms of MACE [37]. However, when the data is pooled in meta-analysis, PES was found to have an increased hazard towards myocardial infarction, TLR/TVR, and stent thrombosis compared to SES utilization (Table 10.4) [62].

On-Label vs. Off-Label Use of DES

The approval of both first-generation drug-eluting stents was based on clinical trials enrolling symptomatic patients treating vessel diameters between 2.5 and 3.5 mm and discrete lesions less than 30 mm in length. These patients did not represent high-risk clinical indications (e.g., acute coronary syndromes) or complex lesion morphologies and therefore constitute the most stable segment of the patient spectrum undergoing PCI yet only make up an estimated 51 % of patients of the NHLBI registry referred for stent implantation [65]. Off-label indications include higher-risk patient and lesion subsets such as acute myocardial infarction, chronic total occlusions, saphenous vein graft lesions, bifurcations, and long stenoses (Table 10.5). The remaining 49 % of patients in the NHLBI Dynamic Registry treated for off-label indications and predictably TVR, MI, stent thrombosis, and death are consistently

Table 10.5 Definitions of on-label and off-label use of drug-eluting stents

On-label indications for DES
Patients with symptomatic CAD of inducible ischemia
Discrete de novo coronary lesions
Vessel diameter ≥2.5 mm to ≤3.5 mm
Lesion length ≤30 mm
Off-label indications for DES
ST-elevation myocardial infarction
Chronic total occlusions
Saphenous vein grafts
Bifurcation lesions
Ostial lesions
Left main stenosis
In-stent restenosis
Long lesions
Small vessels
Large vessels
Multi-lesion percutaneous coronary intervention

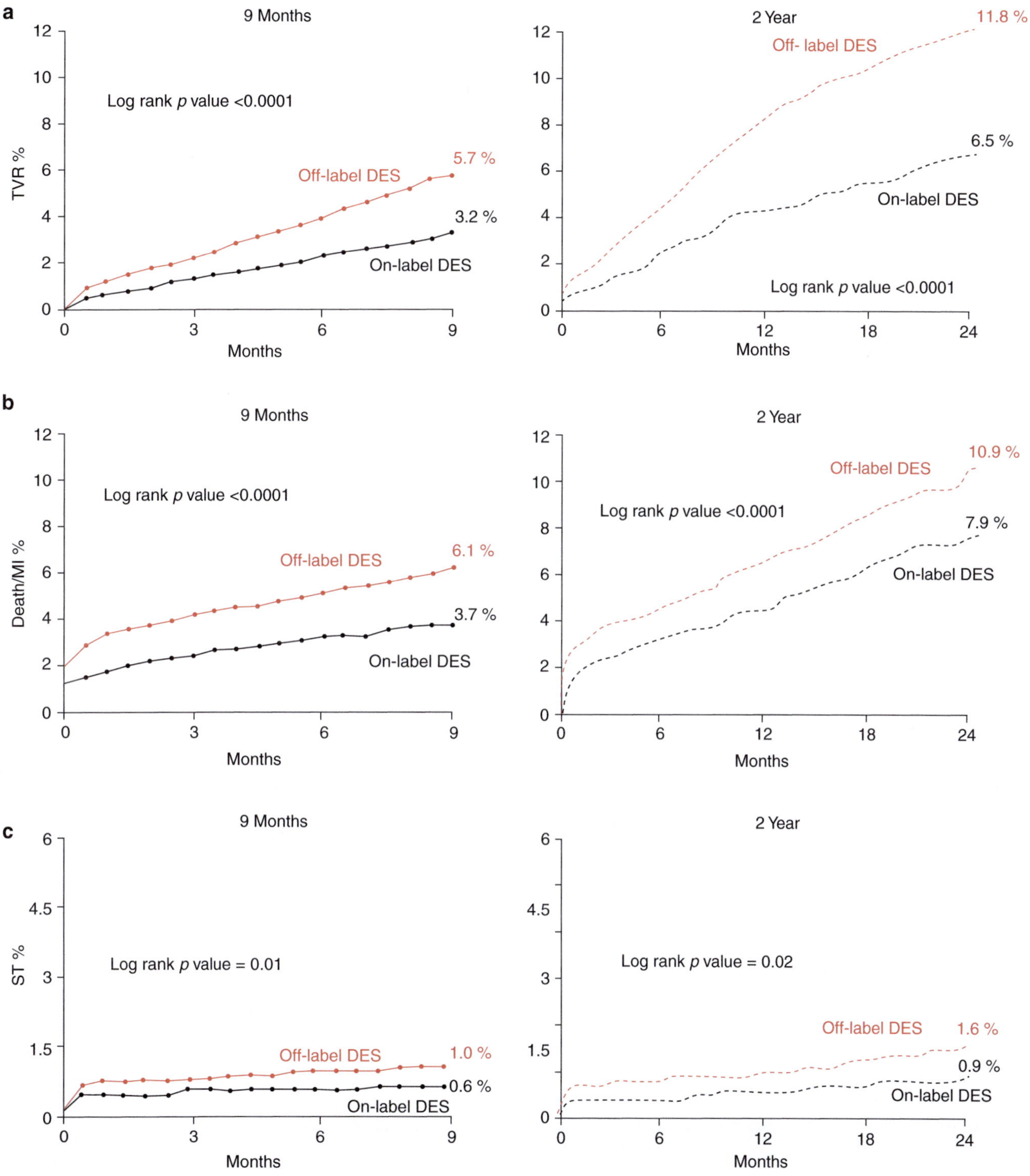

Fig. 10.6 Comparison of event rates between off-label and standard use of drug-eluting stents (*DES*). Kaplan-Meier estimates comparing event rates at 9 months and 2 years between off-label and on-label use of *DES* in the *STENT* (Strategic Transcatheter Evaluation of New Therapies) group, a US multicenter prospective registry. (**a**) Target vessel revascularization (*TVR*), (**b**) death or myocardial infarction (death/MI), and (**c**) stent thrombosis (From Brodie et al. [66], with permission)

worse in the off-label cohort (Fig. 10.6) [66]. The efficacy of DES compared to BMS in off-label use mirrors on-label DES use with improvements in repeat revascularization, but the analysis showed decreased rates for death and MI for DES use (Table 10.6) [65]. High atherosclerotic burden, selection bias towards higher-risk patients (acute myocardial infarction), and more complex anatomy (chronic total occlusions) temper the effectiveness of DES. For instance, in the E-Five Registry,

Table 10.6 Cumulative 1-year rates of safety and efficacy of bare-metal and drug-eluting stents in the NHLBI Dynamic Registry [65]

	Standard			Off-label		
	Bare-metal stent	Drug-eluting stent		Bare-metal stent	Drug-eluting stent	
	N=1,748	N=1,381		N=2,110	N=1,312	
	%		p-Value	%		p-Value
Safety						
Death	2.7	2.8	0.88	6.4	3.7	<0.001
Myocardial infarction	4.1	3.3	0.24	5.9	4.4	0.06
Death or myocardial infarction	6.4	5.8	0.42	11.6	7.5	<0.001
Efficacy						
Repeat percutaneous coronary intervention	10.5	6.5	<0.001	13.6	11.4	0.07
Coronary artery bypass grafting	4.3	1.4	<0.001	5.1	1.5	<0.001
Repeat revascularization	13.4	7.7	<0.001	17.5	12.7	<0.001

DES assessment of safety and efficacy was derived from the 2004–2006 recruitment waves while bare-metal endpoints were abstracted from recruitment waves from 1997 to 2002. Patients receiving only bare-metal stents 2004–2006 were excluded due to significant selection bias (i.e., more cardiogenic shock), and this is essentially a comparison of outcomes between the bare-metal and DES era

Table 10.7 Compiled results of patients receiving zotarolimus-eluting stents (ZES) in major clinical trials and registries

Study	Patient population	Follow-up	N	Cardiac death	MI	TLR/TVR	MACE	ST[a]
ENDEAVOR I [67]	Stable CAD, on-label	12 month	100	0.0 %	1.0 %	1.0 %	2.0 %	1.0 %
ENDEAVOR II[b] [68]	Stable CAD, on-label	270 day	592	1.2 %	2.7 %	4.6 %	7.3 %	0.5 %
ENDEAVOR III[b] [10]	Stable CAD, on-label	3 year	323	3.3 %	0.6 %	17.9 %	18.6 %	0.9 %
ENDEAVOR IV [48]	Stable CAD, on-label	3 year	773	1.7 %	2.1 %	6.5 %	11.3 %	2.2 %
E-Five Registry [69]	Standard use, on-label	12 month	2,125	0.9 %	0.7 %	2.8 %	4.3 %	0.8 %
E-Five Registry [69]	Unrestricted, off-label	12 month	6,189	2.0 %	1.9 %	5.0 %	8.6 %	2.2 %
SORT OUT III [70]	Unrestricted, off-label	18 month	1,162	2.0 %	2.0 %	6.0 %	10.0 %	1.0 %

[a]All ARC defined stent thrombosis including definite, possible, and probable
[b]Study protocol mandated angiographic follow-up

comparison of the on- and off-label use showed increases in stent thrombosis (all ARC ST on-label 0.8 % vs. off-label 2.2 % $P<0.001$), myocardial infarction (MI on-label 0.7 % vs. off-label 1.9 % $p<0.001$), and cardiac death (cardiac death 0.9 % vs. 2.2 % $p<0.001$) (Table 10.7) [69].

Zotarolimus-Eluting Stents

Zotarolimus-eluting stents (ZES) (Endeavor®, Medtronic Vascular, Santa Rosa, California) are composed of a cobalt chromium (Driver®, Medtronic) platform. The stent is coated with phosphorylcholine, a blended composite polymer primarily comprised of hydrophilic monomers engineered to mimic the chemical structure of phospholipid head groups. A basecoat of phosphorylcholine is applied to the stent followed by a layer of zotarolimus, which then overlaid with a final coat of phosphorylcholine. A unique feature of ZES stents is rapid eluting of zotarolimus as 90 % is dispersed within 14 days and should remain within the vessel for 28 days. Zotarolimus (ABT-578, Abbott Pharmaceuticals, Abbott Park, Il) is a tetrazole-containing macrocyclic immunosuppressant that shares structural similarity and biological activity with sirolimus (Fig. 10.4).

Clinical testing of ZES first began in 2003 with ENDEAVOR I trial, a single-arm prospective observational study conducted in patients with stable CAD evaluating the medium- and long-term safety and efficacy in this first-in-man trial. With a low MACE rate of 2 % and 1 year TLR rate of 1 %, this paved the way for subsequent trials (Table 10.7) [67].

Zotarolimus-Eluting Stents vs. Bare-Metal Stents

A prospective multicenter trial outside the United States, the ENDEAVOR II randomized 1,197 patients to ZES or its corresponding Driver bare-metal stent platform (Table 10.7). This study confirmed that ZES successfully decreases rates of TLR and TVR compared to its bare-metal platform without any increase in death, MI, or stent thrombosis [68]. Angiographic and IVUS 8-month follow-up showed that late loss and binary restenosis consistently favored ZES compared to BMS. With regard to the overall safety and efficacy compared to bare-metal stents, a pooled analysis of six studies with a mean follow-up of 4.1 years comparing ZES and BMS in 2,132 and 596 patients, respectively, demonstrated

Table 10.8 Academic Research Consortium (ARC) definitions for stent thrombosis

Academic Research Consortium definitions of stent thrombosis
Definite
Angiographic evidence of thrombosis
Pathological confirmation of stent thrombosis
Probable
Any unexplained death within first 30 days
Irrespective of time after the index procedure, any MI that is related to the documented acute ischemia in the territory of the implanted stent without angiographic confirmation of stent thrombosis
Possible stent thrombosis
Clinical definition of possible stent thrombosis is considered to have occurred with any unexplained death from 30 days after intracoronary stenting until the end of follow-up
Acute stent thrombosis
0 to 24 h after stent implantation
Subacute stent thrombosis
>24 h to 30 days after stent implantation
Late stent thrombosis
>30 days to 1 year after stent implantation
Very late stent thrombosis
>1 year after stent implantation

From Cutlip et al. [72], with permission

equivalence in outcomes with respect to hard endpoints and a 58 % reduction in TLR in patients implanted with ZES compared BMS. A small nonsignificant increase in Academic Research Consortium (ARC)-defined definite/probable stent thrombosis favoring ZES (ZES 0.8 %; BMS 1.7 % P=NS) was observed, signaling that the lower stent thrombosis risk in ZES may confer an advantage to first-generation DES counterparts [71] (Table 10.8).

Zotarolimus-Eluting Stents Compared to Other Drug-Eluting Stents

Clinical development of ZES continued with a non-inferiority comparison of ZES to SES in ENDEAVOR III. Evaluating a primary endpoint of angiographic in-segment late lumen loss at 8 months, the study did not achieve non-inferiority, demonstrating significantly higher late lumen loss and restenosis with the Endeavor stent despite no significant differences in repeat revascularization (SES 0.13±0.32 mm vs. ZES 0.34±0.44 mm $P<0.001$) [10]. Differences in rate of non-Q-wave MI favoring ZES (ZES 0.6 % vs. SES 3.5 % $P=0.04$) were observed largely driven by post-procedure myonecrosis. In spite of initially higher angiographic late lumen loss, rates of clinical restenosis beyond the period of protocol-specified angiographic follow-up remained stable with ZES compared with SES, resulting in similar late-term efficacy [73]. Over 5 years, significant differences in death, MI, and composite endpoints favored treatment with ZES, contesting the notion that less favorable early angiographic surrogates of efficacy accurately predict important clinical events.

ENDEAVOR IV compared ZES to PES in standard de novo coronary stenosis (Table 10.6). ZES compared favorably with PES, with regard to MACE at 1 year, but after extending the follow-up to 3 years, a significant difference in rates of myocardial infarction was observed (ZES 2.1 % vs. PES 4.9 % $p=0.005$) [39]. This was attributed to increased rates in very late stent thrombosis (VLST) observed in the PES cohort (definite/probable ST ZES 0.1 % vs. PES 1.6 % $p=0.004$) with a minimal increase of VLST in ZES during the 2nd and 3rd year of follow-up. Again primary angiographic endpoint at 8 months in the trial showed greater late lumen loss and binary restenosis for ZES; however, this did not confer higher rates of TLR at the 3-year assessment [48, 74].

Zotarolimus-Eluting Stents in Routine Clinical Practice

Results of ZES in routine clinical practice outside stringent clinical trial restrictions on lesion type or patient clinical risk had yet to be tested (e.g., STEMI); therefore, greater than 8,000 patients in post-marketing surveillance were followed for safety and efficacy across a broad spectrum of lesions and patient groups. The 12-month clinical outcomes for ZES implantation showed that implantation in an off-label fashion yielded favorable but less comparable results to on-label utilization of ZES. For instance, higher rates of stent thrombosis (definite/probable ST off-label 1.4 % vs. on-label 0.4 %) and TLR (off-label 5 % vs. on-label 2.8 %) were observed, suggesting that low thrombosis rates previously observed in simple and moderately complexity disease in the ENDEAVOR III/IV trials could not be assumed when treating unselected patients with complex coronary disease [69].

Effectiveness of ZES and SES were directly compared in routine clinical practice in the randomized SORT OUT III trial. A total of 2,332 patients were randomized to receive ZES or SES and followed clinically for 18 months. At 18 months, patients receiving ZES experienced higher rates of TLR (ZES 6 % vs. SES 2 % $P<0.0001$). A slightly higher rate of myocardial infarction was observed in the ZES group (ZES 2 % vs. SES 1 % $P=0.029$), although rates of stent thrombosis were similar between groups at 18 months [70].

New-Generation Zotarolimus-Eluting Stents

The latest generation of zotarolimus-eluting stents is the RESOLUTE® DES (Medtronic Vascular, Santa Rosa, California) which utilizes the identical Driver® platform and

Table 10.9 Clinical results of zotarolimus-eluting Resolute® (Medtronic Cardiovascular, Santa Rosa, California) stents

Study	Patient population	Follow-up	*N*	Cardiac death	MI	TLR/TVR	MACE	ST[a]
RESOLUTE FIM [75]	Stable CAD, on-label	12 month	138	0.7 %	5.8 %	0.7 %	8.7 %	0.7 %
RESOLUTE ALL COMERS [76]	Unrestricted, off-label	12 month	1,119	1.3 %	4.2 %[b]	3.9 %	8.7 %	2.3 %
RESOLUTE ALL COMERS [77]	Unrestricted, off-label	2 year	1,119	2.6 %	5.5 %[b]	8.0 %	12.5 %	1.9 %
RESOLUTE US [78]	Stable CAD, on-label	12 month	1,376	1.3 %	1.4 %	2.8 %	NA	0.1 %

FIM first in man
*Study protocol mandated angiographic follow-up
[a]Definite and probable stent thrombosis
[b]Target vessel myocardial infarction

Table 10.10 Late loss and binary restenosis rates for each drug-eluting stent in pivotal clinical trials

Study	Stent type	Angiographic follow-up	In-stent late loss	Binary restenosis
SIRIUS [79]	SES	240 days	0.17±0.45 mm	3.2 %
TAXUS VI [80]	PES	9 months	0.39±0.57 mm	9.1 %
ENDEAVOR III [10]	ZES	8 months	0.60±0.48 mm	9.2 %
SPIRIT III [81]	EES	8 months	0.16±0.41 mm	2.3 %

SES sirolimus-eluting stent, *PES* paclitaxel-eluting stent, *ZES* zotarolimus-eluting stent, *EES* everolimus-eluting stent

zotarolimus drug but has a different polymer. The Biolinx® (Medtronic Vascular, Santa Rosa, California) polymer is a blend of three polymers: hydrophilic c-19 copolymer, water-soluble polyvinyl pyrrolidinone, and hydrophobic c-10 copolymer [21]. This new polymer extends drug elution to 180 days total in attempts to decrease restenosis rates. RESOLUTE stents showed equivocal outcomes compared to EES with respect to death, ischemia-driven TLR, myocardial infarction, and overall MACE through the 2 years of follow-up (Tables 10.9 and 10.10) in the RESOLUTE ALL COMERS trial. The first year reported rates of definite stent thrombosis favored EES (definite ST RESOLUTE 1.2 % vs. EES 0.3 % $p=0.01$) as did combined definite/probable stent thrombosis rates (definite/probable ST RESOLUTE 1.6 % vs. EES 0.7 % $P=0.05$) [76]. This combined rate of definite/probable stent thrombosis remained numerically higher for the RESOLUTE stent cohort at 2 years but was no longer significantly different (definite/probable ST RESOLUTE 1.9 % vs. EES 1.0 % $P=0.077$) [77]. The RESOLUTE-US study was prospective observational trial enrolling 1,402 patients with stable CAD and demonstrated lower of stent thrombosis relative to RESOLUTE ALL COMERS study (definite/probable ST 0.1 %), likely related to high proportion of patients with myocardial infarction (33–34 %) enrolled in the ALL COMERS study, while the US study excluded acute coronary syndromes [78].

Everolimus-Eluting Stents

The Xience V (Abbott Vascular, Santa Clara, CA) is a next-generation DES consisting of an everolimus-coated Vision (Abbott Vascular, Santa Clara, CA) bare-metal platform. Everolimus is a semisynthetic macrolide analogue of sirolimus substitution at 2-hydroxyethyl group at position 42 (Fig. 10.4). The Vision stent platform is a thin-strutted cobalt chromium open-cell stent coated with a primer layer followed by a drug matrix layer. The primer is an acrylic polymer while the drug matrix layer is a durable copolymer, vinylidene fluoride and hexafluoropropylene (VDF-HFP), blended with everolimus.

Clinical development of the everolimus-eluting stent (EES) began with SPIRIT FIRST, a randomized superiority first-in-man trial enrolling 60 patients. The trial was single-blind 1:1 randomization to Vision bare-metal platform with the primary endpoint of angiographic in-stent late loss at 6 months. EES in-stent late loss of 0.10 mm represented an 88 % reduction compared with bare-metal late loss (0.87 mm), and there was significantly less restenosis in the EES cohort (Table 10.11) [82].

Subsequently the SPIRIT II compared EES to PES with the primary endpoint of angiographic late loss (Table 10.11) [90]. In this study, 6-month angiographic follow-up confirmed superiority to PES with respect to in-stent late loss prompting the larger SPIRIT III trial of EES compared to PES powered for non-inferiority with respect to both angiographic and clinical endpoints. After randomizing 1,002 patients to 2:1 ratio of EES to PES in the SPIRIT III trial, 9-month angiographic follow-up confirmed superiority of EES compared to PES in terms of angiographic late loss (EES 0.14±0.41 vs. PES 0.28±0.48 $P=0.004$) with no difference in target vessel failure at 1 year [91]. At 3-year follow-up, increased late loss translated into higher rates of PES TLR (EES 7.2 % vs. PES 12.8 %, $P=0.008$) with a trend towards higher MI in the PES cohort (EES 3.8 % vs. PES 6.6 % $P=0.07$) [47].

Table 10.11 Published results of patient receiving everolimus-eluting stents in major clinical studies

Study	Patient population	Follow-up	*N*	Cardiac death	MI	TLR/TVR	MACE	ST[a]
SPIRIT I[b] [82]	Stable CAD, on-label	180 day	26	0	3.8 %	3.8 %	7.7 %	0.0 %
SPIRIT II[b] [83]	Stable CAD, on-label	3 year	223	0.5 %	3.6 %	3.1 %	7.2 %	1.0 %
SPIRIT III[b] [81]	Stable CAD, on-label	3 year	669	1.6 %	3.8 %	7.2 %	9.7 %	1.3 %[c]
SPIRIT IV [84]	Stable CAD, on-label	1 year	2,458	0.4 %	1.9 %	2.5 %	4.2 %	0.3 %
SPIRIT IV [85]	Stable CAD, on-label	2 year	2,458	0.9 %	2.5 %	4.5 %	7.1 %	0.42 %
SPIRIT V [86]	Unrestricted, off-label	1 year	2,600	1.1 %	3.5 %	1.8 %	5.1 %	0.66 %
COMPARE [87]	Unrestricted, off-label	1 year	897	1.0 %	3.0 %	2.0 %	6.0 %	0.7 %[c]
COMPARE [88]	Unrestricted, off-label	2 year	897	2.2 %	3.9 %	2.9 %	9.0 %	0.9 %[c]
RESOLUTE[b] [77]	Unrestricted, off-label	2 year	1,126	2.2 %	5.0 %	7.3 %	12.9 %	1.0 %
X-SEARCH [89]	Unrestricted, off-label	6 month	649	5.9 %[d]	NA	3.1 %	9.2 %	0.6 %

[a]All ARC defined stent thrombosis including definite, possible, and probable
[b]Study protocol mandated angiographic follow-up
[c]Definite/probable stent thrombosis
[d]All-cause mortality

SPIRIT IV prospectively randomized EES to PES with more complex lesions with the primary endpoint of ischemia-driven target lesion failure (TLF) at 1 year without angiographic follow-up. Powered for non-inferiority with respect to TLF, 3,690 patients were followed for 1 year and found that PES had an early hazard towards TLF (EES 4.2 %, PES 6.8 % $P=0.001$). In addition rates of MI (MI EES 1.9 % vs. PES 3.1 % $P=0.02$) and stent thrombosis (ST EES 0.3 % vs. PES 1.1 % $p=0.004$) were noted to favor EES significantly. Although TLR rates in this trial were remarkably low, in part due to the absence of protocol-specified angiographic surveillance, a 45 % relative reduction in ischemia-driven TLR was nevertheless demonstrated in the EES (EES 2.5 % vs. PES 4.6 %, $p=0.001$) [84]. The benefits of lower TLR, myocardial infarction, and stent thrombosis of EES implantation compared to PES were durable over a 2-year follow-up [92].

Randomization of EES to PES in unrestricted real-world use recapitulated results from SPIRIT IV with statistically significantly greater myocardial infarctions, ischemia-driven TLR, and stent thrombosis in the PES arm at 1 year and extended into 2-year follow-up in the COMPARE trial (Table 10.11) [86, 88]. Irrespective of treating complex or simple coronary lesions, EES use results in less TLR and stent thrombosis relative to PES. Compiled 3-year data for patients enrolled in SPIRIT II and III showed persistent reductions in ischemia-driven TLR (EES 5.4 % vs. PES 9.1 % $p=0.02$) for EES, but no differences in definite/probable stent thrombosis were observed after 3 years (EES 1.2 % vs. PES 1.9 % $P=0.43$) [93].

DES Safety

Stent Thrombosis

Early clinical experience with bare-metal stents was complicated by a stent thrombosis at a rate of 3–4 % in prospective studies and rates more than doubled (8–16 %) if performed as a rescue from abrupt closure [4, 94–96]. Against the background of aggressive oral vitamin K antagonist (warfarin) use, stent thrombosis rates remained high at 3.4 % while simultaneously incurring excessive vascular complications [97]. Aggressive balloon dilation and use of dual-antiplatelet therapy (DAPT) by adding ticlopidine to aspirin reduced stent thrombosis rates to 0.8 % [7]. Pooled data from prospective stent trials indicate that the 30-day thrombosis rates approximate to 0.9 % that further decline to 0.76 % after 30 days [98, 99]. Preapproval trials of first-generation DES demonstrated acceptably low rates of stent thrombosis rate of 0.4 % for SES and 0.6 % for PES resulting in the initial product labeling recommendation of 3 and 6 months of dual-antiplatelet therapy for SES and PES, respectively [79, 100]. However, implementation of DES in a broader patient population as seen in the BASKET-LATE study using DES in an open-label fashion observed a rate of 1.3 and 2.6 % thrombosis-related clinical events in the BMS and DES cohorts, respectively [101]. Given the dire consequences of stent thrombosis with 25–45 % mortality rate, intensive investigation of late DES safety was launched [102, 103]. This culminated in an FDA advisory panel meeting in December 2006 with patient-level meta-analysis from several sources identifying a numerical excess of late stent thrombosis in both SES and PES but no significant difference with bare-metal controls [104]. Pooled analysis of multiple SES trials showed increased yet low incidence of stent thrombosis beyond 1 year compared to BMS counterparts [29]. Follow-up from unrestricted use of SES and PES in a two-institutional cohort study showed that the late stent thrombosis rate was 1.1 % and a steady late-thrombosis rate of 0.6 % per year with a maximum follow-up of 3 years (Fig. 10.7) [106]. Retrospective analysis of 6,033 patients in the SCAAR Swedish national registry reported a 30 % increase in death after 6 months in the DES population

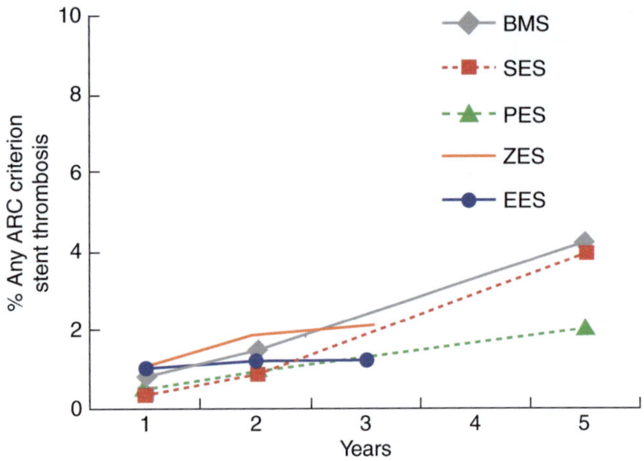

Fig. 10.7 Longitudinal rates of cumulative stent thrombosis for each stent type through long-term follow-up. Event rates included definite, probable, and possible stent thrombosis. Rates for each stent type were derived from the following published trials: (*1*) bare-metal stent (BMS), SIRIUS trial [31, 79, 105]; (*2*) sirolimus-eluting stent (SES), SIRIUS trial [31, 79, 105]; (*3*) paclitaxel-eluting stent (PES), TAXUS IV trial [43, 100]; (*4*) zotarolimus-eluting stent (ZES), ENDEAVOR IV trial [48, 74]; and (*5*) everolimus-eluting stent (EES), SPIRIT III trial [47, 81, 91]

Table 10.12 Factors influencing stent thrombosis

Contributors to stent thrombosis
Patient
Premature antiplatelet therapy discontinuation
Diabetes
Renal failure (acute or chronic)
Left ventricular systolic dysfunction
Malignancy
Acute coronary syndrome
Mechanical
Stent underexpansion or undersizing
Stent malapposition
Incomplete neointimitalization
Bifurcation stenting (especially crush technique)
Stent fracture
Aneurysm formation
Biological
Hypersensitivity
Stenting of highly necrotic plaques

compared to patients receiving BMS with a concurrent increase in myocardial infarction, although such differences were not observed with longer-term and more comprehensive follow-up [107]. In addressing these concerns, multidisciplinary societal guidelines based largely on consensus opinion were released recommending at least 12-month duration of a thienopyridine therapy with indefinite treatment with aspirin despite a paucity of data to assess the efficacy and risks of long-term DAPT [108].

Procedural and biological variables influencing stent thrombosis include inadequate stent expansion, incomplete neointimalization, hypersensitivity, aneurysm formation, stent fracture, and late stent malapposition (Table 10.12). Inadequate stent expansion or stent undersizing has been known to cause for stent thrombosis leading to the practice of high-pressure balloon dilation for optimal procedural results [7, 109–111]. Residual dissections and treatment of bifurcation lesions contribute to the risk of stent thrombosis. Particular stenting techniques, especially the crush technique or leaving stent struts unopposed, predispose to thrombotic complications [112]. The same anti-restenotic agents used to prevent neointimal proliferation likely delay endothelialization, possibly leading to increased fibrin deposition [113, 114]. Stent- or polymer-specific causes of thrombotic events are being identified; pathological analysis of patients with late stent thrombosis demonstrates that those with SES late thrombosis have more inflammation while those with PES have greater amounts of fibrin deposition [115]. Hypersensitivity and aneurysm formation have been implicated in select cases suggesting that allergy to either the drug or polymer may play a role in stent thrombosis [116, 117]. The presence of highly necrotic plaque cores with plaque prolapse is associated with greater rates of stent thrombosis and may also explain relatively high rates of recurrent thrombotic events in patients with acute coronary syndromes [118]. Additionally exposure of stent surface due to loss of stent apposition secondary to positive remodeling or resolution of thrombus has also been implicated in late stent thrombosis [119, 120]. Stent fractures, particularly severe fractures, have also been attributed to stent thrombosis [121, 122]. New pathological studies now reveal formation of atherosclerotic plaques in areas of neointimal hyperplasia, yet it is unclear whether such findings may be associated with late thrombotic events [123].

Patient factors that are independently associated with increased stent thrombosis include early discontinuation of DAPT, diabetes, renal failure, left ventricular systolic dysfunction, malignancy, and acute coronary syndromes (Table 10.12) [102, 124–126]. Patient compliance bears a tremendous impact on the probability of stent thrombosis as early (i.e., <6 months) cessation of DAPT is the most predictive variable in several post hoc analyses and patients stopping clopidogrel early have nearly a ten-fold increase in mortality [126–129]. DES implantation in the setting of acute coronary syndromes, particularly acute myocardial infarction (AMI), increases the incidence of stent thrombosis of 3.4 % range within 1 year, and 1.4 % patients in NSTEMI present with early stent thrombosis as demonstrated in the ACUITY trial [130, 131].

Since stent thrombosis is multifactorial, mitigating its occurrence requires a combination of procedural improvements and recognition of patient variables. First and foremost, the key is appropriate selection of patients with the means to acquire and maintain compliance with antiplatelet medications. Careful ascertainment of patient histories is essential to clarify if susceptibility to bleeding events and possible need for future surgery may lead to premature thienopyridine discontinuation. From a procedural standpoint, appropriate stent sizing and apposition should optimized using high-pressure inflations, and if necessary, the use of intravascular ultrasound. Dissections require early recognition and treatment, usually an additional stent. Although most patient factors are not modifiable (e.g., diabetes, acute coronary syndromes), intensifying antiplatelet therapy to match stent thrombosis risk with agents such as prasugrel may be a strategy helpful in not only decreasing stent thrombosis but also future thrombotic events [132].

Coronary Artery Aneurysm

Coronary aneurysms are defined as a luminal dilation 50 % larger than the adjacent reference vessel diameter, and its appearance post-DES or BMS implantation has an incidence of 0.2–2.3 % in contemporary trials [133, 134]. Dissections or deep arterial wall injury caused by aggressive balloon dilation, oversized stents, or atherectomy has previously been implicated in aneurysm formation [135–137]. Additional mechanisms unique to DES include inflammatory reactions as patients may react to the polymer coating, antiproliferative drug, and alloy of the stent platform. Histological analysis shows extensive inflammation consisting of eosinophils and lymphocytes encompassing stent struts following DES implantation [113, 116]. Incomplete endothelialization has been observed in serial invasive evaluation, and delayed healing may contribute to aneurysm formation [114]. Incomplete stent apposition has been observed in serial follow-up and may be a precursor for aneurysmal dilation; however, these two events have not yet been directly associated with each other. Furthermore, in serial evaluation, some incomplete stent apposition does resolve [138].

Clinical Implications

In the largest reported series of post-DES coronary artery aneurysms, the authors detected 15 (1.25 %) aneurysms in 1,197 consecutive patients undergoing surveillance angiography at 9 months [139]. The investigators reported a 51 % rate of death, MI, and TVR and 33 % rate of death and MI among these 15 patients, in whom 2 events were associated with stent thrombosis.

Management

While there are no guideline recommendations for when to treat aneurysmal dilation of coronary vessels, some investigators advocate individualizing treatment according to rate of expansion, severity of dilation, anatomic location, and symptoms [134]. There are no prospective data to guide practitioners with selection of modalities best at treating aneurysm with respect to observation, balloon overdilation, coils, stent graft implantation, or open surgical procedures. The propensity for adverse outcomes is proportional to aneurysm size, and luminal dimensions may provide the threshold for treatment. Mycotic coronary aneurysms are exceedingly rare but do require immediate surgical intervention as they have typically manifested in critically ill patients [134]. Given the multiple reports of stent thrombosis in association with aneurysms, antiplatelet therapy should likely be extended indefinitely if possible as death and stent thrombosis were consistently associated with platelet discontinuation in the largest reported series [139].

Stent Fracture

Bare-metal stent restenosis was noted in saphenous vein grafts of coronary arteries, and in the intense search to identify safety parameters of drug-eluting stents, stent fracture was found to be a possible contributor to in-stent restenosis and thrombosis. The incidence of stent fracture has been reported to vary between 0.8 and 7.7 % in clinical studies [140]. However, pathological analysis of patients with first-generation drug-eluting stents noted an incidence of 27.5 %, far exceeding those quoted in clinical reports, likely due to improved ability to detect fractures using high-contrast radiography that provides superior resolution compared to fluoroscopy or intravascular ultrasound [121]. The majority of data regarding the incidence of stent fracture originates from single-center studies and published studies from Asian countries and may reflect practice patterns from those regions that incorporate routine angiographic surveillance as part of clinical practice.

Contributors to stent fracture are extreme vessel tortuosity, angulation, calcification, and length of time in the vessel [140]. Given excessive tortuosity and angulation of the right coronary artery, it is not surprising that stents implanted here have the highest fracture rate [141]. Cardiac motion in combination with tortuosity and angulation is certain to cause metal fatigue leading to fracture. Hinge points caused by stent overlap may also contribute, as these segments have the greatest rigidity thus leading to fracture [142].

Stent design is felt to be a factor as most DES stent fractures have been observed in SES [140]. Relatively thick struts combined with a closed-cell design yield a relatively nonconformable, inflexible stent. However, SES are also more radiopaque and constitute the majority of our experience with DES, and these factors may increase the bias towards detecting stent fracture in SES compared to other stent types. Pathological analysis identified stent length, SES use, and duration of implantation as independent predictors of stent fracture [121].

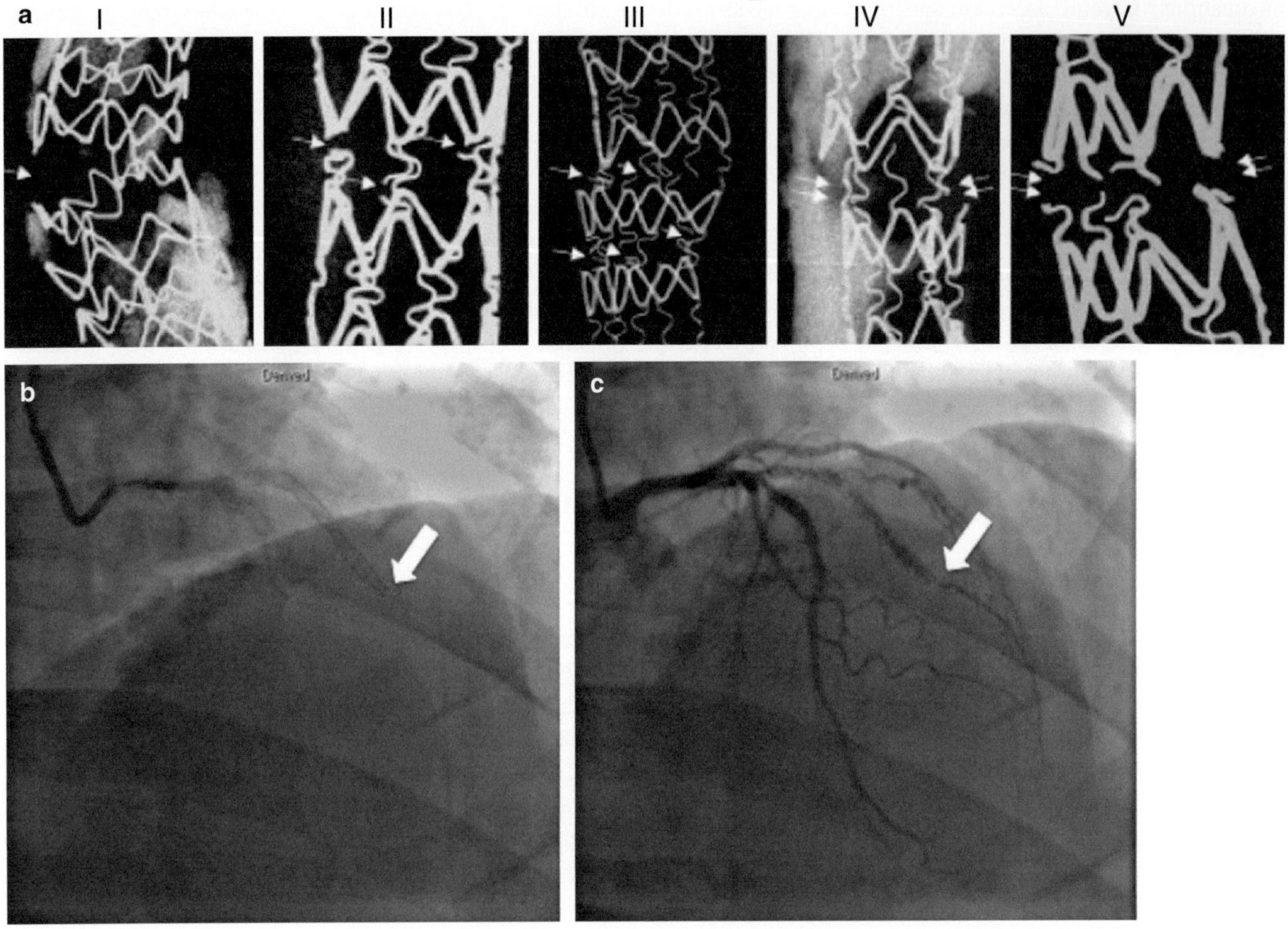

Fig. 10.8 (**a**) Grade I fracture of TAXUS stent (single-strut fracture), grade II fracture of Cypher stent (multiple breaks but alignment is preserved), grade III fracture of Cypher stent (multiple breaks with deformation), grade IV fracture of Cypher stent (multiple breaks with transection of but without gap), and grade V fracture of Cypher stent (total separation) (From Nakazawa et al. [121], with permission). (**b**) High-resolution x-ray of fractured Cypher stent in distal diagonal branch. (**c**) Angiogram of same fractured stent demonstrating severe in-stent restenosis within the fractured segment (*arrows* denote fracture points)

Clinical implications of stent fracture include increased rates of restenosis and stent thrombosis. In the ACROSS Cypher trial evaluating SES treatment in chronic total occlusions, stent fracture was identified in 32/200 patients undergoing 6-month angiographic follow-up [143]. Although stent fracture was associated with a higher likelihood of angiographic restenosis and TLR, when restenosis was identified, its occurrence was seldom at the site of stent fracture, thus raising question as to whether higher TLR are related specifically to fracture or instead greater lesion complexity. In other studies, the rates of restenosis with fracture ranged from 15 to 60 % in published clinical studies. It should be noted that most of these studies included surveillance angiography in the protocol and not necessarily ischemia-driven revascularizations. Pathological analysis reveals that clinical important pathological findings were mostly associated with grade V stent fractures, which defined as complete transection and separation of a stent segment (Fig. 10.8). Associated with greatest amount of inflammation, the investigators documented 6 episodes of stent thrombosis among 51 grade V fractures [121].

Management

Management of stent fracture remains a clinical dilemma with little guidance from any prospective data. Patients presenting with target vessel failure obviously require revascularization, and generally repeat stenting is performed out of practicality and ease. However, operators should consider whether implanting another stent in the milieu responsible for prior stent fracture is wise and bypass surgery should be considered in select cases. In cases of asymptomatic stent fracture, extension of dual-antiplatelet therapy beyond the consensus recommended duration of 1 year should be considered, particularly if associated with disruption of vessel integrity.

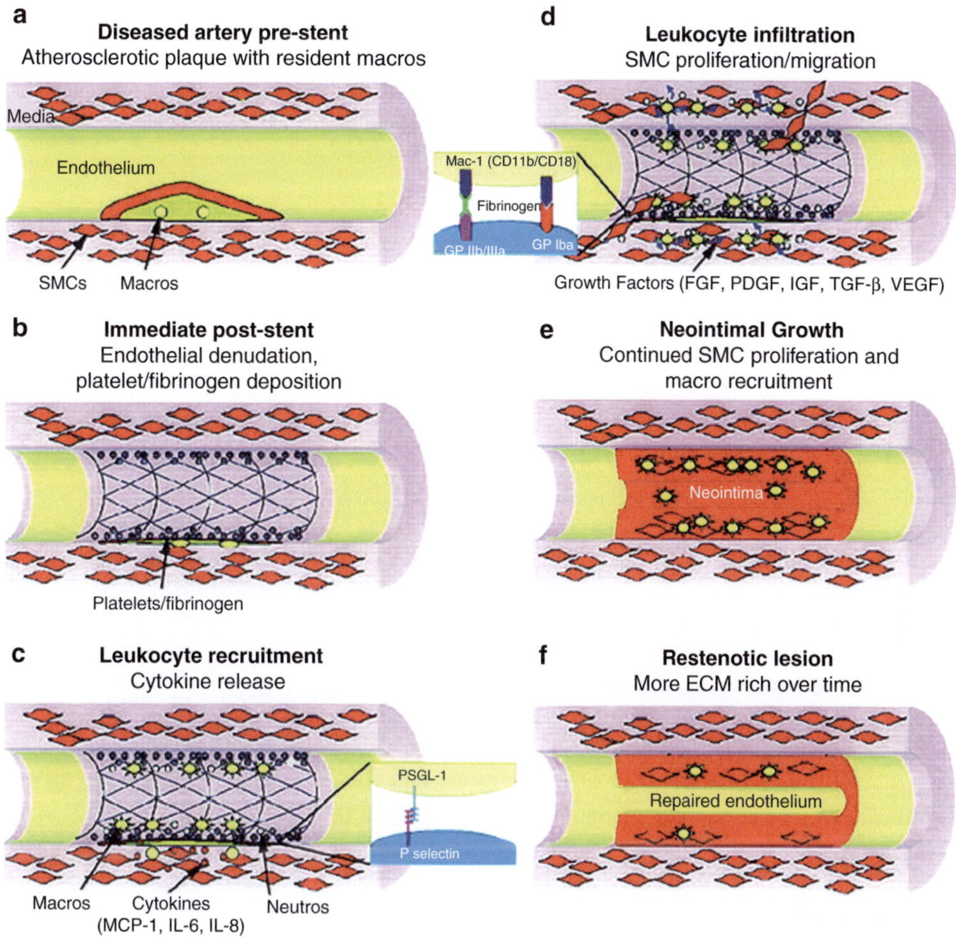

Fig. 10.9 (**a**) Atherosclerotic plaque prior to stent implantation. (**b**) Endothelial denudation and platelet/fibrinogen deposition occur immediately after stenting. (**c**) and (**d**) Days after injury, leukocyte recruitment, infiltration, and smooth muscle cell (*SMC*) proliferation and migration occur within the stented segment. (**e**) Weeks after injury, there is continued SMC proliferation and monocyte recruitment causing neointimal thickening. (**f**) Weeks to months post-stent implantation, the neointima changes from a predominantly cellular to less cellular ECM-rich plaque (From Welt and Rogers [22], with permission)

Restenosis

Comparative trials of PCI and coronary bypass surgery have largely shown that repeat revascularization due to lesion restenosis—rather than death or MI—is responsible for this difference in outcomes between the two revascularization strategies [144]. Restenosis remains the Achilles' heel of percutaneous revascularization, and both balloon angioplasty and stent implantation have distinct mechanisms of restenosis. Vessel recoil and negative remodeling are responsible for restenosis in balloon angioplasty [22]. In contradistinction, stenting mitigates negative remodeling due to greater acute gain, scaffolding, and prevention of vessel recoil; however, late loss due to neointimal hyperplasia causes late ISR. The first model of restenosis was proposed by Forrester consisting of a modified model for wound healing in the endovascular space [145]. The major events in restenosis formation were described as platelet aggregation, inflammatory cell infiltration, release of growth factors, medial smooth muscle cell (SMC) modulation and proliferation, proteoglycan deposition, and extracellular matrix remodeling (Fig. 10.9) [22]. Observations of inflammatory cell deposition and smooth muscle proliferation led to the advances of adding antiproliferative medications to mitigate neointimal hyperplasia. Although ISR in seminal DES trials was minimal (0–4.1 %), subsequent long-term follow-up in unselected patients with more complex pathology has shown restenosis rates greater than 10 % over 5 years [27, 37, 79].

Mechanisms of Restenosis

Biological, mechanical, and technical factors are implicated in restenosis (Table 10.13). Sirolimus and its analogues (zotarolimus, everolimus, biolimus A9) bind to the FK506 binding protein halting the cell cycle. Paclitaxel is a hydrophobic molecule that halts microtubule disassembly and interrupts the cell cycle at G2/mitosis. Several mutations have been identified to binding sites of sirolimus and paclitaxel or to segments of the cell proliferation cascade that render antiproliferative drugs ineffective [147, 148]. Hypersensitivity remains an issue and further inflammation beyond the normal healing response may certainly worsen restenosis. Reactions to nickel and molybdenum in 316 L stainless steel are potential triggering mechanisms for ISR [116]. In the RADAR (Research on Adverse Drug/Device Events and Reports) project, 261 hypersensitivity reactions of 5,783 adverse events were

Table 10.13 Biological, mechanical, and technical variables associated with restenosis

Mechanisms of restenosis
Biological
Drug resistance
Hypersensitivity
Mechanical
Stent underexpansion
Nonuniform drug elution/deposition
Polymer peeling
Stent fracture
Technical factors
Barotrauma outside stented segment
Stent gap
Residual uncovered plaque

Adapted from Dangas et al. [146], with permission

noted, perhaps contributing to ISR formation as well as stent thrombosis [117].

Mechanical factors in ISR formation include stent underexpansion, nonuniform drug distribution, and stent fracture. Suboptimal expansion would simply leave a smaller cross-sectional area and has been implicated in ischemia-driven TLR [110]. Stenting in tortuous segments or arteries with significant mismatch or noncompliant vessels may lead to stent underexpansion and poor drug delivery, especially for longer stents [149]. As mentioned previously, stent fracture, particularly when there is a complete transection and separation of the stent components, is associated with TLR and stent thrombosis [121]. Local blood flow characteristics, stent overlap, and stripping of polymer during stent deliver may also play a role in restenosis formation [150].

Technique-dependent factors include geographic miss, stent gap, and balloon injury outside of stent region. Stent edge restenosis was the major contributor to in-segment binary restenosis early in the DES era [79]. Stent gaps will not receive any drug and furthermore balloon injury may occur in those segments during post-dilation. Finally, geographic miss during the procedure is associated with increased risk of TVR and MI at 1 year as described in the STLLR (Stent Deployment Techniques on Clinical Outcomes of Patients Treated With the Cypher Stent) evaluating the outcomes of suboptimal PCI [151].

Post hoc analyses of real-world, drug eluting stent registries have revealed that many of the predictors of ISR are similar to those in bare-metal stents: diabetes mellitus, complex lesions, small vessels, long lesions, stent underexpansion, and calcified vessels (Table 10.14) [152, 153]. PES was identified to more likely be associated with TVR compared to SES. Certainly, final diameter stenosis and achieving excellent angiographic results are important. Retrospective analysis of IVUS-guided PCI in an unselected patient population showed that a minimal cross-sectional area of 5.5 mm^2 and stented

Table 10.14 Independent predictors of in-stent restenosis (ISR) formation conceptualized as patient, lesion, and procedural attributes

Independent predictors of DES in-stent restenosis
Patient attributes
Age
Female sex
Diabetes mellitus
Multivessel coronary artery disease
Lesion attributes
In-stent restenosis lesion
Bypass graft
Chronic total occlusion
Small vessel diameter
Calcified lesion
Ostial lesion
Lesion length
Procedural attributes
Stent underexpansion
Type of DES
Final diameter stenosis
Bifurcation 2 stent technique

Adapted from Dangas et al. [146]

Table 10.15 Angiographic classification of restenosis based on morphology proposed by Mehran et al.

Angiographic restenosis and classification
Type I focal: ≤10 mm in length
IA articulation or gap
IB margin
IC focal body
ID multifocal
Type 2 diffuse: >10 mm intrastent
Type 3 proliferative : >10 mm extending beyond the stent margins
Type 4 total occlusion: restenotic lesions with TIMI 0 flow

Adapted from Mehran et al. [156], with permission

length less than 40 mm were predictive of decreased future ISR events in SES implantation while a cross-sectional area 5.7 mm^2 was predictive of 9-month patency of PES [154, 155].

In-Stent Restenosis Outcomes

Morphology of ISR varies according to DES vs. bare metal with more diffuse patterns observed in bare-metal restenosis, while DES restenosis tends be more focal (Table 10.15) [149, 157, 158]. Observational studies and randomized trials show that a greater proportion of SES have focal restenosis compared to PES and the restenosis patterns. Morphological differences are predictive of repeat revascularization, analysis of 288 episodes of bare-metal stenting showed that focal restenosis portends better outcomes, and propensity for repeat revascularization increased with diffuse restenosis [156]. These observations were consistent in the DES era as diffuse restenosis and total occlusion of DES resulted in greater rates of repeat revascularization [159].

Table 10.16 Metallic Stents with a biodegradable polymer that are either currently available outside the United States or undergoing clinical evaluation

Stent (manufacturer)	Drug (dosage)	Drug release (%), time (Days)	Stent platform	Strut/max coating thickness, μm	Polymer type (duration of biodegradation, months)
Supralimus (Sahajanand Medical)	Sirolimus (125 μg/19 mm)	50 %, 9–11	316 L SS	80/4–5	PLLA PLGA, PLC, PVP (7)
Excel stent (JW Medical System)	Sirolimus (195–376 μg)	NA	316 L SS	119/15	PLA (6–9)
NEVO (Cordis)	Sirolimus (166 μg/17 mm)	80 %, 30	CoCr	99	Reservoirs of PLGA (3)
BioMatrix (Biosensors)	Biolimus A9 (15.6 μg/mm)	45 %, 30	316 L SS	112/10	Abluminal PLA (6–9)
NOBORI (Terumo)	Biolimus A9 (15.6 μg/mm)	45 %, 30	316 L SS	112/10	Abluminal PLA (6–9)
Axxess (Devax Inc.)	Biolimus A9 (22 μg/mm)	45 %, 30	Nitinol	152/15	Abluminal PLA (6–9)
XTENT (XTENT)	Biolimus A9 (15.6 μg/mm)	45 %, 30	CoCr	NA	Abluminal PLA (6–9)
SYNERGY (Boston Scientific)	Everolimus (LD 56 μg/20 mm)	50 %, 60	PtCr	71/3 (LD)	PLGA Rollcoat
	(SD 113 μg/20 mm)			4 (SD)	Abluminal (3)
Combo (OrbusNeich)	EPC + sirolimus (5 μg/mm)	NA	316 L SS	NA	Abluminal
Elixir Myolimus (Elixir Medical)	Myolimus (3 μg/mm)	90 %, 90	CoCr	80/<3	Abluminal PLA (6–9)
Infinnium (Sahajanand)	Paclitaxel (122 μg/19 mm)	50 %, 9–11	316 L SS	80/4–5	PLL PLGA, PLC PVP (7)
JACTAX Liberte (Boston Scientific)	Paclitaxel (9.2 μg/16 mm)	100 %, 60	316 L SS	97/<1	JAC polymer Abluminal (4)

Adapted from Garg and Serruys [163]
BES biolimus-eluting stent, *BMS* bare-metal stents, *CoCr* cobalt chromium, *EPC* endothelial progenitor capture, *JAC* juxtaposed abluminal coating, *LD* low dose, *NA* not available, *PLC* 75/25 poly-L-lactide-co-caprolactone, *PLGA* 50:50 poly-D,L-lactide-co-glycolide, *PLLA* poly-L-lactic acid, *PtCr* platinum chromium, *PVP* polyvinyl pyrrolidone, *SD* standard dose, *SS* stainless steel

Treatment of In-Stent Restenosis

Therapeutic options for ISR include repeat balloon dilation, vascular brachytherapy, repeat stenting, and coronary artery bypass surgery. Initial treatment of ISR for bare-metal stent restenosis consisted of repeat balloon angioplasty dilation alone; however, up to 44–54 % of patients receiving balloon angioplasty dilation will have restenosis on repeat angiography, and approximately 33 % of patients will require target vessel revascularization at 1 year [59, 160]. Repeat stent implantation is the most common therapy for drug-eluting stent restenosis. Once DES were commercially available, the natural expansion of its use spread to treatment of bare-metal ISR. At the time of their introduction, vascular brachytherapy was the standard of care for treatment of restenosis. Compared to vascular brachytherapy (VBT), SES was found to decrease TVR 50 % (VBT 21.6 % vs. SES 10.8 % $P=0.008$), despite the lack of differences in late loss or binary restenosis at 9 months between SES and VBT [161]. Similarly, PES was shown to decrease rates of TVR (VBT 17.5 % vs. PES 10.5 % $p=0.046$) and binary restenosis (VBT 31.2 % vs. PES 14.5 % $P<0.001$) relative to brachytherapy [162]. ISAR-DESIRE randomized 300 patients to either receive balloon angioplasty, SES, or PES for bare-metal restenosis with repeat angiography at 9 months. SES proved to reduce late loss more effectively than PES, translating into a lower TLR rate of 8 % vs. 19 % ($P<0.001$) at 1-year follow-up. ISAR-DESIRE 2 randomized 483 patients with SES ISR to either repeat PCI with SES or PES. At 9 months, binary restenosis rates were nearly identical (SES 19.0 % vs. PES 20.6 %), and repeat revascularization events were similar at 1 year (SES 16.6 % vs. PES 14.6 %, $P=$NS) [60]. Thus far, the optimal method for treatment of DES ISR has not yet been determined, yet it does not appear that alternating the type of antiproliferative agent (paclitaxel vs. sirolimus) impacts restenosis giving credence to the notion that ISR is a multifactorial process and extends beyond drug sensitivity and resistance.

Future Directions

Developing advances in DES include improvements in platform design and bioresorbable polymers. Prior observations in clinical studies have suggested that polymers while important for regulating drug-release kinetics may play a role in late inflammatory responses and contribute to target lesion failure in the form of stent thrombosis or restenosis. To address this issue, stents with either biodegradable polymers or polymer-free DES systems have emerged as a developing alternative to the current stent design. While several of each type are undergoing concurrent design (Tables 10.16 and 10.17), a discussion limited to one biodegradable polymer and polymer-free stent will serve as an example for each category.

The BioTronix stent is a flexible stainless steel stent that delivers biolimus using a biodegradable polymer [164].

Table 10.17 Polymer-free metallic stents that are either currently available outside the United States or undergoing clinical development

Stent (manufacturer)	Drug (dosage)	Drug release (%), time	Stent platform	Strut/coating thickness, μm	Surface modification
Amazonia Pax (Minvasys)	Paclitaxel (2.5 μg/mm²)	98 %, 30 days	CoCr	73/5[a]	Abluminal microdrop spray crystallization process
BioFREEDOM (Biosensors)	Biolimus A9 (SD) SD† 15.6 μg/mm LD‡ 7.8 μg/mm	90 % 50 h	316 L SS	112	Microporous surface
VESTAsync (MIV Therapeutics)	Sirolimus (total = 55 μg)	100 %, 3 months	316 L SS	65/0.6	Nanoporous hydroxyapatite
Yukon (Transluminal)	Sirolimus (11.7–21.9 μg)	67 %, 7 days	316 L SS	Microporous surface	

Adapted from Garg and Serruys [163]
h hours, *SD* standard dose, *LD* low dose, *SS* stainless steel
[a]Abluminal

Biolimus is a highly lipophilic sirolimus analogue with an alkoxy-alkyl group replacing hydrogen at position 42-O. After submerging the drug in polylactic acid, the combination is applied to the abluminal surface of the stent. In vivo data indicates that polymer absorption should be complete by 6 months [164]. To test the safety and efficacy of the biolimus-eluting stent (BES), 1,757 patients were enrolled in the multicenter European LEADERS study and randomized against SES. A broad patient population was enrolled reflecting "real-world" practice, and at 9 months, outcomes with respect to death (BES 2.6 % vs. SES 2.8 % p = NS), myocardial infarction (BES 5.7 % vs. SES 4.6 % p = NS), and TLR (BES 5.7 % vs. SES 4.6 % p = NS) were similar. Stent thrombosis rates were similar (definite/probable ST BES 2.6 % vs. SES 2.2 % p = NS), although the study follow-up did not extend long enough to detect differences in late stent thrombosis [164].

Another iterative advance in DES technology is to deliver drug without any polymer. While many of these stents are still in preliminary development, a stent-eluting dual DES through micropores has recently undergone clinical testing. YUKON Choice DES contain micropores capable of adsorption of drugs, and once released, the microporous surface favors adhesion of endothelial cells [165]. Several drug combinations may be used, but recently a sirolimus/probucol dual DES stent was randomized against SES and ZES in 1,007 patients in the ISAR-TEST 2 trial. After 2 years of follow-up, all three stent cohorts showed similar rates of MACE endpoints outside of restenosis [166]. However, clinical restenosis in the ZES groups was significantly greater at 1 and 2 years, while the SES and dual DES arms remained similar at 1 year (TLR 2-year SES 10.7 % vs. dual DES 7.7 % vs. ZES 14.3 % P = 0.009). Notably, the dual DES cohort showed less late catch-up restenosis than the SES group at 2 years [166] (Fig. 10.10).

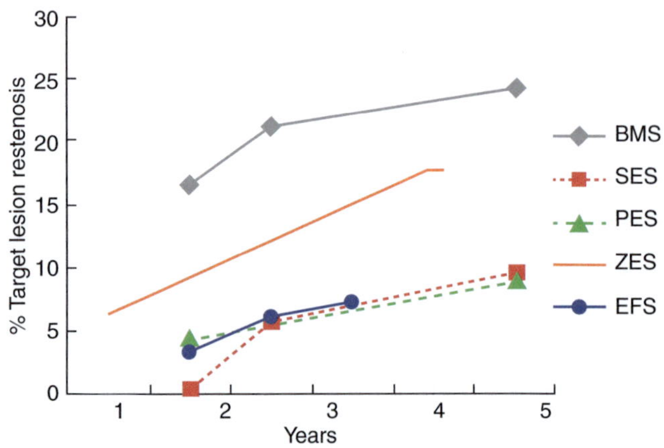

Fig. 10.10 Longitudinal rates of target lesion revascularization (*TLR*) for each stent type through long-term clinical evaluation. Rates of TLR were derived from the following clinical trial data: (*1*) bare-metal stent (*BMS*), SIRIUS trial [31, 79, 105]; (*2*) sirolimus-eluting stent (*SES*), SIRIUS trial [31, 79, 105]; (*3*) paclitaxel-eluting stent (*PES*), TAXUS IV trial [43, 100]; (*4*) zotarolimus-eluting stent (*ZES*), ENDEAVOR III trial [10, 39]; and (*5*) everolimus-eluting stent (*EES*), SPIRIT III trial [47, 81, 91]

Bioresorbable stents (BRS) are constructed of polymers that are sensitive to enzymatic breakdown such as magnesium, tyrosine polycarbonate, poly-L-lactic acid (PLLA), and poly-D,L-lactic acid (PDLLA) (Table 10.18). While the entire development of BRS extends beyond the scope of this chapter, we will briefly discuss the current prototype for this class of stent, the everolimus-eluting BRS. The stent itself is composed of semicrystalline polymer PLLA backbone and coated with a poly-D,lactide acid (PDLLA), a random copolymer of and D- and L-lactic acid. PDLLA prevents crystallization and forms a completely amorphous phase as it solidifies. This coating contains and regulates the release of everolimus. PDLLA and PLLA are both bioresorbable and progressively shortened as ester bonds between repeat units of lactide are hydrolyzed and particles are phagocytized by macrophages. Eventually PDLLA and PLLA are degraded into lactic acid and metabolized by the Krebs cycle.

The macrostructure of the first-generation BRS (Bioresorbable Vascular Scaffold 1.0) is circumferential

Table 10.18 Currently available bioresorbable stents tested in clinical trials

Scaffolds	Strut material	Coating material	Design	Absorption products	Drug elution	Stent radiopacity	Deployment	Total strut thickness (stent + coating) µm	Crossing profile, mm	Stent-to-artery coverage, %	Duration radial support	Absorption time
Igaki-Tamai	PLLA	None	Zigzag helical coils	Lactic acid, CO_2, H_2O	None	Gold markers	Self-expanding with heated balloon	170	?	24	6 mo	2 y
AMS-1	Metal-Mg alloy	None	Sinusoidal in-phase hoops linked by straight bridges	Not applicable	None	None	Balloon	165	1.2	10	Days or weeks	<4 mo
AMS-2	Metal-Mg alloy	None		Not applicable	None	None	Balloon	125	—	—	Weeks	>4 mo
AMS-3	Metal-Mg alloy	None		Not applicable	None	Yes	Balloon	125	—	—	Weeks	>4 mo
REVA	Poly-tyrosine-derived polycarbonate polymer	None	Side and lock	Amino acid, ethanol, CO_2	None	Iodine impregnated	Balloon	200	1.7	55	3–6 mo	6 mo
BTI	Polymer salicylate + linker	Salicylate + different linker	Tube with laser-cut voids	Salicylate, CO_2, H_2O	Sirolimus salicylate	None	Balloon	200	2	65	3 mo	6 mo
BVS 1.0	Poly-L-lactide	Poly-D,L-lactide	Out-of-phase sinusoidal hoops with straight and direct links	Lactic acid, CO_2, H_2O	Everolimus	Platinum markers	Balloon	156	1.4	25	Weeks	2 y
BVS 1.1	Poly-L-lactide	Poly-D,L-lactide	In-phase hoops with straight links	Lactic acid, CO_2, H_2O	Everolimus	Platinum markers	Balloon	156	1.4	25	3 mo	2 y

Adapted from Garg and Serruys [163], with permission
AMS absorbable metallic stent, *BTI* Bioabsorbable Therapeutics Inc., *BVS* bioabsorbable vascular solutions, *D* day, *mo* month, *y* year

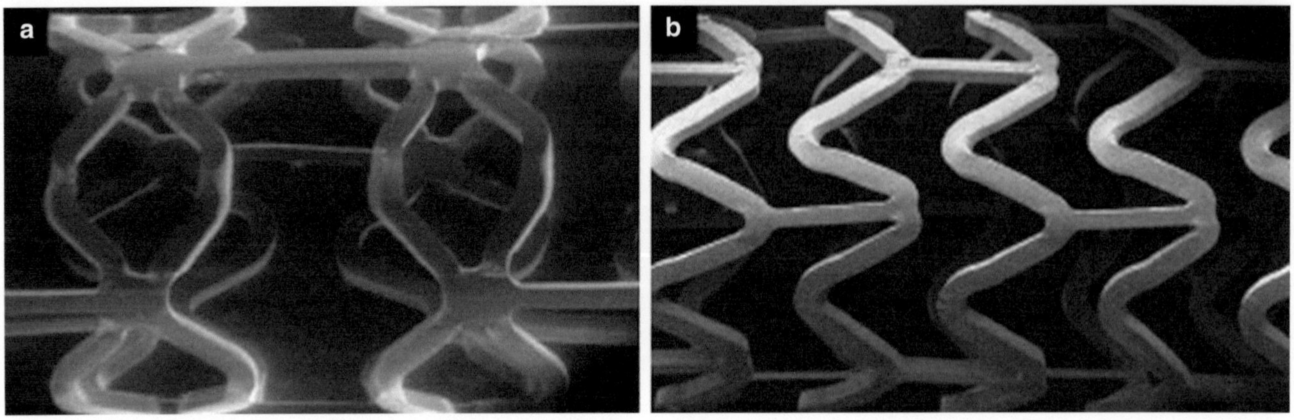

Fig. 10.11 Stent architecture of BioVascular Scaffold (*BVS*) 1.0 and 1.1. (**a**) BVS 1.0 has circumferential out-of-phase zigzag hoops linked together by 3 longitudinal struts between each group. (**b**) BVS 1.1 has in-phase zigzag hoops linked by bridges. Maximum circular unsupported cross-sectional areas are larger in BVS 1.0 than BVS 1.1 (From Garg and Serruys [163], with permission)

hoops of PLLA with struts 150 μm thick either joined or linked by straight bridges (Fig. 10.11). The stent has a crossing profile of 1.4 mm, both ends of the stent of 2 adjacent radiopaque platinum markers, and the stent has comparable radial strength to the Vision bare-metal stent [167]. Everolimus is eluted from the polymer coating, and 80 % of the drug is eluted within 28 days. Arterial tissue concentration is maintained at 0.9–2 ng/mg for 28 days, comparable to the XIENCE V EES.

First-in-human implantation of everolimus-eluting BRS has primarily taken place in the ABSORB A and B cohorts testing the first-generation Bioresorbable Vascular Scaffold (BVS 1.0) and second-generation BVS 1.1, respectively. In ABSORB cohort A, 30 patients were enrolled and followed clinically for 2 years. Serial invasive assessment occurred at 6 months and 2 years, and noninvasive imaging with multislice computed tomography (MSCT) was performed at 18 months. Serial imaging in ABSORB cohort A observed a 11.8 % reduction in stent area and a 24.3 % reduction in minimal luminal area (MLA) at 6 months signaling that there is late recoil of the stent suggesting that the radial strength was lacking [167]. Although in vivo porcine data indicate that the stent is resorbed at 24 months, 2-year optical coherence tomography (OCT) demonstrates a 34.5 % reduction in struts with resolution of any malapposition. Clinically, there was 1 non-Q wave myocardial infarction related to a nonstented lesion [168].

The second iteration BVS 1.1 improved on the original design by adding in-phase zigzag hoops linked by bridges to allow uniform stent distribution as well as a modification in the manufacturing process to slow the in vivo hydrolysis rate (Fig. 10.11) [24]. These revisions that increase the intermediate-term structural integrity to counter the late recoil observed in the ABSORB cohort A were tested in 45 patients to be followed for 2 years. The 6-month results demonstrated a mean scaffold area and MLA loss of 2.0±4.8 % and 5.4±8.7 %, respectively, showing a significant improvement. There were two episodes of TLR (1 related to edge restenosis) and no deaths. One- and 2-year data will elucidate the effects of polymeric stent struts and their rate of degradation.

BRS are in the beginning of clinical development and some unresolved issues will require resolution. Outside of late recoil, another caveat to BVS is the inability to overdilate these stents, as doing so may cause fractures or fissuring of the stent [169]. Therefore, using BVS will be heavily reliant on intravascular imaging for accurate sizing and likely aggressive predilation to ensure good expansion, especially in extremely fibro-calcific lesions. Since the lesion characteristics in the ABSORB trials were carefully selected and fairly simple, it remains uncertain how BRS will perform in "off-label" patients with complex anatomy and more complex pathology.

Conclusion

Drug-eluting stents revolutionized the safety and efficacy of percutaneous coronary intervention and remain the backbone of percutaneous revascularization. Through iterative advances and persistent innovation stent design, vascular biology, and pharmacology, the continued expectation is that advances in design and composition will provide long-term durability and safety for the millions of patients with coronary disease globally.

References

1. Dotter CT, Judklns MP. Transluminal treatment of arteriosclerotic obstruction. Circulation. 1964;30:654–70.
2. Grüntzig A. Transluminal dilation of coronary-artery stenosis. Lancet. 1978;311:263.
3. Venkitachalam L, Kip KE, Selzer F, et al. Twenty-year evolution of percutaneous coronary intervention and its impact on clinical

outcomes: a report from the National Heart, Lung, and Blood Institute-sponsored, multicenter 1985–1986 PTCA and 1997-2006 Dynamic Registries. Circ Cardiovasc Interv. 2009;2:6–13.
4. Schatz R, Baim D, Leon M, et al. Clinical experience with the Palmaz-Schatz coronary stent. Initial results of a multicenter study. Circulation. 1991;83:148–61.
5. Palmaz JC, Richter GM, Noeldge G, et al. Intraluminal stents in atherosclerotic iliac artery stenosis: preliminary report of a multicenter study. Radiology. 1988;168:727–31.
6. Sigwart U, Puel J, Mirkovitch V, Joffre F, Kappenberger L. Intravascular stents to prevent occlusion and restenosis after transluminal angioplasty. N Engl J Med. 1987;316:701–6.
7. Colombo A, Hall P, Nakamura S, et al. Intracoronary stenting without anticoagulation accomplished with intravascular ultrasound guidance. Circulation. 1995;91:1676–88.
8. Kereiakes DJ, Cox D, Hermiller J, et al. Usefulness of a cobalt chromium coronary stent alloy. Am J Cardiol. 2003;92:463–6.
9. Sketch MH, Ball M, Rutherford BD, Popma JJ, Russell C, Kereiakes DJ. Evaluation of the Medtronic (Driver) cobalt-chromium alloy coronary stent system. Am J Cardiol. 2005;95: 8–12.
10. Kandzari DE, Leon M, Popma JJ, et al. Comparison of zotarolimus-eluting and sirolimus-eluting stents in patients with native coronary artery disease. J Am Coll Cardiol. 2006;48:2440–7.
11. Kastrati A, Mehilli J, Dirschinger J, et al. Intracoronary stenting and angiographic results: strut thickness effect on restenosis outcome (ISAR-STERO) trial. Circulation. 2001;103(23):2816–21.
12. Pache J, Kastrati A, Mehilli J, et al. Intracoronary stenting and angiographic results: strut thickness effect on restenosis outcome (ISAR-STERO-2) trial. J Am Coll Cardiol. 2003;41:1283–8.
13. Garasic JM, Edelman ER, Squire JC, Seifer P, Williams MS, Rogers C. Stent and artery geometry determine intimal thickening independent of arterial injury. Circulation. 2000;101:812–8.
14. Kastrati A, Dirschinger J, Boekstegers P, et al. Influence of stent design on 1-year outcome after coronary stent placement: a randomized comparison of five stent types in 1,147 unselected patients. Catheter Cardiovasc Interv. 2000;50:290–7.
15. Joner M, et al. Endothelial cell recovery between comparator polymer-based drug-eluting stents. J Am Coll Cardiol. 2008;53: 333–42.
16. Capelli C, Gervaso F, Petrini L, Dubini G, Migliavacca F. Assessment of tissue prolapse after balloon-expandable stenting: influence of stent cell geometry. Med Eng Phys. 2009;31:441–7.
17. Applegate RJ, Hermiller J, Williams J, et al. Evaluation of the effects of everolimus-eluting and paclitaxel-eluting stents on target lesions with jailed side branches: 2-year results from the SPIRIT III randomized trial. Catheter Cardiovasc Interv. 2010;76: 644–51.
18. Sousa E, Serruys PW, Costa MA. New frontiers in cardiology: drug-eluting stents: Part I. Circulation. 2003;107:2274–9.
19. Virmani R, Liistro F, Stankovic G, et al. Mechanism of late in-stent restenosis after implantation of a paclitaxel derivate-eluting polymer stent system in humans. Circulation. 2002;106:2649–51.
20. Burke SE, Kuntz RE, Schwartz LB. Zotarolimus (ABT-578) eluting stents. Adv Drug Deliv Rev. 2006;58:437–46.
21. Udipi K, Melder RJ, Chen M, et al. The next generation Endeavor Resolute Stent: role of the BioLinx™ Polymer System. EuroIntervention. 2007;3:137–9.
22. Welt FGP, Rogers C. Inflammation and restenosis in the stent era. Arterioscler Thromb Vasc Biol. 2002;22:1769–76.
23. Garg S, Serrrys PW. Coronary stents: current status. J Am Coll Cardiol. 2010;56:S1–42.
24. Serruys PW, Onuma Y, Ormiston J, et al. Evaluation of the second generation of a bioresorbable everolimus drug-eluting vascular scaffold for treatment of de nevo coronary artery stenosis: six-month clinical and imaging outcomes. Circulation. 2010;122:2301–13.
25. Sousa E, Serruys PW, Costa MA. New frontiers in cardiology: drug-eluting stents: Part II. Circulation. 2003;107:2383–9.
26. Al Suwaidi J, Berger PB, Holmes Jr DR. Coronary artery stents. JAMA. 2000;284:1828–36.
27. Morice M-C, Serruys PW, Sousa E, et al. A randomized comparison of a sirolimus-eluting stent with a standard stent for coronary revascularization. N Engl J Med. 2002;346:1773–80.
28. Sousa JE, Costa MA, Abizaid A, et al. Sustained suppression of neointimal proliferation by sirolimus-eluting stents: one-year angiographic and intravascular ultrasound follow-up. Circulation. 2001;104:2007–11.
29. Kastrati A, Mehilli J, Pache J, et al. Analysis of 14 trials comparing sirolimus-eluting stents with bare-metal stents. N Engl J Med. 2007;356:1030–9.
30. Spaulding C, Daemen J, Boersma E, Cutlip DE, Serruys PW. Pooled analysis of data comparing sirolimus-eluting stents with bare-metal stents. N Engl J Med. 2007;356:989–97.
31. Weisz G, Leon M, Holmes Jr DR, et al. Five-year follow-up after sirolimus-eluting stent implantation. J Am Coll Cardiol. 2009;53: 1488–97.
32. Spaulding C, Teiger E, Commeau P, et al. Four-year follow-up of TYPHOON (trial to assess the use of the CYPHer sirolimus-eluting coronary stent in acute myocardial infarction treated with BallOON angioplasty). J Am Coll Cardiol Intv. 2011;4: 14–23.
33. Serruys PW, Onuma Y, Garg S, et al. 5-year clinical outcomes of the ARTS II (Arterial Revascularization Therapies Study II) of the sirolimus-eluting stent in the treatment of patients with multivessel de novo coronary artery lesions. J Am Coll Cardiol. 2010;11: 1093–101.
34. Morice M-C, Serruys PW, Barragan P, et al. Long-term clinical outcomes with sirolimus-eluting coronary stents. J Am Coll Cardiol. 2007;50:1299–304.
35. Kelbaek H, Kløvgaard L, Helqvist S, et al. Long-term outcome in patients treated with sirolimus-eluting stents in complex coronary artery lesions. J Am Coll Cardiol. 2008;51:2011–6.
36. Kawaguchi R, Kimura T, Morimoto T, et al. Safety and efficacy of sirolimus-eluting stent implantation in patients with acute coronary syndrome in the real world. Am J Cardiol. 2010;106: 1550–60.
37. Simsek C, Magro M, Boersma E, et al. The unrestricted use of sirolimus- paclitaxel-eluting stents results in the better clinical outcomes during 6-year follow-up than bare-metal stents: an analysis of the RESEARCH (Rapamycin-Eluting Stent Evaluated At Rotterdam Cardiology Hospital) and T-SEARCH (Taxus Stent Evaluated At Rotterdam Cardiology Hospital) registries. J Am Coll Cardiol Intv. 2010;3:1051–8.
38. Violini R, Musto C, De Felice F, et al. Maintenance of long-term clinical benefit with sirolimus-eluting stents in patients with ST-segment elevation myocardial infarction. J Am Coll Cardiol. 2010;55:810–4.
39. Eisenstein EL, Leon M, Kandzari DE, et al. Long-term clinical and economic analysis of the endeavor zotarolimus-eluting stent versus the cypher sirolimus-eluting stent: 3-year results from the ENDEAVOR III Trial (Randomized Controlled Trial of the Medtronic Endeavor Drug [ABT-578] Eluting Coronary Stent System Versus the Cypher Sirolimus-Eluting Coronary Stent System in De Novo Native Coronary Artery Lesion). J Am Coll Cardiol Intv. 2009;2:1199–207.
40. Kamath KR, Barry JJ, Miller KM. The TAXUS drug-eluting stent: a new paradigm in controlled drug delivery. Adv Drug Deliv Rev. 2006;58:412–36.
41. Colombo A, Drzewiecki J, Banning AP, et al. Randomized study to assess the effectiveness of slow-and moderate-release polymer-based paclitaxel-eluting stents for coronary artery lesions. Circulation. 2003;108:788–94.

42. Silber S, Colombo A, Banning AP, et al. Final 5-year results of the TAXUS II trial: a randomized study to assess the effectiveness of slow- and moderate-release polymer-based paclitaxel-eluting stents for de novo coronary artery lesions. Circulation. 2009;120: 1498–504.
43. Ellis SG, Stone GW, Cox D, et al. Long-term safety and efficacy with paclitaxel-eluting stents: 5-year final results of the TAXUS IV clinical trial (TAXUS IV-SR: treatment of de novo coronary disease using a single paclitaxel-eluting stent). J Am Coll Cardiol Intv. 2009;2:1248–59.
44. Kaltoft A, Jensen LO, Maeng M, et al. 2-year clinical outcomes after implantation of sirolimus-eluting, paclitaxel-eluting, and bare-metal coronary stents. J Am Coll Cardiol. 2009;53: 658–64.
45. Vink MA, Dirksen MT, Suttorp MJ, et al. 5-year follow-up after primary percutaneous coronary intervention with a paclitaxel-eluting stent versus a bare-metal stent in acute ST-segment elevation myocardial infarction: a follow-up study of the PASSION (Paclitaxel-Eluting Versus Conventional Stent in Myocardial Infarction With ST-Segment Elevation) trial. J Am Coll Cardiol Intv. 2011;4:24–9.
46. Stone GW, Witzenbichler B, Guagliumi G, et al. Heparin plus a glycoprotein IIb/IIIa inhibitor versus bivalirudin monotherapy and paclitaxel-eluting stents versus bare-metal stents in acute myocardial infarction (HORIZONS-AMI): final 3-year results from a multicentre, randomised controlled trial. Lancet. 2011;377(9784): 2193–204.
47. Applegate RJ, Yaqub M, Hermiller J, et al. Long-term (three-year) safety and efficacy of *everolimus*-eluting stents compared to *paclitaxel-eluting* stents (from the SPIRIT III Trial). Am J Cardiol. 2011;107:833–40.
48. Leon M, Nikolsky E, Cutlip DE, et al. Improved late clinical safety with zotarolimus-eluting stents compared with paclitaxel-eluting stents in patients with de novo coronary lesions: 3-year follow-up from the ENDEAVOR IV (Randomized Comparison of Zotarolimus- and Paclitaxel-Eluting Stents in Patients With Coronary Artery Disease) trial. J Am Coll Cardiol Intv. 2010;3: 1043–50.
49. Grube E, Silber S, Hauptmann K, et al. TAXUS I: six- and twelve-month results from a randomized, double-blind trial on a slow-release paclitaxel-eluting stent for de novo coronary lesions. Circulation. 2003;107:38–42.
50. Turco M, Ormiston J, Popma JJ, et al. Polymer-based, paclitaxel-eluting TAXUS Liberté stent in de novo lesions. J Am Coll Cardiol. 2007;49:1676–83.
51. Turco M, Ormiston J, Popma JJ, et al. Reduced risk of restenosis in small vessels and reduced risk of myocardial infarction in long lesions with the new thin-strut TAXUS Liberté stent: 1-year results from the TAXUS ATLAS program. J Am Coll Cardiol Intv. 2008;1:699–709.
52. Stone GW, Lansky AJ, Pocock SJ, et al. Paclitaxel-eluting stents versus bare-metal stents in acute myocardial infarction. N Engl J Med. 2009;360:1946–59.
53. Laarman GJ, Suttorp MJ, Dirksen MT, et al. Paclitaxel-eluting versus uncoated stents in primary percutaneous coronary intervention. N Engl J Med. 2006;355:1105–13.
54. Guo N, Maehara A, Mintz G, et al. Incidence, mechanisms, predictors, and clinical impact of acute and late stent malapposition after primary intervention in patients with acute myocardial infarction: an intravascular ultrasound substudy of the Harmonizing Outcomes with Revascularization and Stents in Acute Myocardial Infarction (HORIZONS-AMI) trial. Circulation. 2010;122:1077–84.
55. Windecker S, Remondino A, Eberli FR, et al. Sirolimus-eluting and paclitaxel-eluting stents for coronary revascularization. N Engl J Med. 2005;353:653–62.
56. Galloe A, Thuesen L, Kelbaek H, et al. Comparison of paclitaxel- and sirolimus- eluting stents in everyday clinical practice. JAMA. 2008;299:409–16.
57. Lee CW, Hong M-K, Rhee K-S, et al. A randomized comparison of sirolimus- versus paclitaxel-eluting stent implantation in patients with diabetes mellitus. J Am Coll Cardiol. 2009;53: 812–3.
58. Dibra A, Kastrati A, Mehilli J, et al. Paclitaxel-eluting or sirolimus-eluting stents to prevent restenosis in diabetic patients. N Engl J Med. 2005;353:663–70.
59. Kastrati A, Mehilli J, von Beckerath N, et al. Sirolimus-eluting stent of paclitaxel-eluting stent vs balloon angioplasty for prevention of recurrences in patients with coronary in-stent restenosis. JAMA. 2005;293:165–71.
60. Mehilli J, Byrne RA, Tiroch K, et al. Randomized trial of paclitaxel- versus sirolimus-eluting stents for treatment of coronary restenosis in sirolimus-eluting stents. J Am Coll Cardiol. 2010; 55(24):2710–6.
61. Morice M-C, Colombo A, Meier B, et al. Sirolimus- vs. paclitaxel-eluting stents in de novo coronary artery lesions. JAMA. 2006;295:895–904.
62. Schomig A, Dibra A, Windecker S, et al. A meta-analysis of 16 randomized trials of sirolimus-eluting stents versus paclitaxel-eluting stents in patients with coronary artery disease. J Am Coll Cardiol. 2007;50:1373–80.
63. Lee S-W, Park S-W, Kim Y-H, et al. A randomized comparison of sirolimus- versus paclitaxel-eluting stent implantation in patients with diabetes mellitus. J Am Coll Cardiol. 2008;52:727–33.
64. Mehilli J, Byrne RA, Tiroch K, et al. Sirolimus-eluting stents for treatment of coronary restenosis in sirolimus-eluting stents. J Am Coll Cardiol. 2010;55:2710–6.
65. Marroquin OC, Selzer F, Mulukutla SR, et al. A comparison of bare-metal and drug-eluting stents for off-label indications. N Engl J Med. 2008;358:342–52.
66. Brodie BR, Stuckey T, Downey WE, et al. Outcomes and complications with off-label use of drug-eluting stents: results from the STENT (Strategic Transcatheter Evaluation of New Therapies) group. JACC Cardiovasc Interv. 2008;1:405–14.
67. Meredith I, Ormiston J, Whitbourn R, et al. First-in-human study of the Endeavor ABT-578-eluting phosphorylcholine-encapsulated stent system in *de novo* native coronary artery lesions: Endeavor I trial. EuroIntervention. 2005;1:157–64.
68. Fajadet J, Wijns W, Laarman GJ, et al. Randomized, double-blind, multicenter study of the Endeavor zotarolimus-eluting phosphorylcholine-encapsulated stent for treatment of native coronary artery lesions: clinical and angiographic results of the ENDEAVOR II trial. Circulation. 2006;114:798–806.
69. Lotan C, Meredith I, Mauri L, Liu M, Rothman MT. Safety and effectiveness of the Endeavor zotarolimus-eluting stent in real-world clinical practice: 12-month data from the E-Five registry. J Am Coll Cardiol Intv. 2009;2:1227–35.
70. Rasmussen K, Maeng M, Kaltoft A, et al. Efficacy and safety of zotarolimus-eluting and sirolimus-eluting coronary stents in routine clinical care (SORT OUT III): a randomised controlled superiority trial. Lancet. 2010;375:1090–9.
71. Mauri L, Massaro J, Jiang S, et al. Long-term clinical outcomes with zotarolimus-eluting versus bare-metal coronary stents. J Am Coll Cardiol Intv. 2010;3:1240–9.
72. Cutlip DE, Windecker S, Mehran R, et al. Clinical end points in coronary stent trials: a case for standardized definitions. Circulation. 2007;111(17):2344–51.
73. Kandzari DE, Mauri L, Popma JJ, et al. Late-term clinical outcomes with zotarolimus- and sirolimus-eluting stents: 5-year follow-up of the ENDEAVOR III (A Randomized Controlled Trial of the Medtronic Endeavor Drug (ABT-578) Eluting Coronary Stent System Versus the Cypher Sirolimus-Eluting

Coronary Stent System in De novo Native Coronary Artery Lesions). J Am Coll Cardiol Intv. 2011;4:543–50.
74. Leon MB, Mauri L, Popma JJ, et al. A randomized comparison of the ENDEAVOR zotarolimus-eluting stent versus the TAXUS paclitaxel-eluting stent in de novo native coronary lesions: 12-month outcomes from the ENDEAVOR IV trial. J Am Coll Cardiol. 2010;55:543–54.
75. Meredith I, Worthley S, Whitbourn R, et al. Clinical and angiographic results with the next-generation resolute stent system: a prospective, multicenter, first-in-human trial. J Am Coll Cardiol Intv. 2009;2:977–85.
76. Serruys PW, Silber S, Garg S, et al. Comparison of zotarolimus-eluting and everolimus-eluting coronary stents. N Engl J Med. 2010;363:136–46.
77. Silber S, Windecker S, Vranckx P, Serruys PW. Unrestricted randomised use of two new generation drug-eluting coronary stents: 2-year patient-related versus stent-related outcomes from the RESOLUTE All Comer trial. Lancet. 2011;377:1241–7.
78. Yeung AC, Leon M, Jain A, et al. Clinical evaluation of the resolute zotarolimus-eluting coronary stent system in the treatment of de novo lesions in native coronary arteries. J Am Coll Cardiol. 2011;57:1778–83.
79. Moses JW, Leon MB, Popma JJ, et al. Sirolimus-eluting stents versus standard stents in patients with stenosis in a native coronary artery. N Engl J Med. 2003;349:1315–23.
80. Dawkins KD, Grube E, Guagliumi G, et al. Clinical efficacy of polymer-based paclitaxel-eluting stents in the treatment of complex, long coronary artery lesions from a multicenter, randomized trial: support for the use of drug-eluting stents in contemporary clinical practice. Circulation. 2005;112:3306–13.
81. Stone GW, Midei MG, Newman W, et al. Comparison of an everolimus-eluting stent and a paclitaxel-eluting stent in patients with coronary artery disease. JAMA. 2008;299:1903–13.
82. Serruys PW, Ong ATL, Piek JJ, et al. A randomized comparison of a durable polymer Everolimus-eluting stent with a bare metal coronary stent: the SPIRIT first trial. EuroIntervention. 2005;1:58–65.
83. Garg S, Serruys PW, Onuma Y, et al. 3-year clinical follow-up of the XIENCE V everolimus-eluting coronary stent system in the treatment of patients with de novo coronary artery lesions: the SPIRIT II trial (Clinical Evaluation of the XIENCE V Everolimus Eluting Coronary Stent System in the Treatment of Patients with de novo Native Coronary Artery Lesions). J Am Coll Cardiol Intv. 2009;2:1190–8.
84. Stone GW, Rizvi A, Newman W, et al. Everolimus-eluting versus paclitaxel-eluting stents in coronary artery disease. N Engl J Med. 2010;362:1663–74.
85. Stone GW, Rizvi A, Sudhir K, et al. Randomized comparison of everolimus- and paclitaxel-eluting stents. J Am Coll Cardiol. 2011;58:1–7.
86. Grube E, Chevalier B, Smits P, et al. The Spirit V study: a clinical evaluation of the XIENCE V everolimus-eluting coronary stent system in the treatment of patients with de novo coronary artery lesions. J Am Coll Cardiol Intv. 2011;4:168–75.
87. Kedhi E, Joesef S, McFadden E, et al. Second-generation everolimus-eluting and paclitaxel-eluting stents in real-life practice (COMPARE): a randomised trial. Lancet. 2010;375:201–9.
88. Smits P, Kedhi E, Royaards K-J, et al. 2-year follow-up of a randomized controlled trial of everolimus- and paclitaxel-eluting stents for coronary revascularization in daily practice. J Am Coll Cardiol. 2011;58:2011.
89. Onuma Y, Kukreja N, Piazza N, et al. The everolimus-eluting stent in real-world patients. J Am Coll Cardiol. 2009;54:269–76.
90. Serruys PW, Ruygrok P, Neuzner J, et al. A randomised comparison of an everolimus-eluting coronary stent with a paclitaxel-eluting coronary stent: the SPIRIT II trial. EuroIntervention. 2006;2:286–94.
91. Stone GW, Midei MG, Newman W, et al. Randomized comparison of everolimus-eluting and paclitaxel-eluting stents: two-year clinical follow-up from the Clinical Evaluation of the Xience V Everolimus Eluting Coronary Stent System in the Treatment of Patients with de novo Native Coronary Artery Lesions (SPIRIT) III trial. Circulation. 2009;119:680–6.
92. Ambrosio G, Steinhubl SR, Gresele P, et al. Impact of prior chronic antiplatelet therapy on short- and long-term adverse events in patients presenting with an acute coronary syndrome: insights from the acuity trial. J Am Coll Cardiol. 2010;55:A113. E1059–A113.E.
93. Caixeta A, Lansky AJ, Serruys PW, et al. Clinical follow-up 3 years after everolimus- and paclitaxel-eluting stents: a pooled analysis from the SPIRIT II (A Clinical Evaluation of the XIENCE V Everolimus Eluting Coronary Stents System in the Treatment of Patients With De Novo Native Coronary Artery Stent System in the Treatment of Patients With De Novo Native Coronary Artery Lesions) and SPIRIT III (A Clinical Evaluation of the Investigational Device Xience V Everolimus Eluting Coronary Stent System [EECSS] in the Treatment of Subjects With De Novo Native Coronary Artery Lesions) randomized trials. J Am Coll Cardiol Intv. 2010;3:1220–8.
94. George BS, Voorhees WD, Roubin GS, et al. Multicenter investigation of coronary stenting to treat acute or threatened closure complicating percutaneous transluminal coronary angioplasty. J Am Coll Cardiol. 1993;22:135–43.
95. Roubin GS, Cannon AD, Agrawal SK, et al. Intracoronary stenting for acute and threatened closure complicating percutaneous transluminal coronary angioplasty. Circulation. 1992;85:916–27.
96. Herrman NC, Buchbinder M, Clemen MW, et al. Emergent use of balloon expandable coronary artery stenting for failed percutaneous transluminal coronary angioplasty. Circulation. 1992;86: 812–9.
97. Fischman DL, Leon MB, Baim DS, et al. A randomized comparison of coronary-stent placement and balloon angioplasty in the treatment of coronary artery disease. N Engl J Med. 1994;331: 496–501.
98. Cutlip DE, Baim DS, Ho KKL, et al. Stent thrombosis in the modern era: a pooled analysis of multicenter coronary stent clinical trials. Circulation. 2001;103:1967–71.
99. Wang F, Stouffer GA, Waxman S, Uretsky BF. Late coronary stent thrombosis: early vs. late stent thrombosis in the stent era. Catheter Cardiovasc Interv. 2002;55:142–7.
100. Stone GW, Ellis SG, Cox D, et al. One-year clinical results with the slow-release, polymer-based paclitaxel-eluting TAXUS stent: the TAXUS-IV trial. Circulation. 2004;109:1942–7.
101. Pfisterer M, Brunner-La Rocca HP, Buser PT, et al. Late clinical events after clopidogrel discontinuation may limit the benefit of drug-eluting stents. J Am Coll Cardiol. 2006;48:2584–91.
102. Iakovou I, Schmidt T, Bonizzoni E, et al. Incidence, predictors, and outcome of thrombosis after successful implantation of drug-eluting stents. JAMA. 2005;293:2126–30.
103. Ong ATL, Hoye A, Aoki J, et al. Thirty-day incidence and six-month clinical outcome of thrombotic stent occlusion after bare-metal, sirolimus, or paclitaxel stent implantation. J Am Coll Cardiol. 2005;45:947–53.
104. Laskey WK, Yancy CW, Maisel WH. Thrombosis in coronary drug-eluting stents: report from the meeting of the Circulatory System Medical Devices Advisory Panel of the Food and Drug Administration Center for Devices and Radiologic Health, December 7–8, 2006. Circulation. 2007;115:2352–7.
105. Weisz G, Leon M, Holmes Jr DR, et al. Two-year outcomes after sirolimus-eluting stent implantation. J Am Coll Cardiol. 2006;47: 1350–5.
106. Daemen J, Tsuchida K, Stefanini GG, et al. Two-year clinical follow-up of the unrestricted use of the paclitaxel-eluting stent

compared to the sirolimus-eluting stent as part of the Taxus-Stent Evaluated at Rotterdam Cardiology Hospital (T-SEARCH) registry. EuroIntervention. 2006;2:330–7.
107. James S, Stenestrand U, Lindbäck J, et al. Long-term safety and efficacy of drug-eluting versus bare-metal stents in Sweden. N Engl J Med. 2009;360:1933–45.
108. Grines CL, Bonow RO, Casey Jr DE, et al. Prevention of premature discontinuation of dual antiplatelet therapy in patients with coronary artery stents. J Am Coll Cardiol. 2007;49:734–9.
109. Cheneau E, Leborgne L, Mintz G, et al. Predictors of subacute stent thrombosis: results of a systematic intravascular ultrasound study. Circulation. 2003;108:43–7.
110. Fujii K, Carlier SG, Mintz G, et al. Stent underexpansion and residual reference segment stenosis are related to stent thrombosis after sirolimus-eluting stent implantation. J Am Coll Cardiol. 2005;45:996–8.
111. Alfonso F, Suárez A, Pérez-Vizcayno M-J, et al. Intravascular ultrasound findings during episodes of drug-eluting stent thrombosis. J Am Coll Cardiol. 2007;50(21):2095–7.
112. Hoye A, Iakovou I, Ge L, et al. Long-term outcomes after stenting bifurcation lesions with the "crush" technique. J Am Coll Cardiol. 2006;47:1949–58.
113. Joner M, Finn AV, Mont EK, et al. Pathology of drug-eluting stents in humans. J Am Coll Cardiol. 2006;48:193–202.
114. Awata M, Kotani J-i, Uematsu M, et al. Serial angioscopic evidence of incomplete neointimal coverage after sirolimus-eluting stent implantation: comparison with bare-metal stents. Circulation. 2007;116:910–6.
115. Nakazawa G, Finn AV, Vorpahl M, Ladich E, Kolodgie FD, Virmani R. Coronary responses and differential mechanisms of late stent thrombosis attributed to first-generation sirolimus- and paclitaxel-eluting stents. J Am Coll Cardiol. 2011;57:390–8.
116. Virmani R, Guagliumi G, Farb A, et al. Localized hypersensitivity and late coronary thrombosis secondary to a sirolimus-eluting stent: should we be cautious? Circulation. 2004;109:701–5.
117. Nebeker JR, Virmani R, Bennett CI, et al. Hypersensitivity cases associated with drug-eluting coronary stents. J Am Coll Cardiol. 2006;47:175–81.
118. Farb A, Burke AP, Kolodgie FD, Virmani R. Pathological mechanisms of fatal late coronary stent thrombosis in humans. Circulation. 2003;108:1701–6.
119. Cook S, Wenaweser P, Togni M, et al. Incomplete stent apposition and very late stent thrombosis after drug-eluting stent implantation. Circulation. 2007;115:2426–34.
120. Siqueira DA, Abizaid A, de Ribamar CJ, et al. Late incomplete apposition after drug-eluting stent implantation: incidence and potential for adverse outcomes. Eur Heart J. 2007;28:1304–9.
121. Nakazawa G, Finn AV, Vorpahl M, et al. Incidence and predictors of drug-eluting stent fracture in human coronary artery. J Am Coll Cardiol. 2009;54:1924–31.
122. Umeda H, Gochi T, Iwase M, et al. Frequency, predictors and outcome of stent fracture after sirolimus-eluting stent implantation. Int J Cardiol. 2009;133:321–6.
123. Nakazawa G, Otsuka F, Nakano M, et al. The pathology of neoatherosclerosis in human coronary implants: bare-metal and drug-eluting stents. J Am Coll Cardiol. 2011;57:1–9.
124. Lasala JM, Cox D, Dobies D, et al. Drug-eluting stent thrombosis in routine clinical practice: two-year outcomes and predictors from the TAXUS ARRIVE registries. Circ Cardiovasc Interv. 2009;2:285–93.
125. Kuchulakanti PK, Chu WW, Torguson R, et al. Correlates and long-term outcomes of angiographically proven stent thrombosis with sirolimus- and paclitaxel-eluting stents. Circulation. 2006;113:1108–13.
126. van Werkum JW, Heestermans AA, Zomer C, et al. Predictors of coronary stent thrombosis. J Am Coll Cardiol. 2009;53:1399–409.
127. Park D-W, Park S-W, Park K-H, et al. Frequency of and risk factors for stent thrombosis after drug-eluting stent implantation during long-term follow-up. Am J Cardiol. 2006;98(3):352–6.
128. Roy P, Bonello L, Torguson R, et al. Temporal relation between *Clopidogrel* cessation and stent thrombosis after drug-eluting stent implantation. Am J Cardiol. 2009;103:801–5.
129. Spertus J, Kettelkamp R, Vance C, et al. Prevalence, predictors, and outcomes of premature discontinuation of thienopyridine therapy after drug-eluting stent placement: results from the PREMIER registry. Circulation. 2006;113:2803–9.
130. Spaulding C, Henry P, Teiger E, et al. Sirolimus-eluting versus uncoated stents in acute myocardial infarction. N Engl J Med. 2006;355:1093–104.
131. Aoki J, Lansky AJ, Mehran R, et al. Early stent thrombosis in patients with acute coronary syndromes treated with drug-eluting and bare metal stents: the Acute Catheterization and Urgent Intervention Triage Strategy trial. Circulation. 2009;119:687–98.
132. Montalescot G, Wiviott SD, Braunwald E, et al. Prasugrel compared with clopidogrel in patients undergoing percutaneous coronary intervention for ST-elevation myocardial infarction (TRITON-TIMI 38): double-blind, randomised controlled trial. Lancet. 2009;373:723–31.
133. Demopoulos VP, Olympios CD, Fakiolas CN, et al. The natural history of aneurysmal coronary artery disease. Heart. 1997;78:136–41.
134. Aoki J, Kirtane AJ, Leon MB, Dangas G. Coronary artery aneurysms after drug-eluting stent implantation. J Am Coll Cardiol. 2008;1:14–21.
135. Bell MR, Garratt KN, Bresnahan J, Edwards W, Holmes Jr DR. Relation of deep arterial resection and coronary artery aneurysms after directional coronary atherectomy. J Am Coll Cardiol. 1992;20:1474–81.
136. Baumbach A, Bittl JA, Fleck E, et al. Acute complications of excimer laser coronary angioplasty: a detailed analysis of multicenter results. Coinvestigators of the U.S. and European Percutaneous Excimer Laser Coronary Angioplasty (PELCA) Registries. J Am Coll Cardiol. 1994;23:1305–13.
137. Slota P, Fischman DL, Savage MDMP, Rake BSR, Goldberg MDS. Frequency and outcome of development of coronary artery aneurysm after intra-coronary stent placement and angioplasty. STRESS Trial Investigators. Am J Cardiol. 1997;79:1104–6.
138. Kimura M, Mintz G, Carlier SG, et al. Outcome after acute incomplete sirolimus-eluting stent apposition as assessed by serial intravascular ultrasound. Am J Cardiol. 2006;98:436–42.
139. Alfonso F, Pérez-Vizcayno M-J, Ruiz M, et al. Coronary aneurysms after drug-eluting stent implantation. J Am Coll Cardiol. 2009;53:2053–60.
140. Canan T, Lee MS. Drug-eluting stent fracture: incidence, contributing factors, and clinical implications. Catheter Cardiovasc Interv. 2010;75:237–45.
141. Aoki J, Nakazawa G, Tanabe K, et al. Incidence and clinical impact of coronary stent fracture after sirolimus-eluting stent implantation. Catheter Cardiovasc Interv. 2007;69:380–6.
142. Kereiakes DJ, Wang H, Popma JJ, et al. Periprocedural and late consequences of overlapping Cypher sirolimus-eluting stents. J Am Coll Cardiol. 2006;48:21–31.
143. Kandzari DE, Rao SV, Moses JW, et al. Clinical and angiographic outcomes with sirolimus-eluting stents in total coronary occlusions: ACROSS/TOSCA-4 trial. J Am Coll Cardiol Intv. 2009;2:97–106.
144. Daemen J, Boersma E, Flather M, et al. Long-term safety and efficacy of percutaneous coronary intervention with stenting and coronary artery bypass surgery for multivessel coronary artery disease: a meta-analysis with 5-year patient-level data from the ARTS, ERACI-II, MASS-II, and SoS trials. Circulation. 2008;118:1146–54.

145. Forrester J, Fishbein M, Helfant R, Fagin J. A paradigm for restenosis based on cell biology: clues for the development of new preventive therapies. J Am Coll Cardiol. 1991;17:758–69.
146. Dangas G, et al. In-stent restenosis in the drug-eluting stent era. J Am Coll Cardiol. 2010;56:1897–907.
147. Yusuf RZ, Duan Z, Lamendola DE, Penson RT, Seiden MV. Paclitaxel resistance: molecular mechanisms and pharmacologic manipulation. Curr Cancer Drug Targets. 2003;3:1–19.
148. Huang S, Houghton PJ. Mechanisms of resistance to rapamycins. Drug Resist Updat. 2001;4:378–91.
149. Kang S-J, Mintz G, Park D-W, et al. Mechanisms of in-stent restenosis after drug-eluting stent implantation: intravascular ultrasound analysis. Circ Cardiovasc Interv. 2011;4:9–14.
150. Balakrishnan B, Tzafriri AR, Seifert P, Groothuis A, Rogers C, Edelman ER. Strut position, blood flow, and drug deposition: implications for single and overlapping drug-eluting stents. Circulation. 2005;111:2958–65.
151. Costa MA, Angiolillo DJ, Tannenbaum M, et al. Impact of stent deployment procedural factors on long-term effectiveness and safety of sirolimus-eluting stents (final results of the multicenter prospective STLLR trial). Am J Cardiol. 2008;101:1704–11.
152. Kastrati A, Dibra A, Mehilli J, et al. Predictive factors of restenosis after coronary implantation of sirolimus- or paclitaxel-eluting stents. Circulation. 2006;113:2293–300.
153. Lemos PA, Hoye A, Goedhart D, et al. Clinical, angiographic, and procedural predictors of angiographic restenosis after sirolimus-eluting stent implantation in complex patients: an evaluation from the Rapamycin-Eluting Stent Evaluated At Rotterdam Cardiology Hospital (RESEARCH) study. Circulation. 2004;109:1366–70.
154. Hong M-K, Mintz G, Lee CW, et al. Intravascular ultrasound predictors of angiographic restenosis after sirolimus-eluting stent implantation. Eur Heart J. 2006;27:1305–10.
155. Doi H, Maehara A, Mintz G, et al. Impact of post-intervention minimal stent area on 9-month follow-up patency of paclitaxel-eluting stents: an integrated intravascular ultrasound analysis from the TAXUS IV, V and IV and TAXUS ATLAS Workhorse, Long Lesion, and Direct Stent Trials. JACC Cardiovasc Interv. 2009;2:1269–75.
156. Mehran R, Dangas G, Abizaid AS, et al. Angiographic patterns of in-stent restenosis: classification and implications for long-term outcome. Circulation. 1999;100:1872–8.
157. Lemos PA, Saia F, Ligthart JMR, et al. Coronary restenosis after sirolimus-eluting stent implantation: morphological description and mechanistic analysis from a consecutive series of cases. Circulation. 2003;108:257–60.
158. Iakovou I, Dangas G, Mehran R, et al. Intravascular ultrasound predictors of late recurrence after stent implantation in small coronary arteries. J Am Coll Cardiol. 2003;41:35.
159. Latib A, Mussardo M, Ielasi A, et al. Long-term outcomes after the percutaneous treatment of drug-eluting stent restenosis. J Am Coll Cardiol Intv. 2011;4:155–64.
160. Teirstein PS, Massullo V, Jani S, et al. Catheter-based radiotherapy to inhibit restenosis after coronary stenting. N Engl J Med. 1997;336:1697–703.
161. Holmes Jr DR, Teirstein PS, Satler LF, et al. Sirolimus-eluting stents vs vascular brachytherapy for in-stent restenosis within bare-metal stents. JAMA. 2006;295:1264–73.
162. Stone GW, Ellis SG, O'Shaughnessy CD, et al. Paclitaxel-eluting stents vs vascular brachytherapy for in-stent restenosis within bare-metal stents. JAMA. 2006;295:1253–63.
163. Garg S, Serruys PW. Coronary stents: looking forward. J Am Coll Cardiol. 2010;56:S43–78.
164. Windecker S, Serruys PW, Wandel S, et al. Biolimus-eluting stent with biodegradable polymer versus sirolimus-eluting stent with durable polymer for coronary revascularisation (LEADERS): a randomised non-inferiority trial. Lancet. 2008;372:1163–73.
165. Abizaid A, Costa Jr JR. New drug-eluting stents: an overview on biodegradable and polymer-free next-generation stent systems. Circ Cardiovasc Interv. 2010;3:384–93.
166. Byrne RA, Kastrati A, Tiroch K, et al. 2-year clinical and angiographic outcomes from a randomized trial of polymer-free dual drug-eluting stents versus polymer-based Cypher and Endeavor, drug-eluting stents. J Am Coll Cardiol. 2010;55:2536–43.
167. Ormiston J, Serruys PW, Regar E, et al. A bioabsorbable everolimus-eluting coronary stent system for patients with single de-novo coronary artery lesions (ABSORB): a prospective open-label trial. Lancet. 2008;371:899–907.
168. Serruys PW, Ormiston J, Onuma Y, et al. A bioabsorbable everolimus-eluting coronary stent system (ABSORB): 2-year outcomes and results from multiple imaging methods. Lancet. 2009;373:897–910.
169. Onuma Y, Serruys PW. Bioresorbable scaffold: the advent of a new era in percutaneous coronary and peripheral revascularization? Circulation. 2011;123:779–97.

Adjunctive Pharmacology for Coronary Intervention

11

Osman Faheem and John K. Forrest

This chapter reviews adjunctive pharmacology for coronary interventions focusing on the following: (1) Oral Antiplatelet Agents: Aspirin and Thienopyridines, (2) Heparin and Glycoprotein IIb/IIIa Inhibitors, and (3) Direct Thrombin Inhibitors and Anti-Xa Agents.

Oral Antiplatelet Agents: Aspirin, Thienopyridines, and Ticagrelor

Platelets play a pivotal role in the development of arterial thrombus formation in both the setting of plaque rupture during ST elevation myocardial infarction (STEMI) and in routine PCI through disruption of previously stable coronary plaques. In the setting of acute coronary syndromes, there are critical changes that occur within platelets that promote clot formation. These changes include (1) platelet adhesion mediated by von Willebrand factor and other adhesive proteins; (2) platelet activation, mediated in part by thromboxane A2; and (3) platelet aggregation due to fibrinogen cross-linking of platelets (Fig. 11.1). Many commonly used oral antiplatelet agents discussed subsequently work through mechanisms that disrupt one or more of these pathways.

O. Faheem, MD
Yale University School of Medicine, New Haven, CT, USA
e-mail: osman.faheem@yale.edu

J.K. Forrest, MD (✉)
Assistant Professor of Medicine, Yale University School of Medicine, New Haven, CT, USA
e-mail: john.k.forrest@yale.edu

C.A. Thompson (ed.), *Textbook of Cardiovascular Intervention*,
DOI 10.1007/978-1-4471-4528-8_11, © Springer-Verlag London 2014

Aspirin

Pharmacokinetics

Aspirin, a derivative of salicylic acid whose origins date back to Hippocrates and a powder he made from the bark and leaves of the willow tree, was first commercially produced in 1900 by Felix Hoffmann, a chemist working for Bayer [1]. Aspirin irreversibly inhibits platelet activation through acetylation of the platelet cyclooxygenase-1 enzyme. Blockage of the cyclooxygenase-1 enzyme prevents the conversion of arachidonic acid to prostaglandin H2, which, in normal conditions, is then converted into thromboxane A2. Platelets possess a thromboxane A2 receptor which, upon binding with thromboxane A2, promotes platelet activation. Thus, as a result of inhibited thromboxane A2 production, platelet activation is inhibited. Because the inhibition of the cyclooxygenase-1 enzyme is irreversible and the platelets cannot create more of the enzyme, the effects last for the lifespan of the platelet (7–10 days).

Clinical Evidence for Use

Aspirin (preferably given prior to the procedure) is indicated as an adjunctive pharmacologic therapy in all coronary interventions. In the pre-stent era, Schwartz et al. evaluated aspirin loading prior to PCI in 376 patients undergoing balloon angioplasty. Patients were randomized to receive either a combination of aspirin/dipyridamole (330 mg/75 mg) or placebo 24 h prior to PTCA. Treatment was continued in patients with a successfully dilated vessel until follow-up angiography, which was performed 4–7 months after PTCA. While the investigators had proposed that the combination of aspirin/dipyridamole would reduce restenosis (it did not), they did demonstrate a significant reduction in the incidence of periprocedural Q wave myocardial infarction (6.9 % in placebo vs. 1.6 % in treatment arm; $p = 0.011$) [2].

Similar to pre-PCI loading, there is also a single randomized trial for long-term continuation of aspirin post-PCI. In this study, 752 patients were randomly assigned to aspirin (325 mg daily), the thromboxane A2 receptor antagonist

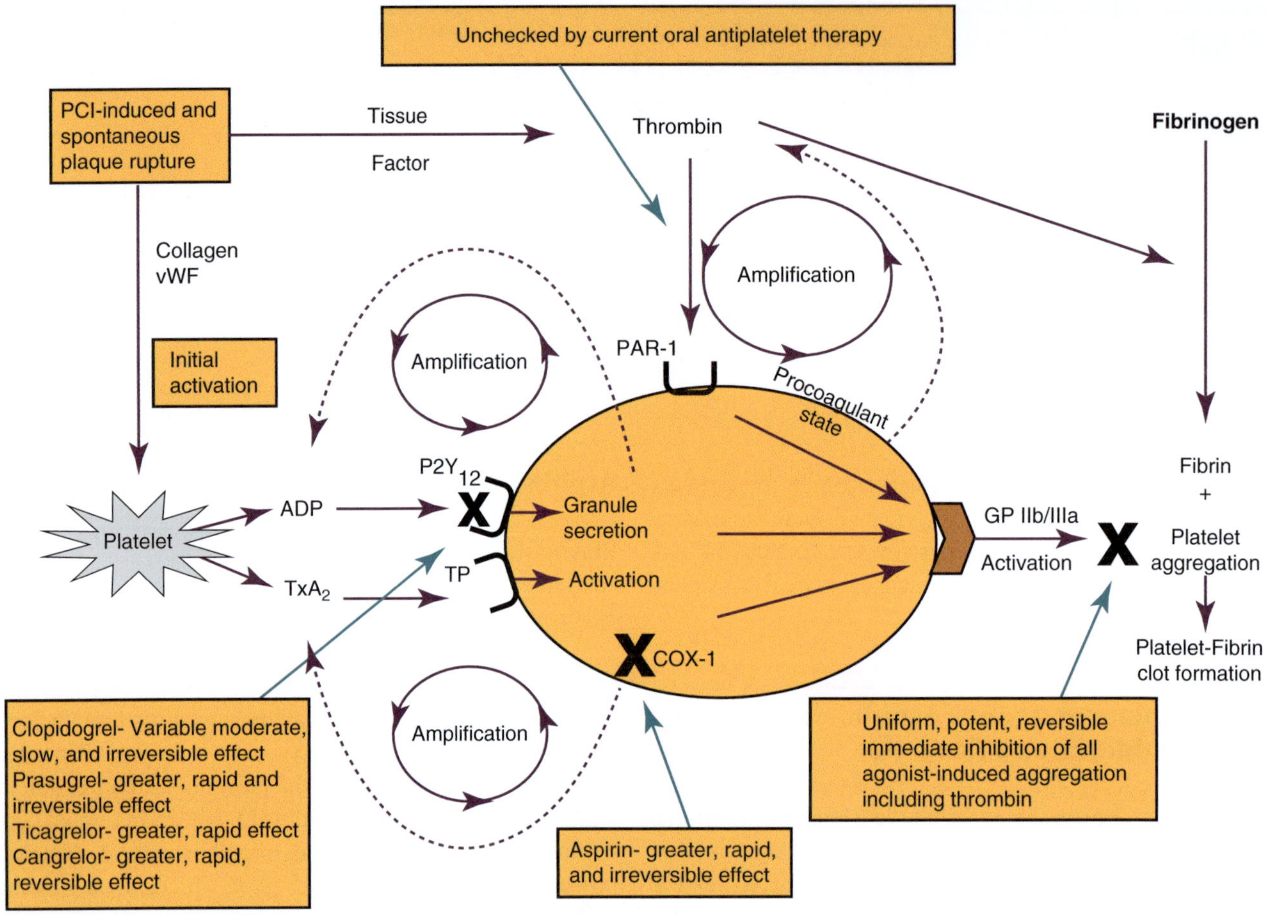

Fig. 11.1 The role of platelets in acute coronary syndrome and targets of platelet inhibitors

sulotroban (800 mg QID), or placebo, started within 6 h before PTCA and continued for 6 months. The results demonstrated that while there was again no difference in restenosis, the rate of myocardial infarction at 6 months was significantly reduced by antithromboxane therapy: 1.2 % in aspirin group, 1.8 % in the sulotroban group, and 5.7 % in the placebo group [3].

The most comprehensive evaluation for dosing of aspirin in the setting of acute coronary syndromes comes from the Antithrombotic Trialists' Collaboration, which made indirect comparisons between either high or low doses of aspirin. This analysis reviewed 287 studies involving both comparisons of antiplatelet therapy versus control and comparisons of different antiplatelet regimens. While a loading dose of at least 150 mg of aspirin was found to be of significant advantage up front, the benefits of long-term aspirin therapy were similarly independent of whether the maintenance dosing was high dose (>150 mg) or low dose (<150) [4]. Higher doses of aspirin are associated with increased rates of both minor as well as major and intracranial bleeding events. In the CURE study, three aspirin dose groups (≤100, 101–199, and ≥200 mg) were evaluated with or without clopidogrel. Results from this study demonstrated an increased incidence of major bleeding associated with increasing aspirin dose both in the group without concomitant clopidogrel (1.9 % for ≤100 mg, 2.8 % for 101–199 mg, and 3.7 % for ≥200 mg; $p=0.0001$) and for the clopidogrel-treated group (3.0 % for ≤100 mg, 3.4 % for 101–199 mg, and 4.9 for ≥200 mg; $p=0.0009$). In addition, there was no benefit in cardiovascular death, myocardial infarction, or stoke associated with the higher dose of aspirin [5].

The ACCF/AHA guidelines recommend a loading dose of 325 mg in the setting of STEMI and pre-PCI, and the most updated guidelines now recommend that after PCI, it is reasonable to use 81 mg of aspirin as the maintenance dose [6] (Table 11.1).

Thienopyridines and Ticagrelor

Pharmacokinetics

In the modern PCI era with both bare-metal and drug-eluting stents, dual antiplatelet therapy with aspirin and a thienopyridine has become the standard of treatment. The thienopyridines

Table 11.1 ACCF/AHA guidelines for oral antiplatelet therapy

Class I
1. Patients already taking daily aspirin therapy should take 81–325 mg before PCI (level of evidence B)
2. Patients not on aspirin therapy should be given nonenteric aspirin 325 mg before PCI (level of evidence B)
3. After PCI, use of aspirin should be continued indefinitely (level of evidence A)
4. A loading dose of a $P2Y_{12}$ receptor inhibitor should be given to patients undergoing PCI with stenting (level of evidence A). Options include:
(a) Clopidogrel 600 mg (ACS and non-ACS patients) (level of evidence B)
(b) Prasugrel 60 mg (ACS patients) (level of evidence B)
(c) Ticagrelor 180 mg (ACS patients) (level of evidence B)
5. The loading dose of clopidogrel for patients undergoing PCI after fibrinolytic therapy should be 300 mg within 24 h and 600 mg more than 24 h after receiving fibrinolytic therapy (level of evidence C)
6. Patients should be counseled on the need for and risks of DAPT before placement of intracoronary stents, especially DES, and alternative therapies should be pursued if patients are unwilling or unable to comply with the recommended duration of DAPT (level of evidence C)
7. The duration of $P2Y_{12}$ inhibitor therapy after stent implantation should generally be as follows:
(a) In patients receiving a stent (BMS or DES) during PCI for ACS, $P2Y_{12}$ inhibitor therapy should be given for at least 12 months. Options include clopidogrel 75 mg daily, prasugrel 10 mg daily, and ticagrelor 90 mg twice daily (level of evidence B)
(b) In patients receiving DES for a non-ACS indication, clopidogrel 75 mg daily should be given for at least 12 months if patients are not at high risk of bleeding (level of evidence B)
(c) In patients receiving BMS for a non-ACS indication, clopidogrel should be given for a minimum of 1 month and ideally up to 12 months (unless the patient is at increased risk of bleeding; then, it should be given for a minimum of 2 weeks) (level of evidence B)
Class IIa
1. After PCI, it is reasonable to use aspirin 81 mg per day in preference to higher maintenance doses (level of evidence B)
2. If the risk of morbidity from bleeding outweighs the anticipated benefit afforded by a recommended duration of $P2Y_{12}$ inhibitor therapy after stent implantation, earlier discontinuation (e.g., <12 months) of $P2Y_{12}$ inhibitor therapy is reasonable (level of evidence C)
Class IIb
1. Continuation of DAPT beyond 12 months may be considered in patients undergoing DES implantation (level of evidence C)
Class III: HARM
Prasugrel should not be administered to patients with a prior history of stroke or transient ischemic attack (level of evidence B)

that are used post-PCI with aspirin are ticlopidine, clopidogrel, and prasugrel. While aspirin inhibits platelet activation, thienopyridines inhibit both platelet activation *and* aggregation. These effects on platelets are due both to their inhibition of the activation of the GPIIb/IIIa receptor responsible for platelet linking and the binding of fibrinogen and to their inhibition of platelet ADP receptor $P2Y_{12}$. The inhibition of the platelet ADP receptor $P2Y_{12}$ prevents platelet activation and aggregation by downregulating platelet degranulation and the subsequent release of prothrombotic and inflammatory mediators [7] (Fig. 11.1). The mechanism of action of ticlopidine, clopidogrel, and prasugrel all involve inhibition of the platelet ADP receptor $P2Y_{12}$ by blocking the ADP binding site. Like aspirin, this results in an irreversible inhibition of the platelet, and thus, the effects last for the 7–10 day lifespan of the platelet. The newest oral antiplatelet agent, ticagrelor, is an exception to this irreversible inhibition. Although ticagrelor also blocks the ADP receptor $P2Y_{12}$ like the thienopyridines, it does so at a different binding site from ADP, and as a result, its effects are reversible [8] .

Clinical Evidence for Use

The evidence in favor of the use of thienopyridines in the setting of STEMI and during PCI is supported by significant clinical evidence. The COMMIT study randomized 45,852 patients presenting with acute myocardial infarction to clopidogrel 75 mg daily with no loading dose vs. placebo, in addition to aspirin 162 mg daily. Within the trial, 93 % of the patients presented with ST segment elevation myocardial infarction. In this study, clopidogrel (or placebo) was continued for the duration of the hospitalization or up to 4 weeks with mean treatment duration of 15 days. The composite end point of death, reinfarction, or stroke was significantly reduced in the group receiving clopidogrel as compared to placebo (9.2 % vs. 10.1 %; $p=0.002$). There was no significant difference in combined rates for fatal bleeds, blood product transfusion, or intracerebral hemorrhage (0.58 % vs. 0.55 %; $p=\text{NS}$) [9].

Clopidogrel loading prior to PCI has also been demonstrated to be beneficial. The PCI-CLARITY trial, a continuation of the CLARITY–TIMI 28 study, prospectively randomized 1,863 patients undergoing PCI after mandatory angiography in the CLARITY–TIMI 28 trial to either clopidogrel (300 mg oral loading dose followed by 75 mg daily) or placebo in addition to aspirin. Pretreatment with clopidogrel led to a significant reduction in the composite end point of cardiovascular death, recurrent MI, or stroke from PCI to 30 days post-randomization (3.6 % in clopidogrel group vs. 6.2 % in the placebo group; $p=0.008$). Pretreatment with clopidogrel also reduced the incidence of

MI or stroke prior to PCI (4.0 % vs. 6.2 %; $p=0.03$). Importantly, as in the COMMIT study, there was no significant difference in both major and minor bleeding risks (2 % vs. 1.9 %; $p=\text{NS}$) [10].

Prasugrel is one of the newer members of the thienopyridine family. Like clopidogrel, prasugrel is a prodrug that requires conversion to an active metabolite in order to become active. What differentiates prasugrel from clopidogrel is that prasugrel is converted to its active form more quickly and inhibits the ADP binding site of the ADP receptor $P2Y_{12}$ more potently. The TRITON–TIMI 38 trial evaluated the safety and efficacy of prasugrel in a double-blinded study involving 13,600 patients presenting with acute coronary syndrome undergoing scheduled percutaneous intervention. Patients were randomized to receive either prasugrel (a 60 mg loading dose followed by 10 mg daily) or clopidogrel (a 300 mg loading dose followed by 75 mg daily) for 6–15 months. The primary end point was death from cardiovascular causes, nonfatal MI, or nonfatal stroke. Of the patients included in the study, 26 % presented with STEMI. The primary end point occurred in 12.1 % of clopidogrel patients and 9.9 % of prasugrel patients ($p<0.001$). This was driven in part by a significant reduction in the rate of myocardial infarction (9.7 % clopidogrel vs. 7.4 % prasugrel; $p<0.001$). Additional benefits of prasugrel included decreased stent thrombosis (3.7 % clopidogrel vs. 2.5 % prasugrel; $p<0.001$), and these benefits carried over to the STEMI subset. The benefit of prasugrel in the primary efficacy end point was seen within the first 24 h of randomization and persisted through 15 months of follow-up. Certain subgroups of patients also had a significant benefit with prasugrel, including diabetics and patients receiving Gp IIb/IIIa inhibitors. These improved efficacy outcomes, presumably due to the more potent pharmacokinetics, were however associated with an increased rate of bleeding. Major bleeding was seen in 2.4 % of prasugrel patients compared to 1.8 % seen in the clopidogrel group, including a significant increase in life-threatening bleeding (1.4 % prasugrel vs. 0.9 % clopidogrel; $p=0.01$) and fatal bleeding events (0.4 % prasugrel vs. 0.1 % clopidogrel; $p=0.002$). Three groups in particular were found to not have a clinical benefit from prasugrel: patients with prior TIA or stroke, patients with a weight <60 kg, and patients >75 years in age. For patients with prior TIA or stroke, there was a net harm from prasugrel administration as compared to clopidogrel [11]. Based on this data, the FDA declared prasugrel to be contraindicated in patients with prior TIA or stroke.

The final current oral antiplatelet agent is ticagrelor, a reversible $P2Y_{12}$ inhibitor. Ticagrelor was recently evaluated in the PLATO trial, which randomized 18,600 patients presenting with ACS to either clopidogrel (300 mg or 600 mg loading dose followed by 75 mg daily) or ticagrelor (180 mg loading dose followed by 90 mg twice daily). A total of 38 % of patients presented with STEMI. The primary end point of death from vascular causes or cerebrovascular causes, or death from an unknown cause, occurred in 9.8 % in the ticagrelor group vs. 11.7 % in the clopidogrel group ($p<0.001$). Furthermore, the composite of all-cause death, MI, or stroke was also reduced in the ticagrelor group (10.2 % vs. 12.3 %; $p<0.001$). Similarly, the rate of stent thrombosis was also lower among those patients receiving ticagrelor (1.3 % vs. 1.9 %; $p=0.009$). While the rates of major bleeding were similar between the two groups, intracranial bleeding episodes were more common among the ticagrelor group. Lastly, there was no significant difference in the incidence of stroke, including hemorrhagic stroke [12]. Based on the PLATO trial, ticagrelor was FDA approved for patients with acute coronary syndromes in July 2011.

Heparin and Glycoprotein IIb/IIIa Inhibitors

According to the most recent ACC/AHA guidelines, use of anticoagulation therapy in addition to antiplatelet therapy is a Class 1 indication in both STEMI (level of evidence B) and NSTEMI (level of evidence B). Unfractionated heparin has historically been the most widely used drug to achieve therapeutic systemic anticoagulation, with low-molecular-weight heparin and fondaparinux being more recent additions [13].

Unfractionated Heparin (UFH)

Pharmacokinetics

Unfractionated heparin has been the standard anticoagulant used for percutaneous coronary interventions around the world. It is relatively safe and inexpensive and, despite some drawbacks, works well in preventing thrombotic complications during PCI. Heparin exerts its action by enhancing the effects of antithrombin III which in turn inactivates factors IIa, IXa, Xa, XIa, and XIIa [14]. It cannot be absorbed orally and is administered parentally either as repeated boluses or infusion. The anticoagulant effects of UFH also vary across patients and require monitoring of the activated clotting time (ACT) in order to achieve the desired level of anticoagulation. Its variable intra- and interpatient effect and the need for monitoring to ensure adequate anticoagulation reflect its most significant limitation. Unfractionated heparin is prepared as polysaccharide chains of variable length and weight with varying affinity for binding with plasma proteins and cells, which limits its bioavailability [15]. In addition, there is a risk of the development of heparin-induced thrombocytopenia and the inability of heparin to inhibit clot-bound thrombin [16].

Clinical Evidence for Use

The 2011 ACC/AHA PCI guidelines have cited use of UFH during elective PCI as a Class 1 indication with level of evidence C (expert consensus). This underscored the absence of randomized controlled trial data supporting routine use of anticoagulation.

Studies during the balloon angioplasty and early stent era have shown a correlation between ACT levels and ischemic events and abrupt vessel closure [17, 18]. A meta-analysis comparing heparin plus aspirin to aspirin alone in patients with unstable angina found a 33 % reduction in mortality and myocardial infarction [19]. Heparin has a narrow therapeutic window and retrospective analysis has not identified a specific ACT value above which ischemic events are prevented without increase in bleeding [20, 21]. ACC/AHA guidelines suggest maintaining an ACT of 200–250 when using UFH + GPI and 250–300 when using UFH alone (300–350 for Hemochron ©). Empiric fixed dose vs. weight-based heparin dosing has also been studied, with both approaches showing equally effective results [22]. The guidelines do not advocate routine prolonged post-PCI use of heparin as it has been shown to be associated with increased risk of access-site bleeding without any benefit in reducing ischemic events [23].

Some recent data has questioned the routine use of anticoagulation in elective PCI. Seven hundred patients undergoing planned PCI and already on aspirin and a thienopyridine were randomized to receive UFH or no anticoagulation during their procedures. The study found decreased bleeding without an increase in ischemic or thrombotic events in the no-UFH arm, suggesting at least the possibility that routine, uncomplicated elective PCI could be performed safely with antiplatelet therapy alone [24].

The use of UFH in ACS is more validated with the guidelines, giving it a Class 1 indication (level of evidence B) for both STEMI and UA/NSTEMI populations undergoing PCI [25, 26]. The thrombotic milieu resulting from an ACS is significantly different from that during elective PCI and justifies the use of systemic anticoagulation. A meta-analysis, which included patients with ACS, found a higher incidence of ischemic and thrombotic events at lower ACTs [20], reinforcing the need for systemic anticoagulation.

LMWH: Enoxaparin

Pharmacokinetics

Low-molecular-weight heparins are fragments of unfractionated heparin with a mean molecular weight of about 5,000. There are several attributes that make LMWH more attractive than UFH: Longer half-life, dose-independent clearance, and better bioavailability allow for a more predictable anticoagulant response. LMWH have a greater ratio of anti-factor Xa activity to anti-factor IIa activity, which reduces the generation and activation of thrombin [27]. LMWH are also less apt to induce platelet activation, release of the von Willebrand factor, and cause inflammation [28]. Of the several LMWH formulations available, enoxaparin is the most widely available and has the strongest level of data backing its use in the catheterization lab. It can be given subcutaneously, or if rapid onset is needed, it may be given intravenously as well. Enoxaparin is renally excreted and its dose must be adjusted for CrCl < 30.

Clinical Evidence for Use

ExTRACT-TIMI 25 was a study comparing enoxaparin to UFH in conjunction with thrombolytic therapy in STEMI patients and found higher bleeding rates with enoxaparin [29]. However, subgroup analysis of patients who underwent PCI demonstrated a reduced risk of 30-day death/recurrent MI with LMWH compared with UFH (10.7 % vs. 13.8 %) without a significant increase in major bleeding (1.4 % vs. 1.6 %) [30]. This finding was duplicated by a prospective single-center nonrandomized comparison of outcomes in STEMI patients undergoing primary PCI with reduced in-hospital mortality with LMWH (OR, 0.32; 95 % CI, 0.12–0.85), as well as a reduction in 30-day mortality (OR, 0.4; 95 % CI, 0.17–0.99) without an increase in major ($p = 0.34$) or minor ($p = 0.65$) bleeding [31]. However, ATOLL, a large study, randomized acute myocardial infarction patients going for primary PCI to enoxaparin or UFH and found no difference in 30-day mortality or MI [32]. The main secondary end point of death, recurrent MI or acute coronary syndrome, or urgent revascularization occurred significantly less often with enoxaparin. Bleeding was similar in both groups.

Recent publication of a meta-analysis has again suggested that enoxaparin use compared to heparin leads to lower mortality and reduced bleeding. The subgroup of patients that were treated with primary PCI had reduced risk of mortality (RR 0.52, 95 % CI, 0.42–0.64) and major bleeding (RR 0.72, 95 % CI, 0.56–0.93) [33].

The majority of data evaluating LMWH use in NSTEMI has been in the conservatively managed population. These data suggest that enoxaparin use may decrease death and MI rates with uncertain effects on bleeding rates. Two studies have evaluated enoxaparin use for inpatients managed with an early invasive strategy. The SYNERGY trial randomized 10,027 patients with NSTEMI to enoxaparin or heparin and found no difference in death or MI at 30 days, 6 months, or 1 year, but there was significantly higher in-hospital bleeding with enoxaparin [34]. In the A to Z trial, enoxaparin was again compared to UFH in the NSTEMI population. The results showed no significant decrease in 30-day death, MI, or recurrent ischemia, but again there was a higher bleeding rate. However, only half of the patients were managed invasively and post hoc analysis suggested the differences were limited to the conservatively managed patients [35].

In elective PCI, STEEPLE, a large trial, randomized patients to either enoxaparin or adjusted UFH with concomitant GPIIb/IIIa and thienopyridine use and found no difference in ischemic outcomes with significantly lower bleeding with enoxaparin [36]. Due to the lack of a rapid assay to evaluate the effect of LMWH, as well as a lack of compelling evidence for its benefits over UFH in the setting of PCI, UFH remains the heparin of choice during both elective and emergent PCI.

Fondaparinux

Pharmacokinetics

Fondaparinux, a synthetic pentasaccharide, indirectly inhibits factor Xa by binding to antithrombin and inhibits thrombin generation. Fondaparinux has complete bioavailability when given subcutaneously and does not undergo metabolism [37]. It exhibits a linear pharmacokinetic profile with little inter- or intrapatient variability. Its elimination half-life is 15 h, allowing once-daily administration [38]. It does not exhibit protein binding, reducing the chances for a variable response and drug interactions [39]. It has rapid onset in 1–3 h and is renally cleared [40].

Clinical Evidence for Use

The use of fondaparinux in the catheterization lab during PCI has been limited due to the results of the OASIS-5 and OASIS-6 trials [37]. Both trials showed increased risk of catheter thrombosis when fondaparinux was used as the sole antithrombotic during PCI. Subsequent trials have shown that addition of dose-adjusted UFH in patients who are already on fondaparinux and going for PCI removed that risk [41]. At present, the use of fondaparinux as a sole antithrombotic agent during PCI is a Class III indication according to the ACC/AHA guidelines and the recommendation is to use additional dose-adjusted UFH in patients going for PCI [42].

GPIIb/IIIa Inhibitors

Pharmacokinetics

GPIIb/IIIa are the most abundant receptors on the platelet surface and have several different binding sites that respond to various stimuli [43]. However, the ones for fibrinogen are the most potent and, once activated, form ligands between platelets, allowing for cross-linking and, ultimately, thrombus formation [44]. As a result, GPIIb/IIIa receptor antagonists that block platelet aggregation and thrombus formation are the most potent antiplatelet agents, much more so than aspirin or thienopyridines [45]. Three main GPIIb/IIIa drugs are widely available: abciximab, eptifibatide, and tirofiban. All three drugs are administered intravenously, and large-scale clinical trials have demonstrated both clinical benefit and safety for adjunctive therapy in percutaneous coronary intervention.

Abciximab was the first to be developed and is a chimeric monoclonal antibody that binds nonspecifically to the GPIIb/IIIa receptor. Despite randomized data supporting its use, concerns regarding immunogenicity and nonspecificity led to development of the so-called small-molecule GPIIb/IIIa receptor inhibitors: eptifibatide and tirofiban. Both are highly specific and have shorter half-lives [43].

Clinical Evidence for Use

The current data has not been able to show clear benefit of GPIIb/IIIa during elective PCI in stable patients. The ambiguity of the timing and appropriate situation for GPIIb/IIIa use during elective PCI is reflected in 2011 ACC/AHA guidelines that give a Class IIa indication for its use in the absence of up-front thienopyridines and Class IIb when the patient has already been pretreated with dual antiplatelet therapy [46]. The TARGET trial found abciximab superior to tirofiban in reducing death, myocardial infarction, and TVR [47]. A large proportion of patients were loaded with clopidogrel 300 mg 6 h pre-procedure and both groups appeared to benefit. Abciximab was widely utilized for elective PCI until both ISAR-REACT and ISAR-SWEET trials evaluated abciximab versus placebo in the setting of preloading with clopidogrel 600 mg and failed to show a reduction in MACE at 30 days, suggesting up-front thienopyridines neutralize the benefit of GPIIb/IIIa administration [48, 49].

Contemporary use of GPIIb/IIIa during elective PCI appears to be based on the presence of high-risk features: coronary thrombus, vessel closure, no reflow/slow flow, and lack of up-front thienopyridines, a practice that is supported by the European guidelines and data from REPLACE-2, where bivalirudin and provisional GPIIb/IIIa had decreased MACE and bleeding as compared to UFH and planned GPIIb/IIIa [50, 51].

The use of GPIIb/IIIa for high-risk patients has extended into the NSTEMI population as well. The 2011 guidelines gave a Class 1 indication to UFH and adjunctive GPIIb/IIIa use in the setting of high-risk features (markedly elevated troponin, anterior MI, large thrombus burden) in the absence of thienopyridine use, and Class IIa when patients were preloaded with clopidogrel [46]. Most trials demonstrating benefit of GPIIb/IIIa in reducing composite ischemic events (EPILOG, CAPTURE, EPIC, RESTORE) were conducted in the era where pretreatment with a thienopyridine was not routine and thus the results may not be directly applicable to contemporary clinical practice [52–56]. As a result, the current guidelines have abandoned up-front treatment with GPIIb/IIIa antagonists in favor of provisional intra-procedure use, based on data that showed lack of benefit and possible increased risk of major bleeding with the former strategy [57].

ISAR-REACT 2 did show abciximab to reduce composite end points in NSTEMI patients going for primary PCI in the setting of preloading with aspirin and clopidogrel 600 mg. However, when analyzed on the basis of positive or negative troponins, the result was clearly limited to the former subset [58]. Tirofiban use during PCI in addition to aspirin and clopidogrel pretreatment also showed decreased ischemic and thrombotic events in diabetics with single vessel disease, multivessel PCI, or NSTEMI patients being treated with early invasive strategy [59].

Data evaluating the use of GPIIb/IIIa inhibitors during PCI for STEMI predates the era of dual antiplatelet therapy as well. The ADMIRAL (platelet glycoprotein IIb/IIIa inhibition with coronary stenting for acute myocardial infarction) study randomized STEMI patients to abciximab or placebo prior to PCI and showed a 51 % relative risk reduction in death and reinfarction at 30 days [60]. Though follow-up of the patients from ADMIRAL showed sustained benefit of adjunctive abciximab use, the study was subject to significant limitations [61]. A similar trial of 400 randomized STEMI patients to abciximab versus placebo demonstrated a significant reduction in mortality, earlier ST segment resolution, and decreased infarct size [62]. However, both studies showed no improvement in TVR or restenosis. Multicenter randomized studies comparing GPIIb/IIIa with placebo in the setting of STEMI and dual antiplatelet therapy have not been done, but the combination of UFH and eptifibatide was inferior to bivalirudin in the HORIZONS-AMI trial [63].

Clinical outcomes in current era of PCI for elective, NSTEMI, or STEMI population have markedly benefited from improved equipment and stent design, early and effective up-front oral antiplatelet therapy (clopidogrel, prasugrel), and improved anticoagulation (bivalirudin). The additional use of GPIIb/IIIa treads a fine line between clinical benefit and increased bleeding and seems to be limited to patients who have clinical or angiographic high-risk features (troponin elevation, large thrombus burden, or acute vessel closure).

Intravenous Direct Thrombin Inhibitors

Hirudin

Hirudin is a naturally occurring 65-amino acid polypeptide originally isolated from the medicinal leech, *Hirudo medicinalis*, and more recently available through recombinant DNA technology. Hirudin blocks the effects of thrombin on the hemostatic system, including the conversion of fibrinogen to fibrin, activation of coagulation factors XI and XIII, positive feedback activation of coagulation factors V and VIII, and thrombin-mediated platelet activation [64]. Administered by intravenous or subcutaneous injection, it has a plasma half-life of approximately 40 min after intravenous injection and 1–3 h after subcutaneous injection. It is primarily excreted renally. The anticoagulant effects of hirudin can be monitored in the laboratory using the activated partial thromboplastin time (aPTT) [65, 66]. Despite having been studied in patients with acute coronary syndromes and percutaneous coronary interventions, it has never assumed use as a frontline therapy.

The OASIS pilot study [67] randomized patients with an acute coronary syndrome without persistent ST elevation to a 72-h infusion of low-dose or medium-dose hirudin infusion or unfractionated heparin (UFH). Hirudin was associated with a reduction in the composite primary outcome of cardiovascular death, myocardial infarction, or refractory angina at 7 days, with a similar incidence of major bleeding. However, the study was not powered for clinical outcomes. In the follow-up OASIS-2 trial, patients with ACS were randomized to medium-dose hirudin or heparin for 72 h. Hirudin was associated with a significantly increased risk of major bleeding compared with UFH [68]. Several large randomized trials followed to evaluate hirudin as an adjunct to thrombolytic therapy in patients with ACS but were terminated because of unacceptably high rates of major hemorrhage [67–71].

Given the bleeding complications, two of the trials, TIMI9A and GUSTO-IIb [67, 68], were restarted with lower doses of hirudin and UFH. The GUSTO-IIb trial showed a small reduction in the primary composite outcome of death or myocardial infarction with hirudin compared with heparin at 30 days. There was a reduction in death or myocardial infarction with hirudin during the first 24 h, and subgroup analysis suggested a highly significant 39 % reduction in death or myocardial infarction at 30 days in the hirudin-treated group. However, in the TIMI-9B trial, no benefit of hirudin over UFH was observed. Neither TIMI-9B nor GUSTO-IIb demonstrated an increase in major or intracranial bleeding with hirudin. Similarly, the HIT-4 trial failed to show any difference between clinical outcomes or major bleeding when comparing hirudin with heparin as adjunctive therapy to streptokinase in acute myocardial infarction [72].

Due to the lack of convincing evidence supporting efficacy of hirudin over heparin and the concern for intracranial bleeding, it was never approved for use in percutaneous coronary interventions. Its only clinical role remains as anticoagulation in patients with heparin-induced thrombocytopenia.

Argatroban

Argatroban is a synthetic, small-molecule direct thrombin inhibitor that is approved in the USA for prophylaxis or treatment of thrombosis in patients with heparin-induced thrombocytopenia (HIT) and for anticoagulation of HIT patients undergoing PCI [73]. Argatroban is parenteral and the polypeptide binds to and inhibits the active site of thrombin. Unlike bivalirudin, argatroban is predominantly eliminated through the liver and plasma concentrations are not influenced by renal function [72]. It has a rapid onset of action and a half-life of 45 min (extended to 2.5 h in patients with hepatic impairment) [74, 75]. Argatroban increases the activated partial thromboplastin time, prothrombin time, and thrombin clotting time in a dose-dependent manner. The activated partial thromboplastin time is commonly used to monitor its anticoagulant effects. Like bivalirudin, argatroban has no known reversal antidote.

Clinical Evidence for Use

There is limited data on the use of argatroban in patients undergoing PCI. The ARGAMI study was a placebo-controlled comparison of argatroban versus heparin as adjunctive therapy to alteplase in patients with acute myocardial infarction. There were no differences in infarct-related artery patency, reocclusion rates up to 10 days (angiographic follow-up), and major bleeding events between the two groups [76]. The ARGAMI-2 study [75] was a phase II trial of patients with acute myocardial infarction receiving thrombolytic therapy who were randomized to one of two doses of argatroban or heparin. Although the data remain unpublished, no difference was reported in clinical outcomes between the randomized groups, including total mortality, recurrent myocardial infarction, pump failure, interventions for ischemia, or stroke. Given the paucity of data supporting the use of argatroban in patients undergoing either elective or urgent percutaneous coronary intervention and the established safety of bivalirudin use in HIT patients, there is very limited role for argatroban in the catheterization lab [77].

Bivalirudin

Bivalirudin, a synthetic analogue of hirudine, is a recombinant protein, and is a specific and reversible inhibitor of thrombin which binds directly with both fluid-phase and clot-bound thrombin [78, 79]. It directly inhibits thrombin by binding simultaneously to its active catalytic site and its substrate recognition site [80]. In addition, bivalirudin has been demonstrated to inhibit thrombin-mediated platelet activation without affecting adenosine 5′-diphosphate (ADP) or collagen-mediated platelet activation and, unlike heparin, does not induce platelet aggregation [81]. The elimination of bivalirudin is through rapid plasma clearance by both renal excretion and proteolytic cleavage. Bivalirudin exhibits linear pharmacokinetics after intravenous administration in patients with normal renal function and in those with mild renal insufficiency (CrCl 60–89 ml/min) and has a half-life of approximately 25 min in patients with normal renal function. The clearance is reduced by approximately 20 % in patients with moderate-to-severe renal insufficiency (CrCl 10–59 ml/min) with an elimination half-life of 34–57 min [82].

Because of its short half-life, bivalirudin rarely requires urgent reversal, but hemodialysis, hemofiltration, and plasmapheresis can be helpful to clear the drug in the event of overdose. Bivalirudin is partially dialyzable, with approximately 25 % of the drug being cleared. In patients dependent on dialysis, clearance is reduced by approximately 80 % and elimination half-life is extended to 3.5 h [83].

Clinical Evidence for Use

Planned Percutaneous Coronary Intervention (PCI) and NSTEMI

Bivalirudin has been comprehensively evaluated in patients with coronary artery disease undergoing PCI. The Hirulog Angioplasty Study compared bivalirudin bolus and infusion with unfractionated heparin in 4,312 patients with ACS who required urgent coronary angioplasty [84]. An on-treatment analysis of 4,098 patients demonstrated similar results between the two groups for the composite outcome of in-hospital death, myocardial infarction, or target-vessel revascularization (11.4 % vs. 12.2 %, relative risk [RR] 0.93, 95 % CI, 0.79–1.10, $p = 0.44$), but significantly reduced rates of major bleeding with bivalirudin (3.8 % vs. 9.8 %, RR 0.39, 95 % CI, 0.30–0.50, $p < 0.001$). The dose of heparin used in this trial was substantially higher than current practice, which may have contributed to increased bleeding. However, based on these results, bivalirudin was approved by FDA for patients with coronary artery disease undergoing PCI.

The use of bivalirudin versus heparin plus a glycoprotein IIb/IIIa inhibitor was initially investigated in the REPLACE (Randomized Evaluation of PCI Linking Angiomax to Reduced Clinical Events) series of trials [51, 83, 85]. REPLACE-1 was an open-label pilot study in which 1,056 patients undergoing PCI were randomized to receive either bivalirudin or heparin. Glycoprotein IIb/IIIa inhibitor was used in 71.1 and 72.5 % of patients randomly allocated to bivalirudin and heparin, respectively. Bivalirudin was associated with a nonsignificant reduction in both the composite outcome of death, MI, or repeat revascularization ($p = 0.41$) and major bleeding ($p = 0.52$).

REPLACE-2 was a blinded, noninferiority, randomized controlled trial of 6,010 patients with planned glycoprotein IIb/IIIa inhibitor use in the heparin group, but provisional in the bivalirudin group. Only 7.2 % of those in the bivalirudin group received either eptifibatide or abciximab. On-treatment analysis showed 7.6 and 7.1 % of patients experienced the 30-day composite outcome of death, MI, or repeat revascularization in the bivalirudin and heparin arms, respectively ($p = 0.40$). Major bleeding was strongly significantly reduced at 30 days in the bivalirudin ($p = 0.0002$). These differences remained significant out to 6 months. Cost analysis of heparin and glycoprotein IIb/IIA against bivalirudin has favored bivalirudin, driven partially by fewer occurrences of major bleeding [86].

Concomitant or prior use of clopidogrel with bivalirudin was evaluated in ISAR-REACT (In the Intracoronary Stenting and Antithrombotic Regimen—Rapid Early Action for Coronary Treatment) [87]. Bivalirudin was compared with heparin in patients undergoing PCI for stable or unstable angina that had been pretreated at least 3 h earlier with 600 mg of clopidogrel. Bivalirudin was noninferior to heparin for the primary composite outcome of death, MI, urgent target-vessel revascularization, or major bleeding ($p=0.57$), and was associated with significantly less major bleeding ($p=0.008$). In a higher risk population, rates of the 30 day net clinical composite outcome of death, large recurrent MI, target-vessel revascularization, or major bleeding were similar in both groups ($p=0.93$). Major bleeding alone was significantly lower in the bivalirudin group ($p=0.02$) [88].

The results have been consistent in patients with diabetes, renal insufficiency, hypertension, or those aged ≥65 years, with a significant reduction in major bleeding with bivalirudin compared to heparin and glycoprotein IIb/IIIA ($p=0.005$) [89, 90].

In the ACUITY trial, 13,819 patients with NSTEMI were enrolled, irrespective of planned management strategy (PCI, medical management, or CABG) [91]. Patients were randomly allocated to bivalirudin alone, or bivalirudin plus a glycoprotein IIb/IIIa inhibitor, or heparin plus a glycoprotein IIb/IIIa inhibitor. All patients undergoing PCI were pretreated with 300 or 600 mg of clopidogrel. Both bivalirudin groups were found noninferior to heparin plus GpIIb/IIIa for the 30-day composite outcome of death, MI, or revascularization. Bivalirudin plus a glycoprotein IIb/IIIa inhibitor was also noninferior for major bleeding. The results were consistent at 12-month follow-up.

In ISAR-REACT 4, NSTEMI patients going for PCI who were treated with bivalirudin had similar 30-day rates of death, recurrent myocardial infarction, or urgent target-vessel revascularization and significantly lower major bleeding as compared to those treated with a combination of abciximab and heparin ($p=0.02$) [88].

ST Segment Elevation MI

There are several trials evaluating the role of bivalirudin in patients undergoing urgent catheterization and PCI for STEMI, the largest and most significant being HORIZONS-AMI [63]. In this study, 3,602 patients with ST segment elevation MI presenting within 12 h of onset of symptoms were randomized to bivalirudin with a provisional glycoprotein IIb/IIIa inhibitor or unfractionated heparin (to achieve an activated clotting time of 200–250 s) plus a glycoprotein IIb/IIIa inhibitor. All patients were pretreated with either 300 or 600 mg of clopidogrel. Ninety-two percent of patients underwent PCI ($n=3,348$) and the remainder had CABG or were managed medically. In the bivalirudin group, 7.2 % of patients received a glycoprotein IIb/IIIa inhibitor. Bivalirudin compared with heparin plus a glycoprotein IIb/IIIa inhibitor significantly decreased the net clinical composite outcome of death, reinfarction, target-vessel revascularization, stroke, or major bleeding not related to CABG surgery ($p=0.005$), driven largely by a reduction in major bleeding ($p<0.001$) and decreased all-cause mortality ($p=0.047$). These results were consistent up to 3 years. However, bivalirudin use was associated with numerically higher stent thrombosis at 30 days, though this difference was not statistically significant ($p=0.30$). HORIZONS-AMI clearly defined the linkage between bleeding-related complications and clinically significant adverse events in this patient population. The results of HORIZONS-AMI supported the use of bivalirudin in STEMI patients as per the trial protocol with a weight-based bolus followed by an infusion that is terminated at completion of the procedure. Prolonged use of bivalirudin up to 4 h post-PCI for stable or unstable angina was evaluated in PROBI VIRI and PROBI VIRI-2 trials, which showed reduced periprocedural myocardial damage and increased ST segment resolution, respectively. An interesting finding in HORIZONS-AMI was the high percentage of patients that received heparin (65.8 %) prior to being switched to bivalirudin. The HORIZONS-SWITCH analysis demonstrated that patients who were switched from heparin to bivalirudin had better outcomes with similar 30-day and 2-year rates of stent thrombosis [92].

Cost analysis has supported the use of bivalirudin as well with 14 % reduced cost as compared to heparin and glycoprotein IIb/IIIa combination, driven largely by reduced bleeding rates and ICU stays [93].

Bivalirudin has been studied extensively in patients with both stable and unstable coronary artery disease undergoing PCI and has demonstrated similar clinical outcomes as compared to the combination of heparin and glycoprotein IIb/IIIA inhibitors. That combined with a consistent finding of reduced bleeding in most major trials and meta-analysis is a major reason why bivalirudin has achieved increased adoption in PCI practice [94].

Oral Direct Thrombin Inhibitors

Dabigatran (Pradaxa)

Dabigatran etexilate is an oral prodrug that is rapidly converted by a serum esterase to dabigatran: a direct, competitive inhibitor of thrombin. It has an absolute bioavailability of 6.5 % (not affected by food) and half-life of 12–17 h and does not require INR monitoring [95]. Inter- and intraindividual variability of dabigatran pharmacokinetics and pharmacodynamics in elderly subjects is low. Renal excretion of unchanged dabigatran is the predominant elimination pathway, with about 80 % of an intravenous dose being excreted in the urine [96]. It is also metabolized by conjugation with glucuronic acid, resulting in the formation of pharmacodynamically active glucuronides, which account for approximately 20 % of total dabigatran in the plasma [97]. In Europe, it is licensed for primary prevention of venous thromboembolism in adults post total hip or knee replacement surgery and for reducing the risk of stroke and systemic embolism in patients with non-valvular atrial fibrillation (AF). In the USA, it is cleared only for use in patients with AF [96].

There is one trial that specifically evaluated the role of dabigatran in the setting of ACS [98, 99]. RE-DEEM was a multicenter, prospective, randomized, double-blind, placebo-controlled, dose-escalation trial. Patients with non-ST or ST segment elevation myocardial infarction within the last 14 days, and receiving treatment with dual antiplatelet therapy (aspirin and clopidogrel or another thienopyridine), were randomized to 50 mg, 75 mg, or placebo. Dose escalation allowed for 110 mg dose in a second stage and the 150 mg dose group in a third stage. The results demonstrated a dose-dependent increase in the risk of bleeding with 50, 75, 110, or 150 mg dabigatran twice daily compared with placebo.

Factor Xa Inhibitors

Apixaban (Eliquis®)

Apixaban is a highly selective and potent inhibitor of free and prothrombinase-bound factor Xa [100]. Although metabolized primarily by CYP3A4, CYP3A5, and sulfotransferase 1A1, more than half of the dose is excreted unchanged. Apixaban does not induce CYP enzymes but is susceptible to interaction with strong CYP enzyme inhibitors and inducers. It is excreted 25 % renally and 75 % through the hepatobiliary system, with a mean half-life of 12 h and onset in 3 h [101].

Several trials have examined the role of apixaban in patients with recent ACS. The apixaban for Prevention of Acute Ischemic and Safety Events (APPRAISE) trial was a phase II, double-blind, placebo-controlled study that compared oral apixaban 2.5 mg bid, 10 mg daily, 10 mg bid, or 20 mg daily, or placebo in patients with recent ACS [102]. Patients were enrolled within 7 days of presentation with ACS (either STEMI or NSTEMI), were clinically stable, and had at least one additional risk factor for recurrent ischemic events. Patients were excluded if they were planned for catheterization or revascularization, had severe renal insufficiency, or were receiving a strong CYP3A4 inhibitor. The primary study outcome was the occurrence of major bleeding and clinically relevant non-major bleeding [101]. Aspirin use was almost 100 %, with 75 % of patients on both aspirin and clopidogrel. This trial had mixed results with a dose-dependent increase in the primary safety end point of ISTH-defined major bleeding or clinically relevant bleeding in the apixaban group. The efficacy end point of cardiovascular death, MI, severe recurrent ischemia, or ischemic stroke was nonsignificantly lower in patients assigned to apixaban 2.5 mg bid and 10 mg daily groups compared with placebo. Bleeding was more frequent in patients receiving concomitant clopidogrel, whereas the dose-dependent reduction in ischemic events was more evident in the apixaban groups not receiving clopidogrel [103].

The unclear role of apixaban in ACS was investigated further in the APPRAISE-2 trial, a randomized, double-blind, placebo-controlled clinical trial comparing apixaban 5 mg twice daily with placebo, in addition to standard antiplatelet therapy, in patients with a recent ACS and at least two additional risk factors for recurrent ischemic events [104]. The trial was terminated prematurely after interim data found an increase in major bleeding events with apixaban plus antiplatelet therapy that was not offset by reductions in ischemic events. The on-treatment analysis for the primary safety outcome of TIMI major bleeding found a more than twofold increase in bleeding with apixaban compared with placebo with higher intracranial and fatal bleeding events. Subgroup analysis showed major bleeding was higher with apixaban regardless of concomitant dual antiplatelet therapy or just aspirin alone. A small study in the Japanese ACS population that aimed to evaluate the role of apixaban 2.5 and 5 mg compared to placebo was terminated early as well. The results from that study have not been yet published (http://clinicaltrials.gov/ct2/show/NCT00852397).

Rivaroxaban

Rivaroxaban (Xarelto®) is a highly selective direct factor Xa inhibitor [105]. It has high plasma protein binding, with serum albumin being the most common [106]. It inhibits free and clot-associated factor Xa in a concentration-dependent manner, preventing thrombin generation by both the intrinsic and extrinsic coagulation pathways [105]. Rivaroxaban exhibits no direct effect on platelet aggregation. The 10 mg dose has bioavailability of 80–100 % and rapidly reaches maximum plasma concentration in 2–4 h. The mean half-life is 11–13 h in elderly patients and 7–11 h for younger patients. One-third of the drug is excreted unchanged in urine; two-thirds is degraded in the liver and excreted in the urine and feces [106, 107]. Rivaroxaban does not affect CYP450 isoforms and is metabolized by CYP34A and CYP2J2. There is no known reversal agent or antidote for rivaroxaban.

There is not a substantial amount of data evaluating the role of rivaroxaban in ACS. ATLAS ACS–TIMI 46 was a phase II, randomized, double-blind, placebo-controlled, multicenter, dose-escalation study evaluating oral rivaroxaban in patients stabilized up to 7 days after the index ACS event [108]. The ACS events were characterized as symptoms lasting at least 10 min with a diagnosis of unstable angina, NSTEMI, or STEMI with one high-risk feature (raised cardiac enzyme markers, ≥1-mm ST segment deviation, or a TIMI risk score of ≥3). Three dose tiers of rivaroxaban were tested in conjunction with aspirin only (5, 10, and 20 mg), and four dose tiers were tested in conjunction with aspirin and a thienopyridine (5, 10, 15, and 20 mg). The primary safety end point was clinically significant bleeding (TIMI major, TIMI minor, or requiring medical attention), and the primary efficacy end point was death, myocardial infarction, stroke, or severe recurrent ischemia requiring revascularization during 6-month follow-up. The risk of clinically significant bleeding with rivaroxaban versus placebo increased in a dose-dependent manner with a nonsignificant reduction in death, myocardial infarction, or stroke compared with placebo.

The follow-up study, ATLAS ACS 2–TIMI 51, was recently published and showed that in patients with a recent acute coronary syndrome, rivaroxaban reduced the risk of the composite end point of death from cardiovascular causes, myocardial infarction, or stroke but increased the risk of major bleeding and intracranial hemorrhage but not the risk of fatal bleeding [109]. This was a double-blind, placebo-controlled trial, randomizing 15,526 patients with recent ACS to receive twice-daily doses of either 2.5 or 5 mg of rivaroxaban or placebo for a mean of 13 months and up to 31 months. Rivaroxaban compared with placebo significantly reduced the primary efficacy composite of cardiovascular death, myocardial infarction, or stroke with respective rates of 8.9 and 10.7 % in the study period ($p=0.008$). Only the 2.5 mg reduced the rates of death during the study period from cardiovascular causes ($p=0.002$) and also from any cause ($p=0.002$), whereas only the 5 mg B.I.D. reduced myocardial infarction. Both doses combined increased the risk of major bleeding ($p<0.001$) and intracranial hemorrhage ($p=0.009$). The 2.5 mg B.I.D. dose resulted in significantly fewer fatal bleeding events than the 5 mg B.I.D. dose. So far, the data is not convincing for routine use of either apixaban or rivaroxaban in post-ACS or PCI population.

Otamixaban

Otamixaban is an intravenous, short-acting, selective, direct factor Xa inhibitor. It has rapid onset after intravenous bolus and infusion (3 min), has an effective half-life of 2–3 h, and is fully eliminated by 12 h [110]. Like rivaroxaban, up to 25 % of otamixaban is excreted unchanged in the urine and the remainder in the bile. Its use in mild renal dysfunction (CrCl 45–80) appears to be safe.

The role of otamixaban in elective PCI was investigated in the SEPIA-PCI trial [111]. This was a double-blind, double-dummy, parallel-group, dose-ranging trial in which the primary end points were change in prothrombin fragments 1 and 2 and anti-factor Xa activity. Although not powered to address clinical end points, there was a lower incidence of 30-day death, MI, and urgent target-vessel revascularization in the intermediate-dose group of 0.120 mg/kg bolus followed by 0.160 mg/kg/h infusion (4 % vs. 9 % in the UFH group). There was no significant difference in the incidence of TIMI bleeding between the otamixaban and UFH groups.

SEPIA-ACS1–TIMI 42 trial (PMID) was a phase II, randomized, double-blind, international trial conducted in 3,241 patients with NSTEMI with 63 % of patients managed with PCI [112]. Patients were randomized to a 0.08 mg/kg bolus followed by one of five otamixaban infusions ranging from 0.035 mg/kg/h to 0.175 mg/kg/h or control consisting of a UFH 60 unit/kg bolus followed by a 12 unit/kg/h infusion plus an eptifibatide 180 μg/kg bolus followed by a 1–2 μg/kg/min infusion. In the PCI subset, there was a higher rate of thrombotic complications (defined as abrupt side branch closure, distal embolization or no/slow reflow, or new thrombus) in the low-dose otamixaban group but no difference between the intermediate-dose (0.105–0.140 mg/kg/h) group and the UFH/eptifibatide group. Intermediate doses of otamixaban 0.08 mg/kg intravenous bolus followed by infusions of 0.1 or 0.14 mg/kg/h compared with a control of intravenous UFH plus eptifibatide in patients with unstable angina or NSTEMI are currently being evaluated in the ongoing TAO trial (the Treatment of Acute Coronary Syndrome with Otamixaban). The primary objective is to demonstrate superior efficacy (composite of all-cause death + myocardial infarction (MI)) of otamixaban to unfractionated heparin (UFH) + eptifibatide. The trial is currently enrolling participants (http://clinicaltrials.gov/ct2/show/NCT01076764).

The role of direct factor Xa inhibitors, both oral and parenteral, is just beginning to be investigated. So far, the data does not support routine use in patients undergoing elective or urgent PCI for unstable angina, NSTEMI, or STEMI. Multicenter randomized clinical trials comparing direct factor Xa inhibitors with either a combination of UFH and glycoprotein IIb/IIIA or bivalirudin need to be performed and the data needs to support clinical efficacy and safety before adoption in routine clinical practice.

References

1. Sneader W. The discovery of aspirin: a reappraisal. BMJ. 2000;321(7276):1591–4.
2. Schwartz L et al. Aspirin and dipyridamole in the prevention of restenosis after percutaneous transluminal coronary angioplasty. N Engl J Med. 1988;318(26):1714–9.
3. Savage MP et al. Effect of thromboxane A2 blockade on clinical outcome and restenosis after successful coronary angioplasty. Multi-Hospital Eastern Atlantic Restenosis Trial (M-HEART II). Circulation. 1995;92(11):3194–200.
4. Antithrombotic Trialists' Collaboration. Collaborative meta-analysis of randomised trials of antiplatelet therapy for prevention of death, myocardial infarction, and stroke in high risk patients. BMJ. 2002;324(7329):71–86.
5. Peters RJ et al. Effects of aspirin dose when used alone or in combination with clopidogrel in patients with acute coronary syndromes: observations from the Clopidogrel in Unstable angina to prevent Recurrent Events (CURE) study. Circulation. 2003;108(14):1682–7.

6. Levine GN et al. 2011 ACCF/AHA/SCAI guideline for percutaneous coronary intervention: executive summary: a report of the American College of Cardiology Foundation/American Heart Association Task Force on practice guidelines and the Society for Cardiovascular Angiography and Interventions. Circulation. 2011;124(23):2574–609.
7. Leon MB et al. A clinical trial comparing three antithrombotic-drug regimens after coronary-artery stenting. Stent anticoagulation restenosis study investigators. N Engl J Med. 1998;339(23):1665–71.
8. Birkeland K, Parra D, Rosenstein R. Antiplatelet therapy in acute coronary syndromes: focus on ticagrelor. J Blood Med. 2010;1:197–219.
9. Chen ZM et al. Addition of clopidogrel to aspirin in 45,852 patients with acute myocardial infarction: randomised placebo-controlled trial. Lancet. 2005;366(9497):1607–21.
10. Sabatine MS et al. Effect of clopidogrel pretreatment before percutaneous coronary intervention in patients with ST-elevation myocardial infarction treated with fibrinolytics: the PCI-CLARITY study. JAMA. 2005;294(10):1224–32.
11. Wiviott SD et al. Prasugrel versus clopidogrel in patients with acute coronary syndromes. N Engl J Med. 2007;357(20):2001–15.
12. Wallentin L et al. Ticagrelor versus clopidogrel in patients with acute coronary syndromes. N Engl J Med. 2009;361(11):1045–57.
13. Kushner FG et al. 2009 focused updates: ACC/AHA guidelines for the management of patients with ST-elevation myocardial infarction (updating the 2004 guideline and 2007 focused update) and ACC/AHA/SCAI guidelines on percutaneous coronary intervention (updating the 2005 guideline and 2007 focused update) a report of the American College of Cardiology Foundation/American Heart Association Task Force on Practice Guidelines. J Am Coll Cardiol. 2009;54(23):2205–41.
14. Morris TA. Heparin and low molecular weight heparin: background and pharmacology. Clin Chest Med. 2003;24(1):39–47.
15. Shriver Z et al. Heparin and heparan sulfate: analyzing structure and microheterogeneity. Handb Exp Pharmacol. 2012;207:159–76.
16. Jang IK, Hursting MJ. When heparins promote thrombosis: review of heparin-induced thrombocytopenia. Circulation. 2005;111(20):2671–83.
17. Ferguson JJ et al. Relation between procedural activated coagulation time and outcome after percutaneous transluminal coronary angioplasty. J Am Coll Cardiol. 1994;23(5):1061–5.
18. Narins CR et al. Relation between activated clotting time during angioplasty and abrupt closure. Circulation. 1996;93(4):667–71.
19. Oler A et al. Adding heparin to aspirin reduces the incidence of myocardial infarction and death in patients with unstable angina. A meta-analysis. JAMA. 1996;276(10):811–5.
20. Chew DP et al. Defining the optimal activated clotting time during percutaneous coronary intervention: aggregate results from 6 randomized, controlled trials. Circulation. 2001;103(7):961–6.
21. Tolleson TR et al. Relationship between heparin anticoagulation and clinical outcomes in coronary stent intervention: observations from the ESPRIT trial. J Am Coll Cardiol. 2003;41(3):386–93.
22. Boccara A et al. A randomized trial of a fixed high dose vs a weight-adjusted low dose of intravenous heparin during coronary angioplasty. Eur Heart J. 1997;18(4):631–5.
23. Friedman HZ et al. Randomized prospective evaluation of prolonged versus abbreviated intravenous heparin therapy after coronary angioplasty. J Am Coll Cardiol. 1994;24(5):1214–9.
24. Stabile E et al. The CIAO (Coronary Interventions Antiplatelet-based Only) Study: a randomized study comparing standard anticoagulation regimen to absence of anticoagulation for elective percutaneous coronary intervention. J Am Coll Cardiol. 2008;52(16):1293–8.
25. Wright RS et al. 2011 ACCF/AHA focused update incorporated into the ACC/AHA 2007 Guidelines for the Management of Patients with Unstable Angina/Non-ST-Elevation Myocardial Infarction: a report of the American College of Cardiology Foundation/American Heart Association Task Force on Practice Guidelines developed in collaboration with the American Academy of Family Physicians, Society for Cardiovascular Angiography and Interventions, and the Society of Thoracic Surgeons. J Am Coll Cardiol. 2011;57(19):e215–367.
26. Levine GN et al. ACCF/AHA/SCAI Guideline for Percutaneous Coronary Intervention. A report of the American College of Cardiology Foundation/American Heart Association Task Force on Practice Guidelines and the Society for Cardiovascular Angiography and Interventions. J Am Coll Cardiol. 2011;58(24):e44–122.
27. Cohen M. The role of low-molecular-weight heparin in the management of acute coronary syndromes. J Am Coll Cardiol. 2003;41(4 Suppl S):55S–61S.
28. Montalescot G et al. Early increase of von Willebrand factor predicts adverse outcome in unstable coronary artery disease: beneficial effects of enoxaparin. French Investigators of the ESSENCE Trial. Circulation. 1998;98(4):294–9.
29. Antman EM et al. Enoxaparin versus unfractionated heparin with fibrinolysis for ST-elevation myocardial infarction. N Engl J Med. 2006;354(14):1477–88.
30. Gibson CM et al. Percutaneous coronary intervention in patients receiving enoxaparin or unfractionated heparin after fibrinolytic therapy for ST-segment elevation myocardial infarction in the ExTRACT-TIMI 25 trial. J Am Coll Cardiol. 2007;49(23):2238–46.
31. Brieger D et al. Heparin or enoxaparin anticoagulation for primary percutaneous coronary intervention. Catheter Cardiovasc Interv. 2011;77(2):182–90.
32. Montalescot G et al. Intravenous enoxaparin or unfractionated heparin in primary percutaneous coronary intervention for ST-elevation myocardial infarction: the international randomised open-label ATOLL trial. Lancet. 2011;378(9792):693–703.
33. Silvain J et al. Efficacy and safety of enoxaparin versus unfractionated heparin during percutaneous coronary intervention: systematic review and meta-analysis. BMJ. 2012;344:e553.
34. Petersen JL et al. Efficacy and bleeding complications among patients randomized to enoxaparin or unfractionated heparin for antithrombin therapy in non-ST-Segment elevation acute coronary syndromes: a systematic overview. JAMA. 2004;292(1):89–96.
35. Blazing MA et al. Safety and efficacy of enoxaparin vs unfractionated heparin in patients with non-ST-segment elevation acute coronary syndromes who receive tirofiban and aspirin: a randomized controlled trial. JAMA. 2004;292(1):55–64.
36. Montalescot G et al. Enoxaparin versus unfractionated heparin in elective percutaneous coronary intervention. N Engl J Med. 2006;355(10):1006–17.
37. Yusuf S et al. Effects of fondaparinux on mortality and reinfarction in patients with acute ST-segment elevation myocardial infarction: the OASIS-6 randomized trial. JAMA. 2006;295(13):1519–30.
38. Donat F et al. The pharmacokinetics of fondaparinux sodium in healthy volunteers. Clin Pharmacokinet. 2002;41 Suppl 2:1–9.
39. Bauer KA et al. Fondaparinux, a synthetic pentasaccharide: the first in a new class of antithrombotic agents - the selective factor Xa inhibitors. Cardiovasc Drug Rev. 2002;20(1):37–52.
40. Tran AH, Lee G. Fondaparinux for prevention of venous thromboembolism in major orthopedic surgery. Ann Pharmacother. 2003;37(11):1632–43.
41. Steg PG et al. Low-dose vs standard-dose unfractionated heparin for percutaneous coronary intervention in acute coronary syndromes treated with fondaparinux: the FUTURA/OASIS-8 randomized trial. JAMA. 2010;304(12):1339–49.
42. Antman EM et al. 2007 focused update of the ACC/AHA 2004 guidelines for the management of patients with ST-elevation myo-

cardial infarction: a report of the American College of Cardiology/American Heart Association Task Force on Practice Guidelines. J Am Coll Cardiol. 2008;51(2):210–47.
43. Meadows TA, Bhatt DL. Clinical aspects of platelet inhibitors and thrombus formation. Circ Res. 2007;100(9):1261–75.
44. Lippi G et al. Glycoprotein IIb/IIIa inhibitors: an update on the mechanism of action and use of functional testing methods to assess antiplatelet efficacy. Biomark Med. 2011;5(1):63–70.
45. Cohen M. Antiplatelet therapy in percutaneous coronary intervention: a critical review of the 2007 AHA/ACC/SCAI guidelines and beyond. Catheter Cardiovasc Interv. 2009;74(4):579–97.
46. Levine GN et al. 2011 ACCF/AHA/SCAI Guideline for Percutaneous Coronary Intervention: a report of the American College of Cardiology Foundation/American Heart Association Task Force on Practice Guidelines and the Society for Cardiovascular Angiography and Interventions. Circulation. 2011;124(23): e574–651.
47. Topol EJ et al. Comparison of two platelet glycoprotein IIb/IIIa inhibitors, tirofiban and abciximab, for the prevention of ischemic events with percutaneous coronary revascularization. N Engl J Med. 2001;344(25):1888–94.
48. Kastrati A et al. A clinical trial of abciximab in elective percutaneous coronary intervention after pretreatment with clopidogrel. N Engl J Med. 2004;350(3):232–8.
49. Mehilli J et al. Randomized clinical trial of abciximab in diabetic patients undergoing elective percutaneous coronary interventions after treatment with a high loading dose of clopidogrel. Circulation. 2004;110(24):3627–35.
50. Hamm CW et al. ESC Guidelines for the management of acute coronary syndromes in patients presenting without persistent ST-segment elevation: the Task Force for the management of acute coronary syndromes (ACS) in patients presenting without persistent ST-segment elevation of the European Society of Cardiology (ESC). Eur Heart J. 2011;32(23):2999–3054.
51. Lincoff AM et al. Bivalirudin and provisional glycoprotein IIb/IIIa blockade compared with heparin and planned glycoprotein IIb/IIIa blockade during percutaneous coronary intervention: REPLACE-2 randomized trial. JAMA. 2003;289(7):853–63.
52. Platelet glycoprotein IIb/IIIa receptor blockade and low-dose heparin during percutaneous coronary revascularization. The EPILOG Investigators. N Engl J Med, 1997;336(24):1689–96.
53. Hamm CW et al. Benefit of abciximab in patients with refractory unstable angina in relation to serum troponin T levels. c7E3 Fab Antiplatelet Therapy in Unstable Refractory Angina (CAPTURE) Study Investigators. N Engl J Med. 1999;340(21):1623–9.
54. Topol EJ et al. Randomised trial of coronary intervention with antibody against platelet IIb/IIIa integrin for reduction of clinical restenosis: results at six months. The EPIC Investigators. Lancet. 1994;343(8902):881–6.
55. McKay RG, Boden WE. Small peptide GP IIb/IIIa receptor inhibitors as upstream therapy in non-ST-segment elevation acute coronary syndromes: results of the PURSUIT, PRISM, PRISM-PLUS, TACTICS, and PARAGON trials. Curr Opin Cardiol. 2001;16(6): 364–9.
56. Effects of platelet glycoprotein IIb/IIIa blockade with tirofiban on adverse cardiac events in patients with unstable angina or acute myocardial infarction undergoing coronary angioplasty. The RESTORE Investigators. Randomized Efficacy Study of Tirofiban for Outcomes and REstenosis. Circulation, 1997;96(5): 1445–53.
57. Giugliano RP et al. Early versus delayed, provisional eptifibatide in acute coronary syndromes. N Engl J Med. 2009;360(21):2176–90.
58. Kastrati A et al. Abciximab in patients with acute coronary syndromes undergoing percutaneous coronary intervention after clopidogrel pretreatment: the ISAR-REACT 2 randomized trial. JAMA. 2006;295(13):1531–8.
59. Valgimigli M et al. The additive value of tirofiban administered with the high-dose bolus in the prevention of ischemic complications during high-risk coronary angioplasty: the ADVANCE Trial. J Am Coll Cardiol. 2004;44(1):14–9.
60. Montalescot G et al. Platelet glycoprotein IIb/IIIa inhibition with coronary stenting for acute myocardial infarction. N Engl J Med. 2001;344(25):1895–903.
61. Admiral Investigators. Three-year duration of benefit from abciximab in patients receiving stents for acute myocardial infarction in the randomized double-blind ADMIRAL study. Eur Heart J. 2005;26(23):2520–3.
62. Antoniucci D et al. A randomized trial comparing primary infarct artery stenting with or without abciximab in acute myocardial infarction. J Am Coll Cardiol. 2003;42(11):1879–85.
63. Stone GW et al. Bivalirudin during primary PCI in acute myocardial infarction. N Engl J Med. 2008;358(21):2218–30.
64. Markwardt F. The development of hirudin as an antithrombotic drug. Thromb Res. 1994;74(1):1–23.
65. Tripodi A et al. Effects of hirudin on activated partial thromboplastin time determined with ten different reagents. Thromb Haemost. 1993;70(2):286–8.
66. Potzsch B et al. Monitoring of r-hirudin anticoagulation during cardiopulmonary bypass–assessment of the whole blood ecarin clotting time. Thromb Haemost. 1997;77(5):920–5.
67. Comparison of the effects of two doses of recombinant hirudin compared with heparin in patients with acute myocardial ischemia without ST elevation: a pilot study. Organization to Assess Strategies for Ischemic Syndromes (OASIS) Investigators. Circulation, 1997;96(3):769–77.
68. Effects of recombinant hirudin (lepirudin) compared with heparin on death, myocardial infarction, refractory angina, and revascularisation procedures in patients with acute myocardial ischaemia without ST elevation: a randomised trial. Organisation to Assess Strategies for Ischemic Syndromes (OASIS-2) Investigators. Lancet, 1999;353(9151):429–38.
69. Randomized trial of intravenous heparin versus recombinant hirudin for acute coronary syndromes. The Global Use of Strategies to Open Occluded Coronary Arteries (GUSTO) IIa Investigators. Circulation, 1994;90(4):1631–7.
70. Antman EM. Hirudin in acute myocardial infarction. Safety report from the Thrombolysis and Thrombin Inhibition in Myocardial Infarction (TIMI) 9A Trial. Circulation. 1994;90(4): 1624–30.
71. Neuhaus KL et al. Safety observations from the pilot phase of the randomized r-Hirudin for Improvement of Thrombolysis (HIT-III) study. A study of the Arbeitsgemeinschaft Leitender Kardiologischer Krankenhausarzte (ALKK). Circulation. 1994; 90(4):1638–42.
72. Neuhaus KL et al. Recombinant hirudin (lepirudin) for the improvement of thrombolysis with streptokinase in patients with acute myocardial infarction: results of the HIT-4 trial. J Am Coll Cardiol. 1999;34(4):966–73.
73. Jeske WP et al. Pharmacology of argatroban. Expert Rev Hematol. 2010;3(5):527–39.
74. Eikelboom JW, French J. Management of patients with acute coronary syndromes: what is the clinical role of direct thrombin inhibitors? Drugs. 2002;62(13):1839–52.
75. Hursting MJ et al. Novastan (brand of argatroban): a small-molecule, direct thrombin inhibitor. Semin Thromb Hemost. 1997;23(6):503–16.
76. Vermeer F et al. Argatroban and alteplase in patients with acute myocardial infarction: the ARGAMI Study. J Thromb Thrombolysis. 2000;10(3):233–40.
77. Alderman EL. Results from late-breaking clinical trials sessions at ACC '98. American College of Cardiology. J Am Coll Cardiol. 1998;32(1):1–7.

78. Carswell CI, Plosker GL. Bivalirudin: a review of its potential place in the management of acute coronary syndromes. Drugs. 2002;62(5):841–70.
79. Lewis BE et al. Argatroban anticoagulation during percutaneous coronary intervention in patients with heparin-induced thrombocytopenia. Catheter Cardiovasc Interv. 2002;57(2):177–84.
80. Gladwell TD. Bivalirudin: a direct thrombin inhibitor. Clin Ther. 2002;24(1):38–58.
81. Weitz JI, Bates SM. Beyond heparin and aspirin: new treatments for unstable angina and non-Q-wave myocardial infarction. Arch Intern Med. 2000;160(6):749–58.
82. Lui HK. Dosage, pharmacological effects and clinical outcomes for bivalirudin in percutaneous coronary intervention. J Invasive Cardiol. 2000;12(Suppl F):41F–52.
83. Koster A et al. An assessment of different filter systems for extracorporeal elimination of bivalirudin: an in vitro study. Anesth Analg. 2003;96(5):1316–9, table of contents.
84. Bittl JA et al. Treatment with bivalirudin (Hirulog) as compared with heparin during coronary angioplasty for unstable or postinfarction angina. Hirulog Angioplasty Study Investigators. N Engl J Med. 1995;333(12):764–9.
85. Lincoff AM et al. Comparison of bivalirudin versus heparin during percutaneous coronary intervention (the Randomized Evaluation of PCI Linking Angiomax to Reduced Clinical Events [REPLACE]-1 trial). Am J Cardiol. 2004;93(9):1092–6.
86. Cohen DJ et al. Economic evaluation of bivalirudin with provisional glycoprotein IIB/IIIA inhibition versus heparin with routine glycoprotein IIB/IIIA inhibition for percutaneous coronary intervention: results from the REPLACE-2 trial. J Am Coll Cardiol. 2004;44(9):1792–800.
87. Kastrati A et al. Bivalirudin versus unfractionated heparin during percutaneous coronary intervention. N Engl J Med. 2008; 359(7):688–96.
88. Kastrati A et al. Abciximab and heparin versus bivalirudin for non-ST-elevation myocardial infarction. N Engl J Med. 2011; 365(21):1980–9.
89. Tavano D et al. Comparison of bivalirudin monotherapy versus unfractionated heparin plus tirofiban in patients with diabetes mellitus undergoing elective percutaneous coronary intervention. Am J Cardiol. 2009;104(9):1222–8.
90. Ebrahimi R et al. Bivalirudin vs heparin in percutaneous coronary intervention: a pooled analysis. J Cardiovasc Pharmacol Ther. 2005;10(4):209–16.
91. Stone GW et al. Bivalirudin for patients with acute coronary syndromes. N Engl J Med. 2006;355(21):2203–16.
92. Dangas GD et al. Effect of switching antithrombin agents for primary angioplasty in acute myocardial infarction: the HORIZONS-SWITCH analysis. J Am Coll Cardiol. 2011;57(23):2309–16.
93. Kessler DP, Kroch E, Hlatky MA. The effect of bivalirudin on costs and outcomes of treatment of ST-segment elevation myocardial infarction. Am Heart J. 2011;162(3):494–500 e2.
94. Lee MS et al. Comparison of bivalirudin versus heparin plus glycoprotein IIb/IIIa inhibitors in patients undergoing an invasive strategy: a meta-analysis of randomized clinical trials. Int J Cardiol. 2011;152(3):369–74.
95. Connolly SJ et al. Dabigatran versus warfarin in patients with atrial fibrillation. N Engl J Med. 2009;361(12):1139–51.
96. Blech S et al. The metabolism and disposition of the oral direct thrombin inhibitor, dabigatran, in humans. Drug Metab Dispos. 2008;36(2):386–99.
97. Stangier J et al. Influence of renal impairment on the pharmacokinetics and pharmacodynamics of oral dabigatran etexilate: an open-label, parallel-group, single-centre study. Clin Pharmacokinet. 2010;49(4):259–68.
98. Posner J. Optimizing the dose of dabigatran etexilate. Br J Clin Pharmacol. 2012;74(5):741–3.
99. Oldgren J et al. Dabigatran vs. placebo in patients with acute coronary syndromes on dual antiplatelet therapy: a randomized, double-blind, phase II trial. Eur Heart J. 2011;32(22):2781–9.
100. Turpie AG. Oral, direct factor Xa inhibitors in development for the prevention and treatment of thromboembolic diseases. Arterioscler Thromb Vasc Biol. 2007;27(6):1238–47.
101. Umer Usman MH et al. Advancement in antithrombotics for stroke prevention in atrial fibrillation. J Interv Card Electrophysiol. 2008;22(2):129–37.
102. Karthikeyan G, Eikelboom JW. Apixaban in acute coronary syndromes. Cardiovasc Ther. 2011;29(5):285–90.
103. Schulman S, Kearon C. Definition of major bleeding in clinical investigations of antihemostatic medicinal products in non-surgical patients. J Thromb Haemost. 2005;3(4):692–4.
104. Alexander JH et al. Apixaban with antiplatelet therapy after acute coronary syndrome. N Engl J Med. 2011;365(8):699–708.
105. Perzborn E et al. Rivaroxaban: a new oral factor Xa inhibitor. Arterioscler Thromb Vasc Biol. 2010;30(3):376–81.
106. Kreutz R. Pharmacodynamic and pharmacokinetic basics of rivaroxaban. Fundam Clin Pharmacol. 2012;26(1):27–32.
107. Weinz C et al. Metabolism and excretion of rivaroxaban, an oral, direct factor Xa inhibitor, in rats, dogs, and humans. Drug Metab Dispos. 2009;37(5):1056–64.
108. Mega JL et al. Rivaroxaban versus placebo in patients with acute coronary syndromes (ATLAS ACS-TIMI 46): a randomised, double-blind, phase II trial. Lancet. 2009;374(9683):29–38.
109. Mega JL et al. Rivaroxaban in patients with a recent acute coronary syndrome. N Engl J Med. 2012;366(1):9–19.
110. Paccaly A et al. Pharmacokinetics of otamixaban, a direct factor Xa inhibitor, in healthy male subjects: pharmacokinetic model development for phase 2/3 simulation of exposure. J Clin Pharmacol. 2006;46(1):37–44.
111. Cohen M et al. Randomized, double-blind, dose-ranging study of otamixaban, a novel, parenteral, short-acting direct factor Xa inhibitor, in percutaneous coronary intervention: the SEPIA-PCI trial. Circulation. 2007;115(20):2642–51.
112. Sabatine MS et al. Otamixaban for the treatment of patients with non-ST-elevation acute coronary syndromes (SEPIA-ACS1 TIMI 42): a randomised, double-blind, active-controlled, phase 2 trial. Lancet. 2009;374(9692):787–95.

Robotic-Assisted Coronary Intervention

12

Jorge C. Magallon and Giora Weisz

The current practice of percutaneous coronary intervention (PCI) lacks standardization and is regarded as an art. As the complexity of the lesions and procedures increase, intervention duration becomes longer, and there is an increased demand for precision and accuracy in device selection and position. Robotic systems have been suggested to enhance the performance of cardiovascular procedures. One of the technical features of a robotic system is the capability to control and accurately position (≤1-mm steps) the stent delivery system. The recent STLLR (Stent deployment Techniques on cLinicaL outcomes of patients treated with the cypheR-stent) trial highlighted the impact of geographic miss and stent misplacement on clinical outcomes [1]. A robotically assisted system may facilitate the positioning of the stent delivery system with a high degree of accuracy. With improved positioning, especially with advanced navigation systems, there is a potential to reduce exposure of patients to radiation and to minimize the volume of contrast media, thereby reducing the risk of contrast-induced nephropathy.

Working in the cath lab may pose occupational hazards on the interventionalist [2]. Remote control robotic systems have been suggested to improve operator safety and comfort. The many hours of standing while wearing a heavy lead apron frequently leads to orthopedic injuries that results in reduced performance and loss of workdays [3, 4]. The RELID (retrospective evaluation study of lens injuries and dose) study revealed that interventional cardiologists are three times more likely to develop cataract-type eye opacities than age-matched control groups [5]. Recently, the interventional community was alarmed about the potential increased risk of brain tumors in interventional cardiologists [6]. Initial studies with robotic systems have been suggested to reduce radiation exposure [7, 8].

The objective of this chapter is to review some of the novel robotic, remote control, navigation, and positioning systems that have been developed in the last decade trying to address the above procedural and safety issues.

Navigation and Positioning Systems

The Medical Positioning System (MPS) has been developed in order to improve the accuracy of coronary imaging and device navigation and positioning without relying on fluoroscopy and contrast media. The system resembles the principles of the Global Positioning System (GPS), which works by having satellites in space that communicate with designed receivers and can calculate its exact location. Similarly, the medical magnetic positioning technology enables continuous positioning and navigation of MPS-enabled devices. A submillimeter MPS sensor (the receiver) can be assembled on a device's tip and sense the low-intensity magnetic field generated by the MPS system (similar to the satellites), generating an electrical signal from which real-time 3D position and orientation information is extracted. The inherent co-registration of the MPS with the angiogram (like the map in the GPS system) provides the anatomical position and orientation of the device tip.

When applied to the cath lab and coronary procedures, the MPS system is designed to create a 3D coronary road map that is superimposed on the angiogram and is not subject to changes in angiographic views or foreshortening. The MPS functions as an adjunct device to the existing X-ray system with the capability of generating 3D reconstruction images of any inspected arterial segment, which can then be superimposed on the coronary angiogram. The

J.C. Magallon
Interventional Cardiology Fellow, Division of Cardiology, Department of Medicine, New York Presbyterian Hospital-Columbia University Medical Center, New York, NY, USA

G. Weisz (✉)
Columbia University, New York, NY, USA

Center for Interventional Vascular Therapy, New-York Presbyterian Hospital – Columbia University Medical Center, New York, NY, USA
e-mail: gw2128@columbia.edu

C.A. Thompson (ed.), *Textbook of Cardiovascular Intervention*,
DOI 10.1007/978-1-4471-4528-8_12, © Springer-Verlag London 2014

system allows continuous tracking (navigation) and projection of the tip's position of the MPS-enabled interventional device onto the 3D road map and live fluoroscopy. By eliminating the factors like vessel tortuosity, vessel overlap, and foreshortening, the system allows for better precision and accuracy when positioning the intravascular device.

Magnetic Positioning System

The MPS comprises hardware and software, which function alongside existing X-ray imaging systems in the catheterization lab. Magnetic transmitters are installed inside the image detector, which generates a low magnetic field less than 200 μTesla around the patient. A magnetic reference sensor is placed on the patient's upper chest to provide information about the spatial relationship between the chest wall and the flat image detector and to adjust for respiratory changes and chest wall movements.

The intravascular device is equipped with a passive magnetic sensor that is assembled on its tip. The sensor senses the low-intensity magnetic field generated by the MPS and provides the real-time three-dimensional position and orientation of the catheter's tip. For the initial human experience with the system, a special investigational device was used, the Guided Measurement Catheters (GMC). The GMC is designed out of a disabled conventional coronary balloon with a passive magnetic sensor assembled on its tip. The catheter is compatible with the 6Fr coronary guiding catheters and conventional 0.014 guidewire. The radio-opaque sensor on the GMC senses the low-intensity magnetic field generated by the MPS to provide real-time three-dimensional position and orientation of the catheter's tip.

Similar to any MPS-enabled device, the GMC catheter is advanced into the coronary artery, and it provides continuous real-time tracking of the catheter tip with projection of images onto fluoroscopy or cineangiography during the manual pullback (Fig. 12.1). In addition, the GMC catheter can generate a color-coded line superimposed on the reference 2D angiogram called the Smart Trace. The Smart Trace is color coded to show the degree of vessel angular foreshortening (Fig. 12.1). By combining the Smart Trace with the angiogram, a 3D model reconstruction is generated (Fig. 12.2). The system provides 3D length measurements of a selected segment based on the trace of the magnetic positioning system (MPS). This model is then utilized to facilitate treatment strategy and equipment selection.

The system also allows the user to place one or more landmarks at points of interest while superimposing them on the angiogram (real-time and cine-loops) and on the 3D model. This mark is intended to point to an anatomical landmark and is displayed on any image and from any viewing angle. This can help the operator to position devices in accurate positions like bifurcations, aorto-ostial, overlapping stents, etc. (Fig. 12.2).

Clinical Experience

The initial preclinical experience demonstrated the safety and clinical potential of the MPS and GMC in pigs [9]. In the first human experience, 20 patients were studied in a single-center study to evaluate the safety and feasibility of the MPS system and GMC catheter. The device met all its expected primary performance end points without any related adverse events in any of the patients [10]. The system performance was evaluated on a semiquantitative one-to-five scale. The

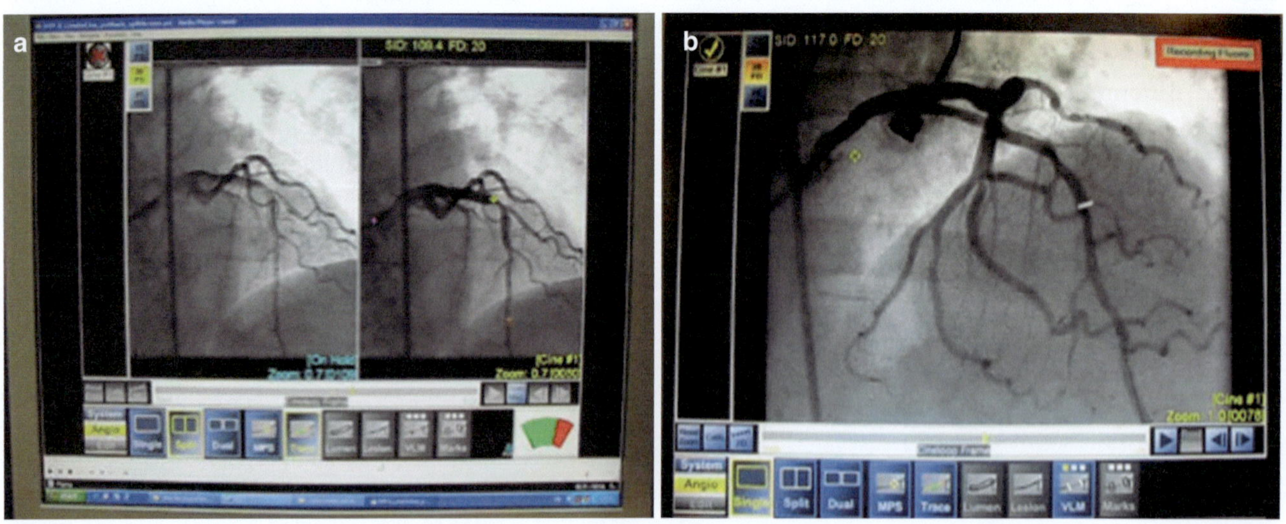

Fig. 12.1 (**a**) Simultaneous projections of live and cine images. (**b**) Virtual landmark tracked on a recorded angiographic loop

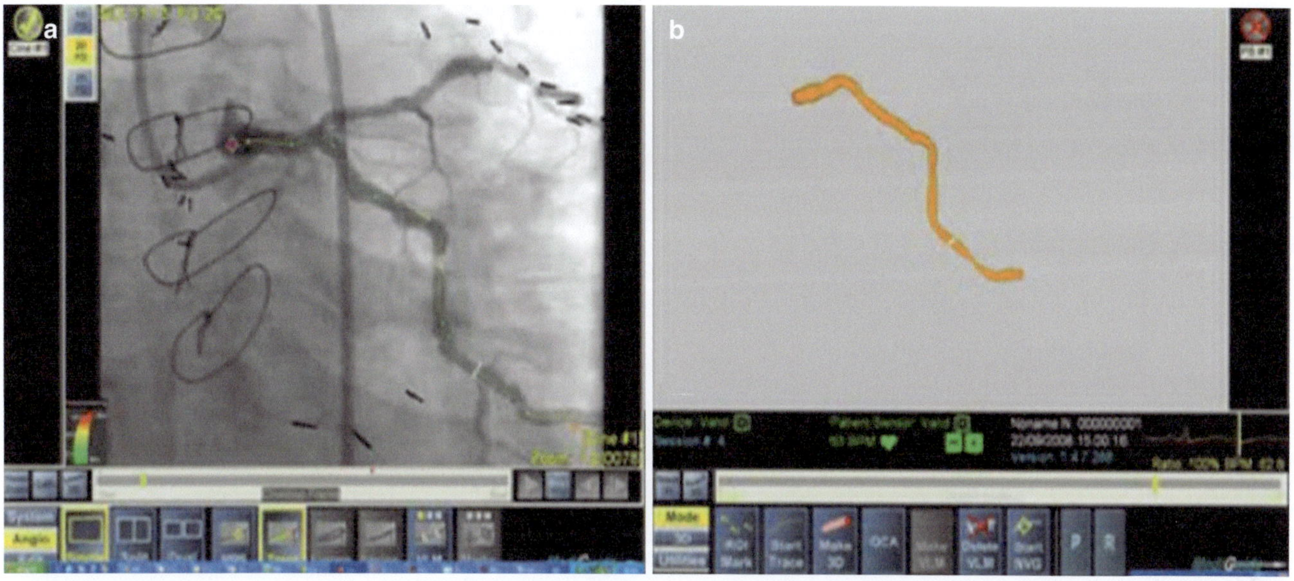

Fig. 12.2 (**a**) Smart trace shown on a recorded cine angiography loop. (**b**) In 3D Image reconstruction, a single cine-loop is used for automatic segmentation of lumen cross-section data

mean scores (out of maximal 5) for tracking as assessed by projection on live fluoroscopy was 4.89 and for tracking as assessed by projection on recorded cine-loop was 3.58. Length measurement of a given 20 mm distance was significantly better with the MPS (mean deviation of 0.6 mm = 3 %) as compared to standard QCA (1.5 mm = 8 %, $p<0.05$). Creating a 3D reconstruction was possible in 13 out of 20 cases with an average score of 4.68.

In a more advanced 2-site study, an additional 40 patients were studied in a safety and feasibility regulatory study evaluating a newer version of the system [11, 12]. There were no complications or adverse events associated with the use of the system. Procedure success (defined as GMC performance success and freedom of MACE at 48 h) was achieved in 90 % of the patients. The GMC catheter was able to reach the distal vessel and perform the necessary measurements (i.e., assessment of minimal luminal diameter (MLD) in patients that underwent PCI) in 97.5 and 95 % of the time, respectively. The MPS accuracy was highest when the target was superimposed on the live fluoroscopy (score of 4.9 out of max 5) and the 3D vessel reconstruction (score 4.7). MLD measurements were not significantly different between the MPS system and conventional QCA. The results confirmed the functional and operational performance of the MPS-enabled GMC while demonstrating an excellent safety profile. Based on this study, the system was cleared by the FDA.

The results of these initial experience studies suggest that the use of this navigation and positioning technology can contribute to PCI procedures. For example, utilizing 3D reconstructions of the coronary tree and lesion minimizes angiographic views thereby potentially reducing radiation exposure and contrast administration. Furthermore, virtual landmarks and interventional devices with sensors can provide the operator with improved accuracy in positioning the interventional device without the need for fluoroscopy or repeat contrast injections.

The inventors of the system suggested combining it with intravascular ultrasound (IVUS) into a system called GIVUS (Guided IVUS). This system may have the potential to collect ultrasound images along their corresponding spatial orientation. GIVUS will use the near real-time segmentation algorithm to automatically identify the vessel's lumen and external elastic membrane on the IVUS images to generate an accurate 3D model of the vessel. The initial GIVUS system was tested in animal models.

In summary, the MediGuide navigation system provides a novel concept of navigation and positioning of intravascular devices. With improved precision, the system has the potential to result in significant reduction in contrast-media volume and radiation exposure. One of its major limitations is the high cost of the system, special installation and occupying space in the cath lab. However, with further development and integration with intravascular devices, the system has the potential to become a prominent tool in treating complex coronary lesions in a robotic-oriented cath lab.

Stereotaxis Magnetic Navigation System

The Stereotaxis Magnetic Navigation System (MNS) introduced a new concept of manipulating devices inside the heart and blood vessels. This technology uses a magnetic field around the patient, affecting the metal devices inside the body. The operator can change the orientation of the

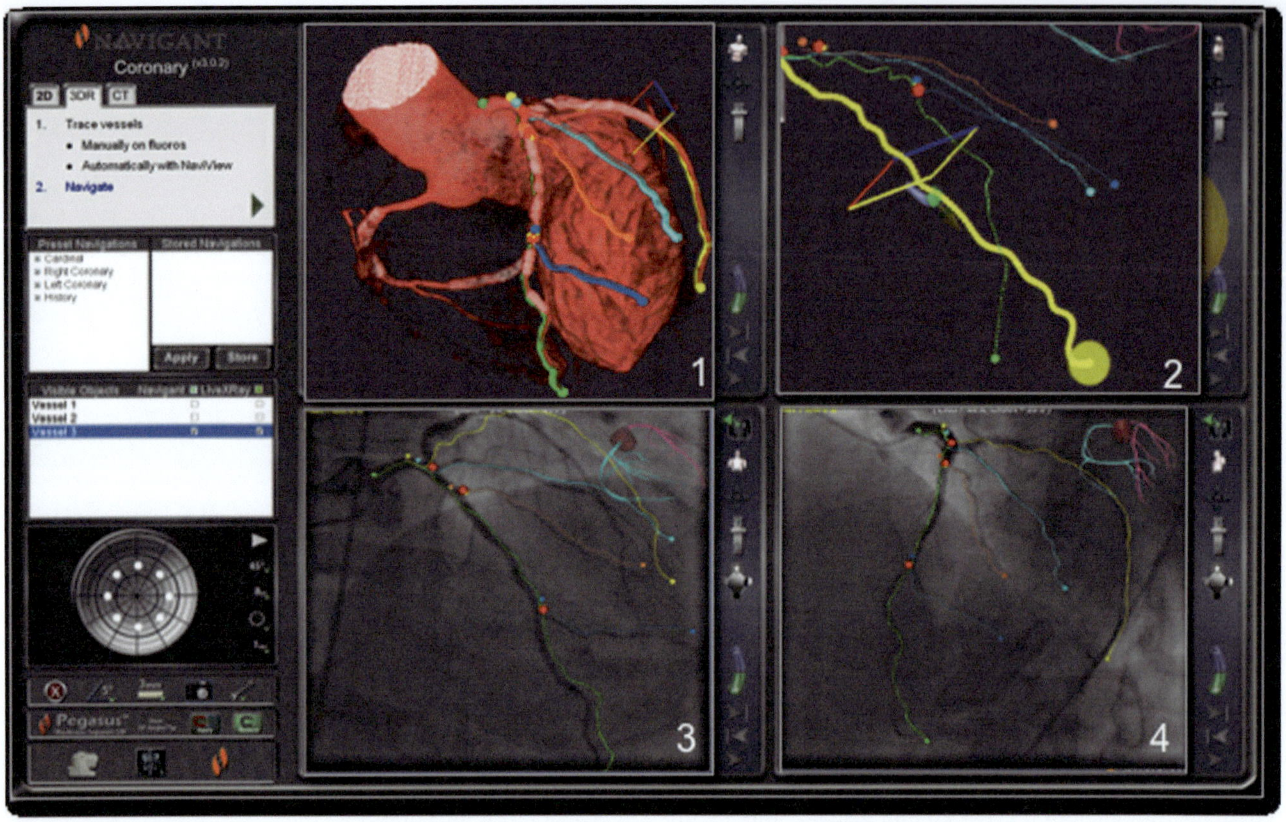

Fig. 12.3 User interface example for left coronary artery. The display shows various options: Three-dimensional navigation using multislice computer tomography (*1*, *2*) and two-dimensional angiography-based navigation (*3*, *4*)

magnetic field, which then changes the position and orientation of the device. By changing the magnetic field, the operator specifically orients the catheter. The MNS has gained wide popularity mainly in the electrophysiology laboratory, combining an ablation catheter with this system, and has been also introduced to the coronary and vascular fields.

Magnetic Navigation System

The MNS is an integrated system consisting of a workstation and magnet control equipment that navigates catheters and guidewires through small magnets placed at their distal tips. These small magnets are then precisely oriented by manipulating the magnetic field generated by two large permanent magnets mounted on mechanical positioners on either side of the fluoroscopy table. Rotation and translation of these magnets maintain a magnetic field of 0.08 T in strength and have a radius of 15 cm over the patient's heart. The magnets can move in three different coordinates, rotate, move toward and from the navigation volume, and tilt. This allows the magnetic field vector to be oriented in full 360°. The two table-side magnets can be rotated into position or parked away when not in use.

The operator uses a navigation workstation that utilizes a software interface that co-registers the coronary imaging with the 3D navigation of the magnetic system. The imaging includes the coronary angiogram as well as a 3D registration of a coronary computerized tomographic scan and the Paieon imaging reconstruction software. These build the 3D vessel road mapping for the magnetic-assisted interventions (Fig. 12.3). With the 3D vessel reconstruction on the screen, the operator can form and direct the device magnetic vector path along the long axis of the coronary arterial vessel (Fig. 12.4) and direct the wire tip longitudinally. The system allows angles of up to 120° from the long axis, facilitating access to very complex coronary angulations.

Magnetic Wires

The magnetic tipped guidewires of the Pegasus family are made in a wide range of shaft support and tip stiffness for different interventional needs. They are blended with nitinol and stainless steel, with the distal 2 mm serving as the magnetic tip. As described above, these wires are precisely oriented through vessels by the MNS. The operator manually

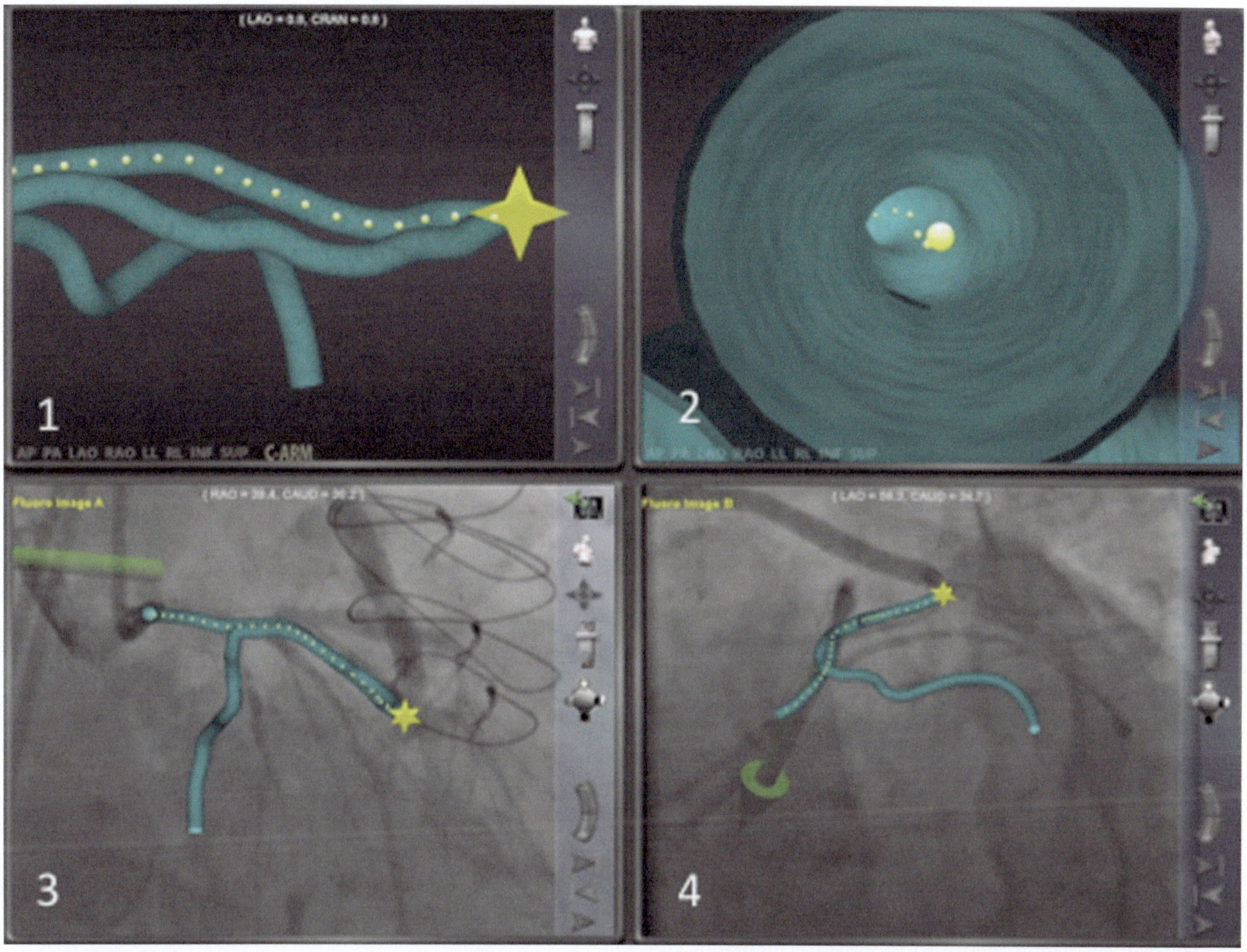

Fig. 12.4 This shows the three-dimensional reconstruction created from the angiogram using the Navigant software system. The system also provides an endoluminal view as well as the opportunity to superimpose the three-dimensional images on the angiographic images

advances the wire but utilizes the software to help guide the direction of the wire. This is particularly important in complex anatomies with severe angulations.

Clinical Experience

The use of the MNS has been shown to be quite effective in several fields other than interventional cardiology. For example, in electrophysiology, the MNS has been successful for mapping and ablating arrhythmias [13] even within complex atrial anatomy [14] with no associated risk of perforation [13, 15].

The initial experience in humans demonstrated the feasibility of the MNS in performing PCI including successful crossing of complex lesions where conventional wires had failed [16, 17]. Additional single-center studies further substantiated the success of the MNS in routine [18, 19] and complex lesions [17, 20–22]. In two large series, which combined over 500 patients undergoing MNS-assisted PCI, procedural success rates were 89 and 93.4 % [17, 23]. These success rates were similar to procedural success rates in standard manual PCI. The MNS system has been reported to be successful in complex coronary lesions like bifurcations [20, 21, 24], bypass grafts with loops [25], and alcohol septal ablation [26]. The big challenge remains, as in standard manual PCI, with chronic total occlusion (CTO). Case reports highlighted the potential of this technology in conquering total occlusions [27]. The use of multislice CT co-registration has importance in planning CTO procedures with the additional benefit of magnetic navigation.

The magnetic navigation system was suggested to reduce fluoroscopy time [20, 23, 25]. By reducing fluoroscopy time, it reduces radiation exposure to both the operator and patient. With further development of remote manipulation of the

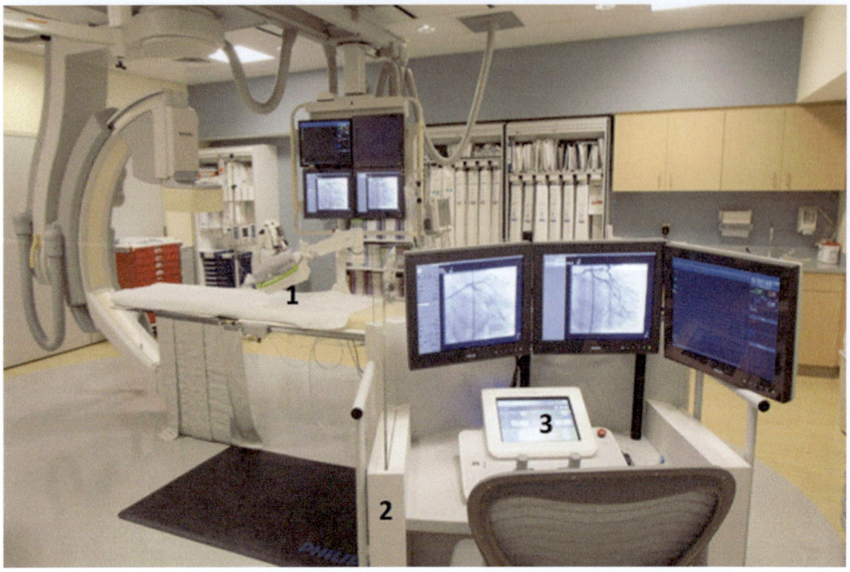

Fig. 12.5 The CorPath 200 robotic system. (*1*) Bedside component-robotic drive hosting the disposable cassette. (*2*) Radiation-protected interventional cockpit. (*3*) Operator console

devices, the radiation exposure will be further reduced, and by controlling the procedure remotely from the control room, the comfort of the operator is improved. Another potential benefit of the MNS is reduction in contrast usage [20, 25], which lowers the risk for contrast-induced nephropathy.

The magnetic navigation system has been also suggested for peripheral arterial procedures. Combined with a radiofrequency ablation catheter, this system has the potential to be successful for long total occlusions with increased success and reduced burden of radiation and orthopedic stress on the operator.

In summary, the Stereotaxis navigation system provides a new avenue for treating challenging and tortuous anatomy, CTO's, and a reduction in contrast, radiation exposure, time, and use of other resources. One of its major limitations is the high cost of the system, occupying a large space in the cath lab, and the inability to be used in patients with metal in their bodies. However, with further development of high-performance dedicated devices, advances in the 3D co-registration, progress in remote manipulation, and development of magnetic resistant pacemakers and ICDs, this system has the potential to become a prominent tool in treating complex coronary lesions in a robotic-oriented cath lab.

CorPath Robotic System

Initially, the CorPath robotic system was developed to provide a remote control radiation-free environment that minimizes the hazardous health effects of radiation and the long-term orthopedic morbidity of wearing the heavy protective lead shielding to the operator. The CorPath robotic system was also designed to be advantageous to the patient by providing improved procedural precision, stability, and accuracy. Addressing the needs of both the patient and the operator, the system has attracted a lot of interest in the interventional world and has become the flagship of robotics in interventional cardiology.

CorPath 200 Robotic System

The system can be assembled in any cath lab. There are two main components to the robotic system: the bedside component and the interventional cockpit (Fig. 12.5).

The interventional cockpit (Fig. 12.6) is a radiation-shielded mobile workstation, which holds the monitors, computerized touch screen control console, and joysticks. The interventional cardiologist can perform the PCI while sitting comfortably at the workstation, with no need for cumbersome lead protection. Since it is a mobile workstation, it can be positioned anywhere inside the cath lab or outside in the control room. The fluoroscopy, electrocardiography, and hemodynamic monitors are duplicated on monitors placed within the cockpit. The intravascular manipulation of devices is controlled by intuitive movements (push, pull, and rotate) of the joysticks in the interventional cockpit console. The operator can manipulate the devices with one hand, while freeing up the other hand to activate the contrast injector. This enables accurate contrast consumption by the interventionalist.

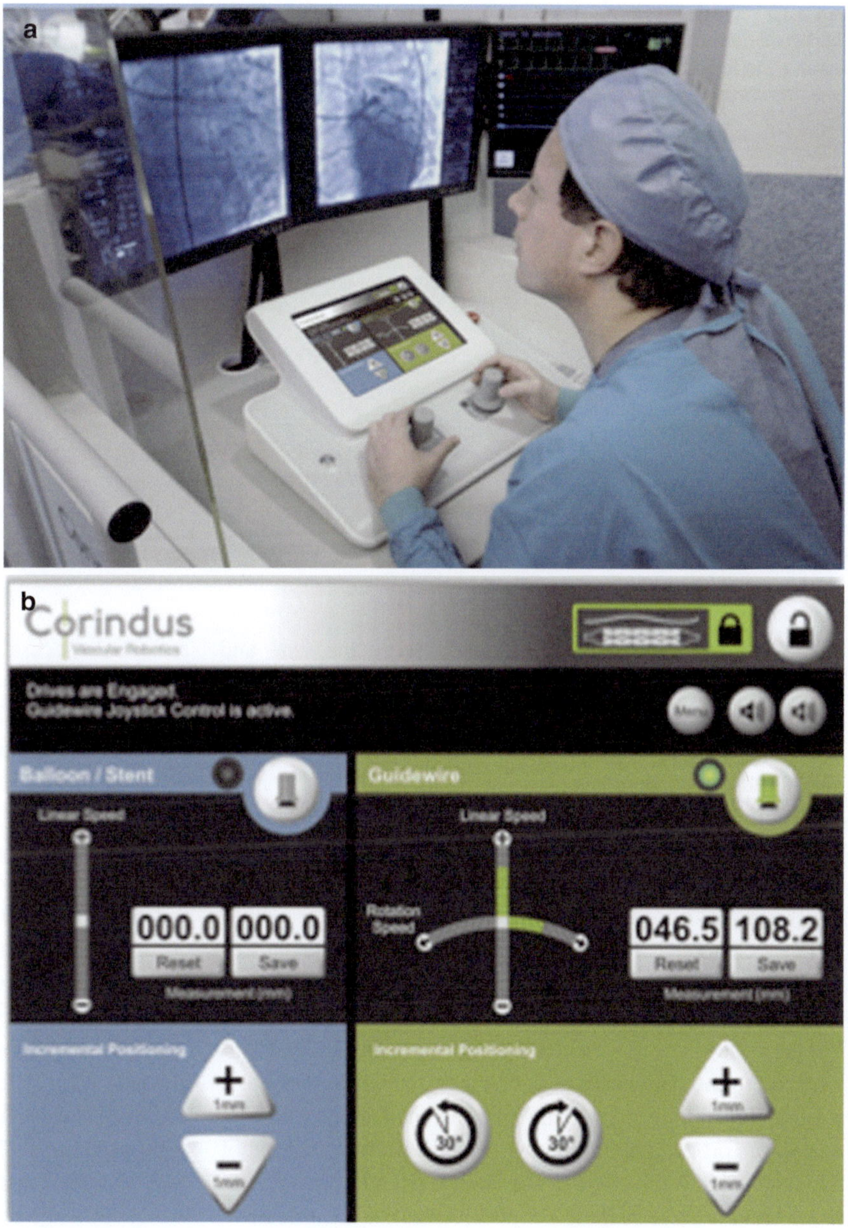

Fig. 12.6 CorPath 200 operator console: (**a**) Operator seated in the interventional cockpit with the control console, angiography, and hemodynamic monitors. The operator manipulates the intravascular devices by operating the two joysticks. (**b**) Touch screen of the console which enable digital control of the linear and rotational movement of the devices. The precise movement enables measurement of the coronary segment of interest

The bedside component (Fig. 12.7) contains a bedrail-mounted articulated arm that contains a robotic drive with an attached single-use cassette. The disposable sterile cassette is connected to the guiding catheter, and after loading the intravascular devices into the cassette, they are held by the cassette components. The cassette manipulates the angioplasty tools (i.e., balloon, stent) in the axial direction by a set of rollers. The guidewire is maneuvered by axial and rotation transmission forces. When the guidewire is manipulated, the device is locked into position and vice versa. The robotic drive is connected to the control console with a communication cable.

The CorPath 200 is an open architecture system, which utilizes standard 0.014-in. rapid-exchange intravascular equipment. There is no need for special catheters, guidewires, balloon, or stents. Every off-the-shelf rapid-exchange interventional device or imaging catheters can be used.

The system provides several potential advantages for the patient. During the procedure, the robotic system enables superior stabilization of the intravascular devices with an arm designed to stabilize the guiding catheter in addition to its connection to the cassette and to the vascular introducer.

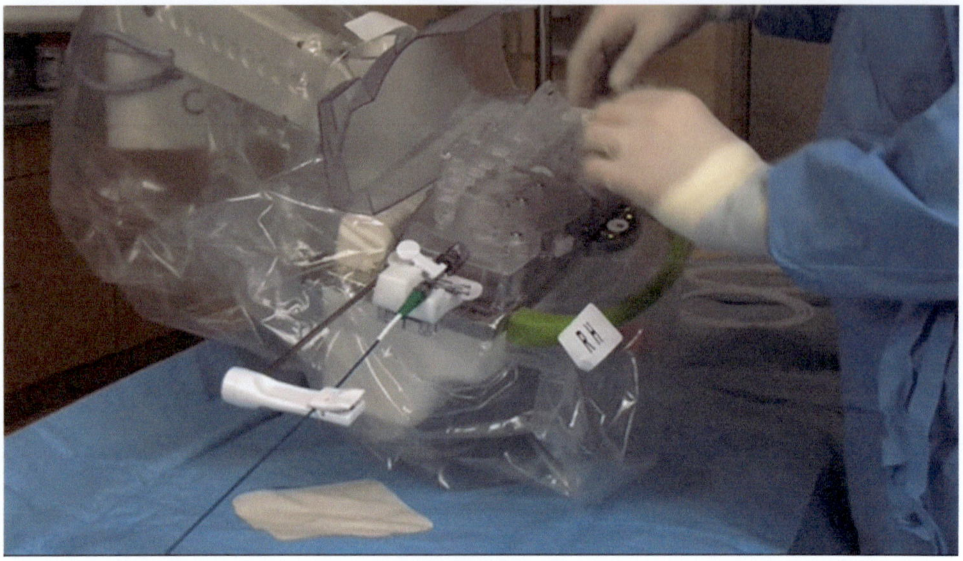

Fig. 12.7 Bedside Unit: A sterile single-use cassette is mounted to the robotic drive and connected to the guide catheter

A locking mechanism differentiates between the wire and the balloon/stent movements, enabling additional stability of the wire while advancing the interventional devices over it, avoiding "telescopic slippage." The intravascular devices can be advanced or retracted in steps as small as 1 mm to control linear movements, enabling precise measurements of the lesion length, unrelated to the angiographic view or foreshortening. This allows for accurate stent selection avoiding the (frequent) need for additional stents because a too-short stent was selected. While having sole control of the contrast-media injector, the operator can decide on the optimal dose and timing of contrast to be injected leading to a more efficient use of contrast media and minimizing excess administration to the patient. For the operator, the CorPath system gives a comfortable ergonomic working environment. Sitting during the procedure without the need for prolonged used of the heavy lead apron frees the interventional cardiologist from accumulative radiation exposure and the accumulative burden of spine problems that are so common in interventional cardiologists. The fluoroscopic monitors, imaging, and hemodynamics are slaved into the interventional cockpit, located closer to the eyes, enabling better vision of the procedure, with potential reduction in the radiation exposure of the patient as well.

Clinical Experience

The initial experience with an experimental intravascular robotic navigation system demonstrated the feasibility and ease of use of a remote control system [28]. Soon after, Bayer et al [29] reported the first in-man pilot clinical study using the robotic system in 18 patients undergoing PCI at three different medical centers. They demonstrated good technical success and excellent clinical results. This clinical first-in-human study demonstrated the safety and feasibility of using even a simple experimental system for successful PCI without complications [29].

After further iterations, the experimental robotic navigation system was redesigned to the current CorPath 200 model. The first-in-human experience study with the CorPath 200 essentially recapitulated the results by Bayer et al with the first system [30]. A total of eight patients with significant coronary artery disease and indications for PCI were studied. All PCIs were done with the CorPath system and commercially available 6 Fr guiding catheters, 0.014″ rapid-exchange wires, and balloons and stents of various types and sizes. Devices were delivered successfully 100 % of the time and retrieved successfully 95.8 % of the time. The overall technical success was 97.9 %. All patients had residual stenosis of <10 %, with TIMI-3 flow at the end of the procedure. There was no inhospital or 30-day MACE. The operators rated the CorPath 200 performance as equal or better than manual procedures 92.5 % of the time. Radiation exposure to the operator in the cockpit was measured and compared to the table position. The radiation exposure to the interventional cardiologist was impressively reduced by 97 % compared to the conventional table position.

The CorPath robotic system was further evaluated in a multicenter, multi-operator study. The CorPath Percutaneous Robotic-Enhanced Coronary Intervention Study (PRECISE) was designed as a prospective, single-arm, multicenter study, to evaluate the clinical and technical performance of the CorPath system. A total of 164 patients were enrolled in 9 sites. The PCI was completed successfully using the robotic system without conversion to manual operation, and device technical success was achieved in 162/164 patients (98.8 %). The advancements of the guidewire proceeded smoothly, without any dissection or perforation. In all patients the predilatation balloon was successfully delivered to the lesion, inflated as clinically indicated, and successfully retrieved by the robotic system back into the guiding catheter. In only two (1.2 %) of the procedures, the operators converted to manual operation due to severe resistance to deliver the stent in the coronary artery. In both cases, the procedure was difficult also manually and completed successfully only after upgrading to a more supportive guiding catheter and use of advance interventional techniques. The conversion to manual operation was immediate and not associated with myocardial ischemia, hemodynamic compromise, or any other complications. There were no device-related complications. Clinical procedural success was achieved in 160/164 patients (97.6 %), while 4 (2.4 %) had periprocedural non-Q wave MI. No death, stroke, Q-wave MI, or revascularization occurred in the 30 days' post-procedures.

The initial and multicenter-wide experience with the CorPath 200 system demonstrated the feasibility, safety, and effectiveness of the remote control robotic system. The learning curve to operate the system was short and simple. There were no adverse events or complications directly related to the system, and the few cases that were converted to manual operation were free of complications. The conversion to manual operation was performed within seconds. The interventional cockpit was reported to be ergonomic and with impressive reduction in radiation exposure to the operators. Although initial experience was limited to coronary interventions, the system can be easily applied to peripheral vascular procedures with stationary vessels that are usually longer in duration and expose the interventionalists to much larger radiation doses.

Conclusion

The development of novel robotic remote control, navigation, and position systems has opened a new era in interventional cardiology. These systems have the potential to improve procedural standardization, precision, safety, and success rate. The navigation and accurate position capabilities can definitely lead to the use of lower volumes of contrast media, reducing the devastating risk of contrast-induced nephropathy. Furthermore, all these systems are associated with reduced exposure to ionizing radiation, for both patients and operators. All the systems described in this chapter have been used in humans with promising initial results. We expect to see the next decade bringing further developments and expansion in the use of robotics systems, with the potential of bringing these technologies into the standard care of interventional cardiology, especially with the development of more complex devices and procedures. Since each of these technologies has different advantages, a pooled effort is needed to combine them into the cath lab of the future.

References

1. Costa MA, Angiolillo DJ, Tannenbaum M, et al. Impact of stent deployment procedural factors on long-term effectiveness and safety of sirolimus-eluting stents (final results of multicenter prospective STLLR trial). Am J Cardiol. 2008;101:1704–11.
2. Kline LW, Miller DL, Balter S, et al. Occupational hazards in the interventional laboratory: time for a safer environment. Catheter Cardiovasc Interv. 2009;73:432–8.
3. Goldstein JA, Balter S, Crowley M, et al. Occupational hazards of interventional cardiologists: prevalence of orthopedic health problems in contemporary practice. Catheter Cardiovasc Interv. 2004;63:407–11.
4. Ross AM, Segal J, Borenstein D, et al. Prevalence of spinal disc disease among interventional cardiologists. Am J Cardiol. 1997; 79:68–70.
5. Duran AD, Duran GD, Ramirez RR, et al. Cataracts in interventional cardiology personnel. Retrospective evaluation study of lens injuries and dose (RELID Study). Eur Heart J. 2009;30:872.
6. Roguin A, Goldstein J, Bar O. Brain tumours among interventional cardiologists: a cause for alarm? Report of four new cases from two cities and a review of the literature. EuroIntervention. 2012;7:1081–6.
7. Garcia-Garcia HM, Tsuchida K, Meulenbrug H, et al. Magnetic navigation in a coronary phantom: experimental results. EuroIntervention. 2005;1:321–8.
8. Steve D, Servatius H, Rostock T, et al. Reduced fluoroscopy during atrial fibrillation ablation: benefits of robotic guided navigation. J Cardiovasc Electrophysiol. 2010;21:6–12.
9. Flugelman M, Shiran A, Nusimovici-Avadis D, et al. Medical positioning system: a technical report. EuroIntervention. 2008;4:158–60.
10. Jeron A, Fredersdorf S, Debl K, et al. First-in-man (FIM) experience with the Magnetic Medical Positioning System (MPS) for intracoronary navigation. EuroIntervention. 2009;5:552–7.
11. Weisz G, Smilowitz NR, Moses JW, Rabbani LE, Collins MB, Herscovici A, Jeron A, Leon MB, Luchner A. Magnetic positioning system in coronary angiography and percutaneous intervention: A feasibility and safety study. Catheterization and cardiovascular interventions: official journal of the Society for Cardiac Angiography and Interventions. 2013
12. Weisz G, Wong D, Laroche V, et al. Intracoronary navigation and positioning using the MediGuide gMPS enabled GMC system. Eurointervention. 2009;5:E11.
13. Ernst S, Ouyang F, Linder C, et al. Initial experience with remote catheter ablation using a novel magnetic navigation system: magnetic remote catheter ablation. Circulation. 2004;109:1472–5.
14. Ernst S, Ouyang F, Linder C, et al. Modulation of the slow pathway in the presence of a persistent left superior caval vein using the novel magnetic navigation system Niobe. Europace. 2004;6: 10–4.
15. Faddis MN, Blume W, Finney J, et al. Novel, magnetically guided catheter for endocardial mapping and radiofrequency catheter ablation. Circulation. 2002;106:2980–5.
16. Tsuchida K, Garcia-Garcia HM, Tanimoto S, et al. Feasibility and safety of guidewire navigation using a magnetic navigation system in coronary artery stenoses. EuroIntervention. 2005;1:329–35.
17. Atmakuri SR, Lev EI, Alviar C, et al. Initial experience with a magnetic navigation system for percutaneous coronary intervention in complex coronary artery lesions. J Am Coll Cardiol. 2006;47: 515–21.
18. Kiemeneij F, Patterson MS, Amoroso G, et al. Use of the stereotaxis Niobe magnetic navigation system for percutaneous coronary intervention: results from 350 consecutive patients. Catheter Cardiovasc Interv. 2008;71:510–6.
19. Hertting K, Ernst S, Stahl F, et al. Use of the novel magnetic system Niobe in percutaneous coronary interventions; the Hamburg experience. EuroIntervention. 2005;1:336–9.

20. Ramcharitar S, Patterson MS, van Genus RJ, et al. Magnetic navigation system used successfully to cross a crushed stent in a bifurcation that failed with conventional wires. Catheter Cardiovasc Interv. 2007;69:852–5.
21. Ramcharitar S, van der Giessen WJ, van der Ent M, et al. Randomized comparison of the magnetic navigation system vs. standard wires in the treatment of bifurcations. Eur Heart J. 2011;32:1479–83.
22. Tsuchida K, Garcia-Garcia HM, van der Giessen WJ, et al. Guidewire navigation in coronary artery stenosis using a novel magnetic navigation system: first clinical experience. Catheter Cardiovasc Interv. 2006;67:356–63.
23. Krause K, Adamu U, Weber M, et al. German stereotaxis-guided percutaneous coronary intervention study group: first multicenter real world experience. Clin Res Cardiol. 2009;98:541–7.
24. Ramcharitar S, van Geuns RJ, Patterson M, et al. A randomized comparison of the magnetic navigation system versus conventional percutaneous coronary intervention. Catheter Cardiovasc Interv. 2008;72:761–70.
25. Ramicharitar S, van Geuns RJ. Magnetic navigation in patients with coronary artery bypass grafting. EuroIntervention. 2009; 5(Supplement D):D58–63.
26. Bach RG, Leach C, Milov SA, et al. Use of magnetic navigation to facilitate transcatheter alcohol septal ablation for hypertrophic obstructive cardiomyopathy. J Invasive Cardiol. 2006;18:E178.
27. Ramcharitar S, van der Giessen WJ, van der Ent M, et al. The feasibility and safety of applying the Magnetic Navigation System to manage chronically occluded vessels: a single centre experience. EuroIntervention. 2011;6:711–6.
28. Beyar R, Wenderow T, Lindner D, et al. Concept, design and preclinical studies for remote control percutaneous coronary interventions. EuroIntervention. 2005;1:340–5.
29. Beyar R, Gruberg L, Deleanu D, et al. Remote-control percutaneous coronary interventions: concept, validation, and first-in-humans pilot clinical trial. J Am Coll Cardiol. 2006;47:296–300.
30. Granada JF, Delgado JA, Uribe MP, et al. First-in-human evaluation of a novel robotic-assisted coronary angioplasty system. JACC Cardiovasc Interv. 2011;4:460–5.

The Transradial Approach for Coronary Angiography and Intervention

13

Michael Mok, Philippe Généreux, and Stéphane Rinfret

Transradial approach (TRA) as a method of accessing the arterial system began in the 1940s [1]. It was not until the late 1980s when the TRA was used in cardiac catheterization [2], and from here it rapidly followed into percutaneous coronary intervention [3]. Recently, the increasing concern of vascular access complications associated with the transfemoral approach has obligated interventional cardiologists to consider training in TRA. With advancements in technology, the array of interventional equipment traditionally compatible only with the transfemoral approach is also available to the TRA operator. The only remaining obstacle to considering a TRA is the "learning curve." In this chapter, we aim to provide insights and techniques, which will help overcome the initial potential difficulties of the TRA.

Assessing the Radial Artery

Patency of the palmar arches is first assessed by either the Allen's test or the Barbeau test (with a pulse oximeter) [4]. It is generally inadvisable to proceed with a TRA in the setting of insufficient hand collateral arterial supply. However, there is significant controversy in this area. Firstly, there is currently no published literature linking an abnormal Allen's test/pulse oximetry result to subsequent hand ischemia. Second, the presence of an adequate collateral arterial supply to the hand does not preclude hand ischemia secondary to other etiologies such as arterial embolism [5].

M. Mok, MBBS, FRACP
Quebec Heart & Lung Institute,
Laval University, Quebec City, QC, Canada

P. Généreux, MD
Angiographic Core Laboratory, Cardiovascular Research Foundation, New York, NY, USA

S. Rinfret, MD, SM, FRCPC (✉)
Multidisciplinary Department of Cardiology, Quebec Heart & Lung Institute, Laval University, Quebec City, QC, Canada
e-mail: stephane.rinfret@criucpq.ulaval.ca

C.A. Thompson (ed.), *Textbook of Cardiovascular Intervention*,
DOI 10.1007/978-1-4471-4528-8_13, © Springer-Verlag London 2014

Right Radial Approach Versus Left Radial Approach

Right radial approach (RRA) is preferred by most operators due to the conventional configuration of catheterization laboratories. The standard setup with monitors on the left of the patient and operators on the right makes the right radial more accessible. However, the left radial approach (LRA) can be made more accessible by adducting and internally rotating the left shoulder over the abdomen of the patient, with support under the left elbow. In the majority of patients, the final location of the left wrist will be close to the right femoral artery. A LRA access is preferred in situations of coronary graft studies with a known left internal mammary artery graft, inaccessible RRA or procedures requiring simultaneous coronary injections.

Puncture Technique (Fig. 13.1)

The patient's upper limb is abducted and external rotated to 90° and supported on an arm board. Gentle extension of the supinated wrist will bring the radial artery to the optimal exposed position. The puncture site is disinfected and draped along with both femoral artery sites. Depending of operator experience/comfort, a seated position may be employed for the radial artery puncture.

The puncture site is identified at approximately 1–2 cm proximal to the radial styloid process. Following infiltration with 2 % lidocaine (without adrenaline), a small skin incision may be made with a No. 11 blade to ease the needle manipulation. The introducing needle is angled at 45° to the horizontal through the prior skin incision. Following insertion of the sheath via a modified Seldinger technique, a cocktail of arterial spasmolytic agents is administered through the side arm of the sheath to prevent radial artery spasm. Kiemeneij et al. demonstrated that an intra-arterial mixture of verapamil (5 mg) and nitroglycerine (200 mcg) resulted in less discomfort during sheath removal and lower rates of

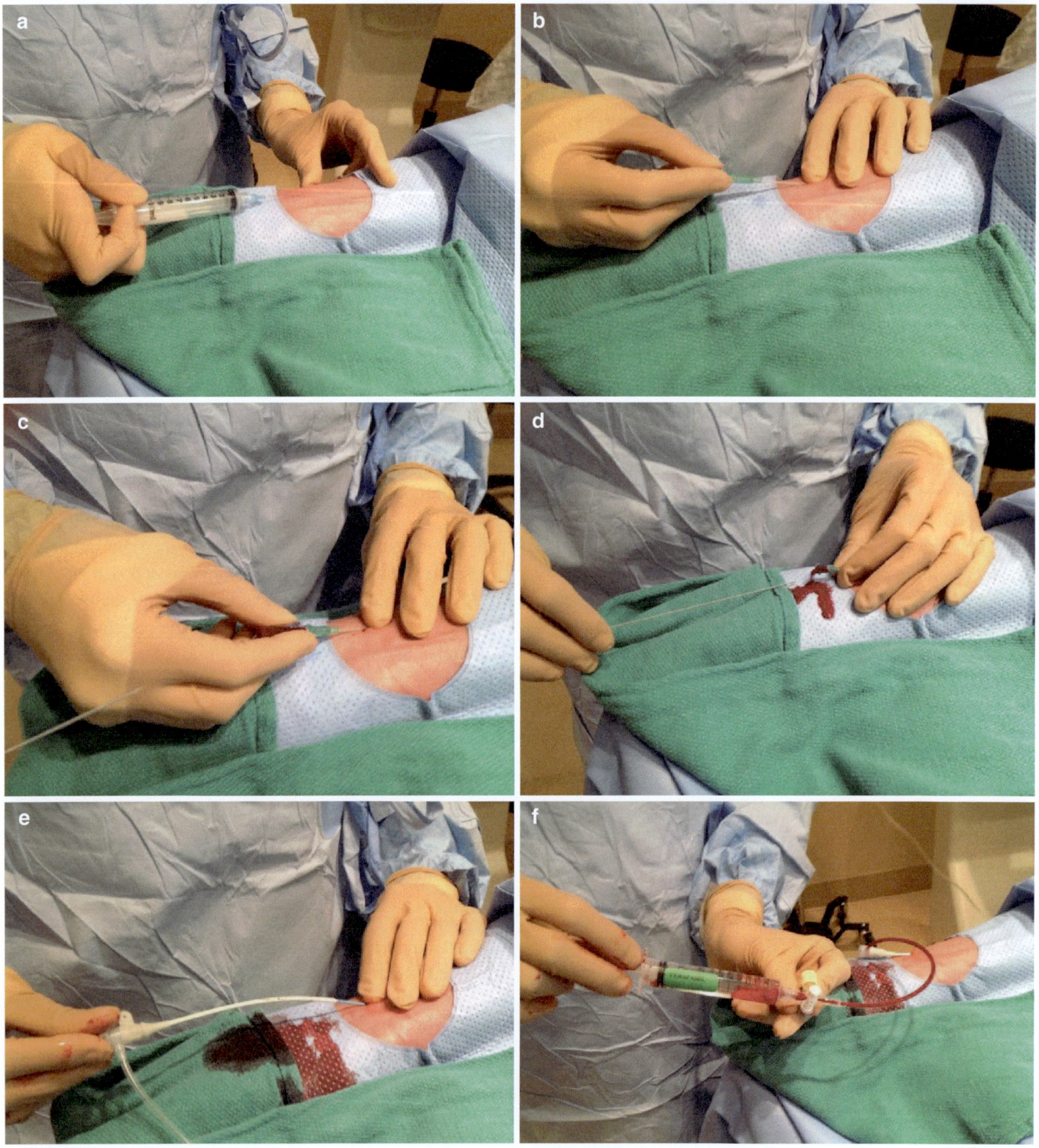

Fig. 13.1 Classical Seldinger technique for radial puncture. (**a**) Local anesthesia, (**b**) puncture of the radial with IV catheter, (**c**) blood back in mandrin, (**d**) 0.035" guidewire inserted into IV sheath, (**e**) regular 5F sheath inserted, (**f**) vasodilator cocktail

radial artery spasm, as compared with patient who received neither [6]. Anticoagulation is recommended to decrease the incidence of radial artery thrombosis (e.g., heparin 50–70 units/kg) [7]. Following successful sheath insertion, the patient's arm is returned to the neutral position (RRA) or the adducted position across the abdomen in a LRA.

Currently, there is a wide array of radial artery sheath kits. At our center, we use standard short femoral non-hydrophilic sheaths. We first puncture the radial artery with an 18-gauge intravenous angiocath catheter, aiming at transfixing the needle through the posterior wall as soon as backflow is noticed through the needle. After removal of the needle, the establishment of a steady pulsatile arterial flow (with careful gentle retraction) from the hub of the IV cannula confirms its location in the true lumen of the artery. Next, a 50-cm straight tip, fixed core 0.035-in. guidewire is introduced to exchange the IV cannula for a 4- to 7-Fr Terumo Pinnacle 10-cm introducer sheath (Terumo Medical Corporation, Elkton, MD, USA). Alternatively, especially if resistance is encountered when wiring the radial, a 0.035 Bentson wire will be used. Our spasmolytic of choice is 2.5 mg of verapamil via the sheath's side arm, although several cocktails have been tested and used with similar effectiveness. The main additional benefit of using an 18-gauge IV catheter over a micropuncture kit is the possibility to introduce a Bentson or a hydrophilic-coated guidewire (such as the Glidewire, Terumo Corporation, Tokyo, Japan) should the fixed core straight guidewire fail to pass due to vessel tortuosity.

Introducing and Exchanging Coronary Catheters

Insertion of the catheter is performed over a 150-cm J-tip fixed core wire. Fluoroscopy is generally advised as there is a risk that the J-tip inadvertently deflects into the common carotid or internal mammary arteries. Further, having the patient perform a breath hold in deep inspiration will aid the entry of the J-tip wire into the ascending aorta. Another maneuver that will assist the passage of the J-tip wire to the coronary cusps is by clocking the catheter (from RRA), which will turn the catheter away from the descending aorta.

Catheter exchanges can be performed over the 150-cm J-tip wire without the need for exchange-length wires. Having the J-tip wire resting in the coronary cusp, withdrawal of the catheter over the wire is performed until the distal end of the wire just disappears into the hub of the catheter. Next, a 10- or 20-mL Luer lock syringe filled with normal saline is attached followed by simultaneous injection of saline and withdrawal of the catheter, leaving the J-tip wire in place. The maneuver can be performed under fluoroscopy, but experienced operators usually do this without monitoring the tip of the wire. Occurrence of premature systolic contractions will indicate passage of the wire though the aortic valve, which will be corrected by retracting the wire under fluoroscopy. The next catheter is introduced over the 150-cm wire while ensuring its stable position in the coronary cusp. In patients with dilated ascending or unfolded aortas, there is a risk that the proximal third of the J-tip wire prolapse towards the descending aorta, resulting in further advancement of the wire, without externalization from the proximal hub of the catheter. Although such situations could lead to an embarrassing situation of "losing" a wire into the patient, a simple withdrawal of the catheter outside the introducer will invariably expose the proximal end of the J-tip wire. The catheter can then be reinserted on the wire, with an alternative technique of proximal wire control. However, occasional fluoroscopy to ensure the J-tip position will help overcome this difficulty.

Inability to Cannulate the Wire or to Advance the First Catheter

First and foremost is to confirm an arterial location of the sheath by connecting the side arm to the arterial monitoring system. Failure to establish pulsatile flow can indicate either distal spasm at the tip of the introducer, radial artery dissection, false lumen catheter insertion, or venous insertion. If the pulsatile flow was established, but the wire cannot progress beyond the forearm, the operator is likely facing a radial loop or a spasm. Alternatively, wire passage into the brachioradial artery (radial artery with a high origin) or the recurrent radial artery [8] can explain why the catheter will not progress, but this is an unusual situation. As loops and spasms explain most of the difficulties, we tend to simply probe the radial with a Bentson guidewire to see if it will successfully traverse the radial to the brachial artery. Alternatively, a Glydewire can be used, keeping in mind that this type of wire is more prone to engage radial artery side braches and cause perforations. The authors prefer the use of a coronary workhorse guidewire, with an atraumatic coil tip, to navigate through loops and spastic segments, usually with success. Micro-perforations commonly occur after extensive wire manipulation, followed by the performance of a forceful angiography to document the etiology of difficult wire cannulation resulting in a hydraulic worsening of any small wire tip perforation. We thus reserve forearm angiography only to situations where all the earlier steps have failed. If an angiography is warranted, a very careful low-pressure injection of contrast should be performed. Vasospasm can also be managed with a further dose of antispasmolytic agents and/or further sedation, especially if noticed on angiography. Changing the catheter to one of a smaller caliber or to one with a gentler curve (e.g., JR, MP) can assist in negotiating tortuosity. Most importantly, the operator should never force the wire or the catheter. On a rare occasion, the operator has to abandon the radial approach and convert to a contralateral access or the femoral approach. During the procedure in the absence of forearm swelling, should a small perforation of the radial or brachial artery be detected, we generally advise to continue as the presence of the catheter helps seal the perforation. Other techniques include inserting a long arterial sheath [9] or sealing it with a prolonged inflation of a peripheral arterial balloon [10].

Choice of Diagnostic Catheters

The full array of catheters designed for the femoral approach can be used in the TRA. In general, a half-size shorter curve will be required for engaging the left coronary ostium from a

RRA, for instance, a JL3.5 instead of a JL4.0. Some operators may prefer a single catheter for right and left coronary angiography to decrease the risk of vasospasm. This can be accomplished with a Multipurpose, Amplatz Left, or radial specific catheters such as the Barbeau, TIG, Tiger, Jacky, Kimny or Fajadet. Operator preference and experience with each catheter will vary, and thus, we will not recommend one catheter over another. We do however recommend smaller caliber diagnostic catheters (5 Fr) to decrease catheter-induced spasm Chap. 7.

Percutaneous Coronary Intervention

Performance of PCI via a TRA is in general limited to 5- and 6-Fr coronary guides and the occasional 7 Fr in a larger patient. The alternative is utilizing the sheathless 6.5-Fr or 7.5-Fr Eaucath guiding catheter (Asahi Intecc, Japan), which has an inner diameter of 1.78 and 2.06 in., respectively. Notwithstanding, a sheathed 6-Fr guiding catheter can permit the performance of most coronary interventions, including PCI, fractional flow reserve (FFR) and intravascular ultrasound (IVUS), rotational atherectomy (up to 1.75-mm burr), aspiration catheter devices, proximal/distal protection devices, and bifurcation stenting. Because of the hydrophilic coating, it is our opinion that Eaucath guiding catheter provides limited support for complex interventions. Use of 5-Fr systems, although potentially decreasing the risk of radial occlusion, substantially reduces options, allowing only for standard angioplasty and stenting. Occasionally, when the radial is large, a 7-Fr catheter can be safely inserted. Some investigators are commonly using radial Doppler echography to guide catheter size selection. In a large proportion of male patients, 7-Fr catheters can be used to improve support and catheter capacitance.

Guide Catheter Selection and Support

Guide catheter selection for TRA PCI is again guided by operator preference. Please refer to Chap. 6 and 7 (vascular access) for more details. Factors to consider for guide selection for TRA include the restriction to smaller guide catheters; lower, passive support offered from the RRA when using catheters designed for femoral approach; and presence of ostial or proximal stenosis precluding deep engagement. At our center, we generally use Backup type or Amplatz for left coronary intervention and Judkins, Amplatz, or Barbeau for right coronary intervention. Further guide support can be obtained from deeper engagement and/or maintaining active torque while advancing equipment into the coronary artery. Other techniques include more distal placement of guidewires, wires with stiffer shafts, buddy wire, the Hi-Torque Wiggle guidewire (Abbott Vascular, CA, USA) anchoring wire/balloon techniques, and "mother and child" techniques. The GuideLiner (Vascular Solutions, Minnesota) is a simplified mother and child technique, providing a 20–25-cm polymer-coated extension to the coronary guide, enabling the distal delivery of balloons/stents.

Bifurcation lesions can be optimally treated though 6-Fr guides, including when a final kissing balloon is needed. The only exception is the inability to introduce two stents simultaneously through a 6-Fr guide. Therefore, the classical crush technique or a V-stenting approach or simultaneous kissing stent technique is not possible. However, a modified crush technique is possible, whereby the side branch stent is crushed with a dilation balloon in the main branch, followed by insertion of the main branch stent.

Chronic total occlusions (CTO) can also be safely and effectively treated from the transradial approach [11].

Examples of Therapeutic Devices Delivered via a Right Radial Artery Approach

Embrella Embolic Deflector System (Edwards Lifesciences, Irvine, CA, USA) is designed to decrease the incidence of cerebrovascular events during transcatheter aortic valve implantation procedures. The device consisting of a membrane mounted on a dual petal nitinol frame attached to a 110-cm shaft. Deployment of the device to cover the ostia of the left subclavian, left common carotid, and brachiocephalic trunk is performed from the right radial artery via a 6-Fr sheath. This device is in current clinical trials.

Claret Montage (Claret Medical, CA) is a dual filter capture device introduced via a 6-Fr right radial system. The first embolic filter is delivered to the brachiocephalic artery and the second to the left common carotid, to capture and remove dislodged debris during vascular procedures.

Conclusion

Radial artery intervention is safe and effective and has a learning curve that can be easily adopted by most experienced transfemoral interventionalists. In the modern era, very complex PCI can routinely be accomplished via transradial technique and improve patient comfort and satisfaction and reduce adverse events largely on the basis of reduction of major vascular complications associated with femoral access.

References

1. Radner S. Thoracic aortography by catheterization from the radial artery. Acta Radiol. 1948;29:178–80.
2. Campeau L. Percutaneous radial artery approach for coronary angiography. Cathet Cardiovasc Diagn. 1989;16:3–7.

3. Kiemeneij F, Laarman GJ. Percutaneous transradial artery approach for coronary stent implantation. Cathet Cardiovasc Diagn. 1993; 30:173–8.
4. Barbeau GR, Arsenault F, Dungas L, Simard S, Lariviere MM. Evaluation of the ulnopalmar arterial arches with pulse oximetry and plethysmography: comparison with the Allen's test in 1010 patients. Am Heart J. 2004;147:489–93.
5. Brzezinski M, Luisetti T, London MJ. Radial artery cannulation: a comprehensive review of recent anatomic and physiologic investigations. Anesth Analg. 2009;109:1763–81.
6. Kiemeneij F, Vajifdar BU, Eccleshall SC, et al. Evaluation of a spasmolytic cocktail to prevent radial artery spasm during coronary procedures. Catheter Cardiovasc Interv. 2003;58:281–4.
7. Spaulding C, Lefevre T, Funck F, et al. Left radial approach for coronary angiography: results of a prospective study. Cathet Cardiovasc Diagn. 1996;39:365–70.
8. Rodriguez-Niedenfuhr M, Vazquez T, Nearn L, Ferreira B, Parkin I, Sunudo JR. Variations of the arterial pattern in the upper limb revisited: a morphological and statistical study, with a review of the literature. J Anat. 2001;199:547–66.
9. Calvino-Santos RA, Vazquez-Rodriquez JM, Salgado-Fernandez J, et al. Management of iatrogenic radial artery perforation. Catheter Cardiovasc Interv. 2004;61:74–8.
10. Rigatelli G, Dell'Avvocata F, Ronco F, Doganov A. Successful coronary angioplasty via the radial approach after sealing a radial perforation. JACC Cardiovasc Interv. 2009;2:1158–9.
11. Rinfret S, Joyal D, Nguyen CM, Bagur R, Hui W, Leung R, Larose E, Love MP, Mansour S. Retrograde recanalization of chronic total occlusions from the transradial approach; early Canadian experience. Catheter Cardiovasc Interv. 2011;78(3):366–74. doi:10.1002/ccd.23140. Epub 2011 May 18.

14 Percutaneous Cell Therapy for Acute and Chronic Cardiac Disease

Abdul M. Mozid, S. Arnous, and Anthony Mathur

Cell therapy continues to evolve as a promising biological therapy for the treatment of cardiovascular disease. This solution relies on finding a therapeutic approach that overcomes overwhelming cell loss. In acute myocardial infarction (AMI), there is a loss of up to a billion cardiomyocytes with subsequent fibrosis and scar formation leading to remodelling and left ventricular dilatation. These processes were thought to be irreversible, and despite the wide variety of contemporary medical and device therapy, there is no current treatment (with the exception of heart transplantation – which is limited by donor availability) that targets the primary problem of myocyte loss. The human heart seems unable to repair itself despite evidence of ongoing cell division and renewal [1], and it is possible that these innate self-repair mechanisms are overwhelmed by the magnitude of cell loss following injury. This is in contrast to nonmammalian vertebrates such as the zebra fish, which are capable of regenerating up to 20 % of myocardium following injury [2]. The aim of cell therapy is to induce cardiac repair, which may occur either through true myogenesis and/or angiogenesis or through upregulation of innate repair mechanisms. In the acute infarct setting, it is hoped that cell therapy may ameliorate the effects of the initial ischemic insult to reduce myocardial infarct size, prevent adverse remodelling, and preserve left ventricular ejection fraction (LVEF). In chronic heart failure, the aim is to reverse adverse remodelling and improve LVEF, which is an important determinant of morbidity and mortality. In refractory angina, it is hoped that cell therapy can improve symptoms by promoting angiogenesis and increasing myocardial perfusion. It is therefore clear that the aims of cell therapy are different according to the patient being treated, and consequently the type of cell and delivery method may need to be tailored to the individual patient according to the underlying pathological process.

The past decade has seen an exponential growth in clinical studies investigating the safety and efficacy of stem cell therapy in different cardiac disease states. New interventional techniques to deliver this therapy have been developed, and there remains an ongoing need for better delivery systems. These specialized systems require that interventional cardiologists acquire the necessary training and proficiency in these techniques if and when cell therapy is established as potentially beneficial therapy in selected patients. Training programs are already being established around the world following guidelines by the International Society for Cardiovascular Translational Research (ISCTR) providing recommendations for successful training in methods of delivery of biological therapeutic material for cardiac regeneration [3]. In this chapter, we will provide a brief overview of relevant stem cell biology, review the available percutaneous techniques, and provide up-to-date clinical trial data in the setting of acute and chronic cardiac disease states.

Stem Cell Biology

Stem cells are defined by unique characteristics: they are unspecialized cells capable of unlimited self-renewal with the ability to differentiate into more specialized cells and organs. The developing embryo contains embryonic stem cells (ESCs), which are pluripotent as they can develop into cells from all three germinal layers (i.e., mesoderm, endoderm, and ectoderm) and produce all the tissue types needed to form a functional organism.

Developed adult organs also contain undifferentiated stem cells, but in far fewer numbers, these are called adult (somatic) stem cells (ASCs). These cells were thought to be limited in differentiation potential and only able to replenish

A.M. Mozid, BMedSci, MRCP (✉) • A. Mathur, PhD, FRCP
NIHR Biomedical Research Unit, Department of Cardiology, London Chest Hospital, London, UK
e-mail: abdul.mozid@bartsandthelondon.nhs.uk

S. Arnous, BSc, MRCP
Department of Cardiology, London Chest Hospital, London, UK

C.A. Thompson (ed.), *Textbook of Cardiovascular Intervention*,
DOI 10.1007/978-1-4471-4528-8_14, © Springer-Verlag London 2014

and repair injured tissue in the organ that they resided in. However, more recently adult stem cells have been shown to "transdifferentiate" into cell types from different germ layers, a property referred to as plasticity, and this has been demonstrated in several landmark studies [4, 5]. Regenerative medicine is an emerging interdisciplinary field of research, which hopes to utilize the properties of ESCs and/or ASCs in clinical applications focusing on the repair and regeneration of cells, tissues, and organs. The potential of cell therapy to improve cardiac function has been demonstrated in animal models of acute myocardial infarction although the molecular mechanisms through which this improvement occurs remain unclear. Initial studies suggested that benefit was due to myogenesis through stem cell transdifferentiation into cardiomyocytes that replaced injured myocardium [6], but this has not been uniformly reproduced by other groups [7, 8]. This has fuelled the ongoing debate regarding the mechanism of action by which stem cell therapy leads to cardiac repair, and it is likely that the beneficial effects seen are multifactorial in origin. Possible explanations include angiogenesis and vascularization by differentiation into an endothelial phenotype, paracrine effects of the cell infusate, cell fusion, as well as myogenesis [9]. Furthermore, the mechanism of benefit is likely to differ depending on the clinical scenario. In the setting of acute myocardial infarction, the key processes may be neoangiogenesis and paracrine effects of the cell infusate in reducing the initial ischemic and reperfusion injuries. In chronic left ventricular systolic dysfunction, true transdifferentiation of the infused cells into cardiac phenotypic cells to produce neoangiomyogenesis is likely to be required to have any major impact on improving preexisting scar tissue, reversing the adverse remodelling process, and ultimately improving LV function. Hence, it is likely that cell therapy will need to be tailored for the individual patient, and different cell types may be required for different conditions. It is partly for this reason that a variety of cell types have been explored for the purposes of cardiac repair (Table 14.1), and some of these will be discussed in more details below.

Table 14.1 Different cell types that have been investigated for use in cardiac repair

Allogeneic	Autologous (adult stem cells)
Embryonic stem cells	Induced pluripotent stem cells (iPSCs)
Fetal cardiomyocytes	Adipose-derived stem cells
Human umbilical cord-derived cells	Resident cardiac stem cells (cardiospheres)
Human allogeneic mesenchymal stem cells	Epicardium-derived stem cells
	Skeletal myoblasts
	Mesenchymal stem cells (MSCs)
	Bone marrow derived:
	Endothelial progenitor cells (EPCs)
	Mononuclear fraction
	CD34+ fraction

Embryonic Stem Cells

Embryonic stem cells (ESCs) have the broadest developmental potential (pluripotent) since they can give rise to cells of all three embryonic germ layers. Functionally intact cardiomyocytes have been generated from human ESCs in vitro [10], and in a mouse model ESC-derived cardiomyocytes, when injection into the infarcted myocardium, formed stable grafts and subsequently contracted in synchrony with adjacent cells [11].

However, the use of ESCs is associated with teratoma formation in animal models [12] which raises concerns regarding their malignant potential. This, together with the ethical and legal issues surrounding the use of human ESCs, has hampered further research efforts, and current focus is on other sources of stem cells for clinical application of cardiac repair.

Unlike ESCs, autologous adult stem cells appear virtually free from the risks of teratoma formation and immune rejection although display more limited differentiation potential. Adult stem cells that have been studied to date include induced pluripotent stem cells, adipose-derived stem cells, tissue-resident cardiac stem cells, skeletal myoblasts, mesenchymal stem cells, circulating endothelial progenitor cells, and most commonly bone marrow-derived mononuclear stem cells.

Induced Pluripotent Stem Cells

An exciting alternative to ESCs is emerging in the form of *inducible pluripotent stem cells* (iPSCs) which are adult somatic cells that have been successfully reprogrammed back to an undifferentiated pluripotent state by inserting four genes, Oct3/4, Sox2, KL4, and c-Myc, into differentiated somatic cells [13–15]. These cells have the morphological phenotype of ES cells and have been demonstrated in vivo and in vitro to have the same differentiation potential as ES cells (able to form all three germ layers). Functioning cardiomyocytes have already been produced from iPSCs [16] demonstrating their potential use in cardiovascular regenerative medicine although there remain theoretical concerns regarding tumor genesis.

Adipose-Derived Stem Cells

Adipose tissue has been investigated as a source of adult progenitor/stem cells for the purposes of cardiac repair as this tissue contains a heterogeneous mixture of endothelial, hematopoietic, and mesenchymal stem cells which can be easily harvested by liposuction [17]. Preclinical studies have shown that adipose-derived stem cells (ADSCs) are associated with improvement in ejection fraction in animal models of myocardial infarction, and neoangiogenesis via paracrine factors has been postulated as a potential mechanism of action of ADSCs [18, 19]. Clinical trials are currently ongoing and include the APOLLO study (ClinicalTrials.gov Identifier: NCT00442806) and PRECISE study (ClinicalTrials.gov Identifier: NCT00426868), which are assessing the safety and efficacy of ADSCs in acute myocardial infarction and chronic myocardial ischemia, respectively.

Resident Cardiac Stem Cells

The heart has been considered a terminally differentiated organ lacking self-renewal capabilities, but this dogma has been challenged recently, particularly with the demonstration of continued cell division within the adult heart following injury such as myocardial infarction [1]. Several independent investigators have now isolated and identified resident cardiac stem cells which are capable of differentiating into multiple cardiac cell lineages such as cardiomyocytes and vascular smooth muscle cells [20, 21]. These cells have been studied in animal models of myocardial infarction with beneficial outcomes in terms of reducing infarct size and improving LV function [22]. Resident cardiac stem cells are clearly an attractive option for cardiac repair although a harvesting technique remains to be perfected and clinical trials of safety and efficacy are still awaited. The ongoing CArdiosphere-Derived aUtologous Stem CElls to Reverse ventricUlar dySfunction (CADUCEUS) study, which is a phase 1 study recruiting 30 patients to receive autologous cardiosphere-derived stem cells, will hopefully answer some of these questions (ClinicalTrials.gov Identifier: NCT00893360).

Epicardium-Derived Progenitor Cells

As mentioned previously the zebra fish can fully regenerate its heart after injuring up to 20 % of the left ventricle [23]. Recent experimental evidence suggests that this regeneration may occur through limited dedifferentiation of existing cardiomyocytes followed by proliferation [24] and through activation and expansion of surrounding epicardial tissue which supports the regenerating myocardium [25]. These studies in zebra fish suggest that the epicardium may play an important role not only in adult heart repair but also during continuous growth of the adult heart [26]. A subset of epicardium-derived cells (EPDCs) expressing known markers of stem cells, c-kit and the CD34, has been identified in the subepicardial space of fetal and adult human hearts [27]. Experimental studies have demonstrated that EPDCs have the potential to differentiate into cardiomyocytes [28] and intramyocardial injection of human EPDCs in a mouse model of myocardial infarction has been shown to improve cardiac function supporting the hypothesis that EPDCs may play an important role in cardiac repair.

Skeletal Myoblasts

Skeletal myoblasts have been widely studied due to several favorable characteristics: (a) their muscle phenotype with hope for contractile function when transplanted into the heart, (b) autologous source of cells avoiding immune rejection, (c) minimal risk of tumor formation after transplantation, (d) and easily harvested, (e) cell numbers can be increased significantly prior to transplantation, and (f) relatively resistant to ischemia which may help long-term survival in the hostile environment within the diseased heart. Early preclinical animal studies have demonstrated the ability for skeletal myoblasts to engraft, form myotubules, and enhance cardiac function after transplantation into infarcted myocardium [29]. However, not all of the preclinical studies have provided positive results. For example, consistently, studies have demonstrated significant cell loss: up to 84 % loss in the first 24 h and death of the transplanted myoblasts within a few days [30, 31]. Furthermore, transplanted cells downregulate the major adhesion and gap junction proteins, N-cadherin and connexin43, of the intercalated disc [32] and are functionally isolated from the host myocardium with no evidence of electromechanical coupling [33]. This may account for the increased incidence of arrhythmias seen in hearts after myoblast transplantation [34]. Another limitation is that they remain committed to the skeletal muscle lineage, and hence interest in the clinical application of these cells is decreasing.

Bone Marrow-Derived Stem/Progenitor Cells

The most widely studied of the adult stem cells has been bone marrow-derived mononuclear/stem cells (BMSCs). Bone marrow-derived cells consist of hematopoietic stem cells (HSCs), mesenchymal stem cells (MSCs), and endothelial progenitor cells (EPCs), all of which have been shown in preclinical studies to have the potential to transdifferentiate to a cardiomyocyte phenotype [35–37]. BMSCs can also be characterized by specific cell surface markers, for example, CD34, which is expressed on primitive stem cells and differentiated progenitor cells and is absent on mature hematopoietic cells. Additionally, cell populations can be further distinguished by the lineage marker (Lin), which if present represents cells committed to a particular lineage, and the stem cell factor receptor c-kit and the stem cell antigen-1 (sca-1), which are both markers of primitive stem cells.

BMSCs have been demonstrated to transdifferentiate into multiple unexpected cell types including neural cells [38], skeletal muscle [4], and hepatic cells [39]. This "plasticity" of BMSCs has led to considerable excitement in their use in cell-based therapies and as vectors to deliver therapeutic agents. This is particularly attractive clinically because bone marrow can be readily obtained from patients by direct aspiration or by indirect peripheral harvest following mobilization with cytokines such as granulocyte colony-stimulating factor (G-CSF). Also, if a patient's own stem cells were taken for ex vivo expansion and directed to differentiate into a cardiac phenotype, immunogenicity issues are unlikely to occur.

In a landmark animal study, $Lin^{-}c\text{-}kit^{+}$ (markers of undifferentiated stem cells) BMSCs were injected directly into the contracting wall bordering a myocardial infarct which had been acutely induced by coronary artery ligation [6]. The transplanted cells appeared to undergo transdifferentiation to cardiomyocytes with newly formed myocardium occupying a significant proportion of the infarcted area with significant improvement in LV ejection fraction just 9 days after cell transplantation. This study at least in part has prompted the rapid translation into clinical trials assessing the safety and efficacy of BMSCs following AMI in humans – these trials are discussed in detail later.

In summary, multiple cell types have been investigated for their potential to be used in cardiac repair. The ideal cell type(s) remains to be identified. However, recent identification and isolation of resident cardiac stem cells offers hope for cardiac-specific stem cell transplantation. Furthermore the cell type to be used may depend on the clinical condition and myocardial substrate being treated. For instance, the angiogenic potential of BMSCs may be most relevant to the AMI setting, while the myogenic potential of skeletal myoblasts may be more applicable to repair of chronically infarcted myocardium. There is ongoing effort to realize the potential of cellular therapy, and scientists together with clinicians continue to work closely to translate the promising preclinical work into meaningful benefits to patients.

Methods of Cell Delivery

There are currently five distinct methods for delivering cell therapy: (1) peripheral infusion, (2) cell mobilization with cytokines such as G-CSF, (3) transvenous via the coronary sinus, (4) intracoronary infusion, and (5) intramyocardial injection – which can be either transepicardial, transendocardial, or trans-coronary-venous injections (Fig. 14.1). All the

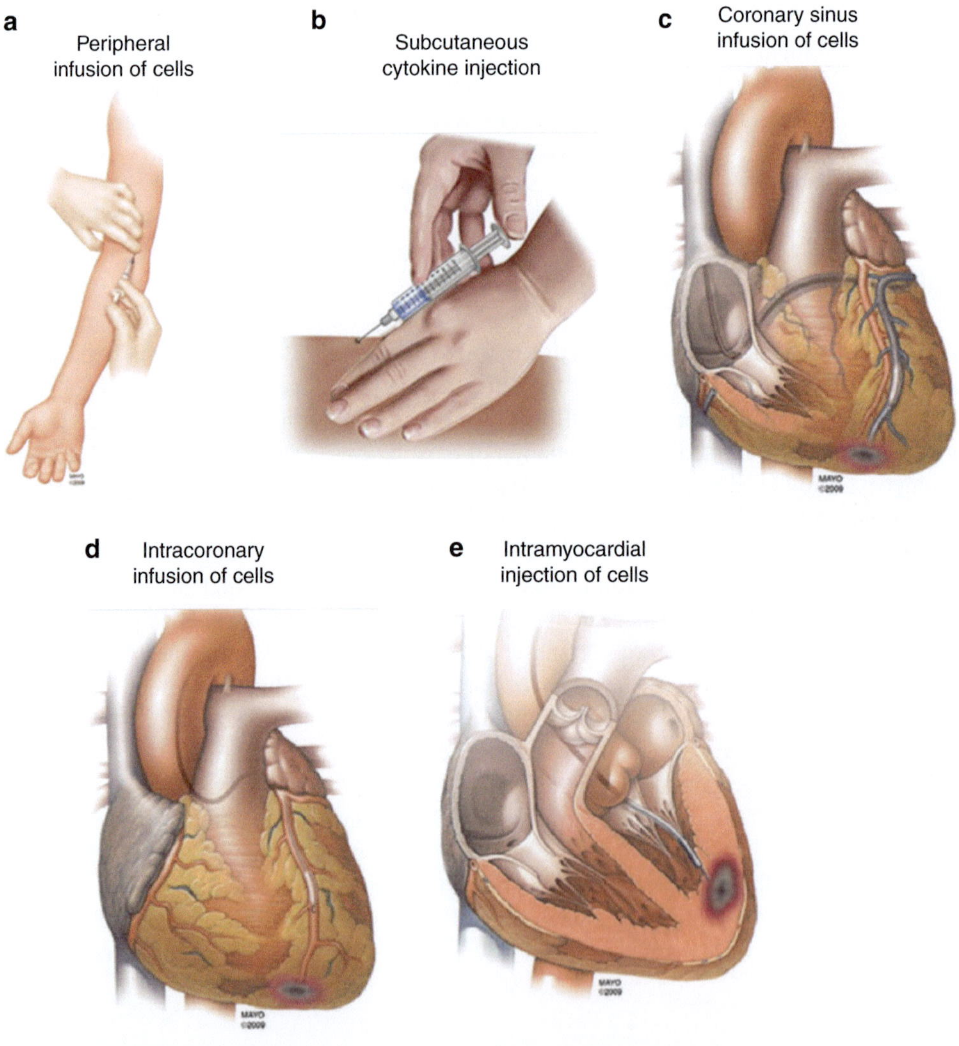

Fig. 14.1 Available methods of delivery for cell therapy. There are currently five different methods for delivering cell therapy: (**a**) peripheral infusion, (**b**) cell mobilization with cytokines such as G-SCF, (**c**) transvenous via the coronary sinus, (**d**) intracoronary infusion, and (**e**) intramyocardial injection – which can be either transepicardial, transendocardial, or trans-coronary-venous injections. Adapted from Gersh et al. [40]

techniques remain in the early stages of clinical investigation, and it remains to be determined which of these will prove to be the most efficacious approach. A limitation common to all current techniques is the low target area cell retention achieved which has been highlighted in a preclinical study [41] that demonstrated maximal cell retention rates within the myocardium of 11 % with intramyocardial injection, 3 % with intracoronary injection, and 3 % with intravenous infusion. There is ongoing work trying to elucidate the reasons for these losses and finding solutions to improve the efficiency of acute cell retention such as combining the cells with a biological scaffold [42]. Numerous scaffold designs have been created for use in cardiac applications using gelatin, fibrin, collagen, and alginates in the form of gels or 3-dimensional (3-D) scaffolds [43, 44].

Peripheral Infusion

Peripheral intravenous infusion of stem cells is an attractive noninvasive method of stem cell delivery due to its simplicity and applicability. Human bone marrow cells have been shown to "home" to peri-infarct areas when infused into the peripheral circulation of a mouse model of acute myocardial infarct [45]. However, this technique may not be suitable in the chronic heart failure setting, which lacks the temporarily upregulated biological homing signals present in the AMI setting. Another significant limitation is that only a few cells appear to reach the affected area due to trapping of the cells in the microvasculature of the lungs, liver, and lymphoid tissues [46]. Peripheral infusion has been extensively used in animal models, but there has been only one human study to date – a placebo-controlled study assessing primarily the safety of peripheral infusion of allogeneic human mesenchymal stem cells (Prochymal™) after acute myocardial infarction [47]. This was confirmed as a safe delivery method, and the treatment group showed significant improvement in symptoms, LV ejection fraction, as well as evidence of reverse remodelling on cardiac MRI. However, given the already small numbers of injected cells that are known to be retained by the heart, it is likely that more direct interventional injection will be more efficacious.

Cell Mobilization

Cell mobilization provides an indirect method of introducing cell therapy to the injured myocardium. In the clinical setting, one of the most studied mobilizing factors is granulocyte-stimulating factor (G-CSF). Endogenous G-CSF is a potent hematopoietic cytokine that affects progenitor cell proliferation, maturation, and functional activation and enhances the mobilization and recruitment of stem cells from the bone marrow to the blood circulation [48]. G-CSF is also proposed to have a range of direct effects on the myocardium, including creating a favorable environment for homing and engraftment of stem cells, inhibiting apoptosis, and promoting cardiomyocyte survival, including angiogenesis and reducing fibrosis associated with adverse cardiac remodelling [49]. G-CSF is generally well tolerated with most common side effects being bone pain and fevers.

Initial preclinical animal studies [50] and phase 1 clinical trials after myocardial infarction showed that G-CSF treatment appeared to be safe with possible beneficial effects on left ventricular systolic function [51, 52]. However, a subsequent randomized placebo-controlled study of subcutaneous G-CSF after primary PCI for AMI showed no additional improvements in left ventricular function when compared to placebo [53]. This was confirmed in a meta-analysis on the effect of G-CSF in AMI which showed no overall benefit although subset analysis showed there may be benefit limited to patients with LV systolic dysfunction and if the infusion is started early [54]. There has also been concerns raised regarding the potential of G-CSF to cause in-stent restenosis (ISR) as it increases the level of circulating neutrophils [55] which may accelerate the process of neointimal proliferation. One of the initial clinical trials reported an unexpectedly high rate of ISR in ten patients treated with G-CSF following an AM [56]. However, a more recent trial involving patients with large infarcts and late revascularization did not show any increased incidence of ISR [57]. Furthermore, an intracoronary intravascular ultrasound (IVUS)-based study, 5 months after stent insertion for AMI, showed no increase in in-stent neointimal hyperplasia in the G-CSF treatment group compared to placebo [58]. Two small, non-randomized, studies have shown possible beneficial effects of G-CSF in chronic ischemic heart failure with regard to patient symptoms and improvement in LV function but also raised concerns regarding worsening of angina during the treatment phase [59, 60]. It remains to be determined if G-CSF treatment could be an effective part of a treatment strategy combining several cytokines and/or local stem cell delivery, and there are ongoing trials of its use (e.g., REGENERATE-IHD [61]) which will provide further data regarding this.

Coronary Sinus Infusion

Retrograde infusion of stem cells through the coronary sinus and coronary venous system has been achieved in experimental models which suggest that this method may provide a more uniform delivery of cells with improved cell retention rates [31]. There have been sporadic case reports [62] demonstrating safety of this technique, but there have not been any published clinical trials of this technique. In this procedure, the coronary sinus is cannulated using a guidewire, and an angioplasty balloon is advanced to the selected cardiac vein related to the coronary artery territory to be treated. The venous blood flow is then halted, by prolonged balloon inflation for approximately 15 min, while the stem cells are infused under pressure. There is yet to be any clinical efficacy data regarding this technique, and the main limitations to this approach are the technical difficulties related to the more variable coronary venous anatomy, which can at times be difficult to negotiate with guidewires and balloons. There are also concerns relating to the potential myocardial injury caused by high-pressure retrograde infusion. This technique may not be possible in patients who already have a coronary sinus device in situ such as a LV lead for resynchronization therapy or a coronary sinus annuloplasty device although cells could be administered as an adjunct to the implantation of such devices.

Intracoronary Infusion

Intracoronary infusion is the method that has been most widely adapted in clinical trials of cell therapy, especially after primary angioplasty for AMI. This method has also been used in patients with heart failure secondary to ischemic heart disease, although in this setting occluded coronary arteries may prevent targeted delivery to the infarcted area. The technique employs the skills of balloon angioplasty and therefore can be performed by an interventional cardiologist with minimal additional training. Cells are infused through the central lumen of an over-the-wire (OTW) balloon catheter during low-pressure balloon inflation for 2–4 min ("stop-flow" technique). Standard short (6–10 mm) balloons are used to minimize endothelial injury, and balloons are also undersized by 0.5 mm less than the reference vessel diameter. Balloon inflation time is empirically chosen, and the purpose is to prolong the contact time between the infused cells and endothelium of the coronary macro-/microcirculation as well as to provide an ischemic stimulus which may improve homing of cells to the target myocardium. Inflation time may need to be curtailed in patients who do not tolerate prolonged occlusion of a clinically important coronary artery. In the AMI setting infusion of cells is limited to the infarct-related artery, while in patients with chronic heart failure, cell infusion may be distributed amongst all patent coronary artery and graft conduits. Some more recent animal work suggests that single bolus infusion may be as effective [63] although stop flow seems to be the prominent method in the published trials.

A preclinical study in dogs raised concerns regarding the possibility of microinfarcts caused by intracoronary injection of mesenchymal stromal cells [64], and there is likely to be a safety threshold with regard to the size and dose of cells delivered using the intracoronary route. Reassuringly, the relative safety of this technique has been confirmed in multiple clinical trials, and a recent meta-analysis of 811 patients confirmed that the relative risks of mortality and morbidity, measured by incidence of reinfarction, arrhythmias, restenosis, hospital readmission, and target vessel revascularization, were not significantly increased in participants who received intracoronary BMSCs following AMI compared with controls [65].

Intramyocardial Injection

Intramyocardial injection is the most direct method of administering cell therapy, and there are several advantages of this technique in patients with heart failure and angina. In contrast to the AMI setting, patients with chronic ischemic cardiomyopathy are unlikely to release signals from damaged myocardium to induce stem cell homing, and theoretically it may be more effective to use intramyocardial injection to deliver the cells to the target area. Also, in the chronic setting the coronary artery subtending the infarct/ischemic area may be occluded without significant collateral formation, and thus intramyocardial delivery provides a means for targeting these areas. Furthermore, experimental data using radionucleotide-labelled BMSCs suggest that target area cell retention may be higher with intramyocardial injection when compared to the intracoronary delivery method [66]. Experience of the intramyocardial route has been mainly limited to chronic conditions due to concerns of myocardial perforation and arrhythmia in the acute setting.

There are currently three methods for intramyocardial injection of cells: open surgical transepicardial injection, percutaneous transendocardial injection, and trans-coronary-venous intramyocardial injection of cells. Earlier clinical trials have relied on surgical transepicardial injection of cells where results are confounded by simultaneous coronary bypass surgery [34, 67–69]. When bypass is not indicated, percutaneous delivery may provide comparable efficacy with reduced risk. Studies in swine models of chronic ischemic heart failure comparing percutaneous and surgical transplantation of skeletal myoblasts have demonstrated that both approaches lead to similar improvements in LVEF and reverse remodelling [70].

Percutaneous transendocardial injection is usually performed via 8Fr femoral access although brachial access for transendocardial injection of stem cells has been reported [71]. A percutaneous approach allows this therapy to be delivered to the higher-risk population and also provides an option for repeated therapy if required. The main additional risks of this approach are ventricular perforation leading to pericardial effusion/tamponade and procedure-related ventricular arrhythmias although the reported incidences of these have been low in the published clinical trials. A deflect-

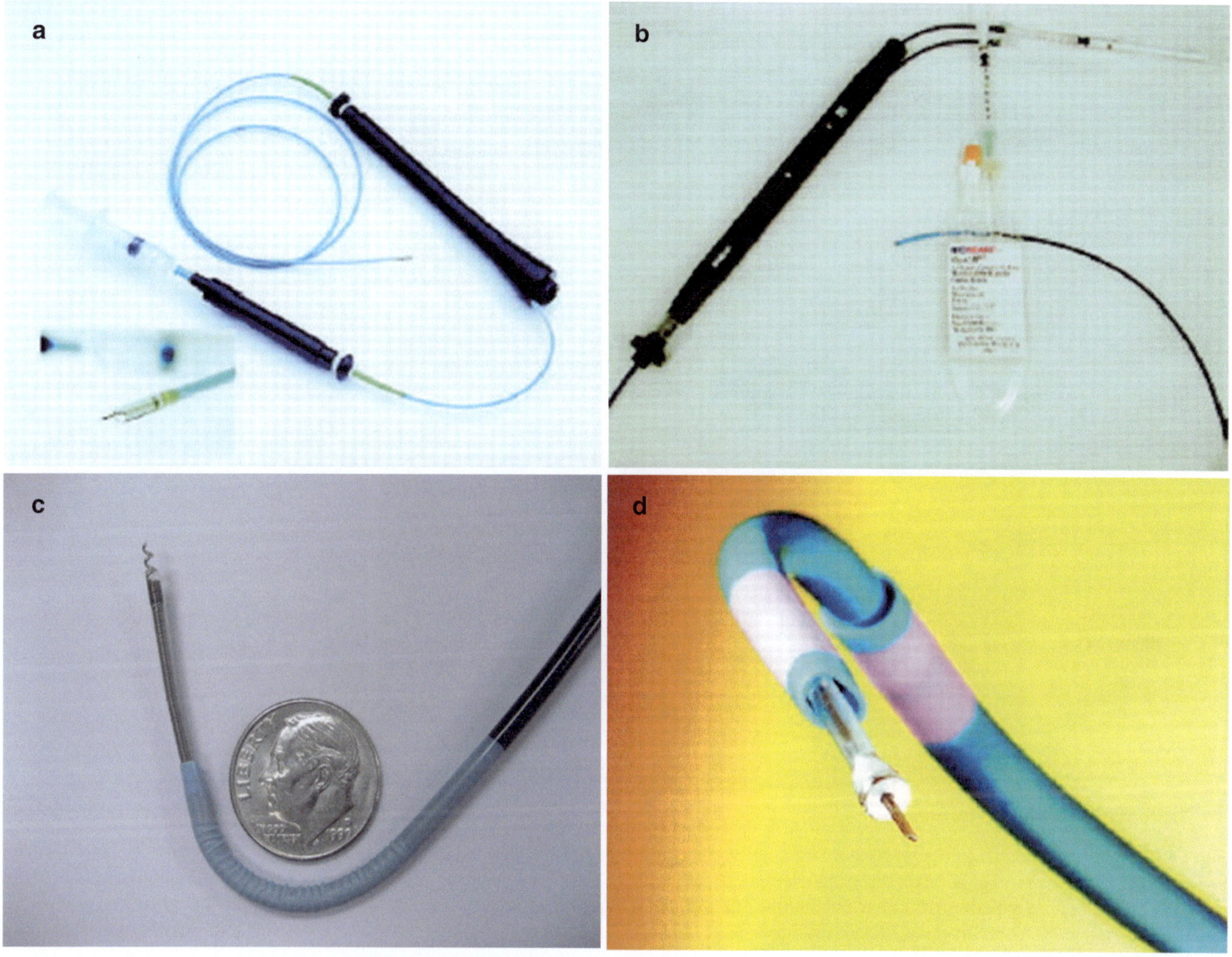

Fig. 14.2 Four commercially available catheters, which are currently under investigational use in clinical trials: (**a**) MyoStar™ (Biosense-Webstar), (**b**) Myocath™ (BioHeart), (**c**) Helix™ (BioCardia), (**d**) Stiletto™ (Boston Scientific)

able tip injection needle catheter is advanced retrogradely across the aortic valve, and cells can be injected directly into any area of the left ventricular endocardium. There are four commercially available catheter systems currently being used for transendocardial cell delivery: the MyoStar™ (Biosense Webster), the MyoCath™ (BioHeart), the Helix™ (BioCardia), and the Stiletto™ (Boston Scientific) catheter delivery systems (Fig. 14.2). The MyoStar™ catheter system utilizes a 3-dimensional (3-D) navigation system to guide injection, and the other three catheters are guided fluoroscopically therefore providing 2-dimensional orientation only. The first two catheter systems are introduced without a guidewire so require manipulation when advanced from the femoral artery and across the aortic valve while the second two catheters are introduced over a traditional guidewire system.

The MyoStar™ mapping catheter system utilizes nonfluoroscopic guidance using the NOGA® (Biosense Webster) magnetic electromechanical system for intramyocardial navigation and mapping (Fig. 14.3). This technique uses ultralow-intensity magnetic fields generated by a triangular magnetic pad positioned beneath the patient and location sensor on the tip of the mapping catheter, which helps determine the real-time location and orientation of the catheter tip inside the left ventricle. The NOGA® system analyzes the movement of the catheter tip at the location of an endocardial point, timed with systole and diastole, and compares it with the movement of neighboring points – the percentage difference represents the degree of mechanical function at that endocardial point. The mapping catheter tip is also capable of measuring endocardial voltage potentials and an electrical map is constructed concurrently with the mechanical map. Healthy endocardium delivers a resting unipolar potential of 15 mV, whereas voltage values less than 6.9 mV reflect scar tissue; potentials between 7 and 15 mV suggest viable myocardium [72]. When the map is complete, all the

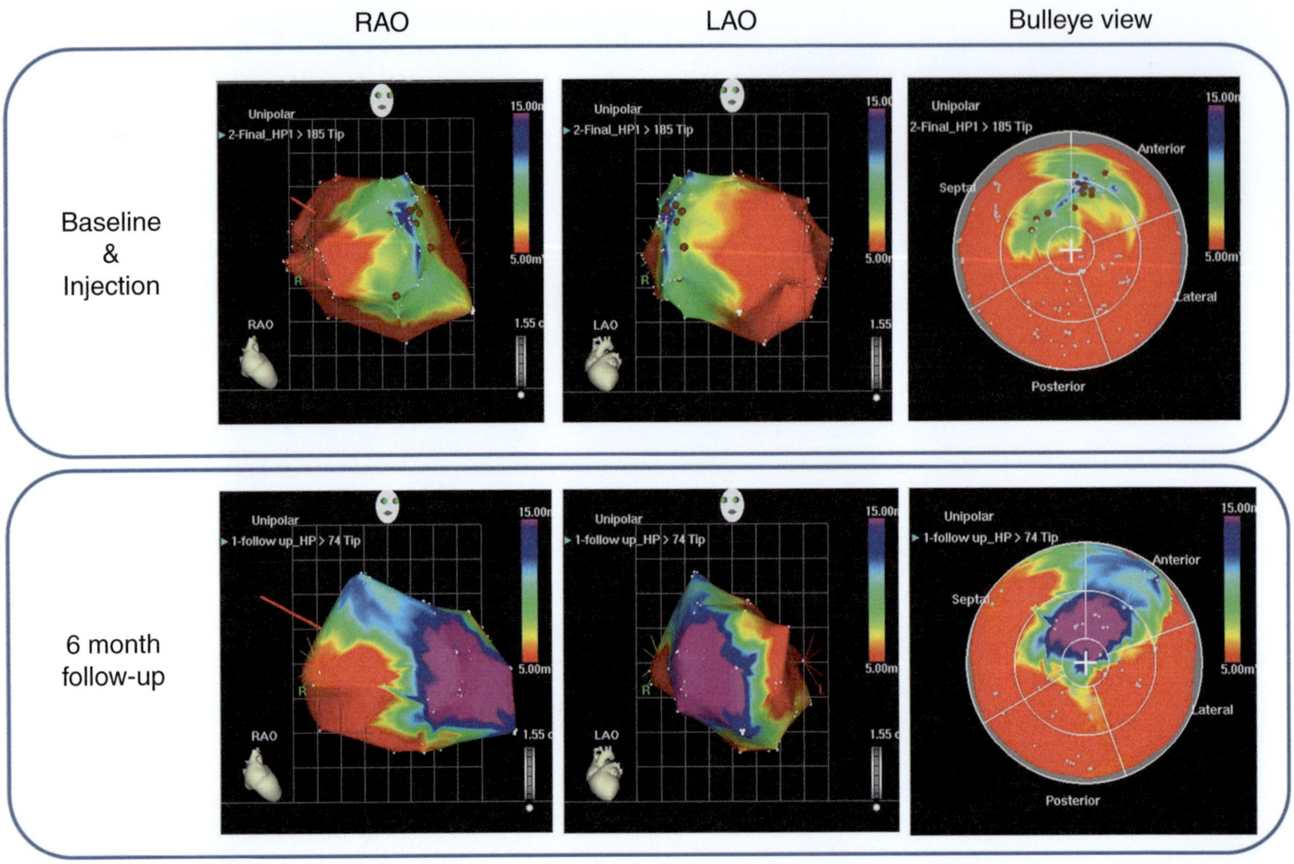

Fig. 14.3 NOGA®-guided injection of bone marrow-derived progenitor/stem cells (BMSCs) using the MyoStar™ catheter in a patient with ischemic cardiomyopathy performed at our institution. The *top panel* represents baseline NOGA® mapping demonstrating a large area of scar tissue (*red*, voltage potential <6.9 mV) and hibernating myocardium (*green-yellow*, voltage potential 7–15 mV) in the anteroseptal regions. The *brown spots* represent injection sites. The *bottom panel* represents repeat NOGA® mapping at 6-month follow-up, and there appears to have been an improvement with more viable myocardium present (*purple*, voltage potential >15 mV)

data points are integrated by the NOGA® workstation and represented in a 3-D color-coded reconstruction of the endocardial surface which is able to distinguish between normal, ischemic (but viable), or infarcted myocardium (Fig. 14.3). Furthermore it allows accurate manipulation of the injection catheter in the left ventricle and therefore precise transendocardial injection. This allows targeted delivery of cells into specific areas, for example, BMSCs tend to be injected into the peri-infarct zone as it has been shown that BMSCs do not engraft well into scarred myocardium compared to skeletal myoblasts which seem capable of engrafting in fibrotic tissue [73]. The main disadvantages of this system are the additional time and costs required to produce an accurate electromechanical map to guide transendocardial injection together with additional operator training.

The MyoStar™ injection catheter (Fig. 14.4) incorporates an integrated injection needle and a location sensor at the tip which interfaces with the NOGA® 3-D mapping system. The 115-cm deflectable tip catheter consists of an outer shaft and inner core lumen, which runs the full length of the catheter and culminates distally in a nitinol 27-gauge needle. The core lumen can be advanced and retracted independently of other catheter movements. The proximal handle contains controls for catheter tip deflection, needle advancement, and the injection port for needle lumen injection. The catheter is prepared by adjusting the retractable needle extension length at 0° and 90° flex, setting the needle length to a maximal needle-to-wall ratio of 0.6. A 1-mL Luer Lock syringe containing the injectate is connected to the injection port, and the catheter "dead space" is filled with the cell suspension prior to introducing the catheter. Multiple injections can be performed at specific sites identified on the 3-D NOGA® electromechanical map – at our institution we perform circumferential 10×0.2-ml injections 1–2 cm apart into the hibernating myocardium around scar tissue. Needle injection into the true apex and myocardial segments with wall thickness less than 0.8 mm should be avoided to minimize the risk of perforation. This technology appears to be associated with a low complication rate in the preclinical and clinical studies performed [72, 74].

The MyoCath™ (BioHeart) injection catheter is similar to the MyoStar™ and consists of a 115-cm long deflectable

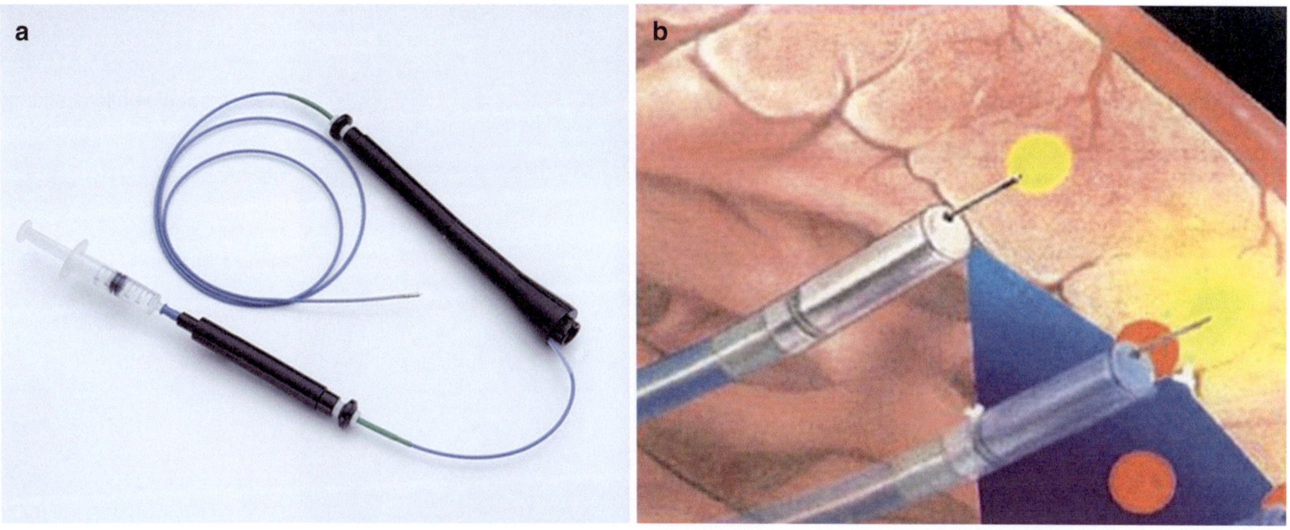

Fig. 14.4 Percutaneous transendocardial injection using the MyoStar™ delivery catheter. (**a**) A flexible, steerable, injection catheter is advanced retrogradely across the aortic valve into the LV cavity, and injections are guided by electromechanical mapping. (**b**) The catheter tip incorporates a fine nitinol 27-gauge needle which is normally retracted (Images courtesy of Biosense Webster, Diamond Bar, CA. © Biosense Webster, Inc., 2012)

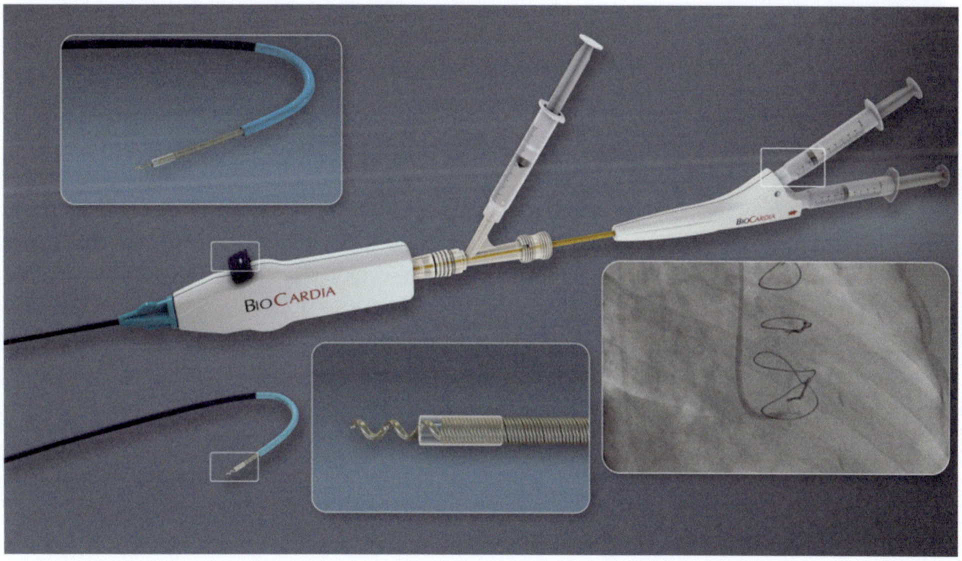

Fig. 14.5 BioCardia Catheter Delivery System. The Helical Infusion Catheter for transendocardial delivery is advanced through the Morph Guide. The therapeutic lumen discharges at the distal tip of the helical needle. A second lumen discharges at the base of the helix for delivering contrast and confirming positioning. The Morph Universal Deflectable Guide Catheter is advanced through the aortic valve over a guidewire and provides the ability to guide the Helical Infusion Catheter (Images courtesy of BioCardia, San Carlos, CA)

injection catheter that also contains an integrated core lumen with a 25-gauge stainless steel needle at its distal end. This can also be advanced and retracted from the tip of the catheter and provides for multiple injections to a predetermined needle insertion depth. The MyoCath™ is however guided by fluoroscopic guidance, and additional imaging such as transesophageal echocardiography is sometimes utilized.

The Stiletto™ (Boston Scientific) catheter (Fig. 14.2d) is also guided fluoroscopically and thus lacks the precision of the NOGA® system although real-time MRI guidance has shown promising results [75]. It contains three separate, independently moveable components: two steerable guiding catheters (9Fr and 7Fr) and an inner spring-loaded needle component. Catheter tip orientation is accomplished by guiding catheter manipulation, and the injection needle is set to a fixed depth (3.5 mm). The spring-loaded advancement mechanism theoretically allows the device to overcome fibrotic scar tissue resistance encountered during needle penetration. This technology is still under investigation; preclinical studies suggest that this is a "safe" technique [76] although higher than expected rates of pericardial effusion has led to the use of the Stiletto™ catheter being halted in the GENASIS investigational trial of VEGF-2 biologic for the treatment of refractory angina.

BioCardia's Helix™ catheter (Fig. 14.5a) has a small, hollow, distal corkscrew needle, which is rotated into the endocardium to provide active fixation (similar to active fixation pacing leads) and to allow local delivery of biological therapeutic products. This catheter is used in combination with the BioCardia Morph® Deflectable (steerable) Guide

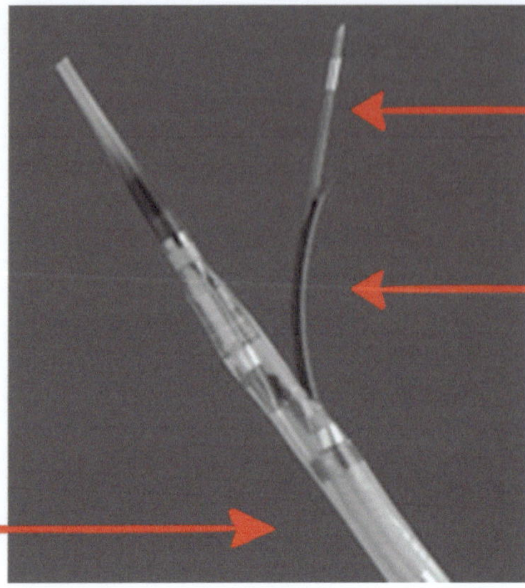

Fig. 14.6 Pioneer (Medtronic, Inc.) catheter tip with IntraLume micro-catheter advanced through the needle tip. IVUS transducer is located at tip of TransAccess catheter

Catheter (Fig. 14.5b) which helps catheter navigation within the LV under fluoroscopic guidance only. By eliminating the process of electromechanical mapping, this technique may have advantages in terms of procedural time and cost. Preclinical studies have proven safety and efficacy of this delivery method [77], and there is preliminary data to suggest that this method may be clinically effective [78].

Trans-coronary-venous intramyocardial (TVIM) injection can be performed using the Pioneer® catheter system (Medtronic Inc., now the Medtronic Pioneer catheter) that is placed percutaneously into the coronary sinus and target vein (Fig. 14.6). Using incorporated intravascular ultrasound (IVUS) guidance, a 24-gauge nitinol needle is extended to perform transvenous myocardial puncture. A 27-guage microinfusion catheter (IntraLume™) is then advanced though the needle to the targeted areas for cell delivery. Initial studies have confirmed the feasibility and safety of this approach in porcine models [79]. A phase 1 clinical trial has confirmed the safety and efficacy of this delivery method of skeletal myoblasts for the treatment of chronic ischemic LV systolic dysfunction [80]. Furthermore, an animal study demonstrated that the TVIM injection of BM-derived mononuclear cells may lead to a greater retention of the cellular product at the target area as compared to intracoronary infusion [81]. The main limitation to this approach is related to the technical difficulties associated with variation in coronary venous anatomy, which can make it difficult to selectively cannulate the target vein.

In summary, several techniques have been trialed for cell delivery in patients with acute and chronic ischemic heart disease. In animal models all routes appear to be equally effective in improving cardiac function although the exact mechanisms of action through which cell therapy may achieve this remains unanswered. There has been translation of all the delivery methods from animal models to humans, and to date the intramyocardial route appears to be the most promising in achieving higher levels of cell retention – whether this translates into improved clinical outcomes is yet to be seen.

Percutaneous Cell Therapy in Acute Myocardial Infarction

The existence of endogenous repair mechanisms as well as the concept of adult stem cell plasticity suggests that cardiac repair may be achieved therapeutically in the setting of AMI. The demonstration of the ability of BMSCs to transdifferentiate into cardiomyocytes and improve LV function following AMI in a mouse model [6] has prompted rapid initiation of human clinical trials. The first-in-man procedure [82] was performed just 1 year after publication of the landmark animal study. A 46-year-old man who had been treated with primary stenting of the LAD for anterior wall myocardial infarction underwent bone marrow aspiration, and after 6 days intracoronary reinfusion of BMSCs was performed during low-pressure balloon inflation in the previously stented segment of the LAD. At 10 weeks after the BMSC infusion, the infarct area had been reduced from 24.6 to 15.7 % and ejection fraction had increased by 20–30 %. There has since been an exponential growth in clinical trials in an attempt to confirm these initial exciting findings. In the following section we discuss some of these trials according to the delivery method employed.

Intracoronary Injection of Cells

Intracoronary delivery of cells has been the preferred method of delivery in the clinical setting, and BMSCs have been the predominant cell type investigated (Table 14.2). In the first human trial, Strauer et al. [83] reinfused intracoronary

Table 14.2 Clinical trials of intracoronary stem cell therapy in acute myocardial infarction

Study name (ref)	Study design	Cell type	*n*	Timing postinfarction	Follow-up period	Primary outcome
Strauer et al. [83] (2002)	NRC	BMSC	20	5–9 days	3 months	Reduction in infarct region from 30±13 to 12±7 %, (*P*=0.005), in cell-treated group
TOPCARE-AMI [84] (2002)	NR	BMSC or PBSC	20	3–6 days	4 months	Improvement in global LVEF from 51.6±9.6 % to 60.1±8.6 % (*P*=0.003)
Fernandez-Aviles et al. [85] (2004)	NR	BMSC	20	8–18 days	6 months	Decrease in end-systolic volume, improvement in regional contractility and global LVEF from 51.3±6.6 % to 57.1±10.4 (*P*=0.002)
BOOST [86] (2004)	RCT	BMSC	60	4.8 days	6 months	Improvement in global LVEF in cell-treated group by 6.7 % compared to 0.7 % in controls (*P*=0.0026), but effect was only maintained in large infarcts at long-term follow-up
Kuethe et al. [87] (2004)	NR	BMSC	5	6 days	3 months	No improvement in global LVEF
Bartunek et al. [88] (2005)	NRC	BMSC	35	12 days	4 months	Reduction in perfusion defect in cell-treated group with improvement in LVEF from 45.0±2.6 % to 52.1±3.5 % (*P*<0.05)
Meluzin et al. [89] (2006)	RCT	BMSC	66	5–9 days	3 months	Dose-dependent improvement of regional myocardial function and global LVEF
LEUVEN-AMI [90] (2006)	RCT	BMSC	69	1 day	4 months	No improvement in global LVEF although there appeared to be significant reduction in myocardial infarct size (BMSC treatment effect 28 %, *P*=0.036)
ASTAMI [91] (2006)	RCT	BMSC	97	6 days	6 months	No improvement in global LVEF
REPAIR-AMI [92] (2006)	RCT	BMSC	204	3–7 days	12 months	Improvement in the global LVEF was significantly greater in the BMSC group than in the placebo group- 5.5±7.3 % vs. 3.0±6.5 % (*P*=0.01)
TCT-STAMI [93] (2006)	RCT	BMSC	20	Immediate	6 months	Improvement in LVEF from 53.8±9.2 % to 58.6±9.9 % (*P*<0.05)
Penicka et al. [94] (2007)	NRC	BMSC	27	9 days	4 months	No improvement global LVEF
Tatsumi et al. [95] (2007)	NRC	PBSC	54	3 days	6 months	Improvement in global LVEF in cell-treated group by 13.4 % compared to 7.4 % in controls (*p*=0.037)
BALANCE [96] (2009)	NRC	BMSC	124	5–9 days	60 months	Reduction in infarct size and improved regional contractility, which was maintained through follow-up. Mortality rate was reduced in cell-treated group
HEBE [97] (2010)	RCT	BMSC or PBSC	200	3–8 days	4 months	No improvement in regional myocardial function or global LVEF

Abbreviations: *BMSCs* bone marrow-derived stem cells, *LVEF* left ventricular ejection fraction, *MSCs* mesenchymal stem cells, *n* number of patients, *NR* nonrandomized, *NRC* nonrandomized with control group, *PBSC* peripheral blood stem cells, *RCT* randomized controlled trial

BMSCs 7 days after AMI. This study appeared to confirm the findings of the earlier animal studies with the cell-treated group showing significant improvement in myocardial perfusion and a reduction in the infarct region compared to controls. Subsequently the TOPCARE-AMI investigators randomized patients into intracoronary infusion of BMSCs or ex vivo expanded circulating progenitor cells 4 days after AMI [84]. This resulted in a significant improvement in global and regional LV function in both groups and a beneficial effect on the postinfarction remodelling process manifest by a profound improvement in wall motion abnormalities in the infarct area and a significant reduction in end-systolic LV volume at 4 months post AMI. The LVEF further improved at 12 months resulting in a total increase of 9.3 % at 1 year [98].

Conversely, the ASTAMI trial, which included only patients with anterior AMI, showed that intracoronary reinfusion of BMSCs 4–8 days after infarction did not have a beneficial effect on LVEF compared to PCI alone at 6 months [91]. This lack of beneficial effect may possibly be explained by the different cell-processing protocols used in this trial. Cell-processing protocols may have a significant impact on the functional capacity of bone marrow-derived stem cells. Comparison of different isolation protocols revealed a vastly reduced recovery of mononuclear cells and nullification of the neovascularization capacity when the ASTAMI cell isolation and storage protocol was used [99].

The BOOST trial included 60 patients that were randomized to receive intracoronary BMSCs or standard therapy 4.8 days post successful PCI following AMI. There was a significant improvement in global LVEF in the cell treatment group at 6 months without an effect on LV remodelling [86]. However, this improvement was only maintained in the largest infarcts at 18 months. The recent HEBE trial, one of the largest trials to date, compared the intracoronary infusion of BMSCs or mononuclear peripheral blood cells to standard therapy alone (without placebo infusion) following an AMI [97]. The intracoronary BMSCs were delivered between 3 and 8 days after AMI. They showed no effect of either treatment on regional or global left ventricular function.

In an attempt to account for the placebo effect, a number of clinical trials have been published where the control group had a bone marrow aspiration procedure and sham placebo reinfusion. In the TCT-STAMI trial, patients who received intracoronary BMSCs immediately after revascularization for AMI had a significant improvement in LVEF at 6 months compared to the control group [93].

The REPAIR-AMI trial, a large randomized double-blind controlled trial which included over 200 patients, showed an improvement in the primary end point in the treatment group which was an absolute change in global LVEF from baseline to 4 months, as measured by quantitative left ventricular angiography [100]. Furthermore, the prespecified cumulative end point of death, MI, or revascularization was significantly reduced, and this benefit was maintained at 1-year follow-up [92]. The mean increase in LVEF in the BMSC group was 2.5 %, and there was an inverse relationship between the baseline EF and the degree of improvement. For example, patients with a baseline EF below the median value (48.9 %) had an absolute increase in global EF that was three times higher than that in the placebo group. In contrast, the improvement in LVEF in patients with a baseline EF that was above the median value was nonsignificant (0.3 %). The timing of cell infusion post PCI also had an effect on the primary end point. Patients in whom the cells were infused ≥5 days post PCI were the only ones who derived benefit.

By contrast, the LEUVEN-AMI study by Janssens et al. showed that intracoronary reinfusion of BMSCs within 24 h of reperfusion, although associated with a greater reduction in infarct size and improvement in regional systolic function, had no effect on the global left ventricular function compared to controls [90]. The very early time point still remains a target for clinical trials. Infusion of BMSCs during the ischemia reperfusion window, i.e., within 6–8 h of reperfusion, may lead to therapeutic benefits seen in the preclinical trials. The REGENERATE-AMI trial (Clinicaltrials.gov Identifier NCT00765453) is currently underway in an attempt to answer this question.

The first long-term study involving patients who underwent intracoronary BMSC transplantation 7 days post AMI not only resulted in an early significant improvement in EF and infarct size, but there was also a trend to significant reduction in mortality and improvement in exercise capacity compared to controls at 5 years [96]. Improved clinical outcome (cumulative end point of death, myocardial infarction, or necessity for revascularization) in the cell treated compared with placebo (hazard ratio, 0.58; 95 % CI, 0.36–0.94; $P = 0.025$) was also seen in the 2-year follow-up data from REPAIR-AMI study (Fig. 14.7) [101].

Meta-analyses [65, 102, 103] of the many randomized controlled trials of intracoronary BMSCs in AMI confirm the technique to be associated with a low complication rate. Using LVEF as a surrogate marker of efficacy, cell therapy appears to be beneficial. The improvement in ejection fraction is comparable in size to that seen in trials of ACEI, thrombolysis, and beta-blockers which have been associated with large reductions in mortality [104]. Larger phase III outcome studies are now needed to assess whether the improvement in surrogate end points translates to a reduction in mortality and morbidity.

Intramyocardial Injection of Stem Cells Following AMI

Cell delivery in the early animal models was performed via direct intramyocardial injection but most of the human studies to date have used intracoronary injection. The first-in-man study of NOGA®-guided intramyocardial injection of BMSCs following AMI (after 10.5 ± 5 days) was performed in 2009 with promising results [105], and there are ongoing studies evaluating this approach. The initial concerns regarding the safety of this technique in the acute setting do not appear to have been realized.

In summary, several trials have now been reported on intracoronary infusion of human BMSCs in the setting of AMI. These studies have uniformly shown that cell therapy is not associated with an increase in adverse events; however, the results on outcome have been heterogeneous. This may be due to a number of reasons including differences in cell isolation and preparation protocols (different number of cells and compositions), the timing of the reinfusion procedure, baseline cardiac fraction, and study design. Interestingly studies with longer-term follow-up have recently demonstrated beneficial effects of BMSC therapy on death and repeat infarction [96, 101] (Fig. 14.7), and the future of this field will depend on large, multicenter, phase III clinical trials that address these hard clinical end points.

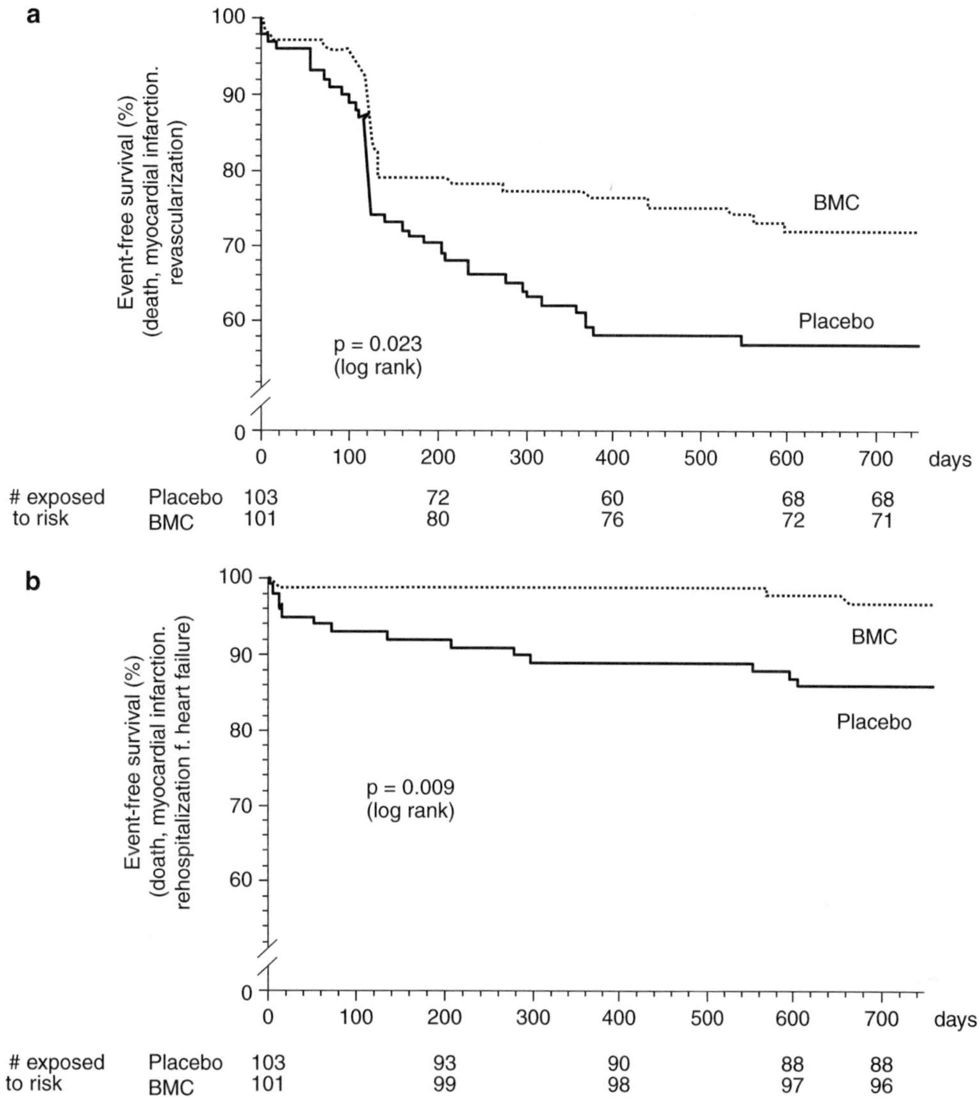

Fig. 14.7 Kaplan–Meier event-free survival analysis in the BALANCE [96] trial of bone marrow-derived progenitor/stem cells (*BMSCs*) in patients with acute myocardial infarction. (**a**) Death, recurrence of myocardial infarction, or revascularization procedures. (**b**) Death, recurrence of myocardial infarction, or rehospitalization for heart failure

Percutaneous Cell Therapy in Chronic Heart Failure

The prevalence of heart failure is ever increasing with an aging population and is estimated that approximately five million people in the USA currently suffer with this condition. The majority of cases are due to ischemic heart disease, and up to 10 % of cases may be due to dilated cardiomyopathy with no evidence of coronary artery disease [106]. Regardless of etiology heart failure is associated with a poor outcome reflected by a 5-year mortality varying from 26 to 75 % [107], a prognosis that is worse than most cancers. These realities have led to intensive efforts to develop novel therapeutic strategies for managing patients with heart failure, and the concept of "interventional treatment of heart failure" has been introduced [108]. Stem cell transplantation has been recognized as one of these emerging therapies with the potential to improve symptoms and long-term prognosis in these patients. Unlike the AMI setting percutaneous transendocardial injection of cells has been the most widely investigated delivery method in patients with heart failure, and skeletal myoblasts have been studied just as extensively as BMSCs. In this section we will review the data from clinical trials of stem cell therapy in patients with heart failure based on method of delivery (Table 14.3).

Table 14.3 Clinical trials of percutaneous stem cell therapy for chronic heart failure

Study name (ref)	Study design	*n*	Cell type	ICM or DCM	Delivery method	Primary outcome
Smits et al. [109]	NR	5	SM	ICM	Transendocardial *MyoStar*™	LVEF increased from 36±11 % to 41±9 % (3 months, $p=0.009$)
CAuSMIC [110] (2009)	NR	23	SM	ICM	Transendocardial *MyoStar*™	Improvement in heart failure symptoms, reduction in LV dimensions, and evidence of improved viability in cell-treated group at 1 year
SEISMIC [111] (2011)	RCT	40	SM	ICM	Transendocardial *MyoCath*™	No change in global LVEF, but there was a trend towards improvement in patient symptoms
Perin et al. [112] (2004)	NRC	20	BMSC	ICM	Transendocardial *MyoStar*™	Improvement in myocardial perfusion and exercise tolerance in cell-treated group but no significant change in LVEF
Beeres et al. [113] (2007)	NR	15	BMSC	ICM	Transendocardial *MyoStar*™	Improvement in regional contractility and global LVEF
Williams et al. [78] (2011)	NR	8	BMSC	ICM	Transendocardial *Helix*™	Improvement in regional contractility and evidence of reverse remodelling
TOPCARE-CHD [114] (2006)	RCT	75	BMSC	ICM	Intracoronary	Improvement in global LVEF by 2.9 % in BMSC-treated group only at 3 months follow-up
DanCell-CHF [114] (2008)	NRC	32	BMSC	ICM	Intracoronary (two infusions 4 months apart)	No improvement in LVEF even with repeated infusions. There was improvement in NYHA class
TOPCARE-DCM [115] (2009)	NR	33	BMSC	DCM	Intracoronary	Improvement in LVEF from 30.2±10.9 to 33.4±11.5 % ($P<0.001$) and microvascular function
STAR-heart [116] (2010)	NRC	391	BMSC	ICM	Intracoronary	Improvement in LVEF and survival in cell-treated group over 5 years follow-up
Vrtovec et al. [117] (2011)	NRC	55	BMSC	DCM	Intracoronary	Improvement in LVEF from 25.5±7.5 % to 30.1±6.7 %, ($P=0.03$) and exercise tolerance

Abbreviations: *ICM* ischemic cardiomyopathy, *DCM* dilated cardiomyopathy, *n* number of patients, *SM* skeletal myoblasts, *BMSCs* bone marrow stem/progenitor cells, *LVEF* left ventricular ejection, *NR* nonrandomized, *NRC* nonrandomized with control group, *RCT* randomized controlled trial

Transendocardial Delivery of Cell Therapy

Percutaneous transcatheter intramyocardial injection of skeletal myoblasts in the treatment of heart failure has shown promise in early phase I/II clinical studies. A pilot study of five patients, published in 2003, demonstrated that NOGA®-guided injection of skeletal myoblasts into the infarcted area of patients with heart failure following previous anterior myocardial infarction was safe with no serious adverse events related to the procedure. There also appeared to be some improvement in regional myocardial thickening as well as global LVEF [109]. The CAuSMIC study also used NOGA®-guided transendocardial injection of skeletal myoblasts into areas of viable myocardium in 12 patients with severe ischemic heart failure. There was improvement in NYHA functional class, quality of life, and evidence of reverse ventricular remodelling when compared to controls after 1-year follow-up [110]. In the SEISMIC trial, a randomized multicenter trial in Europe, 40 patients (14 controls) with ischemic heart failure underwent fluoroscopy-only-guided transendocardial injection of skeletal myoblasts [111] directly into the area of scar using the MyoCath® catheter. Adverse events during follow-up were similar between cell-treated and control groups, and in particular number of arrhythmic events (all patients were required to have an ICD in situ) were also similar. However, although there appeared to be some improvement in patient symptoms, the study failed to show any significant improvement in LVEF. The results of these small studies have prompted the design of larger RCTS including the MARVEL trial (ClinicalTrials.gov Identifier: NCT00526253) which was designed as a randomized, double-blind, placebo-controlled, multicenter phase II/III trial. Enrolment in the MARVEL trial began in October 2007 but unfortunately is currently halted due to limited financial resources.

In view of the underwhelming clinical results with skeletal myoblasts, other cell types are now being investigated. In particular, transendocardial injection of BMSCs has been shown to be safe with potentially beneficial effects. An early nonrandomized trial in 14 patients with severe chronic ischemic heart failure showed that NOGA®-guided intramyocardial injection of BMSCs into viable myocardium appeared to be safe (with no serious adverse events compared to 7 control patients) and was associated with significantly improved regional and global LV systolic function at 6 months [118]. Another nonrandomized study of 20 patients showed that NOGA®-guided intramyocardial injection of BMSCs was again relatively safe and associated with improvements in exercise tolerance and myocardial perfusion [112]. A further small study also showed improvement in patient symptoms and LV function following NOGA®-guided intramyocardial injection of BMSCs [113]. A recent study, using the BioCardia Helix™ catheter system, has confirmed the beneficial effects of BMSCs in chronically infarcted myocardium with improvements seen in regional contractility and evidence of reverse remodelling [78]. There are several ongoing randomized placebo-controlled trials (REGENERATE-IHD [61], TAC-HFT [119], and FOCUS-HF [120]) which will provide important information regarding whether BMSCs provide additional benefit above current optimal therapy.

Intracoronary Delivery of Cell Therapy

There have been relatively few studies assessing intracoronary delivery of BMSCs in chronic ischemic heart failure. In the randomized, crossover design TOPCARE-CHD trial [114], intracoronary delivery of BMSCs showed an improvement in LVEF of 2.9 % with no major adverse cardiac events. In contrast the DanCell-CHF study [116], in which patients received two repeated treatments of intracoronary BMSCs 4 months apart, showed no improvement in LV function at 1-year follow-up although there was significant improvement in patient symptoms. This study adds to the growing belief that using left ventricular ejection fraction (LVEF) as a marker of beneficial effects of cell therapy may be inadequate as patient symptoms do seem to improve without any significant objective change in LVEF. Indeed measures such as VO2 max may be more relevant to patients with heart failure. The STAR-heart study is the largest study to date of BMSC therapy in chronic ischemic heart failure [121]. Of the eligible patients screened, 191 patients underwent intracoronary BMSC therapy, and the control group consisted of 200 patients who declined to have the active intervention. Over a 5-year follow-up period, intracoronary BMSC therapy was associated with significant improvement in LVEF as well as patients' exercise capacity. Interestingly, there was a significant decrease in long-term mortality in the BMSC-treated patients compared with the control group.

There have also been pilot studies of intracoronary BMSC therapy for patients with dilated cardiomyopathy with promising results [115, 117], and randomized controlled trials such as the REGENERATE-DCM [122] and POSEIDON-DCM (ClinicalTrials.gov Identifier NCT01392625) are in progress.

In summary, there have been numerous studies, using different cell types and different delivery methods, assessing whether cell therapy is beneficial in patients with established heart failure secondary to ischemic heart disease and DCM. As in the AMI setting, this early stage of cell therapy appears to be relatively safe with potentially beneficial effects in terms of patient symptoms as well as modest improvements in LV function. Further large multicenter randomized controlled trials are required (and are in process) to define the ideal cell type, delivery method, and patient phenotype that will derive the maximum benefit of this biological therapy.

Percutaneous Cell Therapy in Refractory Angina

Clinical studies are also assessing the safety and efficacy of stem cell therapy for improving symptoms in patients with refractory angina and no further medical or revascularization options (Table 14.4). The end point for these studies has focused on improvement of patient symptoms but has also included objective assessment of changes in myocardial perfusion.

Table 14.4 Clinical trials of stem cell therapy for refractory angina

Study name (ref)	Study design	*n*	Cell type	Delivery method	Primary outcome
Beeres et al. [123] (2006)	NR	20	BMSC	Transendocardial	Improvement in exercise tolerance, CCS class, and myocardial perfusion
Losardo et al. [124] (2007)	RCT	24	BMSC[a] CD34+	Transendocardial	Improvement in exercise tolerance and CCS class. No benefit on myocardial perfusion
PROTECT-CAD [125] (2007)	RCT	28	BMSC	Transendocardial	Improvement in exercise tolerance, CCS class, and myocardial perfusion
Van Ramshorst [126] (2009)	RCT	50	BMSC	Transendocardial	Improvement in exercise tolerance, CCS class, and myocardial perfusion
Losordo et al. [127] (2011)	RCT	167	BMSC[a] CD34+	Transendocardial	Improvement in exercise tolerance in cell-treated group
Lasala et al. [128] (2011)	NR	10	EPC+ MSC	Intracoronary	Improvement in quality of life and myocardial perfusion
Wang et al. [129] (2010)	RCT	112	BMSC	Intracoronary	Improvement in exercise tolerance, CCS class, and myocardial perfusion

Abbreviations: *n* number of patients, *BMSC* bone marrow stem/progenitor cells, *CCS* Canadian Cardiovascular Society functional classification of angina, *NR* nonrandomized, *RCT* randomized controlled study

[a]Bone marrow was mobilized with 5 days of G-CSF prior to cell harvest by peripheral leukapheresis

Intramyocardial Injection of Cells

A nonrandomized study in 2006 involving 20 patients showed that intramyocardial injection of BMSCs was associated with improvement in angina symptoms and also improvement in myocardial perfusion and LV systolic function. There have now been four randomized trials using NOGA®-guided electromechanical mapping to perform intramyocardial injection of stem cells. In a pilot study (24 patients), Losordo et al. [124] showed that intramyocardial injection of autologous peripherally harvested CD34+ BMSCs following bone marrow mobilization was safe and associated with symptomatic improvement in angina class although no clear improvement in myocardial perfusion was demonstrated. The same group has recently published results of a larger follow-up RCT (167 patients) again confirming symptomatic improvement following NOGA®-guided injection of CD34+ cells in patients with refractory angina [127]. The other two studies, PROTECT-CAD [125] and Van Ramhorst et al. [126], have also demonstrated improvements in myocardial perfusion associated with symptomatic improvement following BMSC administration.

Intracoronary Infusion of Cells

Intracoronary administration of stem cells for refractory angina would represent a technically simpler route of administration, and this method has been explored in a large randomized placebo-controlled trial published in 2010 by Wang et al. [129]. In this study 112 patients with intractable angina, diffuse three-vessel coronary artery disease (CAD) not suitable for percutaneous or surgical revascularization, and evidence of perfusion defects on SPECT imaging were randomized to intracoronary injection of BMSCs or placebo. There were no serious adverse events in either group, and the cell-treated group showed reduction in angina episodes and improved myocardial perfusion. Although interesting, intracoronary infusion may be limited to this patient subgroup with diffuse CAD rather than patients with occluded vessels in which intramyocardial injection may be best.

In view of these positive studies showing beneficial effects of cell therapy in patients with refractory angina, larger phase III multicenter trials are now in the planning stages with the hope of establishing whether these results translate into sustained clinical benefit.

Summary

Cell therapy offers an important novel therapeutic strategy for the treatment of a variety of acute and chronic cardiovascular disorders. The potential of many cell types for cardiac repair has been investigated extensively, and it is likely that the ideal candidate will depend on the disease being treated. The advent of biological therapy has also seen the development of novel interventional techniques to deliver this therapy. In the setting of AMI, intracoronary infusion has emerged as the current delivery method of choice, and in more chronic disease states such as heart failure and refractory angina, direct percutaneous intramyocardial injection appears to be possibly the most effective route. New technology is being developed to further improve the ability to target delivery and ensure increased retention of the injected biological product. Educational programs are also being established to provide the training that interventional cardiologists need to ensure standardization and safety. Given that smaller studies using surrogate end points have demonstrated activity, large phase II/III trials with hard clinical end points are awaited. Interventional cardiology will continue to play an important part in this rapidly evolving translational partnership with science.

References

1. Beltrami AP, Urbanek K, Kajstura J, et al. Evidence that human cardiac myocytes divide after myocardial infarction. N Engl J Med. 2001;344(23):1750–7.
2. Chablais F, Veit J, Rainer G, Jazwinska A. The zebrafish heart regenerates after cryoinjury-induced myocardial infarction. BMC Dev Biol. 2011;11:21.
3. Dib N, Menasche P, Bartunek JJ, et al. Recommendations for successful training on methods of delivery of biologics for cardiac regeneration: a report of the International Society for Cardiovascular Translational Research. JACC Cardiovasc Interv. 2010;3(3):265–75.
4. Ferrari G, Cusella-De AG, Coletta M, et al. Muscle regeneration by bone marrow-derived myogenic progenitors. Science. 1998; 279(5356):1528–30.
5. Krause DS, Theise ND, Collector MI, et al. Multi-organ, multi-lineage engraftment by a single bone marrow-derived stem cell. Cell. 2001;105(3):369–77.
6. Orlic D, Kajstura J, Chimenti S, et al. Bone marrow cells regenerate infarcted myocardium. Nature. 2001;410(6829):701–5.
7. Balsam LB, Wagers AJ, Christensen JL, Kofidis T, Weissman IL, Robbins RC. Haematopoietic stem cells adopt mature haematopoietic fates in ischaemic myocardium. Nature. 2004;428(6983): 668–73.
8. Murry CE, Soonpaa MH, Reinecke H, et al. Haematopoietic stem cells do not transdifferentiate into cardiac myocytes in myocardial infarcts. Nature. 2004;428(6983):664–8.
9. Dimmeler S, Zeiher AM, Schneider MD. Unchain my heart: the scientific foundations of cardiac repair. J Clin Invest. 2005;115(3): 572–83.
10. Xu C, Police S, Rao N, Carpenter MK. Characterization and enrichment of cardiomyocytes derived from human embryonic stem cells. Circ Res. 2002;91(6):501–8.
11. Klug MG, Soonpaa MH, Koh GY, Field LJ. Genetically selected cardiomyocytes from differentiating embronic stem cells form stable intracardiac grafts. J Clin Invest. 1996;98(1):216–24.
12. Lee AS, Tang C, Cao F, et al. Effects of cell number on teratoma formation by human embryonic stem cells. Cell Cycle. 2009; 8(16):2608–12.

13. Takahashi K, Yamanaka S. Induction of pluripotent stem cells from mouse embryonic and adult fibroblast cultures by defined factors. Cell. 2006;126(4):663–76.
14. Aasen T, Raya A, Barrero MJ, et al. Efficient and rapid generation of induced pluripotent stem cells from human keratinocytes. Nat Biotechnol. 2008;26(11):1276–84.
15. Takahashi K, Tanabe K, Ohnuki M, et al. Induction of pluripotent stem cells from adult human fibroblasts by defined factors. Cell. 2007;131(5):861–72.
16. Zhang J, Wilson GF, Soerens AG, et al. Functional cardiomyocytes derived from human induced pluripotent stem cells. Circ Res. 2009;104(4):e30–41.
17. Lin K, Matsubara Y, Masuda Y, et al. Characterization of adipose tissue-derived cells isolated with the Celution system. Cytotherapy. 2008;10(4):417–26.
18. Wang L, Deng J, Tian W, et al. Adipose-derived stem cells are an effective cell candidate for treatment of heart failure: an MR imaging study of rat hearts. Am J Physiol Heart Circ Physiol. 2009;297(3):H1020–31.
19. Valina C, Pinkernell K, Song YH, et al. Intracoronary administration of autologous adipose tissue-derived stem cells improves left ventricular function, perfusion, and remodelling after acute myocardial infarction. Eur Heart J. 2007;28(21):2667–77.
20. Beltrami AP, Barlucchi L, Torella D, et al. Adult cardiac stem cells are multipotent and support myocardial regeneration. Cell. 2003;114(6):763–76.
21. Messina E, De AL, Frati G, et al. Isolation and expansion of adult cardiac stem cells from human and murine heart. Circ Res. 2004;95(9):911–21.
22. Oh H, Bradfute SB, Gallardo TD, et al. Cardiac progenitor cells from adult myocardium: homing, differentiation, and fusion after infarction. Proc Natl Acad Sci U S A. 2003;100(21):12313–8.
23. Poss KD, Wilson LG, Keating MT. Heart regeneration in zebrafish. Science. 2002;298(5601):2188–90.
24. Jopling C, Sleep E, Raya M, Marti M, Raya A, Belmonte JC. Zebrafish heart regeneration occurs by cardiomyocyte dedifferentiation and proliferation. Nature. 2010;464(7288):606–9.
25. Lepilina A, Coon AN, Kikuchi K, et al. A dynamic epicardial injury response supports progenitor cell activity during zebrafish heart regeneration. Cell. 2006;127(3):607–19.
26. Wills AA, Holdway JE, Major RJ, Poss KD. Regulated addition of new myocardial and epicardial cells fosters homeostatic cardiac growth and maintenance in adult zebrafish. Development. 2008;135(1):183–92.
27. Limana F, Zacheo A, Mocini D, et al. Identification of myocardial and vascular precursor cells in human and mouse epicardium. Circ Res. 2007;101(12):1255–65.
28. Wessels A, Perez-Pomares J. The epicardium and epicardially derived cells (EPDCs) as cardiac stem cells. Anat Rec A Discov Mol Cell Evol Biol. 2004 Jan;276(1):43–57.
29. Taylor DA, Atkins BZ, Hungspreugs P, et al. Regenerating functional myocardium: improved performance after skeletal myoblast transplantation. Nat Med. 1998;4(8):929–33.
30. Maurel A, Azarnoush K, Sabbah L, et al. Can cold or heat shock improve skeletal myoblast engraftment in infarcted myocardium? Transplantation. 2005;80(5):660–5.
31. Suzuki K, Murtuza B, Fukushima S, et al. Targeted cell delivery into infarcted rat hearts by retrograde intracoronary infusion: distribution, dynamics, and influence on cardiac function. Circulation. 2004;110(11 Suppl 1):II225–30.
32. Reinecke H, MacDonald GH, Hauschka SD, Murry CE. Electromechanical coupling between skeletal and cardiac muscle. Implications for infarct repair. J Cell Biol. 2000;149(3):731–40.
33. Leobon B, Garcin I, Menasche P, Vilquin JT, Audinat E, Charpak S. Myoblasts transplanted into rat infarcted myocardium are functionally isolated from their host. Proc Natl Acad Sci U S A. 2003;100(13):7808–11.
34. Menasché P, Hagège AA, Vilquin J-T, et al. Autologous skeletal myoblast transplantation for severe postinfarction left ventricular dysfunction. J Am Coll Cardiol. 2003;41(7):1078–83.
35. Jackson KA, Majka SM, Wang H, et al. Regeneration of ischemic cardiac muscle and vascular endothelium by adult stem cells. J Clin Invest. 2001;107(11):1395–402.
36. Toma C, Pittenger MF, Cahill KS, Byrne BJ, Kessler PD. Human mesenchymal stem cells differentiate to a cardiomyocyte phenotype in the adult murine heart. Circulation. 2002;105(1):93–8.
37. Badorff C, Brandes RP, Popp R, et al. Transdifferentiation of blood-derived human adult endothelial progenitor cells into functionally active cardiomyocytes. Circulation. 2003;107(7):1024–32.
38. Brazelton TR, Rossi FM, Keshet GI, Blau HM. From marrow to brain: expression of neuronal phenotypes in adult mice. Science. 2000;290(5497):1775–9.
39. Lagasse E, Connors H, Al-Dhalimy M, et al. Purified hematopoietic stem cells can differentiate into hepatocytes in vivo. Nat Med. 2000;6(11):1229–34.
40. Gersh BJ, Simari RD, Behfar A, et al. Cardiac cell repair therapy: a clinical perspective. Mayo Clin Proc. 2009;84(10):876–92.
41. Hou D, Youssef EA, Brinton TJ, et al. Radiolabeled cell distribution after intramyocardial, intracoronary, and interstitial retrograde coronary venous delivery: implications for current clinical trials. Circulation. 2005;112(9 Suppl):I150–6.
42. Dai W, Hale SL, Kay GL, Jyrala AJ, Kloner RA. Delivering stem cells to the heart in a collagen matrix reduces relocation of cells to other organs as assessed by nanoparticle technology. Regen Med. 2009;4(3):387–95.
43. Christman KL, Fok HH, Sievers RE, Fang Q, Lee RJ. Fibrin glue alone and skeletal myoblasts in a fibrin scaffold preserve cardiac function after myocardial infarction. Tissue Eng. 2004;10(3–4):403–9.
44. Masuda S, Shimizu T, Yamato M, Okano T. Cell sheet engineering for heart tissue repair. Adv Drug Deliv Rev. 2008;60(2):277–85.
45. Kocher AA, Schuster MD, Szabolcs MJ, et al. Neovascularization of ischemic myocardium by human bone-marrow-derived angioblasts prevents cardiomyocyte apoptosis, reduces remodeling and improves cardiac function. Nat Med. 2001;7(4):430–6.
46. Gao J, Dennis JE, Muzic RF, Lundberg M, Caplan AI. The dynamic in vivo distribution of bone marrow-derived mesenchymal stem cells after infusion. Cells Tissues Organs. 2001;169(1):12–20.
47. Hare JM, Traverse JH, Henry TD, et al. A randomized, double-blind, placebo-controlled, dose-escalation study of intravenous adult human mesenchymal stem cells (prochymal) after acute myocardial infarction. J Am Coll Cardiol. 2009;54(24):2277–86.
48. Anderlini P, Donato M, Chan KW, et al. Allogeneic blood progenitor cell collection in normal donors after mobilization with filgrastim: the M.D. Anderson Cancer Center experience. Transfusion. 1999;39(6):555–60.
49. Kurdi M, Booz GW. G-CSF-based stem cell therapy for the heart-unresolved issues part A: paracrine actions, mobilization, and delivery. Congest Heart Fail. 2007;13(4):221–7.
50. Orlic D, Kajstura J, Chimenti S, et al. Mobilized bone marrow cells repair the infarcted heart, improving function and survival. Proc Natl Acad Sci U S A. 2001;98(18):10344–9.
51. Kuethe F, Figulla HR, Herzau M, et al. Treatment with granulocyte colony-stimulating factor for mobilization of bone marrow cells in patients with acute myocardial infarction. Am Heart J. 2005;150(1):115.
52. Ince H, Petzsch M, Kleine HD, et al. Prevention of left ventricular remodeling with granulocyte colony-stimulating factor after acute myocardial infarction: final 1-year results of the Front-Integrated Revascularization and Stem Cell Liberation in Evolving Acute Myocardial Infarction by Granulocyte Colony-Stimulating Factor (FIRSTLINE-AMI) Trial. Circulation. 2005;112(9 Suppl):I73–80.

53. Ripa RS, Jorgensen E, Wang Y, et al. Stem cell mobilization induced by subcutaneous granulocyte-colony stimulating factor to improve cardiac regeneration after acute ST-elevation myocardial infarction: result of the double-blind, randomized, placebo-controlled stem cells in myocardial infarction (STEMMI) trial. Circulation. 2006;113(16):1983–92.
54. Abdel-Latif A, Bolli R, Zuba-Surma EK, Tleyjeh IM, Hornung CA, Dawn B. Granulocyte colony-stimulating factor therapy for cardiac repair after acute myocardial infarction: a systematic review and meta-analysis of randomized controlled trials. Am Heart J. 2008;156(2):216–26.
55. Falanga A, Marchetti M, Evangelista V, et al. Neutrophil activation and hemostatic changes in healthy donors receiving granulocyte colony-stimulating factor. Blood. 1999;93(8):2506–14.
56. Kang H-J, Kim H-S, Zhang S-Y, et al. Effects of intracoronary infusion of peripheral blood stem-cells mobilised with granulocyte-colony stimulating factor on left ventricular systolic function and restenosis after coronary stenting in myocardial infarction: the MAGIC cell randomised clinical trial. Lancet. 2004;363(9411):751–6.
57. Engelmann MG, Theiss HD, Hennig-Theiss C, et al. Autologous bone marrow stem cell mobilization induced by granulocyte colony-stimulating factor after subacute ST-segment elevation myocardial infarction undergoing late revascularization: final results from the G-CSF-STEMI (Granulocyte Colony-Stimulating Factor ST-Segment Elevation Myocardial Infarction) trial. J Am Coll Cardiol. 2006;48(8):1712–21.
58. Jorgensen E, Ripa RS, Helqvist S, et al. In-stent neo-intimal hyperplasia after stem cell mobilization by granulocyte-colony stimulating factor Preliminary intracoronary ultrasound results from a double-blind randomized placebo-controlled study of patients treated with percutaneous coronary intervention for ST-elevation myocardial infarction (STEMMI Trial). Int J Cardiol. 2006;111(1):174–7.
59. Joseph J, Rimawi A, Mehta P, et al. Safety and effectiveness of granulocyte-colony stimulating factor in mobilizing stem cells and improving cytokine profile in advanced chronic heart failure. Am J Cardiol. 2006;97(5):681–4.
60. Huttmann A, Duhrsen U, Stypmann J, et al. Granulocyte colony-stimulating factor-induced blood stem cell mobilisation in patients with chronic heart failure–Feasibility, safety and effects on exercise tolerance and cardiac function. Basic Res Cardiol. 2006; 101(1):78–86.
61. Yeo C, Mathur A. Autologous bone marrow-derived stem cells for ischemic heart failure: REGENERATE-IHD trial. Regen Med. 2009;4(1):119–27.
62. Murad-Netto S, Moura R, Romeo LJ, et al. Stem cell therapy with retrograde coronary perfusion in acute myocardial infarction. A new technique. Arq Bras Cardiol. 2004;83(4):352–4.
63. Doyle B, Kemp BJ, Chareonthaitawee P, et al. Dynamic tracking during intracoronary injection of 18F-FDG-labeled progenitor cell therapy for acute myocardial infarction. J Nucl Med. 2007;48(10):1708–14.
64. Vulliet PR, Greeley M, Halloran SM, MacDonald KA, Kittleson MD. Intra-coronary arterial injection of mesenchymal stromal cells and microinfarction in dogs. Lancet. 2004;363(9411):783–4.
65. Martin-Rendon E, Brunskill SJ, Hyde CJ, Stanworth SJ, Mathur A, Watt SM. Autologous bone marrow stem cells to treat acute myocardial infarction: a systematic review. Eur Heart J. 2008; 29(15):1807–18.
66. Makela J, Anttila V, Ylitalo K, et al. Acute homing of bone marrow-derived mononuclear cells in intramyocardial vs. intracoronary transplantation. Scand Cardiovasc J. 2009;43(6): 366–73.
67. Menasche P, Alfieri O, Janssens S, et al. The Myoblast Autologous Grafting in Ischemic Cardiomyopathy (MAGIC) trial: first randomized placebo-controlled study of myoblast transplantation. Circulation. 2008;117(9):1189–200.
68. Ang KL, Chin D, Leyva F, et al. Randomized, controlled trial of intramuscular or intracoronary injection of autologous bone marrow cells into scarred myocardium during CABG versus CABG alone. Nat Clin Pract Cardiovasc Med. 2008;5(10):663–70.
69. Galiñanes M, Loubani M, Davies J, Chin D, Pasi J, Bell PR. Autotransplantation of unmanipulated bone marrow into scarred myocardium is safe and enhances cardiac function in humans. Cell Transplant. 2004;13(1):7–13.
70. Larose E, Proulx G, Voisine P, et al. Percutaneous versus surgical delivery of autologous myoblasts after chronic myocardial infarction: an in vivo cardiovascular magnetic resonance study. Catheter Cardiovasc Interv. 2010;75(1):120–7.
71. Banovic M, Ostojic MC, Bartunek J, Nedeljkovic M, Beleslin B, Terzic A. Brachial approach to NOGA-guided procedures: electromechanical mapping and transendocardial stem-cell injections. Tex Heart Inst J. 2011;38(2):179–82.
72. Kornowski R, Hong MK, Gepstein L, et al. Preliminary animal and clinical experiences using an electromechanical endocardial mapping procedure to distinguish infarcted from healthy myocardium. Circulation. 1998;98(11):1116–24.
73. Agbulut O, Vandervelde S, Al AN, et al. Comparison of human skeletal myoblasts and bone marrow-derived CD133+ progenitors for the repair of infarcted myocardium. J Am Coll Cardiol. 2004;44(2):458–63.
74. Perin EC, Silva GV, Sarmento-Leite R, et al. Assessing myocardial viability and infarct transmurality with left ventricular electromechanical mapping in patients with stable coronary artery disease: validation by delayed-enhancement magnetic resonance imaging. Circulation. 2002;106(8):957–61.
75. Lederman RJ, Guttman MA, Peters DC, et al. Catheter-based endomyocardial injection with real-time magnetic resonance imaging. Circulation. 2002;105(11):1282–4.
76. Goodchild T, Pang W, Tondato F, et al. Safety of intramyocardial injection of autologous bone marrow cells to treat myocardial ischemia in pigs. Cardiovasc Revasc Med. 2006;7(3):136–45.
77. Amado LC, Saliaris AP, Schuleri KH, et al. Cardiac repair with intramyocardial injection of allogeneic mesenchymal stem cells after myocardial infarction. Proc Natl Acad Sci U S A. 2005;102(32):11474–9.
78. Williams AR, Trachtenberg B, Velazquez DL, et al. Intramyocardial stem cell injection in patients with ischemic cardiomyopathy: functional recovery and reverse remodeling. Circ Res. 2011;108(7):792–6.
79. Thompson CA, Nasseri BA, Makower J, et al. Percutaneous transvenous cellular cardiomyoplasty. A novel nonsurgical approach for myocardial cell transplantation. J Am Coll Cardiol. 2003; 41(11):1964–71.
80. Siminiak T, Fiszer D, Jerzykowska O, et al. Percutaneous trans-coronary-venous transplantation of autologous skeletal myoblasts in the treatment of post-infarction myocardial contractility impairment: the POZNAN trial. Eur Heart J. 2005;26(12):1188–95.
81. George JC, Goldberg J, Joseph M, et al. Transvenous intramyocardial cellular delivery increases retention in comparison to intracoronary delivery in a porcine model of acute myocardial infarction. J Interv Cardiol. 2008;21(5):424–31.
82. Strauer BE, Brehm M, Zeus T, et al. [Intracoronary, human autologous stem cell transplantation for myocardial regeneration following myocardial infarction]. Dtsch Med Wochenschr. 2001;126(34–35):932–8.
83. Strauer BE, Brehm M, Zeus T, et al. Repair of infarcted myocardium by autologous intracoronary mononuclear bone marrow cell transplantation in humans. Circulation. 2002;106(15):1913–8.
84. Assmus B, Schächinger V, Teupe C, et al. Transplantation of Progenitor Cells and Regeneration Enhancement in Acute

Myocardial Infarction (TOPCARE-AMI). Circulation. 2002;106(24):3009–17.
85. Fernandez-Aviles F, San Roman JA, Garcia-Frade J, et al. Experimental and clinical regenerative capability of human bone marrow cells after myocardial infarction. Circ Res. 2004;95(7): 742–8.
86. Wollert KC, Meyer GP, Lotz J, et al. Intracoronary autologous bone-marrow cell transfer after myocardial infarction: the BOOST randomised controlled clinical trial. Lancet. 2004;364(9429):141–8.
87. Kuethe F, Richartz BM, Sayer HG, et al. Lack of regeneration of myocardium by autologous intracoronary mononuclear bone marrow cell transplantation in humans with large anterior myocardial infarctions. Int J Cardiol. 2004;97(1):123–7.
88. Bartunek J, Vanderheyden M, Vandekerckhove B, et al. Intracoronary injection of CD133-positive enriched bone marrow progenitor cells promotes cardiac recovery after recent myocardial infarction: feasibility and safety. Circulation. 2005;112(9 Suppl):I178–83.
89. Meluzin J, Mayer J, Groch L, et al. Autologous transplantation of mononuclear bone marrow cells in patients with acute myocardial infarction: the effect of the dose of transplanted cells on myocardial function. Am Heart J. 2006;152(5):975.e9–15.
90. Janssens S, Dubois C, Bogaert J, et al. Autologous bone marrow-derived stem-cell transfer in patients with ST-segment elevation myocardial infarction: double-blind, randomised controlled trial. Lancet. 2006;367(9505):113–21.
91. Lunde K, Solheim S, Aakhus S, et al. Intracoronary injection of mononuclear bone marrow cells in acute myocardial infarction. N Engl J Med. 2006;355(12):1199–209.
92. Schachinger V, Erbs S, Elsasser A, et al. Improved clinical outcome after intracoronary administration of bone-marrow-derived progenitor cells in acute myocardial infarction: final 1-year results of the REPAIR-AMI trial. Eur Heart J. 2006;27(23): 2775–83.
93. Ge J, Li Y, Qian J, et al. Efficacy of emergent transcatheter transplantation of stem cells for treatment of acute myocardial infarction (TCT-STAMI). Heart. 2006;92(12):1764–7.
94. Penicka M, Horak J, Kobylka P, et al. Intracoronary injection of autologous bone marrow-derived mononuclear cells in patients with large anterior acute myocardial infarction: a prematurely terminated randomized study. J Am Coll Cardiol. 2007;49(24): 2373–4.
95. Tatsumi T, Ashihara E, Yasui T, et al. Intracoronary transplantation of non-expanded peripheral blood-derived mononuclear cells promotes improvement of cardiac function in patients with acute myocardial infarction. Circ J. 2007;71(8):1199–207.
96. Yousef M, Schannwell CM, Kostering M, Zeus T, Brehm M, Strauer BE. The BALANCE Study: clinical benefit and long-term outcome after intracoronary autologous bone marrow cell transplantation in patients with acute myocardial infarction. J Am Coll Cardiol. 2009;53(24):2262–9.
97. Hirsch A, Nijveldt R, van der Vleuten PA, et al. Intracoronary infusion of mononuclear cells from bone marrow or peripheral blood compared with standard therapy in patients after acute myocardial infarction treated by primary percutaneous coronary intervention: results of the randomized controlled HEBE trial. Eur Heart J. 2011;32(14):1736–47.
98. Schachinger V, Assmus B, Britten MB, et al. Transplantation of progenitor cells and regeneration enhancement in acute myocardial infarction: final one-year results of the TOPCARE-AMI Trial. J Am Coll Cardiol. 2004;44(8):1690–9.
99. Seeger F, Tonn T, Krzossok N, Zeiher A, Dimmeler S. Cell isolation procedures matter: a comparison of different isolation protocols of bone marrow mononuclear cells used for cell therapy in patients with acute myocardial infarction. Eur Heart J. 2007;28(6):766–72.
100. Schächinger V, Erbs S, Elsässer A, et al. Intracoronary bone marrow-derived progenitor cells in acute myocardial infarction. N Engl J Med. 2006;355(12):1210–21.
101. Assmus B, Rolf A, Erbs S, et al. Clinical outcome 2 years after intracoronary administration of bone marrow-derived progenitor cells in acute myocardial infarction. Circ Heart Fail. 2010;3(1): 89–96.
102. Abdel-Latif A, Bolli R, Tleyjeh I, et al. Adult bone marrow-derived cells for cardiac repair: a systematic review and meta-analysis. Arch Intern Med. 2007;167(10):989–97.
103. Lipinski M, Biondi-Zoccai G, Abbate A, et al. Impact of intracoronary cell therapy on left ventricular function in the setting of acute myocardial infarction: a collaborative systematic review and meta-analysis of controlled clinical trials. J Am Coll Cardiol. 2007;50(18):1761–7.
104. Reffelmann T, Konemann S, Kloner RA. Promise of blood- and bone marrow-derived stem cell transplantation for functional cardiac repair: putting it in perspective with existing therapy. J Am Coll Cardiol. 2009;53(4):305–8.
105. Krause K, Jaquet K, Schneider C, et al. Percutaneous intramyocardial stem cell injection in patients with acute myocardial infarction: first-in-man study. Heart. 2009;95(14):1145–52.
106. Fox KF, Cowie MR, Wood DA, et al. Coronary artery disease as the cause of incident heart failure in the population. Eur Heart J. 2001;22(3):228–36.
107. Cowie MR, Mosterd A, Wood DA, et al. The epidemiology of heart failure. Eur Heart J. 1997;18(2):208–25.
108. Thompson KA, Philip KJ, Barbagelata A, Schwarz ER. Review article: the new concept of interventional heart failure therapy–part 1: electrical therapy, treatment of CAD, fluid removal, and ventricular support. J Cardiovasc Pharmacol Ther. 2010;15(2): 102–11.
109. Smits PC, van Geuns RJ, Poldermans D, et al. Catheter-based intramyocardial injection of autologous skeletal myoblasts as a primary treatment of ischemic heart failure: clinical experience with six-month follow-up. J Am Coll Cardiol. 2003;42(12): 2063–9.
110. Dib N, Dinsmore J, Lababidi Z, et al. One-year follow-up of feasibility and safety of the first U.S., randomized, controlled study using 3-dimensional guided catheter-based delivery of autologous skeletal myoblasts for ischemic cardiomyopathy (CAuSMIC study). JACC Cardiovasc Interv. 2009;2(1):9–16.
111. Duckers HJ, Houtgraaf J, Hehrlein C, et al. Final results of a phase IIa, randomised, open-label trial to evaluate the percutaneous intramyocardial transplantation of autologous skeletal myoblasts in congestive heart failure patients: the SEISMIC trial. EuroIntervention. 2011;6(7):805–12.
112. Perin EC, Dohmann HF, Borojevic R, et al. Improved exercise capacity and ischemia 6 and 12 months after transendocardial injection of autologous bone marrow mononuclear cells for ischemic cardiomyopathy. Circulation. 2004;110(11 Suppl 1): II213–8.
113. Beeres SL, Bax JJ, Dibbets-Schneider P, et al. Intramyocardial injection of autologous bone marrow mononuclear cells in patients with chronic myocardial infarction and severe left ventricular dysfunction. Am J Cardiol. 2007;100(7):1094–8.
114. Assmus B, Honold J, Schachinger V, et al. Transcoronary transplantation of progenitor cells after myocardial infarction. N Engl J Med. 2006;355(12):1222–32.
115. Fischer-Rasokat U, Assmus B, Seeger FH, et al. A pilot trial to assess potential effects of selective intracoronary bone marrow-derived progenitor cell infusion in patients with nonischemic dilated cardiomyopathy: final 1-year results of the transplantation of progenitor cells and functional regeneration enhancement pilot trial in patients with nonischemic dilated cardiomyopathy. Circ Heart Fail. 2009;2(5):417–23.

116. Diederichsen AC, Moller JE, Thayssen P, et al. Effect of repeated intracoronary injection of bone marrow cells in patients with ischaemic heart failure the Danish stem cell study–congestive heart failure trial (DanCell-CHF). Eur J Heart Fail. 2008;10(7):661–7.
117. Vrtovec B, Poglajen G, Sever M, et al. Effects of intracoronary stem cell transplantation in patients with dilated cardiomyopathy. J Card Fail. 2011;17(4):272–81.
118. Perin EC, Dohmann HFR, Borojevic R, et al. Transendocardial, autologous bone marrow cell transplantation for severe, chronic ischemic heart failure. Circulation. 2003;107(18):2294–302.
119. Trachtenberg B, Velazquez DL, Williams AR, et al. Rationale and design of the Transendocardial Injection of Autologous Human Cells (bone marrow or mesenchymal) in Chronic Ischemic Left Ventricular Dysfunction and Heart Failure Secondary to Myocardial Infarction (TAC-HFT) trial: A randomized, double-blind, placebo-controlled study of safety and efficacy. Am Heart J. 2011;161(3):487–93.
120. Willerson JT, Perin EC, Ellis SG, et al. Intramyocardial injection of autologous bone marrow mononuclear cells for patients with chronic ischemic heart disease and left ventricular dysfunction (First Mononuclear Cells injected in the US [FOCUS]): Rationale and design. Am Heart J. 2010;160(2):215–23.
121. Strauer BE, Yousef M, Schannwell CM. The acute and long-term effects of intracoronary Stem cell Transplantation in 191 patients with chronic heARt failure: the STAR-heart study. Eur J Heart Fail. 2010;12(7):721–9.
122. Arnous S, Mozid A, Mathur A. The Bone Marrow Derived Adult Stem Cells for Dilated Cardiomyopathy (REGENERATE-DCM) trial: study design. Regen Med. 2011;6(4):525–33.
123. Beeres SL, Bax JJ, Kaandorp TA, et al. Usefulness of intramyocardial injection of autologous bone marrow-derived mononuclear cells in patients with severe angina pectoris and stress-induced myocardial ischemia. Am J Cardiol. 2006;97(9):1326–31.
124. Losordo DW, Schatz RA, White CJ, et al. Intramyocardial transplantation of autologous CD34+ stem cells for intractable angina: a phase I/IIa double-blind, randomized controlled trial. Circulation. 2007;115(25):3165–72.
125. Tse HF, Thambar S, Kwong YL, et al. Prospective randomized trial of direct endomyocardial implantation of bone marrow cells for treatment of severe coronary artery diseases (PROTECT-CAD trial). Eur Heart J. 2007;28(24):2998–3005.
126. van Ramshorst J, Bax JJ, et al. Intramyocardial bone marrow cell injection for chronic myocardial ischemia: a randomized controlled trial. JAMA. 2009;301(19):1997–2004.
127. Losordo DW, Henry TD, Davidson C, et al. Intramyocardial, autologous CD34+ cell therapy for refractory angina. Circ Res. 2011;109(4):428–36.
128. Lasala GP, Silva JA, Gardner PA, Minguell JJ. Combination stem cell therapy for the treatment of severe limb ischemia: safety and efficacy analysis. Angiology. 2010;61(6):551–6.
129. Wang S, Cui J, Peng W, Lu M. Intracoronary autologous CD34+ stem cell therapy for intractable angina. Cardiology. 2010;117(2):140–7.

Physiologic Evaluation of Patients with Ischemic Heart Disease

15

William F. Fearon

Coronary angiography remains the reference standard for evaluating patients with angina, abnormal noninvasive stress imaging tests, and suspected or known ischemic heart disease. However, numerous studies have revealed the limitations of coronary angiography and, in particular, its inability to accurately detect ischemia-producing coronary artery disease. Recently, more refined methods for invasively determining the functional significance of coronary artery disease have been developed and extensively tested. The goal of this chapter is to review the physiologic evaluation of patients with ischemic heart disease.

Background

The presence of myocardial ischemia is a strong predictor of adverse outcome. The presence and severity of ischemia detected noninvasively with myocardial perfusion imaging correlates directly with the rate of cardiac death during long-term follow-up [1]. Moreover, relieving myocardial ischemia, whether by medical therapy or by coronary revascularization, improves outcomes [2]. Conversely, performing percutaneous coronary intervention on lesions that are not responsible for ischemia does not improve outcomes and may worsen them [3]. Therefore, a primary goal should be to identify patients with a large degree of myocardial ischemia and effectively treat them to reduce their ischemic burden.

Unfortunately, although our noninvasive tests detect the presence or absence of ischemia, their spatial resolution does not provide accurate information regarding the ischemic potential of a particular coronary stenosis in a particular coronary vessel, especially when multivessel coronary disease is present [4]. For these reasons, interventional cardiologists turn to coronary angiography as the reference standard for diagnosing coronary artery disease. However, studies have shown that interventional cardiologists can accurately identify an ischemia-producing lesion when it is angiographically very severe (i.e., >90 % narrowed); however, when it is between 50 and 90 % narrowed on coronary angiography, our ability to determine the lesion's functional significance based on the angiogram alone is poor [5].

The realization that the accurate detection of ischemia-producing lesions and, perhaps as important, nonischemia-producing lesions is critical in determining whether or not to perform percutaneous coronary intervention has led to a shift from the so-called anatomic complete revascularization (i.e., revascularizing all lesions greater than 50 % narrowed) to a new paradigm termed "functional" complete revascularization (i.e., revascularization of only ischemia-producing lesions and medical therapy for nonischemia-producing lesions) [6]. The invasive physiologic evaluation of patients with ischemic heart disease using wire-based techniques to measure indices, such as fractional flow reserve (FFR), allows for a more refined approach to our patients with ischemic heart disease and helps to guide our decisions regarding the need for percutaneous coronary intervention.

Fractional Flow Reserve

FFR is a coronary pressure wire-derived method for assessing the presence of myocardial ischemia. It was described by Pijls and De Bruyne in the early 1990s and is defined as the maximum flow down a vessel in the presence of a stenosis compared to the maximum flow in the hypothetical absence of the stenosis [7]. It is based on the assumption that during maximal hyperemia, myocardial resistance is minimal and constant. In this setting, coronary flow then becomes proportional to coronary pressure.

FFR is easily measured in the cardiac catheterization laboratory by placing a pressure wire in the distal vessel to measure the mean distal coronary pressure during maximal

W.F. Fearon, MD
Division of Cardiovascular Medicine, Stanford University Medical Center, 300 Pasteur Drive, H2103, Stanford, CA 94305, USA
e-mail: wfearon@stanford.edu

C.A. Thompson (ed.), *Textbook of Cardiovascular Intervention*,
DOI 10.1007/978-1-4471-4528-8_15, © Springer-Verlag London 2014

Table 15.1 Unique Aspects of Fractional Flow Reserve

Normal value of 1.0 in all patients and vessels
Independent of the microvasculature
Specific for the epicardial vessel
Not affected by hemodynamic changes
Accounts for collateral flow
Reproducible

vasodilation and dividing this pressure by the mean proximal coronary or aortic pressure, measured with a guiding catheter. The pressure recorded by the guiding catheter in the proximal vessel, or aorta, is a reflection of what the pressure should be in the distal vessel, in the theoretical absence of the stenosis. This is because in a normal epicardial vessel, there is no or minimal loss of pressure and the FFR is 0.94–1.0. In a vessel with significant disease, the FFR may be 0.60, for example, this implies that the myocardium subtended by the vessel being interrogated is receiving only 60 % of the blood flow which it should receive.

FFR is unique because it has an absolute normal value of 1.0 in every vessel and every patient. It is not affected by changes in blood pressure, heart rate, or left ventricular contractility. It is specific for the epicardial vessel and independent of the microvasculature. Finally, FFR has very good reproducibility and is relatively easy to measure (Table 15.1) [8].

Other indices have been introduced for the physiologic assessment of epicardial coronary artery disease. Coronary flow reserve (CFR) preceded FFR and is the best studied. It is defined as peak coronary flow divided by resting coronary flow [9]. CFR is limited by the fact that it interrogates the entire coronary circulation, both the epicardial vessel and the microvasculature. It does not have a clear normal value. It is affected by changes in resting hemodynamics, which limits its reproducibility. For these reasons, FFR has supplanted CFR as the reference standard for the invasively evaluating the physiology of the epicardial coronary artery [10].

Practical Aspects of Measuring FFR

FFR can be measured using one of two commercially available pressure wires. Both the St. Jude Medical and the Volcano Corporation systems use 0.014-in. wires with pressure sensors positioned 3 cm from the tip of the wire at the junction of the radiopaque and radiolucent portion of the wire. One begins by connecting the appropriate pressure wire to the system's console. Most operators use 6-French guiding catheters, but FFR can be measured through 5- and 4-French systems [11].

After administering heparin at a dose of 50–70 units per kilogram and intracoronary nitroglycerin at 100–200 μg, the pressure wire is calibrated and advanced out of the guiding catheter such that the sensor is positioned at the catheter's ostium. In this position the pressure wire recording is equalized to the guiding catheter pressure recording. The wire is then advanced to the distal two-third of the vessel being investigated. If one has difficulty advancing the wire, one can disconnect it from interface connector, to improve torqueability. Rarely, it is necessary to first wire the vessel with another wire and then position the pressure wire through an exchange catheter. If this is the case, the pressure wire must be equalized outside of the exchange catheter in the proximal vessel, removed from the vessel, and then positioned in the distal vessel through the exchange catheter.

Once the pressure wire is in position, hyperemia is achieved usually by administering intracoronary or intravenous adenosine. The dosage and advantages of each hyperemic agent will be discussed below. FFR is then measured as the mean distal pressure divided by the mean proximal pressure, during maximal hyperemia. The lowest value achieved is taken as the FFR.

In many cases, there is a focal lesion with some degree of diffuse coronary disease. In this setting, slowly pulling the pressure wire back during maximal hyperemia allows one to determine exactly where the pressure gradient is being generated and whether or not stenting the focal lesion will have a significant impact on the FFR. If there is a discrepancy between the pressure wire recording and the guiding catheter recording when the pressure sensor has been pulled back and positioned at the ostium of the guiding catheter, then drift in the pressure recording either from the wire or guiding catheter has occurred. Occasionally, flushing the guiding catheter with saline to remove contrast will eliminate this apparent drift. If not, then the FFR can be corrected by taking into account the drift, or the wire can be reequalized, and FFR can be remeasured once the wire is positioned again in the distal vessel.

If the lesion in question is deemed physiologically significant, percutaneous coronary intervention (PCI) can be performed using the pressure wire as the guidewire. After performing PCI, the pressure wire can be reconnected to the interface connector and FFR can be remeasured to assess the effect of PCI. It is important to wipe the distal end of the wire with a wet and then a dry gauze before reconnecting to the interface connector.

Inducing Hyperemia

One of the most important components to the accurate measurement of FFR is insuring that maximal hyperemia has been achieved. In order to fully assess the functional significance of a lesion, it is critical to maximize flow across the lesion and in that way simulates exercise. It is important to remember that the greater the flow across a particular stenosis, the greater the gradient and the lower the FFR.

FFR was originally validated using intravenous adenosine administered at 140 μg/kg/min via a central venous line (typically via the femoral vein); this method has been shown to induce maximal hyperemia, and for these reasons, intravenous adenosine is considered the reference standard and preferred approach [12]. In general, maximal hyperemia is achieved within 1 min after beginning the infusion. Typically, there will be a rise in mean aortic or proximal pressure, followed shortly thereafter by a decline in mean aortic pressure from the baseline. The distal pressure will not rise as much and will then decline more than the mean proximal pressure, depending on how severe the stenosis. FFR is measured at the lowest value during maximal hyperemia. Occasionally, heart block or other arrhythmias can create isolated drops in the FFR, which should be ignored.

When administered from a central vein, there is no advantage to increasing the dose of intravenous adenosine if one suspects inadequate hyperemia [12]. In this case, it is important to recheck the infusion to make sure it has been mixed and dosed correctly and that the stopcock on the venous sheath is positioned appropriately so that the infusion is entering the patient's body. When administered from a peripheral vein, it may take longer before maximal hyperemia is achieved. In addition, there may be respiratory variation in the FFR due to variability of venous return from the peripheral vein. The lowest FFR value should be taken as the true FFR. From the peripheral vein, there may be an advantage to increasing the dose of adenosine to 280 μg/kg/min, if submaximal vasodilation is suspected, because of the short half-life of adenosine.

Intravenous adenosine is advantageous because hyperemia lasts as long as the infusion is continued, which allows for accurate measurement of FFR and the ability to perform a slow pullback of the pressure sensor in order to differentiate focal from diffuse disease or to assess serial stenoses in the same vessel. Intravenous adenosine does usually cause shortness of breath and/or chest discomfort, which is well tolerated, especially if the patient has been forewarned. It is also helpful, in a sense, because if the patient does not have this sensation, one should be concerned about whether maximal hyperemia has occurred, especially if the pressure gradient does not increase. Rarely, intravenous adenosine can cause bronchoconstriction in patients with severe asthma or chronic obstructive pulmonary disease. Another potential drawback to intravenous adenosine is that in the United States, it is more expensive than intracoronary adenosine.

Intracoronary adenosine should be administered through a guide catheter without sideholes and which is well seated in the coronary to insure that the medication is not spilling out into the aorta. Doses of at least 50 μg should be used at first and the operator should readily increase to at least 100 μg [13]. Occasionally, in the right coronary artery or dominant circumflex, transient heart block will occur. Hyperemia occurs immediately after administration so it is important to record pressure right after giving the adenosine. Peak hyperemia lasts on the order of 15–20 s. There are no significant side effects to intracoronary adenosine and in the United States, it is inexpensive. The main drawbacks to using intracoronary adenosine are that in a small portion of patients, maximal hyperemia is not achieved, when compared to intravenous adenosine [13]. In addition, because of the short half-life, a slow pullback of the pressure sensor cannot be performed.

Adenosine, delivered either via an intravenous or intracoronary route, is the most common drug used to achieve hyperemia. Outside of the United States, adenosine triphosphate is commonly used and acts in a similar fashion to adenosine. Papaverine is another medication that has been used in the past. In some respects, it is an ideal hyperemic agent. It is inexpensive and can be given easily using an intracoronary route. Maximal hyperemia lasts about 1 min, which allows one to get an accurate measurement of FFR and to perform a pullback of the pressure sensor. The major drawback to papaverine is that it can cause significant arrhythmias. In 1–2 % of patients, papaverine can cause ventricular tachycardia or torsades de pointes [14]. This side effect has limited the use of papaverine. In small studies, dobutamine and nitroprusside have been tested and shown to be useful hyperemic agents [8, 15]. The main drawback to dobutamine is the time it takes to achieve peak hyperemia, and the main drawback to nitroprusside is hypotension. Finally, there are a number of new selective adenosine 2 receptor agonists being tested or recently approved. These have the advantage of less dyspnea and chest pain when compared to adenosine [16]. More data and experience are necessary with the use of these agents (Table 15.2).

Table 15.2 Hyperemic agents

Agent	Administration	Peak effect	Side effects	Comments
Adenosine (or ATP)	IV at 140 μg/kg/min	Duration of infusion	Dyspnea, chest pain	Reference standard
Adenosine (or ATP)	IC at 40 to >100 μg	15 s	Transient AV block	Does not allow pullback
Papaverine	IC at 10–20 mg	60 s	Torsades de pointes	Not used commonly
Nitroprusside	IC at 0.3–0.9 μg/kg	30 s	Hypotension	Not well studied
Dobutamine	IV at 20–50 μg/kg/min	Duration of infusion	Tachycardia	Slow onset
Regadenoson	IV bolus of 0.4 mg	2–3 min	Dyspnea, chest pain, headache	Not well studied with FFR

ATP adenosine triphosphate, *IV* intravenous, *μg* microgram, *kg* kilogram, *mg* milligram

Common Pitfalls of FFR Measurement

The most common pitfall when measuring FFR is not achieving maximal hyperemia. This usually occurs because the hyperemic agent is not delivered properly, for example, intracoronary adenosine entering the aorta predominantly, instead of the coronary due to poor seating of the guiding catheter or due to use of a guiding catheter with sideholes. Another example can occur when intravenous adenosine is given through a very small peripheral vein, resulting in metabolism before it reaches the heart. One should suspect inadequate hyperemia when the patient does not develop the typical dyspnea and chest heaviness with intravenous adenosine or when there is no change in the resting gradient with intracoronary adenosine.

The guiding catheter can be the source of another potential pitfall. If the coronary ostium is small or if there is some degree of ostial disease, then the guiding catheter, even if only 6 French, can sufficiently obstruct flow down the coronary so that maximal hyperemia does not occur [17]. This can be recognized by a ventricularized pressure tracing from the guiding catheter. It is easily corrected by simply unseating the guiding catheter, thereby allowing maximal hyperemia and an accurate measurement of FFR (Fig. 15.1).

The ingestion of caffeine soon before FFR measurement has been a concern because caffeine is a competitive inhibitor of the adenosine A2a receptor. However, in a small study, FFR was measured before and after patients were exposed to the equivalent of 2–3 cups of caffeine. The average FFR did not change significantly as a result of caffeine ingestion [18].

A final pitfall to consider when concerned about a false negative FFR is exercise-induced vasoconstriction. A patient may have a moderate stenosis, which itself is not ischemia-producing, but which contributes to a significant stenosis when the patient exercises and develops exercise-induced vasoconstriction. This scenario can result in angina and an abnormal exercise test. It is possible that a patient has this condition, but when FFR is measured in the catheterization laboratory with a pharmacologic agent inducing hyperemia, instead of exercise, vasoconstriction does not occur and the residual fixed stenosis is not severe enough to lead to an ischemic FFR [19].

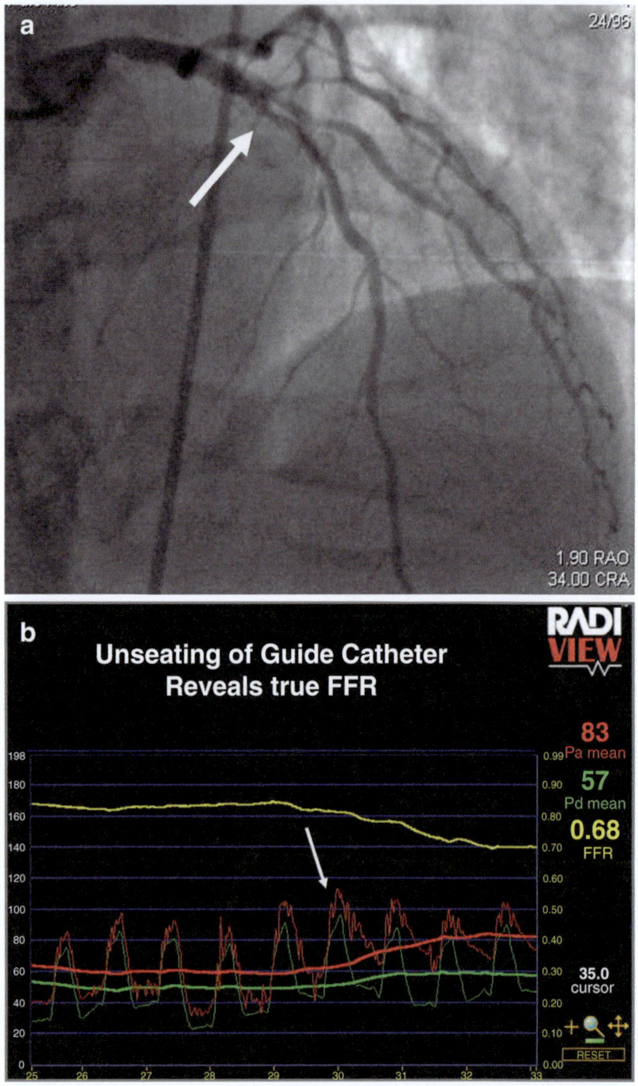

Fig. 15.1 (**a**) Deep-seated guide. Angiogram of the left coronary artery revealing mild ostial left main disease and moderate left anterior descending disease (*white arrows*). (**b**) Deep-seated guide. The *red tracing* represents pressure recorded from the guiding catheter, and the *green tracing* represents pressure recorded from the pressure wire. Initially, the guide is deep seated resulting in ventricularization of the pressure recording and blunting of the gradient and true FFR. After unseating the guiding catheter, maximal flow down the vessel can be achieved and the true FFR is displayed. After stenting the left anterior descending lesion, the FFR was 0.85, indicating that the combination of the ostial left main disease and the residual diffuse disease in the left anterior descending was not causing ischemia

FFR in Intermediate Coronary Disease

FFR was originally validated in patients with intermediate single-vessel coronary disease. In a landmark paper, Pijls and colleagues compared FFR in 45 consecutive patients with an intermediate coronary stenosis to a combination of three different noninvasive stress tests for reversible myocardial ischemia [20]. If anyone of the three stress tests was abnormal, the patient was diagnosed with ischemia. By incorporating all three stress tests into the definition of myocardial ischemia based on noninvasive testing, using Bayesian considerations, the authors established a reference standard with a very high accuracy to which FFR could be compared. In all 21 patients with an FFR < 0.75, at least one stress test was abnormal, giving FFR a specificity of 100 % using this cutoff. Of the 24 patients with an FFR ≥ 0.75, 21 had no ischemia on all 3 noninvasive stress tests, giving a sensitivity of 88 % and a diagnostic accuracy of 93 %.

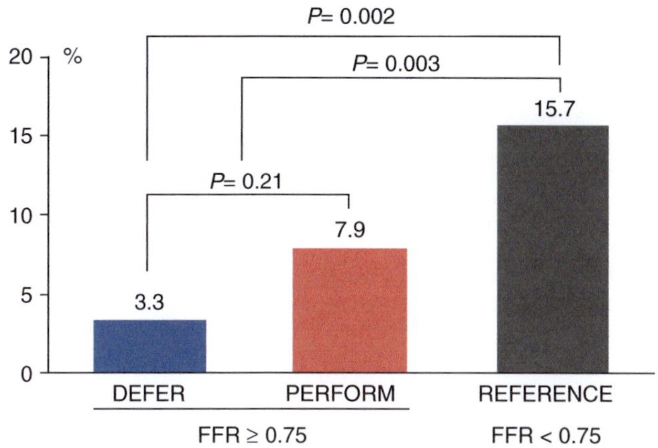

Fig. 15.2 DEFER study: 5-year cardiac death and myocardial infarction. Data from the DEFER trial showing low rates of cardiac death or myocardial infarction in patients with hemodynamically insignificant lesions assigned to medical therapy (DEFER arm), as compared to those subjected to percutaneous coronary intervention (PERFORM arm). The REFERENCE group represents patients with hemodynamically significant lesions treated with PCI (From Pijls et al. [3], with permission)

Another important study establishing the safety of deferring PCI in patients with intermediate coronary disease and FFR values ≥0.75 was a randomized study evaluating 325 patients with moderate coronary lesions [21]. FFR was measured and if ≥0.75, the patient was randomized to either PCI or medical therapy. In the 91 patients randomized to deferral of PCI, the major adverse event rate at 2 years was 11 % compared to 17 % ($p=0.27$) in the 90 patients with FFR ≥ 0.75 who were randomized to performance of PCI. Of note, the percentage of patients free from angina at 2 years was 70 % in the deferral group and 51 % in the performance group ($p=0.02$). These findings were extended to 5-year follow-up in a subsequent publication which demonstrated continued safety of deferring PCI of lesions which are not hemodynamically significant [3]. The cardiac death and myocardial infarction rate at 5 years was 3.3 % in the deferral patients and 7.9 % in the performance group ($p=0.21$) (Fig. 15.2). Other studies have confirmed the excellent outcomes of patients in whom PCI was deferred based on FFR values ≥0.75 [22].

These data confirm that nonischemia-producing lesions when treated medically have a low event rate which is equal to or lower than the event rate when these lesions are revascularized with PCI. Ischemia-producing lesions (FFR < 0.75) appear to have a higher event rate when treated medically. For example, in a study of 107 patients with intermediate lesions and normal nuclear perfusion scans in the region subtended by the vessel with the intermediate lesion, the investigators measured FFR [23]. PCI was deferred on all of the lesions because the nuclear scan was normal. At 1 year, the major adverse event rate in the 14 % of patients in whom the FFR was <0.75 was significantly higher than in the patients in whom the FFR was ≥0.75 (27 % versus 9 %, $p<0.04$). In another study of 407 patients with intermediate coronary lesions, the major adverse event rate was 21 % in the 34 patients with an FFR in the ischemic zone in whom revascularization was deferred compared to 6 % in the 99 patients with an ischemic FFR who were revascularized [24]. These data suggest that ischemia-producing lesions based on FFR measurement are at high risk for causing future events when treated with medical therapy alone.

FFR and the "Grey Zone"

Numerous studies from different investigators comparing FFR to a variety of noninvasive stress tests in a variety of patient populations have established a narrow cutoff value for FFR between 0.75 and 0.80 for identifying ischemia [25]. Most studies found that if the FFR was below 0.75, there is a 100 % specificity for ischemia. However, the sensitivity is less. By extending the cutoff value to 0.80, one loses a small amount of specificity, but gains sensitivity (fewer false negatives). From a practical perspective, if the FFR down a vessel is <0.75, one can be fairly certain myocardial ischemia is inducible, and if there is a focal narrowing, revascularization will improve symptoms and may improve prognosis. If the FFR is >0.80, then one can be fairly certain that significant ischemia is not present and multiple studies have shown excellent outcomes with medical therapy alone. When the FFR falls between 0.75 and 0.80, then one should apply clinical judgment. If the lesion is in the proximal left anterior descending artery and the patient has typical symptoms, then revascularization may be warranted. However, if, for example, the patient has atypical symptoms or no symptoms, an equivocal or negative noninvasive stress test, a diffuse pressure gradient on slow pullback of the pressure sensor without a focal step-up across the lesion, or is undergoing preoperative evaluation for noncardiac surgery, then one might opt for medical therapy.

FFR in Multivessel Coronary Disease

In patients with multivessel coronary disease, the diagnostic accuracy of noninvasive stress imaging studies is worse than in patients with single-vessel disease [4]. One of the advantages of an invasive assessment of coronary physiology with FFR is its unsurpassed spatial resolution. A patient with three-vessel coronary disease may have an unimpressive nuclear perfusion scan because of balanced ischemia [26]. However, FFR assessment of each vessel can determine the contribution of each to the patient's ischemia and symptoms.

Another common scenario is a patient with inferior ischemia on a noninvasive stress test and an occluded right coronary artery, which receives collaterals from a left anterior descending coronary artery, which itself has a moderate proximal lesion. The nuclear scan tends to identify the area of greatest ischemia in the inferior region of the left ventricle and may not detect less severe ischemia in the anterior region. FFR assessment of the left anterior descending artery allows determination of whether the moderate lesion is also contributing to the patient's symptoms and potentially compromising the collaterals to the right coronary artery.

A final scenario highlighting the superior spatial resolution of FFR is the vessel with tandem lesions or a focal lesion within diffuse disease. By performing a slow pullback of the pressure wire, one can often identify the region responsible for the majority of the pressure gradient and thereby focus PCI to the area. This will be discussed in further detail below.

Because of its excellent spatial resolution, one might anticipate that FFR would be useful in guiding PCI in patients with multivessel coronary disease. This was tested in the fractional flow reserve versus Angiography for Multivessel Evaluation (FAME) trial, a prospective, multicenter, international, randomized study comparing an FFR-guided strategy to an angiography-guided strategy for performing PCI in over 1,000 patients with multivessel coronary disease [6, 27]. In order to be included in this study, patients were required to have two or three major epicardial vessels with >50 % stenoses, which the operator felt required PCI with drug-eluting stents based on the angiographic appearance and the clinical scenario. Patients with previous coronary artery bypass graft surgery, significant left main disease, or within 5 days of an ST segment elevation myocardial infarction, were excluded from the study. Once the operator identified which lesions were to be stented, the patient was then randomized to either angiographic guidance or FFR guidance. If randomized to angiographic guidance, the operator stented all of the identified lesions. If randomized to FFR guidance, FFR was measured first and only if <0.80 was the lesion stented. The primary endpoint of the study was 1-year rate of major adverse events including death, myocardial infarction, or the need for repeat revascularization.

At 1 year, the average number of stents placed per patient in the 509 patients randomized to FFR guidance was significantly lower than the number placed in the 496 patients randomized to angiographic guidance (2.7 versus 1.9, $p<0.001$). The amount of contrast required was also significantly less (302 versus 272 mL, $p<0.001$). Yet, the time to perform the procedure was similar in both groups (70 versus 71 min, $p=0.51$), likely because although measuring FFR may add sometime to the procedure, by decreasing the number of lesions which require PCI, it also significantly saves time and contrast.

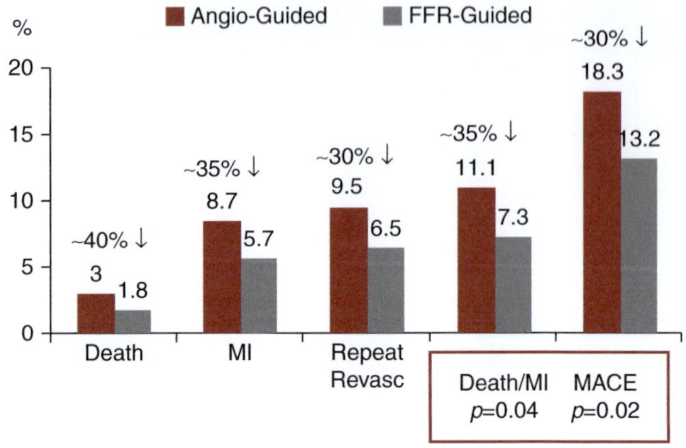

Fig. 15.3 FAME trial: 1-year outcomes. Data from the FAME trial [6] demonstrating a 30–40 % reduction of each endpoint with FFR-guided PCI as compared to angiography-guided PCI. The combination of death and myocardial infarction (*MI*) was significantly reduced, as was the primary endpoint, major adverse cardiac events (*MACE*)

The main finding from the FAME trial, however, was the significant decrease in major adverse events at 1 year; these occurred in 18.3 % of the angiography-guided patients and 13.2 % of the FFR-guided patients ($p=0.02$). This was due to similar relative reductions of 30–40 % in the occurrence of each component of the primary endpoint, death, MI, and the need for repeat revascularization (Fig. 15.3). In addition, the rate of death and MI alone was significantly reduced by FFR guidance from 11.1 to 7.3 %, $p=0.04$. These findings have been extended out to 2 years, in a subsequent publication showing a continued significant decrease in the rate of death and MI by FFR guidance from 12.9 to 8.4 %, $p=0.02$ [28].

The results of the FAME study support a new paradigm termed "functionally complete" revascularization, as opposed to the traditional anatomic complete revascularization. For many years we have focused on revascularizing every angiographically significant coronary stenosis. FAME has taught us that the functional significance of the lesion should dictate whether or not PCI is performed, not the angiographic appearance. In the FFR-guided patients in the FAME study, 20 % of those lesions between 70 and 90 % narrowed had an FFR > 0.80 and did not require PCI [29]. Of the lesions which were 50–70 % narrowed, only 35 % had an FFR ≤ 0.80 and required PCI. This resulted in over 500 angiographically significant appearing lesions being treated medically. At 2 years, the rate of MI and the rate of revascularization for these deferred lesions were only 0.2 and 3.2 %, respectively, providing further reassurance in the safety of this approach [28].

These data also help us to understand why the FFR-guided strategy was superior to the angiography-guided one. If the event rate in functionally nonsignificant lesions is so low with medical therapy, then PCI is unlikely to improve the situation. By performing PCI on these lesions anyway, one incurs the short-term and longer-term risks of PCI, such as myocardial infarction, stent thrombosis, and restenosis, without reaping the reward of relieving myocardial ischemia. FFR guidance allows the operator to achieve complete relief of ischemia (functionally complete revascularization), but avoids unnecessary PCI of nonischemia-producing lesions.

The additional information obtained from FFR may have important implications on our treatment decisions in patients with multivessel disease. The SYNTAX score, an angiography-based grading system, has been advocated as a means for deciding whether or not a patient with multivessel coronary disease would have a better outcome with coronary artery bypass graft surgery or with PCI [30]. This approach stems from data showing that patients with more complex coronary disease resulting in a high SYNTAX score tended to have better outcomes when randomized to coronary artery bypass grafting instead of PCI in the SYNTAX study [31]. However, the SYNTAX score is limited by the fact that it is based on the coronary angiogram. We have a greater appreciation now regarding the inability of one to determine if a stenosis is functionally significant when basing that decision on the angiogram alone.

Recently, a functional SYNTAX score was proposed, in which only lesions with an FFR $\leq$ 0.80 are scored when calculating the SYNTAX score, and functionally insignificant lesions are neglected [32]. The functional SYNTAX score was calculated in the FFR-guided patients in the FAME study and compared to the traditional SYNTAX score. Roughly one-third of the higher risk patients moved to a lower risk group after calculating the functional SYNTAX score. In addition, the functional SYNTAX score was a better predictor of outcomes compared to the SYNTAX score. The functional SYNTAX score will need to be tested prospectively, but it may be a more accurate method for determining the best treatment option and prognosis in patients with multivessel coronary disease.

A final important component to the FFR-guided strategy tested in the FAME study was the economic aspect. Of course, measuring FFR adds costs to a procedure, both for the wire and the hyperemic agent. In a formal analysis incorporating equipment costs as well as follow-up costs in the FAME study, the FFR-guided strategy saved more than $2,000 per patient at 1 year ($14,315 versus $16,700, $p < 0.001$) [33]. A bootstrap simulation showed that the FFR-guided strategy was cost-saving in over 90 % of cases and cost-effective in over 99 % (Fig. 15.4). It is unusual in medicine of a new strategy to not only improve outcomes but to also save resources.

The more recent FAME II study extends the importance of hemodynamic assessment comparing PCI with medical therapy in ischemic heart disease. This trial was halted early after enrollment of 1,220 patients due to a significant reduction in the combined endpoint of death, myocardial infarction, and urgent revascularization in the PCI group (4.3 %) compared with medical therapy (12.7) ($P < 0.001$). These results and subsequent economic analysis continue to support that ischemia reduction with PCI is crucial to improve outcomes [34].

FFR in Particular Patient Subsets

Acute Coronary Syndromes

There are particular patient subsets in which FFR is either contraindicated or should be used with caution. For example, in the setting of ST segment elevation myocardial infarction, FFR should not be used to assess the culprit vessel. Acute myocardial infarction results in microvascular dysfunction. Depending on the scenario, some component of this microvascular dysfunction may be reversible and improve with time. If one measures FFR in the acute setting, the variable degree of microvascular stunning will lead to a maximum achievable flow down the vessel which is lower than normal, a gradient which is smaller and an FFR which is higher than one would expect for a given stenosis. With time, the microvasculature may recover, maximum achievable flow may increase, and a larger gradient with a lower FFR may be measured across a given stenosis. Studies have shown that sometime after 3–6 days, the stunning has resolved in most cases and FFR reliably correlates with the presence of ischemia detected by noninvasive imaging tests [35, 36].

In the setting of an old myocardial infarction, FFR is still reliable. Although the maximum achievable flow down a vessel will be less than normal and the gradient across a stenosis lower than expected resulting in an FFR that is higher than one would expect for a given stenosis, the higher FFR is not falsely elevated, but reflects the smaller amount of viable myocardium supplied by the vessel and still provides information about the expected gain in flow after PCI.

There has been concern about measuring FFR in non-culprit vessels in patients with ST segment elevation myocardial infarction. Some data suggest that global reversible microvascular dysfunction might occur in this setting [37]. This might falsely elevate the FFR in a non-culprit vessel. However, in a recent study, patients presenting with acute coronary syndromes, including ST segment elevation myocardial infarction, had FFR measured in a non-culprit vessel at the time of presentation and again an average of 30 days later [38]. There was no significant difference in the mean FFR value at baseline compared to 30 days later. In only 2 of the 101 patients were FFR > 0.80 at baseline and lower than 0.75 at follow-up.

In patients with non-ST segment elevation myocardial infarction, FFR appears to be reliable in both the culprit

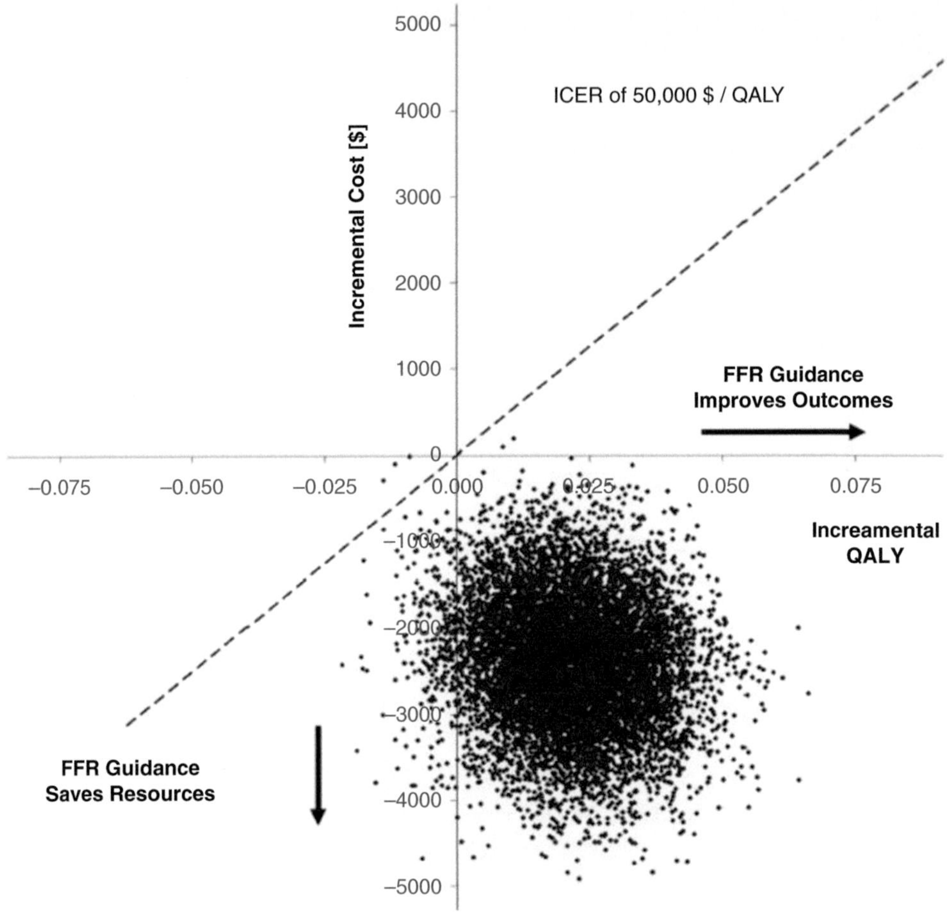

Fig. 15.4 Economic evaluation of an FFR-guided PCI strategy. Bootstrap simulation from data from the FAME trial [33] demonstrating that an FFR-guided strategy is cost-effective in over 99 % and cost-saving in over 90 %

vessel and the non-culprit vessel. In the FAME study, patients with non-ST segment elevation myocardial infarction could be included during the acute setting, as long as the peak creatinine kinase was<1,000 U/L. A substudy demonstrated that the FFR-guided strategy was equally beneficial in patients with acute coronary syndromes as those without in the FAME study [39].

Congestive Heart Failure

Patients with severe left ventricular dysfunction and/or overt congestive heart failure have not been well studied with FFR. The strict definition of FFR is distal coronary pressure minus venous pressure divided by aortic pressure minus venous pressure. In general, venous pressure is ignored because it is usually near zero and much lower than the coronary pressure. However, it is possible that a patient in heart failure might have a venous pressure of 20 mmHg and a mean distal coronary pressure of 40 mmHg and a mean aortic pressure of 60 mmHg. In this case, the calculation of FFR without accounting for the venous pressure would be 0.66, while it would be 0.50 after accounting for the venous pressure. For these reasons, FFR should be used with caution in patients with severe left ventricular dysfunction.

Left Ventricular Hypertrophy

Left ventricular hypertrophy is another condition which might impact FFR assessment. In patients with left ventricular hypertrophy, the myocardium can outgrow the vasculature. This might make myocardial ischemia more easy to induce. Therefore, a moderate lesion resulting in an FFR of 0.83, above the usual ischemia threshold, could potentially be ischemia producing in someone with significant left ventricular hypertrophy. These considerations are theoretical and have not been studied well. It is reassuring that in large trials, like the FAME study, patients with left ventricular hypertrophy were not excluded and FFR remained a useful tool.

Left Main Disease

The role of FFR in assessing patients with left main coronary disease has been studied well. Numerous small studies and one large study have found that using an FFR cutoff value between 0.75 and 0.80 to defer intervention on intermediate left main disease is safe and results in good outcomes [40–42]. Practical considerations when measuring left main disease include the use of intravenous adenosine because it allows the operator to make sure the guide catheter is disengaged from the coronary ostium so that maximal flow down the vessel can be achieved. It also allows the operator to perform a slow pullback of the pressure sensor and better determine to what degree the left main disease is contributing to any observed gradient.

One potential pitfall to using FFR to assess the significance of left main disease is the presence of high-grade downstream disease in either the proximal left anterior descending or in a large circumflex artery. Lesions in either daughter vessel will impact maximal flow across the parent vessel, in this case the left main. So even if one places the pressure wire in a nondiseased circumflex in order to get a "true" assessment of the left main, if there is a high-grade proximal left anterior descending artery lesion, it may decrease the maximum flow across the left main lesion and increase the FFR reading in the circumflex. If one were to remeasure the FFR in the circumflex after stenting the left anterior descending lesion, the flow across the left main might be greater and the FFR lower. This theoretical concern has not been studied well and its clinical importance is not clear.

Serial Stenoses

The presence of tandem or serial stenoses is another clinical situation in which measuring FFR can be quite useful, if performed appropriately. Because each stenosis affects flow across the other, one needs to be careful when interpreting the "FFR" across each lesion. For example, the ratio of the pressure recorded between two stenoses and the proximal coronary pressure may be 0.85 during maximal hyperemia before intervention. After stenting the distal lesion, the flow down the vessel and across the proximal lesion may now be greater because of the decrease in resistance. This may result in a ratio of the pressure recorded just distal to the proximal lesion and the proximal coronary pressure which is now 0.80.

There are complex formulae which were derived and tested by Pijls, De Bruyne, and colleagues and which allow determination of the true FFR of each lesion, separate from the other, before any intervention is performed [43, 44]. But this requires measuring the coronary wedge pressure, and for practical purposes, the equations are not clinically applicable. The practical method for assessing tandem stenoses is to first place the pressure sensor distal to both lesions. If the FFR is above 0.80, then the lesions are not causing ischemia and medical therapy is warranted.

If the FFR is $\leq$0.80, then a slow pullback of the pressure wire should be performed. One should look for at least a 0.10 or greater change in the ratio between the pressure wire and guiding catheter across a focal stenosis before considering stenting. After the pullback, if one of the lesions was more responsible than the other for the abnormal FFR, then the operator should perform PCI on that lesion first. If both were equally responsible, then technical considerations, such as treating the distal lesion first, should dictate which lesion is addressed first. It is critical to then remeasure FFR afterward stenting the first lesion, because with the increased flow down the vessel after removing one lesion, the other lesion may become more significant and also warrant PCI. Certainly, if the FFR across the remaining lesion is $\leq$0.80, then PCI should be performed on the remaining lesion.

FFR After Stenting

There are numerous studies evaluating the role of FFR measurement after stenting. The post-stent FFR appears to correlate with intravascular ultrasound parameters, although FFR normalizes before optimal intravascular ultrasound dimensions are achieved [45]. Despite this, studies have shown that FFR measured after bare-metal stenting predicts major adverse events. In a large registry of 750 patients, the FFR after bare-metal stenting was>0.90 in roughly two-third of the patients, and the death, myocardial infarction, and need for repeat revascularization were between 5 and 6 % at 6 months [46]. In the one-third of patients in whom the FFR was $\leq$0.90, the event rate was 20.3 %. In a small study evaluating FFR measured after drug-eluting stenting in 80 patients, the major adverse event rate, primarily due to repeat revascularization, was significantly higher in the patients with a post-stent FFR $\leq$ 0.90 compared to those with an FFR > 0.90 (12.5 versus 2.5 %, $p<0.01$) [47]. The explanation for the correlation between FFR after stenting and events is likely multifactorial due to stent-related issues, such as underexpansion or edge dissection, and due to the extent of diffuse atherosclerosis outside of the stent, both of which can decrease post-stent FFR and increase the incidence of future events.

A subset of post-stent patients in whom the measurement of FFR has taught us a great deal is the patient with bifurcation disease in which a sidebranch has been "jailed" by a stent. Studies measuring FFR in these "jailed" sidebranches have demonstrated that the coronary angiogram typically overestimates the functional significance, and in most cases, no further intervention on the sidebranch is necessary [48]. Clinical follow-up in these patients demonstrates little change in the functional significance of the sidebranch and excellent outcomes [49].

Assessing the Coronary Microcirculation

Realization of the importance of the coronary microcirculation in determining patient outcomes in a number of settings has occurred as our ability to invasively assess the coronary microcirculation has improved. A number of invasive techniques exist for evaluating the status of the coronary microvasculature, including angiographic ones like the TIMI myocardial perfusion grade and wire-based ones like

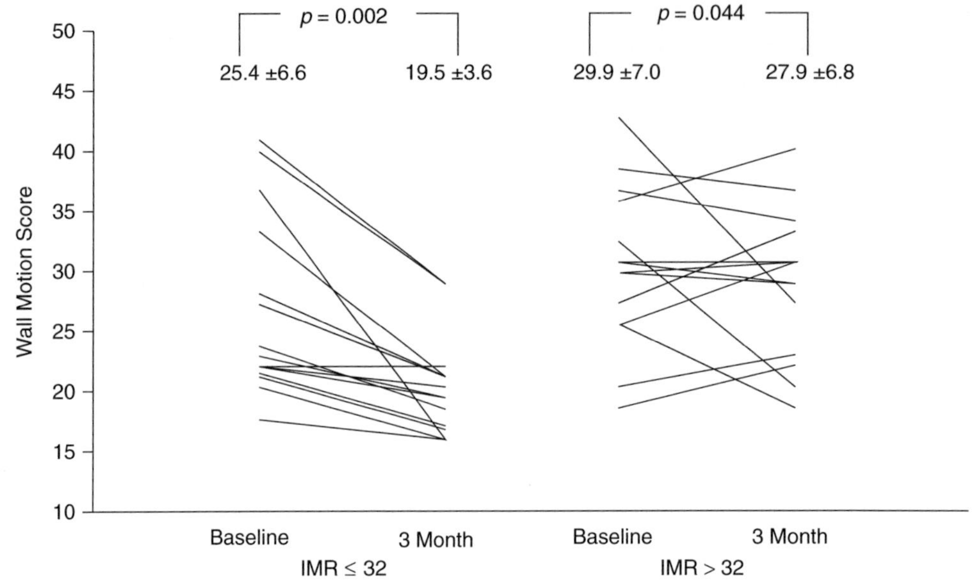

Fig. 15.5 Relationship between IMR and left ventricular function recovery. Data demonstrating that patients with lower IMR immediately after primary PCI for their ST segment elevation myocardial infarction have significant improvement in the left ventricular function as demonstrated by a lower echocardiography-derived wall motion score (lower score implies better left ventricular function). Those with higher IMR, indicative of larger myocardial infarctions, do not have consistent improvement in their wall motion score (From Fearon et al. [61], with permission)

Doppler-derived deceleration time, coronary flow reserve (CFR), and the index of microcirculatory resistance (IMR).

Doppler wire-derived deceleration time has been shown to predict outcomes in patients with acute myocardial infarction; however, its role in stable settings is not clear [50]. TIMI myocardial perfusion grade is a qualitative angiographic score, which is also predictive of outcomes in large populations of patients with acute myocardial infarction [51].

CFR, generally derived with a Doppler velocity wire, is defined as the maximal flow down a vessel divided by the resting flow and is the best studied measure of microvascular function [52]. However, CFR has a number of limitations. In particular, because it interrogates the entire coronary circulation, both the epicardial vessel and the microvasculature, it is not truly specific for microvascular disease. For example, studies have shown that angiographically normal-appearing vessels often have diffuse disease which can be physiologically significant and result in an abnormal FFR [53]. This scenario can lead to an abnormal CFR, even in the setting of normal microvascular function. CFR is also affected by changes in resting hemodynamics, which affects its reproducibility and decreases its utility in situations where these changes commonly occur, like PCI.

To address these limitations of CFR, IMR was recently introduced as a quantitative, reproducible index, which is independent of the epicardial vessel and applicable in stable and unstable patient settings [54]. IMR is defined as the distal coronary pressure minus the venous pressure, all divided by myocardial flow measured during maximal hyperemia. IMR is therefore a measure of the minimum achievable microvascular resistance and felt to be a reflection of microcirculatory function. Because venous pressure is generally low relative to coronary pressure, it is typically neglected and IMR is defined as distal coronary pressure divided by myocardial flow. Coronary pressure is measured with the pressure wire and flow is estimated using a thermodilution technique. With appropriate software, the same pressure sensor can act as a distal thermistor and the shaft of the wire as a proximal thermistor, allowing one to measure the mean transit time of room temperature saline injected into the coronary artery [55, 56]. The mean transit time is inversely proportional to coronary flow, meaning IMR is equal to distal coronary pressure times the mean transit time.

A normal IMR value appears to be less than 25 [57]. IMR has been shown to be more reproducible than CFR and independent of hemodynamic perturbations [58]. When severe epicardial artery disease is present, it remains specific for the microvasculature as long as a more complex equation is used for its calculation, which accounts for collateral flow by measuring the coronary wedge pressure [59, 60]. IMR has been best studied in patients with acute myocardial infarction undergoing primary PCI where it has been shown to be a better predictor of recovery of left ventricular function as compared to CFR, ST segment resolution, and TIMI myocardial perfusion grading (Fig. 15.5) [61]. IMR also correlates with microvascular damage detected by cardiac magnetic resonance imaging [62].

In stable patients, others have found IMR to be a useful predictor of periprocedural myocardial infarction [63]. Studies are ongoing evaluating the role of IMR in conjunction with FFR in patients with chest pain and angiographically normal coronary arteries. This type of patient is seen frequently in the catheterization laboratory, and this type of physiologic evaluation may be particularly useful in diagnosing the etiology of the patient's symptoms.

References

1. Hachamovitch R, Berman DS, Shaw LJ, Kiat H, Cohen I, Cabico JA, Friedman J, Diamond GA. Incremental prognostic value of myocardial perfusion single photon emission computed tomography for the prediction of cardiac death: differential stratification for risk of cardiac death and myocardial infarction. Circulation. 1998;97:535–43.
2. Shaw LJ, Berman DS, Maron DJ, Mancini GB, Hayes SW, Hartigan PM, Weintraub WS, O'Rourke RA, Dada M, Spertus JA, Chaitman BR, Friedman J, Slomka P, Heller GV, Germano G, Gosselin G, Berger P, Kostuk WJ, Schwartz RG, Knudtson M, Veledar E, Bates ER, McCallister B, Teo KK, Boden WE, COURAGE Investigators. Optimal medical therapy with or without percutaneous coronary intervention to reduce ischemic burden: results from the Clinical Outcomes Utilizing Revascularization and Aggressive Drug Evaluation (COURAGE) trial nuclear substudy. Circulation. 2008; 117:1283–91.
3. Pijls NHJ, van Schaardenburgh P, Manoharan G, Boersma E, Bech JW, van't Veer M, Bär F, Hoorntje J, Koolen J, Wijns W, De Bruyne B. Percutaneous coronary intervention of functionally non-significant stenosis: 5-Year follow-up of the DEFER Study. J Am Coll Cardiol. 2007;49:2105–11.
4. Lima RSL, Watson DD, Goode AR, et al. Incremental value of combined perfusion and function over perfusion alone by gated SPECT myocardial perfusion imaging for detection of severe three-vessel coronary artery disease. J Am Coll Cardiol. 2003;42:64–70.
5. Meijboom WB, Van Mieghem CA, van Pelt N, Weustink A, Pugliese F, Mollet NR, Boersma E, Regar E, van Geuns RJ, de Jaegere PJ, Serruys PW, Krestin GP, de Feyter PJ. Comprehensive assessment of coronary artery stenoses: computed tomography coronary angiography versus conventional coronary angiography and correlation with fractional flow reserve in patients with stable angina. J Am Coll Cardiol. 2008;52:636–43.
6. Tonino PAL, De Bruyne B, Pijls NHJ, Siebert U, Ikena F, Van 't Veer M, Klauss V, Manoharan G, Engstrom T, Oldroyd KG, Ver Lee PN, McCarthy PA, Fearon WF. Fractional flow reserve versus angiography for guiding PCI in patients with multivessel coronary disease (FAME study). N Engl J Med. 2009;360:213–24.
7. Pijls NHJ, van Son JAM, Kirkeeide RL, De Bruyne B, Gould KL. Experimental basis of determining maximum coronary, myocardial and collateral blood flow by pressure measurements for assessing functional stenosis severity before and after percutaneous transluminal coronary angioplasty. Circulation. 1993;86:1354–67.
8. de Bruyne B, Bartunek J, Sys SU, Pijls NH, Heyndrickx GR, Wijns W. Simultaneous coronary pressure and flow velocity measurements in humans. Feasibility, reproducibility, and hemodynamic dependence of coronary flow velocity reserve, hyperemic flow versus pressure slope index, and fractional flow reserve. Circulation. 1996;94:1842–9.
9. Gould KL, Lipscomb K, Hamilton GW. Physiologic basis for assessing critical coronary stenosis. Instantaneous flow response and regional distribution during coronary hyperemia as measures of coronary flow reserve. Am J Cardiol. 1974;33:87–94.
10. Kern MJ. Coronary physiology revisited: practical insights from the cardiac catheterization laboratory. Circulation. 2000;101:1344–51.
11. Legalery P, Seronde MF, Meneveau N, Schiele F, Bassand JP. Measuring pressure-derived fractional flow reserve through four French diagnostic catheters. Am J Cardiol. 2003;91:1075–8.
12. De Bruyne B, Pijls NH, Barbato E, Bartunek J, Bech JW, Wijns W, Heyndrickx GR. Intracoronary and intravenous adenosine 5′-triphosphate, adenosine, papaverine, and contrast medium to assess fractional flow reserve in humans. Circulation. 2003;107:1877–83.
13. Casella G, Leibig M, Schiele TM, Schrepf R, Seelig V, Stempfle HU, Erdin P, Rieber J, König A, Siebert U, Klauss V. Are high doses of intracoronary adenosine an alternative to standard intravenous adenosine for the assessment of fractional flow reserve? Am Heart J. 2004;148:590–5.
14. Talman CL, Winniford MD, Rossen JD, Simonetti I, Kienzle MG, Marcus ML. Polymorphous ventricular tachycardia: a side effect of intracoronary papaverine. J Am Coll Cardiol. 1990;15:275–8.
15. Parham WA, Bouhasin A, Ciaramita JP, Khoukaz S, Herrmann SC, Kern MJ. Coronary hyperemic dose responses of intracoronary sodium nitroprusside. Circulation. 2004;109:1236–43.
16. Al Jaroudi W, Iskandrian AE. Regadenoson: a new myocardial stress agent. J Am Coll Cardiol. 2009;54:1123–30.
17. De Bruyne B, Stockbroeckx J, Demoor D, Heyndrickx GR, Kern MJ. Role of side holes in guide catheters: observations on coronary pressure and flow. Cathet Cardiovasc Diagn. 1994;33:145–52.
18. Aqel RA, Zoghbi GJ, Trimm JR, Baldwin SA, Iskandrian AE. Effect of caffeine administered intravenously on intracoronary-administered adenosine-induced coronary hemodynamics in patients with coronary artery disease. Am J Cardiol. 2004;93: 343–6.
19. Pijls NH, Kern MJ, Yock PG, De Bruyne B. Practice and potential pitfalls of coronary pressure measurement. Catheter Cardiovasc Interv. 2000;49:1–16.
20. Pijls NH, De Bruyne B, Peels K, Van Der Voort PH, Bonnier HJ, Bartunek J, Koolen JJ. Measurement of fractional flow reserve to assess the functional severity of coronary-artery stenoses. N Engl J Med. 1996;334:1703–8.
21. Bech GJ, De Bruyne B, Pijls NH, de Muinck ED, Hoorntje JC, Escaned J, Stella PR, Boersma E, Bartunek J, Koolen JJ, Wijns W. Fractional flow reserve to determine the appropriateness of angioplasty in moderate coronary stenosis: a randomized trial. Circulation. 2001;103:2928–34.
22. Bech GJ, De Bruyne B, Bonnier HJ, Bartunek J, Wijns W, Peels K, Heyndrickx GR, Koolen JJ, Pijls NH. Long-term follow-up after deferral of percutaneous transluminal coronary angioplasty of intermediate stenosis on the basis of coronary pressure measurement. J Am Coll Cardiol. 1998;31:841–7.
23. Chamuleau SA, Meuwissen M, Koch KT, et al. Usefulness of fractional flow reserve for risk stratification of patients with multivessel coronary artery disease and an intermediate stenosis. Am J Cardiol. 2002;89:377–80.
24. Legalery P, Schiele F, Seronde MF, et al. One-year outcome of patients submitted to routine fractional flow reserve assessment to determine the need for angioplasty. Eur Heart J. 2005;26:2623–9.
25. Kern MJ, Samady H. Current concepts of integrated coronary physiology in the catheterization laboratory. J Am Coll Cardiol. 2010;55:173–85.
26. Aarnoudse WH, Botman KJ, Pijls NH. False-negative myocardial scintigraphy in balanced three-vessel disease, revealed by coronary pressure measurement. Int J Cardiovasc Intervent. 2003;5:67–71.
27. Fearon WF, Tonino PA, De Bruyne B, Siebert U, Pijls NH, FAME Study Investigators. Rationale and design of the fractional flow reserve versus angiography for multivessel evaluation (FAME) study. Am Heart J. 2007;154:632–6.
28. Pijls NH, Fearon WF, Tonino PA, Siebert U, Ikeno F, Bornschein B, van't Veer M, Klauss V, Manoharan G, Engstrøm T, Oldroyd KG, Ver Lee PN, MacCarthy PA, De Bruyne B, FAME Study Investigators. Fractional flow reserve versus angiography for guiding percutaneous coronary intervention in patients with multivessel coronary artery disease: 2-year follow-up of the FAME (Fractional Flow Reserve Versus Angiography for Multivessel Evaluation) study. J Am Coll Cardiol. 2010;56:177–84.
29. Tonino PA, Fearon WF, De Bruyne B, Oldroyd KG, Leesar MA, Ver Lee PN, Maccarthy PA, Van't Veer M, Pijls NH. Angiographic versus functional severity of coronary artery stenoses in the FAME study fractional flow reserve versus angiography in multivessel evaluation. J Am Coll Cardiol. 2010;55:2816–21.

30. European Association for Percutaneous Cardiovascular Interventions, Wijns W, Kolh P, Danchin N, et al. Guidelines on myocardial revascularization: The Task Force on Myocardial Revascularization of the European Society of Cardiology (ESC) and the European Association for Cardio-Thoracic Surgery (EACTS). Eur Heart J. 2010;31:2501–55.
31. Serruys PW, Morice MC, Kappetein AP, Colombo A, Holmes DR, Mack MJ, Ståhle E, Feldman TE, van den Brand M, Bass EJ, Van Dyck N, Leadley K, Dawkins KD, Mohr FW, SYNTAX Investigators. Percutaneous coronary intervention versus coronary-artery bypass grafting for severe coronary artery disease. N Engl J Med. 2009;360:961–72.
32. Nam CW, Mangiacapra F, Entjes R, Chung IS, Sels JW, Tonino PA, De Bruyne B, Pijls NH, Fearon WF; FAME Study Investigators. Functional SYNTAX Score for Risk Assessment in Multivessel Coronary Artery Disease. J Am Coll Cardiol 2011;58:1211–8.
33. Fearon WF, Bornschein B, Tonino PA, Gothe RM, De Bruyne B, Pijls NH, Siebert U, Fractional Flow Reserve Versus Angiography for Multivessel Evaluation (FAME) Study Investigators. Economic evaluation of fractional flow reserve-guided percutaneous coronary intervention in patients with multivessel disease. Circulation. 2010;122:2545–50.
34. De Bruyne B, Pijls NH, Kalesan B, Barbato E, Tonino PA, Piroth Z, Jagic N, Mobius-Winckler S, Rioufol G, Witt N, Kala P, MacCarthy P, Engstrom T, Oldroyd KG, Mavromatis K, Manoharan G, Verlee P, Frobert O, Curzen N, Johnson JB, Juni P, Fearon WF. Fractional flow reserve-guided PCI versus medical therapy in stable coronary disease. N Engl J Med. 2012;367:991–1001.
35. De Bruyne B, Pijls NH, Bartunek J, Kulecki K, Bech JW, De Winter H, Van Crombrugge P, Heyndrickx GR, Wijns W. Fractional flow reserve in patients with prior myocardial infarction. Circulation. 2001;104:157–62.
36. Samady H, Lepper W, Powers ER, et al. Fractional flow reserve of infarct-related arteries identifies reversible defects on noninvasive myocardial perfusion imaging early after myocardial infarction. J Am Coll Cardiol. 2006;47:2187–93.
37. Uren NG, Marraccini P, Gistri R, de Silva R, Camici PG. Altered coronary vasodilator reserve and metabolism in myocardium subtended by normal arteries in patients with coronary artery disease. J Am Coll Cardiol. 1993;22:650–8.
38. Ntalianis A, Sels JW, Davidavicius G, Tanaka N, Muller O, Trana C, Barbato E, Hamilos M, Mangiacapra F, Heyndrickx GR, Wijns W, Pijls NH, De Bruyne B. Fractional flow reserve for the assessment of nonculprit coronary artery stenoses in patients with acute myocardial infarction. JACC Cardiovasc Interv. 2010;3:1274–81.
39. Sels JW, Tonino PA, Siebert U, Fearon WF, Van't Veer M, De Bruyne B, Pijls NH. Fractional flow reserve in unstable angina and non-ST-segment elevation myocardial infarction experience from the FAME (Fractional flow reserve versus Angiography for Multivessel Evaluation) study. JACC Cardiovasc Interv. 2011;4:1183–9.
40. Bech GJ, Droste H, Pijls NH, et al. Value of fractional flow reserve in making decisions about bypass surgery for equivocal left main coronary artery disease. Heart. 2001;86:547–52.
41. Jasti V, Ivan E, Yalamanchili V, Wongpraparut N, Leesar MA. Correlations between fractional flow reserve and intravascular ultrasound in patients with an ambiguous left main coronary artery stenosis. Circulation. 2004;110:2831–6.
42. Hamilos M, Muller O, Cuisset T, Ntalianis A, Chlouverakis G, Sarno G, Nelis O, Bartunek J, Vanderheyden M, Wyffels E, Barbato E, Heyndrickx GR, Wijns W, De Bruyne B. Long-term clinical outcome after fractional flow reserve-guided treatment in patients with angiographically equivocal left main coronary artery stenosis. Circulation. 2009;120:1505–12.
43. De Bruyne B, Pijls NH, Heyndrickx GR, Hodeige D, Kirkeeide R, Gould KL. Pressure-derived fractional flow reserve to assess serial epicardial stenoses: theoretical basis and animal validation. Circulation. 2000;101:1840–7.
44. Pijls NHJ, De Bruyne B, Bech GJW, et al. Coronary pressure measurement to assess the hemodynamic significance of serial stenoses within one coronary artery: validation in humans. Circulation. 2000;102:2371–7.
45. Fearon WF, Luna J, Samady H, Powers ER, Feldman T, Dib N, Tuzcu EM, Cleman MW, Chou TM, Cohen DJ, Ragosta M, Takagi A, Jeremias A, Fitzgerald PJ, Yeung AC, Kern MJ, Yock PG. Fractional flow reserve compared with intravascular ultrasound guidance for optimizing stent deployment. Circulation. 2001;104: 1917–22.
46. Pijls NH, Klauss V, Siebert U, Powers E, Takazawa K, Fearon WF, Escaned J, Tsurumi Y, Akasaka T, Samady H, De Bruyne B, Fractional Flow Reserve (FFR) Post-Stent Registry Investigators. Coronary pressure measurement after stenting predicts adverse events at follow-up: a multicenter registry. Circulation. 2002;105: 2950–4.
47. Nam CW, Hur SH, Cho YK, Park HS, Yoon HJ, Kim H, Chung IS, Kim YN, Kim KB, Doh JH, Koo BK, Tahk SJ, Fearon WF. Relation of fractional flow reserve after drug-eluting stent implantation to one-year outcomes. Am J Cardiol. 2011;107:1763–7.
48. Koo BK, Kang HJ, Youn TJ, et al. Physiologic assessment of jailed side branch lesions using fractional flow reserve. J Am Coll Cardiol. 2005;46:633–7.
49. Koo BK, Park KW, Kang HJ, Cho YS, Chung WY, Youn TJ, Chae IH, Choi DJ, Tahk SJ, Oh BH, Park YB, Kim HS. Physiological evaluation of the provisional side-branch intervention strategy for bifurcation lesions using fractional flow reserve. Eur Heart J. 2008; 29:726–32.
50. Yamamuro A, Akasaka T, Tamita K, Yamabe K, Katayama M, Takagi T, Morioka S. Coronary flow velocity pattern immediately after percutaneous coronary intervention as a predictor of complications and in-hospital survival after acute myocardial infarction. Circulation. 2002;106:3051–6.
51. Gibson CM, Cannon CP, Murphy SA, Ryan KA, Mesley R, Marble SJ, McCabe CH, Van De Werf F, Braunwald E. Relationship of TIMI myocardial perfusion grade to mortality after administration of thrombolytic drugs. Circulation. 2000;101:125–30.
52. Pepine CJ, Anderson RD, Sharaf BL, Reis SE, Smith KM, Handberg EM, Johnson BD, Sopko G, Bairey Merz CN. Coronary microvascular reactivity to adenosine predicts adverse outcome in women evaluated for suspected ischemia results from the National Heart, Lung and Blood Institute WISE (Women's Ischemia Syndrome Evaluation) study. J Am Coll Cardiol. 2010;55: 2825–32.
53. De Bruyne B, Hersbach F, Pijls NH, Bartunek J, Bech JW, Heyndrickx GR, Gould KL, Wijns W. Abnormal epicardial coronary resistance in patients with diffuse atherosclerosis but "Normal" coronary angiography. Circulation. 2001;104:2401–6.
54. Fearon WF, Balsam LB, Farouque HMO, Caffarelli AD, Robbins RC, Fitzgerald PJ, Yock PG, Yeung AC. Novel index for invasively assessing the coronary microcirculation. Circulation. 2003;107: 3129–32.
55. De Bruyne B, Pijls NH, Smith L, Wievegg M, Heyndrickx GR. Coronary thermodilution to assess flow reserve: experimental validation. Circulation. 2001;104:2003–6.
56. Pijls NH, De Bruyne B, Smith L, et al. Coronary thermodilution to assess flow reserve: validation in humans. Circulation. 2002;105: 2482–6.
57. Melikian N, Vercauteren S, Fearon WF, Cuisset T, MacCarthy PA, Davidavicius G, Aarnoudse W, Bartunek J, Vanderheyden

M, Wyffels E, Wijns W, Heyndrickx GR, Pijls NH, de Bruyne B. Quantitative assessment of coronary microvascular function in patients with and without epicardial atherosclerosis. EuroIntervention. 2010;5:939–45.

58. Ng MK, Yeung AC, Fearon WF. Invasive assessment of the coronary microcirculation: superior reproducibility and less hemodynamic dependence of index of microcirculatory resistance as compared to coronary flow reserve. Circulation. 2006;113:2054–61.
59. Fearon WF, Aarnoudse W, Pijls NHJ, De Bruyne B, Balsam LB, Cooke DT, Robbins RC, Fitzgerald PJ, Yeung AC, Yock PG. Microvascular resistance is not influenced by epicardial coronary artery stenosis severity: experimental validation. Circulation. 2004; 109:2269–72.
60. Aarnoudse W, Fearon WF, Manoharan G, Geven M, van de Vosse F, Rutten M, De Bruyne B, Pijls NHJ. Epicardial stenosis severity does not affect minimal microcirculatory resistance. Circulation. 2004;110:2137–42.
61. Fearon WF, Shah M, Ng M, Brinton T, Wilson A, Tremmel JA, Schnittger I, Lee DP, Vagelos RH, Fitzgerald PJ, Yock PG, Yeung AC. Predictive value of the index of microcirculatory resistance in patients with ST segment elevation myocardial infarction. J Am Coll Cardiol. 2008;51:560–5.
62. McGeoch R, Watkins S, Berry C, Steedman T, Davie A, Byrne J, Hillis S, Lindsay M, Robb S, Dargie H, Oldroyd K. The index of microcirculatory resistance measured acutely predicts the extent and severity of myocardial infarction in patients with ST-segment elevation myocardial infarction. JACC Cardiovasc Interv. 2010;3:715–22.
63. Cuisset T, Hamilos M, Melikian N, et al. Direct stenting for stable angina pectoris is associated with reduced periprocedural microcirculatory injury compared with stenting after pre-dilation. J Am Coll Cardiol. 2008;51:1060–5.

Interventional Management of Acute Myocardial Infarction

16

Nur Jamal, Ron Reiter, and M. Nicholas Burke

Coronary artery disease is the leading cause of death in the United States and was responsible for approximately one of every six deaths in the United States in 2008. Each year, an estimated 785,000 Americans will have an ST segment elevation myocardial infarction (STEMI), and ≈470,000 will have a repeat event. Roughly every 25 s, an American will have a STEMI, and approximately every minute, a STEMI will be the cause of a death [1]. Acute thrombotic occlusion is the predominant pathophysiological cause of STEMI and also forms the rationale for reperfusion therapy, either thrombolysis or primary percutaneous coronary intervention (PCI).

Evolution of Primary PCI in STEMI

PTCA Versus Thrombolysis

An overview of the results of nine trials by the Fibrinolytic Therapy Trialists' Collaborative Group, comparing the outcomes of patients undergoing fibrinolytic therapy and those of controls, demonstrated statistically significant absolute reductions in 35-day mortality rates (of approximately 30 per 1,000 for patients who arrived at the hospital within 6 h of the onset of symptoms and of approximately 20 per 1,000 for patients who arrived 7–12 h after the onset of symptoms) [2]. The greatest benefit was observed among patients with LBBB or anterior STEMI. Despite its universal availability and efficacy, thrombolytic therapy has several limitations including (1) low rates of early and sustained patency of the infarct-related vessel after thrombolysis (90-min TIMI [Thrombolysis in Myocardial Infarction] grade 3 flow rates are restored in only 20–60 % of patients), (2) increased rates of re-infarction, (3) recurrent ischemia in comparison with placebo, (4) hemorrhagic complications of therapy (life-threatening bleeding in 0.5–1.5 %), and (5) limited efficacy in high-risk subgroups [2–4]. These drawbacks to thrombolytic therapy in STEMI resulted in the growth of emergent coronary angiography followed by coronary angioplasty of the infarct-related artery without prior administration of thrombolytic therapy, so-called primary PTCA (percutaneous transluminal coronary angioplasty) or primary PCI (percutaneous coronary intervention).

The publication of large, single-center observational studies; prospective multicenter registries, and multiple, randomized, controlled trials of primary PTCA versus thrombolytic therapy has established the evidence base and role of primary PTCA in acute MI. The first randomized trial was published in 1986, in which 56 patients presenting within 12 h of onset of acute MI were randomly assigned to receive intracoronary streptokinase or undergo primary PTCA [5]. The time to reperfusion (4.8 h vs. 4.1 h) and the degree of patency achieved (85 % vs. 83 %) were similar with both strategies. The residual stenosis, however, was significantly lower in the PTCA group (43 % vs. 83 %; $p<0.001$) and was associated with an improvement in regional wall motion as well as global LVEF.

The Primary Angioplasty in Myocardial Infarction (PAMI) trial was instrumental in establishing the superiority of primary PTCA as a reperfusion modality in STEMI [6] (Table 16.1). This trial randomized 395 patients of any age with acute MI within 12 h of symptom onset to primary PTCA or to an infusion of 100-mg tPA (tissue plasminogen activator) over 3 h. PTCA resulted in lower rates of death and re-infarction, recurrent ischemia, total stroke, and intracranial hemorrhage.

Table 16.1 PAMI trial

	PTCA group ($n=195$)	tPA group ($n=200$)	p value
Re-infarction or death	10(5.1 %)	24(12.0 %)	0.02
Death	5(2.6 %)	13(6.5 %)	0.06
Re-infarction	5(2.6 %)	13(6.5 %)	0.06
Recurrent ischemia	10(5.1 %)	47(23.5 %)	<0.001

N. Jamal, MD • R. Reiter, MD • M.N. Burke, MD (✉)
Department of Cardiology, Minneapolis Heart Institute,
920 East 28th St, Ste. 620, Minneapolis, MN 55417, USA
e-mail: mnicholas.burke@allina.com

C.A. Thompson (ed.), *Textbook of Cardiovascular Intervention*,
DOI 10.1007/978-1-4471-4528-8_16, © Springer-Verlag London 2014

These results were reinforced in the subsequent ZWOLLE trials and GUSTO-IIb angioplasty trial [7–9].

A meta-analysis of 23 randomized trials comparing primary PCI with fibrinolytic therapy demonstrated that PCI was superior to thrombolysis in reducing the incidence of short- and long-term adverse outcomes, including death [10]. Primary PCI has been shown to result in higher rates for infarct artery patency, improved coronary blood flow, and lower rates for recurrent ischemia, re-infarction, emergency repeat revascularization procedures, intracranial hemorrhage, and death when compared to thrombolysis. The survival benefit of primary PCI compared with thrombolytic therapy reported was 21 lives saved per 1,000 patients treated [10]. Early, successful PCI also greatly decreases the complications of STEMI that result from longer ischemic times or unsuccessful fibrinolytic therapy, allowing earlier hospital discharge and resumption of daily activities [11]. The greatest mortality benefit of primary PCI is in high-risk patients such as those with anterior MI, congestive heart failure (CHF), or cardiogenic shock [11, 12]. Primary PTCA outcomes may not be as successful with prolonged time to treatment or when performed either in hospitals or by operators with low PTCA volumes [13, 14].

Stents Versus Thrombolysis

Once primary PTCA became established as the preferred strategy in STEMI patients, the next question was whether PCI with a bare metal stent (BMS) was superior to thrombolysis. Despite the proven benefit of stenting compared to angioplasty in routine PCI, there was a concern that placing a stent in a fresh thrombus would be more likely to result in stent thrombosis. In a meta-analysis of 12 trials comparing primary PCI with stenting to thrombolytic therapy, primary PCI was superior to thrombolytic therapy in terms of lower overall short-term mortality (7 % vs. 9 %; $p=0.0002$), nonfatal re-infarction (3 % vs. 7 %; $p<0.0001$), stroke (1 % vs. 2 %; $p=0.004$), and the combined end point of death, nonfatal re-infarction, and stroke (8 % vs. 14 %; $p<0.0001$) [10].

Stents Versus PTCA

Both PCTA and stenting had been demonstrated to be superior to thrombolytics in the treatment of STEMI, but there remained a question of whether the benefits of less restenosis resulting from the use of stents was offset by the potential increased risk for stent thrombosis if used in a highly thrombotic milieu. The stent-PAMI trial randomized STEMI patients to PCI with either PTCA or stenting and found that stents reduced restenosis, reocclusion, and the need for target vessel revascularization compared with PTCA. Furthermore, the use of stents was not associated with an increase (or reduction) in re-infarction or mortality [9]. These findings were further confirmed in a meta-analysis of STEMI studies comparing PTCA versus stenting [10].

Bare Metal Versus Drug-Eluting Stents

Similar to the finding of decreased restenosis when stents were compared to PTCA, drug-eluting stents (DES) have also been shown to decrease restenosis rates when compared to bare metal stents (BMS) when used in patients with STEMI. Meta-analyses of several small, randomized studies comparing BMS and DES in STEMI patients revealed no differences in death, MI, or stent thrombosis rates between the two groups, but target vessel revascularization (TVR) rates were decreased with DES [15, 16]. The studies included in these meta-analyses were limited by many factors including sample size and duration of follow-up. The most robust evidence comes from the HORIZONS-AMI trial that randomized 3,006 STEMI patients to DES or BMS in a 3:1 ratio. There was no difference in the 12-month composite safety end point of death, re-infarction, stroke, or stent thrombosis. The rates of ischemia-driven target vessel revascularization and target lesion revascularization, however, were significantly lower in the DES group (5.8 % vs. 8.7 % and 4.5 % vs. 7.5 %, respectively; NNT = 33 at 1 year), as was the 13-month binary restenosis rate (10 % vs. 22.9 %) [17]. In conclusion, while there is no difference in terms of mortality, re-infarction, or stent thrombosis with the use of DES as compared to BMS in STEMI patients, there is a benefit associated with the use of DES in STEMI with a reduction in TVR and restenosis.

The Effect of Timing in PCI for STEMI (Door-to-Balloon Time)

It is now generally accepted that STEMI patients presenting to a PCI-capable facility should undergo primary PCI. Guidelines currently call for a time from arrival at the PCI-capable hospital-to-balloon inflation in the infarct-related artery (door-to-balloon or "D2B" time) of less than 90 min. This derives from the assumption that thrombolytic therapy should be able to be administered within 30 min and the fact that a primary PCI strategy may not reduce mortality when a delay of greater than 60 min is anticipated when compared with immediate administration of thrombolytics [18]. According to an analysis of 43,801 patients with STEMI undergoing primary PCI within the National Cardiovascular Data Registry (NCDR), however, any delay in time to reperfusion after arrival at the hospital was associated with a higher adjusted risk of in-hospital mortality in a continuous, nonlinear fashion (30 min = 3 %, 60 min = 3.5 %, 90 min = 4.3 %, 120 min = 5.6 %, 150 min = 7 %, 180 min = 8.4 %; $p<0.001$) [19]. Consequently, rather than a goal of a 90-min D2B time for primary PCI, these data suggest that the standard should be simply as soon as possible.

PCI for Patients Presenting to Non-PCI-Capable Hospitals

Approximately 60 million people (20 % of the US population) live farther than 60 miles from a hospital capable of performing PCI [20]. It is estimated that roughly 175,000 patients per year will have a STEMI within this population and may not have access to timely PCI. According to the NCDR, only 9.9 % of patients transferred from a hospital without PCI capability for primary PCI achieve a door-to-balloon time of less than 90 min [21], and based on the NRMI data, less than 15 % of patients transferred from non-PCI facility are treated in under 2 h [22].

Transfer for PCI Versus Thrombolytics

According to the AHA/ACC guidelines, full-dose thrombolytics is the recommended reperfusion strategy for patients with expected delay [23, 24]. Unfortunately, 26–36 % of patients will ultimately fail to reperfuse and will require transfer for rescue PCI [25]. Two studies published in 2003, the Danish trial in Acute Myocardial Infarction-2 (DANAMI-2) [26] and the Primary Angioplasty in Patients transferred from General Community Hospitals to Specialized PTCA Units with or without Emergency Thrombolysis-2 (PRAGUE-2) [27], compared the outcome of thrombolysis administered immediately at a non-PCI-capable hospital versus emergent transfer for primary PCI (Table 16.2). Patients in DANAMI-2 received tPA in the thrombolytic arm, and bare metal stents were used in 93 % of patients transferred for primary PCI. Mean total door-to-balloon (from referring hospital to balloon in receiving hospital) time was 112 min for patients transferred for PCI. The rate of primary composite end point of death, re-infarction, and disabling stroke at 30 days was lower in the transferred PCI group than in the thrombolysis group (8.0 % vs. 13.7 %, $p=0.002$). This was largely driven by a reduction in the rate of re-infarction (1.6 % vs. 6.3 % in the thrombolytic arm, $p<0.001$), but there was a trend towards lower mortality (6.6 % in the PCI group vs. 7.8 % in thrombolysis group, $p=0.35$) and disabling stroke (1.1 % in the PCI group vs. 2 % in the thrombolysis group, $p=0.15$). The trial was terminated early by the Data Safety and Monitoring Board after observation of a marked improvement in the clinical outcome of patients in the group with transfer for primary PCI.

Table 16.2 DANAMI trial

Outcome at 30 days	Thrombolysis ($n=782$)	Transfer for primary PCI ($n=790$)	p value
Death	61(7.8 %)	52(6.6 %)	0.35
Re-infarction	49(6.3 %)	13(1.6 %)	<0.001
Disabling stroke	16(2.0 %)	9(1.1 %)	0.15
Composite end point	107(13.7 %)	63(8.0 %)	<0.001

Data from Andersen et al. [26]

In PRAGUE-2, patients received streptokinase in the thrombolytic arm and bare metal stents were employed in 63 % of patients transferred for primary PCI. Mean total door-to-balloon time was 97 min. The combined end point of a 30-day incidence of death, re-infarction, and stroke was significantly lower for the transfer for PCI group as compared to thrombolysis (8.4 % vs. 15.2 %, $p<0.003$). This study found a similar trend towards reduction in mortality with transfer for primary PCI (6.8 % vs. 10 %, $p=0.12$). An analysis based on treatment actually received, rather than intention to treat, demonstrated a statistically significant reduction in mortality for patients who were transferred for primary PCI (6 % vs. 10.4 %, $p<0.05$). In addition, the subgroup of patients presenting greater than 3 h from onset of symptoms demonstrated a clear reduction in mortality with transfer for primary PCI (6 % vs. 15.3 %, $p<0.02$) [27]. Both studies reported that interhospital transfer was safe with rare complications. Two deaths and three cases of successfully resuscitated ventricular fibrillation were reported during transportation in PRAGUE-2, while no deaths and eight cases of successfully resuscitated ventricular fibrillation were reported during transportation in DANAMI-2 [26, 27].

The only US randomized transfer trial, AIR-PAMI, randomized high-risk STEMI patients (ST elevation with one of the following criteria: age >70 years, heart rate >100 beats/min, systolic BP <100 mmHg, Killip class II/III, left bundle branch block or anterior MI) presenting to hospitals without PCI capability to either on-site thrombolysis or transfer for primary PCI. The trial was terminated early because of poor enrollment, but there was a trend towards a reduced 30-day mortality with transfer for PCI (8.4 % vs. 12.1 %, $p=0.46$) [28].

A recent meta-analysis confirmed the benefit of transfer for primary PCI over thrombolysis, showing a reduction in 30-day mortality (5.6 % vs. 6.8 %, $p=0.02$), re-infarction (2.1 % vs. 4.7 %, $p<0.001$), and stroke (0.7 % vs. 1.7 %, $p=0.0005$) [29]. These results indicate that transfer for primary PCI from non-PCI centers has advantages over thrombolysis similar to the benefits seen with primary PCI in patients presenting to a PCI center if performed in a timely manner (Table 16.3).

A major concern was whether the results from the European trials could be translated into clinical practice in the United States. The DANAMI-2 and PRAGUE-2 studies were performed in relatively small countries and the transfer

Table 16.3 Meta-analysis of STEMI trials comparing transport for PCI versus lytics

Outcome	Pooled OR (95 % CI)	*p* value
Death	0.77(0.62–0.96)	0.02
Re-infarction	0.42(0.31–0.57)	<0.0001
Stroke	0.40(0.24–0.67)	0.0005

Table 16.4 TRANSFER-AMI

	Standard treatment	Facilitated PCI	*p* value
Death	18(3.4 %)	24(4.5 %)	0.39
Re-infarction	30(5.7 %)	18(3.4 %)	0.06
Recurrent ischemia	11(2.1 %)	1(0.2 %)	0.003
Worsening heart failure	29(5.6 %)	16(3.0 %)	0.04
Cardiogenic shock	16(3.1 %)	24(4.5 %)	0.23
Combined end point at 30 days	90(17.2 %)	59(11.0 %)	0.0004
TIMI major bleeding	47(9.0 %)	40(7.4 %)	0.36

distance ranged from 5 to 74 km in PRAGUE-2 and the mean distance was 35 miles in DANAMI-2 trial. The time for transportation from community hospital to PCI center was 32 min in the DANAMI-2 trial and 48 min in the PRAGUE-2 trial, and the door-to-balloon time averaged 26 min in both studies. Thus, overall time from emergency department admission at the non-PCI hospital to treatment (total door-to-balloon time) in these studies was only 95–108 min [26, 27]. In contrast, in AIR-PAMI, the median total door-to-balloon time was 155 min [28]. Moreover, the median total door-to-balloon time in transfer patients in the US national registry of myocardial infarction 3/4 was 180 min with only 4.2 % of patients treated within 90 min [22]. In 2007, Henry et al. at the Minneapolis Heart Institute reported the results of 1,345 patients treated in a regional program for transfer of patients with STEMI for PCI using a standardized protocol and an integrated transfer system. They demonstrated a median total D2B time of 95 min and transport time of 22 min for patients presenting within 60 miles of the PCI center. Compared to patients presenting at the PCI center (D2B time of 65 min), no difference in mortality, infarct size, or re-infarction was seen in patients transferred for primary PCI [30].

Transfer with Facilitated PCI Versus Thrombolytics

Facilitated PCI for STEMI is a strategy of using full-dose thrombolysis followed by immediate PCI. In the TRANSFER-AMI trial, 1,059 STEMI patients presenting to a non-PCI-capable facility within 12 h of symptom onset who had at least 1 high-risk marker were treated with full-dose fibrinolytic therapy and were then randomized to a facilitated strategy (immediate transfer for PCI within 6 h of fibrinolytic therapy) or to standard therapy which included rescue PCI as needed [31] (Table 16.4). Standard treatment patients who did not require rescue PCI remained at the initial hospital for at least 24 h, and coronary angiography was encouraged within the first 2 weeks. All patients received standard-dose tenecteplase, aspirin, and either unfractionated heparin or enoxaparin. Treatment with clopidogrel was strongly encouraged. Glycoprotein IIb/IIIa inhibitors (GPI) were administered at the PCI-capable hospitals according to institutional practice. The primary end point was a 30-day composite of the first occurrence of death, re-infarction, recurrent ischemia, new or worsening heart failure, or cardiogenic shock. The median time to administration of tenecteplase from onset of symptoms was approximately 2 h in both groups. The median time from tenecteplase to cardiac catheterization was significantly lower in the facilitated arm (2.8 h vs. 32.5 h). Coronary angiography was performed in 98.5 % vs. 88.7 % and PCI in 84.9 % vs. 67.4 % of the facilitated and standard treatment arms respectively. The primary end point occurred in 11.0 % of the facilitated group compared with 17.2 % of the standard therapy group (RR 0.64; 95 % CI 0.47–0.84; $p = 0.004$) Furthermore, there was no significant difference in the rate of TIMI major and minor bleeding or GUSTO moderate and severe bleeding between the groups although there was a higher incidence of GUSTO mild bleeding in the facilitated arm (13 % vs. 9 %; $p = 0.036$). The authors concluded that immediate transfer of high-risk STEMI patients after fibrinolytic therapy at non-PCI hospitals for coronary angiography and PCI resulted in improved outcomes [31].

Transfer with Pharmaco-invasive PCI

As opposed to facilitated PCI, a pharmaco-invasive strategy for STEMI treatment is defined as reduced-dose thrombolysis in conjunction with immediate PCI. The CARESS-in-AMI trial included 600 STEMI patients 75 years of age or younger with at least 1 high risk feature (extensive ST segment elevation, new-onset left bundle branch block, previous MI, Killip class greater than 2, or left ventricular ejection fraction ≤35 %) who were treated initially at non-PCI hospitals with half-dose reteplase, abciximab, heparin, and ASA within 12 h of symptom onset [32] (Table 16.5). These patients were randomized to immediate transfer for PCI or to standard treatment with transfer for rescue PCI if needed. The majority of patients in the immediate transfer group (85.6 %) underwent PCI as compared to only 30.3 % in the rescue PCI group. As expected, there was a shorter median time from fibrinolytic therapy to transfer to a PCI-capable center in the

Table 16.5 CARESS-in-AMI trial

	Pharmaco-invasive ($n=297$)	Standard care ($n=300$)	p value
Death	9(3.0 %)	14(4.7 %)	0.40
Re-infarction	4(1.3 %)	6(2.0 %)	0.75
Refractory ischemia	1(0.3 %)	12(4.0 %)	0.003
Combined end point	13(4.4 %)	32(10.7 %)	0.005
Major bleeding	10(3.4 %)	7(2.3 %)	0.47

Data from Di Mario et al. [32]

immediate versus the rescue PCI group (110 vs. 180 min; $p<0.0001$). Antiplatelet therapy with aspirin and clopidogrel was used less frequently in the rescue arm than in the immediate transfer arm. The primary end point (composite of all-cause mortality, re-infarction, and refractory myocardial ischemia within 30 days) was significantly lower in the immediate PCI group as compared to rescue PCI (4.4 % vs. 10.7 %, $p=0.004$, NNT=17). There were no significant differences in the rates of major bleeding at 30 days (3.4 % vs. 2.3 %; $p=0.47$) or stroke (0.7 % vs. 1.3 %; $p=0.50$) between the two groups. The authors concluded that high-risk STEMI patients presenting at non-PCI hospitals and treated with half-dose fibrinolytic therapy, abciximab, heparin, and aspirin have improved outcomes when transferred for immediate PCI rather than rescue PCI if thrombolysis fails.

STEMI Care Systems

Only 25 % of hospitals in the United States are capable of providing primary PCI and most are located in urban areas [20]. Regional STEMI transfer systems have subsequently been developed to improve timely access to primary PCI. The first of these systems was developed at the Minneapolis Heart Institute (MHI) in 2003, the Level 1 Program [30]. MHI had long-standing referral relationships with 33 hospitals up to 210 miles away. In this system, patients are assigned one of two strategies based on the distance from the PCI center. Zone 1 consists of referral hospitals within 60 miles and Zone 2 consists of referral hospitals 60–210 miles from MHI. A standardized protocol is implemented at each hospital. All patients receive ASA 325 mg, clopidogrel 600 mg, UFH 60U/kg intravenous load (maximum 4000U), and 12U/kg/h intravenous infusion (max 1,000 U/h) in the emergency department at the presenting hospital. Patients who present at the PCI hospital (MHI) or are transferred from a Zone 1 hospital undergo primary PCI. Patients transferred from Zone 2 hospitals undergo a pharmaco-invasive approach with half-dose fibrinolytic (tenecteplase most frequently) followed by emergency transfer for immediate PCI. This strategy was based on the TNK patency results described in TIMI 10A and TIMI 10B [33, 34] and the synergistic effects of clopidogrel with fibrinolytic agents described in CLARITY and COMMIT [35, 36]. Median door-to-balloon times were 62 min for those presenting directly to the PCI hospital, 94 min for those presenting to Zone 1 hospitals, and 122 min for pharmaco-invasively treated patients transferred from Zone 2 hospitals [37]. Pre-PCI patency (TIMI 2 or 3 flow) was found in 73.6 % of the pharmaco-invasive PCI-treated patients versus 40.3 % in primary PCI patients ($p<0.001$). There was no significant difference in 30-day mortality (5.5 % vs. 5.6 %, p=0.94), stroke (1.1 vs. 1.3 %, $p=0.66$), major bleeding (1.5 % vs. 1.8 %, $p=0.65$), or re-infarction/ischemia (1.2 % vs. 2.5 %, $p=0.088$) in patients receiving a pharmaco-invasive strategy compared with patients presenting directly to the PCI center, despite a significantly longer door-to-balloon time.

PCI for Patients Not Receiving Primary Reperfusion

The "late open artery" hypothesis suggested that late patency of an infarct artery is associated with improved LV function, increased electrical stability, and the provision of collateral vessels to other coronary beds for protection against future events. The Occluded Artery Trial (OAT) randomly assigned 2,166 patients with a totally occluded infarct artery 3–28 days after MI (approximately 20 % of whom had received fibrinolytic therapy) to optimal medical therapy and PCI with stenting or to optimal medical therapy alone [38]. Patients with class III or IV heart failure, rest angina, left main or 3-vessel disease, clinical instability, or significant inducible ischemia were excluded. The 4-year cumulative end point (composite of death, re-infarction, or class IV heart failure) was 17.2 % in the PCI group and 15.6 % in the medical therapy group ($p=0.20$). Re-infarction rates tended to be higher in the PCI group. The authors concluded that PCI of a totally occluded infarct artery later than 24 h after STEMI should not be performed in asymptomatic patients with 1- or 2-vessel disease if patients are hemodynamically and electrically stable and do not have evidence of severe ischemia.

Pharmacological Strategies for PCI in STEMI

Thrombolytics

Facilitated PCI (Full-Dose Thrombolytic) Versus PCI

Facilitated PCI is a strategy that involves administration of an initial thrombolytic regimen followed by immediate PCI. It was conceived as an option to fill the time gap between patient presentation and performance of PCI with the objective of improving the patency of coronary arteries before the procedure. Historically, the pharmacological agent in facilitated PCI consists of a full-dose thrombolytic with or without a GPI. The potential advantages of this strategy include earlier time to reperfusion, smaller infarct size, improved patient stability, lower infarct arterial thrombus burden, greater procedural success rates, higher TIMI flow rates, and improved survival rates.

In the ASSENT-4 trial, 1,667 patients presenting with STEMI within 6 h of symptom onset were randomized to receive full-dose tenecteplase and PCI versus primary PCI. All patients received aspirin and a bolus of heparin. The trial was terminated prematurely because patients treated with fibrinolytic therapy before PCI had increased rates of adverse outcomes including in-hospital mortality (6 % vs. 3 %; $p=0.01$) [39]. The primary end point, a composite of death, shock, and congestive heart failure within 90 days, was significantly higher with facilitated PCI than with primary PCI (18.6 % vs. 13.4 %; $p=0.0045$), and there was a trend towards a higher 90-day mortality rate (6.7 % vs. 4.9 %; $p=0.14$). There were more in-hospital strokes (1.8 % vs. 0 %; $p<0.001$) and a higher incidence of ischemic complications such as re-infarction (6 % vs. 4 %; $p=0.0279$) or repeat target vessel revascularization (7 % vs. 3 %; $p=0.0041$) among patients treated with facilitated PCI as compared to primary PCI. The conclusion of the ASSENT-4 trial was that a strategy of facilitated PCI consisting of full-dose thrombolysis plus antithrombotic co-therapy preceding PCI by 1–3 h was associated with worse clinical outcome than a strategy of primary PCI alone [39]. This trial has been criticized because only a minority of patients fit the target population for whom facilitated PCI was designed: patients with an anticipated delay to PCI. Additionally, a facilitated angioplasty regimen would be expected to be of greatest benefit in the early period after infarction when thrombolysis is most effective. A retrospective analysis of the ASSENT-4 trial showed that the group with the shortest time to reperfusion, those patients receiving thrombolysis in the prehospital setting followed by PCI, had the lowest 90-day mortality while complications were increased in the facilitated-PCI arm regardless of timing [40].

Pharmaco-invasive PCI (1/2-Dose Lytics) Versus PCI

The FINESSE (Facilitated Intervention with Enhanced Reperfusion Speed to Stop Events) trial was a randomized double-blind clinical trial of 2,452 patients randomized within 6 h of symptom onset to receive reduced-dose reteplase plus abciximab followed by PCI (combination-facilitated PCI), abciximab alone followed by PCI (abciximab-facilitated PCI), or primary PCI. [41] The primary end point was the composite of all-cause mortality or complications after MI within 90 days. Although on arrival to the catheterization laboratory the percentage of patients with an open artery before PCI was higher in the reteplase plus abciximab group (61 %) than in the abciximab group or the primary PCI group (26 and 25 %, respectively; $p<0.001$, when compared to the combination-facilitated group), there was no difference in the primary end point (9.8 % in the combination-facilitated PCI, 10.5 % in the abciximab-facilitated PCI, and 10.7 % in the primary PCI group; $p=0.55$). TIMI major or minor bleeding was significantly higher in the combination-facilitated PCI group than in either of the other groups ($p<0.001$). Although the study was terminated early because of recruitment challenges, there was less than a 2 % chance that the primary treatment group difference would be significant if the trial had been allowed to continue to its planned completion. A post hoc analysis suggested that high-risk patients presenting to hospitals without PCI capability within 4 h from the onset of symptoms had reduced 1-year mortality with abciximab plus reteplase compared with primary PCI (hazard rate, 0.351; $p=0.01$) [42]. Henry et al. have reported the results of a large regional STEMI transfer program which employs a pharmaco-invasive strategy for patients presenting to referring hospitals where expected D2B times are longer than 90 min. When these patients were compared to patients transferred from closer facilities or to patients presenting to the PCI center with shorter D2B times, no differences in in-hospital, 30-day and 1 year mortality was seen [30].

Rescue PCI

Rescue PCI is defined as PCI within 12 h after thrombolysis for patients with continuing or recurrent myocardial ischemia. The indications for rescue PCI have been defined by a combination of clinical and electrocardiographic clues that an infarct artery has not been reperfused. As the presence or absence of ischemic discomfort may be unreliable for identifying failed reperfusion, ECG criteria of less than 50 % ST segment resolution at 90 min in the lead that showed the greatest degree of ST elevation at presentation is considered indicative of fibrinolytic failure and thus PCI performed at that time would be labeled rescue PCI [43].

The Middlesbrough Early Revascularization to Limit Infarction (MERLIN) trial randomized 307 patients with STEMI and failed thrombolysis to an invasive strategy of emergent coronary angiography and PCI if indicated or to conservative therapy. The primary end point was an all-cause mortality at 30 days and was not different between the two groups (9.8 % in the rescue and 11 % in the in the conservative therapy; $p=0.7$) [44]. The combined incidence of major cardiac adverse events was reduced in the invasive group (37.3 % vs. 50 %; $p=0.02$) largely driven by a decrease in subsequent revascularization (6.5 % vs. 20.1 %; $p=0.01$). In the REACT (Rescue Angioplasty Versus Conservative Treatment or Repeat Thrombolysis) trial, 427 patients with acute MI who had failed thrombolysis at 90 min were randomized to repeat thrombolysis, conservative treatment, or rescue PCI. The primary end point was a composite of death, re-infarction, stroke, or severe heart failure within 6 months. The rate of event-free survival was 84.6 % for patients treated with rescue PCI, 70.1 % for those receiving conservative therapy, and 68.7 % for those undergoing repeat thrombolysis (overall $p=0.004$) [45]. In a meta-analysis of eight trials, an invasive strategy for failed thrombolysis reduced re-infarction rates from 10.7 to 6.1 % (RR 0.58 [95 % CI 0.35–0.97]; $p=0.04$) and reduced heart failure rates from 17.8 to 12.7 % (RR 0.73 [95 % CI 0.54–1.00]; $p=0.05$) when compared with conservative management. There was also a trend towards reduced mortality rates with rescue PCI from 10.4 to 7.3 % (RR 0.69 [95 % CI 0.46–1.05]; $p=0.09$) [46].

Adjunctive Pharmacology for STEMI PCI

Heparin and Low Molecular Weight Heparin (LMWH)

Parenteral anticoagulants include intravenous unfractionated heparin (UFH), bivalirudin, enoxaparin, and fondaparinux. UFH has been a mainstay in the treatment of STEMI for more than 40 years. The 2007 update of the ACC/AHA guidelines recommends an initial UFH bolus of 60 U/kg (maximum, 4000U), followed by an initial infusion of 12 U/kg/h (maximum, 1,000U/h) for 48 h after thrombolysis, with a target APTT of 1.5–2 times the upper limit of normal (approximately 50–70 s) [47]. Limited data exist in the use of UFH or enoxaparin in the setting of primary PCI. The ATOLL trial tested intravenous enoxaparin versus UFH [48]. Enoxaparin did not significantly reduce the composite primary outcome of death, complication of MI, procedure failure, or major bleeding (28 % vs. 34 %, $p<0.07$) but did reduce the main secondary end point of death, recurrent acute coronary syndrome, or urgent revascularization (7 % vs. 11 %, $p=0.015$). This was a small study, however, with an atypical primary end point consisting of clinical, procedural, and angiographic events. Furthermore, as the primary end point was not met, the results of the secondary end point should be seen as hypothesis generating only. In a sub-study of the FINESSE trial, patients were stratified by study center to receive enoxaparin or UFH [49]. Lower non-intracranial TIMI major bleeding was found with enoxaparin (2.6 % vs. 4.4 % for UFH, $p=0.045$). A composite of less death, MI, urgent revascularization, or refractory ischemia through 30 days was also associated with enoxaparin (5,3 % vs. 8.0 %, $p=0.0005$). Li et al. examined a prospective multicenter registry comparing UFH with enoxaparin plus low-dose UFH during PCI. At 8 months both total (4.5 % vs. 7.6 %, $p<0.01$) and cardiac death (3.6 % vs. 5.6 %, $p<0.006$) were reduced in the enoxaparin group [50]. At present there seems to be a trend in favor of enoxaparin over UFH in primary PCI, but in the absence of large randomized trials, no definite statement about the superiority of either drug can be made.

Fondaparinux

The clinical efficacy and safety of fondaparinux was evaluated in the OASIS (Organization for the Assessment of Strategies for Ischemic Syndromes)-6 trial, which randomly assigned 12,092 patients with STEMI to receive either treatment with fondaparinux (2.5 mg/day, started early and given for up to 8 days) or usual care (placebo for those for whom UFH was not indicated or UFH for up to 48 h followed by placebo for up to 8 days) [51]. Patients undergoing primary PCI, however, exhibited a trend towards a higher rate of death or MI with fondaparinux (2.5–5.0 mg administered intravenously) than with UFH. The number of patients with catheter thrombosis was 0 in the UFH group and 22 in the fondaparinux group ($p<0.001$). Thus, fondaparinux should not be used as the sole anticoagulant agent for patient undergoing PCI.

Bivalirudin

The HORIZONS-AMI (Harmonizing Outcomes with Revascularization and Stents in Acute Myocardial Infarction) trial randomly assigned 3,602 patients with STEMI who were undergoing primary PCI to treatment with UFH plus a GPI or to treatment with bivalirudin alone [52]. The incidence of the primary end point of net adverse clinical events, defined as a composite of death, MI, ischemic target vessel revascularization, stroke, or major bleeding at 30 days, was 24 % lower in the group treated with bivalirudin alone (9.2 %) than in the group receiving UFH plus a GPI (12.1 %; $p=0.005$). This difference was driven primarily by a 40 % reduction in the rate of major bleeding (bivalirudin, 4.9 %; UFH/GPI, 8.3 %; $p<0.001$). The incidence of major adverse cardiac events was similar in the two groups (bivalirudin group, 5.4 %; UFH group, 5.5 %; $p>.99$). After a 1-year follow-up period, the rate of cardiac-related mortality was 43 % lower, and the rate of all-cause mortality was 31 % lower (absolute reductions, 1.7 and 1.4 % respectively) in the group receiving bivalirudin monotherapy than in the group receiving UFH plus GPI inhibitors. Although the risk of acute stent thrombosis within 24 h was higher in the bivalirudin group, no statistically significant difference in the incidence of stent thrombosis was seen between the groups at 30 days and at 1 year. Of note, most patients received up-front loading with clopidogrel but not in a randomized fashion. This is likely important as a post hoc analysis of the ACUITY study showed that while patients with an acute coronary syndrome had an improved net clinical benefit when bivalirudin was used instead of UFH and a GPI, this benefit was driven almost entirely by less bleeding. The patients who received bivalirudin but did not receive a thienopyridine beforehand actually had no clinical benefit as they had less bleeding but more ischemic complications. The patients who did receive a thienopyridine and bivalirudin, however, bled less and had the same incidence of ischemic complications as did the UFH/GPI patients [53].

Glycoprotein IIb/IIIa Receptor Antagonists

Much of the evidence that supports the use of GPI in STEMI patients was obtained in an era before the routine use of dual antiplatelet therapy and largely by placebo-controlled trials. The role of these drugs alongside dual antiplatelet therapy and an anticoagulant has been recently been questioned.

The BRAVE-3 study randomized 800 patients presenting within 24 h of a STEMI and treated with 600 mg of clopidogrel and UFH to abciximab or placebo before PCI [54]. The primary end point of infarct size before hospital discharge was not significantly different between the two groups. Moreover, the composite of death, recurrent MI, stroke, or urgent revascularization of the infarct-related artery at 30 days was not significantly different (5 % in abciximab group vs. 3.8 % in placebo group; $p=0.4$). ON-TIME 2 was a multicenter, randomized, European study that randomized 984 STEMI patients to receive high-dose tirofiban (25mcg/kg bolus followed by 0.15 mcg/kg/min for 18 h) or placebo within a median of 76 min from the onset of symptoms [55]. All patients received clopidogrel 600 mg in addition to aspirin and an unfractionated heparin bolus. The primary end point of ST segment resolution before and 1 h after PCI was significantly improved in the tirofiban group ($p=0.003$, NNT 100). There was no difference, however, in TIMI grade 3 flow or blush grade and no difference in death, recurrent MI, or urgent TVR at 30 days between the two groups. Minor and major bleeding was also similar in both groups. The HORIZONS-AMI trial compared unfractionated heparin with a GPI (abciximab or double-bolus eptifibatide) to bivalirudin alone with provisional GPI bailout [52]. All patients received aspirin and clopidogrel loading. The rates of major bleeding and total adverse events were higher among patients treated with UFH and GPI than those of patients treated with bivalirudin.

Data suggest that there is no difference in the efficacy of small-molecule GPI (eptifibatide and tirofiban) and abciximab in STEMI patients. MULTISTRATEGY was a European trial that randomized 745 STEMI patients undergoing primary PCI to high-dose bolus tirofiban or abciximab infusion [56]. All patients received aspirin, clopidogrel 300 mg, and UFH. The prespecified primary end points of 50 % ST segment resolution and rate of major adverse cardiac events at 8 months were not significantly different between the two groups. The incidence of severe or moderate thrombocytopenia was more common with abciximab than with tirofiban (4 % vs. 0.8 %, $p=0.004$). In a meta-analysis of randomized trials, no significant difference was found in the post-procedural TIMI flow grade 3 or ST segment resolution and no difference in 30-day mortality, re-infarction, or major TIMI bleeding when small-molecule GPI was compared with abciximab in primary PCI [57].

The FINESSE trial addressed the issue of up-front initiation of GPI (in the emergency department) as opposed to starting the medication at the time of PCI [41]. It randomized 2,453 STEMI patients to pre-PCI treatment with a half-dose fibrinolytic agent plus abciximab, pre-PCI abciximab alone, or abciximab at the time of PCI. The trial showed no benefit and a tendency towards excess bleeding in the groups receiving prehospital abciximab compared with the group receiving abciximab at the time of PCI.

Oral Antiplatelet Agents for STEMI PCI

There are three oral thienopyridine or thienopyridine-like agents that are routinely used. Clopidogrel was the first thienopyridine to gain wide acceptance for routine use in primary PCI. More recently prasugrel and ticagrelor have been approved for use in US markets.

Given that almost all STEMI patients receive stents thus requiring treatment with a thienopyridine, no studies have been performed comparing clopidogrel to placebo in STEMI PCI. Several studies, however, have examined whether treatment with clopidogrel before PCI for patients with recent STEMI is superior to clopidogrel treatment initiated at the time of PCI in preventing major adverse cardiovascular events. The PCI-CLARITY study was a prospectively planned analysis of the 1,863 patients who underwent PCI after mandated angiography in the CLARITY-TIMI 28 trial [58]. Patients were randomly assigned to receive either clopidogrel or placebo initiated with thrombolysis and given until coronary angiography, which was performed 2–8 days later. Patients undergoing coronary artery stenting were given open-label clopidogrel after diagnostic angiography. Overall, pretreatment with clopidogrel resulted in a statistically significant reduction of 41 % in the incidence of cardiovascular death, MI, or stroke from the time of randomization through 30 days thereafter (7.5 % vs. 12.0 %; odds ratio, 0.59; $p=.001$). No significant difference was found between groups in the rates of TIMI major or minor bleeding. Subsequently, pretreatment with 300–600 mg clopidogrel before PCI in STEMI patients is recommended (class I) [23].

Several investigations have explored various loading doses of clopidogrel before or during PCI. The ISAR-CHOICE trial compared different loading doses of clopidogrel in an elective PCI setting [59]. Compared with a 300-mg loading dose, doses of either 600 mg or 900 mg achieve greater degrees of platelet inhibition with fewer low responders. There is no benefit, however, with increasing the loading dose to 900 mg compared with 600 mg. In a STEMI population, another study suggested that a 600-mg loading dose of clopidogrel is associated with improvements in procedural angiographic end points and 1-year clinical outcomes in patients with STEMI who undergo primary PCI compared with a 300-mg dose [60].

The pivotal trial for the use of prasugrel was the TRITON-TIMI 38 study which randomly assigned 13,608 patients with moderate- to high-risk ACS, 3,534 of whom had STEMI, to receive prasugrel (60 mg loading followed by 10 mg daily) or clopidogrel (300 mg loading followed by 75 mg daily) [61]. Prasugrel was associated with a significant 2.2 % absolute reduction (9.9 % vs. 12.1 %; $p<0.001$) and a 19 % relative reduction in the primary efficacy end point, a composite of the rate of death due to cardiovascular causes, nonfatal MI, or nonfatal stroke during an average follow-up of 145 months. Prasugrel, however, was associated with a significant increase in rate of bleeding (TIMI major hemorrhage [1.8 % vs. 2.4 %, $p=0.03$]). The STEMI results for efficacy and safety are consistent with the main results of the trial. Post hoc analysis suggested that patients with a history of stroke or transient ischemic attack prior to enrollment had net harm from prasugrel and patients older than 75 years of age or patients with body weight less than 60 kg had no clinical benefit [62].

Ticagrelor reversibly binds the $P2Y_{12}$ receptor. Unlike clopidogrel or prasugrel, ticagrelor is not a thienopyridine. It also does not require metabolic conversion to an active metabolite. The PLATO (Platelet Inhibition and Patient Outcomes) trial compared ticagrelor (180-mg loading dose, 90 mg twice daily thereafter) to clopidogrel (300–600-mg loading dose, 75 mg daily thereafter) in over 18,000 patients with ACS (7,000 of whom presented with STEMI) [62]. Ticagrelor was associated with a significant 1.9 % reduction in absolute risk and a 16 % reduction in relative risk in the primary composite end point of vascular death, nonfatal MI, or nonfatal stroke. Importantly, a significant reduction in vascular mortality and all-cause mortality was observed. Although CABG-related bleeding was not significantly increased with ticagrelor compared with clopidogrel, a significantly greater incidence of major bleeding was observed in patients not undergoing CABG. Ticagrelor was associated with higher rates of transient dyspnea and bradycardia compared with clopidogrel, although only a very small percentage of patients discontinued the study drug because of side effects.

Adenosine

Adenosine, acting by stimulating the A_1 and A_3 receptors, has been shown in animal models to mimic ischemic preconditioning responses and to potentially interfere with reperfusion injury. Large-scale clinical trials of adenosine and its analog, however, have failed to demonstrate clinical efficacy. In the pilot Acute Myocardial Infarction Study of Adenosine (AMISTAD)-I trial, intravenous adenosine reduced infarct size in patients treated with thrombolysis, a benefit that was limited to STEMIs involving the anterior wall [63]. The subsequent AMISTAD-II trial was conducted in patients with anterior STEMI receiving either thrombolysis or primary PCI [64]. A 3-h infusion of adenosine did not reduce the primary clinical end point, although in a post hoc subgroup analysis, a benefit was seen in those reperfused within 3 h [65]. In addition, a significant reduction in infarct size was reported in the high-dose adenosine subgroup (median infarct size, 27 % of the left ventricle with placebo vs. 11 % with high-dose adenosine; $p=0.02$) [66].

Technical Aspects of Primary PCI

Thrombus Aspiration

There is concern that conventional STEMI PCI using balloons and stents, by potentially dislodging thrombotic material or atherosclerotic debris into the distal circulation, can cause microvascular obstruction via plugging with secondary spasm and platelet aggregation, resulting in further myocardial necrosis. Sianos et al. reported that a large thrombus burden in acute MI intervention is related to higher rates of distal embolization and no reflow, decreased myocardial perfusion, and lower rates of final TIMI 3 flow which were associated with worse clinical outcomes [67]. Devices which can perform thrombectomy have subsequently been developed in an attempt to improve these outcomes.

TAPAS 1 was a single-center, prospective, non-blinded, randomized trial that enrolled 1,071 patients with STEMI and randomized them before angiography to conventional PCI or thrombectomy using an aspiration catheter before PTCA or stenting [68]. All patients received aspirin, clopidogrel, unfractionated heparin, and abciximab unless contraindicated. The primary end point of myocardial blush grade 0 or 1 occurred in 17.1 % of patients with thrombus aspiration and 26.3 % of patients with conventional PCI ($p<0.001$). Complete ST segment resolution was significantly more frequent in the thrombus aspiration group (56.6 % vs. 44.2 %; $p<0.001$). At 30 days, the incidence of death, re-infarction, and target vessel revascularization was not significantly different between the two groups. At 1 year, however, cardiac death was significantly lower in the thrombus aspiration group (3.6 % with thrombus aspiration vs. 6.7 % with conventional PCI; $p=0.02$) and cardiac death or re-infarction was also reduced (5.6 % with thrombus aspiration vs. 9.9 % with conventional PCI; $p=0.009$) [69]. In a later sub-study, two catheters of differing internal lumen diameters were compared. In this study, the larger catheter did not result in retrieval of larger thrombotic particles or in improved outcomes [70]. EXPIRA was a smaller randomized trial ($n = 175$) that compared thrombus aspiration with conventional PCI, but only in patients with TIMI flow grade 0/1 [71]. There was a significant increase in myocardial blush grade 2 or more (88 % with thrombus aspiration vs. 60 % with conventional, $p < 0.001$) and 90-min ST segment resolution greater than 70 % (64 % with thrombus aspiration vs. 39 % with conventional, $p < 0.001$). Furthermore, infarct size as measured by contrast-enhanced MRI in 75 patients at 3 months was significantly reduced in the thrombus aspiration arm.

In a meta-analysis by Bavry et al. that included 30 studies with 6,415 patients and a weighted mean follow-up of 5 months, manual aspiration thrombectomy with PCI was associated with a reduction in mortality as compared to conventional PCI (2.7 % vs. 4.4 %, $p = 0.018$), while mechanical thrombectomy was associated with an increased mortality (5.3 % vs. 2.8 %, $p = 0.05$) [72].

In ATTEMPT (meta-analysis of 11 trials with over 2,600 patients and a median follow-up of 365 days), manual aspiration with PCI was associated with improved survival, but there was no benefit noted with mechanical thrombectomy [73]. Current guidelines recommend manual aspiration thrombectomy in patients undergoing primary PCI (class IIa) [43].

Rheolytic Thrombectomy

The AngioJet Rheolytic Thrombectomy in Patients undergoing Primary Angioplasty for Acute myocardial infarction (AIMI) trial randomized 480 patients with STEMI presenting within 12 h from symptom onset to treatment with mechanical thrombectomy as an adjunct to primary PCI or PCI alone [74]. Although the device resulted in effective thrombus removal, greater infarct size was seen in patients with rheolytic thrombectomy as compared with PCI alone (12.5 % vs. 9.8 % of the left ventricle, $p = 0.03$). Moreover, major adverse cardiac events at 30 days were significantly higher for the rheolytic thrombectomy group (6.7 % vs. 1.7 %, $p = 0.01$) and mortality was also increased (4.6 % vs. 0.8 %, $p = 0.02$). A later study (JETSTENT) utilized AngioJet mechanical thrombectomy only in patients with large thrombus burden (grade 3–5) [75]. Although the study did not statistically meet its primary end point, there was a trend towards improvement in ST segment resolution at 30 min.

Ischemic Preconditioning

Potential mechanisms that may contribute to further myocardial damage after primary PCI include microvascular dysfunction and lethal reperfusion injury. Activation of the endogenous protective mechanisms against reperfusion injury using a mechanical stimulus has emerged as an attractive approach to limit infarct size. Zhao and Vinten-Johansen demonstrated in dogs that three 30-s cycles of reperfusion interrupted by 30 s of ischemia after sustained lethal ischemia reduced infarct size [76]. The potential clinical application of so-called ischemic preconditioning (IP) in STEMI was recognized early. One of the studies enrolled 30 patients who were randomized to standard primary PCI with direct stenting or direct stenting after IP [77]. IP was performed within 1 min of restoring flow by 4 cycles of balloon inflation in the culprit coronary artery at the site of the lesion for 1 min interspersed with 1 min of deflation. Infarct size, measured as the magnitude of creatine kinase release over 72 h, was reduced by 36 % in the IP-treated patients. Microvascular perfusion, measured by angiographic blush grade, was also significantly improved. In another study of 38 patients, the same group of investigators reported a sustained benefit of IP, with smaller infarct size and a 7 % higher left ventricular ejection fraction at 6 months [78].

Therapeutic Hypothermia

Therapeutic hypothermia (TH) during the treatment of STEMI has been used as an adjunct to PCI in an attempt to limit reperfusion injury. Two small studies demonstrated no significant benefit to TH as an adjunct to PCI [79, 80]. On a post hoc analysis of both studies, patients who reached a core temperature of less than 35 °C demonstrated a significant decrease in the ratio of anterior MI infarct size to percentage of left ventricular surface area [81]. One other small study showed a small but statistically significant decrease in the size of the infarct relative to the myocardium at risk [82].

Embolic Protection

Several studies have utilized embolic or distal protection devices in STEMI patients in an attempt to reduce distal embolization and subsequently improve outcomes. These studies that evaluated different devices failed to demonstrate any significantly beneficial effects of embolic protection devices on myocardial reperfusion or clinical outcomes. The most notable of these studies was the Enhanced Myocardial Efficacy and Recovery by Aspiration of Liberated Debris (EMERALD) trial which enrolled 501 STEMI patients presenting within 6 h and undergoing primary or rescue PCI and randomized them to receive angioplasty with a balloon. Although distal protection was effective in retrieving embolic debris in 73 % of the patients, there was no improvement in microvascular flow and reperfusion success nor was there a reduction in infarct size or enhanced survival [83]. Currently, distal protection devices are not recommended for routine use in STEMI patients except for cases where the culprit is a vein graft where their utility has been demonstrated previously.

Access Route

There has been a great deal of interest in the past few years in the use of radial access over femoral access for PCI, given advantages such as reduced bleeding, patient comfort, etc. Initial studies, however, indicated that radial access is associated with longer procedure times, increased fluoroscopic times, and typically a steep learning curve[84–87]. In addition, it has been felt that certain complex PCIs are perhaps easier or safer to do by the transfemoral route rather than transradially. The RIVAL study randomized 7,021 patients with acute coronary syndrome (including STEMI patients) to radial or femoral access [88]. Interventionalists had to be facile with both access routes and have performed at least 50 radial PCIs in the preceding year. Access site crossover was greater in the radial access arm compared with femoral access (7.6 % vs. 2.0 %, $p<0.0001$). The primary outcome of death, MI, stroke, and non-CABG bleeding was similar between radial and femoral access arms (3.7 % vs. 4.0 %, hazard ratio 0.92, 95 % confidence interval 0.72–1.17, $p=0.5$). Secondary outcomes including death, MI, or stroke (3.2 % vs. 3.2 %, $p=0.9$) and non-CABG major bleeding (0.7 % vs. 0.9 %, $p=0.23$) were similar. Major vascular access site complications (1.4 % vs. 3.7 %, $p<0.0001$) and ACUITY non-CABG major bleeding (1.9 % vs. 4.5 %, $p<0.0001$) were significantly lower in the radial access arm. Although PCI procedure times were similar (35 vs. 34 min, $p=0.62$), fluoroscopy times were higher with radial access (9.3 vs. 8.0 min, $p<0.0001$). Patient-preferred access site for the next procedure was almost twice as high with radial access (90 % vs. 49 %, $p<0.0001$). Of note, in the subgroup of STEMI patients (28 % of the cohort) treated via the radial artery, investigators observed a statistically significant 40 % relative reduction in the risk of death, MI, stroke, or non-CABG-related major bleeding and a significant 61 % relative reduction in the risk of death although the study was not powered to show a mortality benefit in this subgroup analysis. It is clear, however, that there is a reduction in access site complications with radial access, although this was not associated with a reduction in major bleeding or a reduction in major adverse events [88].

Intra-aortic Balloon Pump

The Intra-aortic Balloon Pump (IABP) improves diastolic coronary blood flow and reduces myocardial work. These physiological effects of the IABP have been thought to be especially helpful in patients with STEMI with ongoing or recurrent ischemic discomfort, hypotension from ischemia-mediated LV dysfunction, and cardiogenic shock. The American College of Cardiology and American Heart Association (ACC/AHA) STEMI guidelines list IABP therapy in cardiogenic shock as a class IB recommendation, although there are no randomized studies supporting its use [43]. The SHOCK II trial which randomized 600 patients with acute myocardial infarction complicated by cardiogenic shock to IABP or no standard therapy. There was no difference in the primary end point of a 30-day mortality (39.7 % in the IABP group vs. 41.3 % in the control group, $p=0.69$). There was also no difference in secondary end points including time to hemodynamic stabilization, length of stay in the ICU, dose and duration of catecholamine therapy, and renal function [89].

Impella

The Impella Recover LP 2.5 System (AbioMed, Aachen, Germany/Danvers, Massachusetts) is a 12.5-Fr catheter that is inserted percutaneously through a 13-Fr femoral artery sheath and placed across the aortic valve into the left ventricle, through which a transaxial blood pump provides reported flows of up to 2.5 L/min. This device has been reported to be used successfully in patients with cardiogenic shock due to acute myocardial infarction [90]. The hemodynamic effects of the Impella 2.5 have been studied in high-risk PCI patients, demonstrating beneficial LV unloading effect (decreased end-diastolic pressure and wall stress) with no change in global or systolic LV function [91]. The PROTECT I (A Prospective Feasibility Trial Investigating the Use of the Impella Recover LP 2.5 System in Patients Undergoing High-Risk PCI) trial in 20 patients undergoing high-risk PCI with the Impella 2.5 system concluded that this device was safe, easy to implant, and hemodynamically effective [92]. The randomized PROTECT II (A Prospective, Multicenter, Randomized, Controlled Trial of the Impella Recover LP 2.5 System Versus Intra Aortic Balloon Pump in Patients Undergoing Non Emergent High-Risk PCI) trial, which was designed to demonstrate superiority of Impella over IABP in terms of 1-month adverse events, was halted for futility after interim analysis of study results. There have been no randomized studies on the use of Impella prophylactically in patients with STEMI although it is indicated for use in patients with cardiogenic shock.

Conclusion

In summary, primary PCI in a timely manner has emerged as the current standard of treatment for STEMI patients. Manual thrombus aspiration followed by stent deployment and adjunct pharmacological intervention with dual antiplatelet therapy and an anticoagulant is currently the best treatment option for these patients.

References

1. Roger VL, et al. Heart disease and stroke statistics-2012 update: a report from the American Heart Association. Circulation. 2012;125(1):e2–220.
2. Fibrinolytic Therapy Trialists' (FTT) Collaborative Group. Indications for fibrinolytic therapy in suspected acute myocardial infarction: collaborative overview of early mortality and major morbidity results from all randomised trials of more than 1000 patients. Lancet. 1994;343(8893):311–22.
3. Chesebro JH, et al. Thrombolysis in Myocardial Infarction (TIMI) trial, phase I: a comparison between intravenous tissue plasminogen activator and intravenous streptokinase. Clinical findings through hospital discharge. Circulation. 1987;76(1):142–54.
4. Straznicky IT, White HD. Thrombolytic therapy for acute myocardial infarction in the elderly. Coron Artery Dis. 2000;11(4):299–304.
5. O'Neill W, et al. A prospective randomized clinical trial of intracoronary streptokinase versus coronary angioplasty for acute myocardial infarction. N Engl J Med. 1986;314(13):812–8.
6. Grines CL, et al. A comparison of immediate angioplasty with thrombolytic therapy for acute myocardial infarction. The Primary Angioplasty in Myocardial Infarction Study Group. N Engl J Med. 1993;328(10):673–9.
7. Zijlstra F, et al. A comparison of immediate coronary angioplasty with intravenous streptokinase in acute myocardial infarction. N Engl J Med. 1993;328(10):680–4.
8. de Boer MJ, et al. Immediate coronary angioplasty versus intravenous streptokinase in acute myocardial infarction: left ventricular ejection fraction, hospital mortality and re-infarction. J Am Coll Cardiol. 1994;23(5):1004–8.
9. The Global Use of Strategies to Open Occluded Coronary Arteries in Acute Coronary Syndromes (GUSTO IIb) Angioplasty Substudy Investigators. A clinical trial comparing primary coronary angioplasty with tissue plasminogen activator for acute myocardial infarction. N Engl J Med. 1997;336(23):1621–8.
10. Keeley EC, Boura JA, Grines CL. Primary angioplasty versus intravenous thrombolytic therapy for acute myocardial infarction: a quantitative review of 23 randomised trials. Lancet. 2003;361(9351):13–20.
11. Stone GW, et al. Influence of acute myocardial infarction location on in-hospital and late outcome after primary percutaneous transluminal coronary angioplasty versus tissue plasminogen activator therapy. Am J Cardiol. 1996;78(1):19–25.
12. Henriques JP, et al. Primary percutaneous coronary intervention versus thrombolytic treatment: long term follow up according to infarct location. Heart. 2006;92(1):75–9.
13. Magid DJ, et al. Relation between hospital primary angioplasty volume and mortality for patients with acute MI treated with primary angioplasty vs thrombolytic therapy. JAMA. 2000;284(24):3131–8.
14. Canto JG, et al. The volume of primary angioplasty procedures and survival after acute myocardial infarction. National Registry of Myocardial Infarction 2 Investigators. N Engl J Med. 2000;342(21):1573–80.
15. Kastrati A, et al. Meta-analysis of randomized trials on drug-eluting stents vs. bare-metal stents in patients with acute myocardial infarction. Eur Heart J. 2007;28(22):2706–13.
16. De Luca G, et al. Efficacy and safety of drug-eluting stents in ST-segment elevation myocardial infarction: a meta-analysis of randomized trials. Int J Cardiol. 2009;133(2):213–22.
17. Stone GW, et al. Paclitaxel-eluting stents versus bare-metal stents in acute myocardial infarction. N Engl J Med. 2009;360(19):1946–59.
18. Nallamothu BK, Bates ER. Percutaneous coronary intervention versus fibrinolytic therapy in acute myocardial infarction: is timing (almost) everything? Am J Cardiol. 2003;92(7):824–6.
19. Boersma E. Does time matter? A pooled analysis of randomized clinical trials comparing primary percutaneous coronary intervention and in-hospital thrombolysis in acute myocardial infarction patients. Eur Heart J. 2006;27(7):779–88.
20. Nallamothu BK, et al. Driving times and distances to hospitals with percutaneous coronary intervention in the United States: implications for prehospital triage of patients with ST-elevation myocardial infarction. Circulation. 2006;113(9):1189–95.
21. Chakrabarti A, et al. Time-to-reperfusion in patients undergoing interhospital transfer for primary percutaneous coronary intervention in the U.S: an analysis of 2005 and 2006 data from the National Cardiovascular Data Registry. J Am Coll Cardiol. 2008;51(25):2442–3.
22. Nallamothu BK, et al. Times to treatment in transfer patients undergoing primary percutaneous coronary intervention in the United States: National Registry of Myocardial Infarction (NRMI)-3/4 analysis. Circulation. 2005;111(6):761–7.
23. Kushner FG, et al. 2009 focused updates: ACC/AHA guidelines for the management of patients with ST-elevation myocardial infarction (updating the 2004 guideline and 2007 focused update) and ACC/AHA/SCAI guidelines on percutaneous coronary intervention (updating the 2005 guideline and 2007 focused update) a report of the American College of Cardiology Foundation/American Heart Association Task Force on Practice Guidelines. J Am Coll Cardiol. 2009;54(23):2205–41.
24. Van de Werf F, et al. Management of acute myocardial infarction in patients presenting with persistent ST-segment elevation: the Task Force on the Management of ST-Segment Elevation Acute Myocardial Infarction of the European Society of Cardiology. Eur Heart J. 2008;29(23):2909–45.
25. Ting HH, et al. Regional systems of care to optimize timeliness of reperfusion therapy for ST-elevation myocardial infarction: the Mayo Clinic STEMI Protocol. Circulation. 2007;116(7):729–36.
26. Andersen HR, et al. A comparison of coronary angioplasty with fibrinolytic therapy in acute myocardial infarction. N Engl J Med. 2003;349(8):733–42.
27. Widimsky P, et al. Long distance transport for primary angioplasty vs immediate thrombolysis in acute myocardial infarction. Final results of the randomized national multicentre trial–PRAGUE-2. Eur Heart J. 2003;24(1):94–104.
28. Grines CL, et al. A randomized trial of transfer for primary angioplasty versus on-site thrombolysis in patients with high-risk myocardial infarction: the Air Primary Angioplasty in Myocardial Infarction study. J Am Coll Cardiol. 2002;39(11):1713–9.
29. De Luca G, Biondi-Zoccai G, Marino P. Transferring patients with ST-segment elevation myocardial infarction for mechanical reperfusion: a meta-regression analysis of randomized trials. Ann Emerg Med. 2008;52(6):665–76.
30. Henry TD, et al. A regional system to provide timely access to percutaneous coronary intervention for ST-elevation myocardial infarction. Circulation. 2007;116(7):721–8.
31. Cantor WJ, et al. Routine early angioplasty after thrombolysis for acute myocardial infarction. N Engl J Med. 2009;360(26):2705–18.
32. Di Mario C, et al. Immediate angioplasty versus standard therapy with rescue angioplasty after thrombolysis in the Combined Abciximab REteplase Stent Study in Acute Myocardial Infarction (CARESS-in-AMI): an open, prospective, randomised, multicentre trial. Lancet. 2008;371(9612):559–68.
33. Cannon CP, et al. TNK-tissue plasminogen activator compared with front-loaded alteplase in acute myocardial infarction: results of the TIMI 10B trial. Thrombolysis in Myocardial Infarction (TIMI) 10B Investigators. Circulation. 1998;98(25):2805–14.
34. Cannon CP, et al. TNK-tissue plasminogen activator in acute myocardial infarction. Results of the Thrombolysis in Myocardial Infarction (TIMI) 10A dose-ranging trial. Circulation. 1997;95(2):351–6.

35. Sabatine MS, et al. Addition of clopidogrel to aspirin and fibrinolytic therapy for myocardial infarction with ST-segment elevation. N Engl J Med. 2005;352(12):1179–89.
36. Chen ZM, et al. Addition of clopidogrel to aspirin in 45,852 patients with acute myocardial infarction: randomised placebo-controlled trial. Lancet. 2005;366(9497):1607–21.
37. Larson DM, et al. Safety and efficacy of a pharmaco-invasive reperfusion strategy in rural ST-elevation myocardial infarction patients with expected delays due to long-distance transfers. Eur Heart J. 2012;33(10):1232–40.
38. Hochman JS, et al. Coronary intervention for persistent occlusion after myocardial infarction. N Engl J Med. 2006;355(23):2395–407.
39. Van de Werf F, et al. Primary versus tenecteplase-facilitated percutaneous coronary intervention in patients with ST-segment elevation acute myocardial infarction (Assent-4 PCI): randomized trial. Lancet. 2006;367(9510):569–78.
40. Ross AM, et al. The impact of place of enrollment and delay to reperfusion on 90-day post-infarction mortality in the ASSENT-4 PCI trial: assessment of the safety and efficacy of a new treatment strategy with percutaneous coronary intervention. JACC Cardiovasc Interv. 2009;2(10):925–30.
41. Ellis SG, et al. Facilitated PCI in patients with ST-elevation myocardial infarction. N Engl J Med. 2008;358(8):2205–17 (Is this FINESSE?).
42. Herrmann HC, et al. Benefit of facilitated percutaneous coronary intervention in high-risk ST-segment elevation myocardial infarction patients presenting to nonpercutaneous coronary intervention hospitals. JACC Cardiovasc Interv. 2009;2(10):917–24.
43. Antman EM, et al. ACC/AHA guidelines for the management of patients with ST-elevation myocardial infarction-executive summary. A report of the American College of Cardiology/American Heart Association Task Force on Practice Guidelines (Writing Committee to revise the 1999 guidelines for the management of patients with acute myocardial infarction). J Am Coll Cardiol. 2004;44(3):671–719.
44. Sutton AG, et al. A randomized trial of rescue angioplasty versus a conservative approach for failed thrombolysis in ST-segment elevation myocardial infarction: the Middlesbrough Early Revascularization to Limit INfarction (MERLIN) trial. J Am Coll Cardiol. 2004;44(2):287–96.
45. Gershlick AH, et al. Rescue angioplasty after failed thrombolytic therapy for acute myocardial infarction. N Engl J Med. 2005;353(26):2758–68.
46. Wijeysundera HC, et al. Rescue angioplasty or repeat thrombolysis after failed fibrinolytic therapy for ST-segment myocardial infarction: a meta-analysis of randomized trials. J Am Coll Cardiol. 2007;49(4):422–30.
47. Antman EM, et al. 2007 Focused Update of the ACC/AHA 2004 Guidelines for the Management of Patients With ST-Elevation Myocardial Infarction: a report of the American College of Cardiology/American Heart Association Task Force on Practice Guidelines: developed in collaboration With the Canadian Cardiovascular Society endorsed by the American Academy of Family Physicians: 2007 Writing Group to Review New Evidence and Update the ACC/AHA 2004 Guidelines for the Management of Patients With ST-Elevation Myocardial Infarction, Writing on Behalf of the 2004 Writing Committee. Circulation. 2008;117(2):296–329.
48. Montalescot G, et al. Intravenous enoxaparin or unfractionated heparin in primary percutaneous coronary intervention for ST-elevation myocardial infarction: the international randomised open-label ATOLL Trial. Lancet. 2011;378(9792):693–703.
49. Montalescot G, et al. Enoxaparin in primary and facilitated percutaneous coronary intervention A formal prospective nonrandomized substudy of the FINESSE trial (Facilitated INtervention with Enhanced Reperfusion Speed to Stop Events). JACC Cardiovasc Interv. 2010;3(2):203–12.
50. Li YJ, et al. Low-molecular-weight heparin versus unfractionated heparin in acute ST-segment elevation myocardial infarction patients undergoing primary percutaneous coronary intervention with drug-eluting stents. Am Heart J. 2010;159(4):684–90 e1.
51. Yusuf S, et al. Effects of fondaparinux on mortality and re-infarction in patients with acute ST-segment elevation myocardial infarction: the OASIS-6 randomized trial. JAMA. 2006;295(13):1519–30.
52. Stone GW, et al. Bivalirudin during primary PCI in acute myocardial infarction. N Engl J Med. 2008;358(21):2218–30.
53. Stone GW, et al. Bivalirudin for patients with acute coronary syndromes. N Engl J Med. 2006;355(21):2203–16.
54. Mehilli J, et al. Abciximab in patients with acute ST-segment-elevation myocardial infarction undergoing primary percutaneous coronary intervention after clopidogrel loading: a randomized double-blind trial. Circulation. 2009;119(14):1933–40.
55. Van't Hof AW, et al. Prehospital initiation of tirofiban in patients with ST-elevation myocardial infarction undergoing primary angioplasty (On-TIME 2): a multicentre, double-blind, randomised controlled trial. Lancet. 2008;372(9638):537–46.
56. Valgimigli M, et al. Comparison of angioplasty with infusion of tirofiban or abciximab and with implantation of sirolimus-eluting or uncoated stents for acute myocardial infarction: the MULTISTRATEGY randomized trial. JAMA. 2008;299(15):1788–99.
57. De Luca G, et al. Benefits from small molecule administration as compared with abciximab among patients with ST-segment elevation myocardial infarction treated with primary angioplasty: a meta-analysis. J Am Coll Cardiol. 2009;53(18):1668–73.
58. Sabatine MS, et al. Effect of clopidogrel pretreatment before percutaneous coronary intervention in patients with ST-elevation myocardial infarction treated with fibrinolytics: the PCI-CLARITY study. JAMA. 2005;294(10):1224–32.
59. von Beckerath N, et al. Absorption, metabolization, and antiplatelet effects of 300-, 600-, and 900-mg loading doses of clopidogrel: results of the ISAR-CHOICE (Intracoronary Stenting and Antithrombotic Regimen: Choose Between 3 High Oral Doses for Immediate Clopidogrel Effect) Trial. Circulation. 2005;112(19):2946–50.
60. Mangiacapra F, et al. Comparison of 600 versus 300-mg Clopidogrel loading dose in patients with ST-segment elevation myocardial infarction undergoing primary coronary angioplasty. Am J Cardiol. 2010;106(9):1208–11.
61. Wiviott SD, et al. Prasugrel versus clopidogrel in patients with acute coronary syndromes. N Engl J Med. 2007;357(20):2001–15.
62. Wallentin L, et al. Ticagrelor versus clopidogrel in patients with acute coronary syndromes. N Engl J Med. 2009;361(11):1045–57.
63. Forman MB, Stone GW, Jackson EK. Role of adenosine as adjunctive therapy in acute myocardial infarction. Cardiovasc Drug Rev. 2006;24(2):116–47.
64. Mahaffey KW, et al. Adenosine as an adjunct to thrombolytic therapy for acute myocardial infarction: results of a multicenter, randomized, placebo-controlled trial: the Acute Myocardial Infarction STudy of ADenosine (AMISTAD) trial. J Am Coll Cardiol. 1999;34(6):1711–20.
65. Kloner RA, et al. Impact of time to therapy and reperfusion modality on the efficacy of adenosine in acute myocardial infarction: the AMISTAD-2 trial. Eur Heart J. 2006;27(20):2400–5.
66. Ross AM, et al. A randomized, double-blinded, placebo-controlled multicenter trial of adenosine as an adjunct to reperfusion in the treatment of acute myocardial infarction (AMISTAD-II). J Am Coll Cardiol. 2005;45(11):1775–80.
67. Sianos G, et al. Angiographic stent thrombosis after routine use of drug-eluting stents in ST-segment elevation myocardial infarction: the importance of thrombus burden. J Am Coll Cardiol. 2007;50(7):573–83.
68. Svilaas T, et al. Thrombus aspiration during primary percutaneous coronary intervention. N Engl J Med. 2008;358(6):557–67.

69. Vlaar PJ, et al. Cardiac death and re-infarction after 1 year in the Thrombus Aspiration during Percutaneous coronary intervention in Acute myocardial infarction Study (TAPAS): a 1-year follow-up study. Lancet. 2008;371(9628):1915–20.
70. Vlaar PJ, et al. A comparison of 2 thrombus aspiration devices with histopathological analysis of retrieved material in patients presenting with ST-segment elevation myocardial infarction. JACC Cardiovasc Interv. 2008;1(3):258–64.
71. Sardella G, et al. Thrombus aspiration during primary percutaneous coronary intervention improves myocardial reperfusion and reduces infarct size: the EXPIRA (thrombectomy with export catheter in infarct-related artery during primary percutaneous coronary intervention) prospective, randomized trial. J Am Coll Cardiol. 2009;53(4):309–15.
72. Bavry AA, Kumbhani DJ, Bhatt DL. Role of adjunctive thrombectomy and embolic protection devices in acute myocardial infarction: a comprehensive meta-analysis of randomized trials. Eur Heart J. 2008;29(24):2989–3001.
73. Burzotta F, et al. Clinical impact of thrombectomy in acute ST-elevation myocardial infarction: an individual patient-data pooled analysis of 11 trials. Eur Heart J. 2009;30(18):2193–203.
74. Ali A, et al. Rheolytic thrombectomy with percutaneous coronary intervention for infarct size reduction in acute myocardial infarction: 30-day results from a multicenter randomized study. J Am Coll Cardiol. 2006;48(2):244–52.
75. Migliorini A, et al. Comparison of AngioJet rheolytic thrombectomy before direct infarct artery stenting with direct stenting alone in patients with acute myocardial infarction. The JETSTENT trial. J Am Coll Cardiol. 2010;56(16):1298–306.
76. Zhao ZQ, Vinten-Johansen J. Postconditioning: reduction of reperfusion-induced injury. Cardiovasc Res. 2006;70(2):200–11.
77. Staat P, et al. Postconditioning the human heart. Circulation. 2005;112(14):2143–8.
78. Thibault H, et al. Long-term benefit of postconditioning. Circulation. 2008;117(8):1037–44.
79. Oneill W, et al. A prospective randomized trial of mild systemic hypothermia during percutaneous coronary intervention therapy of ST elevation myocardial infarction. Presented at the transcatheter cariovascular therapeutics conference, Washington, DC; 2004.
80. Grines C, et al. Intravascular cooling adjunctive to PCI. Presented at the transcatheter cardiovascular therapeutics conference, Washington, DC; 2004.
81. Oneill W. Novel myocardial preservation therapies: frustrations and future promise. Presented at the transcatheter cardovascular therapeutics conference, Washington, DC; 2006.
82. Gotberg M, et al. A pilot study of rapid cooling by cold saline and endovascular cooling. Cathet Cardiovasc Interv. 2010;3(5):400–7.
83. Stone GW, et al. Distal microcirculatory protection during percutaneous coronary intervention in acute ST-segment elevation myocardial infarction: a randomized controlled trial. JAMA. 2005; 293(9):1063–72.
84. Brueck M, et al. A randomized comparison of transradial versus transfemoral approach for coronary angiography and angioplasty. JACC Cardiovasc Interv. 2009;2(11):1047–54.
85. Neill J, et al. Comparison of radiation dose and the effect of operator experience in femoral and radial arterial access for coronary procedures. Am J Cardiol. 2010;106(7):936–40.
86. Sciahbasi A, et al. Evaluation of the "learning curve" for left and right radial approach during percutaneous coronary procedures. Am J Cardiol. 2011;108(2):185–8.
87. Looi JL, Cave A, El-Jack S. Learning curve in transradial coronary angiography. Am J Cardiol. 2011;108(8):1092–5.
88. Jolly SS, et al. Radial versus femoral access for coronary angiography and intervention in patients with acute coronary syndromes (RIVAL): a randomised, parallel group, multicentre trial. Lancet. 2011;377(9775):1409–20.
89. Thiele H, et al. Intraaortic balloon support for myocardial infarction with cardiogenic shock. N Engl J Med. 2012;367(14):1287–96.
90. Seyfarth M, et al. A randomized clinical trial to evaluate the safety and efficacy of a percutaneous left ventricular assist device versus intra-aortic balloon pumping for treatment of cardiogenic shock caused by myocardial infarction. J Am Coll Cardiol. 2008;52(19):1584–8.
91. Remmelink M, et al. Effects of mechanical left ventricular unloading by Impella on left ventricular dynamics in high-risk and primary percutaneous coronary intervention patients. Catheter Cardiovasc Interv. 2010;75(2):187–94.
92. Sjauw KD, et al. Supported high-risk percutaneous coronary intervention with the Impella 2.5 device the Europella registry. J Am Coll Cardiol. 2009;54(25):2430–4.

17 Hemodynamic Support in PCI: *From Chronic Heart Failure to Cardiogenic Shock*

Jooby John and Kirk N. Garratt

Atherosclerotic coronary artery disease remains the leading cause of mortality in the USA, accounting for one in six deaths, at a rate of one patient dying per minute [1]. Coronary artery disease also remains a leading cause of heart failure (ischemic cardiomyopathy) [1]. The prevalence of heart failure in the USA is about 6 million with another 23 million patients affected outside the USA [2]. Improvement in survival after myocardial infarction has played a key role in the increased incidence of patients surviving with systolic dysfunction of the left ventricle [3]. This systolic dysfunction has been identified in multiple analyses to be a powerful predictor of amplified risk during percutaneous coronary intervention (PCI) [4, 5]. In an analysis from the National Heart, Lung, and Blood Institute Percutaneous Transluminal Coronary Angioplasty Registry and the Dynamic Registry, patients with systolic dysfunction of the left ventricle had a significantly higher in-hospital and 1-year mortality [6]. The hemodynamic, electrical, and clinical penalties of the transient cessation of coronary blood as a consequence of percutaneous coronary intervention (PCI) are much more severe in a compromised left ventricle with blunted hemodynamic reserve. Even in this age of near universal coronary stent use, the deliverability of stents is not assured and flow-limiting dissections during "pre-dilatation" can immediately impact the clinical course.

The Spectrum of Left Ventricular Dysfunction

Left ventricular (LV) dysfunction can range from minimal systolic dysfunction with no overt clinical signs to fulminant cardiogenic shock with acute decompensation. Cardiogenic shock remains the leading cause of death in patients presenting with acute ST segment elevation myocardial infarction (STEMI) [7], with one in two patients dying from the disease [8]. Extensive research into the pathophysiology of LV systolic dysfunction has revealed myriad complicated pathways with multiple levels of interactions at the cellular and microscopic levels [9–12]. Maladaptive neurohormonal and remodeling mechanisms are thought to play an integral role in the development and deterioration of systolic heart failure. Even minor degrees of LV dysfunction are thought to portend increased periprocedural risk during PCI, with mortality rates for patients in these cohorts ranging from 12 to 33 % in the early days of angioplasty [13].

Percutaneous Coronary Intervention in LV Dysfunction

Risks of intervention increase with reductions in LV function. One of the earlier attempts to define risk with PCI was with the use of a jeopardy score [14]. This score estimates the amount of myocardium at risk based on the location of stenoses in the coronary tree. In conjunction with the LV ejection fraction, the jeopardy score is a powerful stratifier of periprocedural risk. The relatively cumbersome nature of the risk calculation resulted in poor adoption, and it is not in common use today.

Cardiogenic Shock

The prognosis of patients with cardiogenic shock has improved substantially over the last three decades. The incidence of cardiogenic shock in acute myocardial infarction and the associated mortality have both decreased dramatically [15, 16]. Nonetheless, even today mortality from cardiogenic shock remains at around 50 % [17, 18]. Vasopressor and inotrope therapies have long been a mainstay in the

J. John, MD, MPH (✉) • K.N. Garratt, MSc, MD
Interventional Cardiology, Lenox Hill Hospital,
100 E 77th St., New York, NY 10021, USA
e-mail: joobyjohn@gmail.com; kgarratt@lenoxhill.net

C.A. Thompson (ed.), *Textbook of Cardiovascular Intervention*,
DOI 10.1007/978-1-4471-4528-8_17, © Springer-Verlag London 2014

Table 17.1 Comparison of three US approved percutaneous left ventricular support devices

	IABP	TandemHeart™	Impella 2.5®
Mechanism	Pneumatic displacement	Centrifugal flow	Axial flow
Femoral artery access	7–8F	15–17F	13F
Placement time (approx.)	5 min	15 min	30 min
Duration of use	2–5 days	14 days max	6 h max
Additional flow (L/min)	<0.5	4.0–5.0	2.5
Physiologic timing required	Yes	No	No
MAP	↑	↑↑	↑↑
CI	↑	↑↑↑	↑↑
CPO		↑↑	↑

Modified after Cyrus et al. [48], with permission
IABP intra-aortic balloon pump, *MAP* mean arterial pressure, *CI* cardiac index, *CPO* cardiac power output

treatment of cardiogenic shock, despite data that they, in effect, decrease long-term survival [19, 20].

Mechanical Support

Mechanical support with or without PCI has indications ranging from prophylactic to life saving. A useful way to measure the efficacy of mechanical support devices has been the concept of cardiac power output (CPO), which incorporates both parameters: cardiac output and blood pressure [21], and has predictive accuracy in multiple cardiac conditions [22]. CPO in watts = cardiac output in L/min × mean arterial BP/451. A CPO < 0.53 is predictive of mortality in cardiogenic shock. An ideal mechanical support device would therefore augment CPO by increasing cardiac output as well as blood pressure.

Three devices have been approved by US Food and Drug Administration for use in American patients: the intra-aortic balloon pump (IABP) and two percutaneous LV assist devices, the TandemHeart™ device and the Impella® 2.5 device. A review of each follows below; a summary comparison is found in Table 17.1.

Intra-aortic Balloon Pump

The intra-aortic balloon pump (IABP), initially introduced in the 1960s [23], is the most commonly used mechanical support device and has remained a staple in the interventionalist's arsenal [24]. IABPs work by increasing coronary blood flow [25]. Diastolic balloon inflation tends to increase antegrade flow (systemic perfusion), as well as retrograde flow (coronary and cerebral perfusion). Systolic deflation results in decreased afterload and decrease in myocardial oxygen demand. While IABPs do tend to decrease myocardial oxygen demand, there is only a minimal increase in cardiac output, estimated to be about 0.5 L/min [26]. Alleviation of myocardial ischemia thus appears to be the principal benefit accrued from IABP insertion. The IABP is dependent on a minimal baseline left ventricular pump function as well as a stable electrical milieu in order to provide hemodynamic support. Cardiogenic shock is the most common reason for the insertion of IABPs, accounting for about 20 % of all IABP procedures [27]. ACC/AHA and ESC guidelines strongly favor the use of an IABP in cardiogenic shock [28, 29]. Nevertheless, the evidence supporting the use of IABPs in cardiogenic shock is fragile, despite it having become the de facto standard of care for the treatment of cardiogenic shock. Registry data from the National Registry of Myocardial Infarction (NRMI)-2 as well as from the SHOCK (Should We Emergently Revascularize Occluded Coronary Arteries in Shock) trial suggested decreased mortality in cardiogenic shock patients who received IABP and thrombolytics as opposed to just thrombolytics [30, 31]. However, when including PCI, the patients with IABP did not have any benefit in NRMI-2 registry. A recent meta-analysis of randomized and observational date found a similar lack of benefit from the IABP, especially in the setting of optimal care [32]. In one of the earlier reports from the Benchmark Counterpulsation Outcomes Registry, the incidence of both major limb ischemia (0.9 %) and major bleeding (0.8 %) was acceptable compared to much higher prior numbers [33]. Limitations of the IABP lead directly to the development of the novel percutaneous assist devices. The strongest application of the IABP would be in resides in situations requiring reduction in oxygen demand is needed. The results of the CRISP-AMI trial revealed that IABP was not useful in addition to primary PCI for the treatment of STEMI without shock [34]. The recent IABP SHOCK II trial has called the effectiveness of routine IABP use in the setting of cardiogenic shock in question [35]. This randomized, open-label clinical trial evaluated 600 patients presenting with acute myocardial infarction and cardiogenic shock divided into patients receiving and not receiving intra-aortic balloon counterpulsation with intent for early revascularization and optimal medical support. IABP did not reduce mortality (39.7 % vs. 41.3 %, P = NS) or major predefined secondary endpoints. While limitations exist within this investigational setting, this trial supports the need for improved methods to manage this critical patient subset.

Percutaneous Left Ventricular Assist Devices (LVADs)

As opposed to the IABP, percutaneous LVADs provide active hemodynamic support with demonstrable difference in hemodynamic parameters. The two most commonly used percutaneous left ventricular assist devices (LVADs) in the USA are the TandemHeart™ and the Impella®. The TandemHeart™ (TandemHeart, Cardiac Assist, Pittsburgh, PA, USA) is a left atrial-to-femoral artery LVAD, driven by a continuous low-speed centrifugal pump [36]. The Impella® (Impella, Abiomed Europe GmbH, Aachen, Germany) is catheter-based axial-flow pump that pumps blood directly from the left ventricle into the ascending aorta [37]. A meta-analysis of three recent trials of IABP vs. the TandemHeart™ (two trials) and the Impella® (one trial) showed that while these newer devices had better hemodynamic parameters, they did not necessarily improve survival at 30 days [37–39]. Moreover, the TandemHeart™ was found to be associated with significantly worse bleeding and limb ischemia. The recently concluded PROTECT II trial showed in a priori analysis that the Impella® device was similar to the IABP in terms of major outcomes in elective high-risk PCI. It is important to remember that both the TandemHeart and the Impella devices are about ten times as expensive as the IABP. IABPs currently use a 7.5F or 8F sheath, while the Impella requires a 13F arteriotomy and the TandemHeart requires a 17F arteriotomy.

TandemHeart™

The TandemHeart™ is a percutaneous left atrium to iliac artery bypass device. Powered by a centrifugal pump, it can provide up to 4 L/min in forward flow. Insertion technique required venous access and transseptal puncture, with a 21F inflow cannula. Using arterial access a 15F or 17F outflow cannula is placed in the ipsilateral common iliac artery. In the initial human pilot studies, the TandemHeart decreased LV end-diastolic pressure and oxygen demand while simultaneously increasing mean arterial pressure [36]. A small multicenter randomized trial followed comparing the device to the IABP [39]. However, a subsequent meta-analysis of two trials did not show any difference in mortality [32].

Given the demands of transseptal puncture and the large cannulas insertion times in excess of 30 min have been reported in literature [40]. In addition to bleeding and limb ischemia, specific complications of the TandemHeart include arrhythmias, tamponade, atrial perforation, as well as residual atrial septal defects. Specific contraindications include a ventricular septal defect as well as aortic insufficiency or severe peripheral vascular disease. With worsening LV function, hemodynamic support becomes an overriding concern, and it is in this situation that the TandemHeart has definitive indications. The Impella 5.0 may deliver as much support as the TandemHeart but cannot be inserted percutaneously.

Hemodynamic effects of the TandemHeart device include augmentation of both cardiac output as well as blood pressure, effectively raising the cardiac power output. In simulated models, the CPO from a TandemHeart is between the Impella 2.5 and the Impella 5.0 devices, irrespective of the hemodynamic status [41]. Oxygen consumption is directly lowered by the device. In cardiogenic shock the increase in afterload would counter the decrease in myocardial oxygen demand thereby leading to a net neutral effect on myocardial oxygen demand. In animal models of acute myocardial infarction, the device has been demonstrated to restore epicardial as well as microvascular blood flow [42].

At the time of this writing, the US Food and Drug Administration is reviewing a proposal to study the ability of TandemHeart to reduce infarct size when it is placed prior to primary PCI. The TandemHeart to Reduce Infarct Size (TRIS) trial will assign STEMI patients randomly to primary PCI with or without TandemHeart support prior to recanalization of the culprit vessel. Shock patients will be excluded from this trial, but if results are encouraging, additional study in the shock population would be pursued (personal communication, 2011, Howard A. Cohen MD).

Impella®

The Impella consists of a small axial-flow pump that directly unloads the left ventricle by attaching to a pigtail catheter and moving blood from the left ventricle into the ascending aorta. Two devices are currently available with maximal flow rates of 2.5 L/min (Impella 2.5) or 5 L/min (Impella 5.0). The Impella requires a single femoral arteriotomy and the insertion of a 13F (Impella 2.5) catheter. After crossing the aortic valve, an exchange length 0.018″ stiff wire is used to place the device in the LV. Implantation times around 10 min have been documented [43]. A complication specific to the Impella device is hemolysis that can occur in 5–10 % of patients [44]. Aortic valve disease and LV thrombi are specific contraindications to insertion of the Impella device. The Impella has more supportive clinical data for efficacy in the failing ventricle than does the TandemHeart. The first US feasibility trial (PROTECT I) was a multicenter study of

20 sequential patients treated with Impella 2.5 device in a nonrandomized fashion [44]. All patients had poor left ventricular function (ejection fraction ≤35 %) and underwent PCI on an unprotected left main coronary artery or last remaining patent coronary conduit. Patients with acute myocardial infarction or cardiogenic shock were excluded from this study. Two patients died at days 12 and 14, and two patients developed transient hemolysis. The European AMC MACH I trial produced very similar results [37]. The AMC MACH 2 trial looked at patients who were experiencing an acute anterior wall myocardial infarction *without* cardiogenic shock. Compared to IABP, improvement in the LVEF was noted [43]. The ISAR SHOCK trial randomized patients with an acute anterior wall myocardial infarction *with* cardiogenic shock and demonstrated improved hemodynamics when compared to the IABP [45]. In the PROTECT II trial, the Impella 2.5 device was compared to IABP in patients with low LV ejection fractions undergoing non-emergent but high-risk PCI with an expectation that benefit would be seen, using a large composite endpoint made up of ten individual clinical outcomes. [46] The study was terminated prematurely because of futility. An *a priori* analysis showed no difference in mortality between the Impella and the IABP. Despite these disappointing findings, some investigators and many operators appear to believe the results were confounded, as evidenced by the continued (indeed, expanding) use of this device in such patients. In the Europella registry, the Impella device was used in elderly patients with an ejection fraction of less than 30 %. Mortality at 30 days was 5.5 % and hemolysis was seen in about 1 % of patients [47]. It should be noted that the majority of the clinical data are derived from the Impella 2.5 device and that the surgically placed Impella 5.0 device has yet to be subjected to rigorous clinical trial analysis. The IMPRESS in STEMI (European Impella vs. IABP Reduces Infarct Size in STEMI Patients Treated with Primary PCI) is an ongoing clinical trial that compares the Impella 2.5 with the IABP in *pre*-shock STEMI patients. Although these studies do not target overt heart failure or cardiogenic shock patients specifically, the results of these trials will help determine the best populations to target for use of these advanced devices.

Conclusion

Inotrope and vasopressor therapies have been demonstrated to adversely impact infarct size and long term survival in return for a modest increase in short-term survival. Earlier institution of mechanical support devices may allow the heart to rest while simultaneously preserving systemic perfusion. Preliminary study indicates that such a strategy should decrease final infarct sizes, particularly if implemented early, and would lower mortality rates. Clinical trials are ongoing.

References

1. Roger VL, Go AS, Lloyd-Jones DM, et al. Heart disease and stroke statistics–2011 update: a report from the American Heart Association. Circulation. 2011;123(4):e18–209.
2. Bui AL, Horwich TB, Fonarow GC. Epidemiology and risk profile of heart failure. Nat Rev Cardiol. 2011;8(1):30–41.
3. Torabi A, Rigby AS, Cleland JG. Declining in-hospital mortality and increasing heart failure incidence in elderly patients with first myocardial infarction. J Am Coll Cardiol. 2009;55(1):79–81; author reply 81.
4. Wu C, Hannan EL, Walford G, et al. A risk score to predict in-hospital mortality for percutaneous coronary interventions. J Am Coll Cardiol. 2006;47(3):654–60.
5. Singh M, Rihal CS, Selzer F, Kip KE, Detre K, Holmes DR. Validation of Mayo Clinic risk adjustment model for in-hospital complications after percutaneous coronary interventions, using the National Heart, Lung, and Blood Institute dynamic registry. J Am Coll Cardiol. 2003;42(10):1722–8.
6. Holper EM, Blair J, Selzer F, et al. The impact of ejection fraction on outcomes after percutaneous coronary intervention in patients with congestive heart failure: an analysis of the National Heart, Lung, and Blood Institute Percutaneous Transluminal Coronary Angioplasty Registry and Dynamic Registry. Am Heart J. Jan 2006; 151(1):69–75.
7. Hochman JS. Cardiogenic shock complicating acute myocardial infarction: expanding the paradigm. Circulation. 2003;107(24): 2998–3002.
8. Babaev A, Frederick PD, Pasta DJ, Every N, Sichrovsky T, Hochman JS. Trends in management and outcomes of patients with acute myocardial infarction complicated by cardiogenic shock. JAMA. 2005;294(4):448–54.
9. Lowes BD, Minobe W, Abraham WT, et al. Changes in gene expression in the intact human heart. Downregulation of alpha-myosin heavy chain in hypertrophied, failing ventricular myocardium. J Clin Invest. 1997;100(9):2315–24.
10. Meyer M, Schillinger W, Pieske B, et al. Alterations of sarcoplasmic reticulum proteins in failing human dilated cardiomyopathy. Circulation. 1995;92(4):778–84.
11. Liao R, Nascimben L, Friedrich J, Gwathmey JK, Ingwall JS. Decreased energy reserve in an animal model of dilated cardiomyopathy. Relationship to contractile performance. Circ Res. 1996; 78(5):893–902.
12. Dibner-Dunlap ME, Thames MD. Control of sympathetic nerve activity by vagal mechanoreflexes is blunted in heart failure. Circulation. 1992;86(6):1929–34.
13. Vogel RA, Shawl F, Tommaso C, et al. Initial report of the National Registry of Elective Cardiopulmonary Bypass Supported Coronary Angioplasty. J Am Coll Cardiol. 1990;15(1):23–9.
14. Califf RM, Phillips 3rd HR, Hindman MC, et al. Prognostic value of a coronary artery jeopardy score. J Am Coll Cardiol. 1985;5(5): 1055–63.
15. Fang J, Alderman MH, Keenan NL, Ayala C. Acute myocardial infarction hospitalization in the United States, 1979 to 2005. Am J Med. 2010;123(3):259–66.
16. Floyd KC, Yarzebski J, Spencer FA, et al. A 30-year perspective (1975–2005) into the changing landscape of patients hospitalized with initial acute myocardial infarction: Worcester Heart Attack Study. Circ Cardiovasc Qual Outcomes. 2009;2(2):88–95.
17. Cheng JM, Valk SD, den Uil CA, et al. Usefulness of intra-aortic balloon pump counterpulsation in patients with cardiogenic shock from acute myocardial infarction. Am J Cardiol. 2009;104(3):327–32.
18. Goldberg RJ, Samad NA, Yarzebski J, Gurwitz J, Bigelow C, Gore JM. Temporal trends in cardiogenic shock complicating acute myocardial infarction. N Engl J Med. 1999;340(15):1162–8.

19. Dunser MW, Hasibeder WR. Sympathetic overstimulation during critical illness: adverse effects of adrenergic stress. J Intensive Care Med. 2009;24(5):293–316.
20. Petersen JW, Felker GM. Inotropes in the management of acute heart failure. Crit Care Med. 2008;36(1 Suppl):S106–11.
21. Fincke R, Hochman JS, Lowe AM, et al. Cardiac power is the strongest hemodynamic correlate of mortality in cardiogenic shock: a report from the SHOCK trial registry. J Am Coll Cardiol. 2004; 44(2):340–8.
22. Mendoza DD, Cooper HA, Panza JA. Cardiac power output predicts mortality across a broad spectrum of patients with acute cardiac disease. Am Heart J. 2007;153(3):366–70.
23. Kantrowitz A, Tjonneland S, Freed PS, Phillips SJ, Butner AN, Sherman Jr JL. Initial clinical experience with intraaortic balloon pumping in cardiogenic shock. JAMA. 1968;203(2):113–8.
24. Scheidt S, Wilner G, Mueller H, et al. Intra-aortic balloon counterpulsation in cardiogenic shock. Report of a co-operative clinical trial. N Engl J Med. 1973;288(19):979–84.
25. Kern MJ, Aguirre F, Bach R, Donohue T, Siegel R, Segal J. Augmentation of coronary blood flow by intra-aortic balloon pumping in patients after coronary angioplasty. Circulation. 1993; 87(2):500–11.
26. Weber KT, Janicki JS. Intraaortic balloon counterpulsation. A review of physiological principles, clinical results, and device safety. Ann Thorac Surg. 1974;17(6):602–36.
27. Cohen M, Urban P, Christenson JT, et al. Intra-aortic balloon counterpulsation in US and non-US centres: results of the Benchmark Registry. Eur Heart J. 2003;24(19):1763–70.
28. Antman EM, Anbe DT, Armstrong PW, et al. ACC/AHA guidelines for the management of patients with ST-elevation myocardial infarction: a report of the American College of Cardiology/American Heart Association Task Force on Practice Guidelines (Committee to Revise the 1999 Guidelines for the Management of Patients with Acute Myocardial Infarction). Circulation. 2004; 110(9):e82–292.
29. Van de Werf F, Bax J, Betriu A, et al. Management of acute myocardial infarction in patients presenting with persistent ST-segment elevation: the Task Force on the Management of ST-Segment Elevation Acute Myocardial Infarction of the European Society of Cardiology. Eur Heart J. 2008;29(23):2909–45.
30. Barron HV, Every NR, Parsons LS, et al. The use of intra-aortic balloon counterpulsation in patients with cardiogenic shock complicating acute myocardial infarction: data from the National Registry of Myocardial Infarction 2. Am Heart J. 2001;141(6): 933–9.
31. Sanborn TA, Sleeper LA, Bates ER, et al. Impact of thrombolysis, intra-aortic balloon pump counterpulsation, and their combination in cardiogenic shock complicating acute myocardial infarction: a report from the SHOCK Trial Registry. SHould we emergently revascularize Occluded Coronaries for cardiogenic shocK? J Am Coll Cardiol. 2000;36(3 Suppl A):1123–9.
32. Sjauw KD, Engstrom AE, Vis MM, et al. A systematic review and meta-analysis of intra-aortic balloon pump therapy in ST-elevation myocardial infarction: should we change the guidelines? Eur Heart J. 2009;30(4):459–68.
33. Ferguson 3rd JJ, Cohen M, Freedman Jr RJ, et al. The current practice of intra-aortic balloon counterpulsation: results from the Benchmark Registry. J Am Coll Cardiol. 2001;38(5):1456–62.
34. Patel MR, Thiele H, Smalling RW, et al. A multicenter, randomized, controlled study of mechanical left ventricular unloading with counterpulsation to reduce infarct size prepercutaneous coronary intervention for acute myocardial infarction: rationale and design of the Counterpulsation Reduces Infarct Size Acute Myocardial Infarction trial. Am Heart J. 2011;162(1):47–55 e41.
35. Thiele H, Zeymer U, Nuemann FJ, Ferenc M, Olbrich HG, Hausleiter J, Richardt G, Hennersdorf HG, Empen K, Fuernau G, Desch S, Eitel I, Hambrecht R, Fuhrmann J, Bohm M, Ebeit H, Schneider S, Schuler G, Werdan K. Intraaortic balloon support for cardiogenic shock. N Engl J Med. 2012;367:1287–96.
36. Thiele H, Lauer B, Hambrecht R, Boudriot E, Cohen HA, Schuler G. Reversal of cardiogenic shock by percutaneous left atrial-to-femoral arterial bypass assistance. Circulation. 2001;104(24): 2917–22.
37. Henriques JP, Remmelink M, Baan Jr J, et al. Safety and feasibility of elective high-risk percutaneous coronary intervention procedures with left ventricular support of the Impella Recover LP 2.5. Am J Cardiol. 2006;97(7):990–2.
38. Cheng JM, den Uil CA, Hoeks SE, et al. Percutaneous left ventricular assist devices vs. intra-aortic balloon pump counterpulsation for treatment of cardiogenic shock: a meta-analysis of controlled trials. Eur Heart J. 2009;30(17):2102–8.
39. Thiele H, Sick P, Boudriot E, et al. Randomized comparison of intra-aortic balloon support with a percutaneous left ventricular assist device in patients with revascularized acute myocardial infarction complicated by cardiogenic shock. Eur Heart J. 2005; 26(13):1276–83.
40. Al-Husami W, Yturralde F, Mohanty G, et al. Single-center experience with the TandemHeart percutaneous ventricular assist device to support patients undergoing high-risk percutaneous coronary intervention. J Invasive Cardiol. 2008;20(6):319–22.
41. Morley D, Litwak K, Ferber P, et al. Hemodynamic effects of partial ventricular support in chronic heart failure: results of simulation validated with in vivo data. J Thorac Cardiovasc Surg. 2007;133(1): 21–8.
42. Fonger JD, Zhou Y, Matsuura H, Aldea GS, Shemin RJ. Enhanced preservation of acutely ischemic myocardium with transseptal left ventricular assist. Ann Thorac Surg. 1994;57(3):570–5.
43. Sjauw KD, Remmelink M, Baan Jr J, et al. Left ventricular unloading in acute ST-segment elevation myocardial infarction patients is safe and feasible and provides acute and sustained left ventricular recovery. J Am Coll Cardiol. 2008;51(10):1044–6.
44. Dixon SR, Henriques JP, Mauri L, et al. A prospective feasibility trial investigating the use of the Impella 2.5 system in patients undergoing high-risk percutaneous coronary intervention (The PROTECT I Trial): initial U.S. experience. JACC Cardiovasc Interv. 2009;2(2):91–6.
45. Seyfarth M, Sibbing D, Bauer I, et al. A randomized clinical trial to evaluate the safety and efficacy of a percutaneous left ventricular assist device versus intra-aortic balloon pumping for treatment of cardiogenic shock caused by myocardial infarction. J Am Coll Cardiol. 2008;52(19):1584–8.
46. O'Neill WW, Kleiman NS, Moses J, Henriques JP, Dixon S, Massaro J, Palacios I, Maini B, Mulukutla S, Dzavik V, Popma J, Douglas PS, Ohman M. A prospective, randomized clinical trial of hemodynamic support with impella 2.5 versus intra-aortic balloon pump in patients undergoing high-risk percutaneous coronary intervention: the protect ii study. Circulation. 2012;126: 1717–27.
47. Sjauw KD, Konorza T, Erbel R, et al. Supported high-risk percutaneous coronary intervention with the Impella 2.5 device the Europella registry. J Am Coll Cardiol. 2009;54(25):2430–4.
48. Cyrus T, et al. Use of mechanical assist during high-risk PCI and STEMI with cardiogenic shock. Cathet Cardiovasc Interv. 2010;75:S1–6.

18 PCI Considerations in Women: Gender-Specific Outcomes and Challenges

Christopher J. Varughese, Rebecca Pinnelas, Jennifer Yu, and Roxana Mehran

In recent decades, invasive therapy has revolutionized the way cardiovascular disease (CVD) is treated. Percutaneous coronary intervention (PCI) is associated with relief of symptoms, increased quality of life, and longer event-free survival. However, access to invasive care and advantages conferred by PCI may not be equivalent across the population. In particular, of the 1.2 million PCI procedures performed in 2007, only 33 % were performed in women [1]. Historically, there have been discrepancies not only in the number of procedures performed in men and women but also in rates of adverse outcomes for each gender. Female sex was shown to be an independent predictor of mortality in an analysis of data collected in the 1970s and early 1980s for the National Heart, Lung, and Blood Institute (NHLBI) Percutaneous Transluminal Coronary Angioplasty (PTCA) Registry [2]. Though the mortality rate difference decreased over the next decade, it persisted in the 1985–1986 PTCA registry and in subsequent clinical trials [3]. Uncertainty remains as to whether sex is an independent risk factor for present-day PCI outcomes, but trends indicate that gender-related effects are likely confounded by age, comorbidities, and other factors [4–7].

Studies over the last 25 years have sought to understand the difference in outcomes between men and women undergoing PCI by considering both social and biological factors. However, trials investigating new treatments remain underpowered for conclusions about the effect of gender because they usually include no more than 30 % women in their samples. This chapter explores current data and relevant guidelines relating to treatment strategies, outcomes, and barriers to care in women undergoing PCI.

C.J. Varughese, MD
Department of Cardiology, The Mount Sinai Hospital, One Gustave L. Levy Place, New York, NY 10029, USA

R. Pinnelas, BS
Office of Interventional Cardiology Research, Mount Sinai Medical Center, One Gustave L. Levy Place, New York, NY 10029, USA

J. Yu, MBBS, FRACP • R. Mehran, MD, FACC, FACP (✉)
Department of Cardiology, Mount Sinai Medical Center, One Gustave L. Levy Place, New York, NY 10029, USA
e-mail: rmehran@crf.org

C.A. Thompson (ed.), *Textbook of Cardiovascular Intervention*,
DOI 10.1007/978-1-4471-4528-8_18, © Springer-Verlag London 2014

Diagnosing Women Prior to PCI

Clinical Presentation

The primary clinical features of coronary heart disease differ between genders. Women are on average 10 years older than men at the time of presentation of coronary artery disease and demonstrate a longer time from symptom onset to diagnosis and subsequent medical intervention (Table 18.1) [2, 3, 8, 9]. Additionally, the National Registry of Myocardial Infarction Investigators found that women were less likely to receive fibrinolytic agents or undergo invasive procedures and that they also had a substantially increased rate of death during their first hospitalization for coronary artery disease compared to men in the same age decile [3]. Though women more frequently experience noncardiac chest pain than men, their angina is still strongly associated with risk of death. In the Australian Longitudinal Study on Women's Health, elderly women who experienced greater physical limitation and frequency of angina, as assessed by higher scores on the Seattle Angina Questionnaire (SAQ), had higher mortality than those with lower scores [8]. Women are more likely to present with unstable angina (UA) or non-ST elevated myocardial infarction (NSTEMI) [9], while men more frequently present with ST-segment elevated myocardial infarction (STEMI) [10]. Although the initial presentation may differ between sexes, significant morbidity and mortality occur in both populations.

Comorbidities

Women have a higher incidence of comorbidities than men at the time of presentation for acute coronary syndromes (ACS), such as hypertension, hyperlipidemia, and diabetes

Table 18.1 Characteristics and comorbidities of women with cardiovascular disease (CVD)

Characteristics and comorbidities of women with CVD
Older age
Hypertension
Hyperlipidemia
Diabetes
Later presentation
Cardiogenic shock
Renal insufficiency

Table 18.2 Presenting symptoms of cardiovascular disease (CVD) in women

CVD presentation in women
Chest pain[a]
Shortness of breath
Indigestion
Palpitations
Mid-back pain
Pain to jaw, arm, and throat
Attribute pain to noncardiac causes

[a]Most frequent presentation in both men and women

[11]. Women with ACS also tend to present later with dynamic EKG changes, more disabling ischemic symptoms, and even cardiogenic shock, often despite no prior history of MI, PCI, or coronary artery bypass graft surgery [11, 12]. Women are more likely to have renal insufficiency which may have a significant prognostic impact, especially post-STEMI [13]. On the other hand, women are less likely to have a history of smoking, prior MI, and coronary revascularization compared to men [9, 11].

Atypical Presentation

Patient presentation can greatly influence the timeliness of diagnosis and treatment of ACS and MI. Differences in the presenting symptoms between women and men with ST-segment elevation myocardial infarction (STEMI) have been thought to contribute to the rate of 30-day mortality among women [13]. The most common symptom of ACS for both men and women is chest pain (94 % vs. 92 %, respectively), which is frequently accompanied by dizziness and fatigue [14]. Women, however, are more likely to report certain additional symptoms such as indigestion, shortness of breath, palpitations, mid-back pain, and nausea [14] as well as pain in the jaw, arm, and throat (Table 18.2) [15]. Due to the wider variety of symptoms seen in women with ACS, they are more likely than men to assume that these symptoms have noncardiac causes [15]. Such differences in presentation may account for longer symptom onset to treatment times and increased door-to-balloon times in women with STEMI undergoing PCI [16].

Barriers to Optimal Care

Biological Differences

Biological characteristics unique to women play a role in the diagnosis, treatment, and outcome of CVD. Compared to men, women tend to have lower body surface areas, smaller coronary arteries, increased microvascular disease, and different plaque morphology [17]. Younger women, who have higher rates of mortality than age-matched men with ischemic heart disease, are more likely to have erosion of the coronary plaque fibrous cap with intimal exposure [17]. In contrast, older women and men are more likely to have plaques with disrupted caps and necrotic cores [18]. These factors may increase the technical difficulty of coronary artery bypass surgery (CABG) and may partially explain the higher morbidity and mortality experienced in women after CABG.

Cardiovascular events in women are extremely rare before menopause, but become more frequent with age; by the eighth decade of life, the rate for such events is similar for the two sexes [17]. This suggests possible cardioprotective effects for endogenous estrogen in young women. However, exogenous estrogen in the form of hormone replacement therapy appears to have the opposite effect, and in fact, increases the occurrence of CV events in women. The Heart and Estrogen/Progestin Replacement Study (HERS), a secondary prevention trial, found an increased risk of MI in the first few months after initiation of hormone therapy and an increased risk of venous thromboembolic events [19]. The Women's Health Initiative (WHI), a primary prevention trial, found an increased risk of stroke in healthy women taking estrogen plus progestin, without benefit in the incidence of CAD [20]. HRT use was not recommended for CVD prevention in either the WHI (primary) or HERS (secondary) trials. Current AHA/ACC guidelines advise that women with known cardiovascular disease not begin HRT and furthermore that those already on HRT should strongly consider discontinuing its use [21].

Diagnostic Testing

Additional diagnostic challenges exist for women with suspected CAD. Higher percentages of women than men with CAD have normal coronary arteries on diagnostic angiography, highlighting the inaccuracies of proper risk assessment for women prior to testing [16–21]. A combination of differences in clinical presentation and the prevalence of coronary disease prove problematic. Recommendations regarding the use of stress testing in women are often derived from studies performed in men, since there is a paucity of data regarding the best diagnostic strategy for assessment of coronary artery disease in women. In the Coronary Artery Surgery Study (CASS), 50 % of women undergoing coronary angiography for chest pain were found to have nonobstructive disease compared to 17 % of men, yet studies show that women without obstruction may continue to experience cardiac symptoms [22–24].

Electrocardiogram (ECG) stress testing is frequently performed in women, with ACC/AHA guidelines recommending it for those at intermediate and high risk for CAD [25]. However, exercise stress tests alone have decreased sensitivity and specificity in women compared to men, which might be explained by lower ECG voltage or endogenous estrogen in premenopausal women and exogenous estrogen in older women [26, 27]. Alternatively, the addition of imaging to exercise stress testing appears to be both cost-effective and accurate in risk stratification for both sexes [25]. Both stress echocardiography and stress gated myocardial single-photon emission computed tomographic nuclear imaging appear to perform similarly in women [25] . SPECT imaging with dobutamine appears to be another diagnostically accurate tool for detecting CAD in women. Cardiac MRI (CMR) may be useful due to its ability to detect stenosis as well as physiological characteristics such as perfusion and metabolism. CT angiography detects coronary calcification and coronary stenosis. This technique has shown high diagnostic accuracy; however, its diagnostic accuracy in women compare to that for men is uncertain remains to be seen [28–30].

Women have lower rates of revascularization [31, 32], noninvasive testing [31], and arteriography [31] than men despite a similar incidence of ACS. In an ACS registry of 20,290 patients, female sex was a significant predictor for a low likelihood of undergoing PCI [33]. In the USA between 1988 and 2004, men underwent multivessel PCI and CABG twice as often as women [34]. Lower frequency of PCI in women has also been seen in France [35] and Korea [36]. In a study of 32,888 patients with evidence of NSTEMI, men were significantly more likely to undergo intervention [37]. Though most evidence shows differing rates of intervention in ACS between men and women, some have found similar frequency of invasive therapy [38].

Time to admission and intervention is not equivalent between the sexes [39]. In one study of STEMI, women were found to have longer intervals between symptoms and intervention, and there are other reports in the literature of delays at each stage of treatment for STEMI [40, 41]. However, a statewide program focusing on improving STEMI treatment times through regionalization resulted in faster times for women, the elderly, and minorities that were similar to the improved treatment times seen in men. Thus, disparities may be lessened through the use of focused initiatives [33, 42].

Social and Educational Barriers

Social factors also influence treatment and intervention in women with CVD. In a survey of 1,024 women, half correctly named CVD as the number one cause of mortality in women. However, most women could not identify other important CVD risk factors, including smoking and hypertension [43]. Women also have lower documented concern about heart disease as a personal health risk [44]. Lower self-perception of risk may lead to lower acceptance of treatment recommendations [45, 46], with women 6 % less likely to accept a physician recommendation for PCI over medical therapy and 7 % less willing to accept CABG over medical therapy [46].

Table 18.3 Barriers to optimal cardiovascular disease (CVD) diagnosis and care in women

Barriers to optimal CVD diagnosis and care in women
Incomplete understanding of role of estrogen in female CVD
High prevalence of normal coronary arteries on angiography
Healthcare provider bias
Low self-perception of risk

Healthcare Provider Barriers

Healthcare provider behaviors and infrastructure also play a role in gender inequalities. Bias extends to physicians, who are less likely to perceive women's pain as cardiac [23] and less likely to refer women to cardiac rehabilitation [47, 48]. To date the AHA has published three female specific guidelines (2004–2011) for the prevention of CAD [21]. However, physician knowledge and behavior related to gender-specific guidelines is unknown. A national AHA study of 500 physicians revealed that gender disparities in treatment were largely explained by the provider's perception of lower CAD risk in women, although the calculated risk is actually similar for each sex [49]. A survey of internists and obstetrician/gynecologists on major barriers towards preventive care identified lack of physician time with patients and low reimbursement for lifestyle change interventions as major reasons for lack of primary prevention education [49]. Restructuring health care systems and reimbursement models may narrow the gender gap in preventive care. Gender-related factors related to barriers of care are summarized in Table 18.3.

Outcomes in Women Post-PCI

Since the advent of PCI, women have experienced a higher frequency of adverse clinical outcomes compared to men, including reinfarction, emergency coronary artery bypass graft surgery, restenosis, mortality, bleeding, and vascular complications. Improvements in technology have decreased sex differences in outcomes, but discrepancies remain.

Mortality

Trends

Women continue to experience increased in-hospital mortality after PCI compared to men, but the phenomenon frequently disappears following multivariate adjustment.

This can be largely explained by women's increased age and incidence of comorbidities on presentation, rather than inherent sex differences. In a 25-year, single-center study of 18,885 consecutive PCI at the Mayo Clinic, mortality was reduced significantly between an early group of PCI patients (1979–1995) and more recent group (1996–2004) in both men and women [50]. Such improvements in survival rates have been attributed to newer technology, operator technical experience, and improved medical therapy [51].

Short Term

In recent studies which assess the in-hospital mortality after PCI in UA, NSTEMI and STEMI combined, there was usually no difference between men and women after multivariate adjustment [9, 52, 53], though there were some exceptions [10]. In studies of PCI in UA/NSTEMI alone, female sex was not an independent predictor of mortality after adjustment for other factors [4, 5]. In studies of elective procedures alone, there was also no difference in early mortality between men and women [54].

However, controversy regarding the impact of female sex on in-hospital mortality, post-PCI still persists in studies of STEMI. In some studies, in-hospital mortality was higher in women even after multivariate adjustment [35, 55], yet in others the difference disappeared after adjustment [6, 7]. Some evidence exists for higher in-hospital mortality post-acute myocardial infarction (AMI) in certain female subpopulations, such as women under 50 years of age [56], elderly women within 48 h of STEMI [57], and women over 75 [12]. Furthermore, in the *Get with the Guidelines*-CAD registry, higher in-hospital mortality for women in the STEMI population remained even after adjustment for baseline characteristics, with a high incidence of early deaths [58]. It is possible that underutilization of treatments for women and delayed reperfusion is responsible for the high incidence of early deaths observed [59]. Thirty-day mortality has also been reported to be higher in women in univariate analysis, but sex was not an independent predictor [10, 60].

Long Term

Despite some evidence of persistent early mortality in women undergoing PCI, sex-specific mortality appears to decrease with time. In trials of consecutive PCI patients as well as in studies of PCI registries, there was no adjusted difference in long-term mortality at 6 months, 1 year [10, 53, 61], 3 years [53], or 5 years [62]. In fact, some studies even found that women had decreased mortality compared to men in long-term analysis [53, 63]. On the other hand, D'Ascenzo et al. recently found that although major adverse cardiac events (MACE) following PCI for ACS are similar in men and women, women had a higher long-term mortality rate in PCI following STEMI (20 % vs. 8.1 % at 5 years) [62].

Drug-Eluting (DES) Versus Bare-Metal Stents (BMS) in Women

Stenting is a safe and effective intervention in women with the ability to reduce rates of restenosis and revascularization [64]. In trials of bare-metal stents (BMS) compared to balloon angioplasty, BMS use resulted in reduced in-hospital mortality and subsequent restenosis [65, 66]. BMS use was also more effective than balloon angioplasty when used in smaller coronary arteries [67]. Due to the lack of sex-specific data published in the earlier years of stenting versus balloon angioplasty, the advantages of stenting were generalized to women [1]. With the advent of drug-eluting stents, restenosis and mortality rates have decreased even further. In a randomized trial of BMS versus DES, there were no differences in stent thrombosis or other outcomes between men and women, although DES as an independent predictor for low risk of repeat PCI in both sexes [68]. Solinas et al. evaluated gender-specific outcomes in a pooled analysis of four trials that randomized sirolimus-eluting stents (SES) versus BMS [69]. They found that women, who comprised 28 % of the combined study populations, had significant reductions in rates of in-segment binary restenosis (6.3 % vs. 43.8 %) and significant reductions in 1-year major cardiac events ($P<0.0001$) with SES. Others have found similar in-hospital outcomes between men and women following DES [70], decreased long-term target vessel revascularization (TVR) and MACE in women receiving DES [71], and reduced restenosis in both men and women despite less favorable baseline presentations for women [72].

Restenosis and Revascularization

Data on restenosis in women following PCI is conflicting, with some evidence showing increased restenosis in women compared to men, especially in the short term [73–75]. This is due in part to the small sample size of women in the earlier bare-metal stent (BMS) prospective trials. However, studies of newer DES continue to show promise in women.

Both taxus and sirolimus drug-eluting stents have been associated with favorable outcomes in women. The TAXUS IV trial and the SIRIUS trials revealed reductions in target vessel revascularization (TVR) rates, restenosis, and MACE in both sexes at 1 year. In the TAXUS IV trial ($n=1,314$, 27.9 % women) women (7.6 %) and men (8.6 %) had comparable rates of restenosis ($P=0.80$). When compared to BMS stents, women treated with TAXUS stents had significant reductions in 9-month restenosis (29.2 % vs. 8.6 %, $P<0.001$) and 1-year target lesion revascularization rates (TLR) (14.9 % vs. 7.6 %, $P=0.02$), (61.5). In a substudy of the SPIRIT III trial ($n=1,001$, women 31.4 %), the XIENCE V everolimus-eluting stent was superior to TAXUS at preventing restenosis in women, confirming the observations seen in men [76]. However, compared to men also receiving the XIENCE V, women did have higher rates of MACE and restenosis.

A recent meta-analysis (n = 156,798, women 31.3 %) found that 30-day target vessel revascularization (TVR) was present in 4.25 % of female patients and 3.83 % of male patients, with male sex significantly associated with a reduction in short-term TVR [75]. Although improvements in stent technology have improved overall outcomes, increased rates of diabetes, aspirin resistance, and smaller vessel size among women may be responsible for higher short-term TVR observed in women [75]. Small artery size has been shown to predict restenosis [74]. Estrogen may also be protective against restenosis [74], but this explanation appears insufficient given the older age of many female PCI patients [77]. Further investigation is needed to see how these factors might play a role in short-term TVR, without extending long-term risk. Long-term outcomes for DES in women are also encouraging. A pooled analysis of DES-treated patients from randomized trials (n = 2,271, women 29.3 %) and real-world registries (n = 7,492, women 32.7 %) found that women with DES had lower TLR than women with BMS stents (11.5 % vs. 22.6 %, $p < 0.001$) and found no difference in 5-year outcomes between DES-treated women versus men [73]. Findings of similar outcomes in men and women with DES may indicate a trend towards reducing disparities among the sexes in gender outcomes post-PCI [78, 79]. It should be noted, however, that access to DES may not be equal between men and women, and thus, outcomes may still differ by sex [62].

Bleeding and Vascular Complications

Despite progress in reducing MACE in the female PCI population, bleeding and vascular complications remain significant sources of morbidity and mortality post-intervention. Recent analysis combining three PCI trials – REPLACE-2, ACUITY, and HORIZONS (n = 17,034, 4,366 women) – found that female sex was one of six main predictors of non-CABG-related TIMI (thrombolysis in myocardial infarction criteria) major bleeding, which was strongly associated with 1-year mortality [80]. Bleeding complications, including access site hematomas and transfusions, remain higher in women compared to men even after adjustment for baseline factors [9, 10, 52, 60, 76, 81–84]. In a study of consecutive PCI in African-Americans (n = 835, female 443), women had higher adjusted major and minor bleeding than men, despite similar in-hospital outcomes [85]. Still, some evidence remains that bleeding risk is partially attributed to comorbidities. In a substudy of the REPLACE-2 trial, sex was associated with in-hospital bleeds in univariate analysis but not after multivariate adjustment [86]. Given the higher risk of bleeding in women, physicians and researchers must continue to find ways to reduce the occurrence of this adverse outcome.

Progress has been made in lowering bleeding and vascular complications. In a study of 45,987 patients (13,653 women) from the Northern New England PCI Registry, there was a 50 % decrease in absolute bleeding and vascular complications from 2002 to 2007 [87]. Protective factors included fluoroscopy-guided access, use of closure devices, and use of direct thrombin inhibitor bivalirudin [87]. Bivalirudin has been shown to decrease major and minor bleeding in women, including access site bleeding, compared to heparin + glycoprotein IIb/IIIa inhibitor [86]. Similarly, in an 8-year study of CATH and PCI from 1998 to 2005 (n = 18,467, 7,922 women), the vascular complication rate was 3.2 % in women undergoing PCI compared with 1.3 % in men. Up until the last year of the trial, female sex remained a strong predictor of vascular complications. Notably, during the study period the vascular complication rates decreased significantly in both men and women, which might be attributed to the use of smaller sheath sizes in later years [88]. In the large-scale ACC-NCDR registry (n = 199,690 patients, 68,026 women), women retained higher rates of vascular complications even after adjusting for confounders [9]. Possible explanations for increased vascular complications in women include aggressive anticoagulation and smaller vessel size. To date, there has been no gender-specific data on arterial vascular closure devices.

Increased use of radial access for PCI may help prevent access site bleeding [89, 90]. In the Radial versus Femoral access for coronary intervention (RIVAL) trial, 7,021 ACS patients (1,861 women) were randomized to femoral or radial access and similar rates of adverse outcomes were observed. Notably, vascular complications were less common in patients undergoing PCI with radial access [89]. In a study of 3,261 PCI (900 in women), there was no major bleeding in women who underwent radial access for PCI, although an alternative access site was used more often in women than men [90]. Procedure failure might be explained by the presence of smaller and tortuous vessels which are more prone to spasm in women [91]. In another study, men and women undergoing radial access did not differ in MACE after 1 year of follow-up, but female sex remained a predictor of mild to moderate access site hematomas even after baseline adjustment [92].

In summary, short-term in-hospital mortality in women following PCI is largely explained by later presentation with the presence of additional comorbidities, while long-term mortality occurs at similar rates in both sexes. Some increased mortality in women with STEMI may remain. Restenosis and revascularization rates may be higher in women in the short term, but may actually be lower in the long term, and these rates continue to decline in the DES era. Bleeding and vascular complications, while declining in frequency, are still more likely to occur in women; however, these outcomes might be mitigated by the use of bivalirudin or the use of radial access.

Other Outcomes

Despite increased comorbidities at presentation, women and men have similar procedural success rates [81, 82, 93]. In one recent study of STEMI patients, women had lower success rates compared to men (94.7 % vs. 95.9 %, $p=0.002$) [12], but other studies have found no difference in STEMI success [7]. In a study in Korea, the opposite was true. PCI success rates were similar in STEMI but were higher in men versus women with NSTEMI [36].

Following PCI, women also have higher incidence of cardiogenic shock [9], contrast-induced nephropathy (CIN) [52], and increased likelihood of a rise in serum creatinine greater than 1 mg/dl rise in creatinine [81]. Female sex has been reported as an independent predictor of CIN in some studies [52, 94]. Other studies have shown only a univariate association between female sex and CIN, thus attributing part of the observed sex disparity to differences in baseline conditions [95, 96]. Although female sex is not one of the variables in the Mehran CIN risk score, it is noteworthy that females experience higher rates of certain comorbidities (e.g., CHF, diabetes) that are included in the model [97].

Women are more likely to have lower health-related quality of life following PCI than men. At both 6 [98] and 12 months [98, 99], women had lower scores on the Short Form Health Survey (SF-36), though both men and women have shown trends in improvement over time (at 6 and 12 months) [98].

Treatment of Acute Coronary Syndrome in Women

Invasive Versus Conservative Strategies

Randomized trials have demonstrated the benefit of an invasive strategy over conservative treatment in ACS, but it has been difficult to reach conclusions regarding gender-specific strategies. The current AHA/ACC 2007 guidelines for treatment of NSTEMI/UA distinguish between high- and low-risk women for early invasive versus conservative treatment [100]. Invasive therapy is recommended for high-risk men and women, whereas conservative treatment is recommended for low-risk women (Class I, level of evidence B). Low-risk men did not show significant advantages or disadvantages with early invasive strategy. Medical therapy guidelines are the same for both genders, but consideration should be given to correct dosage for body weight [101]. Notably, the 2011 update contained comorbidity recommendations that may especially apply to women. Treatment decisions should be made similarly in patients with and without diabetes. Regarding renal function, consideration should be given to pre-procedure hydration in order to prevent CIN and caution exercised in the use of renally cleared medications [102].

Though randomized trials uniformly favor aggressive therapy for ACS in men, results in women are mixed [103]. The TACTICS-TIMI 18 trial ($n=2{,}220$, 34 % women) randomized patients to receive early invasive therapy or conservative medical therapy, with a primary endpoint of death, MI, or rehospitalization within 30 days. In women who received early invasive therapy, there were similar reductions in the primary composite endpoint to men, and these observed reductions were further increased after accounting for baseline conditions [38]. In the RITA-3 trial, only men derived a significant benefit from early invasive treatment [104]. Similarly, the FRISC II study, which randomized patients to early invasive or noninvasive treatment, found no difference in MI or death at 12 months for women (12.4 % vs. 10.5 %), whereas men had a significantly reduced incidence of the primary endpoint in the invasive arm (9.6 % invasive vs. 15.8 % noninvasive) [105]. FRISC II found an interaction between early intervention and gender on the occurrence of MI and death ($p=0.008$), which indicates a different response of men and women to invasive therapy [105]. Recent data from the Berlin Myocardial Infarction Registry ($n=2{,}808$) for years 2004–2008 also indicate that after baseline adjustment that men (0.41, 0.21–0.78) benefited from early invasive therapy, while women (1.24, 0.53–2.91) did not. Possible reasons for the lack of agreement among trials include differences in the baseline procedure risk for women enrolled in each trial difference in definition of MI among the trials and beneficial use of tirofiban with PCI in TACTICS-TIMI 18 [104].

Treatment of Acute Myocardial Infarction in Women

PCI Versus Fibrinolytic Strategies

AHA/ACC STEMI guidelines for both men and women recommend PCI over fibrinolytic therapy, with door-to-balloon time within 90 min [106]. In the GUSTO-IIb PTCA trial, both men and women who underwent PTCA versus tissue plasminogen activator (tPA) administration experienced lower rates of the composite endpoint (death, nonfatal MI, nonfatal disabling stroke) [107]. For women, 56 events per 1,000 women treated with PTCA were prevented compared to 42 events per 1,000 men [108]. In a subanalysis of the PAMI trial which also randomized AMI patients to tPA or PTCA, women had higher mortality than men with tPA but no significant mortality difference with PTCA. In-hospital survival in women was independently predicted by PTCA [109], demonstrating the efficacy of invasive therapy in STEMI for women.

Studies have also compared PTCA with primary stenting in STEMI patients. In the CADILLAC trial, women who had primary stenting experienced a reduction in 1-year MACE (28.1 % in PTCA to 19.1 % in stenting) and ischemic TVR (20.4–10.8 %, $P=0.002$) compared to the PTCA arm [64].

Despite evidence of the effectiveness of invasive therapy for STEMI in women, studies have found underuse of reperfusion therapy. In GUSTO V, angiography and subsequent PCI were less frequently performed in women [110]. Similarly, the *Get with the Guidelines*-CAD Registry found that women in the STEMI population were less likely to undergo revascularization [59].

Adjunctive Pharmacotherapy

Substantial evidence exists for adjunctive pharmacotherapy in PCI, but women receive medical therapy with lower frequency than men following interventions [111, 112]. A study of Canadian ACS Registry patients found that although women received similar antiplatelets to men at discharge, they received fewer lipid-lowering medications and ACE inhibitors, even after multivariate adjustment [112]. Similarly, analysis from the CRUSADE trial ($n=35{,}875$, 41 % women) found that women were less likely to be discharged with aspirin, statins, and ACE inhibitors than men [113]. Others have found lower rates of beta-blockers [114] or glycoprotein IIb/IIIa inhibitors and clopidogrel [115] at discharge. Still, others have found comparable rates of aspirin, lipid-lowering agents, and beta-blockers at discharge [115]. In a study of secondary prevention in women, beta-blockers and statins were underutilized according to current guidelines for patients with CHD [110–112, 116].

Antiplatelet Agents

Aspirin

Large-scale clinical trials such as the Physician's Health Study and Primary Prevention Project have demonstrated the benefit of aspirin use in men for the prevention of cardiovascular events, but evidence for primary prevention in women is less robust [23]. A recent meta-analysis including 51,342 women [117] found that aspirin reduces the frequency of MI in men by 32 % but does not significantly reduce MI in women. On the other hand, aspirin was associated with a stroke rate decrease of 17 % in women.

Nevertheless, aspirin remains an integral part of AHA 2011 guidelines for the prevention of CVD in women. A daily dose of 75–325 mg/day is recommended in high-risk women with CHD (Class I, Level of Evidence A) as well as women with diabetes mellitus (Class IIa, Level of Evidence B). If aspirin is contraindicated in high-risk women, clopidogrel should be prescribed (Class I, Level of Evidence B). In healthy women over the age of 65, aspirin therapy (81 mg/day or 100 every other day) is recommended for stroke and MI prevention if the benefits outweigh the risk of bleeding (Class IIa, Level B) [118]. In women under the age of 65, aspirin may be reasonable for the prevention of stroke (Class IIb, level of evidence B), but it is not indicated for MI prevention (Class III, Level of evidence B). For women with atrial fibrillation, daily aspirin is recommended if warfarin cannot be used or if they are at low risk for stroke [118].

Evidence for the use of aspirin in secondary prevention is strong but has not been fully assessed by stratifying according to gender [23]. The Antithrombotic Trialists' Collaboration saw a significant reduction in cardiovascular events (22 %) after the use of aspirin in patients with CVD or at high risk [119]. In light of the lack of evidence saying that secondary prevention in women is not warranted, it is concerning that aspirin is underused as secondary prevention in women [116].

Aspirin use in women may also be complicated by new evidence suggesting that aspirin resistance is up to four times more prevalent in women than men [23]. In a study of healthy drug naïve patients, women were less likely to respond to platelet inhibition therapy by aspirin and were more likely to have higher platelet aggregation at baseline [120]. Others have found that women have the same level of direct COX-1 pathway suppression as men with aspirin, but may maintain some higher level of indirect COX-1 activation [121]. Further studies on gender-based responsiveness to antiplatelet therapy, including alternative options, are necessary.

For the treatment of ACS, ACC/AHA 2011 guidelines recommend administering aspirin immediately upon presentation for UA/NSTEMI and maintaining therapy lifelong. For patients who cannot tolerate aspirin, clopidogrel should be substituted. Patients receiving initial invasive therapy should receive dual antiplatelet therapy before PCI with ASA + clopidogrel or GP IIb/IIIA inhibitors, with additional anticoagulation administered at the time of PCI. Aspirin is also indicated in conservative therapy, with ASA + clopidogrel given for 1-month to 1-year post-event [102].

Thienopyridines

Clopidogrel

Clopidogrel is utilized as part of dual antiplatelet therapy in CAD patients. In a recent meta-analysis that analyzed studies of elective PCI, UA/NSTEMI, and STEMI [122], clopidogrel was beneficial in reducing composite endpoints as well as MI alone in both sexes. In 8.3 months of treatment with clopidogrel, there were 9 fewer CV events per 1,000 women treated and 12 fewer CV events per 1,000 men treated. It should be noted that clopidogrel added to aspirin therapy raised major bleeding risk by 43 % in women and 21 % in men [122].

Clopidogrel's ability to reduce MACE in elective PCI was tested in Clopidogrel for the Reduction of Events During Observation (CREDO) trial. Patients were randomized to receive a 300 mg loading dose of placebo, followed by clopidogrel through day 28, and then randomized to clopidogrel or placebo for the remainder of 12 months. Aspirin was given to both groups. Subjects who received long-term clopidogrel therapy experienced a 26.9 % decrease in MACE. Risk reduction rate of death, MI, and stroke at 1 year was 32.1 % in women and 24.5 % in men. Pretreatment did not lower the risk of 28-day events. Risk of bleeding was not significantly increased at 1 year [123].

Prasugrel

Prasugrel, a thienopyridine approved in 2009, has stronger effects and more rapid onset than its predecessor, clopidogrel, which demonstrated superiority to clopidogrel in the TRITON-TIMI 38 trial ($n=3{,}524$, 22 % women) [124, 125]. In subgroup analysis, women demonstrated a 12 % decrease in the primary MACE endpoint., while men revealed a 21 % reduction [126]. Recent subgroup findings of TRITON-TIMI 38 showed that women and men had similar rates of non-CABG TIMI major bleeding, but only women had higher non-CABG minor bleeding [127].

The latest guidelines from the AHA/ACC do not comment on the use of prasugrel in elective PCI, but guidelines for UA/NSTEMI [102] and STEMI [128] were updated to include the administration of 60 mg prasugrel upon presentation in patients with a planned PCI. Those updates also describe patients in whom prasugrel may cause harm: patients with a history of stroke or transient ischemic attack, weight below 60 kg, and age above 75 years. Given the increased likelihood women have of presenting at older age, lower weight, and with more comorbidities, these criteria are particularly relevant for determining appropriate prasugrel use in women.

Ticagrelor

Unlike the irreversible platelet inhibitors prasugrel and clopidogrel, ticagrelor is a reversible P2Y12-receptor antagonist recently approved in the United States. In the Ticagrelor versus Clopidogrel in Patients with Acute Coronary Syndromes (PLATO) trial ($n=18{,}624$, 28.4 % women ticagrelor arm and 28.3 % women clopidogrel arm), there were no differences in the primary composite endpoint of death from vascular causes, MI, or stroke between the sexes for patients who were hospitalized for ACS [129]. However, within each sex, there was a gender-specific risk reduction; low-weight men and women were less likely to benefit from ticagrelor than higher weight men and women.

Notably, ticagrelor approval in the United States was delayed compared to Europe due to increased adverse outcomes in the North American cohort in patients randomized to ticagrelor [130]. The increase in complications has been attributed to a higher dosage of aspirin prescribed in the United States compared to other sites [131]. Upon examination of other sites with high aspirin dosage, similar increased outcomes were noted. The Food and Drug Administration (FDA) has approved ticagrelor with a black box warning regarding concomitant high-dose aspirin.

Substudies of PLATO for ACS patients with planned invasive therapy (both STEMI and NSTEMI) showed similar results [132], with no difference in the primary endpoint between men and women. In an STE-ACS subpopulation of PLATO ($n=7{,}544$; women$=1{,}796$), primary outcomes did not differ significantly between men and women.

Thienopyridine use is effective in both men and women, and newer agents such as prasugrel and ticagrelor may be beneficial in both sexes. However, women compromise only 30 % of the cohort populations in each of the studies in which these findings are based (CURE, TRITON-TIMI 38, PLATO). Given the increased risk of bleeding in women with the use of any antiplatelet therapy, studies targeted at women should be conducted prior to extrapolating conclusions from these trials.

Glycoprotein IIb/IIIa Inhibitors

For patients undergoing early invasive treatment for UA/NSTEMI, ACC/AHA guidelines indicate that glycoprotein IIb/IIIa antagonists may be used as part of dual antiplatelet therapy alongside aspirin, instead of clopidogrel. Glycoprotein IIb/IIIa antagonists may also be used in place of clopidogrel for initial conservative strategy patients who are undergoing angiography for recurrent symptoms, heart failure, or arrhythmias [102]. However, in lower-risk patients, antagonists should be used with caution due to the bleeding risks associated with triple antiplatelet therapy [102]. In STEMI, the use of abciximab in patients undergoing PCI is recommended regardless of stent use [128].

Pooled analysis with a composite endpoint of death, MI, or urgent revascularization within 1-month primary endpoint of death, MI, or urgent revascularization within 30 days and 2 months showed significant reduction in both men (12.7–6.5 %) and women (11.3–5.8 %) who were treated with abciximab for PCI. Female sex was associated with greater major and minor bleeding, but the use of abciximab was not a predictor of an increased bleeding risk [133]. In a study of 32,601 patients with NSTE-ACS, women treated with tirofiban or eptifibatide had higher rates of bleeding than treated men (15.7 % vs. 7.3 %) and higher rates than untreated women (8.5 % vs. 5.4 %). The observed bleeding risk was partially explained by excess dosing in women [134]. Despite evidence of efficacy of glycoprotein IIb/IIIa inhibitors in women with definite ACS [135, 136], like other medical therapies, they remain underused in women presenting for invasive therapy [137].

Anticoagulants

Unfractionated Heparin and Low Molecular Weight Heparin

In the 2007 ACC/AHA guidelines update for UA/NSTEMI, unfractionated heparin (UFH) and enoxaparin (LMWH) were recommended for both invasive and conservative therapies [101]. Enoxaparin is the recommended therapy unless CABG is scheduled within 24 h [138]. Two randomized studies, A to Z and SYNERGY, found non-inferiority with enoxaparin compared to UFH in both sexes, but increased risk of bleeding with enoxaparin was observed [1, 101]. Updated guidelines for STEMI recommended that patients receiving fibrinolytics receive anticoagulation including UFH, enoxaparin, or fondaparinux, but UFH should not be given for more than 48 h [101]. Due to renal clearance of LWMH, attention should be paid to renal function in patients receiving these drugs, which may especially impact women.

Direct Thrombin Inhibitors

Bivalirudin

Bivalirudin is a direct thrombin inhibitor that is frequently used in PCI. In a trial comparing bivalirudin + glycoprotein IIb/IIIa inhibitors with heparin + glycoprotein IIb/IIIa inhibitors (REPLACE-2), the bivalirudin combination was non-inferior to heparin treatment. Subgroup analysis ($n=6{,}010$, 1.537) showed that women who had received either therapy did not have significantly different rates of death, MI, and revascularization. However, women who had been treated with bivalirudin experienced significantly less major and minor bleeding than those who had received heparin [86].

Subgroup analysis of women was also performed in the ACUITY trial of ACS patients ($n=13{,}819$, 30.1 % women). Women experienced similar event rates with bivalirudin, bivalirudin + GPI, and heparin + GPI, but experienced lowest rates of bleeding with bivalirudin alone [139]. These results were supported by the HORIZONS-AMI study which found that bivalirudin monotherapy significantly improved mortality and bleeding in AMI patients. Notably, bivalirudin therapy was not superior to UFH + GPI in patients with anemia [16].

Statins

It is well established that there is an absolute benefit in reduction of low density lipoprotein cholesterol (LDL) levels in secondary prevention of CAD. However, the impact of lipid management in women without CAD is a topic of ongoing controversy [139]. In 2008, two large randomized trials: the Management of Elevated Cholesterol in the Primary Prevention Group of Adult Japanese (MEGA) study and the Justification for the Use of Statins in Primary Prevention (JUPITER) trial, provided insight into the role of lipid-lowering therapy in primary prevention of CAD among women [140, 141]. The MEGA study, which enrolled 5,356 women and 2,476 men, revealed that pravastatin was associated with a significant benefit only in men [142]. Women had a 37 % reduction in risk of all CVD, but this difference was not statistically significant. The lack of a clear effect in women was thought to be due to the inherent lower cardiovascular risk among women at low risk for CAD. The JUPITER study randomized 6,801 women age > 60 years old and 11,001 men age > 50 years old without CAD and LDL < 130 with CRP > 2 to rosuvastatin 20 mg versus placebo with a combined primary endpoint of MI, stroke, revascularization, UA, or death by CVD [141]. Due to a significant reduction (44 %) in the primary endpoint, the trial was stopped after a median of just 1.9 years. While the hazard reduction was similar for both men and women, the absolute benefit in women was lower, which may be a reflection of the cohort's overall lower baseline risk profile, as seen in the MEGA trial. Subsequently, a Cochrane Database review published in 2011 revealed that the evidence is not in favor of the use of statins in individuals with an annual all-cause mortality risk of < 1 % or an annual CAD risk event rate of < 2 % [143].

Although current guidelines recommend the use of statins after PCI, studies have revealed that women are less likely to receive statins post-intervention and are not treated as aggressively [144]. A protective benefit of high-dose statin therapy prior to elective PCI has been shown to be beneficial regardless of gender [145].

CABG

Coronary artery bypass grafting is another viable revascularization option for many women. Women who initially present for CABG are typically older, have increased comorbidities, have decreased diameter of coronary arteries, have lower body surface area, and have a greater requirement for urgent or emergent procedures [146]. Historically, increased rates of operative mortality have been reported in women (relative risk from 1.4 to 4.4 compared to men) [131–134]. However, following adjustment for covariates, gender has not proven to be an independent risk factor for

Table 18.4 Gender differences from presentation to treatment strategy in patients with ACS

	Women	Men
Clinical presentation	More frequently present with UA/NSTEMI On average, 10 years older than men Often present with atypical symptoms[a] Longer door-to-treatment times	More frequently present with STEMI
Comorbidities	Higher incidence of multiple cardiovascular disease risk factors Less likely to have prior cardiovascular disease	More likely to be smokers, have prior myocardial infarction (MI), and coronary revascularization
Mortality post-PCI	Similar rates of mortality as physician experience and technology improves Some higher mortality for women may persist in STEMI	
Drug-eluting stents (DES) versus Bare-metal stents (BMS)	Limited date on BMS due to small sample size but long-term benefits of stenting generalizable DES reduces restenosis and MACE at 1 year	Similar outcomes in men and women treated with DES
Bleeding and vascular complications	Significantly higher risk of non-CABG related TIMI major bleeding	Lower risk of bleeding/vascular complications as compared to women
ACS treatment strategy UA/NSTEMI (Early invasive vs. conservative strategy)	Invasive strategy with stenting and GPIIb/IIIA inhibition recommended for high-risk women Conservative management recommended for low-risk women	Trials suggest reduced incidence of adverse outcomes (MI and death) with early invasive strategy in men as compared with women
ACS treatment strategy STEMI (Early invasive vs. conservative strategy)	Timely PCI results in improved outcomes as compared with fibrinolysis	

Table 18.2 summarizes the findings from the literature and should serve as a convenient point of reference. Refer to text for full discussion and citations

MACE major adverse cardiac event, *CABG* coronary artery bypass surgery, *GPIIB/IIIA* glycoprotein IIB/IIIA inhibitor, *PCI* percutaneous coronary intervention

[a]See Table 18.2

operative mortality. Long-term survival has been shown to be equal between genders, but postoperative long-term quality of life has shown to be significantly different between sexes. Women exhibit worse functional status, are more symptomatic, have increased rates of depression and anxiety, and have a higher incidence of graft occlusion with increased rates of repeat revascularization [135, 136]. The type of CABG, on-pump versus off-pump, has also revealed significant differences in postoperative mortality in women compared to men [147]. Two large studies to date have revealed off-pump surgeries had lower mortality rates and reductions in respiratory complications and hospital stay [146, 147]. Furthermore, women undergoing conventional on-pump CABG tended to have higher mortality rates and complications due to bleeding [137, 138].

Conclusions

Despite major advancements in therapies aimed at reducing the dreaded complications of heart disease, cardiovascular disease still remains the leading cause of death among women accounting for more deaths than cancer, Alzheimer's disease, and pneumonia combined [148]. Furthermore, differences in presentation, treatment, and outcome exist between men and women (summarized in Table 18.4), but these difference are often difficult to quantify, partly due to an underrepresentation of women in clinical trials. As life expectancy increases, the prevalence of CAD among women will increase thereby necessitating a more thorough understanding of treatment differences between genders. Current advances in research and therapies show promise to elucidate the inherent gender differences and improve outcomes.

References

1. Lansky AJ, Hochman JS, Ward PA, et al. Percutaneous coronary intervention and adjunctive pharmacotherapy in women: a statement for healthcare professionals from the American Heart Association. Circulation. 2005;111(7):940–53.
2. Cowley MJ, Mullin SM, Kelsey SF, et al. Sex differences in early and long-term results of coronary angioplasty in the NHLBI PTCA Registry. Circulation. 1985;71(1):90–7.
3. Kelsey SF, James M, Holubkov AL, Holubkov R, Cowley MJ, Detre KM. Results of percutaneous transluminal coronary angioplasty in women. 1985–1986 National Heart, Lung, and Blood Institute's Coronary Angioplasty Registry. Circulation. 1993;87(3):720–7.
4. Elkoustaf RA, Mamkin I, Mather JF, et al. Comparison of results of percutaneous coronary intervention for non-ST-elevation acute myocardial infarction or unstable angina pectoris in men versus women. Am J Cardiol. 2006;98(2):182–6.

5. Heer T, Gitt AK, Juenger C, et al. Gender differences in acute non-ST-segment elevation myocardial infarction. Am J Cardiol. 2006; 98(2):160–6.
6. Heer T, Schiele R, Schneider S, et al. Gender differences in acute myocardial infarction in the era of reperfusion (the MITRA registry). Am J Cardiol. 2002;89(5):511–7.
7. Suessenbacher A, Doerler J, Alber H, et al. Gender-related outcome following percutaneous coronary intervention for ST-elevation myocardial infarction: data from the Austrian acute PCI registry. EuroIntervention. 2008;4(2):271–6.
8. Berecki-Gisolf J, Humphreyes-Reid L, Wilson A, Dobson A. Angina symptoms are associated with mortality in older women with ischemic heart disease. Circulation. 2009;120(23):2330–6.
9. Akhter N, Milford-Beland S, Roe MT, Piana RN, Kao J, Shroff A. Gender differences among patients with acute coronary syndromes undergoing percutaneous coronary intervention in the American College of Cardiology-National Cardiovascular Data Registry (ACC-NCDR). Am Heart J. 2009;157(1):141–8.
10. Al-Fiadh AH, Andrianopoulos N, Farouque O, et al. Contemporary outcomes in women undergoing percutaneous coronary intervention for acute coronary syndromes. Int J Cardiol. 2011;151(2): 195–9.
11. O'Donoghue M, Boden WE, Braunwald E, et al. Early invasive vs conservative treatment strategies in women and men with unstable angina and non-ST-segment elevation myocardial infarction: a meta-analysis. JAMA. 2008;300(1):71–80.
12. Benamer H, Tafflet M, Bataille S, et al. Female gender is an independent predictor of in-hospital mortality after STEMI in the era of primary PCI: insights from the greater Paris area PCI Registry. EuroIntervention. 2011;6(9):1073–9.
13. Lawesson SS, Stenestrand U, Lagerqvist B, Wallentin L, Swahn E. Gender perspective on risk factors, coronary lesions and long-term outcome in young patients with ST-elevation myocardial infarction. Heart. 2010;96(6):453–9.
14. Milner KA, Funk M, Richards S, Wilmes RM, Vaccarino V, Krumholz HM. Gender differences in symptom presentation associated with coronary heart disease. Am J Cardiol. 1999;84(4): 396–9.
15. Philpott S, Boynton PM, Feder G, Hemingway H. Gender differences in descriptions of angina symptoms and health problems immediately prior to angiography: the ACRE study. Appropriateness of Coronary Revascularisation study. Soc Sci Med. 2001;52(10):1565–75.
16. Tsujita K, Nikolsky E, Lansky AJ, et al. Impact of anemia on clinical outcomes of patients with ST-segment elevation myocardial infarction in relation to gender and adjunctive antithrombotic therapy (from the HORIZONS-AMI trial). Am J Cardiol. 2010; 105(10):1385–94.
17. Blum A, Blum N. Coronary artery disease: are men and women created equal? Gend Med. 2009;6(3):410–8.
18. Timoteo AT, Mota Carmo M, Ferreira RC. Carotid intima-media thickness and carotid plaques improves prediction of obstructive angiographic coronary artery disease in women. Angiology. 2013;64(1):57–63.
19. Simon JA, Hsia J, Cauley JA, et al. Postmenopausal hormone therapy and risk of stroke: the Heart and Estrogen-progestin Replacement Study (HERS). Circulation. 2001;103(5): 638–42.
20. Rossouw JE, Anderson GL, Prentice RL, et al. Risks and benefits of estrogen plus progestin in healthy postmenopausal women: principal results from the Women's Health Initiative randomized controlled trial. JAMA. 2002;288(3):321–33.
21. Mosca L, Benjamin EJ, Berra K, et al. Effectiveness-based guidelines for the prevention of cardiovascular disease in women–2011 update: a guideline from the American Heart Association. Circulation. 2011;123(11):1243–62.
22. Kennedy JW, Killip T, Fisher LD, Alderman EL, Gillespie MJ, Mock MB. The clinical spectrum of coronary artery disease and its surgical and medical management, 1974–1979. The Coronary Artery Surgery study. Circulation. 1982;66(5 Pt 2):III16–23.
23. Xhyheri B, Bugiardini R. Diagnosis and treatment of heart disease: are women different from men? Prog Cardiovasc Dis. 2010;53(3):227–36.
24. Sullivan AK, Holdright DR, Wright CA, Sparrow JL, Cunningham D, Fox KM. Chest pain in women: clinical, investigative, and prognostic features. BMJ. 1994;308(6933):883–6.
25. Gibbons RJ, Balady GJ, Beasley JW, et al. ACC/AHA guidelines for exercise testing: executive summary. A report of the American College of Cardiology/American Heart Association Task Force on Practice Guidelines (Committee on Exercise Testing). Circulation. 1997;96(1):345–54.
26. Kwok Y, Kim C, Grady D, Segal M, Redberg R. Meta-analysis of exercise testing to detect coronary artery disease in women. Am J Cardiol. 1999;83(5):660–6.
27. Lokhandwala JO, Skelding KA. Sex differences in percutaneous coronary interventions. J Cardiovasc Transl Res. 2009;2(3): 300–5.
28. Mieres JH, Shaw LJ, Arai A, et al. Role of noninvasive testing in the clinical evaluation of women with suspected coronary artery disease: Consensus statement from the Cardiac Imaging Committee, Council on Clinical Cardiology, and the Cardiovascular Imaging and Intervention Committee, Council on Cardiovascular Radiology and Intervention, American Heart Association. Circulation. 2005;111(5):682–96.
29. Scheffel H, Alkadhi H, Plass A, et al. Accuracy of dual-source CT coronary angiography: first experience in a high pre-test probability population without heart rate control. Eur Radiol. 2006;16(12): 2739–47.
30. Mollet NR, Cademartiri F, van Mieghem CAG, et al. High-resolution spiral computed tomography coronary angiography in patients referred for diagnostic conventional coronary angiography. Circulation. 2005;112(15):2318–23.
31. de Gevigney G, Mosnier S, Ecochard R, et al. Are women with acute myocardial infarction managed as well as men? Does it have consequences on in-hospital mortality? Analysis of an unselected cohort of 801 women and 1,718 men. Acta Cardiol. 2001;56(3): 169–79.
32. Doyle F, De La Harpe D, McGee H, Shelley E, Conroy R. Gender differences in the presentation and management of acute coronary syndromes: a national sample of 1365 admissions. Eur J Cardiovasc Prev Rehabil. 2005;12(4):376–9.
33. Radovanovic D, Erne P, Urban P, Bertel O, Rickli H, Gaspoz JM. Gender differences in management and outcomes in patients with acute coronary syndromes: results on 20,290 patients from the AMIS Plus Registry. Heart. 2007;93(11):1369–75.
34. Movahed MR, Ramaraj R, Jamal MM, Hashemzadeh M. Nationwide trends in the utilization of multivessel percutaneous coronary intervention (MVPCI) in the United States across different gender and ethnicities. J Interv Cardiol. 2009;22(3):247–51.
35. Milcent C, Dormont B, Durand-Zaleski I, Steg PG. Gender differences in hospital mortality and use of percutaneous coronary intervention in acute myocardial infarction: microsimulation analysis of the 1999 nationwide French hospitals database. Circulation. 2007;115(7):833–9.
36. Lee KH, Jeong MH, Ahn YK, et al. Gender differences of success rate of percutaneous coronary intervention and short term cardiac events in Korea Acute Myocardial Infarction Registry. Int J Cardiol. 2008;130(2):227–34.

37. Tavris D, Shoaibi A, Chen AY, Uchida T, Roe MT, Chen J. Gender differences in the treatment of non-ST-segment elevation myocardial infarction. Clin Cardiol. 2010;33(2):99–103.
38. Glaser R, Herrmann HC, Murphy SA, et al. Benefit of an early invasive management strategy in women with acute coronary syndromes. JAMA. 2002;288(24):3124–9.
39. Carrabba N, Santoro GM, Balzi D, et al. In-hospital management and outcome in women with acute myocardial infarction (data from the AMI-Florence Registry). Am J Cardiol. 2004;94(9): 1118–23.
40. Bufe A, Wolfertz J, Dinh W, et al. Gender-based differences in long-term outcome after ST-elevation myocardial infarction in patients treated with percutaneous coronary intervention. J Womens Health (Larchmt). 2010;19(3):471–5.
41. Sadowski M, Gasior M, Gierlotka M, Janion M, Polonski L. Gender-related differences in mortality after ST-segment elevation myocardial infarction: a large multicentre national registry. EuroIntervention. 2011;6(9):1068–72.
42. Glickman SW, Granger CB, Ou FS, et al. Impact of a statewide ST-segment-elevation myocardial infarction regionalization program on treatment times for women, minorities, and the elderly. Circ Cardiovasc Qual Outcomes. 2010;3(5):514–21.
43. Mosca L, Ferris A, Fabunmi R, Robertson RM. Tracking women's awareness of heart disease: an American Heart Association national study. Circulation. 2004;109(5):573–9.
44. Mosca L, Jones WK, King KB, et al. Awareness, perception, and knowledge of heart disease risk and prevention among women in the United States. Arch Fam Med. 2000;9(6):506–15.
45. Takakuwa KM, Shofer FS, Limkakeng Jr AT, Hollander JE. Preferences for cardiac tests and procedures may partially explain sex but not race disparities. Am J Emerg Med. 2008;26(5): 545–50.
46. Mumma BE, Baumann BM, Diercks DB, et al. Sex bias in cardiovascular testing: the contribution of patient preference. Ann Emerg Med. 2011;57(6):551–560 e554.
47. Taggu W, Lloyd G. Treating cardiovascular disease in women. Menopause Int. 2007;13(4):159–64.
48. Allen JK, Scott LB, Stewart KJ, Young DR. Disparities in women's referral to and enrollment in outpatient cardiac rehabilitation. J Gen Intern Med. 2004;19(7):747–53.
49. Mosca L, Linfante AH, Benjamin EJ, et al. National study of physician awareness and adherence to cardiovascular disease prevention guidelines. Circulation. 2005;111(4):499–510.
50. Singh M, Rihal CS, Gersh BJ, et al. Mortality differences between men and women after percutaneous coronary interventions. A 25-year, single-center experience. J Am Coll Cardiol. 2008;51(24):2313–20.
51. Singh IM, Holmes Jr DR. Myocardial revascularization by percutaneous coronary intervention: past, present, and the future. Curr Probl Cardiol. 2011;36(10):375–401.
52. Duvernoy CS, Smith DE, Manohar P, et al. Gender differences in adverse outcomes after contemporary percutaneous coronary intervention: an analysis from the Blue Cross Blue Shield of Michigan Cardiovascular Consortium (BMC2) percutaneous coronary intervention registry. Am Heart J. 2010;159(4):677–683 e671.
53. Berger JS, Sanborn TA, Sherman W, Brown DL. Influence of sex on in-hospital outcomes and long-term survival after contemporary percutaneous coronary intervention. Am Heart J. 2006;151(5): 1026–31.
54. Kovacic JC, Mehran R, Karajgikar R, et al. Female gender and mortality after percutaneous coronary intervention: results from a large registry. Catheter Cardiovasc Interv. 2012;80(4):514–21.
55. Vakili BA, Kaplan RC, Brown DL. Sex-based differences in early mortality of patients undergoing primary angioplasty for first acute myocardial infarction. Circulation. 2001;104(25):3034–8.
56. Srinivas VS, Garg S, Negassa A, Bang JY, Monrad ES. Persistent sex difference in hospital outcome following percutaneous coronary intervention: results from the New York State reporting system. J Invasive Cardiol. 2007;19(6):265–8.
57. Roncalli J, Elbaz M, Dumonteil N, et al. Gender disparity in 48-hour mortality is limited to emergency percutaneous coronary intervention for ST-elevation myocardial infarction. Arch Cardiovasc Dis. 2010;103(5):293–301.
58. Mehta RH, Montoye CK, Gallogly M, et al. Improving quality of care for acute myocardial infarction: the Guidelines Applied in Practice (GAP) Initiative. JAMA. 2002;287(10):1269–76.
59. Jneid H, Fonarow GC, Cannon CP, et al. Sex differences in medical care and early death after acute myocardial infarction. Circulation. 2008;118(25):2803–10.
60. Cheng CI, Yeh KH, Chang HW, et al. Comparison of baseline characteristics, clinical features, angiographic results, and early outcomes in men vs women with acute myocardial infarction undergoing primary coronary intervention. Chest. 2004;126(1): 47–53.
61. Jacobs AK, Johnston JM, Haviland A, et al. Improved outcomes for women undergoing contemporary percutaneous coronary intervention: a report from the National Heart, Lung, and Blood Institute Dynamic registry. J Am Coll Cardiol. 2002;39(10): 1608–14.
62. D'Ascenzo F, Gonella A, Quadri G, et al. Comparison of mortality rates in women versus men presenting with ST-segment elevation myocardial infarction. Am J Cardiol. 2011;107(5):651–4.
63. Mehilli J, Kastrati A, Dirschinger J, et al. Sex-based analysis of outcome in patients with acute myocardial infarction treated predominantly with percutaneous coronary intervention. JAMA. 2002;287(2):210–5.
64. Lansky AJ, Pietras C, Costa RA, et al. Gender differences in outcomes after primary angioplasty versus primary stenting with and without abciximab for acute myocardial infarction: results of the Controlled Abciximab and Device Investigation to Lower Late Angioplasty Complications (CADILLAC) trial. Circulation. 2005;111(13):1611–8.
65. Fischman DL, Leon MB, Baim DS, et al. A randomized comparison of coronary-stent placement and balloon angioplasty in the treatment of coronary artery disease. Stent Restenosis Study Investigators. N Engl J Med. 1994;331(8):496–501.
66. Serruys PW, de Jaegere P, Kiemeneij F, et al. A comparison of balloon-expandable-stent implantation with balloon angioplasty in patients with coronary artery disease. Benestent Study Group. N Engl J Med. 1994;331(8):489–95.
67. Savage MP, Fischman DL, Rake R, et al. Efficacy of coronary stenting versus balloon angioplasty in small coronary arteries. Stent Restenosis Study (STRESS) Investigators. J Am Coll Cardiol. 1998;31(2):307–11.
68. Abbott JD, Vlachos HA, Selzer F, et al. Gender-based outcomes in percutaneous coronary intervention with drug-eluting stents (from the National Heart, Lung, and Blood Institute Dynamic Registry). Am J Cardiol. 2007;99(5):626–31.
69. Solinas E, Nikolsky E, Lansky AJ, et al. Gender-specific outcomes after sirolimus-eluting stent implantation. J Am Coll Cardiol. 2007;50(22):2111–6.
70. Presbitero P, Belli G, Zavalloni D, et al. "Gender paradox" in outcome after percutaneous coronary intervention with paclitaxel eluting stents. EuroIntervention. 2008;4(3):345–50.
71. Onuma Y, Kukreja N, Daemen J, et al. Impact of sex on 3-year outcome after percutaneous coronary intervention using bare-metal and drug-eluting stents in previously untreated coronary artery disease: insights from the RESEARCH (Rapamycin-Eluting Stent Evaluated at Rotterdam Cardiology Hospital) and T-SEARCH (Taxus-Stent Evaluated at Rotterdam Cardiology Hospital) Registries. JACC Cardiovasc Interv. 2009;2(7):603–10.

72. Brown RA, Williams M, Barker CM, et al. Sex-specific outcomes following revascularization with zotarolimus-eluting stents: comparison of angiographic and late-term clinical results. Catheter Cardiovasc Interv. 2010;76(6):804–13.
73. Mikhail GW. Coronary revascularisation in women. Heart. 2006;92 Suppl 3:iii19–23.
74. Mehilli J, Kastrati A, Bollwein H, et al. Gender and restenosis after coronary artery stenting. Eur Heart J. 2003;24(16):1523–30.
75. Chen Z, Qian J, Ma J, Ge L, Ge J. Effect of gender on repeated coronary artery revascularization after intra-coronary stenting: a meta-analysis. Int J Cardiol. 2012;157(3):381–5.
76. Lansky AJ, Ng VG, Mutlu H, et al. Gender-based evaluation of the XIENCE V™ everolimus-eluting coronary stent system. Catheter Cardiovasc Interv. 2009;74(5):719–27.
77. Funakoshi S, Furukawa Y, Ehara N, et al. Clinical characteristics and outcomes of Japanese women undergoing coronary revascularization therapy. Circ J. 2011;75(6):1358–67.
78. Mikhail GW, Gerber RT, Cox DA, et al. Influence of sex on long-term outcomes after percutaneous coronary intervention with the paclitaxel-eluting coronary stent: results of the "TAXUS Woman" analysis. JACC Cardiovasc Interv. 2010;3(12):1250–9.
79. Jacobs AK. The efficacy of drug-eluting stents in women: a window of opportunity. JACC Cardiovasc Interv. 2009;2(7):611–3.
80. Mehran R, Pocock S, Nikolsky E, et al. Impact of bleeding on mortality after percutaneous coronary intervention: results from a patient-level pooled analysis of the REPLACE-2 (randomized evaluation of PCI linking angiomax to reduced clinical events), ACUITY (acute catheterization and urgent intervention triage strategy), and HORIZONS-AMI (harmonizing outcomes with revascularization and stents in acute myocardial infarction) trials. J Am Coll Cardiol Intv. 2011;4(6):654–64.
81. Chiu JH, Bhatt DL, Ziada KM, et al. Impact of female sex on outcome after percutaneous coronary intervention. Am Heart J. 2004;148(6):998–1002.
82. Argulian E, Patel AD, Abramson JL, et al. Gender differences in short-term cardiovascular outcomes after percutaneous coronary interventions. Am J Cardiol. 2006;98(1):48–53.
83. Peterson ED, Lansky AJ, Kramer J, Anstrom K, Lanzilotta MJ. Effect of gender on the outcomes of contemporary percutaneous coronary intervention. Am J Cardiol. 2001;88(4):359–64.
84. Thompson CA, Kaplan AV, Friedman BJ, et al. Gender-based differences of percutaneous coronary intervention in the drug-eluting stent era. Catheter Cardiovasc Interv. 2006;67(1):25–31.
85. Poludasu S, Cavusoglu E, Clark LT, Marmur JD. Impact of gender on in-hospital percutaneous coronary interventional outcomes in African-Americans. J Invasive Cardiol. 2007;19(3):123–8.
86. Chacko M, Lincoff AM, Wolski KE, et al. Ischemic and bleeding outcomes in women treated with bivalirudin during percutaneous coronary intervention: a subgroup analysis of the Randomized Evaluation in PCI Linking Angiomax to Reduced Clinical Events (REPLACE)-2 trial. Am Heart J. 2006;151(5):1032 e1031–1037.
87. Ahmed B, Piper WD, Malenka D, et al. Significantly improved vascular complications among women undergoing percutaneous coronary intervention: a report from the Northern New England Percutaneous Coronary Intervention Registry. Circ Cardiovasc Interv. 2009;2(5):423–9.
88. Applegate RJ, Sacrinty MT, Kutcher MA, et al. Vascular complications in women after catheterization and percutaneous coronary intervention 1998–2005. J Invasive Cardiol. 2007;19(9):369–74.
89. Jolly SS, Yusuf S, Cairns J, et al. Radial versus femoral access for coronary angiography and intervention in patients with acute coronary syndromes (RIVAL): a randomised, parallel group, multicentre trial. Lancet. 2011;377(9775):1409–20.
90. Pristipino C, Pelliccia F, Granatelli A, et al. Comparison of access-related bleeding complications in women versus men undergoing percutaneous coronary catheterization using the radial versus femoral artery. Am J Cardiol. 2007;99(9):1216–21.
91. Bertrand OF, Rao SV, Pancholy S, et al. Transradial approach for coronary angiography and interventions: results of the first international transradial practice survey. JACC Cardiovasc Interv. 2010;3(10):1022–31.
92. Tizon-Marcos H, Bertrand OF, Rodes-Cabau J, et al. Impact of female gender and transradial coronary stenting with maximal antiplatelet therapy on bleeding and ischemic outcomes. Am Heart J. 2009;157(4):740–5.
93. Glaser R, Selzer F, Jacobs AK, et al. Effect of gender on prognosis following percutaneous coronary intervention for stable angina pectoris and acute coronary syndromes. Am J Cardiol. 2006; 98(11):1446–50.
94. Iakovou I, Dangas G, Mehran R, et al. Impact of gender on the incidence and outcome of contrast-induced nephropathy after percutaneous coronary intervention. J Invasive Cardiol. 2003;15(1): 18–22.
95. Jackson EA, Moscucci M, Smith DE, et al. The association of sex with outcomes among patients undergoing primary percutaneous coronary intervention for ST elevation myocardial infarction in the contemporary era: insights from the Blue Cross Blue Shield of Michigan Cardiovascular Consortium (BMC2). Am Heart J. 2011; 161(1):106–112 e101.
96. Mueller C, Buerkle G, Perruchoud AP, Buettner HJ. Female sex and risk of contrast nephropathy after percutaneous coronary intervention. Can J Cardiol. 2004;20(5):505–9.
97. Mehran R, Aymong ED, Nikolsky E, et al. A simple risk score for prediction of contrast-induced nephropathy after percutaneous coronary intervention: development and initial validation. J Am Coll Cardiol. 2004;44(7):1393–9.
98. Pedersen SS, Ong AT, Lemos PA, Erdman RA, Serruys PW, van Domburg RT. Risk factors for impaired health status differ in women and men treated with percutaneous coronary intervention in the drug-eluting stent era. J Psychosom Res. 2006;61(1):11–7.
99. Mortensen OS, Bjorner JB, Newman B, et al. Gender differences in health-related quality of life following ST-elevation myocardial infarction: women and men do not benefit from primary percutaneous coronary intervention to the same degree. Eur J Cardiovasc Prev Rehabil. 2007;14(1):37–43.
100. Anderson JL, Adams CD, Antman EM, et al. ACC/AHA 2007 guidelines for the management of patients with unstable angina/ non ST-elevation myocardial infarction: a report of the American College of Cardiology/American Heart Association Task Force on Practice Guidelines (Writing Committee to Revise the 2002 Guidelines for the Management of Patients With Unstable Angina/ Non ST-Elevation Myocardial Infarction): developed in collaboration with the American College of Emergency Physicians, the Society for Cardiovascular Angiography and Interventions, and the Society of Thoracic Surgeons: endorsed by the American Association of Cardiovascular and Pulmonary Rehabilitation and the Society for Academic Emergency Medicine. Circulation. 2007;116(7):e148–304.
101. Anderson JL, Adams CD, Antman EM, et al. ACC/AHA 2007 guidelines for the management of patients with unstable angina/ non-ST-Elevation myocardial infarction: a report of the American College of Cardiology/American Heart Association Task Force on Practice Guidelines (Writing Committee to Revise the 2002 Guidelines for the Management of Patients With Unstable Angina/ Non-ST-Elevation Myocardial Infarction) developed in collaboration with the American College of Emergency Physicians, the Society for Cardiovascular Angiography and Interventions, and the Society of Thoracic Surgeons endorsed by the American Association of Cardiovascular and Pulmonary Rehabilitation and the Society for Academic Emergency Medicine. J Am Coll Cardiol. 2007;50(7):e1–157.

102. Wright RS, Anderson JL, Adams CD, et al. 2011 ACCF/AHA focused update incorporated into the ACC/AHA 2007 Guidelines for the Management of Patients with Unstable Angina/Non-ST-Elevation Myocardial Infarction: a report of the American College of Cardiology Foundation/American Heart Association Task Force on Practice Guidelines developed in collaboration with the American Academy of Family Physicians, Society for Cardiovascular Angiography and Interventions, and the Society of Thoracic Surgeons. J Am Coll Cardiol. 2011;57(19):e215–367.
103. Kumbhani DJ, Shishehbor MH, Willis JM, et al. Influence of gender on long-term mortality in patients presenting with non-ST-elevation acute coronary syndromes undergoing percutaneous coronary intervention. Am J Cardiol. 2012;109(8):1087–91.
104. Clayton TC, Pocock SJ, Henderson RA, et al. Do men benefit more than women from an interventional strategy in patients with unstable angina or non-ST-elevation myocardial infarction? The impact of gender in the RITA 3 trial. Eur Heart J. 2004;25(18):1641–50.
105. Lagerqvist B, Safstrom K, Stahle E, Wallentin L, Swahn E. Is early invasive treatment of unstable coronary artery disease equally effective for both women and men? FRISC II Study Group Investigators. J Am Coll Cardiol. 2001;38(1):41–8.
106. Antman EM, Hand M, Armstrong PW, et al. 2007 focused update of the ACC/AHA 2004 guidelines for the management of patients with ST-elevation myocardial infarction. Circulation. 2008;117(2):296–329.
107. Berger PB, Ellis SG, Holmes DR, et al. Relationship between delay in performing direct coronary angioplasty and early clinical outcome in patients with acute myocardial infarction : results from the global use of strategies to open occluded arteries in acute coronary syndromes (GUSTO-IIb) trial. Circulation. 1999;100(1):14–20.
108. Tamis-Holland JE, Palazzo A, Stebbins AL, et al. Benefits of direct angioplasty for women and men with acute myocardial infarction: results of the global use of strategies to open occluded arteries in acute coronary syndromes (GUSTO II-B) Angioplasty Substudy. Am Heart J. 2004;147(1):133–9.
109. Collins SD, Ahmad S, Waksman R. Percutaneous revascularization in women with coronary artery disease: we've come so far, yet have so far to go. Nutr Metab Cardiovasc Dis. 2010;20(6):436–44.
110. Reynolds HR, Farkouh ME, Lincoff AM, et al. Impact of female sex on death and bleeding after fibrinolytic treatment of myocardial infarction in GUSTO V. Arch Intern Med. 2007;167(19):2054–60.
111. Enriquez JR, Pratap P, Zbilut JP, Calvin JE, Volgman AS. Women tolerate drug therapy for coronary artery disease as well as men do, but are treated less frequently with aspirin, [beta]-blockers, or statins. Gend Med. 2008;5(1):53–61.
112. Bugiardini R, Yan AT, Yan RT, et al. Factors influencing underutilization of evidence-based therapies in women. Eur Heart J. 2011;32(11):1337–44.
113. Blomkalns AL, Chen AY, Hochman JS, et al. Gender disparities in the diagnosis and treatment of non-ST-segment elevation acute coronary syndromes: large-scale observations from the CRUSADE (Can Rapid Risk Stratification of Unstable Angina Patients Suppress Adverse Outcomes With Early Implementation of the American College of Cardiology/American Heart Association Guidelines) National Quality Improvement Initiative. J Am Coll Cardiol. 2005;45(6):832–7.
114. Anand SS, Xie CC, Mehta S, et al. Differences in the management and prognosis of women and men who suffer from acute coronary syndromes. J Am Coll Cardiol. 2005;46(10):1845–51.
115. Moriel M, Tzivoni D, Behar S, et al. Contemporary treatment and adherence to guidelines in women and men with acute coronary syndromes. Int J Cardiol. 2008;131(1):97–104.
116. Vittinghoff E, Shlipak MG, Varosy PD, et al. Risk factors and secondary prevention in women with heart disease: the Heart and Estrogen/progestin Replacement Study. Ann Intern Med. 2003;138(2):81–9.
117. Berger JS, Roncaglioni MC, Avanzini F, Pangrazzi I, Tognoni G, Brown DL. Aspirin for the primary prevention of cardiovascular events in women and men: a sex-specific meta-analysis of randomized controlled trials. JAMA. 2006;295(3):306–13.
118. Mosca L, Benjamin EJ, Berra K, et al. Effectiveness-based guidelines for the prevention of cardiovascular disease in women–2011 update: a guideline from the American Heart Association. J Am Coll Cardiol. 2011;57(12):1404–23.
119. Antithrombotic Trialists Collaboration. Collaborative meta-analysis of randomised trials of antiplatelet therapy for prevention of death, myocardial infarction, and stroke in high risk patients. BMJ. 2002;324(7329):71–86.
120. Shen H, Herzog W, Drolet M, et al. Aspirin resistance in healthy drug-naive men versus women (from the Heredity and Phenotype Intervention Heart Study). Am J Cardiol. 2009;104(4):606–12.
121. Becker DM, Segal J, Vaidya D, et al. Sex differences in platelet reactivity and response to low-dose aspirin therapy. JAMA. 2006;295(12):1420–7.
122. Berger JS, Bhatt DL, Cannon CP, et al. The relative efficacy and safety of clopidogrel in women and men a sex-specific collaborative meta-analysis. J Am Coll Cardiol. 2009;54(21):1935–45.
123. Steinhubl SR, Berger PB, Mann JT, et al. Early and sustained dual oral antiplatelet therapy following percutaneous coronary intervention. JAMA. 2002;288(19):2411–20.
124. Montalescot G, Wiviott SD, Braunwald E, et al. Prasugrel compared with clopidogrel in patients undergoing percutaneous coronary intervention for ST-elevation myocardial infarction (TRITON-TIMI 38): double-blind, randomised controlled trial. Lancet. 2009;373(9665):723–31.
125. Sugidachi A, Ogawa T, Kurihara A, et al. The greater in vivo antiplatelet effects of prasugrel as compared to clopidogrel reflect more efficient generation of its active metabolite with similar antiplatelet activity to that of clopidogrel's active metabolite. J Thromb Haemost. 2007;5(7):1545–51.
126. Wiviott SD, Braunwald E, McCabe CH, et al. Prasugrel versus clopidogrel in patients with acute coronary syndromes. N Engl J Med. 2007;357(20):2001–15.
127. Mega JL, Close SL, Wiviott SD, et al. Genetic variants in ABCB1 and CYP2C19 and cardiovascular outcomes after treatment with clopidogrel and prasugrel in the TRITON-TIMI 38 trial: a pharmacogenetic analysis. Lancet. 2010;376(9749):1312–9.
128. Kushner FG, Hand M, Smith SC, et al. 2009 focused updates: ACC/AHA guidelines for the management of patients with ST-elevation myocardial infarction (updating the 2004 guideline and 2007 focused update) and ACC/AHA/SCAI guidelines on percutaneous coronary intervention (updating the 2005 guideline and 2007 focused update). Circulation. 2009;120(22):2271–306.
129. Wallentin L, Becker RC, Budaj A, et al. Ticagrelor versus clopidogrel in patients with acute coronary syndromes. N Engl J Med. 2009;361(11):1045–57.
130. AstraZeneca replies to the US FDA complete response letter for BRILINTA (Ticagrelor Tablets). 2011; Press Release. Available at: http://www.astrazeneca.com/Media/Press-releases/Article/20110121CRL-to-US-FDA-for-Brilinta (2012). Accessed 14 Apr 2012.
131. Mahaffey KW, Wojdyla DM, Carroll K, et al. Ticagrelor compared with clopidogrel by geographic region in the Platelet Inhibition and Patient Outcomes (PLATO) trial. Circulation. 2012;124(5):544–54.
132. Cannon CP, Harrington RA, James S, et al. Comparison of ticagrelor with clopidogrel in patients with a planned invasive strategy for acute coronary syndromes (PLATO): a randomised double-blind study. Lancet. 2010;375(9711):283–93.

133. Cho L, Topol EJ, Balog C, et al. Clinical benefit of glycoprotein IIb/IIIa blockade with abciximab is independent of gender: pooled analysis from EPIC, EPILOG and EPISTENT trials. J Am Coll Cardiol. 2000;36(2):381–6.
134. Alexander KP, Chen AY, Newby LK, et al. Sex differences in major bleeding with glycoprotein IIb/IIIa inhibitors. Circulation. 2006;114(13):1380–7.
135. Boersma E, Harrington RA, Moliterno DJ, et al. Platelet glycoprotein IIb/IIIa inhibitors in acute coronary syndromes: a meta-analysis of all major randomised clinical trials. Lancet. 2002; 359(9302):189–98.
136. Fernandes LS, Tcheng JE, O'Shea JC, et al. Is glycoprotein IIb/IIIa antagonism as effective in women as in men following percutaneous coronary intervention?: Lessons from the ESPRIT study. J Am Coll Cardiol. 2002;40(6):1085–91.
137. Ebbinghaus J, Maier B, Schoeller R, Schuhlen H, Theres H, Behrens S. Routine early invasive strategy and in-hospital mortality in women with non-ST-elevation myocardial infarction results from the Berlin Myocardial Infarction Registry (BMIR). Int J Cardiol. 2012;158(1):78–82.
138. Coons JC, Battistone S. 2007 guideline update for unstable angina/non–ST-segment elevation myocardial infarction: focus on antiplatelet and anticoagulant therapies. Ann Pharmacother. 2008;42(7):989–1001.
139. Lansky AJ, Mehran R, Cristea E, et al. Impact of gender and antithrombin strategy on early and late clinical outcomes in patients with non-ST-elevation acute coronary syndromes (from the ACUITY trial). Am J Cardiol. 2009;103(9):1196–203.
140. Nakamura H, Arakawa K, Itakura H, et al. Primary prevention of cardiovascular disease with pravastatin in Japan (MEGA Study): a prospective randomised controlled trial. Lancet. 2006;368(9542): 1155–63.
141. Ridker PM, Danielson E, Fonseca FA, et al. Rosuvastatin to prevent vascular events in men and women with elevated C-reactive protein. N Engl J Med. 2008;359(21): 2195–207.
142. Mizuno K, Nakaya N, Ohashi Y, et al. Usefulness of pravastatin in primary prevention of cardiovascular events in women. Circulation. 2008;117(4):494–502.
143. Taylor F, Ward K, Moore TH, et al. Statins for the primary prevention of cardiovascular disease. Cochrane Database Syst Rev. 2011;1, CD004816.
144. Corbelli JA, Corbelli JC, Bullano MF, et al. Gender bias in lipid assessment and treatment following percutaneous coronary intervention. J Gend Specif Med. 2003;6(3):21–6.
145. Patti G, Cannon CP, Murphy SA, et al. Clinical benefit of statin pretreatment in patients undergoing percutaneous coronary intervention: a collaborative patient-level meta-analysis of 13 randomized studies. Circulation. 2011;123(15):1622–32.
146. Brown PP, Mack MJ, Simon AW, et al. Outcomes experience with off-pump coronary artery bypass surgery in women. Ann Thorac Surg. 2002;74(6):2113–9; discussion 2120.
147. Mack MJ, Brown P, Houser F, et al. On-pump versus off-pump coronary artery bypass surgery in a matched sample of women: a comparison of outcomes. Circulation. 2004;110(11 Suppl 1): II1–6.
148. Leading causes of death in females United States, 2007. [Webpage]. 2011; leading causes of death in females for 2007. Available at: http://www.cdc.gov/women/lcod/ (2012). Accessed 14 Apr 2012.

Percutaneous Coronary Interventions in the Elderly

19

Emmanouil S. Brilakis and Subhash Banerjee

The definition of elderly varies from study to study: Klein proposed a classification of elderly into (a) the "young old" (patients between the ages of 65 and 70 years, who are near the end of the working careers and are relatively healthy), (b) the "retired old" (patients between the ages of 70 and 80 years, who are increasingly less independent but still enjoy their retirement), and (c) the "old old" (patients >80 years old, who often live in nursing homes) [1]. The 2011 ACC/AHA guidelines update for the management of non-ST segment elevation acute coronary syndromes (ACS) uses the term "older patients" or "elderly" to refer to those who are 75 years and older [2].

Percutaneous coronary intervention (PCI) is frequently performed in elderly patients: in an analysis of 1,410,069 undergoing PCI between 2001 and 2006 in the NCDR, 52 % were aged 60–79 years and 11 % were aged ≥80 years. Moreover, the number of PCIs performed in elderly patients has been increasing over time: in the Scottish Coronary Revascularization Register, there was an increase in the number and percentage of PCIs undertaken in elderly patients, from 196 (8.7 %) in 2000 to 752 (13.9 %) in 2007 [3]. The number of elderly patients needing PCI and cardiac care is expected to further increase in the coming years: in the USA, elderly patients are estimated to increase from 12.9 to 20 % between 2000 and 2030, as baby boomers enter their senior years [4].

There are few studies examining the optimal PCI strategies for elderly patients [5]. The current European Society of Cardiology coronary revascularization guidelines state that "although subgroups of patients such as women and the elderly may be at higher risk of bleeding, there are no data supporting the suggestion that they should be treated differently from other patients included in randomized controlled trials" [6].

In this chapter we review various aspects of PCI in the elderly: the increased risk of PCI in these patients and the causes underlying this increased risk, strategies for approaching various anatomic and clinical subgroups commonly encountered in elderly patients, and the adjunctive pharmacologic strategy.

PCI in the Elderly

Risk

PCI in the elderly carries lower success rates and higher risk compared to PCI in younger patients [7–9]. There is increased risk for bleeding, myocardial infarction, death, stroke, renal failure, and vascular access complications, both during elective PCI and during PCI for acute coronary syndromes [10]. Batchelor et al. compared the in-hospital outcomes of 7,472 octogenarians (mean age 83 years) with those of 102,236 younger patients (mean age 62 years) who underwent PCI between 1994 and 1997 [3]. Octogenarians had more comorbidities, more extensive coronary disease, and a two- to fourfold increased risk of complications, including death (3.8 % vs. 1.1 %), Q wave myocardial infarction (1.9 % vs. 1.3 %), stroke (0.58 % vs. 0.23 %), renal failure (3.2 % vs. 1.0 %), and vascular complications (6.7 % vs. 3.3 %) ($p<0.001$ for all comparisons).

The risk of PCI among the elderly has been decreasing over time [3]. In the Scottish Coronary Revascularization Register between 2000 and 2007, there was a significant increase in the proportion of elderly patients who had multiple comorbidities, yet the underlying risk of complications did not change significantly over time [8]. An analysis of 1,410,069 patients undergoing PCI between 2001 and 2006

E.S. Brilakis, MD, PhD (✉)
UT Southwestern Medical School, Dallas, TX, USA

Cardiac Catherterization Laboratories,
VA North Texas Healthcare, Dallas, TX, USA
e-mail: esbrilakis@gmail.com

S. Banerjee, MD
UT Southwestern Medical School, Dallas, TX, USA

Division of Cardiology,
VA North Texas Healthcare System, Dallas, TX, USA

C.A. Thompson (ed.), *Textbook of Cardiovascular Intervention*,
DOI 10.1007/978-1-4471-4528-8_19, © Springer-Verlag London 2014

in the National Cardiovascular Data Registry showed that a significant temporal improvement in the adjusted in-hospital mortality of patients aged 60–79 years (odds ratio, 0.94; 95 % CI, 0.92 to 0.96) and those aged ≥80 years (odds ratio, 0.95; 95 % CI, 0.92 to 0.97) [9]. These improvements are likely a reflection of better angiographic techniques (such as use of transradial access), equipment developments (such as routine stent and drug-eluting stent implantation), and application of evidence-based medical therapies (such as statin and thienopyridine use [11]).

Pathophysiology of Increased Risk

There are many reasons underlying the higher PCI risk among elderly patients (Fig. 19.1) [12]:

- More extensive and complex coronary artery disease: elderly patients often have multivessel disease, multiple lesions, tortuosity and calcification (Fig. 19.2), and chronic total occlusions and often have had prior coronary artery bypass graft surgery [8].
- Vascular endothelial changes, with reduced nitric oxide production and prostacyclin synthesis.
- Decrease in circulating endothelial progenitor cells [13].
- High frequency of myocardial disease, due prior myocardial infarction, hypertension, or other causes.
- Multiple comorbidities, such as peripheral arterial disease, renal disease, chronic lung disease, anemia, and frailty. Frailty is characterized by vulnerability to acute stressors and is a consequence of decline in overall function and physiologic reserves and is estimated to be present in 30 % of octogenarians [14].
- Altered hemostasis: elderly patients have increased coagulation factors levels and increased platelet reactivity [15].
- Decrease in lean body mass and increase in adipose tissue.
- Impaired drug metabolism that may frequently lead to medication overdosing. Among non-ST segment elevation ACS patients in the CRUSADE (Can Rapid Risk Stratification of Unstable Angina Patients Suppress Adverse Outcomes With Early Implementation of the American College of Cardiology/American Heart Association Guidelines), National Quality Improvement Initiative Registry patients aged ≥75 years or older were more likely to receive excess doses of antithrombotic agents compared with patients younger than 65 years (16.5 % vs. 12.5 % for low molecular weight heparin, 38.4 % vs. 28.7 % for unfractionated heparin, and 64.5 % vs. 8.5 % for glycoprotein IIb/IIIa inhibitors) [16]. Those receiving excess doses had higher risk for bleeding (15 % of all bleeding events were attributed to excess dosing) [16].

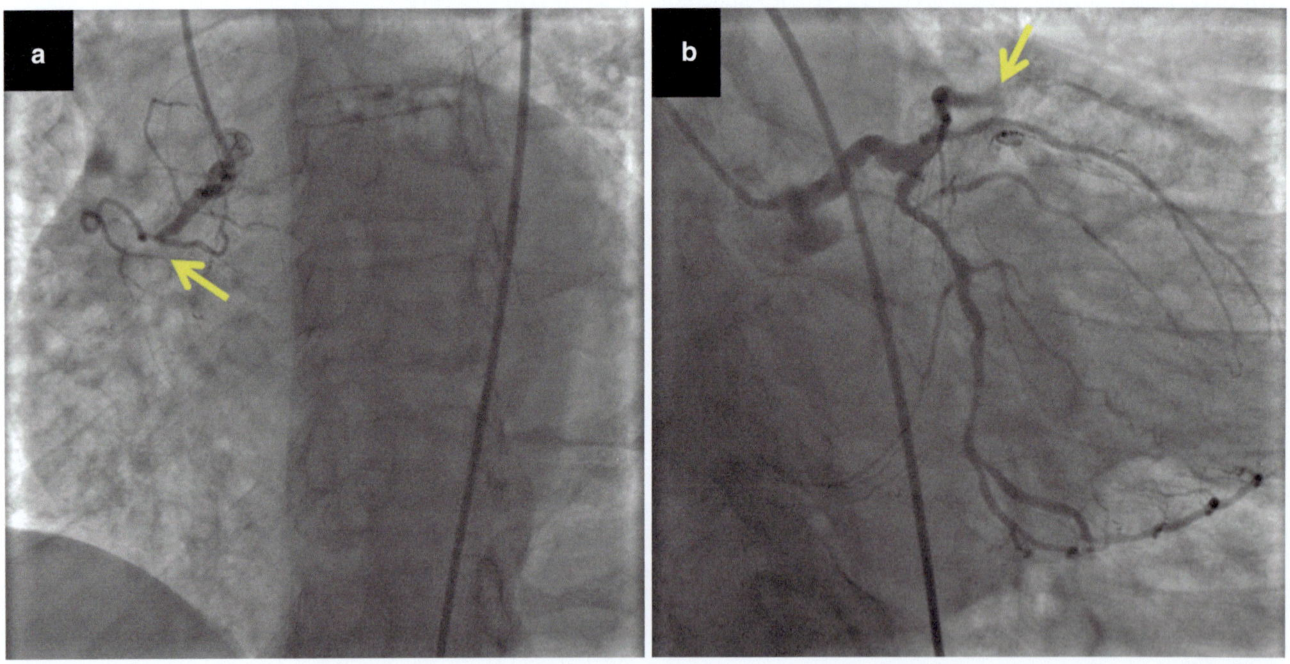

Fig. 19.1 Illustrative case of multivessel disease, calcification, and tortuosity in an 83-year-old man presenting with acute ST segment elevation anterior myocardial infarction. Coronary angiography demonstrating 100 % occlusion of the proximal right coronary artery (*arrow*, *panel* **a**) and of the mid-left anterior descending artery (*arrow*, *panel* **b**), as well as diffuse disease in the circumflex artery (*panel* **b**). The left anterior descending artery was wired with difficulty due to marked tortuosity and calcification, and balloon angioplasty was performed (*arrow*, *panel* **c**), resulting in restoration of antegrade flow (*panel* **d**). Severe calcification was also presenting the right common femoral artery (*arrows*, *panel* **e**)

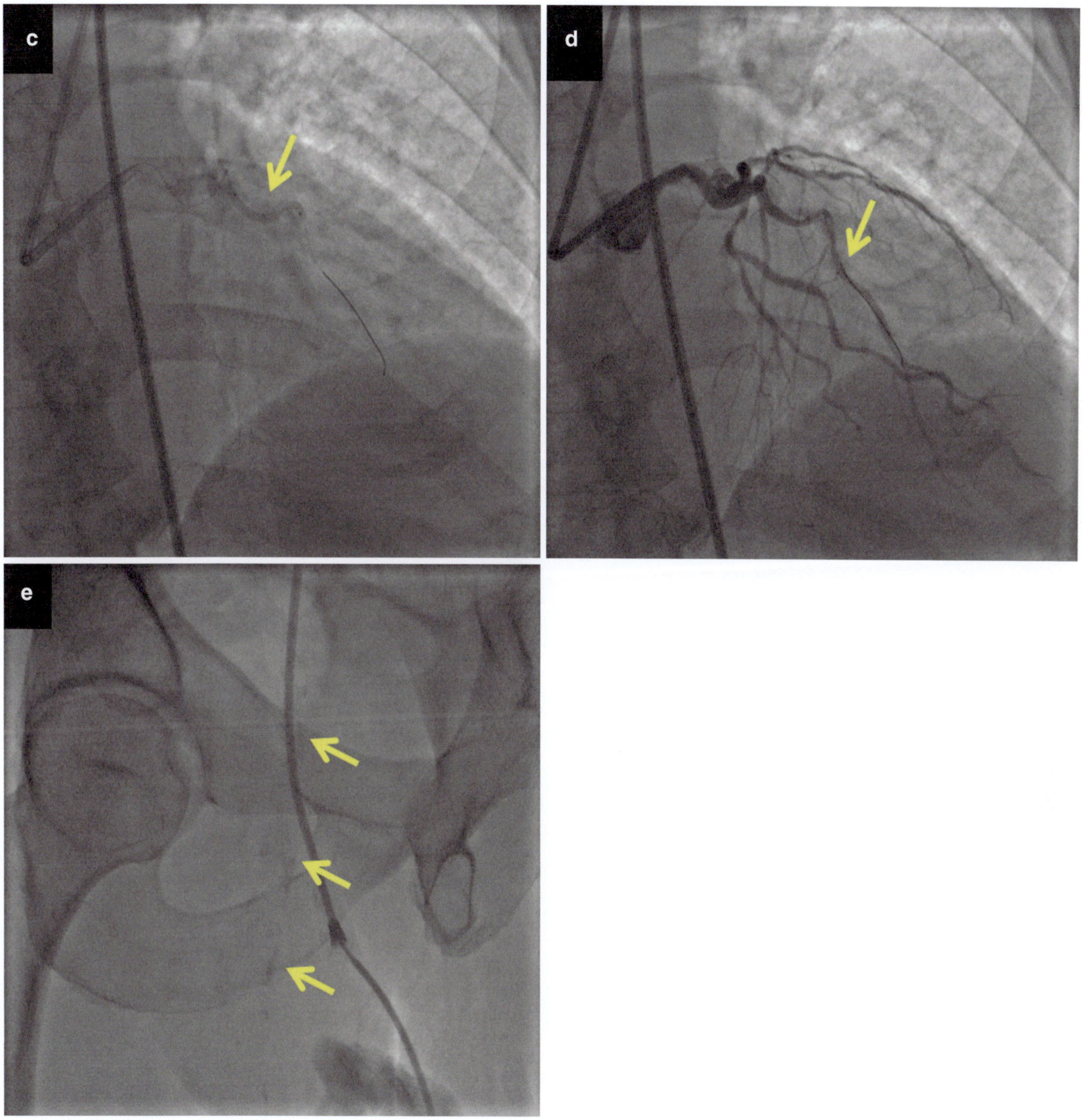

Fig. 19.1 (continued)

- Polypharmacy: surveys of community-based elderly patients show that 2–9 prescription medications on average are taken per day [17]. Many elderly patients are also taking supplements, further increasing the risk for drug-to-drug interactions [18].

Careful attention to modifiable risk factors, such as polypharmacy medication dosage adjustment based on the patients' renal function and comorbidities, is important for optimizing the PCI outcomes in elderly patients.

Technical Aspects

Vascular Access

Older patients are more likely to develop vascular complications for various reasons [19]. First, female gender is the predominant gender among older age groups, and women are known to have higher risk for vascular access complications. Second, peripheral vasculature is thickened and has increased stiffness, in part due to chronic hypertension, which is also

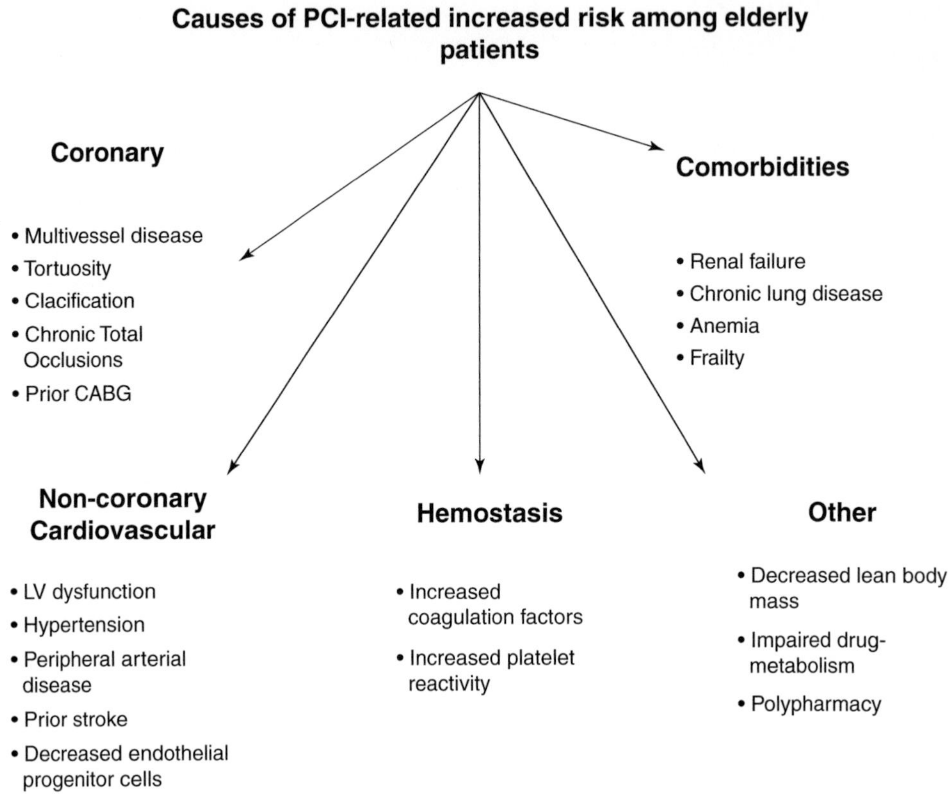

Fig. 19.2 Pathophysiology of increased risk associated with percutaneous coronary interventions in elderly patients

very prevalent in this age group. Third, peripheral vessels are often calcified, predisposing to dissection, and fourth there is reduced nitric oxide production predisposing patients to vasoconstriction.

A major advantage of the radial over the femoral access is the very low risk of bleeding and vascular access complications, which is particularly important among elderly patients. In a series of 323 patients aged ≥70 years, radial access was successful in 98.8 % of the patients, and the cannulation and total procedural time were similar to those of patients <70 years old. Only one access bleeding (0.4 %) occurred in the elderly patient group [20]. Similar results were observed in a series of 103 octogenarians undergoing left main PCI [21]. In the largest transradial vs. transfemoral comparative trial performed to date, the RadIal Vs femorAL access for coronary intervention (RIVAL) trial, patients aged ≥75 years with acute coronary syndromes had similarly favorable outcomes using the radial approach with patients <75 years old [1]. The radial approach may also be used for performing coronary angiography and angiography in anticoagulated patients safely, without needing to discontinue warfarin [22].

Use of the radial artery in the elderly also has limitations: (1) advancing the catheters to the coronary ostia may be challenging due to subclavian artery tortuosity [20] but may be assisted by use of hydrophilic 0.035 in. guidewires and having the patient take deep breaths during wire and catheter advancement; (2) guide catheter support is less than that offered by the femoral approach, especially in patients with prior coronary artery bypass graft surgery who need saphenous vein graft interventions [23]; (3) similarly large (such as 8 French) guide catheter may not be used with the radial approach, providing fewer options for treating complex lesions, such as bifurcations; and (4) there is more radiation exposure for the patient and the operator, although the patients may not have long enough life expectancy to manifest complications (such as cancer) due to radiation exposure.

In summary, the radial approach is appealing for PCI in elderly patients due to improved safety profile. Using the left radial artery may be advantageous compared to the right radial artery in the elderly: in a recent randomized trial, the left radial approach was associated with shorter procedural and fluoroscopy times in patients ≥70 years old [24].

Elective PCI

Elective PCI is one of the few areas in which a dedicated study involving the elderly has been performed. In the Trial of Invasive versus Medical Therapy in the Elderly (TIME), an invasive strategy was compared with an optimized medical strategy among 305 patients aged ≥75 years. All patients had Canadian Cardiac Society (CCS) class II or greater angina, despite being medicated with at least 2 antianginal drugs. Coronary revascularization was performed in 74 % of the invasive group patients vs. 37 % of the optimized medical strategy group patients. Six months post enrollment angina severity decreased and measures of quality of life increased in both treatment groups, but these improvements were significantly greater in the revascularization group [25]. Major adverse cardiac events occurred in 72 (49 %) of patients in the medical group and 29 (19 %) in the invasive group ($p<0.0001$) [25]. The benefit with the invasive strategy persisted after 4 years of follow-up [26].

In the Alberta Provincial Project for Outcomes Assessment in Coronary Heart Disease (APPROACH) cohort, adjusted 4-year mortality rates for coronary artery bypass graft surgery (CABG), PCI, and medical therapy in patients 70–79 years of age ranged between 13 and 21 % and in patients ≥80 years of age, from 23 % for CABG surgery, to 28 % for PCI, and to 40 % for medical therapy [27]. More importantly, quality of life improved to a similar or higher extent with coronary revascularization among patients aged 70–79 years and ≥80 years compared to patients aged <70 years [28].

The more contemporary Clinical Outcomes Utilizing Revascularization and Aggressive Drug Evaluation (COURAGE) trial proved that PCI did not reduce the risk of death, nonfatal MI, and hospitalization for ACS in patients with stable angina compared to optimal medical therapy alone, in patients <65 years old or in patients ≥65 years old [29]. However PCI improved the quality of life more than medical therapy [30], which may be the more important than prolongation of life for elderly patients, especially for the "old old" (>80 years old) patients [1]. In a study of 624 ACS patients undergoing PCI, elderly patients experienced the most improvement in physical health compared to younger patients [31].

Given the complex coronary anatomy often found in elderly patients, PCI of the most important culprit lesion rather than complete revascularization may provide the most favorable risk/benefit ratio.

PCI in Acute Coronary Syndromes

Primary PCI is preferred to thrombolytic administration in elderly patients presenting with ST segment elevation acute myocardial infarction, in part because of the high intracranial hemorrhage rates with thrombolytic administration in elderly patients [32]. The largest prospective trial of primary PCI vs. thrombolytics is the Senior Primary Angioplasty in Myocardial Infarction (PAMI) study (presented at the 2005 Transcatheter Cardiovascular Therapeutics conference, Washington DC), enrolled 481 patients aged ≥70 years. The composite endpoint of death, reinfarction, and stroke was reduced by 55 % ($p=0.009$), but no difference was observed among patients aged ≥80 years. In the Global Registry of Acute Coronary Events (GRACE), a 38 % relative decrease in adjusted mortality ($p=0.03$) was observed with primary PCI among patients ≥70 years old, although most elderly patients did not receive any reperfusion therapy [33]. In a meta-analysis of 22 randomized trials comparing primary PCI with fibrinolysis, a similar relative mortality reduction favoring primary PCI was observed in all age strata (except in patients ≤50 years of age) [34]. Moreover, due to higher risk of older patients, the absolute risk reduction was strongly and positively associated with age: at age 60 years, primary PCI was associated with 1.4 fewer deaths/100 patients treated compared with fibrinolytic therapy, whereas the risk reduction amounted to 5.1/100 patients at age 80 years [34]. In the Thrombolysis Versus Primary Angioplasty for AMI in Elderly Patients (TRIANA) trial (NCT00257309), primary PCI reduced recurrent ischemia compared to thrombolysis (0.8 % vs. 9.7 %, $p<0.001$) in patients over 75 years of age.

Elderly patients presenting with non-ST segment elevation ACS appear to have improved outcomes with an early invasive approach. In the Treat Angina with Aggrastat and Determine Cost of Therapy with an Invasive or Conservative Strategy–Thrombolysis in Myocardial Infarction (TACTICS–TIMI) 18 trial compared to an early conservative strategy, an early invasive strategy provided greater absolute reduction in the composite of death or myocardial infarction with increasing age: 1.5 % among patients 55–65 years old, 2.5 % among patients >65–75 years old, and 10.8 % among patients >75 years old [10]. However, major bleeding rates were higher with an early invasive strategy in patients older than 75 years of age (16.6 % vs. 6.5 %, $p=0.009$) [10]. Similar results were seen in the German Acute Coronary Syndromes Registry [35].

In summary primary PCI is the preferred mode of reperfusion for elderly STEMI patients, and an early invasive strategy is preferred for elderly with non-ST segment elevation acute coronary syndromes, with careful attention to antithrombotic regimens utilized to minimize the risk of bleeding (discussed in the Adjunctive Pharmacotherapy section below).

Multivessel Disease, Tortuosity, and Calcification

Elderly are more likely to have multivessel disease, which increases the complexity of coronary revascularization. Moreover, their coronary vessels are more likely to have tortuosity and calcification.

Calcification and tortuosity (Fig. 19.2) are associated with significantly increased technical difficulty and risk, related to equipment delivery to the target lesion and to optimal stent expansion. Careful lesion preparation by predilation and/or use of rotational atherectomy may be needed to facilitate stent delivery [36] and minimize the risk for stent loss [37]. Post-stenting invasive imaging with intravascular ultrasonography or optical coherence tomography is also important to ascertain adequate procedural result and minimize the risk for subsequent complications.

Drug-Eluting vs. Bare-Metal Stents

Although there are no randomized controlled trials comparing bare-metal stents (BMS) with drug-eluting stents (DES) specifically in elderly patients, observational studies have shown encouraging results with lower mortality and repeat revascularization rates with DES [38, 39]. A meta-analysis of five randomized trials of paclitaxel-eluting stents showed that compared to patients receiving BMS, patients receiving paclitaxel DES aged >70 years had comparable rates of death, myocardial infarction, and stent thrombosis but a significantly lower target lesion revascularization rate (22.2 vs. 10.2, $P<0.001$) [40]. Moreover, although the mortality rate of patients aged >70 years was higher than those of younger patients, it was comparable with age- and gender-matched norms in the general population [40]. Therefore, DES can be utilized in older patients, provided they can receive at least 12 months of dual antiplatelet therapy.

Prior Coronary Bypass Graft Surgery

Elderly patients in need for PCI are more likely to have prior coronary artery bypass graft surgery, which increases their risk for subsequent events [41]. Although most PCIs are still performed on native coronary artery lesions in prior CABG patients, the proportion of interventions performed in saphenous vein grafts increases with increasing time interval from CABG [42]. Saphenous vein graft PCI carries high risk for periprocedural myocardial infarction (usually due to distal embolization) and in-stent restenosis. The risk of myocardial infarction can be reduced by using embolic protection devices (EPDs), which have a class I indication for use in SVGs "when technically feasible" in both American [43] and European [6] guidelines. However, EPDs are currently used in only 22–23 % of SVG interventions in the USA [44, 45]. Although there have been conflicting results on the benefit of DES in SVG lesions in early studies [46–49], in the largest trial performed to date (ISAR-CABG [50]), DES use was associated with lower need for repeat revascularization with similar incidence of death and myocardial infarction compared to BMS. DES are currently utilized in the majority of SVG PCI in the USA [45].

Left Main

Treatment of left main disease remains controversial with CABG recommended for most patients in the USA. However, based on the promising results of the Synergy Between Percutaneous Coronary Intervention with TAXUS and Cardiac Surgery (SYNTAX) trial that showed similar outcomes at 1 year post PCI or CABG for left main disease [51], in the European coronary revascularization guidelines, left main PCI carries a class IIa indication for isolated left main or left main and one-vessel disease, IIb indication for left main with 2- or 3-vessel disease, and SYNTAX score ≤32 but class III indication for left main with 2- or 3-vessel disease and SYNTAX score ≥33 [6]. Considering the potentially higher rate of perioperative complications with CABG in elderly patients, PCI may be particularly useful in elderly patients with left main disease and high surgical risk. A retrospective analysis of 259 elderly patients (≥75 years old) with unprotected left main coronary artery disease demonstrated similar incidence of death and myocardial infarction but higher need for repeat revascularization among patients treated with DES compared to those treated with CABG [52]. However, more studies such as the ongoing Evaluation of Xience Prime versus Coronary Artery Bypass Surgery for Effectiveness of Left Main Revascularization trial (EXCEL, NCT01205776), in which the outcomes of PCI with a second-generation drug-eluting stent are compared with those of CABG in patients with unprotected left main coronary artery stenosis, are needed to allow for better decisions on the risks and benefits associated with left main stenting.

Adjunctive Pharmacotherapy

Periprocedural Antithrombotic Therapy

Elderly patients have higher risk of bleeding compared to younger patients. This is related to several factors, such as decreased drug metabolism, overdosing, and higher susceptibility to bleeding for anatomic reasons, such as peripheral arterial tortuosity and calcification.

Apart from use of the radial access, bleeding may be reduced by use of less aggressive anticoagulant and antiplatelet regimens. In the Randomized Evaluation in PCI Linking Angiomax to Reduced Clinical Events (REPLACE) 2 trial, patients >75 years old had lower mortality with bivalirudin compared to heparin + glycoprotein IIb/IIIa inhibitors [53]. Similarly, in the Acute Catheterization and Urgent Intervention Triage Strategy (ACUITY) trial, non-ST segment elevation acute coronary syndrome patients aged ≥75 years undergoing PCI had similar incidence of ischemic events but higher risk of bleeding compared to younger patients. The risk of non-CABG-related bleeding was 6.1 % with bivalirudin vs. 12.3 % with heparin and glycoprotein IIb/IIIa inhibitors (number needed to treat = 16) [54].

Compared to younger patients, the administration of glycoprotein IIb/IIIa inhibitors in elderly patients carries decreased efficacy and increased bleeding risk: in a meta-analysis of six randomized controlled trials of glycoprotein IIb/IIIa inhibitors that included 31,402 patients, those who

Table 19.1 Outcomes among elderly patients in contemporary studies of antiplatelet therapy in acute coronary syndromes

Study	Description	Elderly patients	Efficacy endpoint for elderly	Bleeding overall/elderly
ISAR-REACT-2 [55]	Non-ST segment elevation ACS	40 %>70 year	Abciximab 10.9 % UFH 9.9 %	1.4 % vs. 1.4 %/2.7 % vs. 1.9 %
Early ACS [56]	Non-ST segment elevation ACS	25 %>75 year	Eptifibatide Early 11.4 % Late 11.4 %	2.6 % vs. 1.8 %/not reported
ACUITY [53]	Non-ST segment elevation ACS	18 %>75 year	Bivalidurin 11.7 % UFH/GPI 9.6 %	3.0 % vs. 5.7 %/5.8 % vs. 10.1 %
CURE [57]	Non-ST segment elevation ACS	49 %>65 year	Clopidogrel 13.3 % Placebo 15.3 %	3.7 % vs. 2.7 %/not reported
TRITON-TIMI 38 [58]	ST segment elevation and Non-ST segment elevation ACS	13 %>75 year	Prasugrel 17.2 % Clopidogrel 18.3 %	2.4 % vs. 1.8 %/not reported
PLATO [59]	ST segment elevation and Non-ST segment elevation ACS	15 %>75 year	Ticagrelor 16.8 % Clopidogrel 18.3 %	11.6 % vs. 11.2 %/14.2 % vs. 13.3 %

ISAR-REACT 2 = Intracoronary Stenting and Antithrombotic: Regimen Rapid Early Action for Coronary Treatment 2
ACUITY = Acute Catheterization and Urgent Intervention Triage Strategy
EARLY-ACS = Early Glycoprotein IIb/IIIa Inhibition in Non-ST Segment Elevation Acute Coronary Syndrome trial
CURE = Clopidogrel in Unstable angina to prevent Recurrent Events
TRITON-TIMI 38 = Trial to Assess Improvement in Therapeutic Outcomes by Optimizing Platelet Inhibition with Prasugrel-Thrombolysis in Myocardial Infarction 38
PLATO = Platelet Inhibition and Patient Outcomes trial
ACS acute coronary syndromes

were ≥70 years old (35 % of the overall patient population) had a nonsignificant 4 % relative reduction in the 30-day risk of death or myocardial infarction but had 62 % increase in major bleeding [55].

In summary, bivalirudin use may reduce the bleeding risk among elderly patients undergoing PCI without decreased efficacy in preventing ischemic events. When more aggressive antiplatelet therapy is needed, such as administration of glycoprotein IIb/inhibitors for cases of large coronary thrombus, careful attention should be paid to avoid overdosing (by careful measurement of patient's weight and creatinine clearance) and minimize the risk for bleeding [16].

Post-procedural Antithrombotic Therapy

The preferred antiplatelet therapy post PCI in elderly patients is low-dose aspirin and clopidogrel (Table 19.1).

Aspirin

Aspirin is beneficial in reducing ischemic events post PCI, but can cause complications, mainly bleeding [61]. The Clopidogrel and Aspirin Optimal Dose Usage to Reduce Recurrent Events–Seventh Organization to Assess Strategies in Ischemic Syndromes (CURRENT–OASIS 7) trial demonstrated that higher-dose aspirin (300–325 mg daily) provided similar outcomes to lower-dose aspirin (75–100 mg daily) in patients with acute coronary syndromes referred for an early invasive strategy [62]. There was a small increase in the incidence of major gastrointestinal bleeding among patients who received higher-dose aspirin, as compared with those who received lower-dose aspirin (0.4 % vs.0.2 %, $P=0.04$) [62]. Similar results were seen in a meta-analysis of 192,036 patients enrolled in 31 clinical trials, in which daily doses of >100 mg of aspirin were associated with higher rates of minor, gastrointestinal, and total bleeding and stroke [63]. Aspirin use can also cause renal dysfunction among elderly patients [64].

Given that post PCI aspirin is combined with an adenosine diphosphate P2Y12 receptor antagonist, use of low-dose aspirin (81 mg daily) is recommended in the elderly.

Adenosine Diphosphate P2Y12 Receptor Antagonists

The use of an adenosine diphosphate P2Y12 receptor antagonist is critical for reducing the risk of stent thrombosis [65]. Clopidogrel is most commonly utilized, although prasugrel has recently become available for clinical use in the USA.

In the PCI-CURE (Clopidogrel in Unstable angina to prevent Recurrent Events) trial, the combination of clopidogrel and aspirin was associated with a 31 % relative reduction in the combined ischemic endpoint (composite of cardiovascular death, nonfatal myocardial infarction, or stroke) at 8 months, as compared with aspirin alone [58]. Compared with patients <65 years old, patients ≥65 years old had smaller relative reduction (21 % vs. 41 %) but similar absolute reduction (3.5 % vs. 3.9 %) of the composite ischemic endpoint with clopidogrel [58].

In the Trial to Assess Improvement in Therapeutic Outcomes by Optimizing Platelet Inhibition with Prasugrel-Thrombolysis in Myocardial Infarction 38 (TRITON-TIMI 38) [59], ACS patients were randomized to prasugrel or placebo [59]. In the entire study cohort, prasugrel at a dose of 10 mg daily reduced the risk of major adverse cardiovascular events by 19 % (from 12.1 to 9.9 %, $p<0.001$) but at the cost of a 32 % relative increase in major bleeding (from 1.8 to 2.4 %, $p=0.03$). Patients aged ≥75 years had only 6 % relative ischemic event risk reduction that was counterbalanced by an increase in bleeding [59]. Whether a lower dose of prasugrel (5 mg daily) is equally efficacious and safer in elderly patients is currently being evaluated (NCT00699998).

In the study of Platelet Inhibition and Patient Outcomes (PLATO), ticagrelor, a reversible and direct-acting oral antagonist of the adenosine diphosphate receptor P2Y12, reduced the incidence of major adverse events by 16 % in the overall patient population, but only by 6 % among patients ≥75 years in age, that was counterbalanced by a 4 % increase in major bleeding [60].

In summary, clopidogrel is the preferred adenosine diphosphate P2Y12 receptor antagonists post PCI in elderly patients. Prasugrel is currently not recommended in patients ≥75 years old, except possibly among such patients who do not have any contraindication (such as prior transient ischemic attack or stroke or active bleeding) and also have high-risk features, such as either diabetes or a past history of myocardial infarction [61].

Older patients undergoing PCI may often have other comorbidities, such as atrial fibrillation requiring use of oral anticoagulation with warfarin or dabigatran. Considering the significantly increased bleeding risk with use of triple antithrombotic therapy (aspirin, adenosine diphosphate P2Y12 receptor antagonist, and warfarin) [66], use of bare-metal stents should be strongly considered in such patients, especially when treating noncomplex coronary lesions.

Conclusions

A new paradigm was recently proposed for the care of elderly patients with cardiovascular disease encompassing a patient-centered approach to care, screening for coexisting geriatric syndromes and comorbidities, purposeful management of pharmacologic regimen, and emphasis on the importance of transitions of care [4].

More research is required on identifying the optimal timing and techniques for PCI in the elderly as well as for adjunctive pharmacologic therapy. This should include increased participation of elderly patients in ongoing and future PCI-related research studies and in studies examining hybrid surgical and percutaneous revascularization techniques.

PCI in elderly patients carries higher risk but can also provide significant benefits. In-depth communication with the patients about the goals, risks, benefits, and alternatives of PCI and careful attention to the procedural technique and to the selection of adjunctive medical therapy are key for optimizing the PCI outcomes in this large and expanding group of patients.

References

1. Jolly SS, Yusuf S, Cairns J, et al. Radial versus femoral access for coronary angiography and intervention in patients with acute coronary syndromes (RIVAL): a randomised, parallel group, multicentre trial. Lancet. 2011;377:1409–20.
2. Anderson JL, Adams CD, Antman EM, et al. 2011 ACCF/AHA focused update incorporated into the ACC/AHA 2007 guidelines for the management of patients with unstable angina/non-ST-elevation myocardial infarction: a report of the American College of Cardiology Foundation/American Heart Association Task Force on Practice Guidelines. Circulation. 2011;123(18):e426–579.
3. Batchelor WB, Anstrom KJ, Muhlbaier LH, et al. Contemporary outcome trends in the elderly undergoing percutaneous coronary interventions: results in 7,472 octogenarians. National Cardiovascular Network Collaboration. J Am Coll Cardiol. 2000;36:723–30.
4. Forman DE, Rich MW, Alexander KP, et al. Cardiac care for older adults: time for a new paradigm. J Am Coll Cardiol. 2011;57:1801–10.
5. Dauerman HL, Bhatt DL, Gretler DD, French PA, Smyth SS, Becker RC. Bridging the gap between clinical trials of antiplatelet therapies and applications among elderly patients. Am Heart J. 2010;159:508-17 e1.
6. Wijns W, Kolh P, Danchin N, et al. Guidelines on myocardial revascularization: The Task Force on Myocardial Revascularization of the European Society of Cardiology (ESC) and the European Association for Cardio-Thoracic Surgery (EACTS). Eur Heart J. 2010;31:2501–55.
7. Kiatchoosakun S, Keelapang P, Kaewsuwana P, Chotinaiwattarakul C, Piumsomboon C. Percutaneous coronary intervention in the elderly: results from the Thai National Percutaneous Coronary Intervention Registry (TPCIR). EuroIntervention. 2010;6:611–5.
8. Johnman C, Oldroyd KG, Mackay DF, et al. Percutaneous coronary intervention in the elderly: changes in case-mix and periprocedural outcomes in 31,758 patients treated between 2000 and 2007. Circ Cardiovasc Interv. 2010;3:341–5.
9. Singh M, Peterson ED, Roe MT, et al. Trends in the association between age and in-hospital mortality after percutaneous coronary intervention: National Cardiovascular Data Registry experience. Circ Cardiovasc Interv. 2009;2:20–6.
10. Bach RG, Cannon CP, Weintraub WS, et al. The effect of routine, early invasive management on outcome for elderly patients with non-ST-segment elevation acute coronary syndromes. Ann Intern Med. 2004;141:186–95.
11. Jaber WA, Lennon RJ, Mathew V, Holmes Jr DR, Lerman A, Rihal CS. Application of evidence-based medical therapy is associated with improved outcomes after percutaneous coronary intervention and is a valid quality indicator. J Am Coll Cardiol. 2005;46:1473–8.
12. Wang TY, Gutierrez A, Peterson ED. Percutaneous coronary intervention in the elderly. Nat Rev Cardiol. 2011;8:79–90.
13. Scheubel RJ, Zorn H, Silber RE, et al. Age-dependent depression in circulating endothelial progenitor cells in patients undergoing coronary artery bypass grafting. J Am Coll Cardiol. 2003;42:2073–80.
14. Singh M, Alexander K, Roger VL, et al. Frailty and its potential relevance to cardiovascular care. Mayo Clin Proc. 2008;83:1146–53.
15. Franchini M. Hemostasis and aging. Crit Rev Oncol Hematol. 2006;60:144–51.
16. Alexander KP, Chen AY, Roe MT, et al. Excess dosing of antiplatelet and antithrombin agents in the treatment of non–ST-segment elevation acute coronary syndromes. JAMA. 2005;294:3108–16.
17. Hajjar ER, Cafiero AC, Hanlon JT. Polypharmacy in elderly patients. Am J Geriatr Pharmacother. 2007;5:345–51.
18. Tachjian A, Maria V, Jahangir A. Use of herbal products and potential interactions in patients with cardiovascular diseases. J Am Coll Cardiol. 2010;55:515–25.

19. Dick P, Barth B, Mlekusch W, et al. Complications after peripheral vascular interventions in octogenarians. J Endovasc Ther. 2008;15:383–9.
20. Valsecchi O, Musumeci G, Vassileva A, et al. Safety and feasibility of transradial coronary angioplasty in elderly patients. Ital Heart J. 2004;5:926–31.
21. Bertrand OF, Bagur R, Costerousse O, Rodes-Cabau J. Transradial vs femoral percutaneous coronary intervention for left main disease in octogenarians. Indian Heart J. 2010;62:234–7.
22. Hildick-Smith DJ, Walsh JT, Lowe MD, Petch MC. Coronary angiography in the fully anticoagulated patient: the transradial route is successful and safe. Catheter Cardiovasc Interv. 2003;58:8–10.
23. Cooper L, Banerjee S, Brilakis ES. Crossover from radial to femoral access during a challenging percutaneous coronary intervention can make the difference between success and failure. Cardiovasc Revasc Med. 2010;11:266 e5-8.
24. Sciahbasi A, Romagnoli E, Burzotta F, et al. Transradial approach (left vs right) and procedural times during percutaneous coronary procedures: TALENT study. Am Heart J. 2011;161:172–9.
25. TIME investigators. Trial of invasive versus medical therapy in elderly patients with chronic symptomatic coronary-artery disease (TIME): a randomised trial. Lancet 2001;358:951–7.
26. Pfisterer M. Long-term outcome in elderly patients with chronic angina managed invasively versus by optimized medical therapy: four-year follow-up of the randomized Trial of Invasive versus Medical therapy in Elderly patients (TIME). Circulation. 2004;110:1213–8.
27. Graham MM, Ghali WA, Faris PD, Galbraith PD, Norris CM, Knudtson ML. Survival after coronary revascularization in the elderly. Circulation. 2002;105:2378–84.
28. Graham MM, Norris CM, Galbraith PD, Knudtson ML, Ghali WA. Quality of life after coronary revascularization in the elderly. Eur Heart J. 2006;27:1690–8.
29. Boden WE, O'Rourke RA, Teo KK, et al. Optimal medical therapy with or without PCI for stable coronary disease. N Engl J Med. 2007;356:1503–16.
30. Weintraub WS, Spertus JA, Kolm P, et al. Effect of PCI on quality of life in patients with stable coronary disease. N Engl J Med. 2008;359:677–87.
31. Li R, Yan BP, Dong M, et al. Quality of life after percutaneous coronary intervention in the elderly with acute coronary syndrome. Int J Cardiol. 2012;155:90–6.
32. Simoons ML, Maggioni AP, Knatterud G, et al. Individual risk assessment for intracranial haemorrhage during thrombolytic therapy. Lancet. 1993;342:1523–8.
33. Mehta RH, Sadiq I, Goldberg RJ, et al. Effectiveness of primary percutaneous coronary intervention compared with that of thrombolytic therapy in elderly patients with acute myocardial infarction. Am Heart J. 2004;147:253–9.
34. de Boer SP, Westerhout CM, Simes RJ, Granger CB, Zijlstra F, Boersma E. Mortality and morbidity reduction by primary percutaneous coronary intervention is independent of the patient's age. JACC Cardiovasc Interv. 2010;3:324–31.
35. Bauer T, Koeth O, Junger C, et al. Effect of an invasive strategy on in-hospital outcome in elderly patients with non-ST-elevation myocardial infarction. Eur Heart J. 2007;28:2873–8.
36. Saeed B, Banerjee S, Brilakis ES. Percutaneous coronary intervention in tortuous coronary arteries: associated complications and strategies to improve success. J Interv Cardiol. 2008;21:504–11.
37. Brilakis ES, Best PJ, Elesber AA, et al. Incidence, retrieval methods, and outcomes of stent loss during percutaneous coronary intervention: a large single-center experience. Catheter Cardiovasc Interv. 2005;66:333–40.
38. Groeneveld PW, Matta MA, Greenhut AP, Yang F. Drug-eluting compared with bare-metal coronary stents among elderly patients. J Am Coll Cardiol. 2008;51:2017–24.
39. Douglas PS, Brennan JM, Anstrom KJ, et al. Clinical effectiveness of coronary stents in elderly persons: results from 262,700 Medicare patients in the American College of Cardiology-National Cardiovascular Data Registry. J Am Coll Cardiol. 2009;53:1629–41.
40. Forman DE, Cox DA, Ellis SG, et al. Long-term paclitaxel-eluting stent outcomes in elderly patients. Circ Cardiovasc Interv. 2009;2:178–87.
41. Brilakis ES, de Lemos JA, Cannon CP, et al. Outcomes of patients with acute coronary syndrome and previous coronary artery bypass grafting (from the Pravastatin or Atorvastatin Evaluation and Infection Therapy [PROVE IT-TIMI 22] and the Aggrastat to Zocor [A to Z] trials). Am J Cardiol. 2008;102:552–8.
42. Brilakis ES, Rao SV, Banerjee S, et al. Percutaneous coronary intervention in native arteries vs. bypass grafts in prior coronary bypass grafting patients: a report from NCDR. J Am Coll Cardiol Intv. 2011;4:844–50.
43. Smith Jr SC, Feldman TE, Hirshfeld Jr JW, et al. ACC/AHA/SCAI 2005 guideline update for percutaneous coronary intervention–summary article: a report of the American College of Cardiology/American Heart Association Task Force on Practice Guidelines (ACC/AHA/SCAI Writing Committee to update the 2001 Guidelines for Percutaneous Coronary Intervention). Catheter Cardiovasc Interv. 2006;67:87–112.
44. Mehta SK, Frutkin AD, Milford-Beland S, et al. Utilization of distal embolic protection in saphenous vein graft interventions (an analysis of 19,546 patients in the American College of Cardiology-National Cardiovascular Data Registry). Am J Cardiol. 2007;100:1114–8.
45. Brilakis ES, Wang TY, Rao SV, et al. Frequency and predictors of drug-eluting stent use in saphenous vein bypass graft percutaneous coronary interventions: a report from the American College of Cardiology National Cardiovascular Data CathPCI Registry. J Am Coll Cardiol Intv. 2010;3:1068–73.
46. Brilakis ES, Lichtenwalter C, de Lemos JA, et al. A randomized controlled trial of a paclitaxel-eluting stent versus a similar bare-metal stent in saphenous vein graft lesions the SOS (Stenting of Saphenous Vein Grafts) trial. J Am Coll Cardiol. 2009;53:919–28.
47. Brilakis ES, Lichtenwalter C, Abdel-karim A-rR, et al. Continued benefit from paclitaxel-eluting compared with bare-metal stent implantation in saphenous vein graft lesions during long-term follow-up of the SOS (Stenting of Saphenous Vein Grafts) Trial. J Am Coll Cardiol Intv. 2011;4:176–82.
48. Vermeersch P, Agostoni P, Verheye S, et al. Randomized double-blind comparison of sirolimus-eluting stent versus bare-metal stent implantation in diseased saphenous vein grafts: six-month angiographic, intravascular ultrasound, and clinical follow-up of the RRISC Trial. J Am Coll Cardiol. 2006;48:2423–31.
49. Vermeersch P, Agostoni P, Verheye S, et al. Increased late mortality after sirolimus-eluting stents versus bare-metal stents in diseased saphenous vein grafts: results from the randomized DELAYED RRISC Trial. J Am Coll Cardiol. 2007;50:261–7.
50. Mehilli J, Pache J, Abdel-Wahab M, et al. Drug-eluting versus bare-metal stents in saphenous vein graft lesions (ISAR-CABG): a randomised controlled superiority trial. Lancet 2011;378:1071–8.
51. Morice MC, Serruys PW, Kappetein AP, et al. Outcomes in patients with de novo left main disease treated with either percutaneous coronary intervention using paclitaxel-eluting stents or coronary artery bypass graft treatment in the Synergy Between Percutaneous Coronary Intervention with TAXUS and Cardiac Surgery (SYNTAX) trial. Circulation. 2010;121:2645–53.
52. Palmerini T, Barlocco F, Santarelli A, et al. A comparison between coronary artery bypass grafting surgery and drug eluting stent for the treatment of unprotected left main coronary artery disease in elderly patients (aged>or =75 years). Eur Heart J. 2007;28:2714–9.
53. Lincoff AM, Kleiman NS, Kereiakes DJ, et al. Long-term efficacy of bivalirudin and provisional glycoprotein IIb/IIIa blockade vs

heparin and planned glycoprotein IIb/IIIa blockade during percutaneous coronary revascularization: REPLACE-2 randomized trial. JAMA. 2004;292:696–703.
54. Lopes RD, Alexander KP, Manoukian SV, et al. Advanced age, antithrombotic strategy, and bleeding in non-ST-segment elevation acute coronary syndromes: results from the ACUITY (Acute Catheterization and Urgent Intervention Triage Strategy) trial. J Am Coll Cardiol. 2009;53:1021–30.
55. Boersma E, Harrington RA, Moliterno DJ, et al. Platelet glycoprotein IIb/IIIa inhibitors in acute coronary syndromes: a meta-analysis of all major randomised clinical trials. Lancet. 2002;359: 189–98.
56. Kastrati A, Mehilli J, Neumann FJ, et al. Abciximab in patients with acute coronary syndromes undergoing percutaneous coronary intervention after clopidogrel pretreatment: the ISAR-REACT 2 randomized trial. JAMA. 2006;295:1531–8.
57. Giugliano RP, White JA, Bode C, et al. Early versus delayed, provisional eptifibatide in acute coronary syndromes. N Engl J Med. 2009;360:2176–90.
58. Mehta SR, Yusuf S, Peters RJ, et al. Effects of pretreatment with clopidogrel and aspirin followed by long-term therapy in patients undergoing percutaneous coronary intervention: the PCI-CURE study. Lancet. 2001;358:527–33.
59. Wiviott SD, Braunwald E, McCabe CH, et al. Prasugrel versus clopidogrel in patients with acute coronary syndromes. N Engl J Med. 2007;357:2001–15.
60. Wallentin L, Becker RC, Budaj A, et al. Ticagrelor versus clopidogrel in patients with acute coronary syndromes. N Engl J Med. 2009;361:1045–57.
61. Capodanno D, Angiolillo DJ. Antithrombotic therapy in the elderly. J Am Coll Cardiol. 2010;56:1683–92.
62. Mehta SR, Bassand JP, Chrolavicius S, et al. Dose comparisons of clopidogrel and aspirin in acute coronary syndromes. N Engl J Med. 2010;363:930–42.
63. Serebruany VL, Steinhubl SR, Berger PB, et al. Analysis of risk of bleeding complications after different doses of aspirin in 192,036 patients enrolled in 31 randomized controlled trials. Am J Cardiol. 2005;95:1218–22.
64. Segal R, Lubart E, Leibovitz A, et al. Early and late effects of low-dose aspirin on renal function in elderly patients. Am J Med. 2003;115:462–6.
65. Leon MB, Baim DS, Popma JJ, et al. A clinical trial comparing three antithrombotic-drug regimens after coronary-artery stenting. Stent Anticoagulation Restenosis Study Investigators. N Engl J Med. 1998;339:1665–71.
66. Khurram Z, Chou E, Minutello R, et al. Combination therapy with aspirin, clopidogrel and warfarin following coronary stenting is associated with a significant risk of bleeding. J Invasive Cardiol. 2006;18:162–4.

Left Main PCI: Patient Selection and Technique

20

Seung-Jung Park and Duk-Woo Park

Left main coronary artery (LMCA) disease is associated with increased mortality and morbidity than other sites of coronary artery disease (CAD) [1]. Therefore, traditional and standard treatment for such complex lesions has been a coronary artery bypass surgery (CABG), ensuring more complete and safe revascularization to either the left anterior descending or circumflex artery [2]. However, due to improved techniques, skills, and concomitant pharmacotherapy, percutaneous coronary intervention (PCI) for LMCA disease has been an attractive and challenging field to the interventional cardiologist worldwide [3]. Even alongside of the advent of drug-eluting stents (DES) with markedly improved efficacy, the revascularization option of unprotected LMCA disease is no longer purely surgical place in routine clinical practice. This chapter summarizes cumulative evidence of CABG, PCI with stenting, and comparative outcomes of two active procedures for the optimal treatment of LMCA disease.

CABG for LMCA Disease

In patients with multivessel disease and receiving CABG, the presence of a significant LMCA stenosis is one of major determinants of morbidity and mortality after surgery. Based on large surgical databases, perioperative and long-term mortality was significantly higher in patients with LMCA disease than those without LMCA disease having the relative risk ratio of 1.3:1.5 [4]. The outcomes of patients with left main disease treated with CABG have improved over time. There were numerous efforts during the previous decade to improve operative mortality for patients receiving CABG. Based on a recent Medicare data report, risk-adjusted mortality associated with CABG operation was significantly reduced during the previous decade (4.3–3.4 %, approximately 21 % risk reduction) and also fell steadily [5]. To continuously improve surgical outcomes, strategies such as operating room checklists, outcomes measurement and feedback programs, and collaborative quality improvement initiatives might be essential.

As a surgical technique, the presence of LMCA disease in patients with multivessel CAD has been considered to be a relative contraindication to off-pump CABG due to intraoperative hemodynamic instability. However, to coincide with improvement of surgical devices and of surgical and anesthetic experience, outcomes of off-pump CABG for LMCA disease have much been improved. A meta-analysis of nine clinical studies comparing off-pump ($n=1,036$; 23.5 %) and on-pump CABG ($n=3,375$; 76.5 %) for 4,411 patients with significant LMCA disease showed that the incidence of stroke was lower in the off-pump CABG group (odd ratio 0.17, 95 % CI 0.05–0.60) and early mortality, length of hospital stay, blood loss, and inotropic requirements were also significantly favored by off-pump CABG [6]. In addition, alongside of mandatory use of internal mammary artery, additional conduits are needed for complete revascularization in patients with LMCA disease, in whom more than 70–80 % of cases have other concomitant major coronary artery involvement. Arterial grafts are thought to be better conduits than saphenous vein grafts based on experience with using the left internal mammary artery to bypass the left anterior descending coronary artery. Recent randomized trial suggested that there was no significant difference in angiographic graft patency at 1 year after CABG (radial artery, 89 % vs. saphenous vein, 89 %) [7]. However, the important question still remained for long-term patency of these patients more than 5 years. In addition, the risk of arterial graft spasm in the immediate postoperative period has been problematic in use for total arterial complete revascularization of LMCA disease. Therefore, more studies regarding intraoperative or postoperative adjuncts pharmacologic

S.-J. Park, MD, PhD (✉) • D.-W. Park, MD, PhD
Division of Cardiology, Department of Medicine,
University of Ulsan College of Medicine,
Asan Medical Center, 388-1 Poongnap-dong,
Songpa-gu, Seoul 138-736, South Korea
e-mail: sjpark@amc.seoul.kr

C.A. Thompson (ed.), *Textbook of Cardiovascular Intervention*,
DOI 10.1007/978-1-4471-4528-8_20, © Springer-Verlag London 2014

preparation (i.e., vasodilator, calcium channel blocker, or papaverine) and improved surgical harvesting techniques to minimize arterial injury and spasm might be needed.

Stenting for LMCA Disease

Early Clinical Experience

In the era of bare-metal stents (BMS), LMCA intervention has demonstrated technical feasibility and acceptable short- and midterm outcomes [3]. However, considerable rates of angiographic restenosis and its expected clinical impact in critical LMCA zone have been problematic and burdened to the treating physician for routine use of BMS in elective patients. Based on studies demonstrating a marked improvement of efficacy of DES compared to BMS in simple and complex lesions, most interventional cardiologists currently use DES for PCI intervention for patients with unprotected LMCA disease. Several observational studies, although limited by a non-randomized nature, small number of patients, and short follow-up periods, have shown promising PCI outcomes using DES compared with BMS [8–10]. Recently, summated, large meta-analysis data comparing outcome for DES and BMS in PCI for unprotected LMCA disease was reported [11]. A total of 44 studies, 10,342 patients who received BMS or DES were included for merged analysis. At long-term follow-up of 3 years, adjusted risks for mortality (hazard ratio [HR] 0.70, 95 % CI 0.53–0.93, $p=0.01$), MI (HR 0.49, 95 % CI 0.26–0.92, $p=0.03$), target-lesion (TLR) or target-vessel revascularization (TVR) (HR 0.46, 95 % CI 0.30–0.69, $p=0.01$), and major adverse cardiac events (MACE) (HR 0.78, 95 % CI 0.57–1.07, $p=0.12$) uniformly favored for DES than for BMS.

Safety and Efficacy Issues

In patients with unprotected LMCA intervention with DES, there has been a propensity for late stent thrombosis, which has catastrophic consequences such as sudden death. However, beyond initial negative expectations, cumulative large and long-term clinical data provide a backup support to alleviate serious concerns about the safety of PCI with DES for these patients. Recent "real-world" clinical data reported rates of stent thrombosis ranging between 1 and 2 % up to 3 years in patients receiving LMCA stenting with DES [12, 13]. As evidence, LMCA intervention with DES resulted in lower or, at worst, similar rates of stent thrombosis than those reported in other coronary lesions. In addition, since second- or newer-generation DES show superior safety and efficacy to first-generation DES [14, 15], the clinical results of newer DES for LMCA intervention would be better and reassessed for optimal LMCA revascularization as compared to standard CABG.

Clinical consequence of in-stent restenosis (ISR) in LMCA has been expected to be more severe and sometimes critical as compared to ISR in non-LMCA coronary lesions. However, recent two registry data suggested that ISR in LMCA lesions could be safely retreated medically, surgically, or percutaneously and long-term clinical prognosis of patients with DES-ISR associated with LMCA stenting was benign regardless of treatment type, which was mainly dependent on physician discretion [16, 17].

Use of Fractional Flow Reserve (FFR) or Intravascular Ultrasound Guidance (IVUS)

In clinical practice, there are some cases showing intermediate LMCA disease by coronary angiography and definite treatment for this lesion is not yet determined. For these ambiguous LMCA lesions, several studies suggested the functionally guided role of FFR to treat or not. In these studies, FFR >0.75–0.80 was a strong predictor of favorable clinical outcomes in patients with intermediate LM disease [18–20]. One study reported that 3-year long-term survival rate in patients with intermediate LMCA disease and corresponding FFR value ≥ 0.75 were 100 % [18]. In another study using FFR to guide surgical revascularization or medical treatment (<0.80 referred to CABG vs. ≥0.80 deferred for medical treatment), long-term survival rates were similar between surgical and nonsurgical groups (85.4 % vs. 89.8 %, $p=0.48$) [20]. Based on these evidences, FFR measurement could identify patients with intermediate LM stenosis in whom deferral of revascularization is associated with excellent survival and cardiovascular event rates.

Considering procedural complexity and highly demanding technical completeness, the IVUS-guided PCI with stent implantation would be essential to perform LMCA intervention [3]. IVUS evaluation might be helpful to measure the degree of stenosis, plaque characteristics, and anatomic configuration (with delineation of major side branches), to select the appropriate diameter and length of the stent as well as the optimal stenting strategy, and to detect post-procedural stent underexpansion, incomplete lesion coverage, residual plaque, and stent inapposition. Recent long-term observational registry data suggested that elective DES implantation with IVUS guidance might reduce the long-term mortality rate for unprotected LMCA as compared with conventional angiography-alone guidance [21].

LMCA Intervention in Different Lesion Subsets

Ostial or Shaft Lesions

Clinical Data

The feasibility and success of PCI with stent implantation for LMCA disease require a careful evaluation of lesion complexity, in which a major component is whether the atherosclerotic plaque just involves the ostium/shaft of the LMCA or distally involves the distal bifurcation lesions. With remarkably improved device efficacy with DES and technically easy accessibility of innate LMCA, ostial/shaft disease might be the attractive target for the interventional cardiologists. By data, favorable outcome was documented. In a multicenter observational registry evaluating 147 consecutive patients who had a stenosis in the ostium and/or the midshaft of an unprotected LMCA (treatment of the bifurcation not required), procedural success rate was 99 % and there was no case of in-hospital Q-wave MI or death [22]. In available angiographic follow-up, mean late lumen loss of 0.01 mm and binary restenosis rate was very low (0.9 %). During long-term clinical follow-up of median 2.4 years, cumulative clinical events were relatively low (3.4 % cumulative mortality and 4.7 % TVR).

Techniques for Left Main Ostial Stenting

Selection of Guiding Catheter

Relatively large-lumen guiding catheters such as 7 F or 8 F are preferred because the end of the guiding catheter may suddenly advance into the lesion at some point, which may damage the plaque or may induce global ischemia. A guiding catheter with side holes is also preferred to maintain the flow during the procedure.

Type of Stent

Slotted-tube stents, instead of coil stents, are preferred for the treatment of the LMCA ostial disease, because of their strong radial force. The stent size is selected based on the reference-artery size and lesion length.

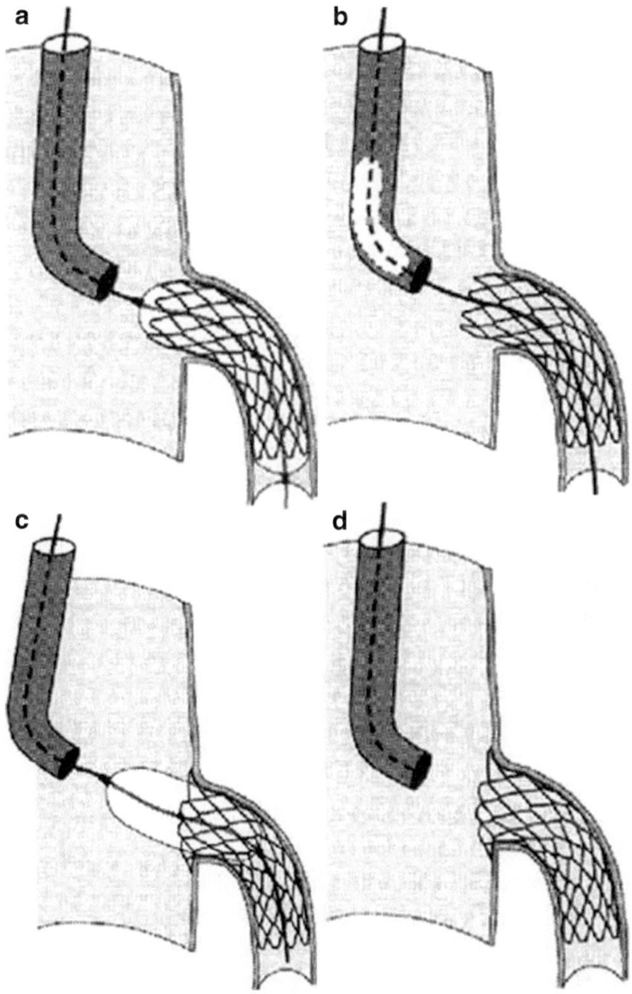

Fig. 20.1 The proper stenting technique for the treatment of left main ostial lesions

Technical Tips

In general, the stenting procedure can be performed safely, as with other ostial coronary lesions, only if meticulous guiding or careful hemodynamic monitoring is undertaken. Each important step for left main ostial stenting was illustrated in Fig. 20.1. As with other ostial coronary lesions, the coaxial alignment of the guiding catheter is important to minimize ostial injury and to position the stent properly. As long as the coaxial alignment is maintained, it is usually easy to advance the balloon and to position it at the target lesion. Once the balloon is properly positioned, the guiding catheter can be gently retracted 1–2 cm into the aorta with a gentle forward pressure on the balloon catheter. The ostial LMCA lesion is dilated and stented with the guide tip positioned in the aortic sinus. The left proximal end of the stent protrudes outside the ostium and is expanded against the aortic wall, as in the standard stenting of an aorto-ostial lesion. The stent is usually deployed slightly to protrude into the aorta (1–2 mm) for the treatment of an LMCA ostial lesion. The balloon inflation is brief (<30s) and multiple (>3) to avoid prolonged global ischemia and ischemia-related complications. Stenting for LMCA shaft stenosis is technically simple, similar to non-LMCA lesions, except for the large vessel size.

Guidance of Intravascular Ultrasound (IVUS)

IVUS provides much quantitative and qualitative information regarding coronary artery lesions. It is often difficult to evaluate the actual size of the LMCA via angiography. Often, the left main trunk is short and lacks a normal segment for comparison purposes. In addition, the contrast in the aortic cusp sometimes obscures the ostium, and "streaming" of the contrast may result in a false impression of luminal narrowing. Furthermore, angiography underestimates the stenosis severity. IVUS before stenting, therefore, provides useful information regarding the selection of the adequate size of balloons and stents and regarding the accurate amounts and extent of calcification, which contribute to the change in the treatment modality in 40 % of non-LMCA lesions.

Distal Bifurcation Lesions

Due to the technical difficulties involved, stenting for the ULMCA bifurcation disease should be performed only by highly skilled interventional cardiologist working with patients who understand the risk to benefit ratio of the percutaneous approach. During the procedure, the occlusion of the side branch resulting from plaque shifting or stent strut indicates the acute closure of the ostium of the left anterior descending artery or left circumflex artery, which can lead to disastrous clinical events. Park et al. reported that stenting with or without debulking for LMCA bifurcation stenosis was performed in selected patients with safety and technical feasibility.

Clinical Data

By contrast to excellent long-term angiographic and clinical outcomes of LMCA ostial/shaft lesions treated by PCI with stenting, distal LMCA bifurcation lesions are still challenging to the treating physician and showed less favorable outcomes with PCI. Cumulative evidence suggested that results are less favorable when distal LMCA lesions are treated by two-stent complex techniques as compared to single-stent crossover technique [23, 24]. Even with distal bifurcation treatment, single crossover techniques with optional kissing balloon showed favorable outcomes of low TLR rate less than 5 % equivalent to results obtained with DES for ostial or mid-left main lesions. In contrast, two-stent complex techniques are still challenging with a high TLR rate more than 20 %, mainly related to side-branch restenosis. In large observational study comparing the outcomes between ostial/shaft and distal bifurcation lesion in 1,111 patients with LMCA stenting with DES, distal left main bifurcations were associated with a 50 % excess risk of adverse outcomes, which was mainly driven by bifurcation lesions that were treated with complex stenting, as compared to ostial or midshaft lesions [25]. There was no difference in each and composite clinical outcomes were observed between patients with single-stent bifurcation treatment and those with ostial or midshaft LMCA lesions.

Techniques for Left Main Distal Bifurcation

For treating distal LMCA bifurcation lesions, the relative benefits of provisional stenting of bifurcation lesions, in which a single main-vessel stent is deployed and side-branch stenting is only used in cases of suboptimal angiographic results, as compared with a complex approach, in which stenting is performed in both the main and side branch, have been a long-standing debate for which there is now a general consensus [3]. A single-stent technique, in which a stent is placed across the side branch (usually the circumflex coronary artery), is preferred in patients with diminutive or normal-appearing side branches [26]. However, if the operators decide on a single-stent approach, it is almost always possible to place second stent on the side branch if stenting crossover does not yield an optimal result. A number of two-stent techniques, various levels of complexity and indications, can be used to treat distal LMCA bifurcation stenosis (Fig. 20.2).

Single-Stent Techniques with Optional T-Stenting

For bifurcation lesions, the single-stent technique, in which a stent is placed across the side branch (SB, usually the LCX), is preferred in patients with diminutive or normal-appearing side branches. If the operators decide to use the single-stent approach, however, there is almost always the possibility of placing a second stent on the LCX in case the result is not optimal or adequate. This condition is defined as provisional

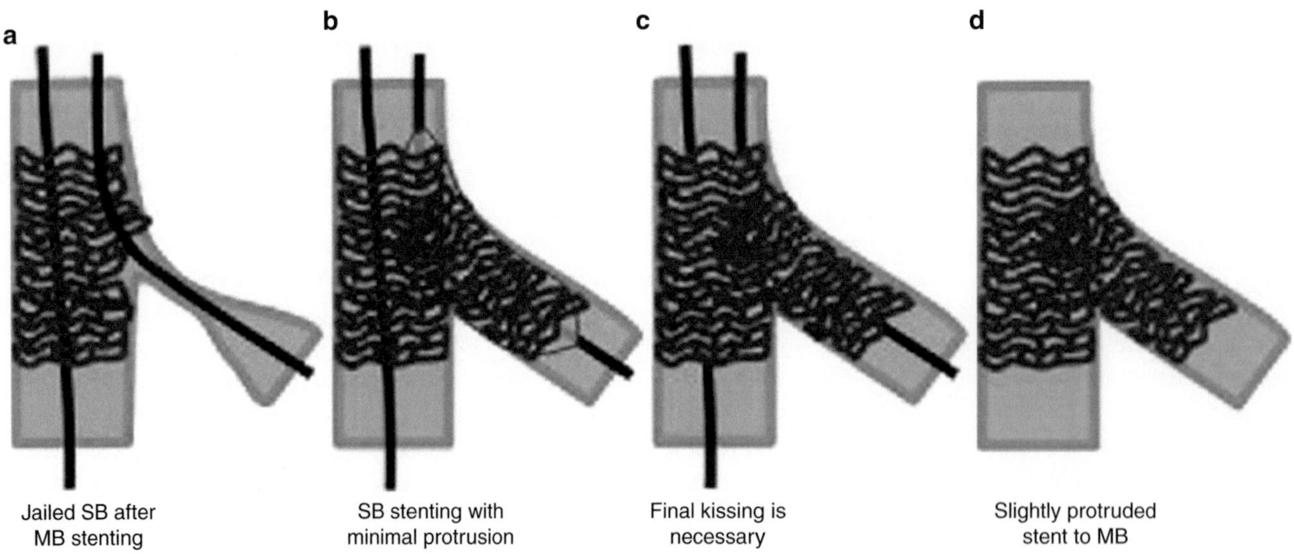

Fig. 20.2 Stenting crossover with optional T-stenting

stenting. A wire in the LCX before stenting is usually needed in the cases with (1) narrowing at the ostial LCX; (2) severe stenosis of the main branch (MB), with a large plaque burden at risk for plaque shifting; (3) narrow angle of the SB origination; and (4) deterioration of the SB ostium after the predilatation of the MB. The predilatation of the MB is usually recommended to ensure optimal balloon expansion and easy stent delivery. The predilatation of the SB is performed only if it is diseased or if it significantly deteriorates after the dilatation of the MB (threatened SB occlusion). Many SBs without a significant disease do not require predilatation. If the procedural result of the SB after MB stenting is not satisfactory, dilatation of the SB and kissing balloon inflation are performed. If the results are not acceptable (suboptimal results, plaque shifting with 75 % residual stenosis, or flow-limiting dissection) after kissing balloon inflation, SB stenting is then performed. Like kissing balloon inflation, provisional stenting in the LCX is selectively used when suboptimal dilatation or significant dissection occurs after kissing balloon inflation. As a bailout procedure for suboptimal results or significant dissection at the ostial LCX, the provisional T-stenting and reverse-crush techniques are commonly used. The provisional T-stenting technique is a strategy involving T-stenting in the LCX with the second stent after MB stenting, as shown in Fig. 20.2. Final kissing balloon dilatation after T-stenting is a mandatory step for the optimal final result. Reverse crush is a variation of the crush technique, in which provisional LCX stenting with a T-shape configuration is performed after MB stenting, which is similar to provisional T-stenting (Fig. 20.3). After the removal of the LCX wire and the balloons, however, the LCX stent is crushed within the MB stent. The final step of kissing balloon inflation after sequential high pressure in both branches with noncompliant balloons is also mandatory for successful results. Furthermore, in both provisional SB stenting strategies, the minimal protrusion of the LCX stent into the MB may be beneficial to minimize the destruction and underexpansion of the stents. An attempt should also be made, however, to avoid incomplete lesion coverage.

Complex Two-Stent Techniques

A number of two-stent techniques applicable to the treatment of distal LMCA bifurcation stenosis are available, with various levels of complexity and indications. These techniques fall mainly into four broad categories: T-stenting, crush stenting, culotte stenting, and simultaneous kissing stenting (SKS) or Y-stenting (Fig. 20.4). There is little consensus and data on which of these two-stent techniques is the best. As restenosis or stent thrombosis can be catastrophic in LMCA locations, all measures for achieving an optimal final result should be considered.

The Classic T-Stenting Technique

The LAD and LCX are wired. A stent is positioned at the ostium of the SB (LCX) without protruding into the MB (LMCA to LAD). Once the SB stent is deployed, the balloon and wire are removed from the SB, and a second stent is deployed in the MB (LMCA to LAD). The SB is rewired, and final kissing balloon dilatation is performed. The modified T-stent technique involves the simultaneous placement of the stents in the two vessels, but with the SB stent being deployed first.

The Crush Techniques

The MB and SB are wired and predilated. Stents are placed in both vessels, with the SB stent slightly protruding (2–3 mm) proximal to its ostium and the LMCA stent extending into the MB to fully cover the lesion. The SB stent is

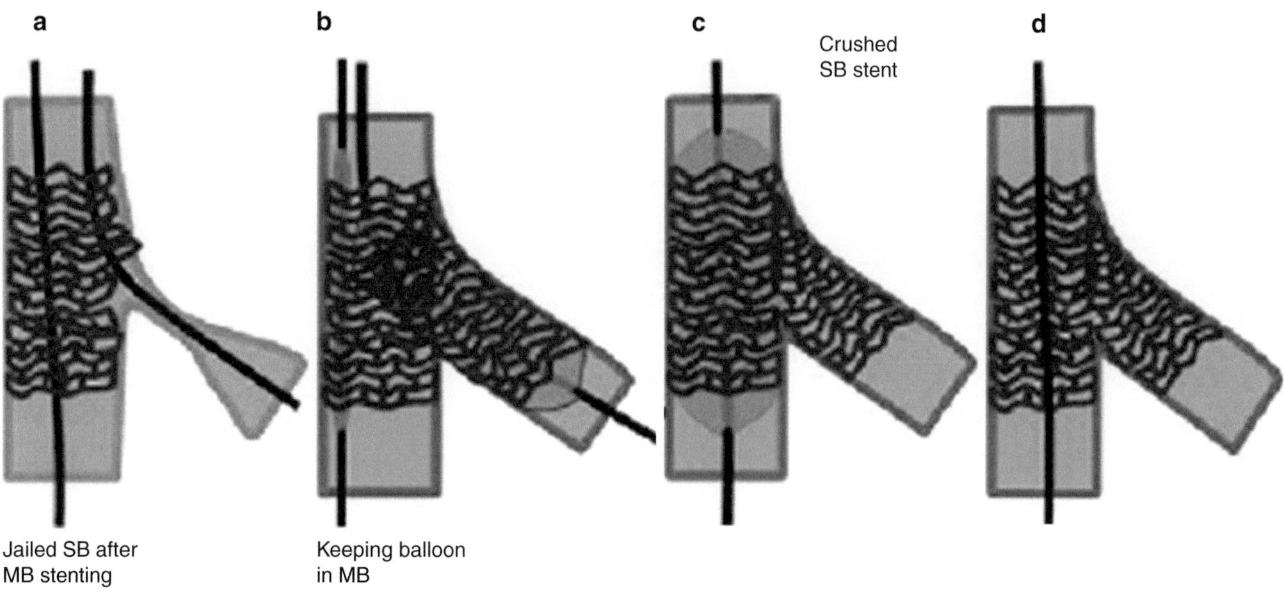

Fig. 20.3 Stenting crossover with optional reverse-crush stenting

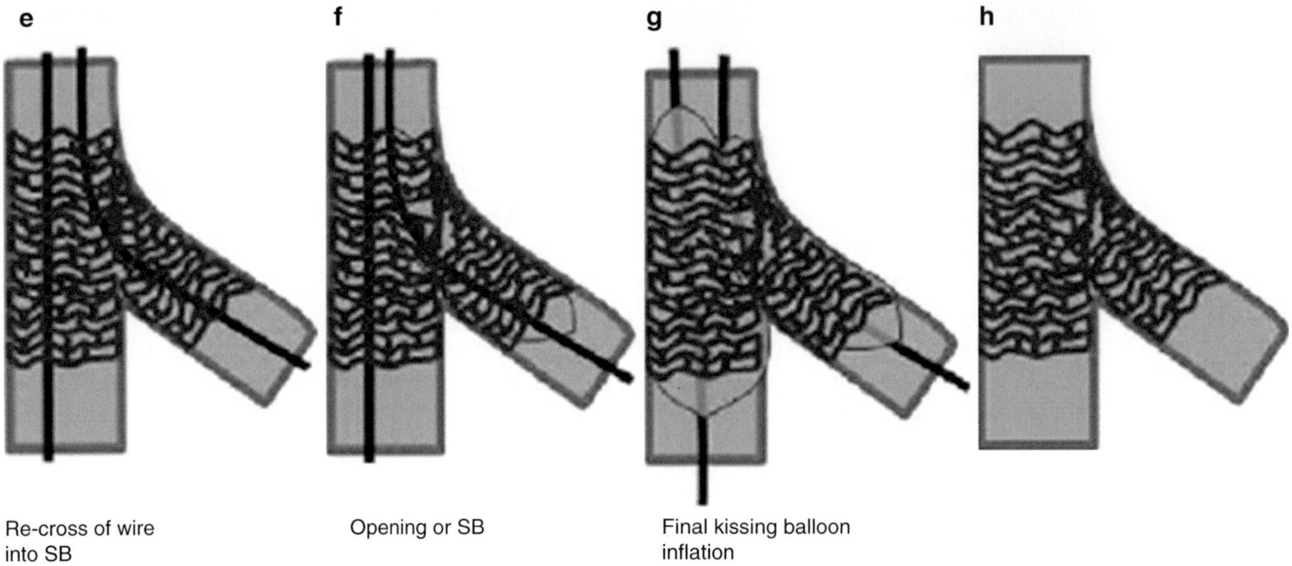

Fig. 20.3 (continued)

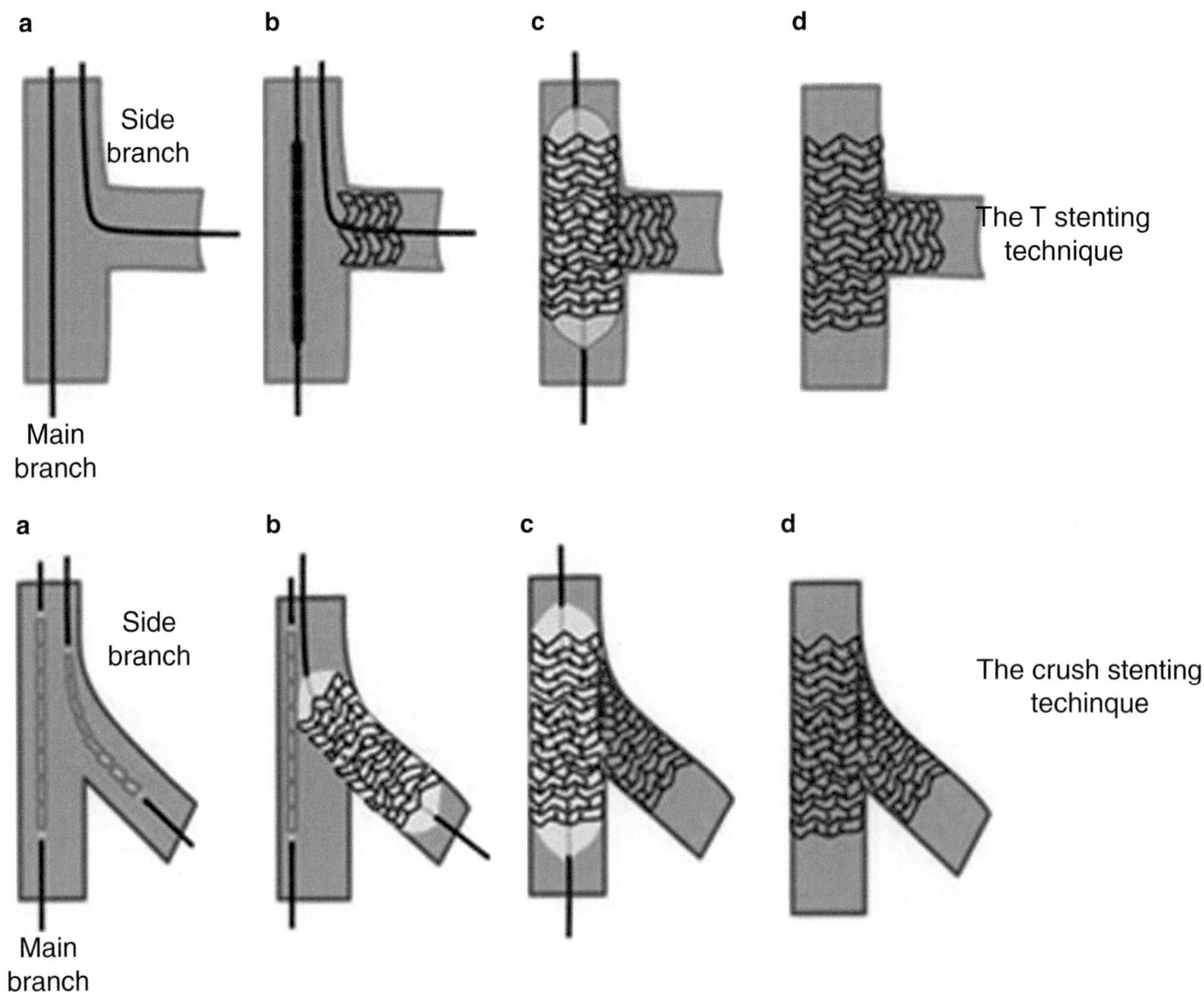

Fig. 20.4 Complex stenting techniques used to treat left main coronary artery stenosis involving distal true bifurcation lesions

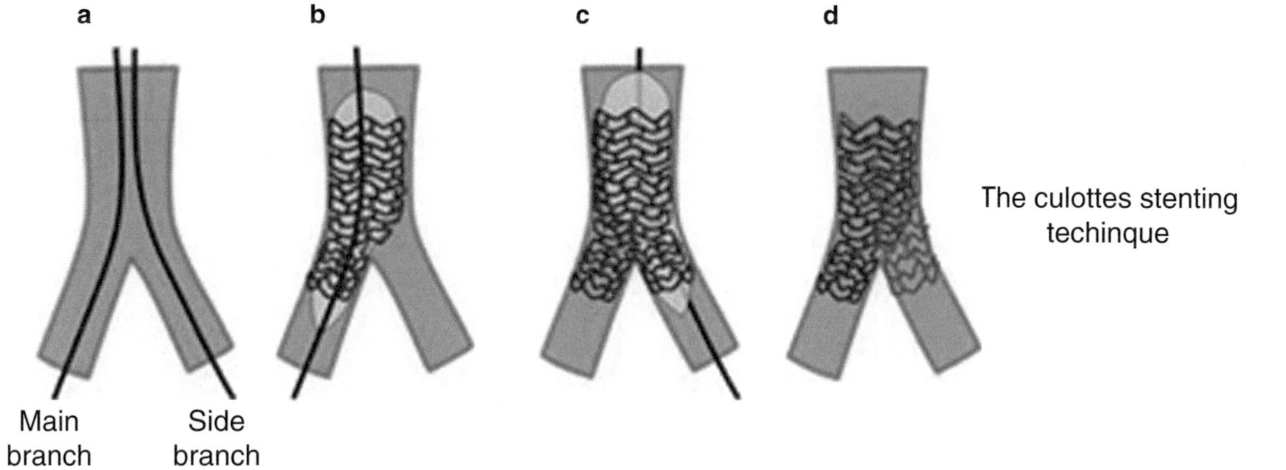

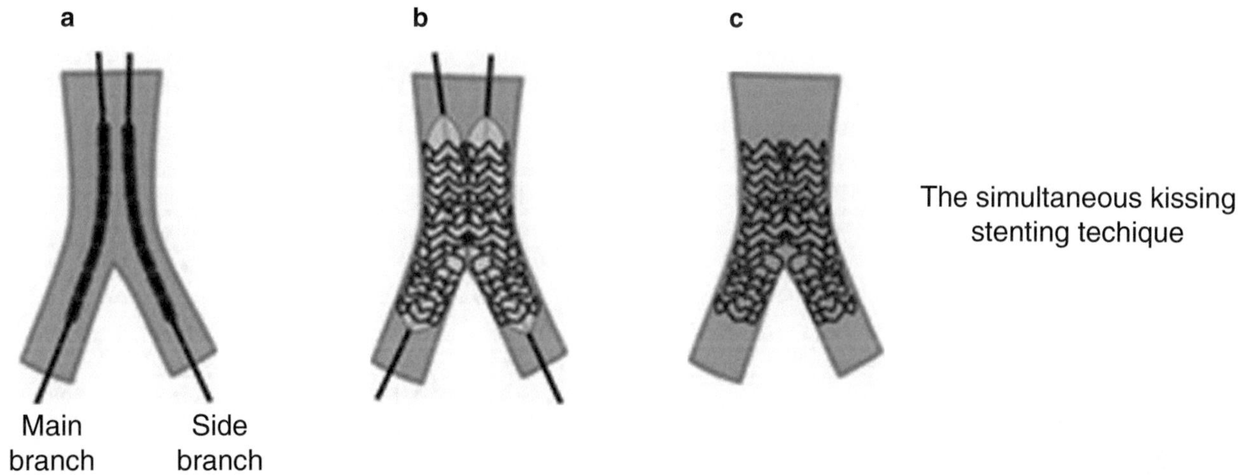

Fig. 20.4 (continued)

deployed, the balloon and wire are removed from the SB, the MB stent is deployed, the SB is rewired, and final kissing balloon inflations are performed.

The Culotte Technique

The more angulated branch (usually the LCX) is stented first, with the stent protruding back into the LMCA; the MB (usually the LAD) is wired through the SB stent, the struts of the SB stent are dilated, and the MB is stented; the wire is removed from the SB and the SB is rewired; and final kissing balloon dilatations are performed. The disadvantage of this technique is that there is a heavy concentration of metal due to the double layer of stents in the LMCA proximal to the carina. The initial results of the use of the culotte technique with BMS were discouraging, but better results were achieved with DES.

The SKS Technique

This technique includes V- or Y-stenting. In V-stenting, stents are advanced into both the LAD and LCX and are pulled back to touch each other, forming a proximal carina. If the stents extend proximal to the bifurcation and into the LMCA, they form a double lumen; this is then considered SKS or Y-stenting, or double-barrel stenting. Sequential followed by final kissing balloon dilatation is performed for optimal results. The main advantage of this technique is that access to both branches is never lost during the PCI. On the other hand, its main disadvantages are (1) the difficulty of placing a stent (if necessary) proximal to this double barrel, (2) subsequently engaging the ostium of the LMCA with a diagnostic or guiding catheter, (3) rewiring the LAD or LCX, and (4) the large amount of metal that is left in the LMCA exposed to the free lumen without direct wall contact. Another variation is the skirt technique, which involves V-stenting the ostia of the LAD and LCX and placing a third stent in the distal LMCA. In the classical Y-stent approach, one stent is crimped over two balloons, but a gap is inevitable at the transition zone between the stents.

Dedicated Bifurcation Stents

Because of the measurable risk of restenosis and revascularization after complex stenting, the use of dedicated LMCA bifurcation stents is currently being explored [27]. The Axxess Plus LM system is currently an available dedicated LMCA device.

Current Evidence of CABG vs. Stents Therapy

Patient Selection: Possible Indication or Contraindication for PCI or CABG

The choice of PCI or CABG for treatment of unprotected LMCA disease depends on several clinical and anatomic features, making optimal patient selection crucial for appropriate treatment of LMCA disease and achievement of favorable long-term outcomes. In patients with very complex anatomic features, which are not feasible for stenting, and concomitant diffuse multivessel disease, CABG is preferred so as to avoid procedural and future thrombotic risks and to provide more complete revascularization. However, in patients with relatively simple LMCA disease, such as ostial/shaft LMCA disease or isolated LMCA disease (with or without one- or two-vessel involvement), PCI is an alternative and in some cases a preferred strategy in order to reduce surgical risks (e.g., stroke and in-hospital events following major surgery).

LMCA lesion characteristics (severe calcification, distal LMCA involvement with relation to major branches), the extent of extra LMCA (concomitant multivessel disease, the status of distal runoff), and patient clinical characteristics (age, diabetes, ejection fraction, and other comorbidities) are important in patient selection. Patient/physician preference is also influential. Several clinical and angiographic factors generally considered for proper choice of patients for the PCI or CABG treatment are listed in Table 20.1.

Table 20.1 Relative indication or contraindication of PCI and CABG for treatment of unprotected left main coronary artery disease

Possible indication of PCI
Ostium or midshaft lesions
Distal left main disease anatomically suitable for stenting with intact left ventricular function
Isolated left main disease
Unstable hemodynamic conditions requiring urgent revascularization: bailout procedure, acute myocardial infarction, or cardiogenic shock due to left main stenosis
Serious comorbidity (high surgical risk): chronic lung disease, poor general performance status, advanced age such that major surgery cannot be tolerated, limited life expectancy, prior bypass surgery, unsuitable coronary anatomy for bypass grafting
Patient refusal of surgery
Strong recommendation of CABG
Complex coronary anatomy unsuitable for stenting: severe calcification, severe tortuosity, total occlusions at other major epicardial coronary arteries (≥ 2), multiple and diffuse long coronary lesions, complex in-stent restenosis unsuitable for repeat stenting procedure
Severely compromised left ventricular function
Extensive peripheral vascular disease unsuitable for placement of a guiding catheter or intra-aortic balloon pump
Contraindication to antiplatelet therapy including aspirin, heparin, or thienopyridine
Patient refusal of stenting

Registry and Meta-analysis Data

Several small-sized observational studies comparing stents and CABG for unprotected LMCA disease showed that in-hospital or early clinical outcomes favored for stenting due to relatively higher incidence of periprocedural MI or stroke by CABG, but mortality or composite hard end points (death, Q-wave MI, or stroke) were similar in the PCI and the CABG groups. The risk of TVR was consistently higher with PCI than with CABG [28–31]. The MAIN-COMPARE registry was the largest, multicenter observational study comparing stenting and CABG for unprotected LMCA disease [32], in which a total of 2,240 patients with unprotected LMCA disease who underwent stenting (BMS, 318, and DES, 784) or CABG (1,138) were analyzed. Up to 5 years, the adjusted, long-term risks of death and the composite outcome of death, Q-wave MI, or stroke were not significantly different for patients undergoing stenting vs. CABG, but repeat revascularization was significantly higher in patients receiving stenting [33]. Despite of these cumulative data, whether or not the results achieved with coronary stenting would be stable for 5–10 years remains to be determined in unprotected LMCA disease. Recently, very long-term comparative clinical data with follow-up durations of 5–10 years has been reported. The ASAN–MAIN (ASAN Medical Center–Left MAIN Revascularization) registry is the longest follow-up study to report 10-year results of BMS and 5-year results of DES as compared to concurrent CABG [34]. In these two follow-up cohorts, the adjusted risks of death and the composite of death, Q-wave MI, or stroke were similar between the two groups. However, the rate of TVR was significantly higher in the stenting group.

Several meta-analyses or merged analyses comparing two primary revascularization therapies for LMCA disease are currently available. Systemic review conducted by Taggart et al. suggested that early (in-hospital, to 30 days) and longer-term (1–2 year) mortality rates were better after CABG (early, 2–4 %, average 3 %; late, 5–6 %, average 5 %) than PCI with BMS (early, 0–14 %, average 6 %; late, 3–31 %, average 17 %) or DES (early, 0–10 %, average 2 %; late, 0–14 %, average 7 %) [35]. Takagi et al. reported a meta-analysis of 2,181 patients with unprotected LMCA disease

Table 20.2 Four randomized trials of stenting and coronary artery bypass grafting for left main coronary artery disease

	LE MANS [38]		SYNTAX [39]		Boudriot et al. [40]		PRECOMBAT [41]	
Participating center	Single center		Multicenter		Multicenter		Multicenter	
Revascularization group	PCI	CABG	PCI	CABG	PCI	CABG	PCI	CABG
Number of subjects, n	52	53	348	357	100	101	300	300
Age (mean, years)	61	61	66	65	66	69	62	63
Diabetes (%)	19	17	26	24	40	33	34	30
Bifurcation involvement (%)	56	60	58	64	74	69	70	62
Stent type (%)	DES		PES		SES		SES	
Ejection fraction (%)	54	54	NA	NA	65	65	62	61
SYNTAX score (mean)	25	25	30	30	24	23	24	26
Follow-up duration	1 year		1 year		1 year		2 year	
Clinical outcomes								
Safety outcomes (%)								
Death	1.9	7.5	4.2	4.4	2.0	5.0	2.4	3.4
Myocardial infarction	1.9	5.6	4.3	4.1	3.0	3.0	1.7	1.0
Stroke	0	3.7	0.3	2.7	NA	NA	0.4	0.7
Efficacy outcomes (%)								
Repeat revascularization	28.8	9.4	12.0	6.7	14.0	7.9	9.0[a]	4.2[a]

Abbreviations: *BMS*, bare-metal stent, *CABG* coronary artery bypass grafting, *DES* drug-eluting stents, *NA* not available, *MACCE* major adverse cardiac or cerebrovascular events, *PES* paclitaxel-eluting stents, *SES* sirolimus-eluting stents

[a]In PRECOMBAT trial, repeat revascularization means ischemic-driven target-vessel revascularization. Others mean any repeat revascularization

who received stenting ($n=1{,}006$) or CABG ($n=1{,}175$) from six studies (one randomized and five observational studies) [36]. Analytic results demonstrated no significant difference in death rate between stenting and CABG, but a statistically significant increase in repeated revascularization with stenting. Lee et al. also performed a similar meta-analysis (2,905 patients from eight clinical studies; two randomized trials and six observational studies) comparing CABG and PCI with DES for unprotected LMCA disease [37]. Consistent with previous findings, there was no significant difference between the CABG and DES groups in the risk for death or the composite end point of death, MI, or stroke, but the risk for repeat revascularization was significantly lower in patients undergoing CABG.

Randomized Trials

Although there have been cumulative large data evidence comparing PCI and CABG for unprotected LMCA disease, most of these are derived from real-world registry database. In addition, results of systemic review and meta-analysis should be interpreted with caution and regarded as only exploratory findings, given the limited number of patients, selection or publication bias in the literature reviewed, and caveats on internal validity of the included clinical studies. Therefore, pure treatment effects among two primary revascularization methods can be achieved from randomized clinical trials, although the use of composite end point, the small number of patients, and the limited duration of follow-up have biased the study findings. Table 20.2 summarizes the currently available randomized trials comparing PCI with stent implantation and standard bypass surgery for unprotected LMCA disease [38–41]. In the future, over these available findings, larger, ongoing, international randomized trial of EXCEL (Evaluation of Xience Prime vs. Coronary Artery Bypass Surgery for Effectiveness of Left Main Revascularization) might provide more confirmative information regarding the relative efficacy and safety of PCI with DES and CABG for patients with unprotected LMCA disease.

Current Guideline for LMCA Revascularization

Currently, the guideline of optimal revascularization of LMCA disease has been updated to reflect an increasing off-label experience with stenting and clinical studies (Table 20.3). Based on cumulative data, previous strong guideline to regard PCI as a contraindication of unprotected LMCA disease has been modified to partly approve PCI as a viable alternative (in level of class IIb) in carefully selected patients with LMCA disease [42, 43]. It is likely that further discussion will ensue as to whether the current knowledge basis for LMCA stenting justifies a IIa rather than a IIb recommendation.

Table 20.3 Current guideline for appropriate revascularization for unprotected left main coronary artery disease

Guideline	Current recommendation
2009 Updated guideline on percutaneous coronary intervention of the evidence, the American College of Cardiology Foundation/ American Heart Association/ Society for Cardiovascular Angiography and Interventions (ACCF/AHA/SCAI) [42]	*Class IIb* Comments: PCI of the left main coronary artery with stents as an alternative to CABG may be considered in patients with anatomic conditions that are associated with a low risk of PCI procedural complications and clinical conditions that predict an increased risk of adverse surgical outcomes (*Level of Evidence: B*)
2010 Updated guideline on myocardial revascularization of the European Society of Cardiology (ESC) and the European Association for Cardio-Thoracic Surgery (EACTS) [43]	*Class IIaB–IIIB* Comments: (1) Left main (isolated or single-vessel disease, ostium/shaft) – Class IIa B (2) Left main (isolated or single-vessel disease, distal bifurcation involvement) – Class IIb B (3) Left main plus two-vessel or triple-vessel disease, SYNTAX score ≤32 – Class IIb B (4) Left main plus two-vessel or triple-vessel disease, SYNTAX score >33 – Class III B

Conclusions

Current evidences from several real-practice registry data and some clinical trials suggested that PCI with stenting would achieve similar rates of safety outcomes such as death, MI, or stroke as compared to standard CABG for patients with unprotected LMCA disease. Inferior efficacy outcome with stenting should be revolutionized with newer-generation DES. Ongoing large randomized clinical trials using newer-generation DES can provide more confirmative answers. In the upcoming future, these cumulative evidences might have prompted the physicians to choose PCI with DES as an alternative or replaceable treatment option for patients with LMCA disease instead of CABG.

References

1. Caracciolo EA, Davis KB, Sopko G, Kaiser GC, Corley SD, Schaff H, Taylor HA, Chaitman BR. Comparison of surgical and medical group survival in patients with left main equivalent coronary artery disease. Long-term CASS experience. Circulation. 1995;91:2335–44.
2. Eagle KA, Guyton RA, Davidoff R, Edwards FH, Ewy GA, Gardner TJ, Hart JC, Herrmann HC, Hillis LD, Hutter Jr AM, Lytle BW, Marlow RA, Nugent WC, Orszulak TA. ACC/AHA 2004 guideline update for coronary artery bypass graft surgery: a report of the American College of Cardiology/American Heart Association Task Force on Practice Guidelines (Committee to Update the 1999 Guidelines for Coronary Artery Bypass Graft Surgery). Circulation. 2004;110:e340–437.
3. Park SJ, Park DW. Percutaneous coronary intervention with stent implantation versus coronary artery bypass surgery for treatment of left main coronary artery disease: is it time to change guidelines? Circ Cardiovasc Interv. 2009;2:59–68.
4. Chikwe J, Kim M, Goldstone AB, Fallahi A, Athanasiou T. Current diagnosis and management of left main coronary disease. Eur J Cardiothorac Surg. 2010;38:420–8.
5. Finks JF, Osborne NH, Birkmeyer JD. Trends in hospital volume and operative mortality for high-risk surgery. N Engl J Med. 2011;364:2128–37.
6. Panesar SS, Chikwe J, Mirza SB, Rahman MS, Warren O, Rao C, Negus J, Zacharakis E, Darzi A, Athanasiou T. Off-pump coronary artery bypass surgery may reduce the incidence of stroke in patients with significant left main stem disease. Thorac Cardiovasc Surg. 2008;56:247–55.
7. Goldman S, Sethi GK, Holman W, et al. Radial artery grafts vs saphenous vein grafts in coronary artery bypass surgery: a randomized trial. JAMA. 2011;305:167–74.
8. Park SJ, Kim YH, Lee BK, Lee SW, Lee CW, Hong MK, Kim JJ, Mintz GS, Park SW. Sirolimus-eluting stent implantation for unprotected left main coronary artery stenosis: comparison with bare metal stent implantation. J Am Coll Cardiol. 2005;45:351–6.
9. Valgimigli M, Malagutti P, Aoki J, Garcia-Garcia HM, Rodriguez Granillo GA, van Mieghem CA, Ligthart JM, Ong AT, Sianos G, Regar E, Van Domburg RT, De Feyter P, de Jaegere P, Serruys PW. Sirolimus-eluting versus paclitaxel-eluting stent implantation for the percutaneous treatment of left main coronary artery disease: a combined RESEARCH and T-SEARCH long-term analysis. J Am Coll Cardiol. 2006;47:507–14.
10. Chieffo A, Stankovic G, Bonizzoni E, Tsagalou E, Iakovou I, Montorfano M, Airoldi F, Michev I, Sangiorgi MG, Carlino M, Vitrella G, Colombo A. Early and mid-term results of drug-eluting stent implantation in unprotected left main. Circulation. 2005;111:791–5.
11. Pandya SB, Kim YH, Meyers SN, Davidson CJ, Flaherty JD, Park DW, Mediratta A, Pieper K, Reyes E, Bonow RO, Park SJ, Beohar N. Drug-eluting versus bare-metal stents in unprotected left main coronary artery stenosis a meta-analysis. JACC Cardiovasc Interv. 2010;3:602–11.
12. Chieffo A, Park SJ, Meliga E, Sheiban I, Lee MS, Latib A, Kim YH, Valgimigli M, Sillano D, Magni V, Biondi-Zoccai G, Montorfano M, Airoldi F, Rogacka R, Carlino M, Michev I, Lee CW, Hong MK, Park SW, Moretti C, Bonizzoni E, Sangiorgi GM, Tobis J, Serruys PW, Colombo A. Late and very late stent thrombosis following drug-eluting stent implantation in unprotected left main coronary artery: a multicentre registry. Eur Heart J. 2008;29:2108–15.
13. Meliga E, Garcia-Garcia HM, Valgimigli M, Chieffo A, Biondi-Zoccai G, Maree AO, Cook S, Reardon L, Moretti C, De Servi S, Palacios IF, Windecker S, Colombo A, van Domburg R, Sheiban I, Serruys PW. Longest available clinical outcomes after drug-eluting stent implantation for unprotected left main coronary artery disease: the DELFT (Drug Eluting stent for LeFT main) registry. J Am Coll Cardiol. 2008;51:2212–19.
14. Stone GW, Rizvi A, Newman W, Mastali K, Wang JC, Caputo R, Doostzadeh J, Cao S, Simonton CA, Sudhir K, Lansky AJ, Cutlip DE, Kereiakes DJ. Everolimus-eluting versus paclitaxel-eluting stents in coronary artery disease. N Engl J Med. 2010;362:1663–74.
15. Kedhi E, Joesoef KS, McFadden E, Wassing J, van Mieghem C, Goedhart D, Smits PC. Second-generation everolimus-eluting and paclitaxel-eluting stents in real-life practice (COMPARE): a randomised trial. Lancet. 2010;375:201–9.

16. Sheiban I, Sillano D, Biondi-Zoccai G, Chieffo A, Colombo A, Vecchio S, Margheri M, Gunn JP, Raina T, Liistro F, Bolognese L, Lee MS, Tobis J, Moretti C. Incidence and management of restenosis after treatment of unprotected left main disease with drug-eluting stents 70 restenotic cases from a cohort of 718 patients: FAILS (Failure in Left Main Study). J Am Coll Cardiol. 2009;54:1131–6.
17. Lee JY, Park DW, Kim YH, Yun SC, Kim WJ, Kang SJ, Lee SW, Lee CW, Park SW, Park SJ. Incidence, predictors, treatment, and long-term prognosis of patients with restenosis after drug-eluting stent implantation for unprotected left main coronary artery disease. J Am Coll Cardiol. 2011;57:1349–58.
18. Jasti V, Ivan E, Yalamanchili V, Wongpraparut N, Leesar MA. Correlations between fractional flow reserve and intravascular ultrasound in patients with an ambiguous left main coronary artery stenosis. Circulation. 2004;110:2831–6.
19. Courtis J, Rodes-Cabau J, Larose E, Potvin JM, Dery JP, Larochelliere RD, Cote M, Cousterousse O, Nguyen CM, Proulx G, Rinfret S, Bertrand OF. Usefulness of coronary fractional flow reserve measurements in guiding clinical decisions in intermediate or equivocal left main coronary stenoses. Am J Cardiol. 2009;103: 943–9.
20. Hamilos M, Muller O, Cuisset T, Ntalianis A, Chlouverakis G, Sarno G, Nelis O, Bartunek J, Vanderheyden M, Wyffels E, Barbato E, Heyndrickx GR, Wijns W, De Bruyne B. Long-term clinical outcome after fractional flow reserve-guided treatment in patients with angiographically equivocal left main coronary artery stenosis. Circulation. 2009;120:1505–12.
21. Park SJ, Kim YH, Park DW, Lee SW, Kim WJ, Suh J, Yun SC, Lee CW, Hong MK, Lee JH, Park SW. Impact of intravascular ultrasound guidance on long-term mortality in stenting for unprotected left main coronary artery stenosis. Circ Cardiovasc Interv. 2009;2: 167–77.
22. Chieffo A, Park SJ, Valgimigli M, Kim YH, Daemen J, Sheiban I, Truffa A, Montorfano M, Airoldi F, Sangiorgi G, Carlino M, Michev I, Lee CW, Hong MK, Park SW, Moretti C, Bonizzoni E, Rogacka R, Serruys PW, Colombo A. Favorable long-term outcome after drug-eluting stent implantation in nonbifurcation lesions that involve unprotected left main coronary artery: a multicenter registry. Circulation. 2007;116:158–62.
23. Valgimigli M, Malagutti P, Rodriguez-Granillo GA, et al. Distal left main coronary disease is a major predictor of outcome in patients undergoing percutaneous intervention in the drug-eluting stent era: an integrated clinical and angiographic analysis based on the Rapamycin-Eluting Stent Evaluated At Rotterdam Cardiology Hospital (RESEARCH) and Taxus-Stent Evaluated At Rotterdam Cardiology Hospital (T-SEARCH) registries. J Am Coll Cardiol. 2006;47:1530–7.
24. Kim YH, Park SW, Hong MK, Park DW, Park KM, Lee BK, Song JM, Han KH, Lee CW, Kang DH, Song JK, Kim JJ, Park SJ. Comparison of simple and complex stenting techniques in the treatment of unprotected left main coronary artery bifurcation stenosis. Am J Cardiol. 2006;97:1597–601.
25. Palmerini T, Sangiorgi D, Marzocchi AT. Ostial and midshaft lesions vs. bifurcation lesions in 1111 patients with unprotected left main coronary artery stenosis treated with drug-eluting stents: results of the survey from the Italian Society of Invasive Cardiology. Eur Heart J. 2009;30:2087–94.
26. Park S-J, Lee CW, Kim Y-H, Lee J-H, M-Ki H, Kim J-J, Park S-W. Technical feasibility, safety, and clinical outcome of stenting of unprotected left main coronary artery bifurcation narrowing. Am J Cardiol. 2002;90:374–8.
27. Baim DS, Mauri L, Cutlip DC. Drug-eluting stenting for unprotected left main coronary artery disease: are we ready to replace bypass surgery? J Am Coll Cardiol. 2006;47: 878–81.
28. Chieffo A, Morici N, Maisano F, Bonizzoni E, Cosgrave J, Montorfano M, Airoldi F, Carlino M, Michev I, Melzi G, Sangiorgi G, Alfieri O, Colombo A. Percutaneous treatment with drug-eluting stent implantation versus bypass surgery for unprotected left main stenosis: a single-center experience. Circulation. 2006;113: 2542–7.
29. Lee MS, Kapoor N, Jamal F, Czer L, Aragon J, Forrester J, Kar S, Dohad S, Kass R, Eigler N, Trento A, Shah PK, Makkar RR. Comparison of coronary artery bypass surgery with percutaneous coronary intervention with drug-eluting stents for unprotected left main coronary artery disease. J Am Coll Cardiol. 2006;47:864–70.
30. Palmerini T, Marzocchi A, Marrozzini C, Ortolani P, Saia F, Savini C, Bacchi-Reggiani L, Gianstefani S, Virzi S, Manara F. Comparison between coronary angioplasty and coronary artery bypass surgery for the treatment of unprotected left main coronary artery stenosis (the Bologna registry). Am J Cardiol. 2006;98:54–9.
31. Sanmartin M, Baz JA, Claro R, Asorey V, Duran D, Pradas G, Iniguez A. Comparison of drug-eluting stents versus surgery for unprotected left main coronary artery disease. Am J Cardiol. 2007;100:970–3.
32. Seung KB, Park DW, Kim YH, Lee SW, Lee CW, Hong MK, Park SW, Yun SC, Gwon HC, Jeong MH, Jang Y, Kim HS, Kim PJ, Seong IW, Park HS, Ahn T, Chae IH, Tahk SJ, Chung WS, Park SJ. Stents versus coronary-artery bypass grafting for left main coronary artery disease. N Engl J Med. 2008;358:1781–92.
33. Park DW, Seung KB, Kim YH, et al. Long-term safety and efficacy of stenting versus coronary artery bypass grafting for unprotected left main coronary artery disease: 5-year results from the MAIN-COMPARE (Revascularization for Unprotected Left Main Coronary Artery Stenosis: Comparison of Percutaneous Coronary Angioplasty Versus Surgical Revascularization) registry. J Am Coll Cardiol. 2010;56:117–24.
34. Park DW, Kim YH, Yun SC, et al. Long-term outcomes after stenting versus coronary artery bypass grafting for unprotected left main coronary artery disease: 10-year results of bare-metal stents and 5-year results of drug-eluting stents from the ASAN-MAIN (ASAN Medical Center-Left MAIN Revascularization) Registry. J Am Coll Cardiol. 2010;56:1366–75.
35. Taggart DP, Kaul S, Boden WE, et al. Revascularization for unprotected left main stem coronary artery stenosis stenting or surgery. J Am Coll Cardiol. 2008;51:885–92.
36. Takagi H, Kawai N, Umemoto T. Stenting versus coronary artery bypass grafting for unprotected left main coronary artery disease: a meta-analysis of comparative studies. J Thorac Cardiovasc Surg. 2009;137:e54–7.
37. Lee MS, Yang T, Dhoot J, Liao H. Meta-analysis of clinical studies comparing coronary artery bypass grafting with percutaneous coronary intervention and drug-eluting stents in patients with unprotected left main coronary artery narrowings. Am J Cardiol. 2010;105:1070–5.
38. Buszman PE, Kiesz SR, Bochenek A, et al. Acute and late outcomes of unprotected left main stenting in comparison with surgical revascularization. J Am Coll Cardiol. 2008;51: 538–45.
39. Morice MC, Serruys PW, Kappetein AP, Feldman TE, Stahle E, Colombo A, Mack MJ, Holmes DR, Torracca L, van Es GA, Leadley K, Dawkins KD, Mohr F. Outcomes in patients with de novo left main disease treated with either percutaneous coronary intervention using paclitaxel-eluting stents or coronary artery bypass graft treatment in the Synergy Between Percutaneous Coronary Intervention with TAXUS and Cardiac Surgery (SYNTAX) trial. Circulation. 2010;121:2645–53.
40. Boudriot E, Thiele H, Walther T, et al. Randomized comparison of percutaneous coronary intervention with sirolimus-eluting stents versus coronary artery bypass grafting in unprotected left main stem stenosis. J Am Coll Cardiol. 2011;57:538–45.

41. Park SJ, Kim YH, Park DW, et al. Randomized trial of stents versus bypass surgery for left main coronary artery disease. N Engl J Med. 2011;364:1718–27.
42. Kushner FG, Hand M, Smith Jr SC, et al. Focused updates: ACC/AHA guidelines for the management of patients with ST-elevation myocardial infarction (updating the 2004 guideline and 2007 focused update) and ACC/AHA/SCAI guidelines on percutaneous coronary intervention (updating the 2005 guideline and 2007 focused update): a report of the American College of Cardiology Foundation/American Heart Association task force on practice guidelines. Circulation. 2009;120:2271–306.
43. Wijns W, Kolh P, Danchin N, et al. Guidelines on myocardial revascularization: the task force on myocardial revascularization of the European Society of Cardiology (ESC) and the European Association for Cardio-Thoracic Surgery (EACTS). Eur Heart J. 2010;31:2501–55.

Multivessel Disease

21

Vishal Kapur, Ajay J. Kirtane, and Jeffrey W. Moses

The treatment of multivessel coronary artery disease involves some of the most prognostically important decisions a cardiologist can face. While there has been a movement to simplify the treatment of multivessel disease using scoring systems that lead to a "one-size-fits-all approach," at its essence, the treatment of MVD must be individualized to the patient and clinical scenario. Thus, the clinical presentation, extent and severity of coronary artery disease, left ventricular function, and associated comorbid conditions all influence the choice of initial management of a patient with MVD.

The incidence of MVD in patients undergoing percutaneous intervention has remained relatively stable since 1980s [1–4]. As noted in the National Heart, Lung, and Blood Institute (NHBLI) PCI registry from 1985 to 1986, 32 % of the patients had two-vessel disease and 21 % had three-vessel disease; these numbers remained unchanged a decade later (from 1997 to 1998) and the trend remains stable in the last decade (from 1997 to 2006) with 31 % having two-vessel disease and 32 % having three-vessel disease [5]. Despite some claims to the contrary, prior studies have shown significant advantages in reducing morbidity as well as mortality with revascularization over medical therapy in cases of MVD [4]. Both coronary artery bypass surgery and PCI when judiciously applied are safe and effective treatment modalities for patients in this group [3, 4].

The initial use of CABG for treatment of coronary artery disease dates back almost 50 years when Garrett, Dennis, and DeBakey pioneered the use of CABG to treat coronary artery disease in 1964 [6]. In the 1970s, the indications for coronary revascularization (specifically establishing the role of CABG vs. medical therapy) became a major focus of clinical investigation [7, 8]. Percutaneous transluminal coronary angioplasty (PTCA) was introduced by Dr. Andreas Gruentzig only in 1977 as a technique for the treatment of proximal, noncalcified, concentric lesions involving a single coronary artery with use of balloon dilation [9]. As equipment and techniques improved, the popularity of PTCA rapidly increased due to its less invasive nature compared to CABG. Provided that the acute results of the procedure did not lead to abrupt vessel closure, balloon angioplasty was generally acutely effective, but restenosis was frequent, occurring in ~40–50 % of cases, usually within the first year after dilation. It was not until after 1986 when Puel and Sigwart implanted the first coronary stents in patients that the acute results of angioplasty became more predictable, demonstrating a significant reduction in restenosis as well. Several trials in the 1990s demonstrated the superiority of stent placement over balloon angioplasty [10, 11]. While the incidence of restenosis was reduced by the elimination of acute and chronic recoil [12], stents that prevented abrupt closure of the coronary artery (and the requirement for emergency CABG) were also improving safety and further opening the door to multi-lesion and multivessel treatments [13]. By 1999, following the introduction of the Palmaz-Schatz stent and several additional iterative technological advances in stent and delivery system design, stents were used in the vast majority of PCI procedures. The advent of drug-eluting stents provided a further reduction in the rate of restenosis and subsequently enhanced the desire to investigate the utility of more aggressive use of PCI in MVD [14]. Recent years have witnessed improvements in both percutaneous and surgical revascularization. The use of stents, arterial bypass conduits, minimally invasive coronary artery surgery, and hybrid procedures all have modified the approach to the management of patients with complex MVD. Additional pharmacological advances in antiplatelet medications, direct thrombin inhibitors, and aggressive lipid lowering have also aided in improving PCI outcomes.

V. Kapur, MD • A.J. Kirtane, MD, SM • J.W. Moses, MD (✉)
Division of Cardiology, Department of Medicine,
Columbia University Medical Center,
New York-Presbyterian Hospital,
161 Fort Washington Avenue, 6th Floor,
New York, NY 10032, USA
e-mail: jmoses@crf.org

C.A. Thompson (ed.), *Textbook of Cardiovascular Intervention*,
DOI 10.1007/978-1-4471-4528-8_21, © Springer-Verlag London 2014

CABG vs. POBA (Plain Old Balloon Angioplasty)

The debate regarding the use of PCI vs. CABG as the preferred treatment modality for MVD began in the balloon angioplasty era. Initial trials comparing the two strategies enrolled relatively low-risk patients, mainly with two-vessel disease and normal left ventricular function. The use of adjunctive antiplatelet therapies such as glycoprotein IIb/IIIa inhibition or dual antiplatelet therapies was very limited. One of the landmark trials initiated by the National Heart, Lung, and Blood Institute (NHLBI) was the Bypass Angioplasty Revascularization Investigation (BARI) [15], which was aimed at ascertaining the efficacy of PCI as an alternative method of revascularization to CABG in patients with MVD. A total of 1,829 patients were randomized and followed for an average of 5.4 years. Initial results of this trial demonstrated rates of in-hospital mortality for CABG and PTCA of 1.3 % vs. 1.1 %, respectively, rates of Q-wave myocardial infarction of 4.6 % vs. 2.1 % ($p<0.01$), and rates of stroke of 0.8 % vs. 0.2 %, respectively. Longer-term follow-up of this trial has been reported at 5 and 10 years [16, 17]. The five-year survival rate was 89.3 % for those assigned to CABG and 86.3 % for those assigned to PTCA ($p=0.19$) and 73.5 and 71.0 % at 10 years ($p=0.18$). The respective 5-year survival rates free from Q-wave myocardial infarction were 80.4 and 78.7 %. Despite similarities in the rates of death and Myocardial Infarction (MI), striking differences were observed in the rates of repeat revascularization procedures. By 5 years after study entry, 8 % of the patients assigned to CABG had undergone additional revascularization procedures, as compared with 54 % of those assigned to PTCA; 31 % of those assigned to PTCA subsequently underwent CABG. Among diabetic patients who were being treated with insulin or oral hypoglycemic agents at baseline, 5-year survival was higher for the CABG group as compared with the PTCA group (80.6 % vs. 66.5 %, $p=0.003$). At 10 years, survival in diabetic patients was 45.5 % for PCI and 57.9 % for CABG ($p=0.025$) but the interaction term was negative. At 10-year follow-up, overall survival rate was similar in both arms (71 % in PCI arm and 73.5 % in CABG, $p=0.18$). However, PCI had significantly higher subsequent revascularization as compared to CABG (76.8 % vs. 20.3 %, $p<0.001$). There were significantly lower rates of revascularization in patients with treated diabetes in the CABG arm (20.3 %) when compared to the PCI arm (81.7 %). The 10-year rates of persistent angina were similar between the two groups (23.1 % vs. 25.1 %).

Smaller trials comparing CABG and PTCA including ERACI [18], EAST [19], GABI [20], and CABRI [21] have not demonstrated any significant difference in mortality between the two strategies, but observed significantly greater rates of repeat revascularization in the PTCA arm as compared to the CABG arm. However, given the current use of stents (particularly drug-eluting stents) as well as more contemporary adjunctive pharmacological therapies, the relevance of these earlier POBA studies to contemporary practice is questionable. In summary, even in early PTCA vs. CABG studies, in the absence of diabetes mellitus, rates of survival and of survival free of myocardial infarction (MI) were very similar among patients with MVD with follow-up ranging for 6.5–10 years (Table 21.1). Additional revascularization procedures were required 2.5–4.5 times more frequently in PTCA-treated compared to CABG-treated patients.

Bare Metal Stenting vs. CABG

As the era of balloon angioplasty gave way to stent placement, several clinical trials of bare metal stenting vs. CABG in MVD were initiated (Table 21.2). The ARTS (Arterial Revascularization Therapies Study) [22] enrolled 1,205 patients with mean age of 61 years, with diabetics comprising 19 % of the Bare Metal Stent (BMS) group and 16 % of the Coronary Artery Bypass Graft (CABG) group. The extent of disease between the two groups was well matched, with approximately 2/3 of patients having double-vessel disease and 1/3 of patients having triple-vessel disease. Left anterior descending artery involvement was present in 90 % of patients. There were no significant differences between the PCI and CABG groups in the 1-year rates of death (2.5 % vs. 2.8 %), stroke (1.7 % vs. 2.1 %), Q-wave MI (5.3 % 4.3 %),

Table 21.1 CABG vs. PTCA

Trial	No. of patients	Follow-up	Mortality (%)	MI (%)	Repeat revascl (%)
BARI	CABG – 914	5.4 year	1.3	4.6	8
	PTCA – 915		1.1	2.1	54
EAST	CABG – 194	3 year	6.2	19.6	13
	PTCA – 198		7.1	14.6	54
ERACI	CABG – 64	1 year	3.2	3.2	32
	PCI – 63		0	1.8	3.2
GABI	CABG – 177	1 year	2.5	8.1	44
	PCI – 182		1.1	2.3	6
CABRI	CABG – 531	1 year	2.7	3.5	6.5
	PCI – 548		3.9	4.9	33.6

Table 21.2 CABG vs. BMS

Trial	No. of patient	Follow-up	MACCE (%)	Mortality (%)	MI (%)	Repeat revascl (%)
ARTS	CABG – 605	5 year	21.8	8	–	8.8
	PCI – 600		41.7	7.6	–	30
AWESOME	CABG – 232	3 year	–	21	–	–
	PCI – 222		–	20	–	–
MASS II	CABG – 203	10 year	–	25.1	10.3	7.4
	PCI – 205		–	24.9	13.3	41.9
	Med t/t– 203		–	31	20.7	39.4
SOS	CABG – 500	6 year	–	6.8	–	6 (2 year)
	PCI – 488		–	10.9	–	21 (2 year)
ERAC II	CABG – 225	5 year	24.6	11.5	6.2	7.2
	PCI – 225		34.7	7.1	2.8	28.4

or non-Q-wave MI (0.8 % vs. 0.5 %). Among patients who survived without stroke or MI, a higher proportion of the BMS group than the CABG group (16.8 % vs. 3.5 %) needed repeat revascularization. Thus, the survival free of Major Cardiac and Cerebrovascular Events (MACCE) (a composite of death, stroke, myocardial infarction, or repeat revascularization) at 1 year was 73.8 % in the BMS group compared with 87.8 % in the CABG group ($p<0.001$). At 5 years, the mortality rate was 8 % in the PCI group as compared to 7.6 % in the CABG group ($p=0.83$). The incidence of composite death, stroke, or MI was numerically greater, but not significantly different between the PCI (18.2 %) and CABG (14.9 %) groups ($p=0.14$). However, repeat revascularization was significantly more frequent in the stent group compared to CABG (30.3 % vs. 8.8 %, $p<0.001$); additionally, there was a small excess of patients reporting persistent angina in the PCI group as compared to the CABG group (21.2 % vs. 15.5 %, $p<0.05$).

The second Argentine Randomized Study: Coronary Angioplasty with Stenting Versus Coronary Bypass Surgery in patients with MVD (ERACI II) compared BMS with CABG in patients with symptomatic MVD. Out of a total of 2,759 patients screened, 450 were randomized to either PCI ($n=225$) or CABG ($n=225$). Initially (for the first month), the MACCE was lower in the PCI arm as compared to the CABG arm (12.3 % vs. 36 %, $p=0.02$), and at 1-year follow-up [23], there was a favorable survival benefit in the PCI arm as compared to CABG arm (freedom from mortality: 96.9 % vs. 92.5 %, $p<0.017$). However, at 5-year follow-up [24], freedom from MACE was significantly lower with CABG compared with PCI (76.4 % vs. 65.3 %; $p=0.013$), again driven mainly by repeat revascularization [24].

The MASS-II (Medicine, Angioplasty, or Surgery Study II) trial was a single-center study designed to compare the long-term effects of medical therapy, angioplasty, or surgical strategies among 611 patients with chronic angina, multivessel Coronary Artery Disease (CAD), and preserved left ventricular function who were appropriate candidates for all three therapies [4]. MASS II was the first randomized clinical trial with long-term follow-up (10 year) comparing all three treatment strategies for patients with MVD. Overall mortality was similar between the medical therapy, PCI, and CABG arms (2, 4, 4 %, respectively, p=nonsignificant), whereas nonfatal MI occurred in 20.7, 13.2, and 10.3 % of patients, respectively ($p=0.016$), and repeat revascularization in 39.4, 41.5, and 7.4 %, respectively ($p<0.001$). Patients who underwent CABG (64 %) and PCI (59 %) were more likely to be angina-free at the end of 10 years when compared to medical therapy (43 %). The incidence of stroke was similar in all three groups: 6.9 % with medical therapy, 5.4 % with PCI, and 6.9 % with CABG ($p=0.55$). Notably, the occurrence of the composite of cardiac death, MI, and Cerebrovascular Accident (CVA) was similar with both PCI and CABG, but more frequent with medical therapy, refuting the contention that these early trials enrolled patients that would have done just as well with medical therapy alone.

Two other trials comparing CABG vs. BMS for MVD were the AWESOME (Angina with Extremely Serious Operative Mortality Evaluation) and SOS trials. AWESOME [25] screened high-risk patients from 16 VA centers and then randomized them to CABG ($n=232$) or PCI ($n=222$). The 30-day survival for CABG and PCI were 95 and 97 %, respectively. Survival rates for CABG vs. PCI were 90 % vs. 94 % at 6 months, 79 % vs. 80 % at 36 months ($p=0.46$), and 73 % vs. 78 % at 5 years ($p=0.46$). Similarly, 5-year survival free of unstable angina was comparable in both groups. The Stent or Surgery (SOS) trial involved 988 patients ($n=488$ PCI, $n=500$ CABG) randomized at 53 centers during the period from 1996 to 1999 [26]. At the end of 2 years, patients randomized to PCI had a higher rate of repeat revascularization than patients randomized to CABG (20.7 % vs. 6.0 %; $p<0.001$). While the incidence of death or nonfatal Q-wave myocardial infarction was similar in both groups, death occurred in 4.5 % of the PCI group compared with 1.6 % of the CABG group ($p=0.01$). At a median follow-up of 6 years, 53 patients (10.9 %) died in the PCI group compared with 34 (6.8 %) in the CABG group (hazard ratio 1.66, 95 % confidence interval 1.08–2.55, $p=0.022$) driven by an excess of noncardiac deaths (25 patients in PTCA arm and 11 patients in the CABG arm), the majority being cancer related.

Among diabetic patients, 17.6 % of patients died in the PCI group compared with 5.4 % in the CABG group; among non-diabetic patients, 9.8 % of patients died in the PCI group compared with 7.0 % in the CABG group.

Meta-analyses of PCI and CABG (Pre-DES (Drug Eluting Stents))

Several attempts have been made to synthesize the existing prior studies of PCI vs. CABG for MVD. A meta-analysis by Bravata et al. [27] evaluated 23 randomized trials comparing 5,019 patients treated with PCI and 4,944 with CABG. Overall, the difference in survival between the two groups was less than 1 % at 10-year follow-up. Of the six trials, which reported data on the diabetic subpopulation, there was no significant survival benefit noted with the overall rate of survival with CABG being higher by just 0.2 %. Procedure-related stroke was more common after CABG than after PCI (1.2 % vs. 0.6 %, $p=0.002$). When segregating the PCI arm and comparing balloon angioplasty vs. CABG and stenting vs. CABG, there were no significant differences in the 5-year survival in either group. However, 90.2 % of CABG patients were free of repeat revascularization at 5 years compared to 53.9 % with balloon angioplasty and 59.9 % with stent placement ($p<0.001$).

A pooled analysis of 3,051 patients in four randomized stent trials – ARTS, ERACI-II, MASS-II, and SOS trials – was performed by Daemen et al. [28] to evaluate the relative safety and efficacy of PCI with stenting vs. CABG at 5 years for treatment of MVD. At the end of 5 years, the cumulative incidence of death, MI, and stroke was similar between the two groups (16.7 % PCI vs. 16.9 % CABG, $p=0.69$). However, the rate of repeat vascularization was significantly higher in the stent arm (29 % vs. 8 %, $p<0.0001$). As a result, overall MACCE was significantly higher in the stent arm (39 % vs. 23 %, $p<0.0001$). Among diabetics, there were no statistically significant differences noted in the rate of death (12.4 % vs. 7.9 %, $p=0.09$) or the composite end point of death, MI, or stroke (21.4 % PCI vs. 20.9 % CABG, $p=0.9$).

Hlatky performed a meta-analysis [29] of ten randomized trials of both PTCA and PCI with BMS compared to CABG for MVD. This patient-level analysis included at a total of 7,812 patients and the PCI arm included six angioplasty trials and four bare metal stent trials. After a mean follow of 5.9 years, overall death was similar in both arms (15 % CABG vs. 16 % PCI, $p=0.12$). The composite end point of death or MI was also nonsignificantly different (15.4 % CABG vs. 16.7 % PCI, $p=0.47$), while the rate of death or repeat revascularization was significantly lower for CABG (9.9 % vs. 24.5 %, $p<0.0001$). In patients with diabetes (CABG $n=615$, PCI $n=618$), mortality was substantially lower in patients treated with CABG when compared to PCI (23 % vs. 29 %, $p=0.014$).

Overall, these three meta-analyses of early PCI (prior to the introduction of drug-eluting stents) vs. CABG for MVD highlight the fact that when comparing "hard" clinical end points, PCI performs similarly to CABG. The main driver of differences between the two therapies is the rate of repeat revascularization, which is expectedly higher among PCI-treated patients.

Drug-Eluting Stenting vs. CABG

The use of drug-eluting stents has dramatically reduced the rate of restenosis and repeat revascularization procedures and revolutionized the field of interventional cardiology, making PCI possible for an expanding range of patient and lesion subsets [14, 30]. By slowly releasing a drug which can be either immunosuppressive/antiproliferative (sirolimus/everolimus/zotarolimus) or antiproliferative (paclitaxel), drug-eluting stents reduce the amount of neointimal hyperplasia within implanted stents, thereby reducing rates of restenosis and rates of repeat revascularization by 20–70 % when compared to BMS [30] (Table 21.3). Given that the primary observed disadvantage of BMS over CABG for MVD related to the rate of repeat revascularization procedures, soon after their introduction, DES were tested in the setting of MVD in several clinical trials in the hope of narrowing that difference.

ARTS II Trial

ARTS II was a multicenter, nonrandomized, open-label trial designed to compare the safety and efficacy of the sirolimus-eluting stent (SES) in patients with de novo multivessel coronary artery disease using the surgical group of ARTS I as a historical control. ARTS II enrolled 607 patients with the same inclusion and exclusion criteria, end points, and protocol definitions as ARTS I. Despite enrolling a higher-risk population than ARTS I trial, the 5-year MACCE (a composite of death, MI, stroke, and repeat revascularization) rate with SES in ARTS II (27.5 %), while significantly higher than ARTS I CABG (21.1 %, $p=0.02$), was significantly lower than among BMS-treated patients in ARTS (41.5 %, $p<0.001$). At 5 years, the death/stroke/myocardial infarction event-free survival rate was 87.1 % in ARTS II SES vs. 86.0 % ($p=0.1$) and 81.9 % ($p=0.007$) in the ARTS I CABG and BMS cohorts, respectively. Interestingly, approximately one-third of the adverse events seen with SES in ARTS II could be attributed to early, late, and very late stent thrombosis with SES.

Using an angiographic scoring system derived from the subsequently conducted SYNTAX trial (the SYNTAX score, see below), the ARTS II investigators sought to further stratify the patients enrolled in ARTS II to assess the risk/benefit of PCI vs. CABG [31, 32]. Patients with lowest-tercile SYNTAX scores had MACCE-free survival rates greater than that of patients in the middle or highest terciles, and the

Table 21.3 CABG vs. DES

Trial	No. of patients	Follow-up	MACCE (%)	Mortality (%)	MI (%)	Repeat revascl
SYNTAX	CABG – 897	4 year	23.6	8.8	3.8	11.9
	PCI – 903		33.5	11.7	8.3	23
ARTS II	CABG – 605	5 year	20.8	7.1	4.0	7.0
	DES – 607		27.2	5.4	4.4	14.5
	BMS – 600		41.2	7.8	6.8	23.3
ERAC III	CABG – 225	3 year	22.7	9.8	6.2	5.8
	PCI – 225		22.7	5.7	6.2	14.2
CARDia	CABG – 254	1 year	11.3	3.2	5.7	2.0
	PCI – 256		19.3	3.2	9.8	11.8

SYNTAX score was an independent predictor of 5-year stent thrombosis and MACCE. Among patients with lowest-tercile SYNTAX scores, the MACCE rate was similar between SES-treated patients in ARTS II and the entire surgical cohort from ARTS I, suggesting that patients with MVD and a low SYNTAX score may be adequately treated with PCI.

ERACI-III Trial

This was a multicenter, prospective, nonrandomized, open-labeled registry that compared the various treatment options in patients with MVD; ERAC III [33] was aimed at comparing patients who received DES ($n=225$) with the patients who received BMS ($n=225$) and CABG ($n=225$) in the ERACI-II trial after meeting similar clinical and angiographic inclusion criteria. However, when comparing the baseline characteristics between the three groups, patients in DES group were older, more often smokers, and higher risk (by EuroSCORE); had more type C lesions; and received more stents but had less frequent angina. Nevertheless, at the end of 3 years, the occurrence of the primary end point (MACCE) was similar in both DES and CABG groups (22.7 % for each, $p=1.0$) and lower when compared to BMS group (29.8 %, $p=0.015$) mainly due to reduced repeat revascularization in the DES group (14.2 % DES vs. 24.4 % BMS, $p=0.009$). The DES group had nonsignificantly higher rates of death or MI when compared to BMS (10.2 % vs. 6.2 %, $p=0.08$) but nonsignificantly lower rates than CABG (15.1 %, $p=0.07$ %). Among diabetics, there was no significant difference in MACCE between the three groups (DES, 36.2 %; BMS, 43.6 %; CABG, 30.8 %; $p=0.49$); however, the rate of repeat vascularization was significantly different between the three groups with lowest rates observed among patients treated with CABG (DES, 21.3 %; BMS, 38.5 %; CABG, 15.4 %; $p=0.048$).

CARDia (Coronary Artery Revascularization in Diabetes) Trial

This study [34] was designed as non-inferiority trial to assess the safety and efficacy of PCI against CABG for patients with diabetes and MVD. 510 diabetic patients with MVD were randomized to PCI with stenting and routine use of abciximab ($n=256$) or CABG ($n=254$). Initially BMS were used for PCI (in 31 % of the overall cohort) but with the advent of DES, SES stents were ultimately used in 69 % of patients. At the end of 1 year, the rate of the composite primary end point of death, stroke, or MI was 10.5 % with CABG vs. 13 % with PCI ($p=0.39$). There were no differences in rates of all-cause mortality (3.2 % vs. 3.2 %), but repeat vascularization rates were lower with CABG vs. PCI (2.0 % vs. 11.8 %, $p<0.0001$). The trial did not meet non-inferiority criteria due to early termination and thus reduced sample size; however, CARDia did demonstrate that PCI was a viable option in diabetic patients with follow-up to 1 year. The upcoming results of the FREEDOM trial will hopefully add some further clarity to this issue.

The SYNTAX Trial

The Synergy Between Percutaneous Coronary Intervention with TAXUS and Cardiac Surgery (SYNTAX) trial, conducted from 2005 to 2007, has shaped much of the current thinking regarding the treatment of MVD in the era of drug-eluting stents [35]. Prior to this trial, as stated in the 2005 ACC/AHA/SCAI guideline update for PCI, CABG remained the treatment of choice for patients with severe coronary artery disease, including those with left main coronary artery disease and three-vessel disease. Due to the lack of data from adequately powered randomized trials of DES-PCI in such patients, the SYNTAX trial sought to assess the optimal revascularization strategy for patients with MVD and/or left main coronary artery disease and to define the populations of patients for whom only one or the other revascularization method would be most effective. SYNTAX was a prospective, randomized clinical trial conducted at 62 European and 23 US sites. Inclusion criteria included treatment of de novo lesions with ≥50 % target vessel stenosis in symptomatic patients (or with the evidence of myocardial ischemia in asymptomatic patients). Patients were screened for both CABG and PCI suitability by an interventional cardiologist and a cardiac surgeon at each site (a concept termed the "heart team") and if suitable for both were randomized. Patients considered eligible for only one form of treatment were assigned to the equivalent registry. The primary analysis was non-inferiority comparison of MACCE between the two groups with the hypothesis that PCI with DES would be non-inferior to CABG at 1 year. A total of 1,800 patients were randomized to undergo CABG ($n=897$) or PCI with the TAXUS Express paclitaxel-eluting stent (PES) ($n=903$). Of the patients included LM disease was prevalent in 38.8 % of CABG patients and 39.5 % of PCI patients. At the end of 12 months, the primary outcome of MACCE was significantly higher with PCI (17.6 % vs. 12.3 %, $p=0.002$) mainly driven by increased rates of revascularization (13.5 % vs. 5.9 %, $p<0.001$); as such, the primary non-inferiority hypothesis was rejected. Interestingly, the incidence of composite death, MI, or stroke was similar in both arms at the end of 12 months (7.6 % PCI vs. 7.7 % CABG, $p=0.98$), and the rate of stroke was significantly higher with CABG (2.2 % vs. 0.6 %, $p=0.003$). The 12-month rate of symptomatic graft occlusion in CABG group and stent thrombosis in the PCI group was similar among both arms of the trial (3.4 % vs. 3.3 %: $p=0.89$).

Several exploratory sub-analyses of the SYNTAX data have been performed in order to attempt to further define the suitability of specific subgroups of the trial for PCI vs. CABG. When comparing the two groups based on SYNTAX score terciles, MACCE at 12 months was similar in the lowest (13.6 % PCI vs. 14.7 % CABG, $p=0.71$) and intermediate terciles (16.7 % PCI vs. 12.0 % CABG, $p=0.1$). However, there was a statistically significant difference in highest tercile in favor of CABG (23.4 % PCI vs. 10.9 % CABG, $p<0.001$). In the left main subset, there was no significant difference in MACCE at 12 months (15.8 % PCI vs. 13.7 % CABG, $p=0.44$). In the 3-vessel disease subset, when comparing PCI and CABG, all-cause death (4.4 % vs. 2.9 %, $p=0.18$), CVA (0.8 % vs. 1.9 %, $p=0.09$), and symptomatic graft occlusion or stent thrombosis (3.7 % vs. 3.3 %, $p=0.73$) were non-statistically different among the study arms. However, the rates of MI (2.6 % vs. 5.2 %, $p=0.04$) and repeat revascularization (5.4 % vs. 14.7 %, $p<0.001$) favored CABG.

SYNTAX at 4 Years

The 4-year results of SYNATX trial [36] have been reported on 819 patients in the CABG arm (91.3 %) and 879 in the PCI arm (97.3 %) with 78 CABG patients and 24 PCI patients lost to follow-up. The benefit of CABG continued over to the fourth year, with the MACCE rate being significantly lower when compared to PCI (23.6 % vs. 33.5 %, $p<0.001$). There remain no significant differences in the rate of death, stroke, or MI between the two groups, although the rate is numerically lower with CABG (14.6 vs. 18 % with PCI, $p=0.07$). At 4 years, patients treated with CABG had a significantly lower rate of all-cause mortality when compared to PCI (8.8 % vs. 11.7 %, $p=0.048$), with a similar significant difference observed for cardiac death (4.3 % vs. 7.6 %; $p=0.004$), MI (3.8 % vs. 8.3 %; $p<0.001$), and also the rate of repeat revascularization (11.9 % vs. 23 %; $p<0.001$). When comparing the stroke rates at 4-year follow-up, there was no significant difference noted (3.7 % CABG vs. 2.3 % PCI).

Due to the difference in ascertainment of follow-up between the two study arms, a sensitivity analysis was conducted assuming that all non-evaluable patients had died. In this analysis, there was still a significant difference favoring CABG for MACCE ($p=0.04$), but no difference in death/stroke/MI. When analyzing the data according to the three terciles of SYNTAX scores, at the end of 4 years, there was no significant difference in MACCE between CABG and PCI in those with a SYNTAX score of 0–22 (lowest tercile) (26.1 % vs. 28.6 %; $p=0.57$) but the rates of revascularization were higher with PCI (20 % vs. 13.6 %, $p=0.04$). In the intermediate tercile (score: 23–32), MACCE was significantly lower with CABG (21.5 % vs. 32.2 %, $p=0.006$) with no difference noted between the two groups in regard to death, CVA, or MI (CABG (17.3 %) vs. PCI (14.9 %), $p=0.44$). In the highest tercile group (score ≥33), CABG maintained its superiority consistently with MACCE being significantly lower (23.6 % vs. 40.1 %, $p<0.001$) as well as death, CVA, or MI (CABG (14.6 %) vs. PCI (22.7 %), $p=0.01$).

Limitations of the SYNTAX Trial

While the SYNTAX trial represents the most current head-to-head comparison of CABG vs. PCI with DES for the treatment of MVD, there are several caveats that should be noted limiting its applicability to current-day clinical practice. The SYNTAX trial tested the use of PCI with the first-generation TAXUS PES vs. CABG. This stent has largely been supplanted by second-generation stents, which have been associated with lower rates of target-lesion revascularization, MI, and stent thrombosis compared to PES, [37–39] findings that become more evident (on an absolute scale) as lesion complexity increases. Also, the definition of myocardial infarction was based on a surgical definition (the finding of a new Q wave on electrocardiography, in association with a value for the creatine kinase-MB fraction that was five times the upper limit of the normal range), which may have resulted in underreporting of myocardial infarction. Although randomization was conducted in a blinded manner, it was not possible to blind the performance of the treatment. Additionally, in SYNTAX, complete revascularization was attempted based upon angiography and only occurred in 50 % of patients with chronic total occlusions [35]. The FAME trial [40] has demonstrated lower rates of adverse events with similar long-term outcomes among patients selected for a functionally guided as opposed to a purely anatomic revascularization strategy. In fact, in FAME, the use of fractional flow reserve has been demonstrated to allow operators to "downgrade" the severity of MVD, therefore allowing operators to perform less complex procedures in order to effect functionally complete revascularization [41]. Additionally, in SYNTAX, the use of adjunctive medical therapies differed between the groups, reflecting variations in the standard care of patients between the two treatment groups. Optimal medical therapy has been demonstrated to be critically important in the treatment of patients with chronic coronary artery disease [42]. With regard to interpretation of the longer-term follow-up data, more patients withdrew after randomization from the CABG group than from the PCI group.

The SYNTAX Score and Other Risk-Stratification Schemes

The SYNTAX trial employed a novel scoring system to grade the angiographic complexity of coronary artery disease (the SYNTAX score) [32]. The score is an additive score consisting of 9 components: dominance, number of lesions, left main disease, triple-vessel disease, total occlusion, tortuosity, bifurcation, thrombus, and calcification. The SYNTAX score reflects a comprehensive anatomic assessment, with higher scores indicating more complex coronary disease thus stratifying risk when applied to PCI with DES but not with CABG.

While the SYNTAX score represents a comprehensive angiographic assessment of the severity and complexity of CAD, it does have limitations. The calculation of the SYNTAX score can be cumbersome and time-consuming and marked inter-observer and intra-observer variability is seen when it is calculated by individuals without sufficient training [43]. Additionally, the SYNTAX score algorithm does not include lesions associated with previous revascularization such as in-stent restenosis and stenotic bypass grafts. Angiographic findings such as patent bypass grafts, coronary anomalies, muscular bridges, and aneurysms are not accounted for. Finally the weight of some angiographic variables might be overemphasized. For example, an ostial left main lesion is assigned a score of 11; however, a lesion in distal left main lesion involving the ostial left anterior descending and the left circumflex arteries (obviously much more complex to treat) is assigned a similar score of 12.

In its essence, the SYNTAX score is a measure of the technical difficulty of PCI with a given anatomic profile and thus correlates with adverse outcomes after PCI. Importantly, it is a measure of relative but not an absolute risk as different stents have been shown to have different outcomes with a given score [44]. Most importantly, the SYNTAX score does not account for clinical variables that are known to impact outcomes with both PCI and CABG such as left ventricular ejection fraction, serum creatinine, associated valvular abnormalities, and the use of antiplatelet therapy. Factors which perhaps affect the adverse outcomes of patients with high SYNTAX score such as diabetes, incomplete revascularization, early stent thrombosis, chronic kidney disease, and stent number are not incorporated in the assessment of SYNTAX score and have never been subjected to multivariate analysis to define their contribution to adverse PCI outcomes relative to the score. The combination of clinical variables and SYNTAX score has the potential to partially address these issues with improved discrimination ability but needs to be placed in context of the patient and the overall CABG risk as well.

Clinical SYNTAX Score (CSS), Global Risk Score (GRC), and NERS Score

One of the most discussed critiques about SYNTAX score is the absence of clinical characteristics assessment during its calculation. This prompted the idea for a new scoring system such as the Clinical SYNTAX Score (CSS) [44]. CSS is a combination of the SYNTAX and ACEF score. ACEF score includes parameters – age, serum creatinine, and ejection fraction – and is calculated as follows: age (years)/ejection fraction (%) +1 (if serum creatinine value was >2 mg/dL). CSS is calculated as = SYNTAX score × (age/ejection fraction + 1) (if creatinine >2 mg/dL). In order to assess the ability of CSS to predict long-term mortality and MACCE, Serruys et al. [45] calculated the score on 512 patients enrolled in ARTS II trial who had 2- or 3-vessel disease and underwent PCI. The clinical outcomes were stratified according to the CSS terciles: low (<15.6), mid (15.6–27.5), and high (>27.5). At the end of 12 months, overall mortality was comparable in each tercile (low, 0.6 %; mid, 0 %; high, 2.3 %; $p=0.09$); however, MACCE (6.5 % low, 7.6 % mid, and 18.7 % high, $p=0.001$) and repeat revascularization were significantly higher in the highest tercile (5.3 % low, 6.4 % mid, and 15.8 % high, $p=0.002$). When comparing CSS and SYNTAX score, the ROC curves for mortality (0.69 vs. 0.62, $p<0.05$) and MACCE (0.62 vs. 0.57, $p<0.05$) favored CSS. Hence, CSS was found to be superior to SYNTAX score in its ability to predict MACCE and mortality at 5 years, and the log of CSS was an independent predictor of long-term MACCE. Similarly, a substudy of the SIRTAX (sirolimus-eluting stent compared with paclitaxel-eluting stent for coronary revascularization) trial investigated the ability of the SYNTAX score and CSS to predict long-term outcomes in patients receiving DES [44]. Terciles for SYNTAX score and CSS were defined as follows: SS (low ≤7, mid 7–14, and high >14) and CSS (low ≤8.0, mid 8–17, and high >17.0). The rate of MACCE was significantly higher in high SYNTAX score compared with low scores at 5-year follow-up (24.2 % vs. 12.5 %, $p<0.01$). Similar results were noted between higher and lower terciles of CSS (28 % vs. 14.1 %, $p<0.01$). Both the SYNTAX score and CSS were found to be independent predictors of 5-year MACE, and CSS was an independent predictor of 5-year mortality. The C statistics for CSS and SYNTAX score for 5-year mortality were 0.69 and 0.62, respectively ($p<0.05$).

In present-day clinical practice, the EuroSCORE and the SYNTAX score are two of the most used scores for surgical risk stratification in patients with MVD/left main disease. Capodanno et al. [46] proposed a risk model including both clinical and angiographic information known as the Global Risk Classification (GRC). By combining the EuroSCORE and SYNTAX score, three categories of risk were identified: high (EuroSCORE >6 and SYNTAX score >26), intermediate (EuroSCORE >6 or SYNTAX score >26), and low (EuroSCORE <6 and SYNTAX score <26). The GRC demonstrated the best predictability and discriminative ability in terms of predicting 24-month cardiac mortality (HR 3.4, $p<0.01$; c-statistic 0.756) when compared to SYNTAX score alone (HR 2.87, $p=0.006$; c-statistic 0.747) or EuroSCORE alone (HR 3.04, $p=0.005$; c-statistic 0.708).

The NERS score system [47] consists of 17 clinical, four procedural, and 33 angiographic variables. Among the clinical variables that contribute to a high score includes acute MI with the highest predicted score, followed by cardiogenic shock, previous MI, and intra-aortic balloon pump requirement. Of angiographic variables, complex LM lesions, including distal stenosis, CTO, restenosis, severe calcification, and thrombotic lesions, result in higher scores. Among procedural variables, failure of non-left main CTO recanalization was associated with the highest predicted score. When compared with the SYNTAX score, NERS score had increased sensitivity and specificity for prediction of cumulative MACE, stent thrombosis, cardiogenic death, TVR, and MI. Also, NERS higher score had significantly greater predictive value over SYNTAX intermediate, SYNTAX higher, and SYNTAX high-risk scores. Its extreme complexity, however, limits its overall utility and applicability.

Complete vs. Incomplete Revascularization in MVD

Early observational studies with CABG demonstrated a mortality benefit in patients who were completely revascularized as compared to those who underwent "incomplete revascularization" [48–50]. While subsequent observational data have largely supported these findings, there is no well-defined standard definition for "complete" revascularization with different studies employing different definitions, and hence comparisons between studies must be interpreted with caution. On the whole, complete revascularization can be broadly divided into anatomic or functional. Anatomic complete revascularization also has variable definitions; some define it as all stenotic vessels being revascularized, irrespective of size and territory supplied, while others employ a minimum diameter criteria, and others differentiate between main vessels and branch vessels. When employing functional classification, revascularization is considered complete if all ischemic myocardial territories are reperfused excluding areas of infarction with no viable myocardium. Data from various retrospective analysis, trials, and registries suggest that complete revascularization can have beneficial effects over incomplete revascularization [48–51]. The only randomized trial [52] comparing patients with MVD with PCI limited to culprit vessel vs. PCI of all vessels >50 % involved 219 patients followed for 5 years. The study had a mean follow-up of 4.6 years and demonstrated that target-lesion revascularization rates were similar in the completely revascularized and the culprit vessel-treated group (17.3 % vs. 12.0 %, $p=0.3$), with a nonsignificant difference in overall repeat revascularization (21.2 % vs. 31.2 %, $p=0.06$). Also, overall long-term MACCE rates were similar between groups (34.6 % vs. 40.4 %, respectively, $p=0.4$).

Several recent observational analyses, however, have supported a goal of more complete revascularization if PCI is performed. In the ARTS trial, [22] true anatomic complete revascularization occurred in 70.5 % of patients. It was observed that stented patients who were incompletely revascularized had a significantly higher requirement for subsequent CABG in the first year of follow-up compared to those who were completely revascularized (10 % vs. 2 %, $p<0.05$). This resulted in a lower overall MACCE-free rate for incompletely revascularized patients (69.4 % vs. 76.6 %, $p<0.05$). Further strengthening the argument in favor of complete revascularization with PCI was data from New York State's Percutaneous Coronary Intervention Reporting System [53] including data collected between October 1, 2003, and December 31, 2004, on 11,294 MVD patients who received a stent. This analysis demonstrated that incomplete revascularization was associated with higher 18-month mortality and death/MI compared to complete revascularization. Finally, data from the Alberta Provincial Project for Outcome Assessment in Coronary Heart Disease (APPROACH) involved identifying long-term outcomes of 1,308 patients undergoing multivessel PCI with complete revascularization as compared to those of 648 patients with incomplete revascularization [54]. With a median follow-up time of 3.0 +/− 1.8 years, the adjusted hazard ratio (HR) for the association between complete revascularization and outcome was

0.75 (0.54–1.04) for death, 0.55 (0.37–0.84) for subsequent CABG, and 0.93 (0.65–1.34) for repeat PCI. In conclusion, while none of the current guidelines formally discuss the issue of complete revascularization in detail, strong consideration should be given to which technique (e.g., PCI or CABG) affords the highest likelihood of complete revascularization of major viable territories when long-term prognosis is considered paramount. Unfortunately there are at present very limited data pertaining to how quality of life is affected by a strategy of complete vs. incomplete revascularization.

Fractional Flow Reserve (FFR)-Guided PCI in MVD

FFR is an index of the physiological significance of a coronary stenosis measured as ratio of pressure distal to and proximal to a stenosis under conditions of maximum hyperemia. FFR is a measurement of flow dynamics and is readily measured at the time of coronary angiography using a pressure wire. Hyperemia is achieved most commonly by using adenosine at 140 μg/kg/min administered via peripheral or central venous access. An FFR value of 0.80 is the most common cutoff used to identify an ischemia-causing coronary stenosis with an accuracy of 75–90 % [40]. The advantage of FFR over noninvasive perfusion studies is that FFR is lesion specific and each region of the coronary tree can be individually analyzed. FFR can also be used to differentiate between a hemodynamically significant epicardial stenosis and microvascular dysfunction, [55, 56] but FFR does not ordinarily produce definitive data about myocardial viability in the region subserved by the culprit artery. According to the 2011 guidelines for PCI [57], in cases with intermediate coronary lesions (50–70 %), FFR can be helpful to determine stenosis severity and to guide revascularization decisions in patients with stable ischemic heart disease (Class IIa).

The FAME Trial

The FAME trial aimed to evaluate a strategy of FFR-guided vs. angiography-guided PCI for the treatment of MVD. [40] Out of 1,905 screened patients, based on the inclusion criteria of having at least lesions with ≥50 % in two of the three epicardial vessels, 1,005 patients were randomized to angiography-guided ($n=496$) vs. FFR-guided ($n=509$) PCI. After a successful 98.1 % follow-up at 1 year, the rate of the primary MACCE end point favored FFR-guided PCI over an angiography alone-based approach (13.2 % vs. 18.3 %, $p=0.02$). Though not significant, there was a trend towards lower all-cause mortality (1.8 % FFR vs. 3.0 % angiography, $p=0.19$), MI (5.7 % FFR vs. 8.7 % angiography, $p=0.07$), and repeat revascularization (6.5 % FFR vs. 9.5 % angiography, $p=0.08$). The number of stents used per patient was significantly lower in the FFR-guided arm (1.9±1.3 vs. 2.7±.1.2, $p<0.001$). At 2-year follow-up [58], there was a significantly reduced occurrence of death or myocardial infarction in the FFR-guided PCI arm the angiography-guided group (8.4 % vs. 12.9 %, $p=0.02$). The combined rates of death, nonfatal MI, and revascularization were 17.9 and 22.4 %, respectively ($p=0.08$). A noteworthy finding from the 2-year follow-up was that for the lesions deferred on the basis of FFR >0.80, the rate of subsequent MI was only 0.2 % and the rate of subsequent revascularization was 3.2 %. More recently, the FAME II study was halted prematurely by the data safety monitoring board after enrollment of 1,220 patients due to a significant reduction in the combined end point of death, myocardial infarction, and urgent revascularization in the PCI group (4.3 %) compared with medical therapy (12.7 %) ($p<0.001$) [59]. These results and subsequent economic analysis continue to support that ischemia reduction with PCI is crucial to improve outcomes.

Considerations for Performing Multivessel PCI

Treating MVD with PCI is a complex medical decision that involves careful consideration and planning before executing the actual procedure. The treatment of MVD with PCI may involve single-vessel or multivessel interventions, performed in one or more stages depending on many considerations such as safety, functional goals, patient comfort and convenience, and cost (Tables 21.3, 21.4, and 21.5). In some cases, careful consideration and evaluation may lead to single-vessel PCI with other lesions managed medically while, in others, multivessel PCI with complete revascularization may be considered in the same sitting or in multiple stages. In order to determine the significance of coronary disease – specifically that of borderline 50–70 % lesions – the use of adjunctive IVUS and FFR can be used which help reduce inter-observer variability by giving an objective evaluation to the lesion. According to a recently published consensus document by the SCAI,[60] the recommended approach to a patient with MVD is the "heart team" approach. This approach involves the interaction of interventionalist, cardiac surgeon, medical cardiologist, and patient with an opportunity to discuss various revascularization strategies. Typically, this discussion should involve the risk and benefits of various revascularization strategies and is recommended to occur either before the beginning of the diagnostic procedure itself or after the diagnostic procedure is completed except in urgent/emergent cases. Depending on the complexity of the disease and patient characteristics, treatment strategies can be divided into single-stage or multiple-stage PCI. One-stage multivessel PCI is reasonable when the first lesion

Table 21.4 Factors favoring PCI or CABG in MVD

Factors favoring PCI in MVD
Patient refusing to undergo surgery
Low- to intermediate-risk SYNTAX score
High risk for surgery (high STS score or EuroSCORE)
History of prior CABG
Coronary anatomy unsuitable for bypass (poor targets)
Suitable coronary anatomy
Serious comorbid conditions (e.g., severe COPD)
Factors favoring CABG in MVD
Patient refusing to undergo PCI
Contraindication to antiplatelet therapy (aspirin, thienopyridine)
History of bleeding disorders
High SYNTAX score
Unfavorable coronary anatomy
Comorbid conditions (peripheral vascular disease, chronic kidney disease)
Associated decreased LV systolic function

Table 21.5 Summary of Treatment of MVD

Define the coronary anatomy and complexity of lesion(s)
With and without left main disease
Scoring systems – SYNTAX, GRC, NERS, EuroSCORE, STS, and FFR of intermediate lesions
Use of stress test to assess extent of ischemia
Assess LV function
Assess patient comorbid conditions
Chronic kidney disease
Diabetes mellitus
Bleeding diathesis
Allergies or intolerance to medications (specially dual antiplatelet therapy)
Other contraindications to PCI or CABG
Heart team approach
Integration of inputs from patients, interventional cardiologist, and CT surgeon
Timing of PCI/CABG – emergent vs. urgent vs. elective
Consider staging vs. single-setting multivessel PCI
Consider complete vs. incomplete revascularization strategy
Consider use of support devices during PCI: IABP, Impella, Tandem Heart – based on LV function and lesion complexity and location
Special consideration for CTO interventions in multivessel disease; CTO first or after simpler lesions

treatment is uncomplicated, without excessive radiation or contrast doses, and treatment of the remaining lesion(s) is unlikely to risk a cumulative excess of either. Single staging can have an advantage of convenience and cost. Multiple staging of PCI in MVD is preferred in cases when certain patient factors like compromised renal function, complexity of the lesions to be treated, or anticipated high doses of radiation may be limiting factors.

As a part of treatment strategy for MVD, the expert consensus report recommends [60] six important points taken into consideration before, during, and after planning of MVD PCI.

1. Medical therapy: It is recommended that patients be on "optimal" medical therapy including antianginal therapy before planning PCI. If PCI is staged, the optimal medical therapy should be continued to control any residual anginal symptoms.
2. Informed consent: It is very important that as a part of heart team approach, the patient should understand in advance the risks and benefits of various treatment strategies including one-stage vs. multi-stage PCI.
3. PCI strategy: When proceeding with the PCI, the interventionalist should develop a strategy of and order of lesion treatment, the timing of possible staging of PCI (time period between two procedures) and what technique to exercise for each individual lesion.
4. Flexibility of PCI strategy: The interventionalist should be flexible in his/her approach to MVD. Planned PCI of additional lesions should be performed only after success of the first PCI with adequate time in between for the patient to recover. If there are complications during the first PCI, then it is reasonable for the interventionalist to defer the staged PCI.
5. Reassessment between stages of multivessel PCI: The need for subsequent PCI of additional lesions should be reviewed after the first procedure using patient symptoms and residual ischemic burden as a guide.
6. Regulatory and reimbursement status: Treatment of patients with multistaging PCI should be purely based on clinical decisions and in the best interest of the patient and not on any financial/reimbursement motive. Payers should realize that the staging of PCI is not an indicator of poor technical quality and rather is a strategy to minimize patient risk.

Conclusion: An Integrated Approach to the Patient with Multivessel Disease

The decision to treat MVD with PCI requires careful consideration and an orderly approach. An initial thorough assessment of MVD starts with defining the coronary anatomy and the extent of disease, for example, the number and characteristics of lesions involved including attention to calcification, tortuosity, and bifurcation involvement. An assessment of left ventricular ejection fraction is essential to understanding the overall clinical picture. Other comorbid clinical conditions including chronic kidney disease, diabetes mellitus, presence of a bleeding diathesis, and intolerance to or nonadherence to medications can be confounding factors in determining the mode of revascularization. In addition to the gross angiographic assessment of the number and degree of stenosis, objective evaluation of disease extent and its prognostic significance should be assessed. Various scoring systems, including, for example, the SYNTAX score, GRC, NERS, EuroSCORE, and STS, can help us better evaluate the relative risks of revascularization strategies and help determine the most appropriate revascularization approach. For example, while a patient with low SYNTAX score may preferably be directed to PCI, and a high-tercile SYNTAX score would direct one towards CABG, the presence of high surgical risk based upon patient comorbidities could substantially modify that initial recommendation. Lesions with intermediate severity should routinely be assessed with the fractional flow reserve or IVUS at the time of diagnostic angiography so as to better inform the decision of which vessels to revascularize. Decisions regarding the use of supportive devices such as an intra-aortic balloon pump, Impella, or Tandem heart depend on the extent of disease and the underlying left ventricular function. A patient with low ejection fraction and left main and/or proximal epicardial vessel disease subserving a large area of residual viable myocardium may occasionally benefit from such devices [61, 62] though routine use is not recommended. In conclusion, the management of patients with MVD involves an integrated, multidisciplinary approach, keeping in mind not only the extent and prognosis of the disease, the available management options, and knowledge of the relative risks of various therapeutic strategies but, most importantly, the wants and needs of an informed patient.

References

1. Hilliard AA, et al. Percutaneous revascularization for stable coronary artery disease temporal trends and impact of drug-eluting stents. JACC Cardiovasc Interv. 2010;3(2):172–9.
2. Curtis JP, et al. All-cause readmission and repeat revascularization after percutaneous coronary intervention in a cohort of medicare patients. J Am Coll Cardiol. 2009;54(10):903–7.
3. Yusuf S, et al. Effect of coronary artery bypass graft surgery on survival: overview of 10-year results from randomised trials by the Coronary Artery Bypass Graft Surgery Trialists Collaboration. Lancet. 1994;344(8922):563–70.
4. Hueb W, et al. Ten-year follow-up survival of the Medicine, Angioplasty, or Surgery Study (MASS II): a randomized controlled clinical trial of 3 therapeutic strategies for multivessel coronary artery disease. Circulation. 2010;122(10):949–57.
5. Venkitachalam L, et al. Twenty-year evolution of percutaneous coronary intervention and its impact on clinical outcomes: a report from the National Heart, Lung, and Blood Institute-sponsored, multicenter 1985–1986 PTCA and 1997–2006 Dynamic Registries. Circ Cardiovasc Interv. 2009;2(1):6–13.
6. Garrett HE, Dennis EW, DeBakey ME. Aortocoronary bypass with saphenous vein graft. Seven-year follow-up. JAMA. 1973;223(7):792–4.
7. Eighteen-year follow-up in the Veterans Affairs Cooperative Study of Coronary Artery Bypass Surgery for stable angina. The VA Coronary Artery Bypass Surgery Cooperative Study Group. Circulation. 1992;86(1)121–30.
8. Alderman EL, et al. Ten-year follow-up of survival and myocardial infarction in the randomized Coronary Artery Surgery Study. Circulation. 1990;82(5):1629–46.
9. Gruntzig AR, Senning A, Siegenthaler WE. Nonoperative dilatation of coronary-artery stenosis: percutaneous transluminal coronary angioplasty. N Engl J Med. 1979;301(2):61–8.
10. Serruys PW, et al. A comparison of balloon-expandable-stent implantation with balloon angioplasty in patients with coronary artery disease. Benestent Study Group. N Engl J Med. 1994;331(8):489–95.
11. Fischman DL, et al. A randomized comparison of coronary-stent placement and balloon angioplasty in the treatment of coronary artery disease. Stent Restenosis Study Investigators. N Engl J Med. 1994;331(8):496–501.
12. Gordon PC, et al. Mechanisms of restenosis and redilation within coronary stents–quantitative angiographic assessment. J Am Coll Cardiol. 1993;21(5):1166–74.
13. Frutkin AD, et al. Drug-eluting stents and the use of percutaneous coronary intervention among patients with class I indications for coronary artery bypass surgery undergoing index revascularization: analysis from the NCDR (National Cardiovascular Data Registry). JACC Cardiovasc Interv. 2009;2(7):614–21.
14. Stone GW, et al. One-year clinical results with the slow-release, polymer-based, paclitaxel-eluting TAXUS stent: the TAXUS-IV trial. Circulation. 2004;109(16):1942–7.
15. Comparison of coronary bypass surgery with angioplasty in patients with multivessel disease. The Bypass Angioplasty Revascularization Investigation (BARI) Investigators. N Engl J Med. 1996;335(4):217–25.
16. Berger PB, et al. Survival following coronary angioplasty versus coronary artery bypass surgery in anatomic subsets in which coronary artery bypass surgery improves survival compared with medical therapy. Results from the Bypass Angioplasty Revascularization Investigation (BARI). J Am Coll Cardiol. 2001;38(5):1440–9.
17. Investigators B. The final 10-year follow-up results from the BARI randomized trial. J Am Coll Cardiol. 2007;49(15):1600–6.
18. Rodriguez A, et al. Argentine randomized trial of percutaneous transluminal coronary angioplasty versus coronary artery bypass surgery in multivessel disease (ERACI): in-hospital results and 1-year follow-up. ERACI Group. J Am Coll Cardiol. 1993;22(4):1060–7.
19. King 3rd SB, et al. A randomized trial comparing coronary angioplasty with coronary bypass surgery. Emory Angioplasty versus Surgery Trial (EAST). N Engl J Med. 1994;331(16):1044–50.
20. Hamm CW, et al. A randomized study of coronary angioplasty compared with bypass surgery in patients with symptomatic multivessel coronary disease. German Angioplasty Bypass Surgery Investigation (GABI). N Engl J Med. 1994;331(16):1037–43.
21. First-year results of CABRI (Coronary Angioplasty versus Bypass Revascularisation Investigation). CABRI trial participants. Lancet. 1995;346(8984)1179–84.
22. Serruys PW, et al. Five-year outcomes after coronary stenting versus bypass surgery for the treatment of multivessel disease: the final analysis of the Arterial Revascularization Therapies Study (ARTS) randomized trial. J Am Coll Cardiol. 2005;46(4):575–81.
23. Rodriguez A, et al. Argentine randomized study: coronary angioplasty with stenting versus coronary bypass surgery in patients with multiple-vessel disease (ERACI II): 30-day and one-year follow-up results. ERACI II investigators. J Am Coll Cardiol. 2001;37(1):51–8.
24. Rodriguez AE, et al. Five-year follow-up of the Argentine randomized trial of coronary angioplasty with stenting versus coronary bypass surgery in patients with multiple vessel disease (ERACI II). J Am Coll Cardiol. 2005;46(4):582–8.
25. Morrison DA, et al. Percutaneous coronary intervention versus coronary artery bypass graft surgery for patients with medically refractory myocardial ischemia and risk factors for adverse outcomes with bypass: a multicenter, randomized trial. Investigators of the Department of Veterans Affairs Cooperative Study #385, the Angina With Extremely Serious Operative Mortality Evaluation (AWESOME). J Am Coll Cardiol. 2001;38(1):143–9.
26. Booth J, et al. Randomized, controlled trial of coronary artery bypass surgery versus percutaneous coronary intervention in patients with multivessel coronary artery disease: six-year follow-up from the Stent or Surgery trial (SoS). Circulation. 2008;118(4):381–8.
27. Bravata DM, et al. Systematic review: the comparative effectiveness of percutaneous coronary interventions and coronary artery bypass graft surgery. Ann Intern Med. 2007;147(10):703–16.

28. Daemen J, et al. Long-term safety and efficacy of percutaneous coronary intervention with stenting and coronary artery bypass surgery for multivessel coronary artery disease: a meta-analysis with 5-year patient-level data from the ARTS, ERACI-II, MASS-II, and SoS trials. Circulation. 2008;118(11):1146–54.
29. Hlatky MA, et al. Coronary artery bypass surgery compared with percutaneous coronary interventions for multivessel disease: a collaborative analysis of individual patient data from ten randomised trials. Lancet. 2009;373(9670):1190–7.
30. Moses JW, et al. Sirolimus-eluting stents versus standard stents in patients with stenosis in a native coronary artery. N Engl J Med. 2003;349(14):1315–23.
31. Serruys PW, et al. 5-year clinical outcomes of the ARTS II (Arterial Revascularization Therapies Study II) of the sirolimus-eluting stent in the treatment of patients with multivessel de novo coronary artery lesions. J Am Coll Cardiol. 2010;55(11):1093–101.
32. Sianos G, et al. The SYNTAX score: an angiographic tool grading the complexity of coronary artery disease. EuroIntervention. 2005;1(2):219–27.
33. Rodriguez AE, et al. Late loss of early benefit from drug-eluting stents when compared with bare-metal stents and coronary artery bypass surgery: 3 years follow-up of the ERACI III registry. Eur Heart J. 2007;28(17):2118–25.
34. Kapur A, et al. Randomized comparison of percutaneous coronary intervention with coronary artery bypass grafting in diabetic patients. 1-year results of the CARDia (Coronary Artery Revascularization in Diabetes) trial. J Am Coll Cardiol. 2010;55(5):432–40.
35. Serruys PW, et al. Percutaneous coronary intervention versus coronary-artery bypass grafting for severe coronary artery disease. N Engl J Med. 2009;360(10):961–72.
36. Four-year follow-up of the SYNTAX trial: optimal revascularization strategy in patients with three-vessel disease and/or left main disease. TCT 2011. 2011.
37. Stone GW, et al. Everolimus-eluting versus paclitaxel-eluting stents in coronary artery disease. N Engl J Med. 2010;362(18):1663–74.
38. Kedhi E, et al. Second-generation everolimus-eluting and paclitaxel-eluting stents in real-life practice (COMPARE): a randomised trial. Lancet. 2010;375(9710):201–9.
39. Baber U, et al. Impact of the everolimus-eluting stent on stent thrombosis: a meta-analysis of 13 randomized trials. J Am Coll Cardiol. 2011;58(15):1569–77.
40. Tonino PA, et al. Fractional flow reserve versus angiography for guiding percutaneous coronary intervention. N Engl J Med. 2009;360(3):213–24.
41. Nam CW, et al. Functional SYNTAX score for risk assessment in multivessel coronary artery disease. J Am Coll Cardiol. 2011;58(12):1211–18.
42. Boden WE, et al. Optimal medical therapy with or without PCI for stable coronary disease. N Engl J Med. 2007;356(15):1503–16.
43. Genereux P, et al. SYNTAX score reproducibility and variability between interventional cardiologists, core laboratory technicians, and quantitative coronary measurements. Circ Cardiovasc Interv. 2011;4(6):553–61.
44. Girasis C, et al. SYNTAX score and Clinical SYNTAX score as predictors of very long-term clinical outcomes in patients undergoing percutaneous coronary interventions: a substudy of SIRolimus-eluting stent compared with pacliTAXel-eluting stent for coronary revascularization (SIRTAX) trial. Eur Heart J. 2011;32(24):3115–27.
45. Garg S, et al. A new tool for the risk stratification of patients with complex coronary artery disease: the clinical SYNTAX score. Circ Cardiovasc Interv. 2010;3(4):317–26.
46. Capodanno D, et al. EuroSCORE refines the predictive ability of SYNTAX score in patients undergoing left main percutaneous coronary intervention. Am Heart J. 2010;159(1):103–9.
47. Chen SL, et al. Comparison between the NERS (New Risk Stratification) score and the SYNTAX (Synergy between Percutaneous Coronary Intervention with Taxus and Cardiac Surgery) score in outcome prediction for unprotected left main stenting. JACC Cardiovasc Interv. 2010;3(6):632–41.
48. Buda AJ, et al. Long-term results following coronary bypass operation. Importance of preoperative actors and complete revascularization. J Thorac Cardiovasc Surg. 1981;82(3):383–90.
49. Jones EL, et al. Importance of complete revascularization in performance of the coronary bypass operation. Am J Cardiol. 1983;51(1):7–12.
50. Bell MR, et al. Effect of completeness of revascularization on long-term outcome of patients with three-vessel disease undergoing coronary artery bypass surgery. A report from the Coronary Artery Surgery Study (CASS) registry. Circulation. 1992;86(2): 446–57.
51. Kleisli T, et al. In the current era, complete revascularization improves survival after coronary artery bypass surgery. J Thorac Cardiovasc Surg. 2005;129(6):1283–91.
52. Ijsselmuiden AJ, et al. Complete versus culprit vessel percutaneous coronary intervention in multivessel disease: a randomized comparison. Am Heart J. 2004;148(3):467–74.
53. Hannan EL, et al. Incomplete revascularization in the era of drug-eluting stents: impact on adverse outcomes. JACC Cardiovasc Interv. 2009;2(1):17–25.
54. McLellan CS, et al. Association between completeness of percutaneous coronary revascularization and postprocedure outcomes. Am Heart J. 2005;150(4):800–6.
55. Lima RS, et al. Incremental value of combined perfusion and function over perfusion alone by gated SPECT myocardial perfusion imaging for detection of severe three-vessel coronary artery disease. J Am Coll Cardiol. 2003;42(1):64–70.
56. Pijls NH. Optimum guidance of complex PCI by coronary pressure measurement. Heart. 2004;90(9):1085–93.
57. Levine GN, et al. ACCF/AHA/SCAI Guideline for Percutaneous Coronary Intervention. A report of the American College of Cardiology Foundation/American Heart Association Task Force on Practice Guidelines and the Society for Cardiovascular Angiography and Interventions. J Am Coll Cardiol. 2011;58(24): e44–122.
58. Pijls NH, et al. Fractional flow reserve versus angiography for guiding percutaneous coronary intervention in patients with multivessel coronary artery disease: 2-year follow-up of the FAME (Fractional Flow Reserve Versus Angiography for Multivessel Evaluation) study. J Am Coll Cardiol. 2010;56(3):177–84.
59. De Bruyne B, Pijls NH, Kalesan B, et al. Fractional flow reserve-guided PCI versus medical therapy in stable coronary disease. N Engl J Med. 2012;367:991–1001.
60. Blankenship JC, et al. Staging of multivessel percutaneous coronary interventions: an expert consensus statement from the Society for Cardiovascular Angiography and Interventions. Catheter Cardiovasc Interv. 2012;79(7):1138–52.
61. Dixon SR, et al. A prospective feasibility trial investigating the use of the Impella 2.5 system in patients undergoing high-risk percutaneous coronary intervention (The PROTECT I Trial): initial U.S. experience. JACC Cardiovasc Interv. 2009;2(2):91–6.
62. Schwartz BG, et al. High-risk percutaneous coronary intervention with the TandemHeart and Impella devices: a single-center experience. J Invasive Cardiol. 2011;23(10):417–24.

Coronary Bifurcation Lesions

22

James T. DeVries and Aaron V. Kaplan

Coronary artery intervention for bifurcation lesions remains a hotly contested topic, mainly because of the heterogeneity of bifurcation lesions and the paucity of large randomized trials to guide decision making. Functionally, coronary bifurcation lesions are defined as angiographically significant lesions which involve a branch point or the immediate vicinity of a branch point between two coronary arteries larger than 2 mm in diameter (Fig. 22.1). Consensus societies have simplified this definition to "a coronary artery narrowing adjacent to and/or involving a significant side branch [1]." The larger of the two vessels (either in size or territory supplied) is referred to as the parent or main branch, while the smaller vessel is designated as the side branch. Although many classification systems exist, in general bifurcation lesions are defined by the location of the intraluminal stenosis relative to site of the bifurcation – either before the bifurcation, after the bifurcation, or at the bifurcation (involving the side branch). While a stenosis must be present either before, after, or at a side branch, it is possible to have a complex bifurcation lesion which involves all three locations. It is estimated that as a whole, coronary bifurcation lesions involve about 15–20 % of all coronary interventions [2], and bifurcation stenting has been linked to adverse events including stent thrombosis [3]. Various techniques involving complex angioplasty plus one or more stents can be employed for treating bifurcation lesions, making the development of a standardized approach difficult. The situation has been further complicated by the use of confusing bifurcation-specific terminology such as "crush stenting," "mini-crush," "double barrel," "culotte stenting," "T-stenting," and "provisional stenting." Moreover, it has been recognized that rates of stent thrombosis, restenosis, and target-lesion revascularization are all higher in bifurcation lesions when compared with non-bifurcation lesions [4, 5], making the stakes for intervention higher. The advent of drug-eluting stents has mitigated this effect somewhat, but significant variability exists in clinical practice and outcomes with respect to bifurcation stenting [6].

High complexity and lesion variability, high rates of restenosis and thrombosis, and a myriad of approaches to treating bifurcation lesions have left the field with many unanswered questions. Small trials, case series, and registries

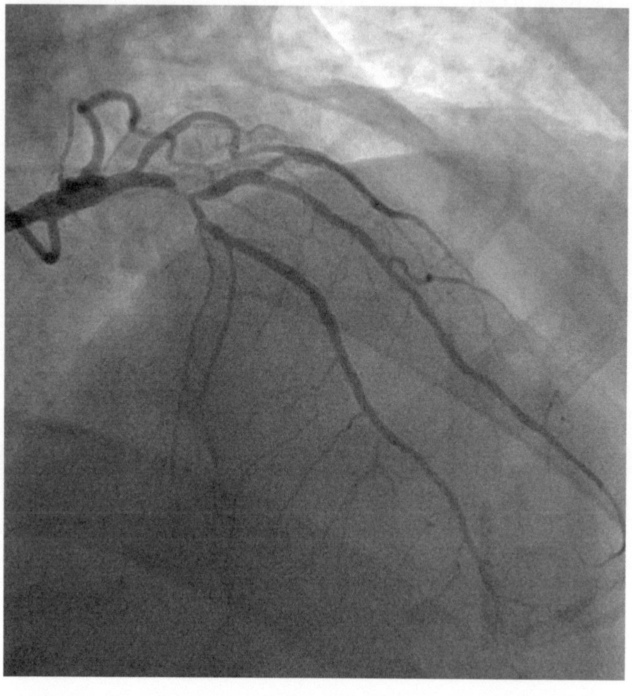

Fig. 22.1 Functionally, coronary bifurcation lesions are defined as angiographically significant lesions which involve a branch point or the immediate vicinity of a branch point between two coronary arteries larger than 2 mm in diameter

J.T. DeVries, MD, FACC, FSCAI (✉)
Department of Medicine, Dartmouth Medical School, Lebanon, NH, USA

Division of Cardiology, Dartmouth Hitchcock Medical Center, Lebanon, NH, USA
e-mail: James.T.DeVries@Hitchcock.ORG

A.V. Kaplan, MD
Device Development and Research, Geisel School of Medicine at Dartmouth, Dartmouth Hitchcock Medical Center, Lebanon, NH, USA

C.A. Thompson (ed.), *Textbook of Cardiovascular Intervention*,
DOI 10.1007/978-1-4471-4528-8_22, © Springer-Verlag London 2014

have reported on specialized techniques including dedicated bifurcation-specific stents, but for now interventional cardiologists are left choosing an approach based on personal preference and anecdotal experience rather than rigorous randomized data. Ongoing randomized trials with dedicated stent platforms [7] for treating bifurcation disease may ultimately provide the needed data to guide appropriate therapies, but clearly there remains significant knowledge deficit in the management of these challenging lesions.

Classification

There are multiple classification systems, which can be used to characterize bifurcation lesions (Fig. 22.2). One of the more complex systems is the Lefevre system [8], which attempts to characterize the lesions by the location of the stenosis and angulation of the lesion (Fig. 22.3). Although descriptive, it is rather cumbersome to use for day-to-day practice and consensus societies such as the European Bifurcation Club (EBC) have proposed using the simpler Medina classification system [1]. With the Medina classification system, lesions can be easily characterized using a three-number designation system where the first number represents the presence or absence of disease in the proximal main branch, the second number represents the presence or absence of disease in the distal main branch, and the third number represents the presence or absence of disease in the side branch (Fig. 22.4). For each of the three locations, a zero (0) is designated for less than 50 % stenosis, and a one (1) is designated for a greater than or equal to a 50 % stenosis. Each of the three numbers is then listed in order separated by a comma to create a classification schema for the lesion. For example, a bifurcation lesion, which spares the proximal main branch but involves the distal main branch as well as the side branch, would be designated [0,1,1]. In practice, the Medina system is both easy to calculate and has been shown to have excellent inter-observer agreement for classification of lesion subtypes [9].

Despite its strengths, the Medina system has several weaknesses, including that it does not account for the side branch angle or side branch size, two factors which may impact an interventional approach and the number of stents which are utilized [10]. Additionally, it does not quantify the percent stenosis, but uses a binary "present or not present" approach, which can lead to the same classification for a 50 % stenosis as a 99 % stenosis in a main vessel or side branch, despite the difference in interventional risks which may be present with these disparate lesions. Nevertheless, the trade-off in ease of use may be justified, especially when considering that complex lesion subsets are easily identified with the Medina classification despite its simplistic formulation [11, 12].

Current Treatment Options for Bifurcation Lesions

When considering intervention on a bifurcation lesion, there are two general tactics that can be employed. The more conservative, or provisional, approach involves the intent to only

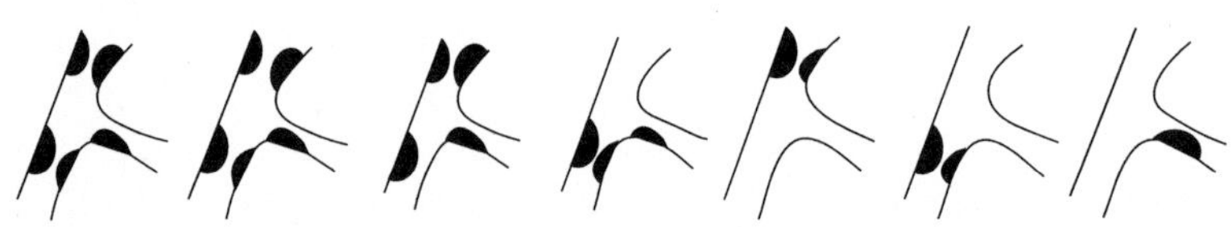

Medina	1,1,1	1,1,0	1,0,1	0,1,1	1,0,0	0,1,0	0,0,1
Duke (modified)	D	C	E	G	A	B	E
Sanborn	I	_	_	III	IV	II	IV
Lefevre	1	2	-	4	3	4a	4b
Safian	IA	IB	IIA	IIIA	IIIB	IIIB	IV
Movahed	L	S	2	1m	1s	V	T
Staico-Feres	3	2A	2B	2C	1A	1B	1C

Fig. 22.2 Multiple classification systems can be used to characterize bifurcation lesions

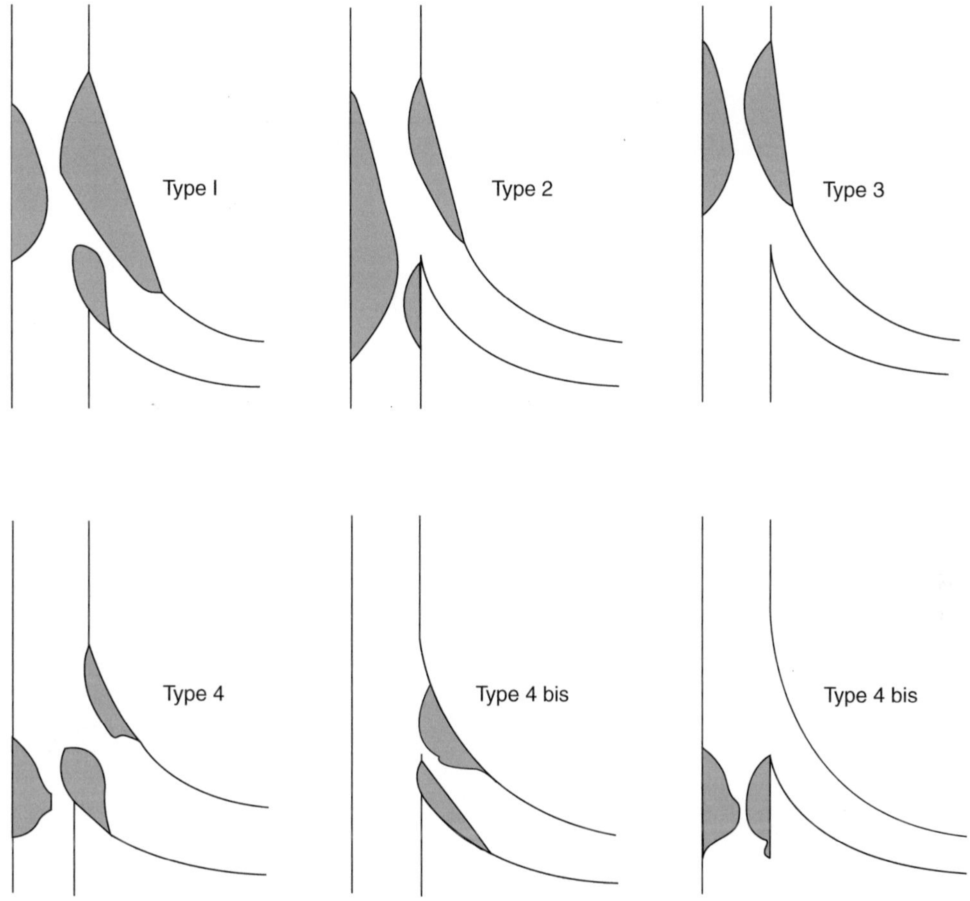

Fig. 22.3 The Lefevre system attempts to characterize the lesions by the location of the stenosis and angulation of the lesion

use one stent to treat the stenosis (typically the main branch is stented). Frequently, balloon angioplasty is used to "bail out" the side branch using a "kissing balloon" inflation, which involves simultaneous inflation of two balloons in the coronary which are touching ("kissing"), with one in the main branch and one in the side branch. The operator can elect to use a second stent, but usually this would only be performed if there was significant compromise to the side branch (residual high-grade stenosis, dissection, or reduced distal flow) which could not be rectified with additional balloon angioplasty. The goal of the provisional approach is to minimize the complexity of the procedure, reduce the fluoroscopic time and contrast volume required, and reduce the resource (stent) utilization. In contradistinction to a provisional approach, a dedicated approach implies the planned use of two stents, one in the main branch and one in the side branch.

In choosing a dedicated approach, a number of techniques can be used to address the main branch and side branch plaque adequately with stents. The most straightforward two-stent technique is the T-stent [5]. In this approach, the side branch stent is deployed just across the ostium of the vessel, and the main branch stent is then deployed across the side branch to complete the "T." It is best suited for side branches which have a 90-degree angle of intersection with the main branch. Typically, the side branch stent is deployed first, at which point the guidewire and stent-delivery equipment is then removed from the branch (to avoid jailing). Next, the main vessel stent is positioned and deployed, after which the side branch can be recrossed with a guidewire and final kissing balloon angioplasty can be performed. Modifications of this technique exist which dictate inflation of a balloon in the main vessel at the time of deployment of the side branch stent, which allows the side branch stent to be retracted back against the main vessel balloon at the time of deployment to ensure coverage of the true ostium [2, 5, 13]. There are various comparative studies of the T-technique, but a more recent comparison of T-stenting and crush stenting (discussed below) demonstrated that crush stenting had significantly less restenosis in the side branch than T-stenting, provided a final kissing balloon inflation was performed [13]. Interestingly, there was no evidence that final kissing balloon angioplasty improved restenosis in the side branch of T-stents, and overall, T-stenting had lower overall target-lesion revascularization-free survival out to 1 year when compared to crush stenting [13].

Crush stenting is another dedicated approach to dealing with complex coronary bifurcation lesions [14]. In a crush,

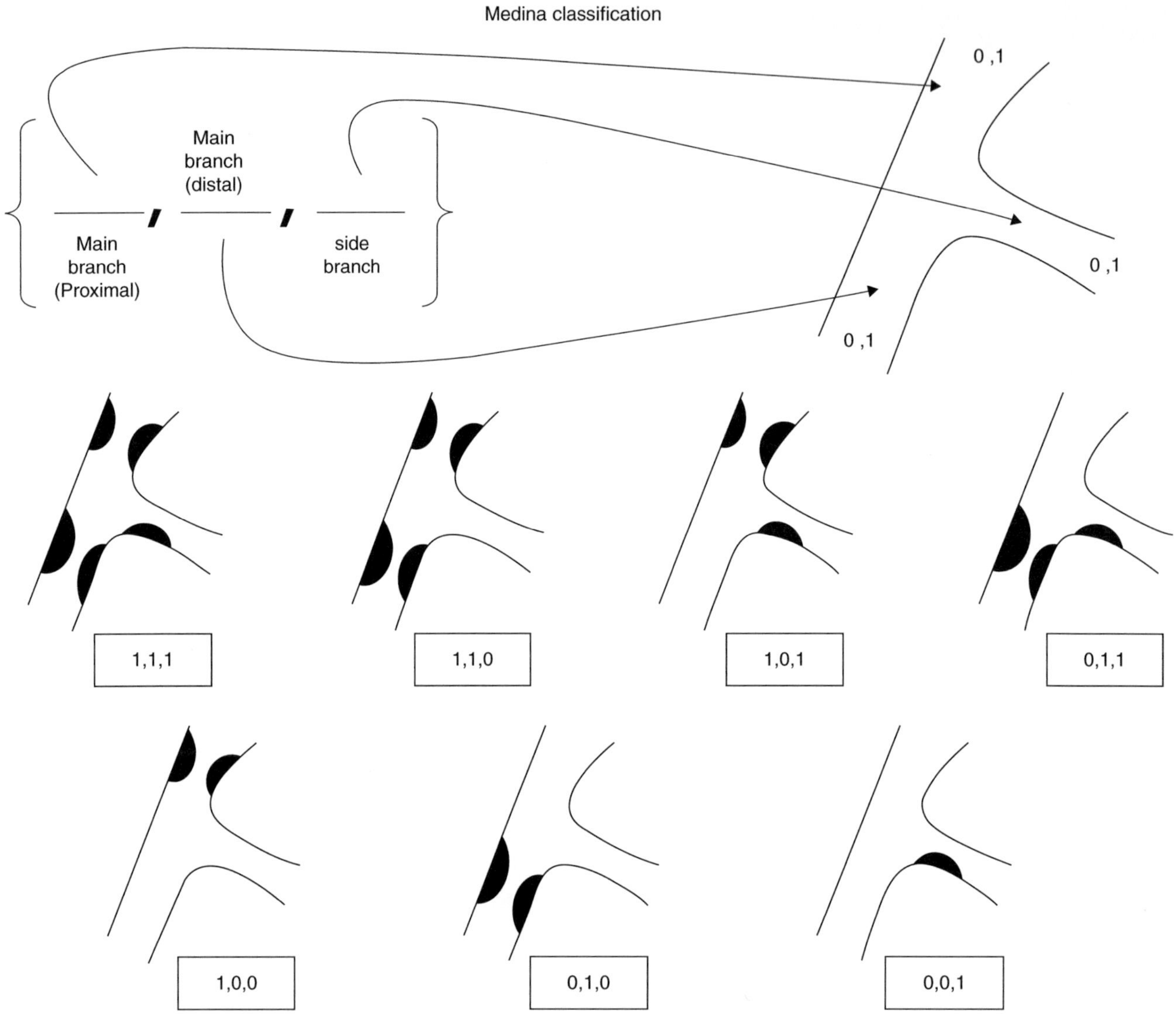

Fig. 22.4 Medina classification system for bifurcation lesions

the side branch stent is deployed so that the proximal end of the stent extends into the main vessel 3–5 mm beyond the ostium of the side branch alongside the un-deployed main vessel stent. The side branch stent is then deployed, and the guidewire and delivery system is removed. Next, the main vessel stent is deployed, which effectively "crushes" the portion of the side branch stent which extended into the main vessel against the vessel wall. In effect, this results in three layers of stent on one side of the vessel just proximal to the side branch carina and one layer on the opposite side. A guidewire is then used to recross into the side branch and final kissing angioplasty is performed with a balloon in the side branch and the main branch inflated simultaneously. Final kissing angioplasty has been demonstrated to be particularly important in crush stenting to lower the risk of restenosis at the side branch [15, 16]. Downsides to using the crush technique include the need for larger guiding catheters which can accommodate two stents simultaneously (although modified crush techniques can be performed with a 6Fr guide) and the occasional difficulty of recrossing the side branch through the multiple layers of stent. With experience, the crush technique can be performed quickly and effectively, and long-term restenosis rates are acceptable when using DES [17].

Another dedicated stent strategy is the double barrel or simultaneous kissing stent (SKS) technique. This involves the use of two stents positioned side by side in the main branch, with the proximal edge of both stents aligned (Fig. 22.5) [18]. The side branch stent extends into the side branch to cover the ostium and extends beyond any stenosis in the proximal side branch, while the main branch stent continues past the side branch origin and extends further down the main vessel.

Fig. 22.5 The double barrel or simultaneous kissing stent technique

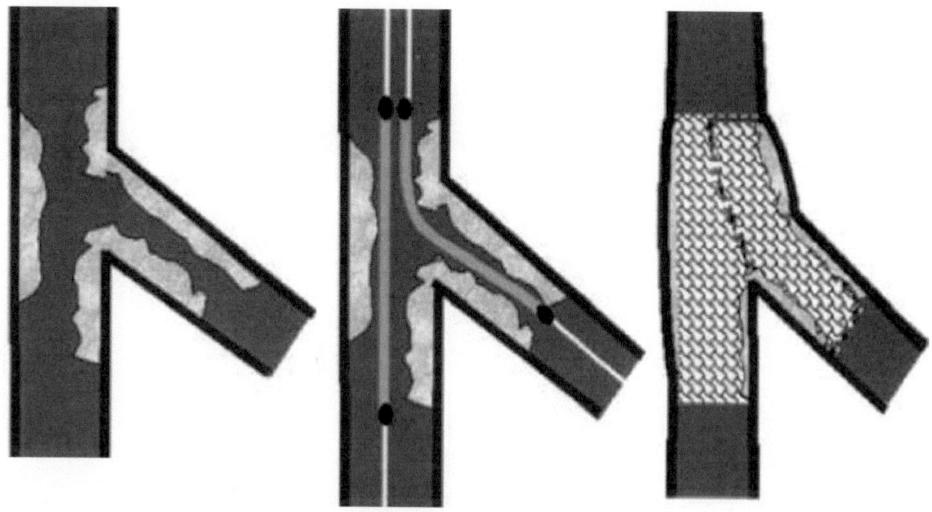

Importantly, this technique requires a guiding catheter large enough to accommodate two stents simultaneously (usually 7Fr or greater). Once both stents have been positioned and care has been given to making certain the proximal edges are lined up, both stents are simultaneously inflated and deployed at the same pressures. The difference between an SKS and a crush, which often positions the stents in the same manner, is the way the stents are deployed. In a crush, the stents are deployed sequentially, whereas in an SKS, they are deployed simultaneously. Essentially, simultaneous deployment creates a new carina which extends from the side branch to the proximal extent of the stented main branch. If one were to look down the main vessel, the previous single lumen would be converted into two lumens side by side, each outlined with stent. Because of the similarity to a shotgun barrel when visualized in this manner, this technique is also referred to as the double barrel technique. Advantages include the ability to maintain guidewire control of both the side branch and the main vessel at all times during the intervention (no need to recross). Additionally, this technique can be performed quickly in patients with compromised hemodynamics, allowing rapid reperfusion of threatened coronary distributions. However, dealing with restenosis at a later date can be an issue, as recrossing the double lumen cleanly with a guidewire can be tricky, as the guidewire often inadvertently crosses into the carina between the two stents (which does not allow passage of equipment or disrupts the architecture if the equipment crosses). Occasionally, if the vessel cannot be cleanly recrossed, the initial SKS can be converted to a crush, where either the main vessel or side vessel stent is crushed to the side and then recrossed. Overall, SKS's main advantage is that it allows for rapid stent deployment with favorable intermediate outcomes when compared to the provisional approach [18].

V-stenting is another method of dedicated stenting for bifurcation lesions. In this technique, which is best suited for moderate to narrowly angulated lesions, two stents are aligned with the proximal edges just proximal to the side branch and both stents are deployed together simultaneously (Fig. 22.6). The difference between V-stenting and double barrel stenting is that in the former, there is minimal to no overlap of the proximal stent portions, whereas in the latter, there is formation of a length new carina between the stents. V-stenting can be performed quickly and relatively easily, with no need for recrossing, but is really ideally suited to bifurcation lesions that have the bulk of the disease at or beyond the bifurcation (Medina classification 0, x, x).

Culotte (or "Y") stenting is a dedicated approach for bifurcation lesions. First described in 1998 by Chevalier [19], this technique takes its name from the French word for trousers. Much like a trouser leg, in this technique two stent "legs" are extended down the main vessel and side branch, with the proximal portions of the stents deployed concentrically inside one another. In practice, this results in the proximal portion of the vessel having two layers of stent and the area distal to the bifurcation having just one layer. The technique for performing a culotte technique is perhaps the most demanding of all dedicated approaches, both in terms of wire technique and deployment sequence of the stents. Despite this challenge, the procedure times, fluoroscopic times, and contrast volumes are similar between this dedicated approach and others [20]. To perform a culotte, both the main vessel and side branch are wired and predilation is performed. Next, the side branch stent is deployed so it extends back across the ostium of the side branch into the main vessel. This traps the wire which was in the main branch outside the side branch stent. An additional wire is then used to cross into the lumen side

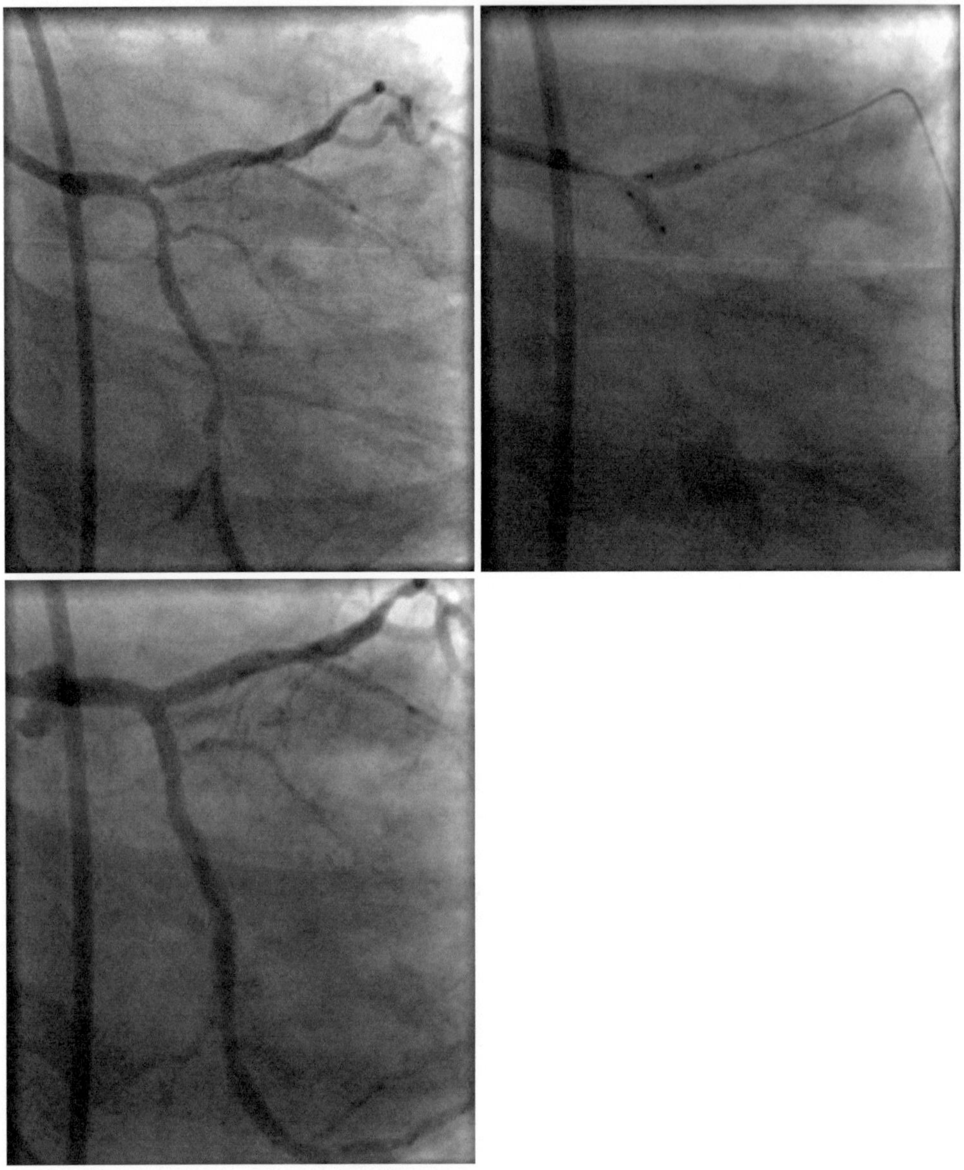

Fig. 22.6 V-stenting is another method of dedicated stenting for bifurcation lesions

branch stent, exiting the stent via a side cell into the downstream main vessel. At this point the trapped wire can be removed and the main branch stent can be delivered over the newly placed main vessel guidewire. Note that the proximal portion of the main vessel will now have two stents concentrically positioned. Prior to deployment of the main vessel stent, the wire should be removed from the side branch so as not to pin it between two layers of stent. Once the side branch wire is out and the main vessel stent is deployed, the side branch can be recrossed and final kissing balloon angioplasty is then performed (Fig. 22.7). Functionally, the culotte technique has been shown to have less in-stent restenosis when compared with the crush technique, with no difference in overall major adverse cardiac events [20].

Randomized Data for Bifurcation Approaches

Since the availability of drug-eluting stents, a number of randomized trials have been performed to assess an optimal approach to bifurcation stenosis, primarily comparing the provisional approach to a dedicated two-stent strategy (Table 22.1) [15]. Although there is significant heterogeneity between the trial end points, stenting strategies used, lesion characteristics, and side branch bailout approaches, general wisdom holds that for most bifurcations, there is no disadvantage to a provisional approach in terms of clinical outcomes. Moreover, a provisional approach allows for potentially less resource utilization, less procedure time, and less procedure complexity. However, interventionalists need

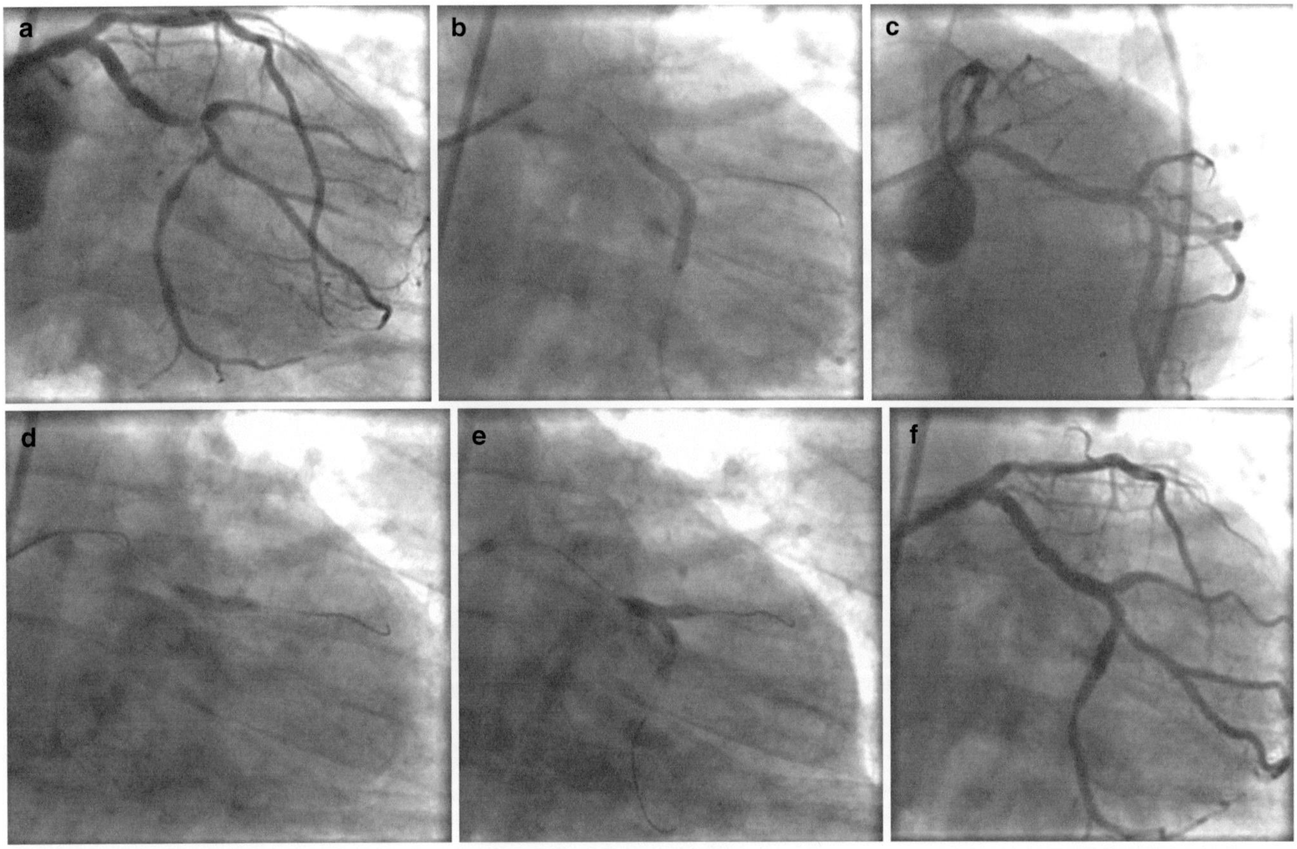

Fig. 22.7 (a–f) Culotte (or "Y") stenting is a dedicated approach for bifurcation lesions

Table 22.1 Outcomes of patients with bifurcation lesions randomized to Elective Double Stenting (*EDS*) Versus Provisional Stenting (*PS*)

	NORDIC [7]		BBK [8]		CACTUS [9]		BBC-ONE [10]	
Study	Elective (*N*=206)	Provisional (*N*=207)	Elective (*N*=101)	Provisional (*N*=101)	Elective (*N*=177)	Provisional (*N*=173)	Elective (*N*=250)	Provisional (*N*=250)
Clinical Outcome	6 months		1 year		6 months		9 months	
Primary end point	Death, MI, TVR, or Stent thrombosis		% DS of the SB		Death, MI, TVR		Death, MI, TVF	
	3.4 %	2.9 %	27.7 ± 24.8	23.0 ± 20.2	15.8 %	15 %	15.2 %*	8 %*
Death (%)	1.5	1	1	2	0.0	0.5	0.8	0.4
Non- fatal MI (%)	0.5	0.0	2	1	10.7	8.6	11.2*	3.6*
Peri-procedure	18	8	NA	NA	8.5	6.9	6.8	1.6
TVR (%)	1.9	1.9	8.9	10.9	7.9	7.5	6.8	5.6
Stent thrombosis (%)	0.0	0.5	2	1	1.7	1.1	2.4	0.4
Angiographic outcome	8 months		9 months		6 months		NA	
Re stenosis (%)								
MV	5.1	4.6	3.1	7.3	4.6	6.7	NA	NA
SB		19.2	12.5	9.4	13.2	14.7	NA	NA
%DS in SB	24 ± 21*	31 ± 22*	27.7 ± 24.8	23.0 ± 20.2	30 ± 19	31 ± 22	NA	NA

From Moussa [15], with permission

The CACTUS trial: Peri-procedural and non-Q-wave MI was defined as an elevation of postprocedural CK levels >2 times normal levels with elevated CK-MB in the absence of pathological Q waves.

The NORDIC trial: Peri-procedural cardiac biomarker elevation was defined as a CK-MB or troponin increase to ≥3 times the upper limit of normal with or without clinical manifestations.

BBC ONE: Peri-procedure non-Q-wave myocardial infarction was defined as a CK-MB or troponin increase to ≥3 times the upper limit of normal.

BBK: Peri-procedure Non-Q-wave myocardial infarction was defined as. an elevation of creatine kinase or its MB isoenzyme to at least three times the upper limit of normal in two samples during hospitalization.

*$p < 0.05$

to remember that randomized data is not a substitute for keen clinical judgment in approaching the more complex bifurcation lesions, many of which were not well represented in the randomized trials and may be better served with a dedicated two-stent approach [15].

One of the first randomized trials of a provisional versus dedicated approach to bifurcation lesions was the Nordic trial [21] in which 413 patients with bifurcation lesions were assigned to one of the two treatments, with the patients assigned to a two-stent approach undergoing culotte or crush stenting at the discretion of the operator. Primary end points were cardiac death, myocardial infarction, target-vessel revascularization, or stent thrombosis assessed at 6 months. Overall, there was no difference in the primary outcome to 6 months in the trial, with rates of 2.9 % in the provisional group and 3.4 % in the dedicated group. A subset of these patients underwent angiographic follow-up at 8 months, which revealed very similar outcomes in the two arms. There was a slight advantage to a two-stent strategy in minimal lumen diameter of the side branch (1.90 mm versus 1.76 mm, $p=0.018$) and SB stenosis or occlusion at follow-up (11.5 % vs. 19.2 %, $p=0.062$), but all other angiographic parameters were similar. Of note, the "cost" of a dedicated approach was higher contrast volume, fluoroscopy time, and procedure time with a higher incidence of biomarker elevation in the dedicated two-stent group. Overall, the authors concluded that the data support a de facto provisional approach, although they concede that certain bifurcation lesions (such as those with large side branches and complex disease) may in fact be better served with a dedicated strategy.

The BBK trial [22] randomly assigned 202 patients with bifurcation lesions to a provisional or T-stent strategy with a primary outcome of percent angiographic diameter stenosis of the side branch at 9-month follow-up. Additional end points were clinical outcomes at 1- and 2-year intervals, including death and myocardial infarction. Overall, there were no statistical differences between the two groups for the primary end point, nor were there any clinical differences between the groups at follow-up. Encouragingly in this trial which used sirolimus-eluting stents, the rates of stent thrombosis and death were very low in both groups, suggesting a safety signal in this patient population who historically have had higher incidences of adverse cardiac events [3]. In parallel to the Nordic trial, results from the BBK trial suggest that a provisional stent strategy is the optimal approach for most bifurcation lesions [21, 22].

Shortly after the publication of the Nordic and BBK trials, the Cactus trial was reported [23]. In this randomized trial, 350 patients with bifurcation lesions were assigned to a dedicated crush-stenting approach or to a provisional strategy using sirolimus-eluting stents. Of note, final kissing balloon inflation was mandated in the patients randomized to the dedicated arm (crush stenting). The primary angiographic outcome measure was in-segment restenosis at 6 months, and the primary clinical outcome was MACE defined as cardiac death, myocardial infarction, or target-vessel revascularization at 6 months. The results demonstrated a statistically identical, but numerically lower, rate of restenosis in the side branch of 13.2 % in patients who received the dedicated crush versus 14.7 % in those with provisional stenting [23]. Clinical outcomes as measured by MACE at 6 months were also identical between the two approaches. Notably, about a third of the patients assigned to the provisional stent arm crossed over and had a second stent (T-stent), which suggests that a significant portion of lesion subsets will not yield acceptable angiographic results with a provisional approach. Yet despite this finding, this trial again supported the preceding trials (Nordic, BBK) in finding that a provisional approach, while not producing better angiographic or clinical results than a dedicated two-stent strategy, at least results in outcomes which are no worse with the added benefit of shorter procedure time, less contrast administration, and less equipment usage.

The BBC-One trial [24] is another randomized trial to compare a provisional and dedicated approach in bifurcation lesions. In this trial, which used paclitaxel-eluting stents, 500 patients were randomly assigned to provisional stenting or dedicated two-stent strategies (using crush or culotte) and were followed for the primary end point of death, myocardial infarction, or target-vessel failure at 9 months. Contrary to previous trials, the 9-month primary outcome was statistically more likely to occur in the dedicated two-stent strategy (15.2 % vs. 8.0 %, $p=0.009$) [24]. This was driven largely by a higher incidence of periprocedural myocardial infarction in the dedicated two-stent arm of the trial. It is very possible that the choice of stent/polymer drug, in this case paclitaxel, may have influenced this outcome, as previous studies have also found superior results with sirolimus stents in bifurcation lesions when compared to paclitaxel stents [25, 26].

The DKCrush-II trial[27] is the most recent randomized trial comparing a double kissing crush technique with provisional stenting. In this trial, 370 patients were assigned to either the double kissing crush technique or the provisional technique. Of the patients assigned to the provisional technique, about 28 % crossed over to a 2-stent technique. Double kissing crush technique [28] involves deploying the side branch stent, balloon crushing that stent, then performing a kissing balloon inflation in the side branch and main vessel. Next, the main vessel stent is deployed and a final kissing balloon angioplasty is performed. In the DKCrush trial, the primary end point was MACE at 12 months and the secondary end point was angiographic restenosis at 8 months. Results of the study demonstrated a lower rate of target-lesion revascularization in the two-stent group (4.3 % vs. 13.0 %, $p=0.005$) and lower target-vessel revascularization in the two-stent approach (6.5 % vs .14.6 %, $p=0.017$) [27]. Moreover, the restenosis in the side branch was 4.9 vs. 22.2 % ($p=0.001$) when comparing the two-stent approach to the provisional approach, respectively. Taken together, the trial stands alone by offering the first randomized evidence that a dedicated two-stent strategy has statistically significant benefit over a provisional approach.

Dedicated Bifurcation Stents

The vast data generated with drug-eluting stents demonstrates their ability to address straight lesions with high procedural success, minimal complications, and durable long-term results. The quest to achieve similar results when addressing bifurcation lesions has been more elusive. This is felt to be in large part due to the inability of "workhorse" DES to achieve similar stent coverage and radial strength at the carina of a bifurcation lesion as is possible with straight lesions. This is understandable, in that "workhorse" DES's were designed to treat straight lesions. This has led industry to design and develop stents designed specifically for bifurcation lesions.

When examining the various bifurcation-specific stents, it is logical to group stents by their design using two parameter sets: balloon expandable versus self-expanding and main branch versus side branch as depicted in Fig. 22.8.

Balloon Expandable/Main Branch Stent

The most common approach attempted has been to intercalate into the standard "workhorse" design a design feature, typically an aperture, which can accommodate the side branch ostium. The challenge with this approach is that for the stent to provide side branch origin, scaffolding requires it to be tracked to the lesion site and rotated such that the aperture and the side branch origin are aligned. There are many example stents designed using this of this approach including the TAXUS® *Petal*™ (*Boston Scientific* Corporation, Natick, MA, USA), Antares (TriReme Medical, Inc., Pleasanton, CA, USA), Xience Side Branch Access Stent (Abbott Vascular, Santa Clara, CA, USA), and Nile Paclitaxel-Eluting SideBranch Access Stent (Minvasys, Gennevilliers, France). The strength of this design approach is that it is consistent with a "provisional" approach allowing the main branch to be stented initially followed by side branch stent if there is high-grade residual stenosis or decreased flow. Furthermore, this approach allows for a device manufacturer to leverage much of what has been developed for its main branch stent including basic design and drug-drug delivery polymer and balloon delivery systems. For stents with this design feature to work, it requires both axial and radial alignment of the side branch feature with the side branch origin. The addition of radial alignment requires new design features to the stent-delivery balloon. These designs have universally required the addition of a second wire lumen and typically an additional dilation balloon. In addition to the larger size and mass associated with

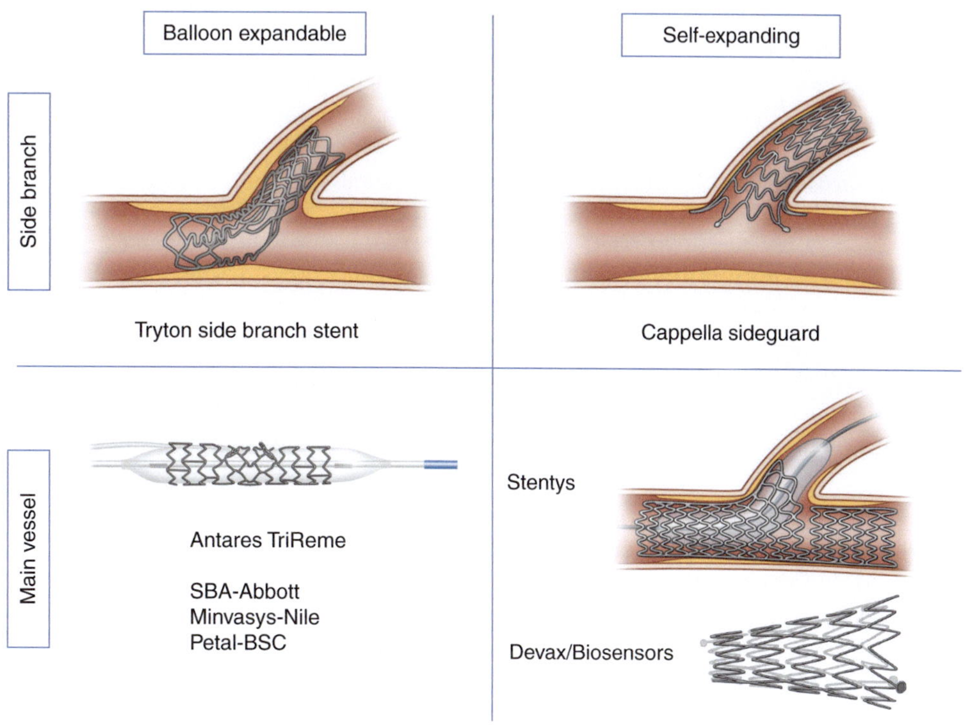

Fig. 22.8 Dedicated bifurcation stents

this delivery system, they limit rotational freedom of the devices which has resulted in tracking difficulties. The combination of the difficult manufacturing, marginal performance, and an uncertain regulatory pathway in the USA had led to the largest medical device manufacturers to abandon these projects.

Self-Expanding/Main Branch Stent

Another approach is to utilize a self-expanding design to address this problem. Unlike the balloon expandable main branch designs discussed above, self-expanding main branch designs do not require rotational orientation for side branch ostium alignment. There have been two designs, which fall into this category: STENTYS stent (STENTYS SA, Paris, France) and the Devax-Axxess Plus (BioSensors International, Ltd., Singapore).

The Devax-Axxess Plus stent is a slotted tube self-expanding stent with a reverse taper intended to be placed in the proximal main branch after which the distal main branch and side branch segments can be treated. The Devax stent is coated with Biolomus A9 and has been studied most notably in the Diverge Trial, a single-arm study in which 305 patient were treated with an impressive procedural success rate of 96.7 %, a 9-month restenosis rate of 6.4 %, and a MACE rate of 14 % at 2 years [29].

The STENTYS stent is tubular self-expanding stent with small detachable interconnectors. The stent is tracked to the lesion site across the side branch ostium. When side branch access is desired, the operator wires the ostium and tracks balloon through a side cell. The interconnectors are disconnected allowing for side branch access. The STENTYS stent has been developed both in a bare metal and with DES (paclitaxel-eluted via a biostable polysulfone polymer). This platform has been studied in Open I Trial in which 60 stents were implanted in 63 patients (33 BMS, 27 DES) with a procedural success of 95.2 %, a 6-month MACE rate of 3.75 for DES (3.7 %), and 27.3 % BMS [30]. The bare metal STENTYS is the focus of the APPOSITION IV Trial, an 880 US IDE Trial focused on a STEMI (not bifurcation lesions) indication. Further bifurcation studies are in the planning stages.

Self-Expanding/Side Branch Stent

Specialized side branch stent design strategy has been utilized using both a balloon expandable and self-expanding formats. The Sideguard Stent (Cappella Medical Devices, Ltd., Galway, Ireland) utilizes a trumpet-shaped design made of nitinol, a shape memory alloy that returns to its original shape when unconstrained. The Cappella Stent is mounted on a specialized delivery system, which utilizes a balloon-facilitated, split-sheath system. The Sideguard is delivered to the side branch with the proximally flared trumpet design feature at the side branch ostium. The stent is secured within the side branch with balloon inflation which also releases the split sheath allowing the unconstrained stent to conform to the side branch ostium. The balloon-sheath delivery system is then removed after which a "workhorse" main vessel stent is tracked to the lesion site covering the now stented side branch ostium. This procedure is typically completed with a simultaneous kiss. The Cappella Sideguard 1 and 2 studies ($n=83$) with 12 month MACE 9.6 % and TLR 9.6 % with a late loss of 0.58 mm [31].

Balloon Expandable/Side Branch Stent

The final approach to be discussed is the balloon expandable/ side branch stent design strategy, which has been utilized by the Tryton Side Branch Stent (Tryton Medical, Inc., Durham, NC). The strength of this design approach is that it allows for utilization of an established slotted tube technology as well as a standard balloon delivery system without the need for rotational orientation. The Tryton Side Branch Stent is a slotted tube thin strut CoCr (L605) stent comprised of three zones: a side branch zone which has features (coverage and radial strength) typical of "workhorse" stent, a transition zone which is specifically designed to provide ostial coverage which can accommodate the wide range of angles and geometries encountered clinically, and a proximal zone with minimal metal to provide access for the "workhorse" DES. The system is mounted on a standard rapid-exchange stepped balloon delivery system and is deployed like a standard stent. The Tryton has received CE Mark and was studied in the initial first-in-man trial which demonstrated a high procedural success (93.3 %) and with a low 6-month TVR of 3.3 % and late loss of 0.17 ± 0.35 mm [32]. These results have been replicated in many different settings with similar results. Grundeken and colleagues recently presented a pooled patient level analysis from 9 studies involving 905 patients with a 4.0 % TLR rate and a stent thrombosis rate of 0.5 %[33]. The Tryton Side Branch Stent is being compared to balloon angioplasty (provisional) stenting in the treatment complex bifurcation disease in a Pivotal IDE Study randomizing 704 patients involving >60 centers in the USA, Europe, and Israel. This trial is scheduled to be completed with data available by the end of 2013.

Conclusions

Bifurcation lesions are relatively common and intervention on them is associated with higher rates of MACE, more complexity, and longer procedure times. Overall, the last 10 years since the advent of drug-eluting stents, cardiologists have become more aggressive in their treatment for these difficult lesions. Most randomized data (with the exception of DKCRUSH trial) have demonstrated parity in outcomes using a provisional approach to bifurcation work. Nevertheless, there are certain situations where a two-stent approach seems logical, including large side vessels, high-grade disease in either branch of the bifurcation, and heavily angulated lesions. Many techniques for dedicated approaches to treating bifurcations exist, but available evidence suggests that either the culotte technique or DK crush technique is probably the preferred method of intervention. Over the coming years, more information will become available about the newer bifurcation-specific stent designs and how they perform compared to current options. Until then, interventional cardiologists must use common sense and good clinical judgment to help shape decision making for treating bifurcation lesions.

References

1. Louvard Y, et al. Classification of coronary artery bifurcation lesions and treatments: time for a consensus! Catheter Cardiovasc Interv. 2008;71(2):175–83.
2. Freed E, Safian R, Grines C. Manual of interventional cardiology. In: Koller P, Safian R, editors. Bifurcation stenosis. 1st ed. Birmingham: Physician Press; 1997. p. 229–41.
3. Iakovou I, et al. Incidence, predictors, and outcome of thrombosis after successful implantation of drug-eluting stents. JAMA. 2005;293(17):2126–30.
4. Al Suwaidi J, et al. Immediate and one-year outcome in patients with coronary bifurcation lesions in the modern era (NHLBI dynamic registry). Am J Cardiol. 2001;87(10):1139–44.
5. Sheiban I, et al. Immediate and long-term results of "T" stenting for bifurcation coronary lesions. Am J Cardiol. 2000;85(9):1141–4. A9.
6. Movahed MR, et al. Coronary artery bifurcation lesions: a review and update on classification and interventional techniques. Cardiovasc Revasc Med. 2008;9(4):263–8.
7. Onuma Y, et al. Tryton I, First-In-Man (FIM) study: six month clinical and angiographic outcome, analysis with new quantitative coronary angiography dedicated for bifurcation lesions. EuroIntervention J EuroPCR Collab Work Group Interv Cardiol Eur Soc Cardiol. 2008;3(5):546–52.
8. Lefèvre T, et al. Stenting of bifurcation lesions: classification, treatments, and results. Catheter Cardiovasc Interv. 2000;49(3): 274–83.
9. Zlotnick DM, et al. Classification and treatment of coronary artery bifurcation lesions: putting the Medina classification to the test. Cardiovasc Revasc Med. 2012;13(4):228–33.
10. Dzavik V, et al. Predictors of long-term outcome after crush stenting of coronary bifurcation lesions: importance of the bifurcation angle. Am Heart J. 2006;152(4):762–9.
11. Latib A, Colombo A. Bifurcation disease: what do we know, what should we do? JACC Cardiovasc Interv. 2008;1(3):218–26.
12. Ong AT, et al. Thirty-day incidence and six-month clinical outcome of thrombotic stent occlusion after bare-metal, sirolimus, or paclitaxel stent implantation. J Am Coll Cardiol. 2005;45(6):947–53.
13. Ge L, et al. Treatment of bifurcation lesions with two stents: one year angiographic and clinical follow up of crush versus T stenting. Heart. 2006;92(3):371–6.
14. Colombo A, et al. Modified T-stenting technique with crushing for bifurcation lesions: immediate results and 30-day outcome. Catheter Cardiovasc Interv. 2003;60(2):145–51.
15. Moussa ID. Coronary artery bifurcation interventions: the disconnect between randomized clinical trials and patient centered decision-making. Catheter Cardiovasc Interv. 2011;77(4):537–45.
16. Ge L, et al. Clinical and angiographic outcome after implantation of drug-eluting stents in bifurcation lesions with the crush stent technique: importance of final kissing balloon post-dilation. J Am Coll Cardiol. 2005;46(4):613–20.
17. Colombo A, et al. Randomized study to evaluate sirolimus-eluting stents implanted at coronary bifurcation lesions. Circulation. 2004;109(10):1244–9.
18. Sharma SK, et al. Simultaneous kissing stents (SKS) technique for treating bifurcation lesions in medium-to-large size coronary arteries. Am J Cardiol. 2004;94(7):913–17.
19. Chevalier B, et al. Placement of coronary stents in bifurcation lesions by the "culotte" technique. Am J Cardiol. 1998;82(8):943–9.
20. Erglis A, et al. Randomized comparison of coronary bifurcation stenting with the crush versus the culotte technique using sirolimus eluting stents: the Nordic stent technique study. Circ Cardiovasc Interv. 2009;2(1):27–34.
21. Steigen TK, et al. Randomized study on simple versus complex stenting of coronary artery bifurcation lesions: the Nordic bifurcation study. Circulation. 2006;114(18):1955–61.
22. Ferenc M, et al. Randomized trial on routine vs. provisional T-stenting in the treatment of de novo coronary bifurcation lesions. Eur Heart J. 2008;29(23):2859–67.
23. Colombo A, et al. Randomized study of the crush technique versus provisional side-branch stenting in true coronary bifurcations: the CACTUS (Coronary bifurcations: application of the crushing technique using sirolimus-eluting stents) study. Circulation. 2009;119(1):71–8.
24. Hildick-Smith D, et al. Randomized trial of simple versus complex drug-eluting stenting for bifurcation lesions: the British Bifurcation Coronary Study: old, new, and evolving strategies. Circulation. 2010;121(10):1235–43.
25. Chen S, et al. Crush stenting with paclitaxel-eluting or sirolimus-eluting stents for the treatment of coronary bifurcation lesions. Angiology. 2008;59(4):475–83.
26. Pan M, et al. Drug-eluting stents for the treatment of bifurcation lesions: a randomized comparison between paclitaxel and sirolimus stents. Am Heart J. 2007;153(1):15e1–7.
27. Chen S-L, et al. A Randomized Clinical Study comparing double kissing crush with provisional stenting for treatment of coronary bifurcation lesions results from the DKCRUSH-II (Double kissing crush versus provisional stenting technique for treatment of coronary bifurcation lesions) trial. J Am Coll Cardiol. 2011;57(8):914–20.
28. Chen S-L, et al. DK crush technique: modified treatment of bifurcation lesions in coronary artery. Chin Med J. 2005;118(20):1746–50.
29. Verheye S. The DIVERGE trial (DES intervention for treating side branches effectively): 3-year clinical results. EuroIntervention J EuroPCR Collab Work Group Interv Cardiol Eur Soc Cardiol. 2011;7(Supplement M):428–33.
30. Verheye S, et al. Six-month clinical and angiographic results of the STENTYS(R) self-apposing stent in bifurcation lesions. EuroIntervention. 2011;7(5):580–7.
31. Latib A. Procedural outcomes from the European Sideguard Registry. EuroIntervention J EuroPCR Collab Work Group Interv Cardiol Eur Soc Cardiol. 2010;6(Supplement J):143–46.
32. Onuma Y, et al. Tryton I, First-In-Man (FIM) study: six month clinical and angiographic outcome, analysis with new quantitative coronary angiography dedicated for bifurcation lesions. EuroIntervention. 2008;3(5):546–52.
33. Grundeken MJ, et al. Six-month clinical outcomes of the Tryton Side Branch Stent for the treatment of bifurcation lesions. Neth Heart J. 2012;20(11):439–46.

Chronic Total Occlusion Angioplasty: Indications, Appropriateness, and Strategy

23

J. Aaron Grantham and Craig A. Thompson

Chronic total occlusions (CTOs) are commonly encountered complex coronary lesions that can be associated with symptoms, ischemia, LV dysfunction, and excess mortality. The decision to offer percutaneous coronary intervention (PCI) as part of the therapeutic regimen for patients with chronic total occlusions is complex and should include a detailed discussion with patients about the indications, goals, risks, and alternatives to PCI that also includes a comprehensive review of all of the available data. In this chapter, we will review the evidence for the benefits of CTO PCI, a deep understanding of which is fundamentally important to the selection of patients for whom this therapy is to be offered.

CTO Prevalence and Current Practice in North America

CTOs are commonly encountered complex coronary lesions discovered in approximately one of every six patients referred for coronary angiography [1]. Fefer and colleagues evaluated 14,439 patients entered into the Canadian CTO Registry. Among the three participating centers, 2,630 CTOs were discovered (18.3 %). Among those with prior bypass and those presenting with ST elevation myocardial infarction (STEMI), who were eventually excluded from subsequent analyses, CTO was discovered in 54 and 10 %, respectively. Prior studies have suggested that the prevalence of CTO among patients referred for coronary angiography was between 15 and 50 % [2, 3]. The variability is attributable to the varying definitions of both CTO and population being evaluated. For instance, some studies were restricted to only those who were discovered to have coronary artery disease. Nonetheless CTOs are discovered as a part of the routine practice of diagnostic coronary angiography. Yet CTO PCI rates are low.

Abbott and colleagues found that only 5 % of PCIs in the NHLBI registry were performed for CTO [4]. We used the National Cardiovascular Disease Registry (NCDR) Catheterization and PCI registries and found that when a CTO is discovered it is attempted only 13.7 % of the time [5]. Further, we identified operator characteristics (specifically operator PCI volume) that were independently associated with the likelihood of attempting a CTO PCI. Using the same definition of attempt rate, Fefer and colleagues [1] identified variability in the attempt rate between institutions ranging from 1 to 16 %. While referral rates for coronary artery bypass surgery remained consistent between institutions. Variability can be a sign of over or underutilization. In the case of CTO PCI, it would be hard to argue that over utilization exists given the very low attempt rates overall and the barriers to CTO PCI that have impeded widespread adoption of contemporary CTO PCI techniques. Taken together these observations both from Canada and the United States suggest that patients with chronic total occlusions are more likely to be offered therapy based on where and from whom they receive care rather than on which therapy might benefit them the most.

Determining the optimal CTO PCI attempt rate would ultimately require an assessment of the appropriateness of CTO PCI which examines the appropriate, uncertain, and inappropriate use of PCI in this setting. No effort, as yet, has been made to examine underutilization of PCI in patients with CTOs.

J.A. Grantham, MD, FACC
Department of Medicine, University of Missouri School of Medicine, Columbia, MO, USA

St. Luke's Mid America Heart Institute, Kansas City, MO, USA
e-mail: jgrantham@saint-lukes.org

C.A. Thompson, MD, MMSc (✉)
Director, Cardiovascular Catheterization and Intervention, Yale New Haven Hospital, New Haven, CT, USA

Cardiology Section, Department of Medicine, Director, Invasive Cardiology and Vascular Medicine, Yale University School of Medicine, 789 Howard Avenue, Dana 305, New Haven, CT 06520, USA
e-mail: craig.a.thompson99@icloud.com

C.A. Thompson (ed.), *Textbook of Cardiovascular Intervention*,
DOI 10.1007/978-1-4471-4528-8_23, © Springer-Verlag London 2014

Appropriateness and CTO PCI

Recently the American College of Cardiology Foundation, joined by multiple stake holders in coronary revascularization, released the Appropriate Use Criterion (AUC) for revascularization [6]. The AUC represent an attempt to codify clinical decision-making. The rational for AUC are at least in part, based upon observed variability in the treatment of patients with coronary artery disease between operators, institutions, and Medicare recipients (Dartmouth Atlas Project. Available at: http://www.dartmouthatlas.org). AUC potentially serve multiple roles. According the AUC document for revascularization, "Appropriateness criteria are developed to serve as a supplement to ACC/AHA guideline documents. Appropriateness criteria are designed to examine the use of diagnostic and therapeutic procedures to support efficient use of medical resources during the pursuit of quality medical care…they cannot act as substitutes for sound clinical judgment and practice experience. Rather, the aim of these criteria is to allow assessment of utilization patterns for a test or procedure. Comparing utilization patterns across a large subset of provider's patients can allow for an assessment of a provider's management strategies with those of his/her peers. The ACCF and its collaborators believe that an ongoing review of one's practice using these criteria will help guide a more effective, efficient, and equitable allocation of health care resources, and ultimately, better patient outcomes."

The AUC technical panel, none of whom had expertise in CTO PCI at the time, rated a multitude of clinical scenarios. Within those clinical scenarios were 18 rankings that included hypothetical patients with single-vessel chronic total occlusions (Fig. 23.1). An examination of these AUC technical panel recommendations on the appropriateness of coronary revascularization of patients with CTOs is worthwhile.

There were four scenarios which were deemed to be appropriate for revascularization in the setting of the single-vessel CTO. These four scenarios included patients with severe angina (CCS Class 3 or 4) who were treated with maximum medical therapy (two or more antiangina drugs), regardless of the risk associated with noninvasive imaging (low, intermediate, or high). One additional scenario included patients with mild angina (CCS Classes 1 and 2) who were on maximal therapy and found to have high-risk noninvasive imaging features. There were six clinical scenarios deemed to be inappropriate. These included patients that were asymptomatic, not on maximal medical therapy, regardless of the noninvasive risk assessment and those who were found to have low risk stress testing and on less than two anti-ischemic drugs regardless of their symptom classification (none, mild, or severe). The remaining nine clinical scenarios were deemed to be of uncertain appropriateness.

Single vessel

	Class 0	Class I/II	Class III/IV
High Risk Max Rx	U	A	A
Int Risk Max Rx	U	U	A
Low Risk Max Rx	U	U	A
High Risk No Rx	I	U	U
Int Risk No Rx	I	U	U
Low Risk No Rx	I	I	I

Fig. 23.1 Single-vessel chronic total occlusions

Recall that appropriate is defined as highly likely to confer benefit to the patient, inappropriate was unlikely to confer benefit to the patient, and uncertain was uncertainty based upon a lack of data, to confer benefit to the patient. While these criteria were intended to inform physicians, payers and patients as to the appropriateness of "revascularization," these criteria have been used and in the future will be used to address the appropriateness of PCI specifically [7].

Figure 23.2 illustrates the eighteen clinical scenarios that include patients with one- or two-vessel disease not involving the proximal LAD. It is particularly interesting to note that there are five down codes in the appropriateness of the single-vessel chronic total occlusion in comparison to one- or two-vessel disease not involving the proximal LAD (i.e., non-CTO disease).

Symptomatic Patients

Considering the four scenarios where appropriateness is downgraded among patients with symptoms and a single-vessel CTO compared to a subtotal lesion, it is difficult to imagine that a patient with a chronic total occlusion would derive less benefit from revascularization than patients with a chronic subtotal occlusion. Take for instance two patients with mild angina on maximal medical therapy with intermediate risk noninvasive imaging studies. One has a 70 % mid right coronary artery lesion and receives PCI or bypass surgery. That procedure would be graded as appropriate. The other patient has a 100 % mid right coronary artery lesion. Revascularization with either PCI or CABG surgery in this case would be considered of uncertain appropriateness. While an uncertain rating does not preclude revascularization, it does imply less certainty over benefit. This can no longer be argued in light of several studies, some recent and some not so recent [8–10].

Whether assessed by physician reported (CCS class) or patient reported methods (e.g., the Seattle Angina Questionnaire [11]), successful CTO PCI is associated with improvements in symptoms and quality of life as compared to unsuccessful CTO PCI. Recently, Safley and colleagues [12] have shown that CTO PCI was as effective at alleviating symptoms and restoring physical function and quality of life as non-CTO disease (Table 23.1). In this study, the final Seattle Angina (SAQ) scores and Rose dyspnea scale scores among the CTO group were equal to the non-CTO group despite lower success rates in the CTO groups (86 % vs. 96 %, $p<0.05$).

1 or 2VD no proximal

	Class 0	Class I/II	Class III/IV
High Risk Max Rx	A	A	A
Int Risk Max Rx	U	A	A
Low Risk Max Rx	U	A	A
High Risk No Rx	I	U	A
Int Risk No Rx	I	U	U
Low Risk No Rx	I	I	U

Fig. 23.2 Eighteen clinical scenarios that include patients with one- or two-vessel disease not involving the proximal LAD

One scenario does preclude revascularization for CTO but not non-CTO disease. Consider the patient with Class 3 or 4 angina on less than two anti-ischemic drugs and a low risk noninvasive imaging study. Revascularization in a patient with these characteristics and a 70 % mid right coronary artery lesion would be of uncertain appropriateness, whereas if the lesion were a chronic total occlusion, revascularization would be deemed inappropriate. Again, it is inconceivable that the patient with a symptom causing CTO would be less likely to benefit from revascularization than one with a symptom causing non-CTO. It cannot be argued that concerns over procedural safety drove this inconsistency because revascularization could have been done by CABG surgery, which carries the same risk no matter what the severity of occlusion.

Especially among those patients who are symptomatic, the systematic down coding in the appropriateness of revascularization for patients with chronic total occlusions is illogical, even when applying the AUC solely to percutaneous revascularization. There is no doubt that revascularization confers the benefit of angina relief among patients with CTOs, especially when the revascularization method is PCI. These logical incongruities violate the principle that revascularization should be offered based upon the patient's needs as reflected in their symptoms, not the angiogram, and should be corrected in future AUC updates.

Asymptomatic Patients

It can be argued that PCI outside of the setting, acute coronary syndrome does not confer a survival advantage. This contention however is being challenged by a plethora of data suggesting a potential of survival benefit no matter what method of ischemic burden reduction is used. There is now sufficient equipoise to warrant a randomized controlled trial

Table 23.1 Success of CTO vs. no CTO

	CTO $n=124$	No CTO $n=1833$	
Baseline health status			
SAQ physical limitation score	72.1 ± 26.9	77.9 ± 23.4	0.016
SAQ angina frequency score	70.1 ± 28.1	72.9 ± 23.6	0.212
SAQ quality of life score	54.3 ± 25.5	56.0 ± 25.4	0.487
Rose dyspnea score	1.9 ± 1.5	1.7 ± 1.5	0.209
6-month health status			
SAQ physical limitation score	96.2 ± 12.8	95.7 ± 12.9	0.742
SAQ angina frequency score	91.0 ± 19.0	93.2 ± 15.1	0.126
SAQ quality of life score	80.6 ± 21.4	80.5 ± 19.9	0.951
Rose dyspnea score	1.0 ± 1.4	0.9 ± 1.3	0.497

of PCI vs. medical therapy based on the baseline ischemic burden (ISCHEMIA trial www.NIH.gov).

It has long been suggested that among patients with a CTO successful PCI, compared to unsuccessful CTO PCI, there is associated survival advantage. Among patients who are asymptomatic, with a high-risk stress test, on maximal medical therapy and with a subtotal culprit lesion, revascularization is deemed appropriate. However, when the culprit is a CTO, revascularization is rated of uncertain appropriateness.

CTO PCI and Survival

In 2001, Suero and colleagues published the first retrospective analysis that suggested there may be an association between successful CTO PCI and survival [13]. These findings have been reproduced by several other groups and institutions and have also been challenged. In a recent meta-analysis of 13 reports of success vs. failed CTO PCI, Joyal et al. found that the odds ratio of death during the variable time of follow-up among the reports was 0.56 with a 95 % confidence interval of 0.43–0.72 and $p<0.0001$ [9]. While retrospective analyses are potentially confounded and can only be used in hypothesis generation there is no potential for a US randomized controlled trial (RCT) to definitively address this hypothesis. There are two efforts to test the hypothesis through an RCT outside the United States, one in Southeast Asia (DISCOVER CTO, www.NIH.gov) and the EuroCTO trial. It will be 5–10 years before these trial results are known, and until then practicing cardiologists will face the difficult decision of whether or not to offer CTO PCI to asymptomatic patients with CTOs. To say that there is no evidence to support CTO PCI among asymptomatic patients is as dishonest as claiming that there is irrefutable evidence supporting CTO PCI. Therefore, patients must be informed about ALL of the data that exists and must be engaged in the decision to proceed with revascularization or medical therapy alone.

In order for a hypothesis to warrant testing, there must be biological plausibility. There are, indeed, several studies in CTO patients where specific mechanism of benefit are suggested, and the findings corroborate the survival hypothesis.

Ischemia is associated with adverse event and many CTOs, even those that are "well collateralized result in ischemia [14]. Hachamvitch and colleagues described a linear relationship between ischemic burden and mortality [15]. This was confirmed and extended in the nuclear substudy of the COURAGE trial where baseline ischemic burden was again linearly related to 3-year death and MI rates [16]. Further, Shaw et al. reported that among patients in the COURAGE trial with moderate to large ischemic burden, PCI was more effective than medical therapy at reducing the ischemic burden by at least 5 % and amount previously shown to be prognostically significant.

Safley and colleagues evaluated the ischemic burden reduction among 312 patients with CTO who were successfully treated [17]. They found that the baseline ischemic burden was associated with the likelihood of reducing the ischemic burden by 5 % or more. Using a receiver operator model, they found that a baseline ischemic burden of greater than 12.5 % of the LV mass was predictive of a 5 % reduction in ischemia, whereas a baseline ischemic burden of less than 6.25 % was associated with an increase in ischemic burden by 5 %. A 5 % reduction in ischemic burden was associated with improved survival as compared to those with minimal or no reduction in ischemia.

Another plausible mechanism of increased mortality due to a CTO is the "double jeopardy" theory. Multivessel disease in the setting of an acute myocardial infarction (AMI) is associated with excess mortality as compared to single-vessel disease. Dutch investigators have demonstrated that this excess mortality is mostly attributable to the presence of a CTO [18]. They confirmed and extended this observation in a subsequent study landmarked at 30 days and showed continued divergence of the survival curves over time with the highest mortality among patients who present with AMI and are found to have a CTO in a nonculprit vessel (18 % at 5 years after 30-day landmarking), followed by those with AMI and significant non-CTO disease (11 % at 5 years after 30-day landmarking) and then those who present with AMI and no other significant CAD (10 % at 5 years after 30-day landmarking) [19]. Further, CTO was associated with the development of left ventricular dilation and/or a fall in ejection fraction (HR 3.5 95 % CI 1.6–7.8, $p<0.01$). These observations lead to the initiation of the EXPLORE trial. The EXPLORE trial will test the hypothesis that early CTO PCI (within the index hospitalization) as compared to no CTO PCI will result in improved ejection fraction and less LV remodeling as assessed by MRI at 4 months after AMI. It is not powered for testing a mortality endpoint.

Recently, the VACTO study demonstrated that among patients who had undergone AICD implantation for primary prevention and had incomplete revascularization, the appropriate arrhythmia therapy (antitachycardia pacing or defibrillation) during the 3 year follow-up timeframe was 30 % among those with a CTO and 15 % among those with non-CTO incomplete revascularization, $p<0.01$ [20].

Taken together, these observations suggest that CTOs are associated with adverse events including death, MI, potentially fatal arrhythmias, and adverse LV remodeling regardless of the symptom status. There is only one randomized controlled trial designed to test the hypothesis that CTO PCI will alter the course of adverse events among asymptomatic patients based on any of these hypotheses, the EXPLORE trial. Hopefully results from that trial will be available in the next 3–4 years to help guide decision-making. Unfortunately that trial is not powered for a mortality endpoint, so these surrogates for survival (LV remodeling and EF) will have to suffice. Again, fully informed consent, which includes a discussion of these nuances and incorporates the patient's wishes, should precede CTO PCI procedures.

In summary, CTO PCI is noninferior to non-CTO PCI when it comes to relief of symptoms (including dyspnea), restoration of physical function, and restoration of quality of life. In the absence of symptoms, there are compelling data supporting the hypothesis that CTO PCI is associated with a mortality benefit. Without a full armamentarium of techniques to enhance procedural success and safety, interventional cardiologists are likely to deny their patients access to this form of effective therapy. When faced with a patient who has a CTO, the operator need only ask himself, "if it were 90 %, would I perform PCI?" If the answer is affirmative, there is an obligation to perform the procedure or refer the patient to a competent CTO operator.

Classic Technique and the Myth of the True Lumen

There has been great historical, and current, interest from many operators to make efforts to heroic levels to "stay in the true lumen" when wiring the CTO segment. The primary cited reasons are a theoretic improvement in healing and better safety-durability profile for drug-eluting stents placed during the procedure and safety concerns when exploiting the subadventitial space as a treatment pathway. It is this author's and editor's view that the practical ramification of this philosophy as a dogmatic approach is reduced success rates and prolonged procedures. Furthermore, methodical wire technique is perhaps the most difficult of skillsets to teach and learn and cannot resolve the issues of best approaches to highly complex anatomy. Both technique and technologies designed to cross the true lumen or provide subintimal return don't consistently work by that mechanism (IVUS of wire only, true-to-true technique reveals subadventitial pathways ~30–50 % of the time). So if the end goal is to have more open arteries and treat all patients irrespective of anatomy with appropriate indications, then we should recognize that singular strategies will not adequately serve the public need.

Physicians have a tendency to reflect to intellectual comfort zones in interventional cardiology. Management of CTO challenges these constructs in several ways. Technology and techniques in 2013 for optimal CTO PCI can be counterintuitive to standard PCI procedures…, e.g., (a) crossing catheters or looped wires in the subadventitial space provide greater safety than standard wire techniques, (b) retrograde methods can be more safe and effective in selected patients, and (c) in a "standard" antegrade approach, Ellis grade 1–3 "perforations" are typically dissections and do not constitute a safety hazard or stopping point for many procedures. Another such construct is "the true lumen." We recall vascular morphology and biology and classification of endothelial, intima, media, and adventitial layers and internal and external elastic membranes. Within a completely occluded segment, histopathologic survey often demonstrates a destruction of the integrity of these layers, and we can speculate a disconnection with standard nondiseased vascular biologic function [19]. The strength of the adventitia and its elasticity are the only layer to provide security in the vessel structure. If one can accept a "clinical utility" model that there are two effective layers in CTO: (1) adventitia and (2) plaque, then therapeutic options abound and opportunities to effectively manage patients will increase accordingly. Finally, we should recognize that negative remodeling occurs in these vessels, and many that are considered "small" or "poor targets" in fact will enlarge (~30 %) over time with restoration of flow and can provide fine clinical results for the patients.

Prerequisites to the Hybrid Technique

The remainder of this manuscript will be devoted to summarizing hybrid approach for CTO PCI. The requisite knowledge base and skillsets assumed include CTO wiring strategies (wire shaping, selection, characteristics, and handling), antegrade dissection reentry (practically speaking, the Stingray technology, though IVUS-guided intralesional rewiring would be included in this category) [20, 21], and retrograde techniques including the reverse controlled antegrade-retrograde tracking (reverse CART) and CART methods [22–29]. These techniques have been described in detail elsewhere, so the nuances will be omitted in this manuscript to highlight practical application of the hybrid technique, "what to do when." During the learning phase, it is appropriate to leverage experience in a given strategy when technique overlap exists and net safety is neutral. The initial experiences with the more advanced strategies, dissection-reentry, and retrograde methods are best suited for new operators and programs to have an experienced proctor onsite in an advisory capacity. Proctors can be identified at national/regional training programs and also at www.ctofundamentals.org.

The Hybrid Approach for CTO PCI

The goal of the hybrid approach is to combine technologies and techniques in a manner that facilitates opportunities to attempt CTO PCI in patients with appropriate clinical indications irrespective of anatomy. The technical merits and emphasis are on procedural success and importantly, procedural efficiency with an acceptable safety profile [30]. Efficient procedures and a process can help drive CTO PCI adoption (and therefore lead to primary initiative of more open arteries) and likely reduce complications specific to better management of radiation and contrast exposure and perhaps reduce bleeding/thrombotic complications that have higher frequency rates in prolonged cases.

Hybrid CTO PCI refers to (1) a standard, simplified process to approach CTO PCI based on anatomy, (2) harmonizing antegrade and retrograde techniques, and (3) harmonizing lesion wire or device-based crossing with dissection-reentry methods. Hybrid CTO PCI exploits the phenomenon of conditional probability and attempts to employ high reward strategies at a point in the procedure that they are most likely to be successful and endorses rapid change to alternate methods when failure modes dictate that secondary and bailout strategies have more probable positive outcome than the current strategy.

Anatomy Dictates Strategy

The initial angiogram is reviewed, and initial strategy with provisional strategies is developed before entering the procedure. Occasionally, additional angiography with the second catheter is required to completely inform this decision. Virtually all CTO PCI procedures with contralateral or multiple collateral beds should have the second catheter (a guide catheter if any possibility for retrograde exists) for optimal imaging. Remember that collateral patterns often shift during the course of these procedures.

Four variables are considered:

1. Ambiguity of the proximal cap (can the proximal CTO cap be clearly identified with angiography or by use of an IVUS catheter in nearby sidebranch)
2. Lesion length ≥20 mm (longer lesions can be successfully wired with standard techniques, but success rates dramatically decline at this point and case times are prolonged) [31]
3. Quality of the distal target (size, imaging, degree of disease, and sidebranches of clinical interest)
4. Interventional collaterals (perceived likelihood of successful crossing of collaterals to employ retrograde techniques in safe and efficient manner)

Based on these results, initial strategy is determined (Fig. 23.3):

1. Antegrade, wire escalation – clear proximal cap, short lesion <20 mm, good target, and interventional collaterals irrelevant
2. Antegrade dissection reentry – clear proximal cap, long lesion, good target, and interventional collaterals irrelevant
3. Retrograde, wire escalation – ambiguous proximal cap, short lesion, good or poor target, and suitable interventional collaterals
4. Retrograde dissection reentry – ambiguous proximal cap, long lesion, good or poor target, and suitable interventional collaterals.

One should note that the driver for primary retrograde technique, in order of relevance, is ambiguity of the proximal cap and poor target in patients with suitable collaterals. Nuanced methods to troubleshoot patients not in these anatomic bins exist but are outside the scope of this manuscript.

Secondary strategies are developed in advance in anticipation of failed or failing primary strategies. Generally, the secondary strategy for antegrade or retrograde wire escalation is dissection-reentry method in the same direction. Remember that the initial directional choice was determined by characteristics favoring success and efficiency with that direction (antegrade vs. retrograde). Failed dissection reentry

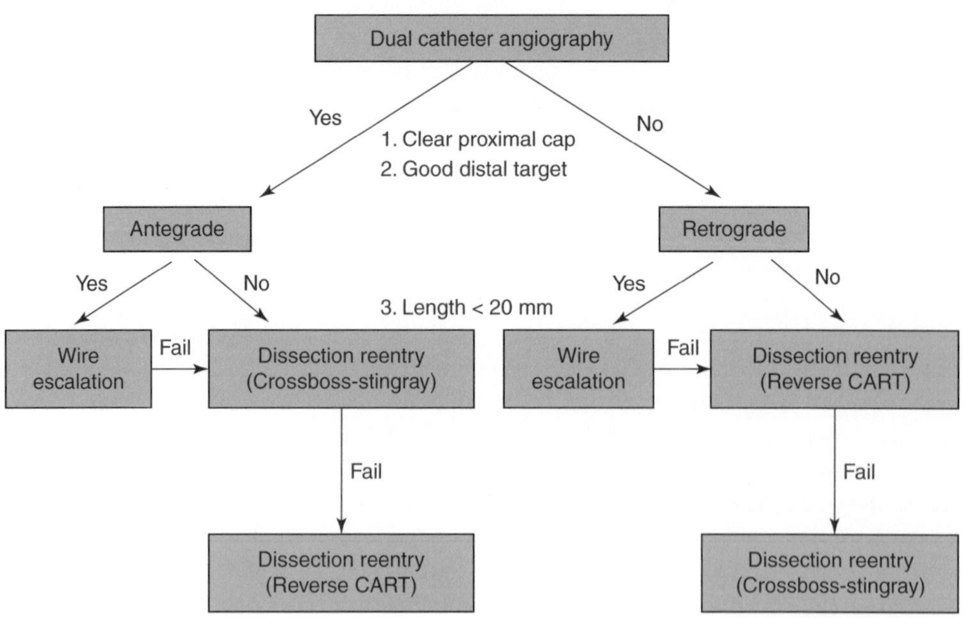

Fig. 23.3 Hybrid algorithm for CTO PCI with initial and provisional strategies determined by baseline coronary anatomy

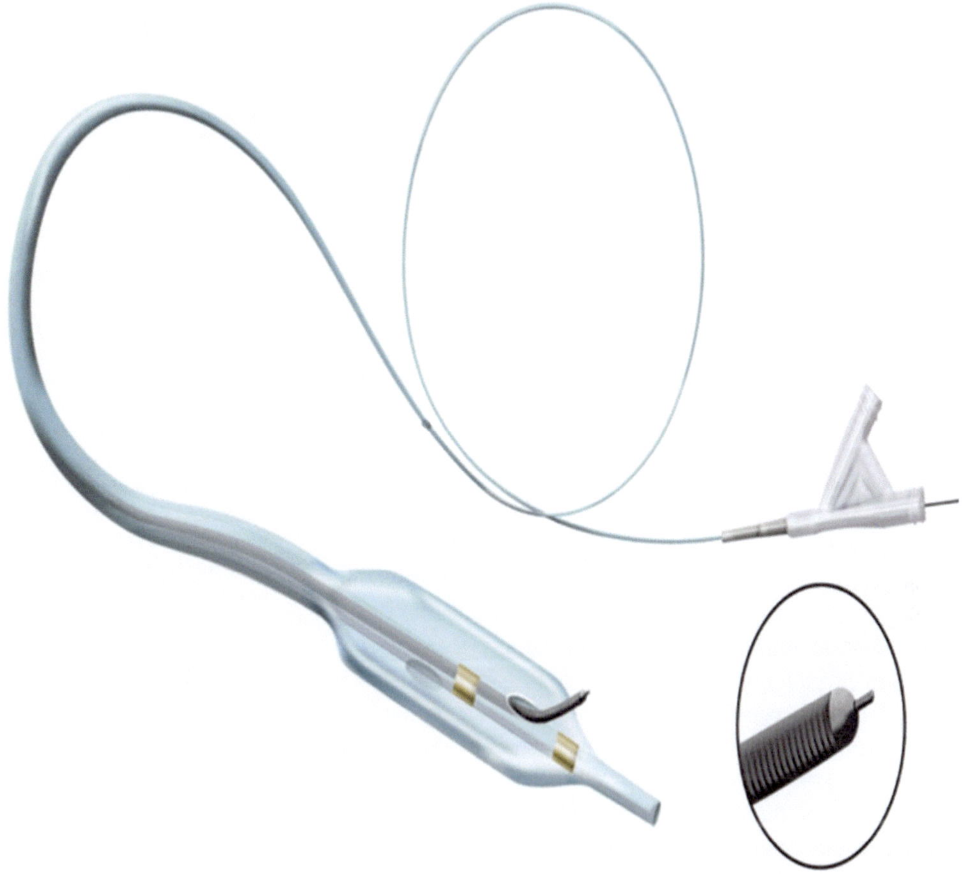

Fig. 23.4 Stingray orienting balloon and Stingray guidewire technology for coronary reentry (Courtesy of BridgePoint Medical/Boston Scientific, Natick, MA)

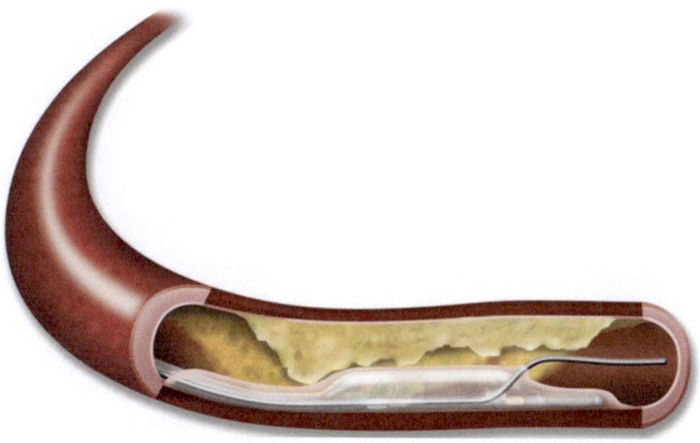

Fig. 23.5 Reentry using Stingray balloon and guidewire in diseased artery distal to CTO segment (Courtesy of BridgePoint Medical/Boston Scientific, Natick, MA)

in one direction favors dissection reentry in the other direction as secondary or as final bailout strategy (e.g., failed dissection reentry antegrade, then go retrograde and utilize reverse CART; for failed retrograde techniques, go antegrade with intent for stingray reentry).

The "toolkit" for this approach is previously described in articles specific for the specific techniques employed but includes:

- Wires:
  - Soft tapered polymer jacketed wire for lesion probing and knuckle wire techniques (example includes Fiedler XT (Asahi Intecc))
  - Soft non-tapered polymer jacketed or hydrophilic wire for retrograde collateral crossing and lesion probing (examples include Fiedler FC and Sion (Asahi Intecc), pilot 50 (Abbott Vascular))
  - Stiff polymer jacketed wire for complex lesion wiring, dissection reentry, and knuckle wire technique (example includes pilot 200 (Abbott Vascular))
  - Stiff tapered wire for lesion penetration (example includes Confianza pro 12 g (Abbott Vascular))
- Antegrade reentry tools:
  - Stingray orienting balloon and Stingray guidewire (BridgePoint Medical/Boston Scientific) (Figs. 23.4 and 23.5)
- Retrograde tools:
  - Corsair microcatheter (Asahi Intecc)

In addition, other devices that are useful in CTO PCI not specific to the hybrid approach include the guideliner catheter (vascular solutions), Tornus microcatheter (Asahi Intecc), large and small snares, covered stents, and coils, among others.

In general, wire escalation is chosen for short lesions (<20 mm) with nonambiguous proximal caps and good distal target. We advocate a soft polymer jacketed wire to explore the lesion. Should this not be successful in lesion crossing, escalation is performed to the stiff jacketed wire (e.g., Pilot 200) if the lesion is long, dissected, or tortuous or to the Confianza pro 12 g if penetration is required or the remainder of the vessel course is short and obvious.

For longer lesions, with clear proximal caps and good targets or if wire strategy leads to subintimal position, the stingray reentry system can be utilized to gain true lumen access and successful result. A variety of techniques for optimal reentry exist which are beyond the scope of this chapter. In addition, retrograde techniques as primary and provisional strategies will be discussed in the next chapter.

Conclusion

Coronary CTO PCI has been limited historically by poor success rates and clinical uptake. Recent technique and technology advances have provided a platform to create a systematic method to improve success rates and efficiency and importantly to extend therapy to a broader group of patients with need, by addressing consistency and training needs and overcoming anatomic hurdles. This process is summarized in this chapter by the method known as "hybrid CTO PCI." While CTO PCI is rapidly evolving and these methods may, in turn, adapt over time, this method can provide a starting point to expand the pool of operators and ideally, achieve the goal of "more open arteries" worldwide.

References

1. Fefer P, Knudtson ML, Cheema AN, et al. Current perspectives on coronary chronic total occlusions the Canadian multicenter chronic total occlusions registry. J Am Coll Cardiol. 2012;59:991–7.
2. Kahn JK. Angiographic suitability for catheter revascularization of total coronary occlusions in patients from a community hospital setting. Am Heart J. 1993;126:561–4.
3. Christofferson RD, Lehmann KG, Martin GV, Every N, Caldwell JH, Kapadia SR. Effect of chronic total coronary occlusion on treatment strategy. Am J Cardiol. 2005;95:1088–91.
4. Abbott JD, Kip KE, Vlachos HA, et al. Recent trends in the percutaneous treatment of chronic total coronary occlusions. Am J Cardiol. 2006;97:1691–6.
5. Grantham JA, Marso SP, Spertus JA, House J, Holmes DR, Rutherford BD. State of the art: chronic total occlusion angioplasty in the United States. JACC Int. 2009;2:479–86.
6. Patel MR, Dehmer GJ, Hirshfeld JW, Smith PK, Spertus JA. ACCF/SCAI/STS/AATS/AHA/ASNC 2009 Appropriateness Criteria for Coronary Revascularization: a report by the American College of Cardiology Foundation Appropriateness Criteria Task Force, Society for Cardiovascular Angiography and Interventions, Society of Thoracic Surgeons, American Association for Thoracic Surgery, American Heart Association, and the American Society of Nuclear Cardiology Endorsed by the American Society of Echocardiography, the Heart Failure Society of America, and the Society of Cardiovascular Computed Tomography. J Am Coll Cardiol. 2009;53:530–53.
7. Chan PS, Patel MR, Klein LW, et al. Appropriateness of percutaneous coronary intervention. JAMA. 2011;306:53–61.
8. Grantham JA, Jones PG, Cannon L, Spertus JA. Quantifying the early health status benefits of successful chronic total occlusion recanalization. Circ Qual Care Outcomes Res. 2010;3:284–90.
9. Joyal D, Afilalo J, Rinfret S. Effectiveness of recanalization of chronic total occlusions: a systematic review and meta-analysis. Am Heart J. 2010;160:179–87.
10. Borgia F, Viceconte N, Ali O, et al. Improved cardiac survival, freedom from mace and angina-related quality of life after successful percutaneous recanalization of coronary artery chronic total occlusions. Int J Cardiol. 2012;161(1):31–8.
11. Spertus JAWJ, Dewhurst TA, Deyo RA, Prodzinski J, McDonell M, Fihn SD. Development and evaluation of the Seattle angina questionnaire: a new functional status measure for coronary artery disease. J Am Coll Cardiol. 1995;25:333–41.
12. Safley DS, Grantham JA, Jones PA, Spertus J. Health status benefits of angioplasty for chronic total occlusions: an analysis from the OPS/PRISM studies. J Am Coll Cardiol. 2012;59:e101.
13. Suero JA, Marso SP, Jones PG, et al. Procedural outcomes and long-term survival among patients undergoing percutaneous coronary intervention of a chronic total occlusion in native coronary arteries: a 20-year experience. J Am Coll Cardiol. 2001;38:409–14.
14. Werner GS, Surber R, Ferrari M, Fritzenwanger M, Figulla HR. The functional reserve of collaterals supplying long-term chronic total coronary occlusions in patients without prior myocardial infarction. Eur Heart J. 2006;27:2406–12.
15. Hachamovitch R, Hayes SW, Friedman JD, Cohen I, Berman DS. Comparison of the short-term survival benefit associated with revascularization compared with medical therapy in patients with no prior coronary artery disease undergoing stress myocardial perfusion single photon emission computed tomography. Circulation. 2003;107:2900–7.
16. Shaw LJ, Berman DS, Maron DJ, et al. Optimal medical therapy with or without percutaneous coronary intervention to reduce ischemic burden: results from the Clinical Outcomes Utilizing Revascularization and Aggressive Drug Evaluation (COURAGE) trial nuclear substudy. Circulation. 2008;117:1283–91.
17. Safley DM, Koshy S, Grantham JA, et al. Changes in myocardial ischemic burden following percutaneous coronary intervention of chronic total occlusions. Catheter Cardiovasc Int. 2011;78:337–43.
18. van der Schaaf RJ, Vis MM, Sjauw KD, et al. Impact of multivessel coronary disease on long-term mortality in patients with ST-elevation myocardial infarction is due to the presence of a chronic total occlusion. Am J Cardiol. 2006;98:1165–9.
19. Sumitsuji S, Inoue K, Ochiai M, Tsuchikane E, Ikeno F. Fundamental wire technique and current standard strategy of percutaneous intervention for chronic total occlusion with histopathological insights. JACC Cardiovasc Interv. 2011;4:941–51.
20. Whitlow PL, Burke MN, Lombardi WL, et al. Use of a novel crossing and ee-entry system in coronary chronic total occlusions that have failed standard crossing techniques: results of the FAST-CTOs (Facilitated Antegrade Steering Technique in Chronic Total Occlusions) trial. JACC Cardiovasc Interv. 2012;5:393–401.
21. Whitlow PL, Lombardi WL, Araya M, et al. Initial experience with a dedicated coronary re-entry device for revascularization of chronic total occlusions. Catheter Cardiovasc Interv. 2012;80(5):807–13.
22. Brilakis ES, Grantham JA, Thompson CA, et al. The retrograde approach to coronary artery chronic total occlusions: a practical approach. Catheter Cardiovasc Interv. 2012;79:3–19.
23. Jones DA, Weerackody R, Rathod K, et al. Successful recanalization of chronic total occlusions is associated with improved long-term survival. JACC Cardiovasc Interv. 2012;5:380–8.
24. Joyal D, Thompson CA, Grantham JA, Buller CE, Rinfret S. The retrograde technique for recanalization of chronic total occlusions: a step-by-step approach. JACC Cardiovasc Interv. 2012;5:1–11.

25. Thompson CA, Jayne JE, Robb JF, et al. Retrograde techniques and the impact of operator volume on percutaneous intervention for coronary chronic total occlusions an early U.S. experience. JACC Cardiovasc Interv. 2009;2:834–42.
26. Kimura M, Katoh O, Tsuchikane E, et al. The efficacy of a bilateral approach for treating lesions with chronic total occlusions the CART (controlled antegrade and retrograde subintimal tracking) registry. JACC Cardiovasc Interv. 2009;2:1135–41.
27. Rathore S, Katoh O, Matsuo H, et al. Retrograde percutaneous recanalization of chronic total occlusion of the coronary arteries: procedural outcomes and predictors of success in contemporary practice. Circ Cardiovasc Interv. 2009;2:124–32.
28. Rathore S, Matsuo H, Terashima M, et al. Procedural and in-hospital outcomes after percutaneous coronary intervention for chronic total occlusions of coronary arteries 2002 to 2008: impact of novel guidewire techniques. JACC Cardiovasc Interv. 2009;2:489–97.
29. Surmely JF, Tsuchikane E, Katoh O, et al. New concept for CTO recanalization using controlled antegrade and retrograde subintimal tracking: the CART technique. J Invasive Cardiol. 2006;18:334–8.
30. Brilakis ES, Grantham JA, Rinfret S, et al. A percutaneous treatment algorithm for crossing coronary chronic total occlusions. JACC Cardiovasc Interv. 2012;5:367–79.
31. Morino Y, Abe M, Morimoto T, et al. Predicting successful guidewire crossing through chronic total occlusion of native coronary lesions within 30 min: the J-CTO (Multicenter CTO Registry in Japan) score as a difficulty grading and time assessment tool. JACC Cardiovasc Interv. 2011;4:213–21.

The Retrograde Approach to Chronic Total Occlusion PCI

24

David V. Daniels and William L. Lombardi

The advent of retrograde techniques to facilitate chronic total occlusion (CTO) PCI has improved overall success rates from 50 to 70 % with antegrade only approaches to greater than 90 % in contemporary series with very low complication rates [1–3]. Kahn and Hartzler first described the concept of retrograde PCI in 1990 using saphenous vein grafts as the retrograde conduit [4]. Since then, the technique has evolved utilizing septal or epicardial collaterals for CTO access [5, 6]. We define retrograde PCI broadly as any technique utilizing a donor collateral artery for the delivery of interventional equipment that ultimately facilitates successful CTO recanalization. Barriers to the widespread adoption of CTO PCI include excessive procedural time translating to higher radiation, contrast, and institutional costs when compared to routine PCI, coupled with relatively low success rates when restricted to antegrade only techniques. We have demonstrated that with the addition of a retrograde option, dramatically higher success rates are achievable with lower procedural time and contrast utilization when retrograde operators are compared to non-retrograde operators [3]. This chapter will focus on indications for a retrograde approach, setting up for success, techniques for achieving reproducible results, and the recognition and management of retrograde-specific complications.

D.V. Daniels, MD
Stanford University,
Palo Alto Medical Foundation,
Palo Alto, CA, USA

W.L. Lombardi, MD (✉)
Peacehealth St. Joseph Hospital,,
2979 Squalicom Parkway, Suite 101,
Bellingham, WA 98225, USA
e-mail: wllombardi@peacehealth.org

Indications for a Retrograde Approach and Case Selection

Retrograde CTO PCI can be employed either as a bailout strategy for a failed antegrade attempt or, in the right circumstances, as a primary approach [7]. In patients with a failed antegrade attempt, retrograde success rates are significantly higher than another antegrade only procedure. The presence of a suitable collateral and a predictor of low antegrade success could be considered as an indication for primary retrograde approach and is associated with a high success rate [8]. Predictors of antegrade failure include long occlusions (>20 mm), apparent small distal target, side branch at a flush proximal cap, and distal cap at a bifurcation. Predictors of retrograde success include visible collateral connections, <90° collateral body tortuosity, and <90° angle between the distal collateral anastomosis with the CTO vessel [9]. Figure 24.1 illustrates a proposed algorithm for an approach to CTO PCI incorporating the retrograde option in selected cases. To maximize the safety, efficiency, and potential benefits of the retrograde approach, we suggest the following guidelines: (1) An operator should have performed at least 100 antegrade CTO procedures prior to a retrograde attempt. (2) Initially only septal collaterals should be traversed, and operators should avoid epicardial collaterals until they are sufficiently comfortable with retrograde wire and equipment handling. (3) On-site proctoring with an experienced retrograde operator is strongly recommended during the initial cases. (4) An array of retrograde-specific equipment should be stocked including devices for managing specific complications (see section "Retrograde Operators Toolbox" below).

Setting Up for Success

Review of the Diagnostic Angiogram

A very careful review of the diagnostic angiogram is important, and it is not unusual to spend up to 30 min scrutinizing

C.A. Thompson (ed.), *Textbook of Cardiovascular Intervention*,
DOI 10.1007/978-1-4471-4528-8_24, © Springer-Verlag London 2014

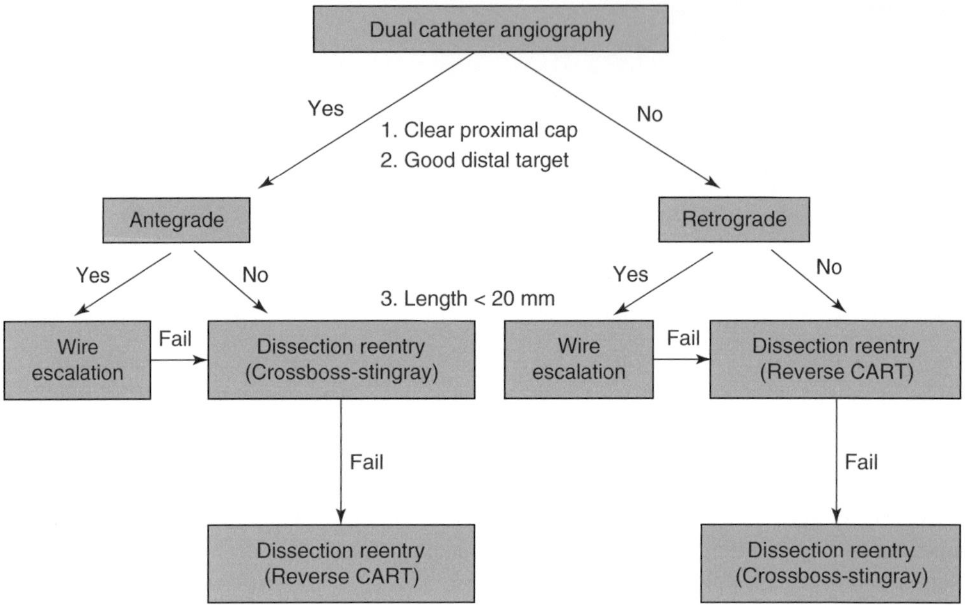

Fig. 24.1 A hybrid algorithm in the approach to CTO PCI

every aspect of the available information, especially when first attempting retrograde procedures. Focus initially on antegrade and retrograde ostial diameters and orientations for selecting the proper guiding catheters. The length of the CTO is often overestimated based upon single catheter injection, but one should attempt to get a sense of length to formulate a strategy ahead of time. Collateral sources both epicardial and septal should be carefully assessed as potential retrograde conduits, paying particular attention to tortuosity, location, entrance, and exit angles as discussed later in this chapter. Both collateral size and distal vessel filling will often be more prominent with injections through large-caliber guiding catheters, so be aware that all usable options may not be fully delineated until one performs dual-injection guiding catheter angiography.

Vascular Access

All procedures start with proper vascular access, and while considered a footnote in many texts on CTO PCI, we should emphasize the importance of starting with the right access for the right job. In fact, a theme of our approach is to bring every advantage to bear at each step along the way, both in terms of enhancing procedural efficiency and success. The first choice is radial versus femoral, and while CTO PCI has traditionally been performed via the femoral route, reasonable technical success with perhaps lower access site complications has been described with radial access [10, 11]. The principal limitation of radial access for retrograde PCI is not only the operators comfort with radial procedures in general but also the requirement for double-guide access with a lot of support, especially for the retrograde catheter as we will describe. It is for this reason that we will focus our discussion on the femoral approach. For those wishing to pursue the radial approach, it is highly recommended that the operator currently perform greater than 90 % of the procedures radially and understand the limitations of smaller guiding catheters.

Seven or ideally eight French sheaths should be placed in each femoral based on the choice of guiding catheter size as described below. We advocate long, reinforced sheaths to improve passive support to the guiding catheters as well as torque ability in patients with peripheral vascular disease. The use of long sheaths increases passive support and comes with minimal consequences.

Guiding Catheter Selection and Setup

Support-type guides including the “extra backup” for the left coronary and Amplatz shape for the right coronary are useful, but guide selection should not be dogmatic, and careful scrutiny of the diagnostic angiogram is important in this respect. For example, Judkins right guides may be more appropriate for a very proximal RCA occlusion in which a more aggressive guide has a higher risk of proximal dissection. We recommend at least seven and if allowable by ostial size 8 French guiding catheters both for support considerations and equipment delivery. While 6

French catheters can certainly be used successfully for CTO PCI, one is somewhat more limited in the ability to use trapping techniques, multiple over-the-wire (OTW) devices, and with respect to overall guide support especially for the retrograde guide [12]. If review of the diagnostic angiogram suggests a small ostium, the use of side holes should be considered for the antegrade guide. There are two reasons for considering an antegrade side-hole guide: First, although damping during the procedure is not likely to be clinically relevant because the vessel is chronically occluded, hydraulic coronary dissection from injections can occur with a "damped" guide. This becomes increasingly more likely once an antegrade subintimal dissection has been created when performing reverse CART, which will be discussed later in this chapter. The use of side holes may not be justified with the retrograde guide. Any damping should be recognized promptly as donor vessel ischemia puts a large territory of myocardium at risk (including the collateralized territory), and hemodynamic compromise may ensue. The need for active retrograde guide management during delivery of devices, as well as the tendency for it to deep seat during removal of equipment, makes quick recognition of donor vessel ischemia important. If bilateral guides are engaged into the two native coronary ostia, it is advisable to place the left coronary guide first and then the right to avoid displacing the RCA catheter. "Access/guide consistency," such as always putting the antegrade guide in the right femoral and retrograde guide in the left femoral, can help to avoid accidentally injecting via the antegrade guide at the wrong time, e.g., after antegrade subintimal ballooning but prior to distal recanalization, and creating a hydraulic dissection. Acquiring short guides or the ability to shorten a guide is important for retrograde procedures especially when planning to externalize a guidewire (see section "Retrograde Operators Toolbox" below).

Although many cardiac catheterization laboratories use the Tuohy-Borst hemostatic valve, retrograde procedures in particular use devices such as the Corsair Catheter and Tornus, which require rotational motions for advancement. This can lead to significant blood loss because of the need for an open valve for free rotation of the devices. Therefore, we recommend the COPILOT (Abbott) or Guardian II (Vascular Solutions) valves, both of which allow free rotation of OTW devices while maintaining hemostasis. Power injectors, though useful for improving efficiency and possibly contrast utilization, can be potentially dangerous when injecting into the antegrade guide at high pressure and can result in hydraulic dissections. Therefore, we feel a manifold, at least for the antegrade guide, should be considered when performing CTO procedures.

Table 24.1 Vascular access and guiding catheter quick tips

7 or 8 French access depending on guide catheter size
Consider 8 French guiding catheters based on ostial coronary diameter
Side holes are useful for the antegrade guide, avoid for retrograde
Practice "Access/Guide Consistency" – antegrade right, retrograde left
Use a plunger-type hemostatic valve to decrease blood loss
Avoid power injectors
Use heparin alone for procedural anticoagulation – ACT >300

Procedural Anticoagulation

Patients should be preloaded with aspirin and clopidogrel in advance of the procedure. Most CTO operators advocate unfractionated heparin (UFH) as the sole anticoagulation strategy and avoidance of GP IIB/IIIA inhibitors or bivalirudin because of the intrinsically higher risk of perforation compared to traditional PCI and the ability to rapidly reverse UFH with protamine if needed. The retrograde or antegrade guide may be dormant for prolonged periods of time depending on the stage of the procedure. This increases the risk of thrombus formation in the guide, and for this reason, we recommend keeping the activated clotting time (ACT) above 350 s, and the staff systematically alert the operator every 30 min to obtain another sample. Donor vessel thromboembolism from the retrograde guide can be particularly disastrous as a large area of myocardium is at risk (both donor and recipient territories). Additionally, when drawing an ACT, it is advisable to do so from the most recently dormant guiding catheter as that will provide an opportunity to flush that guide and thus decrease the risk of thrombus formation within the guide catheter (Table 24.1).

Collateral Angiography

A careful evaluation of collaterals is critical to the planning and success of the retrograde approach. Ideally, good collateral angiography should be performed at the time of diagnostic angiography in all patients with a CTO. This will allow the operator the time to carefully review candidate collaterals offline. Collaterals can be classified according to the Rentrop classification: grade 0 = no visible filling of any collateral channel, grade 1 = filling of the side branch of the occluded artery, grade 2 = partial filling of the occluded vessel, or grade 3 = complete collateral filling of the occluded vessel up to its occlusion [13].

Werner et al. have also described a collateral connection (CC) classification: CC0 = collateral with no visible connection to the recipient artery, CC1 = tiny or faint CC connections, and CC2 = small vessel-like connections

(Fig. 24.2) [14]. Whether dedicated collateral angiography is performed during the diagnostic or at the time of intervention, some basic guidelines apply. Cineangiograms should be acquired in angulations intended to maximize the exposure of the collateral origin from the donor vessel and associated side branches, course of the collateral, and distal anastomosis with the CTO vessel (Table 24.2) (Fig. 24.3). During acquisition, low magnification and the avoidance of panning improve the resolution of very faint collaterals.

Retrograde Operators Toolbox

While we could generate an extensive list of equipment used by experts in retrograde CTO, our goal is to focus on a tenable amount of options for one lab to stock and retrograde-specific needs. Short retrograde guides are a necessity for these procedures, as standard length guides will often not allow the Corsair or other support catheters to reach the antegrade guide via collaterals. Full reach of the support catheter from retrograde guide to antegrade guide is required if one wishes to externalize the guidewire to facilitate recanalization.

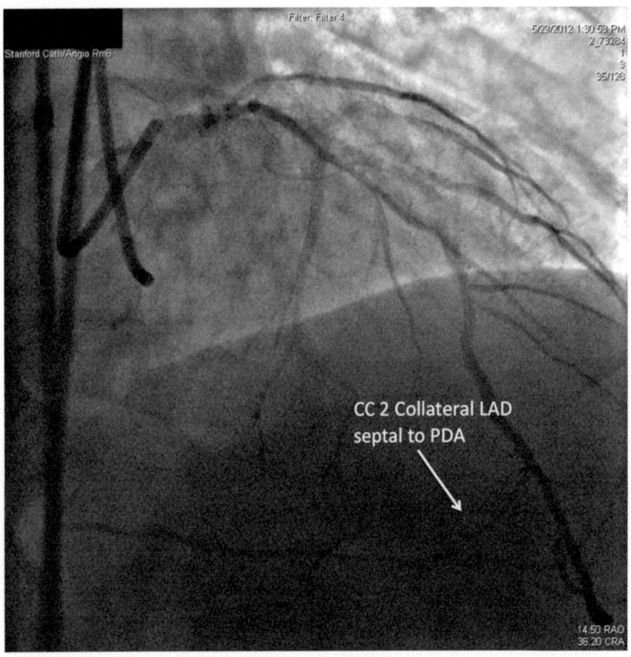

Fig. 24.2 An example of a CC2 or "side branch-like" collateral. In this case, a distal LAD septal which provided excellent access to the PDA for retrograde CTO PCi

90 cm guides are available for most curves, or alternatively a standard guide can be shortened (Fig. 24.4). With respect to guidewires, we advocate simplifying the inventory to five classes of wires as these will provide you with all the tools needed to successfully navigate a CTO, will improve your familiarity with a limited amount of equipment, and are more feasible from an inventory and purchasing perspective. The five classes of wires required include a soft-tipped tapered polymer-jacketed wire (i.e., Fielder XT), a soft-tipped non-tapered polymer-jacketed wire (i.e., Fielder FC), a stiff tipped non-tapered polymer-jacketed wire (i.e., Pilot 200), a stiff-tipped tapered unjacketed wire (i.e., Confianza Pro 12), and an externalization wire (RG 3 or ViperWire Advance). The Fielder XT can be used to probe for microchannels within the CTO, or it can be used as a "knuckle" wire to facilitate subintimal tracking. Wires specific to retrograde collateral crossing are non-tapered polymer-jacketed wires such as the Fielder FC, Whisper, or Pilot 50 and occasionally a tapered polymer-jacketed wire such as the Fielder XT. Recently, a new dedicated collateral wire has been developed, Sion and Sion Blue; these wires have a unique double-core, core-to-tip design with exposed wire coils that may improve access through epicardial collaterals. The Pilot 200 is useful for crossing the CTO and if it enters the subintimal space can also be knuckled to allow for subintimal tracking. The Confianza Pro 12 should be used for directed puncture when anatomic ambiguity is minimal or during a wire-based reentry technique. For wire externalization techniques, the RG3 is a dedicated 330 cm 0.010″ wire developed for this purpose but may not be available globally. Other choices include a long stiff wire such as the ViperWire Advance (335 cm). The rota-floppy wire (325 cm) is long enough and can be used for this purpose but is more prone to kinking and therefore should only be used if another more suitable wire is not available. In addition to an externalization wire, a snare may be needed to grab the retrograde wire tip from the aortic root or retrograde guide to help externalize a guidewire.

In order to assist with collateral wire manipulation and allow for subsequent wire exchange, an OTW support catheter should be used. Many advocate a dedicated exchange catheter such as the Terumo FineCross or a 1.25 mm/1.5 mm OTW balloon catheter. Standard microcatheters have largely been supplanted by the Corsair catheter, which is an OTW hybrid support catheter and channel dilator specifically designed for retrograde PCI. It consists of an array of eight thin wires wound together with two larger wires in a spiral

Table 24.2 Collateral angiography

Artery	Artery	Collateral	Primary angulation	Secondary angulation
LAD	PDA	Septal-septal	RAO cranial	RAO caudal
LAD	PDA	Apical epicardial	LAO caudal	LAO/AP cranial
CTX	RCA	AV groove epicardial	LAO cranial	RAO caudal
OM	Diagonal	Epicardial	RAO caudal	LAO cranial

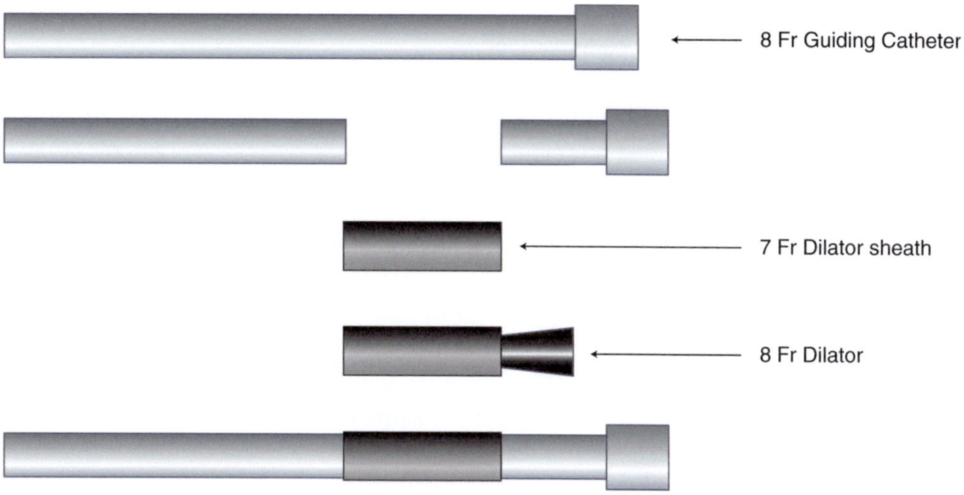

Fig. 24.3 Guide shortening. In order to shorten an 8 Fr guide, we start with trimming and cutting the appropriate length, usually at least 10 cm from the guiding catheter near the proximal hub. Then, cut out a 2–3 CM section from a 7 Fr sheath. An 8 Fr dilator is used to flare out the 7 Fr sheath on both ends in order to accept the 8 Fr guiding catheter. Finally, the 7 Fr sheath joint is pushed over both ends of the cut guiding catheter to make the shortened guide

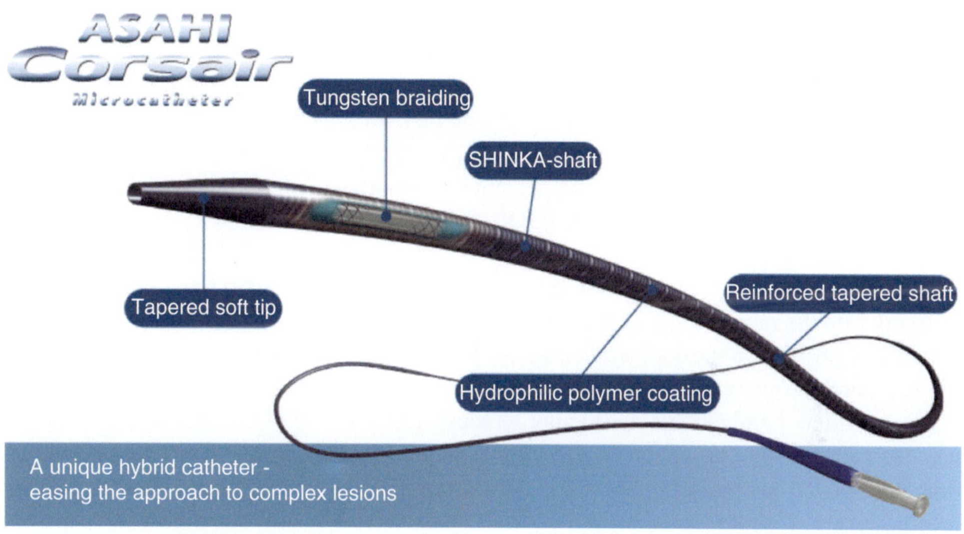

Fig. 24.4 Corsair microcatheter. The Corsair is a tungsten braided lubricious over-the-wire microcatheter that greatly facilitates retrograde collateral crossing (Courtesy of ASAHI INTECC USA, INc., Santa Ana, CA, USA)

structure allowing torque to be transmitted from shaft to tip, and advancement is facilitated by rotation similar to the Tornus catheter. It has a hydrophilic polymer coating on the distal 60 cm to facilitate channel crossing. In a recent study, procedural retrograde CTO PCI success in cases in which the retrograde channel was successfully crossed with a guidewire was 99 % with the Corsair versus 92.5 % with standard techniques ($p = 0.030$). There was also a strong trend toward lower fluoroscopy and procedural time [15]. 1.25 and 1.5 mm OTW balloon catheters should also be available for septal dilatation if needed for the advancement of retrograde equipment.

Collateral Wiring

After bilateral guide engagement, baseline angiography and procedural anticoagulation with UFH collateral wiring can be performed. Initially septal collaterals should be attempted primarily as epicardial vessels have a higher risk of perforation and subsequent complications. Optimal septal collaterals associated with a higher success rate are those with <90° of tortuosity and good visibility of the collateral to recipient vessel connection [9]. For septal collaterals, a straight course is more important than size in achieving procedural success, and even "invisible" septal channels can be crossed, whereas for epicardial collaterals, size is more important than tortuosity. Once a candidate collateral is identified, a non-jacketed workhorse wire with a standard working curve is loaded into a Corsair catheter and maneuvered via the antegrade guide to the origin of the collateral identified for retrograde crossing. As above, another microcatheter or a 1.25–1.5 OTW balloon could be used for this purpose, but the Corsair has proven to be more efficient, and our practice has evolved to using this device almost exclusively to support retrograde crossing. The tip of the catheter is brought down to the origin of the collateral, and then the working wire is exchanged for a non-tapered polymer-jacketed wire such as the Fielder FC. The tip should be shaped with a very short 1< mm 70–90° bend to facilitate collateral engagement and maneuvering. Once the collateral is engaged, the wire should be gently advanced with close attention paid to insuring free tip movement and preventing wire buckling, as collaterals are very susceptible to injury. With septal collaterals, a blind probing technique, so-called septal surfing, can often facilitate efficient crossing while minimizing contrast utilization. If after a few minutes little progress has been made, the support catheter can be advanced into the proximal collateral channel to perform a selective angiogram as a road map. After removal of the guidewire, a 3 cc syringe with contrast should be attached and air aspirated from the catheter prior to angiography. Prior to guidewire replacement, this should be flushed with saline, particularly with the Corsair catheter, to prevent guidewire sticking and problems with maneuverability. Different wire shapes may be needed to progress through the collateral, and the Corsair catheter may need to be advanced for support depending on the collateral tortuosity. The operator should rapidly progress through different wire shapes and paths through the collateral network, and one should not get stuck attempting to cross one particular collateral connection. Forward progress resulting in the guidewire appearing to have crossed the collateral can be the result of successful retrograde crossing into the recipient artery true lumen, dissection and subintimal position in the collateral or recipient vessel, vessel exit into the pericardial space, or vessel exit into the ventricle often heralded by ventricular ectopy. Prior to advancement of the Corsair or OTW balloon catheter, the operator MUST be confident of the wire position in the distal true lumen. If there are other ipsilateral or contralateral collaterals, this can be achieved with an angiogram from the appropriate guiding catheter. Orthogonal views, guidewire feel and tracking the recipient vessel anatomy, are the best predictors of crossing into the true lumen of the recipient vessel. At this point, the Corsair catheter should be advanced across the collateral into the distal CTO artery using gentle pressure and fast rotations alternating 4–5 counterclockwise and clockwise. The Corsair catheter moves forward better in the counterclockwise rotation but will move forward in either direction. The Corsair is also limited to ten rotations maximally without movement before the torque must be relieved. The key is momentum, and once the catheter gets moving, it is important to continue alternating high-speed rotations while advancing. If an OTW balloon is employed, gentle low-pressure inflations (2–6 atms depending on the 1.25/1.5 mm balloon compliance curves) may be needed to dilate the septal. The catheter should be advanced to the area of the distal cap to facilitate lesion crossing (Fig. 24.5).

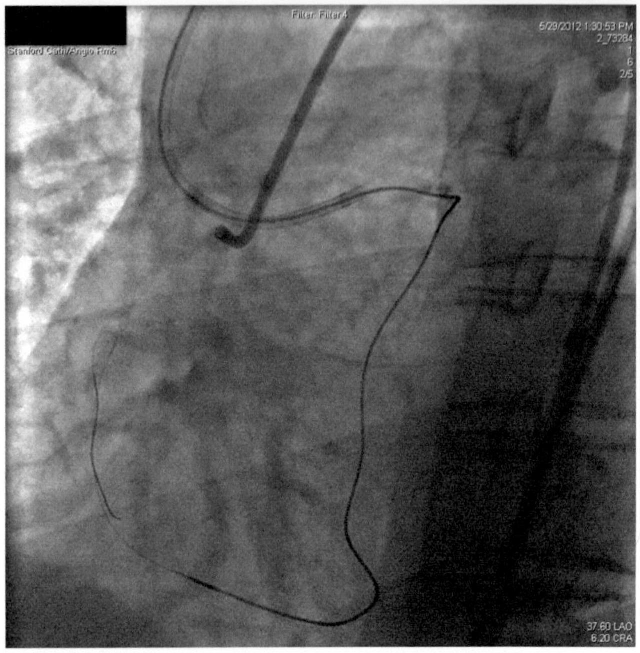

Fig. 24.5 RCA CTO PCI. Corsair catheter positioned at the distal cap with a Pilot 200 knuckle wire dissecting up the mid-RCA

Lesion Crossing

Once a "base of operations" has been established at the distal cap, there are several techniques available for crossing the CTO retrograde. The simplest technique is retrograde wiring, and it has been observed that the distal cap is often softer and more penetrable than the proximal cap.

We can position an antegrade wire as well and proceed with the simple "landmark" and "kissing wire" techniques, which are variation of the same technique. The "landmark" technique simply uses the retrograde wire as a landmark. The retrograde wire is positioned at the distal cap of the occlusion to help navigate the antegrade wire in the proper direction. If the retrograde wire had initially advanced substantially within the occlusion, the technique is called "kissing" as both wires are advanced toward each other. The meeting point can be either within the lumen or in the subintimal space, as both wires are clearly within true lumen distally and proximally. The antegrade wire can initially serve as a marker for retrograde wiring attempts using the "kissing wire" approach and, if unsuccessful, subsequently as setup for reverse controlled antegrade and retrograde tracking (CART) as we will describe. With our support catheter at the distal cap, the collateral crossing wire should be removed and replaced with a CTO crossing wire. If the path of the CTO segment is well defined, unambiguous, and short, we advocate using a stiff tapered non-jacketed guidewire such as a Confianza Pro 12 as this combines steer ability with maximal puncture force. If the path is ill defined initially, a tapered soft jacketed guidewire (i.e., Fielder XT), or a stiff jacketed guidewire like the Pilot 200 is more likely to stay within the vessel architecture. Advancing through the lesion should be expeditious but steady, and any significant progress should be checked with contrast injections from the appropriate guide; but in general, we discourage injections through the microcatheter once out of the collaterals as if it is in the subintimal space, a large hydraulic dissection will be created which can complicate further progress. If the retrograde wire passes into the proximal true lumen, as confirmed by two angiographic views, see section "Retrograde Recanalization Techniques" below. If the retrograde jacketed guidewire is difficult to advance and forms a loop or a "knuckle," this can be used to dissect up the subintimal space and is often easier to cross the lesion in this subintimal plane. This approach was originally described by Colombo et al. as an adjunct to antegrade CTO PCI and is referred to as the subintimal tracking and reentry (STAR) technique [16]. Stiffed tapered non-jacketed wires and stiff non-tapered jacketed wires can be used to enter the distal cap in a resistant lesion but can be exchanged for a softer wire once they have served their purpose. The Pilot 200 can be an effective knuckle wire but tends to make larger loops. The Fielder XT is the initial wire used for this technique, as the tapered hydrophilic tip often easily enters the subintimal space, and it tends to form a smaller controllable knuckle. Once the retrograde wire is knuckled and advanced into the CTO, the objective is to get the knuckle and microcatheter to the proximal cap in the subintimal space so that we are set up for reverse CART.

CART

The controlled antegrade and retrograde tracking (CART) technique was originally described by Surmely and colleagues in 2006 and consists of advancing the retrograde wire into the occlusion segment and deploying a retrograde balloon in the subintimal space to connect the subintimal retrograde wire with the antegrade wire in the true lumen (Figs. 24.6 and 24.7) [17]. This technique has an advantage over the STAR technique where subintimal dissections can be extensive and side branches distal to the occlusion segment can be compromised. Subintimal wire passage and reentry to the true lumen followed by "true-false-true" stenting can facilitate CTO recanalization by bypassing challenging intraluminal fibrocalcific plaque. Since its first description in the treatment of coronary CTOs, there is some controversy as to its efficacy and safety [18–20]. Recently, however, a large series of CART stenting was presented demonstrating re-occlusion rates of only 6 % and a 12-month TVR rate of 13 %, which is comparable to traditional antegrade CTO outcomes with DES [21–23]. Since the advent of the Corsair septal dilator and support catheter, reverse CART has gained popularity. In this case, wires are advanced both retrograde and antegrade, and subintimal balloon inflations are carried out over the antegrade wire, which serves to facilitate retrograde crossing into the true lumen. Prior to inflating a balloon, you must be certain the catheter is within the vessel architecture. Confirmation of this is made easier with the retrograde technique as both wires can be seen lying adjacent to each other in multiple views. Once you have dilated the antegrade subintimal balloon, you should be very careful not to inject via the antegrade guide until recanalization has been performed as this can lead to a hydraulic dissection that can make the procedure more challenging. Large balloons sized to the reference vessel diameter will increase the chances of connecting the luminal and subintimal spaces. Recoil of the subintimal space can prevent retrograde wiring, and larger balloons may improve the chances of connecting the spaces. Recently, a case series of intravascular ultrasound (IVUS)-guided reverse CART has been published showing high success rates in the hands of very experienced operators [24]. IVUS was utilized to size antegrade balloons to the reference vessel and to evaluate the relative position of the retrograde and antegrade wires. Although the technical success rate of IVUS-guided reverse CART was 100 % in this series, the added complexity and cost of adding IVUS to routine retrograde procedures has not been evaluated. After successful retrograde wiring into the true lumen, we can proceed with any number of recanalization techniques.

Retrograde Recanalization Techniques

Once the retrograde wire is apparently proximal to the occlusion segment, the wire should advance easily to the aorta and appear to freely flop into the aortic root. Failure to observe this free motion suggests the wire may still be subintimal, and withdrawal and readvancement should be attempted until the result is satisfactory. Additionally, IVUS may be performed at this point over the antegrade wire to confirm the intraluminal position of the retrograde wire if there is any concern. CTO recanalization may be performed via number of techniques, the most popular include the following: (1) wire externalization and subsequent antegrade balloon and stent delivery, (2) retrograde ballooning with or without retrograde wire trapping followed by antegrade wiring and stent delivery, (3) retrograde ballooning and stenting with or without retrograde wire trapping, and (4) antegrade snaring of the retrograde wire with pull-through and subsequent antegrade ballooning and stenting.

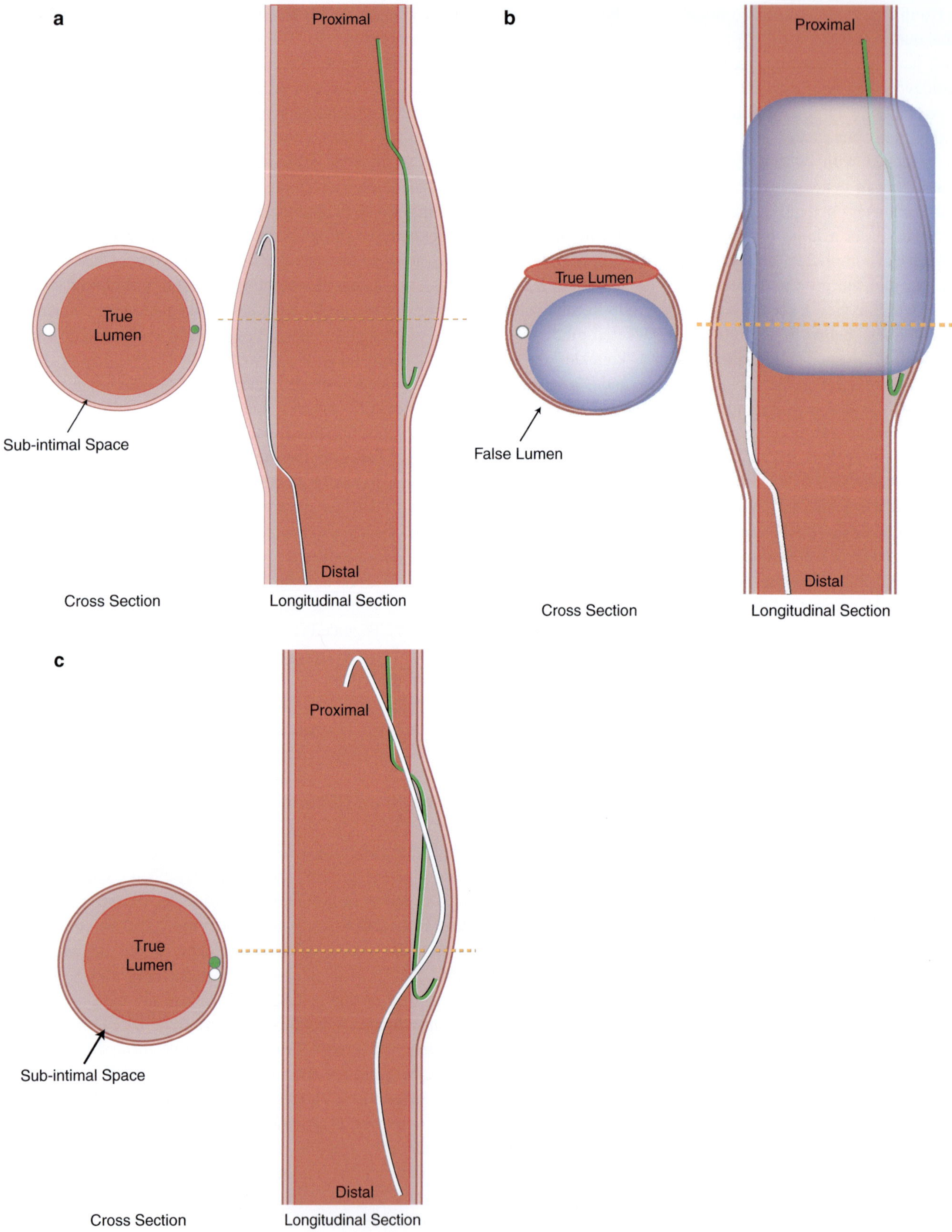

Fig. 24.6 (**a**) Concept of reverse CART. In this example, both the antegrade (*green*) and retrograde (*white*) wires are in the subintimal (*black*) space. (**b**) A large antegrade monorail balloon sized to the estimated vessel reference diameter is dilated over the antegrade wire to reorient the wires into the same space. (**c**) Since the retrograde and antegrade wires both originate in the true lumen, and the antegrade balloon dilatation provides a large connection between the subintimal space and the true lumen proximally, the retrograde wire can now be easily advanced into the true lumen proximally. The retrograde wires pass from true to false to true lumen all within the CTO segment. One advantage of reverse CART is the natural restriction of the subintimal dissection and reentry within the boundaries of the CTO segment

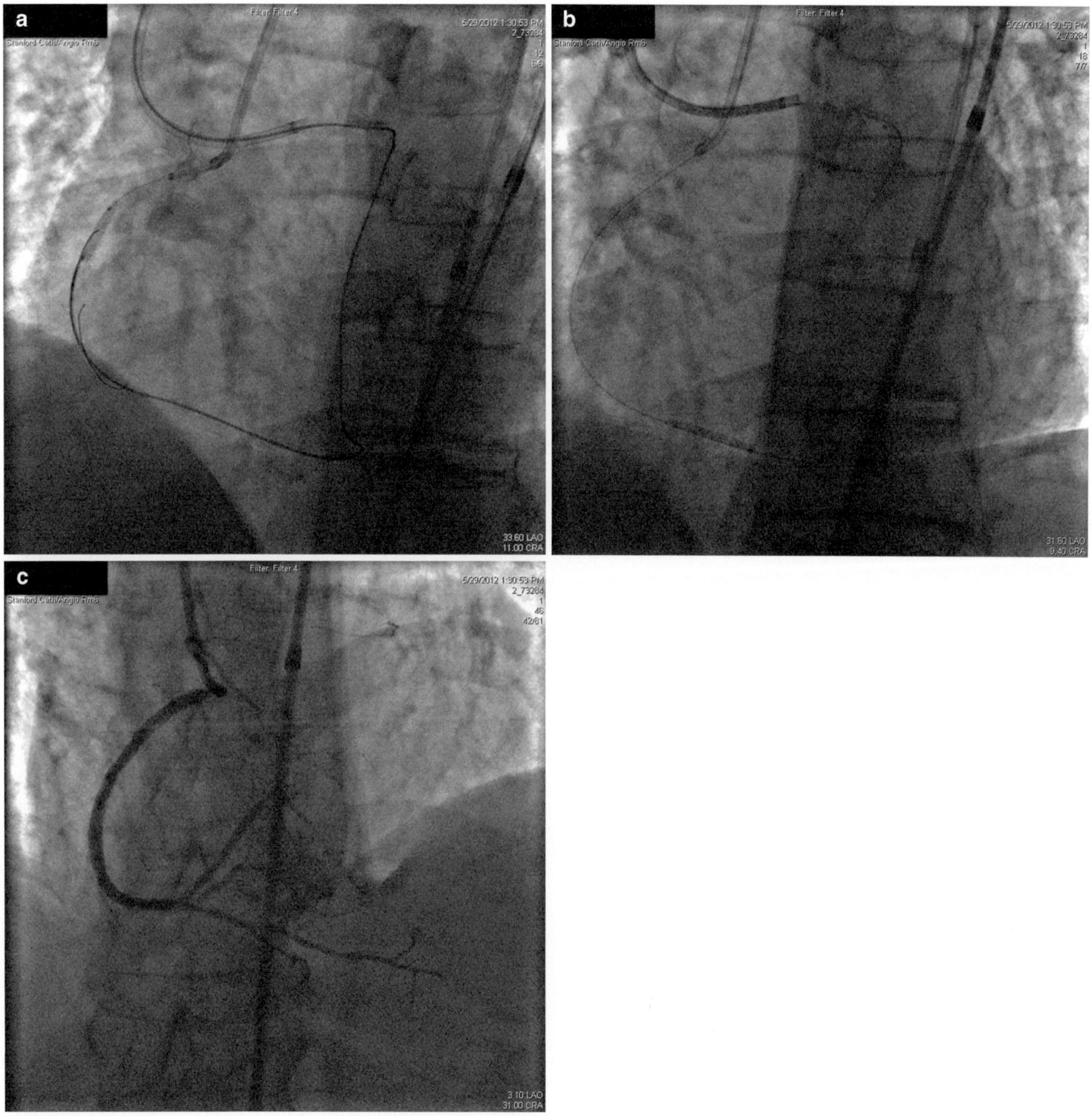

Fig. 24.7 (**a**) Guideliner reverse CART being performed in the proximal RCA. A 3.0 balloon is dilated on the antegrade wire with the tip of the Corsair and retrograde wire in the adjacent subintimal space. The balloon is then deflated and the retrograde wire is easily advanced into the Guideliner. In this case, a Guideliner shortens the distance the retrograde wire needs to travel within the heavily diseased proximal segment. Once the guidewire is in the Guideliner, the wire is easily advanced to allow for subsequent externalization. (**b**) Once the wire was externalized, we performed antegrade PCI over the externalized retrograde wire. (**c**) Final result

Of these approaches, we advocate wire externalization as the primary technique that most effectively facilitates efficient recanalization and provides the most support for balloon and stent delivery in complex CTOs [25]. We start by advancing our retrograde wire into the antegrade guide. If this cannot be easily achieved, and the retrograde wire is in the aorta, we employ a Merit EN Snare (18/30), 3-loop snare via the antegrade guide to trap the wire (Fig. 24.8). This is often easier to accomplish in the ascending aorta or the arch and may require pulling back the antegrade guide to facilitate capture and then carefully reseating the guide once the retrograde wire is pulled inside. You must be careful to snare the wire distally with stiff wires as prolapsing the wire into the guide on the stiff portion may not be

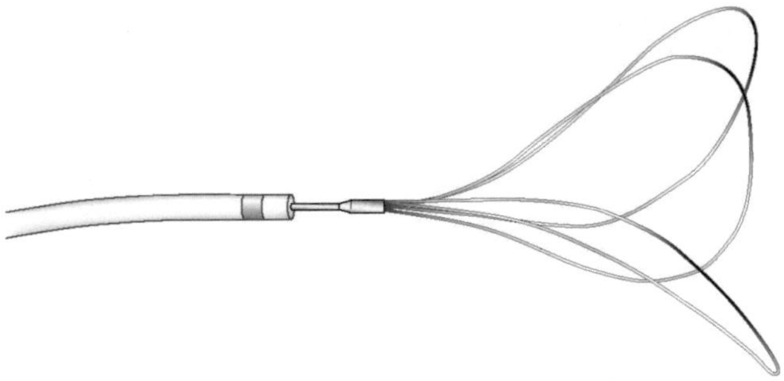

Fig. 24.8 18-3 Merit EN Sare. This large snare can be used directly in the guiding catheter without a collar to retrieve wires in the aorta. Care should be taken not to fold over a stiff wire such as the Confianza Pro 12 on the body of the wire as these will not pull through into the guide

possible. It is not recommended to snare the rota-floppy guidewire as the weld at the distal transition can snap. Once in the antegrade guide, the Corsair catheter is advanced until in the antegrade guide and then the retrograde wire is removed if not snared. This is the point at which if you did not use a short retrograde guide, the Corsair catheter may not have the length to reach the antegrade guide. We then use a dedicated externalization wire; examples are the RG3 available outside the United States which is the preferred option as it is a dedicated 330 cm externalization wire. Alternatively, the ViperWire Advance, a 335 cm stiff peripheral wire or R350 (Vascular Solutions), a 350 cm moderate stiffness wire, have sufficient length and support to be easily externalized. An alternative is the rota-floppy wire, which is a 325 cm wire. This wire can be more challenging as the reverse taper to 0.008″ can lead to kinking, and the lack of support can make advancing through the system painstakingly slow. Once the retrograde wire is approaching the antegrade hemostatic valve, this should be removed and the retrograde wire advanced with sufficient length protruding from the antegrade guide to reload the hemostatic valve over the wire. Retention of the introducer needle in the valve can make this step easier. From this point forward, great care should be exercised when pulling on the retrograde wire or when backing out any retrograde gear as this can cause deep seating of the retrograde guide and subsequent donor vessel ischemia and/or dissection. In order to use the retrograde wire for antegrade equipment delivery, we need to back out our microcatheter to a position distal to the CTO. The microcatheter should remain across the collaterals to protect them from injury as balloons, and stents are passed antegrade on the retrograde wire. The floppy tip of the wire can be cut off to facilitate easily loading of balloons and stents. At this point, we can advance an appropriately sized Rx balloon antegrade over our externalized retrograde wire and perform angioplasty of the occlusion segment. Again, care must be taken when withdrawing any gear over the retrograde wire as this can cause deep seating of the retrograde guide and both fluoroscopic supervision, as well as attention to retrograde pressure is paramount to preventing a complication at this stage. The likelihood of inadvertent guide displacement is higher in calcified or tortuous CTO segments as with traditional PCI. Stenting and post-dilatation can then be performed in the same fashion. At this point, a gentle angiogram should be performed via the antegrade guide to document the result, and further stenting and post-dilatation can be performed as indicated. In general, we favor restricting stenting to the occlusion segment and any uncovered dissections and not stenting the distal vessel if diffusely small. Often the distal vessel size will improve with blood flow as often is documented in follow-up of these patients.

Once the PCI is complete, retrieval of the retrograde equipment needs to be performed. The first step is to readvance the microcatheter to the antegrade guide or minimally into the stented segment in order to protect the vessel from the distal tip, especially if you cut the tip of the guidewire off to facilitate balloon and stent loading. Then, the retrograde wire should be pulled back completely through the microcatheter followed by removal of the microcatheter from the collaterals with attention to preventing deep seating of the retrograde guide. A final retrograde injection should be made to document there is no dissection in the ostium and to assess collaterals for damage. The collateral flow may be weak or reversed at this point depending on the acute flow increase in the CTO.

Another option for retrograde wire PCI is the delivery of stents via the collaterals which is achieved by overdilation of the septal (and only septals) with a 2.0 × 40 mm or 2.0 × 100 mm length balloons at 4–6 atm to overstretch the septal. A stent can then be passed retrograde through this overdilated septal. This technique has not gained widespread adoption as it is rare that recanalization with externalization of the guidewire cannot be achieved with currently available technologies. It has also been proposed, however, in cases of failure that overdilating the septal to promote a large collateral to reduce ischemic burden could be performed. Data in regard to safety and efficacy are pending at the time of this submission.

Conclusion

Retrograde CTO PCI has becoming increasingly popular among a growing number of interventionalists as the technologies and procedural methodologies have improved. It is clear in the current CTO PCI era retrograde techniques are critical to achieving a high degree of success and efficiency. As the number of "retrograde" operators and the understanding of this procedure grow, we expect this will become a standard technique for the treatment of CTOs.

References

1. Joyal D, Afilalo J, Rinfret S. Effectiveness of recanalization of chronic total occlusions: a systematic review and meta-analysis. Am Heart J. 2010;160:179–87.
2. Morino Y, Kimura T, Hayashi Y, et al. In-hospital outcomes of contemporary percutaneous coronary intervention in patients with chronic total occlusion insights from the J-CTO Registry (Multicenter CTO Registry in Japan). JACC Cardiovasc Interv. 2010;3:143–51.
3. Thompson CA, Jayne JE, Robb JF, et al. Retrograde techniques and the impact of operator volume on percutaneous intervention for coronary chronic total occlusions an early U.S. experience. JACC Cardiovasc Interv. 2009;2:834–42.
4. Kahn JK, Hartzler GO. Retrograde coronary angioplasty of isolated arterial segments through saphenous vein bypass grafts. Cathet Cardiovasc Diagn. 1990;20:88–93.
5. Surmely J-F, Katoh O, Tsuchikane E, Nasu K, Suzuki T. Coronary septal collaterals as an access for the retrograde approach in the percutaneous treatment of coronary chronic total occlusions. Catheter Cardiovasc Interv. 2007;69:826–32.
6. Zhang B, Liao H-T, Jin L-J, et al. Retrograde percutaneous recanalization of chronic total occlusion of the coronary arteries via epicardial coronary collateral artery in 5 patients. Zhonghua Xin Xue Guan Bing Za Zhi. 2010;38:794–7.
7. Barlis P, Di Mario C. Retrograde approach to recanalising coronary chronic total occlusions immediately following a failed conventional attempt. Int J Cardiol. 2009;133:e14–17.
8. Hsu JT, Tamai H, Kyo E, Tsuji T, Watanabe S. Traditional antegrade approach versus combined antegrade and retrograde approach in the percutaneous treatment of coronary chronic total occlusions. Catheter Cardiovasc Interv. 2009;74:555–63.
9. Rathore S, Katoh O, Matsuo H, et al. Retrograde percutaneous recanalization of chronic total occlusion of the coronary arteries: procedural outcomes and predictors of success in contemporary practice. Circ Cardiovasc Interv. 2009;2:124–32.
10. Rathore S, Hakeem A, Pauriah M, Roberts E, Beaumont A, Morris JL. A comparison of the transradial and the transfemoral approach in chronic total occlusion percutaneous coronary intervention. Catheter Cardiovasc Interv. 2009;73:883–7.
11. Rinfret S, Joyal D, Nguyen CM, et al. Retrograde recanalization of chronic total occlusions from the transradial approach; Early Canadian experience. Catheter Cardiovasc Interv. 2011;78(3):366–74.
12. Di Mario C, Ramasami N. Techniques to enhance guide catheter support. Catheter Cardiovasc Interv. 2008;72:505–12.
13. Rentrop KP, Cohen M, Blanke H, Phillips RA. Changes in collateral channel filling immediately after controlled coronary artery occlusion by an angioplasty balloon in human subjects. J Am Coll Cardiol. 1985;5:587–92.
14. Werner GS, Ferrari M, Heinke S, et al. Angiographic assessment of collateral connections in comparison with invasively determined collateral function in chronic coronary occlusions. Circulation. 2003;107:1972–7.
15. Tsuchikane E, Katoh O, Kimura M, Nasu K, Kinoshita Y, Suzuki T. The first clinical experience with a novel catheter for collateral channel tracking in retrograde approach for chronic coronary total occlusions. JACC Cardiovasc Interv. 2010;3:165–71.
16. Colombo A, Mikhail GW, Michev I, et al. Treating chronic total occlusions using subintimal tracking and reentry: the STAR technique. Catheter Cardiovasc Interv. 2005;64:407–11. discussion 12.
17. Surmely J-F, Tsuchikane E, Katoh O, et al. New concept for CTO recanalization using controlled antegrade and retrograde subintimal tracking: the CART technique. J Invasive Cardiol. 2006;18: 334–8.
18. Reimers B, Di Mario C, Colombo A. Subintimal stent implantation for the treatment of a chronic coronary occlusion. G Ital Cardiol. 1997;27:1158–63.
19. Erlich I, Strauss BH, Butany J. Stent thrombosis following the STAR technique in a complex RCA chronic total occlusion. Catheter Cardiovasc Interv. 2006;68:708–12.
20. Miyazaki S, Hiasa Y, Kishi K. Very late thrombosis after subintimal sirolimus-eluting stent implantation during percutaneous coronary intervention for chronic total occlusion. J Invasive Cardiol. 2010; 22:E162–5.
21. Masashi Kimura ET, Osamu Katoh, Nobuyoshi Tanaka, Kenya Nasu, Yoshihisa Kinoshita, Yasushi Asakura, Tatsuya Ito, Suzuki T. The safety and efficacy of sub-intimal stenting after retrograde approach for chronic total occlusions: a sub-analysis of the CARTTM registry. In: I2 Summit April 3, 2011.
22. Liu W, Wagatsuma K, Toda M, et al. Short- and long-term follow-up of percutaneous coronary intervention for chronic total occlusion through transradial approach: tips for successful procedure from a single-center experience. J Interv Cardiol. 2011;24:137–43.
23. Rahel BM, Laarman GJ, Kelder JC, Ten Berg JM, Suttorp MJ. Three-year clinical outcome after primary stenting of totally occluded native coronary arteries: a randomized comparison of bare-metal stent implantation with sirolimus-eluting stent implantation for the treatment of total coronary occlusions (Primary Stenting of Totally Occluded Native Coronary Arteries [PRISON] II study). Am Heart J. 2009;157:149–55.
24. Rathore S, Katoh O, Tuschikane E, Oida A, Suzuki T, Takase S. A novel modification of the retrograde approach for the recanalization of chronic total occlusion of the coronary arteries intravascular ultrasound-guided reverse controlled antegrade and retrograde tracking. JACC Cardiovasc Interv. 2010;3:155–64.
25. Ge J-B, Zhang F, Ge L, Qian J-Y, Wang H. Wire trapping technique combined with retrograde approach for recanalization of chronic total occlusion. Chin Med J. 2008;121:1753–6.

Intravascular Ultrasound Applications for Chronic Total Occlusion Percutaneous Intervention

25

Satoru Sumitsuji

There are primary two roles for intravascular ultrasound (IVUS) in chronic total occlusion percutaneous intervention (CTO-PCI). One is to facilitate lesion access and wire crossing and the other is for optimization of the PCI result such as optimal stent expansion and lesion coverage. In this chapter, we will briefly focus on the former: how to use IVUS for wire crossing in CTO-PCI.

A major point of IVUS use for wire crossing in CTO-PCI relates to understanding of histopathology. We will introduce the relationships between IVUS findings and histopathology and then demonstrate how to apply IVUS information for CTO-PCI with case reviews.

Understanding Histopathologic Features and IVUS Images in Chronic Total Occlusion

Two important anatomic factors in the CTO segment are "intimal plaque" and "subintimal space." IVUS can confirm this relationship and determine equipment position in clinical practice. Figure 25.1 shows histopathologic and IVUS imaging that demonstrates the lumen segment and subintimal/subadventitial space. In histopathology, the subintimal space locates between intimal plaque and adventitia and is weaker and more easily dissected than those two adjacent components. In the corresponding IVUS image, the subintimal space is located around external elastic membrane (EEM), which can be dissected and cause intramural hematoma. Thus, a wire or device located near EEM means it is located in subintimal space and subsequently has a higher possibility of subintimal tracking.

S. Sumitsuji, MD
Advanced Cardiovascular Therapeutics,
Osaka University, 1-1 Yamadaoka, Suita, Osaka 565-0871, Japan
e-mail: sumi2g@sea.plala.or.jp

IVUS in CTO-PCI

The options of IVUS use in CTO-PCI are (1) identifying the optimal point for wiring at CTO entry, (2) IVUS-guided reentry from false lumen to true lumen, and (3) to determine appropriate strategy to cross wire to true lumen in retrograde approaches.

Identifying Optimal Position for CTO Entry

The entry point of the CTO segment is one of risk area where the wire can inadvertently migrate into the subintimal space or exit the vessel architecture altogether, especially in abrupt-/blunt-type CTO located at side branches. The IVUS catheter can be advanced into the side branch near the proximal cap and identify the intimal plaque position and center of intimal plaque (sweet spot) in angiogram (Fig. 25.2).

In practice:

1. Advance IVUS catheter to proximal side branch of CTO.
2. Move transducer manually examining the IVUS image in real time.
3. Stop transducer when IVUS shows entry of main branch occlusion.
4. 1 mm pull back transducer (mostly transducer advances 1 mm with dye injection) and take image to identify where is the correlated position in the angiogram.

Depending on the IVUS system and vessel-lesion characteristics, the IVUS catheter may remain inside the coronary for live imaging or withdrawn into the guide catheter during CTO wiring. Simultaneous IVUS observation during wire manipulation is useful, but sometimes the IVUS catheter disturbs CTO wire control. Once the proximal cap is penetrated, confirmatory IVUS can be performed easily by reinserting the IVUS into the coronary to reassure that the starting point is correct.

A case using IVUS to identify the sweet spot in CTO entry was shown in Fig. 25.3.

C.A. Thompson (ed.), *Textbook of Cardiovascular Intervention*,
DOI 10.1007/978-1-4471-4528-8_25, © Springer-Verlag London 2014

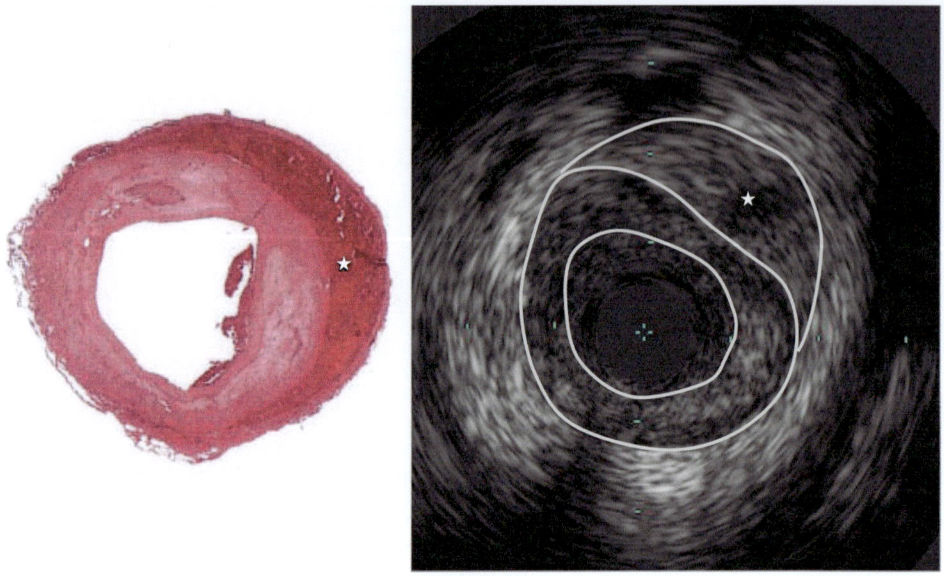

Fig. 25.1 Comparison images of coronary cross section. Histopathology (Lt) and IVUS (Rt) show quite similar findings; lumen, intimal plaque, and subintima space.* subintimal space

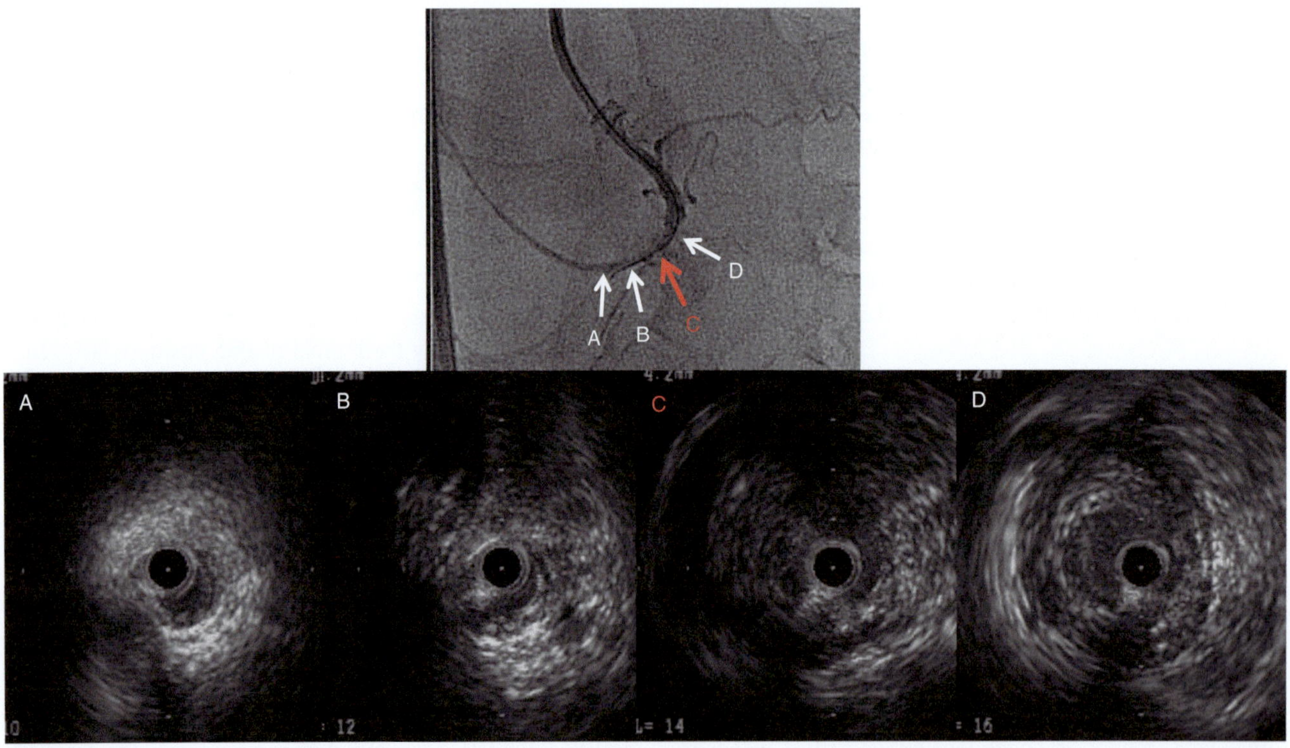

Fig. 25.2 IVUS demonstrates where is the best point (sweet spot) for wire advancement at entry of CTO lesion. In this RCA CTO case, *second image* from the *right* shows the sweet spot. *arrows* indicate IVUS images with corresponding area of the angiogram

The target lesion was in the proximal to mid RCA with a proximal side branch and a tiny channel. The first guide wire (GW) was advanced into the channel without IVUS; however, the GW went beside the distal true lumen. Next, an IVUS catheter was advanced to the proximal side branch, and we confirmed the first GW was already positioned near EEM area at entry point which suggest high risk of subintimal tracking. After confirmation of position of sweet spot of CTO entry, we intentionally advanced second GW, and IVUS clearly showed the difference in position of those two wires and the correct position of the second GW position in the intimal plaque. The second wire was relatively easily crossed to distal true lumen.

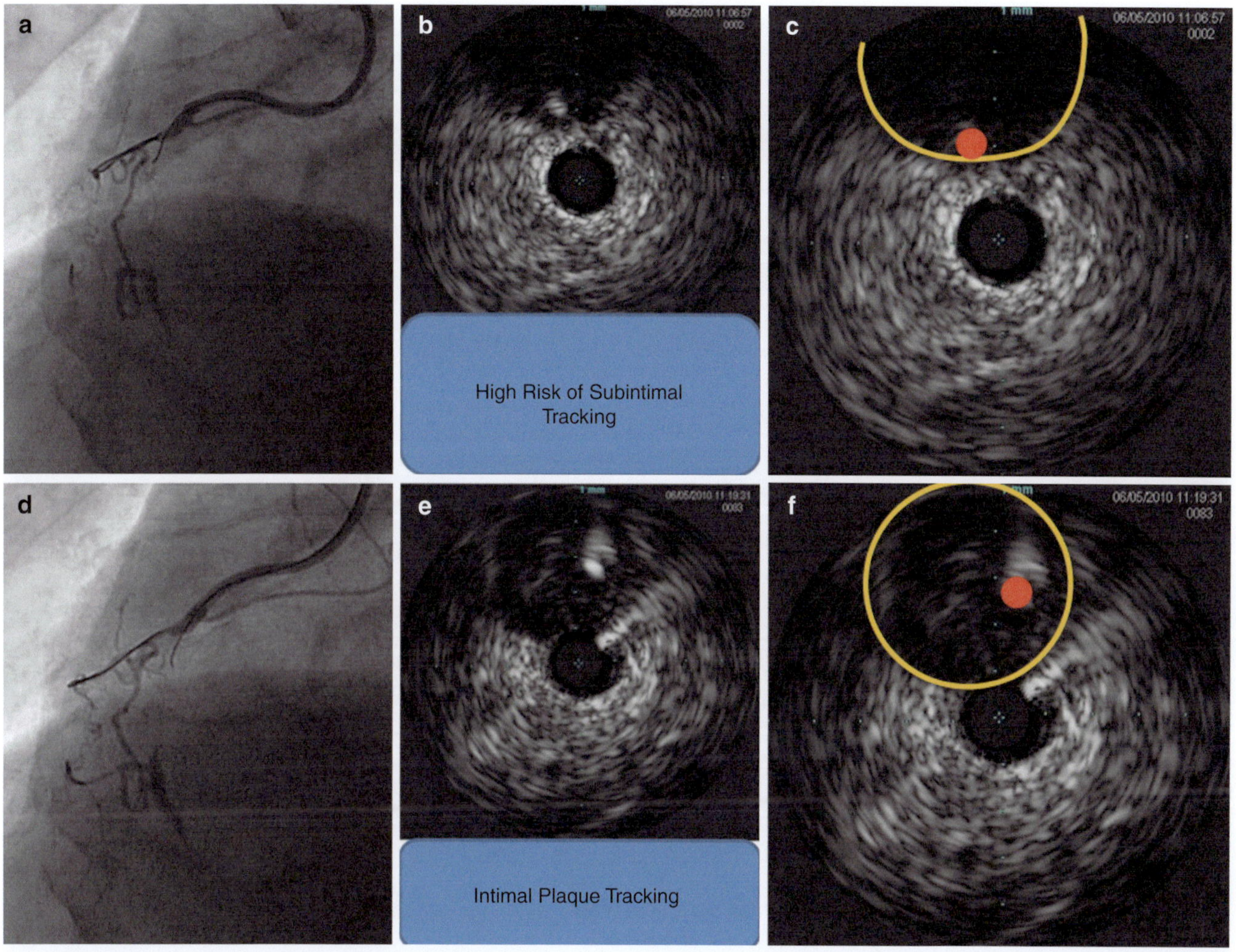

Fig. 25.3 RCA proximal – mid CTO case. First guide wire was advanced around EEM; on the other hand, second guide wire was clearly more inside and intra- intimal plaque. Using this IVUS information, we could avoid subintimal tracking. (**a**) the first guide wire was advanced into remaining channel, (**b**) high risk of subintimal tracking, (**c**) guide wire was clearly positioned around EEM which means high risk of subintimal tracking, (**d**) the second wire directed into more inside in LAO view, (**e**) intimal plaque tracking, and (**f**) the second guide wire located more center which means intimal plaque tracking

IVUS-Guided Reentry from False Lumen to True Lumen

Another IVUS use in antegrade approach for CTO-PCI is using IVUS for wire reentry from false lumen to true lumen. With recent development of sophisticated reentry devices, this option may not be used for many cases, but still we have situations without reentry device availability or poor candidate reentry device.

The target is a large obtuse marginal branch of the left circumflex artery, total occluded lesion without good retrograde channel or reentry device options. After failure of usual antegrade parallel wire technique, we finally tried to perform IVUS-guided reentry. To advance the IVUS catheter distally, the false lumen was carefully dilated with small size balloon (1.5 mm as usual, 2.0 mm in maximum). Then, the IVUS catheter could be advanced to the lesion and demonstrate position of the wire (Fig. 25.4). According to the IVUS information, we could identify the site the wire migrated into subintimal space and advanced another GW to intimal plaque and finally distal true lumen. One tip for this technique is to minimize contrast injection so as not to make the false lumen larger because subintimal hematoma can decrease the chance of successful wire crossing.

IVUS for Retrograde Approach

In retrograde approaches for CTO-PCI, IVUS can be used to confirm retrograde wire position and to decide appropriate strategy for wire crossing.

A case of proximal LAD CTO with diseased SVG graft is shown in Fig. 25.5. Retrograde approach was performed through the diseased SVG, and retrograde wire was

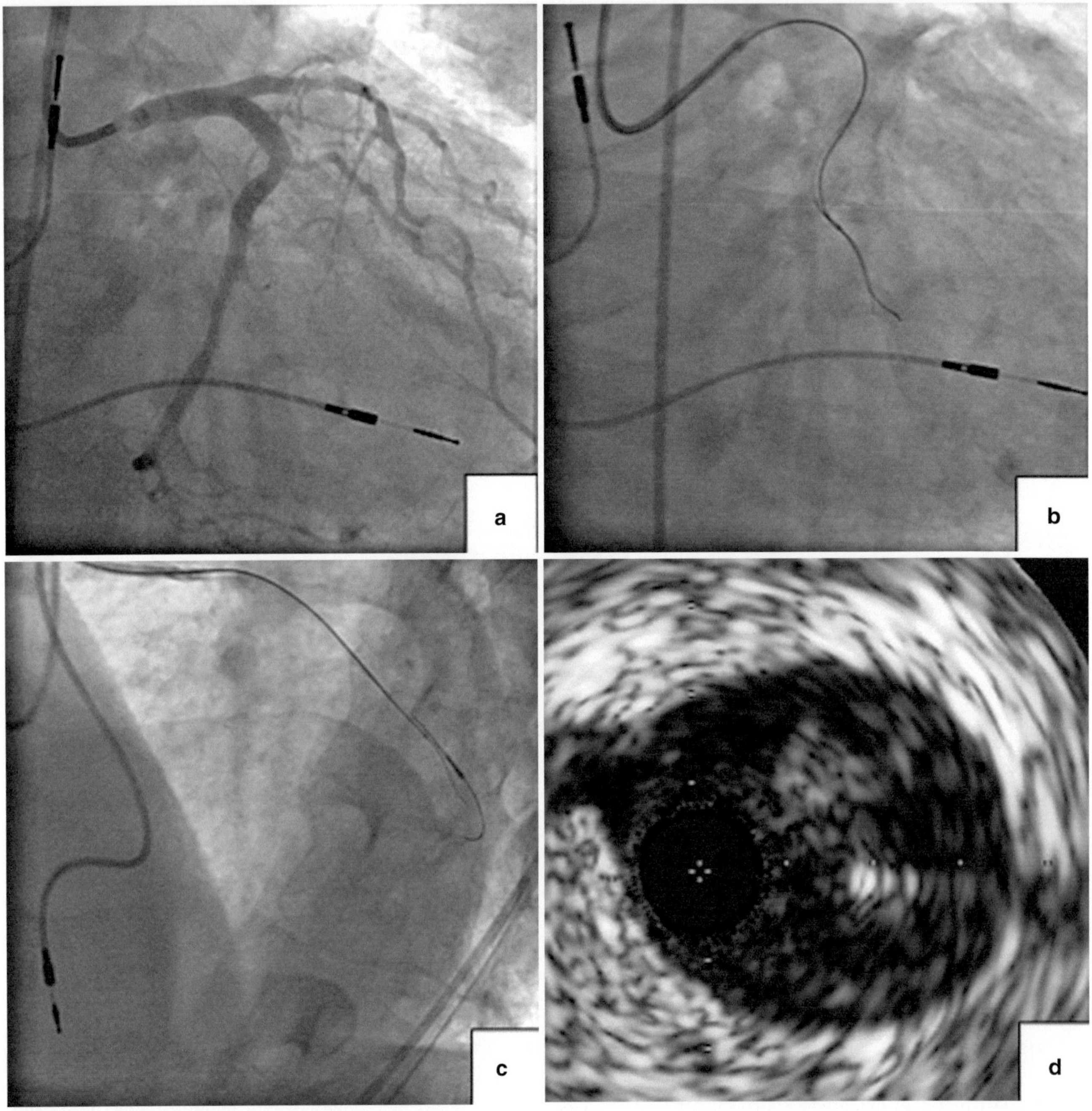

Fig. 25.4 IVUS-guided reentry in OM CTO-PCI case. (**a**) pre-angiogram, (**b**) failure with parallel wire technique, (**c**) fluoro-image of IVUS-guided reentry, (**d**) IVUS was in the subintimal space and 2nd CTO wire was in the intimal plaque. The 2nd CTO wire was subsequently crossed into the distal true lumen. (**e**) final angiogram

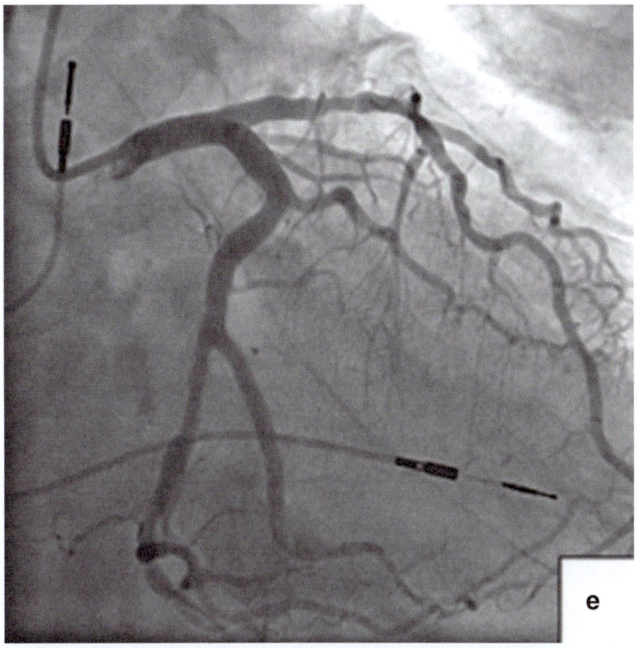

Fig. 25.4 (continued)

confirmed by IVUS advanced into the proximal diagonal branch. The position of the retrograde wire was very close to the proximal true lumen but still in the intimal plaque and at point 2 was the closest site to the proximal true lumen. Next, we directed the wire toward the proximal true lumen from point 2 and finally a stiff wire (Confianza Pro 9 g) successfully crossed to the proximal true lumen.

A case of reverse CART with a reattempted distal RCA CTO is shown in Fig. 25.6. Both the antegrade and retrograde wire were advanced into the CTO lesion. It is an important point for success with this technique to advance both wires with enough length of overlap for confirmation by IVUS. In this case, IVUS imaging demonstrated separation of the two wires (IVUS at 6 o'clock and the retrograde wire at 12 o'clock) as angiogram showed. With careful investigation of IVUS, however, position of the retrograde wire tip was very close to the proximal lumen after antegrade balloon dilation. According to the IVUS information, the best strategy must be simply advancing the retrograde wire, and the retrograde wire easily crossed to proximal true lumen.

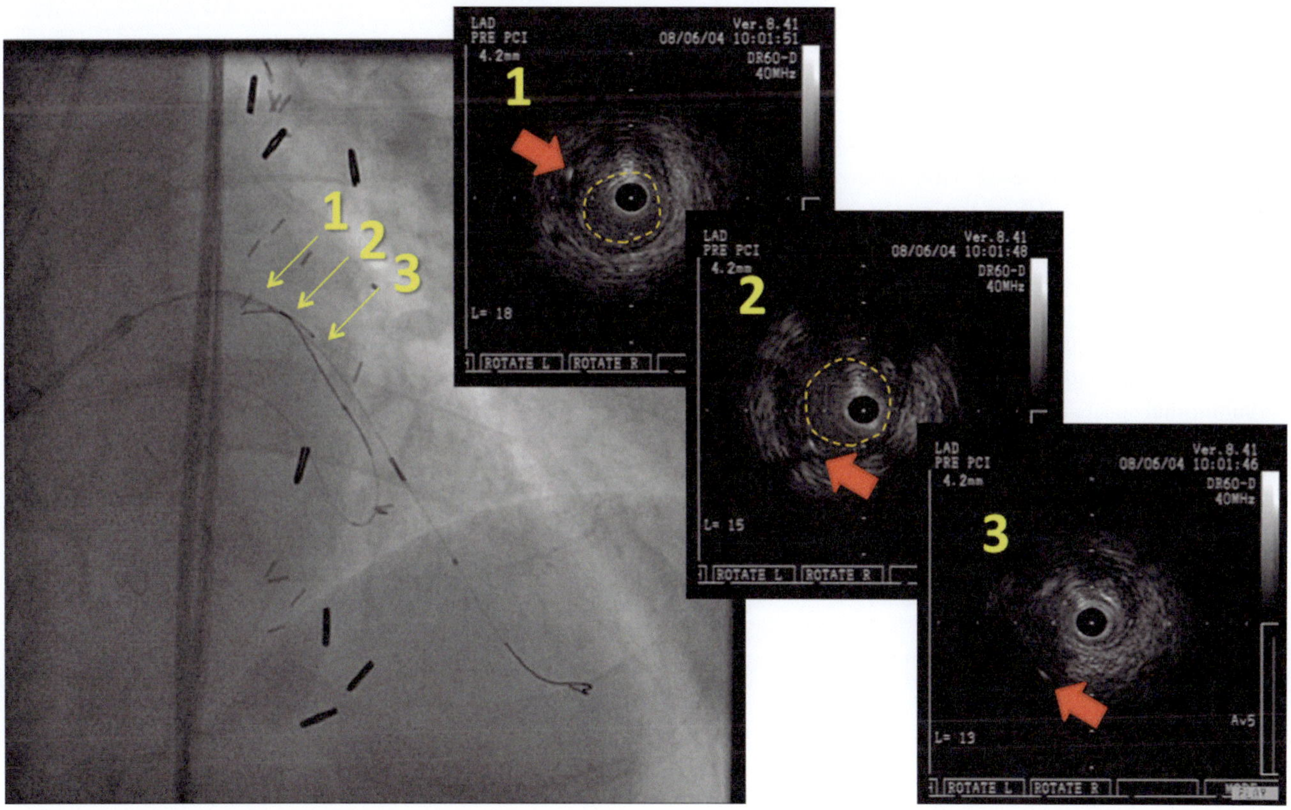

Fig. 25.5 IVUS-guided retrograde wire crossing. IVUS was advanced into diagonal branch, and IVUS showed position of retrograde wire clearly (*red arrow*). Retrograde wire was closest to the proximal true lumen at point 2. *Yellow arrows* shows positions of IVUS cross sections (1–3) and *yellow dashed* line in IVUS image 1 and 2 is proximal true lumen, also *red arrow* in IVUS image 1 and 2 means position of retrograde wire

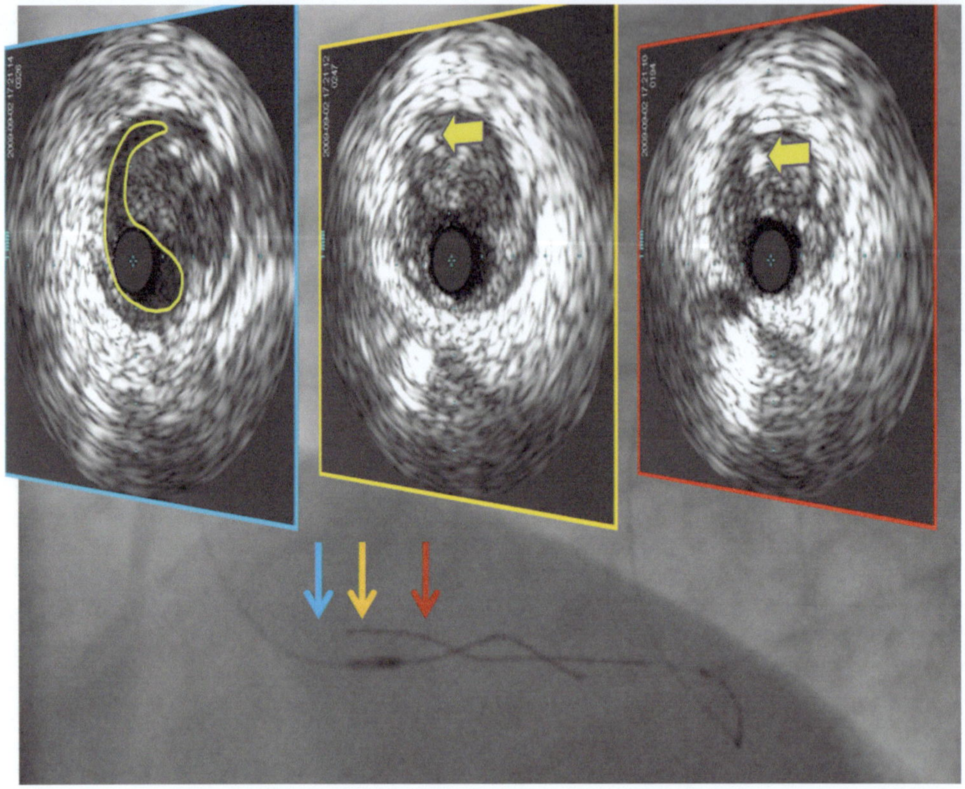

Fig. 25.6 IVUS images in reverse CART case. As with angiogram, positions of two wires (antegrade and retrograde) were distantly positioned in cross section (*yellow*, retrograde wire in 11–12 o'clock and antegrade wire and IVUS in 6 o'clock). However, with careful assessment of IVUS, in long axis position of retrograde, wire's tip was close to the proximal lumen which was created by antegrade balloon (*blue*, *yellow line*)

The last case example is from an LCX CTO-PCI procedure, and both the antegrade and retrograde wires were advanced into the CTO lesion after failure of conventional antegrade approach. IVUS on the antegrade wire showed the following images:

1. In distal CTO site, both the antegrade wire and retrograde wire were positioned in same lumen.
2. In the mid- to proximal CTO site, the antegrade wire was in an intimal plaque, but the retrograde wire was in the subintimal space, and the tip of retrograde wire was positioned behind calcium.

According to the IVUS information, what we should do next is to direct the retrograde wire to the proximal true lumen. In this particular case, the retrograde wire made a dissection space, but with IVUS information, the redirection of the retrograde wire to the proximal true lumen was simple.

Conclusion

In this section, we described several patterns of IVUS use during CTO-PCI. Key points of IVUS use are understanding of histopathologic features of the CTO lesion and getting accurate information of device position.

Percutaneous Mitral and Aortic Balloon Valvuloplasty

26

Igor F. Palacios, Sammy Elmariah, and Dabit Arzamendi

Mitral Valvuloplasty

Before 1982, cardiac surgery was the conventional form of treatment for symptomatic stenotic valvular heart disease lesions. Today, percutaneous balloon dilatation of stenotic cardiac valves is being used in many centers for the treatment of patients with pulmonic, mitral, aortic, and tricuspid stenosis. Since its introduction in 1984 by Inoue et al. [1–11] percutaneous mitral balloon commissurotomy (PMV) has been used successfully as an alternative to open or closed surgical mitral commissurotomy in the treatment of patients with symptomatic rheumatic mitral stenosis [12–34]. PMV produces good immediate hemodynamic outcome, low complication rate, and clinical improvement in the majority of patients with mitral stenosis. PMV is safe and effective and provides sustained clinical and hemodynamic improvement in patients with rheumatic mitral stenosis. The immediate and long-term results appear to be similar to those of surgical mitral commissurotomy [12–34]. Today, PMV is the preferred form of therapy for relief of mitral stenosis for a selected group of patients with symptomatic mitral stenosis.

I.F. Palacios, MD
Department of Medicine, Division of Cardiology, Harvard Medical School, Boston, MA, USA

Interventional Cardiology, Massachusetts General Hospital, 55 Fruit Street, Boston, MA 02114, USA

S. Elmariah, MD
Division of Cardiology, Department of Medicine, Massachusetts General Hospital, 55 Fruit Street, Boston, MA, USA

D. Arzamendi, MD, MSc (✉)
Interventional Cardiology & Structural Heart Disease, Cardiology Division, Massachusetts General Hospital, 55 Fruit Street, GBR 800, Boston, MA 02114, USA
e-mail: darzamendi@partners.org

Patient Selection

Selection of patients for PMV should be based on symptoms, physical examination, and two-dimensional and Doppler echocardiographic findings [35]. PMV is usually performed electively. However, emergency PMV can be performed as a lifesaving procedure in patients with mitral stenosis and severe pulmonary edema refractory to medical therapy and/or cardiogenic shock. Patients considered for PMV should be symptomatic (NYHA $\geq$ II), should have no recent thromboembolic events, have less than 2 grades of mitral regurgitation by contrast ventriculography (using the Sellers' classification) [36], and have no evidence of left atrial thrombus on 2D and transesophageal echocardiography (Table 26.1). Transthoracic and transesophageal echocardiography should be performed routinely before PMV. Patients in atrial fibrillation and patients with previous embolic episodes should be anticoagulated with warfarin with a therapeutic prothrombin time for at least 3 months before PMV. Patients with left atrium thrombus on 2D echocardiography should be excluded. However, PMV could be performed in these patients if left atrium thrombus has resolved after warfarin therapy.

Percutaneous mitral valvuloplasty (PMV) success depends on appropriate patient selection. A multifactorial score derived from clinical, anatomic/echocardiographic, and hemodynamic variables would predict procedural success and clinical outcome (Fig. 26.1). Demographic data, echocardiographic parameters (including echocardiographic score, Fig. 26.2), and procedure-related variables recorded from 1,085 consecutive patients who underwent PMV at the MGH and their long-term clinical follow-up (death, mitral valve replacement, redo PMV) were used to derive this clinical score. Multivariate regression analysis of the first 800 procedures was performed to identify independent predictors of procedural success. Significant variables were formulated into a risk score and validated prospectively. Six independent predictors of PMV success were identified: age less than 55 years, New York Heart

C.A. Thompson (ed.), *Textbook of Cardiovascular Intervention*,
DOI 10.1007/978-1-4471-4528-8_26, © Springer-Verlag London 2014

Table 26.1 Recommendations for percutaneous mitral valvuloplasty

Current indication	Class	Level of evidence
Symptomatic patients (NYHA functional class II, III, or IV), moderate or severe mitral stenosis (area <1.5 cm^2), and valve morphology favorable for percutaneous balloon valvuloplasty in the absence of left atrial thrombus or moderate to severe mitral regurgitation	I	Grade A
Asymptomatic patients with moderate or severe mitral stenosis (area <1.5 cm^2) and valve morphology favorable for percutaneous balloon valvuloplasty who have pulmonary hypertension (pulmonary artery systolic pressure >50 mmHg at rest or 60 mmHg with exercise) in the absence of left atrial thrombus or moderate to severe mitral regurgitation	IIa	Grade C
Patients with NYHA functional classes III–IV, moderate or severe mitral stenosis (area <1.5 cm^2), and a nonpliable calcified valve who are at high risk for surgery in the absence of left atrial thrombus or moderate to severe mitral regurgitation	IIa	Grade B
Asymptomatic patients, moderate or severe mitral stenosis (area <1.5 cm^2), and valve morphology favorable for percutaneous balloon valvuloplasty who have new onset of atrial fibrillation in the absence of left atrial thrombus or moderate to severe mitral regurgitation	IIb	Grade B
Patients in NYHA functional classes III–IV, moderate or severe mitral stenosis (area <1.5 cm^2), and a nonpliable calcified valve who are low-risk candidates for surgery	IIb	Grade C
Patients with mild mitral stenosis	III	Grade C

Adapted from current American College of Cardiology/American Heart Association and European Guidelines for the management of patients with valvular heart disease

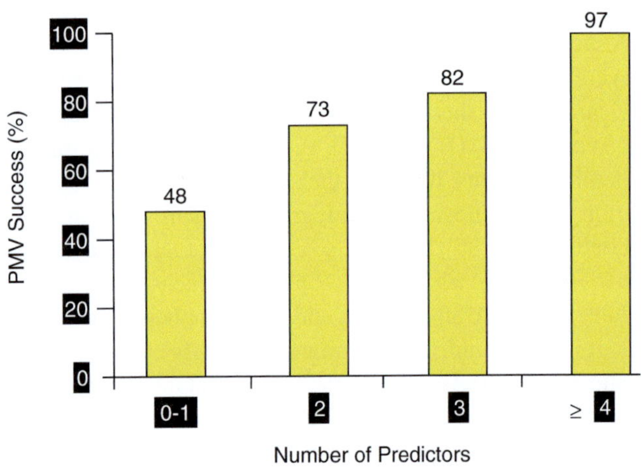

Fig. 26.1 A multifactorial score derived from clinical, anatomic/echocardiographic, and hemodynamic variables would predict procedural success and clinical outcome

Association classes I and II, pre-PMV mitral area of 1 cm^2 or greater, pre-PMV mitral regurgitation grade less than 2, echocardiographic score of 8 or greater, and male sex. A score was constructed from the arithmetic sum of variables present per patient. Procedural success rates increased incrementally with increasing score (0 % for 0/6, 39.7 % for 1/6, 54.4 % for 2/6, 77.3 % for 3/6, 85.7 % for 4/6, 95 % for 5/6, and 100 % for 6/6; $P<.001$). In a validation cohort ($n=285$ procedures), the multifactorial score remained a significant predictor of PMV success ($P<.001$). Comparison between the new score and the echocardiographic score confirmed that the new index was more sensitive and specific ($P<.001$). This new score also predicts long-term outcomes ($P<.001$). Clinical, anatomic, and hemodynamic variables predict PMV success and clinical outcome and may be formulated in a scoring system that would help to identify the best candidates for PMV.

PMV Technique

PMV is performed in the fasting state under mild sedation. Antibiotics (dicloxacillin 500 mg p.o. q/6 h for four doses started before the procedure or cefazolin 1 g i.v. at the time of the procedure) are used. Patients allergic to penicillin should receive vancomycin 1 g i.v. at the time of the procedure.

All patients carefully chosen as candidates for mitral balloon valvuloplasty should undergo diagnostic right and left and transseptal left heart catheterization. Following transseptal left heart catheterization, systemic anticoagulation is achieved by the intravenous administration of 100 units/Kg of heparin. In patients older than 40 years, coronary arteriography is recommended and should also be performed.

Hemodynamic measurements, cardiac output, and cine left ventriculography are performed before and after PMV. Cardiac output is measured by thermodilution and Fick method techniques. Mitral valve calcification and angiographic severity of mitral regurgitation (Sellers' classification) are graded qualitatively from 0 to 4 grades as previously described [36]. An oxygen diagnostic run is performed before and after PMV to determine the presence of left to right shunt across the atrial septum after PMV.

There is not a unique technique of percutaneous mitral balloon valvuloplasty. Most of the techniques of PMV require transseptal left heart catheterization and use of the antegrade approach [12–22, 24–28]. Antegrade PMV can be accomplished using a single- (Fig. 26.3a) or a double-balloon technique (Fig. 26.3b). In this later approach, the two balloons

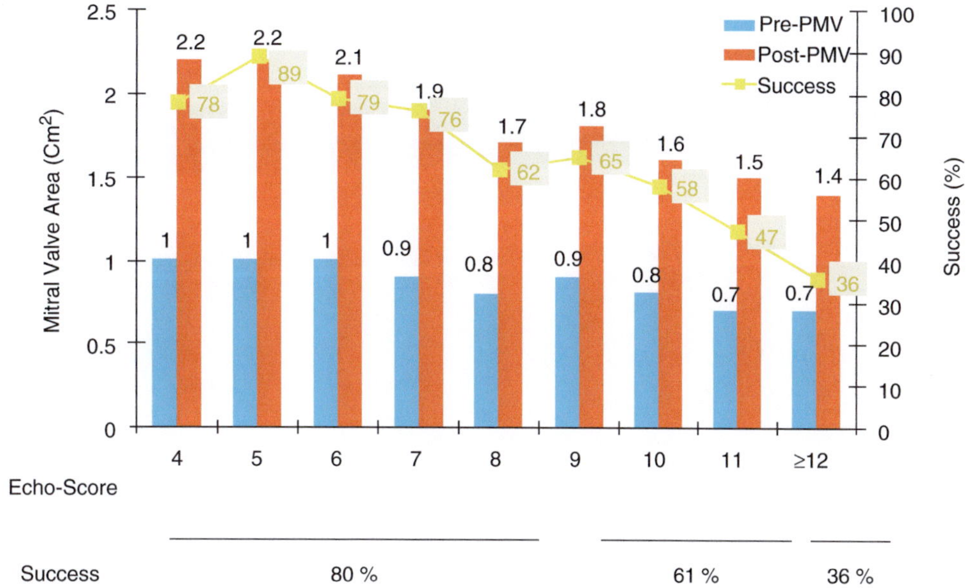

Fig. 26.2 Relationship between the echo score, the pre- and post-PMV MVA, and immediate success after PMV

could be placed through a single femoral vein and single transseptal punctures or through two femoral veins and two separate atrial septal punctures. In the retrograde technique of PMV, the balloon dilating catheters are advanced percutaneously through the right and left femoral arteries over guide wires that have been snared from the descending aorta. These guide wires have been advanced transseptally from the right femoral vein into the left atrium, the left ventricle, and the ascending aorta [37]. A retrograde nontransseptal technique of PMV has also been described [38]. Recently a technique of PMV using a newly designed metallic valvulotome was introduced [24]. The device consists of a detachable metallic cylinder with two articulated bars screwed onto the distal end of a disposable catheter whose proximal end is connected to an activating pliers. Squeezing the pliers opens the bars up to a maximum of 40 mm (Fig. 26.3c). The results with this device are at least comparable to those of the other balloon techniques of PMV [27]. However, multiple uses after sterilization should markedly decrease procedural costs.

The Antegrade Double-Balloon Technique

In performing PMV using the antegrade double-balloon technique (Fig. 26.3a), two 0.0038 in., 260 cm long Teflon-coated exchange wires are placed across the mitral valve into the left ventricle, through the aortic valve into the ascending and then the descending aorta [14–16]. Care should be taken to maintain large and smooth loops of the guide wires in the left ventricular cavity to allow appropriate placement of the dilating balloons. If a second guide wire cannot be placed into the ascending and descending aorta, a 0.038 in. Amplatz-type transfer guide wire with a preformed curlew at its tip can be placed at the left ventricular apex. In patients with aortic valve prosthesis, both guide wires with performed curlew tips should be placed at the left ventricular apex. When one or both guide wires are placed in the left ventricular apex, the balloons should be inflated sequentially. Care should be taken to avoid forward movement of the balloons and guide wires to prevent left ventricular perforation. Two balloon dilating catheters, chosen according to the patients' body surface area, are then advanced over each one of the guide wires and positioned across the mitral valve parallel to the longitudinal axis of the left ventricle. The balloon valvotomy catheters are then inflated by hand until the indentation produced by the stenotic mitral valve is no longer seen. Generally one but occasionally two or three inflations are performed. After complete deflation, the balloons are removed sequentially.

The Inoue Technique of PMV

PMV can also been performed using the Inoue technique (Fig. 26.3b) [12]. The Inoue balloon is a 12 French shaft, coaxial, double-lumen catheter. The balloon is made of a double layer of rubber tubing with a layer of synthetic micromesh in between. Following transseptal catheterization, a stainless steel guide wire is advanced through the transseptal catheter and placed with its tip coiled into the left atrium and the transseptal catheter removed. A 14 French dilator is advanced over the guide wire and used to dilate the femoral vein and the atrial septum. A balloon catheter chosen according to the patient's height is advanced over the guide wire into the left atrium. The distal part of the balloon is inflated and advanced into the left ventricle with the help of the spring wire stylet, which has been inserted through the inner lumen of the catheter. Once the catheter is in the left ventricle, the partially inflated balloon is moved back and forth inside the left ventricle to assure that it is free of the chordae tendineae.

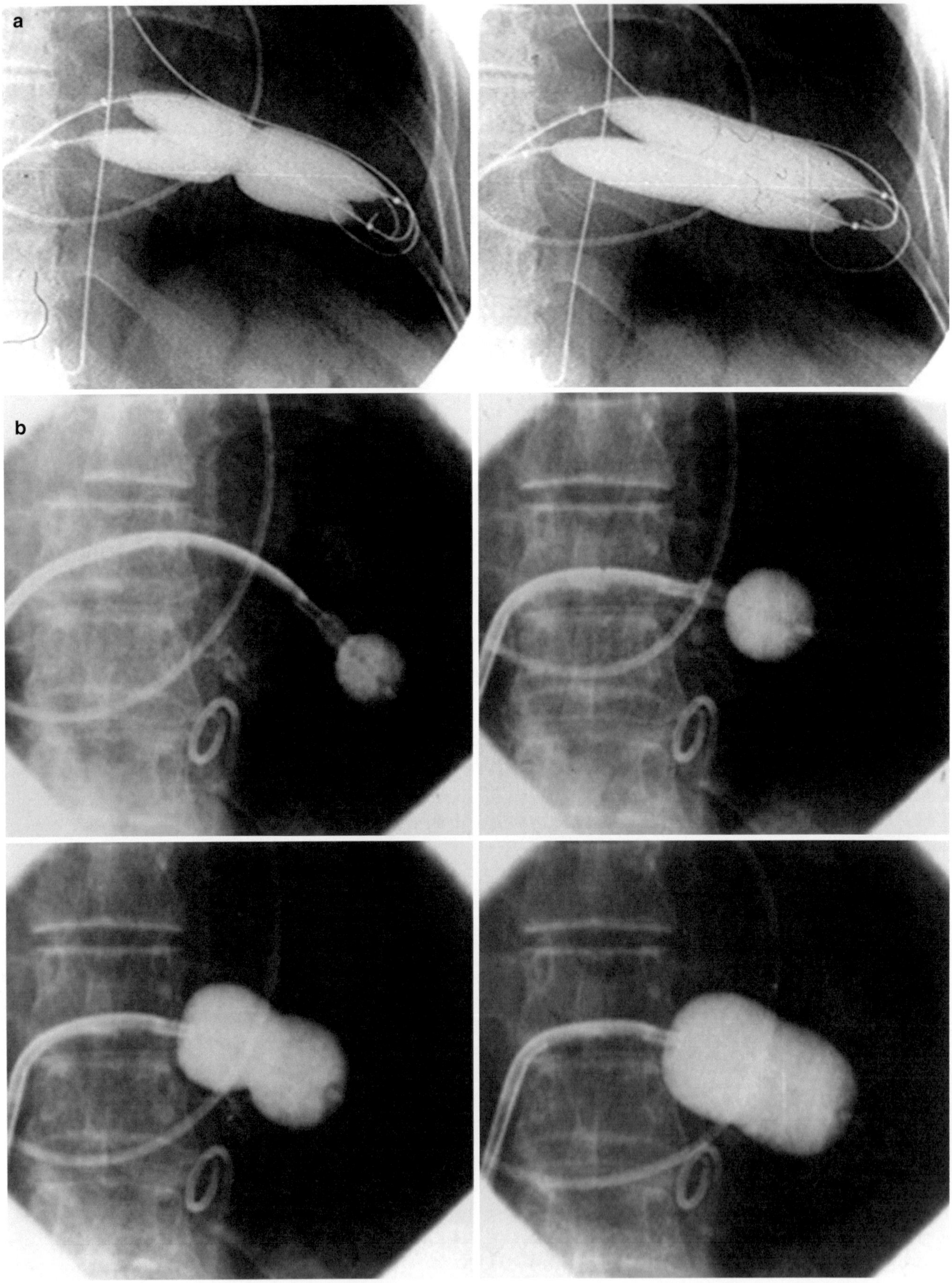

Fig. 26.3 Different percutaneous approaches of PMV: the double-balloon technique (**a**), the Inoue technique (**b**), and the metallic valvulotome (**c**)

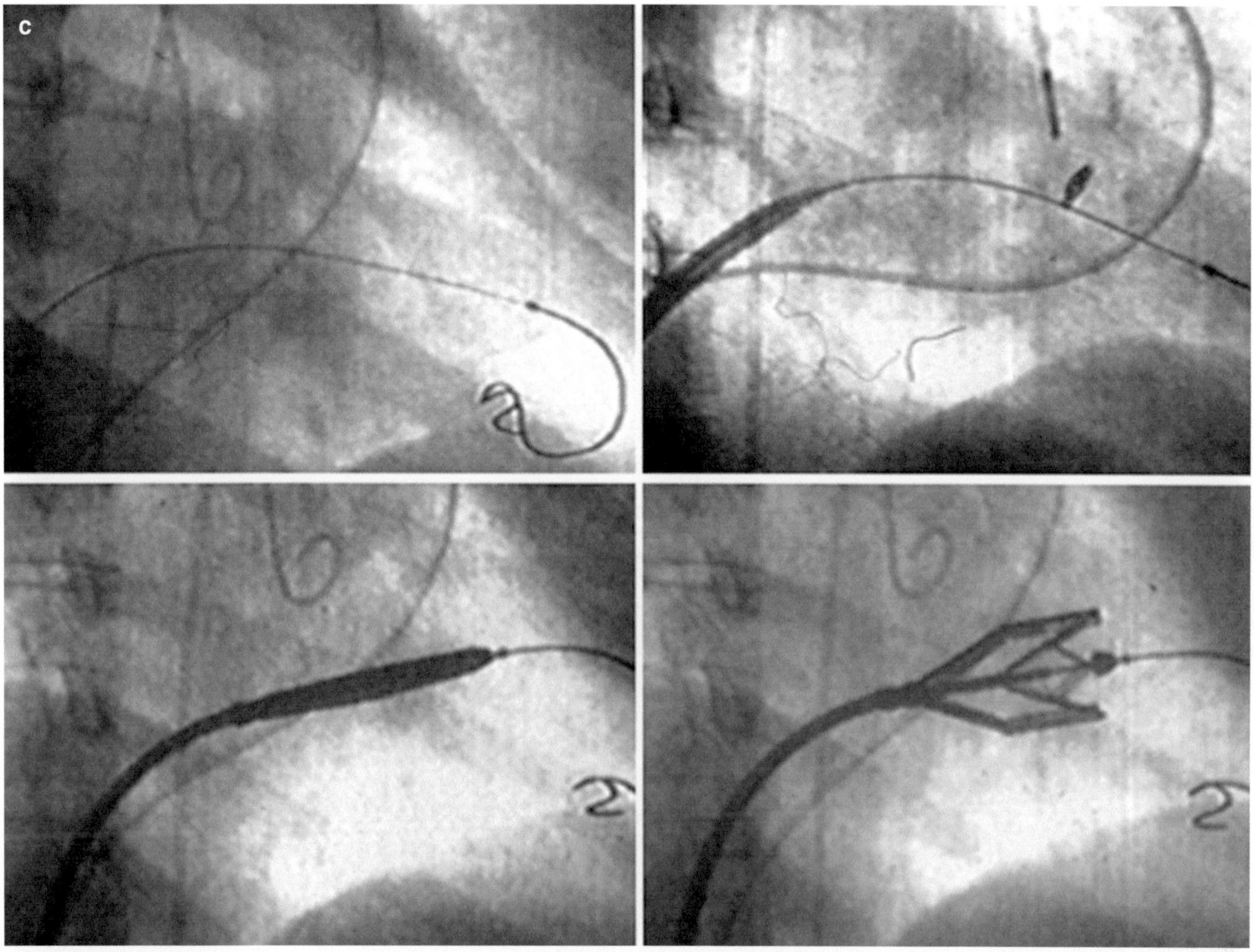

Fig. 26.3 (continued)

The catheter is then gently pulled against the mitral plane until resistance is felt. The balloon is then rapidly inflated to its full capacity and then deflated quickly. During inflation of the balloon, an indentation should be seen in its mid-portion. The catheter is withdrawn into the left atrium and the mitral gradient and cardiac output measured. If further dilatations are required, the stylet is introduced again and the sequence of steps described above repeated at a larger balloon volume. After each dilatation, its effect should be assessed by pressure measurement, auscultation, and 2D echocardiography. If mitral regurgitation occurs, further dilation of the valve should not be performed.

Mechanism of PMV

The mechanism of successful PMV is splitting of the fussed commissures toward the mitral annulus, resulting in commissural widening. This mechanism has been demonstrated by pathological, surgical, and echocardiographic studies [39–43]. In addition in patients with calcific mitral stenosis, the balloons could increase mitral valve flexibility by the fracture of the calcified deposits in the mitral valve leaflets [44]. Although rare, undesirable complications such as leaflet tears, left ventricular perforation, tear of the atrial septum, and rupture of chordae, mitral annulus, and papillary muscle could also occur.

Immediate Outcomes

Figure 26.3 shows the hemodynamic changes produced by PMV in one patient. PMV resulted in a significant decrease in mitral gradient, mean left atrium pressure, and mean pulmonary artery pressure and an increase in cardiac output and mitral valve area. Table 26.2 shows the changes in mitral valve area reported by several investigators using different techniques of PMV. In most series, PMV is reported to increase mitral valve area from less than 1.0 cm^2 to approximately 2.0 cm^2 [18–20, 23, 25–28, 34].

Table 26.2 Immediate changes in mitral valve area after percutaneous mitral valvuloplasty (*PMV*)

Author	Institution	No. patients	Age	Pre-PMV	Post-PMV
Palacios et al.	MGH[a]	879	55±15	0.9±0.3	1.9±0.7
Vahanian et al.	Tenon	1,514	45±15	1.0±0.2	1.9±0.3
Hernández et al.	Clínico Madrid	561	53±13	1.0±0.2	1.8±0.4
Stefanadis et al.	Athens University	438	44±11	1.0±0.3	2.1±0.5
Chen et al.	Guangzhou	4,832	37±12	1.1±0.3	2.1±0.2
NHLBI	Multicenter	738	54±12	1.0±0.4	2.0±0.2
Inoue et al.	Takeda	527	50±10	1.1±0.1	2.0±0.1
Inoue Registry	Multicenter	1,251	53±15	1.0±0.3	1.8±0.6
Ben Farhat et al.	Fattouma	463	33±12	1.0±0.2	2.2±0.4
Arora et al.	G.B. Pan	600	27±8	0.8±0.2	2.2±0.4
Cribier et al.	Ruen	153	36±15	1.0±0.2	2.2±0.4

[a]Massachusetts General Hospital

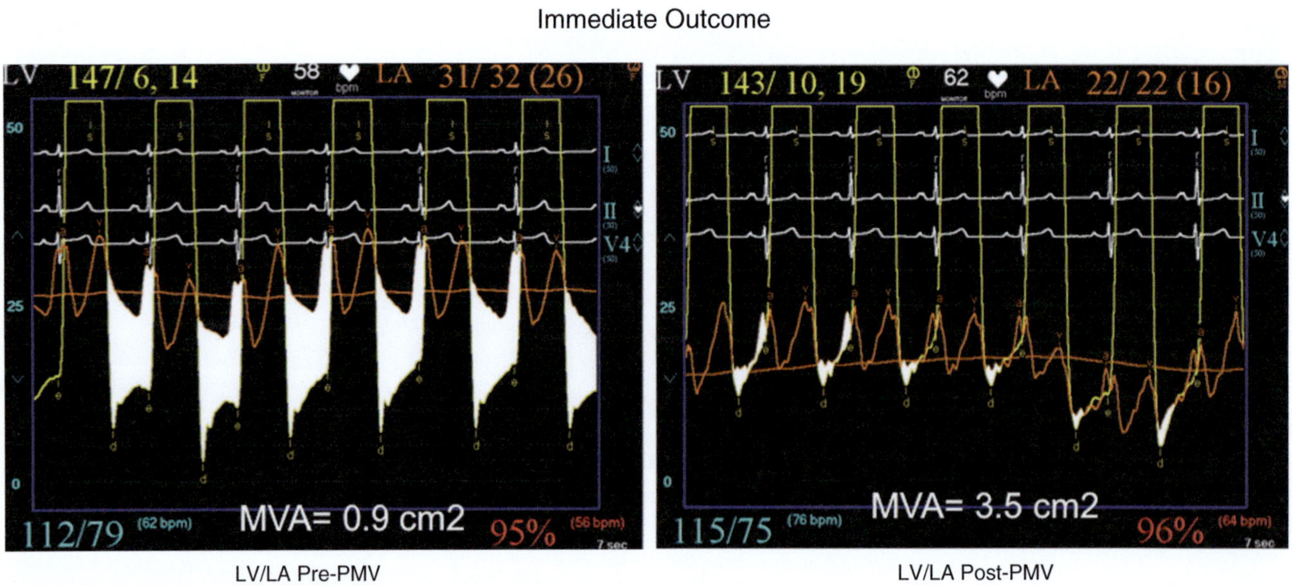

Fig. 26.4 Hemodynamic changes produced by a successful PMV in one patient with severe mitral stenosis. At the *top panels*, simultaneous left atrium and left ventricular pressures before (*upper-right panel*) and after (*upper-left panel*) PMV. The phasic and mean pulmonary artery pressures before (*lower-right panel*) and after (*lower-left panel*) PMV are shown at the *bottom*. The corresponding cardiac outputs and calculated mitral valve areas are also displayed (*LV* left ventricle, *LA* left atrium, *PA* pulmonary artery pressure, *PMV* percutaneous mitral balloon valvuloplasty)

Eight hundred and seventy-nine consecutive patients with mitral stenosis have undergone 939 PMVs at the Massachusetts General Hospital between July 1986 and July 2000 [28]. As shown in Fig. 26.4, in this group of patients, PMV resulted in a significant decrease in mitral gradient from 14±6 to 6±3 mmHg. The mean cardiac output significantly increased from 3.9±1.1 to 4.5±1.3 L/min. and the calculated mitral valve area from 0.9±0.3 to 1.9±0.7 cm^2. In addition, mean pulmonary artery pressure significantly decreased from 36±13 to 29±11 mmHg and the mean left atrial pressure decreased from 25±7 to 17±7 mmHg and, consequently, the calculated pulmonary vascular resistance decreased significantly following PMV.

A successful hemodynamic outcome (defined as a post-PMV mitral valve area ≥1.5 cm^2 and post-PMV MR <3 Sellers' grade) was obtained in 72 % of the patients. Although a suboptimal result occurred in 28 % of the patients, a post-PMV mitral valve area ≤1.0 cm^2 (critical mitral valve area) was present in only 8.7 % of these patients.

Predictors of Increase in Mitral Valve Area and Procedural Success

Univariate analysis demonstrated that the increase in mitral valve area with PMV is directly related to the balloon size employed as it reflects in the effective balloon dilating area

Table 26.3 The echocardiographic score. Echocardiographic grading of the severity and extent of the anatomic abnormalities in patients with mitral stenosis

Grade	Leaflet mobility	Valvular thickening	Valvular calcification	Subvalvular thickening
0	Normal	Normal	Normal	Normal
1	Highly mobile valve with restriction of only the leaflet tips	Leaflet near normal (4–5 mm)	A single area of increased echo brightness	Minimal thickening of chordal structures just below the valve
2	Middle portion and base of leaflets have reduced mobility	Mid-leaflet thickening, marked thickening of the margins	Scattered areas of brightness confined to leaflet margins	Thickening of chordae extending up to one third of chordal length
3	Valve leaflets move forward in diastole mainly at the base	Thickening extending through the entire leaflets (5–8 mm)	Brightness extending into the mid-portion of leaflets	Thickening extending to the distal third of the chordae
4	No or minimal forward movement of the leaflets in diastole	Marked thickening of all leaflet tissue (>8–10 mm)	Extensive brightness throughout most of the leaflet tissue	Extensive thickening and shortening of all chordae extending down to the papillary muscles

The total score is the sum of each of these echocardiographic features (maximum 16)

(EBDA) and inversely related to the echocardiographic score (Fig. 26.2), the presence of atrial fibrillation, the presence of fluoroscopic calcium, the presence of previous surgical commissurotomy, older age, NYHA pre-PMV, and presence of mitral regurgitation before PMV. Multiple stepwise regression analysis identified balloon size ($p<.02$), the echocardiographic score ($p<.0001$), and the presence of atrial fibrillation ($p<.009$) and mitral regurgitation before PMV ($p<0.03$) as independent predictors of the increase in mitral valve area with PMV.

Univariate predictors of procedural success included age, pre-PMV MVA, mean pre-PMV pulmonary artery pressure, male sex, echocardiographic score, pre-PMV mitral regurgitation ≥2+, history of previous surgical commissurotomy, presence of atrial fibrillation, and presence of mitral valve calcification under fluoroscopy.

Multiple stepwise logistic regression analysis identified larger pre-PMV MVA (odds ratio [OR] 13.05, 95 % confidence interval [CI]: 7.74–22.51; $p<0.001$), less degree of pre-PMV mitral regurgitation (OR 3.85, CI: 2.27–6.66; $p<0.001$), younger age (OR 3.33, CI: 1.41–7.69; $p=0.006$), absence of previous surgical commissurotomy (OR 1.85, CI: 1.20–2.86; $p=0.004$), male sex (OR 1.92, CI: 1.19–3.13; $p=0.008$), and echocardiographic score ≤8 (OR 1.69, CI: 1.18–2.44; $p=0.004$).

The Echocardiographic Score

The echocardiographic examination of the mitral valve can accurately characterize the severity and extent of the pathological process in patients with mitral stenosis. The most utilized score to identify the anatomic abnormalities of the stenotic mitral valve is that described by Wilkins et al. (Table 26.3, Fig. 26.2) [42]. This echocardiographic score is an important predictor of the immediate and long-term outcome of PMV. In this morphologic score, each of the following: leaflet rigidity, leaflet thickening, valvular calcification, and subvalvular disease, is scored from 0 to 4. A higher score would represent a heavily calcified, thicken, and immobile valve with extensive thickening and calcification of the subvalvular apparatus. The increase in mitral valve area with PMV is inversely related to the echocardiographic score. The best outcome with PMV occurs in those patients with echocardiographic scores ≤8. The increase in mitral valve area is significantly greater in patients with echocardiographic scores ≤8 than in those with echocardiographic score >8. Among the four components of the echocardiographic score, valve leaflets thickening and subvalvular disease correlate the best with the increase in mitral valve area produced by PMV [44]. Therefore, suboptimal results with PMV are more likely to occur in patients with valves which are more rigid, more thickened, and those with more subvalvular fibrosis and calcification.

Balloon Size and EBDA

The increase in mitral valve area with PMV is directly related to balloon size. This effect was first demonstrated in a subgroup of patients who underwent repeat PMV [45]. They initially underwent PMV with a single balloon resulting in a mean mitral valve area of 1.2 ± 0.2 cm^2. They underwent repeat PMV using the double-balloon technique, which increased the effective balloon dilating area (EBDA) normalized by body surface area (EBDA/BSA) from 3.41 ± 0.2 to 4.51 ± 0.2 cm^2/m^2. The mean mitral valve area in this group after repeat PMV was 1.8 ± 0.7 cm^2. The increase in mitral valve area in patients who underwent PMV at the Massachusetts General Hospital using the double-balloon technique (EBDA of 6.4 ± 0.03 cm^2) was significantly greater than the increase in mitral valve area achieved in patients who underwent PMV using the single-balloon technique (EBDA of 4.3 ± 0.02 cm^2). The mean mitral valve areas were 1.9 ± 0.7 cm^2 and 1.4 ± 0.1 cm^2 for patients who underwent PMV with the double-balloon and the single-balloon techniques, respectively. However, care should be taken in the

Table 26.4 Complications following percutaneous mitral valvuloplasty

Author	No. patients	Mortality (%)	Tamponade (%)	Severe MR[a] (%)	Embolism (%)
Palacios et al.	879	0.6	1.0	3.4	1.8
Vahanian et al.	1,514	0.4	0.3	3.4	0.3
Hernández et al.	561	0.4	0.6	4.5	
Stefanadis et al.	438	0.2	0.0	3.4	0.0
Chen et al.	4,832	0.1	0.8	1.4	0.5
NHLBI	738	3.0	4.0	3.0	3.0
Inoue et al.	527	0.0	1.6	1.9	0.6
Inoue Registry	1,251	0.6	1.4	3.8	0.9
Ben Farhat et al.	463	0.4	0.7	4.6	2.0
Arora et al.	600	1.0	1.3	1.0	0.5
Cribier et al.	153	0.0	0.7	1.4	0.7

[a]MR denotes mitral regurgitation

selection of dilating balloon catheters so as to obtain an adequate final mitral valve area and no change or a minimal increase in mitral regurgitation.

Mitral Valve Calcification

The immediate outcome of patients undergoing PMV is inversely related to the severity of valvular calcification seen by fluoroscopy. Patients without fluoroscopic calcium have a greater increase in mitral valve area after PMV than patients with calcified valves. Patients with either no or 1 + fluoroscopic calcium have a greater increase in mitral valve area after PMV (1.1 ± 0.6 cm^2 and 0.9 ± 0.5 cm^2, respectively) than those patients with 2, 3, or 4+of calcium (0.8 ± 0.6 cm^2, 0.8 ± 0.5 cm^2, and 0.6 ± 0.4 cm^2, respectively).

Previous Surgical Commissurotomy

Although the increase in mitral valve area with PMV is inversely related to the presence of previous surgical mitral commissurotomy, PMV can produce a good outcome in this group of patients. The post-PMV mean mitral valve area in 154 patients with previous surgical commissurotomy was 1.8 ± 0.7 cm^2 compared with a valve area of 1.9 ± 0.6 cm^2 in patients without previous surgical commissurotomy ($P<0.05$). In this group of patients, an echocardiographic score ≤ 8 was an important predictor of a successful hemodynamic immediate outcome.

Age

The immediate outcome of PMV is directly related to the age of the patient. The percentage of patients obtaining a good result with this technique decreases as age increases. A successful hemodynamic outcome from PMV was obtained in only less than 50 % of patients ≥65 years old [46]. This inverse relationship between age and the immediate outcome from PMV is due to the higher frequency of atrial fibrillation, calcified valves, and higher echocardiographic scores in elderly patients.

Atrial Fibrillation

The increase in mitral valve area with PMV is inversely related to the presence of atrial fibrillation; the post-PMV mitral valve area of patients in normal sinus rhythm was 2.0 ± 0.7 cm^2 compared with a valve area of 1.7 ± 0.6 cm^2 of those patients in atrial fibrillation. The inferior immediate outcome of PMV in patients with mitral stenosis who are in atrial fibrillation is more likely related to the presence of clinical and morphological characteristics associated with inferior results after PMV. Patients in atrial fibrillation are older and present more frequently with echocardiographic scores >8, NYHA functional class IV, calcified mitral valves under fluoroscopy, and with a previous history of surgical mitral commissurotomy.

Mitral Regurgitation Before PMV

The presence and severity of mitral regurgitation before PMV is an independent predictor of unfavorable outcome. The increase in mitral valve after PMV is inversely related to the severity of mitral regurgitation determined by angiography before the procedure. This inverse relationship between presence of mitral regurgitation and immediate outcome of PMV is in part due to the higher frequency of atrial fibrillation, higher echocardiographic scores, calcified mitral valves under fluoroscopy, and older age in patients with mitral regurgitation before PMV.

Complications

Table 26.4 shows the complications reported by several investigators after PMV [18–20, 23, 25–28, 34]. Mortality and morbidity with PMV are low and similar to surgical commissurotomy. Overall, there is less than 1 % mortality. Severe mitral regurgitation (4 grades by angiography) has been reported in 1–5.2 % of the patients. Some of these patients required inhospital mitral valve replacement. Thromboembolic episodes and stroke have been reported in 0–3.1 % and pericardial tamponade in 0.2–4.6 % of cases in these series. Pericardial tamponade can occur from transseptal catheterization and more rarely from ventricular perforation. PMV is associated with a 3–16 % incidence of left to right shunt immediately after the procedure. However, the pulmonary to systemic flow ratio is ≥2:1 in only a minimum number of patients.

We have demonstrated that severe mitral regurgitation (4 grades by angiography) occurs in about 3 % of patients undergoing PMV [28]. An undesirable increase in mitral regurgitation (≥2 grades by angiography) occurred in 10.1 % of patients. This undesirable increase in mitral regurgitation is well tolerated in most patients. Furthermore, more than half of them have less mitral regurgitation at follow-up cardiac catheterization. We have demonstrated that the ratio of the effective balloon dilating area to body surface area (EBDA/BSA) is the only predictor of increased mitral regurgitation after PMV [47–49]. The effective balloon dilating area (EBDA) is calculated using standard geometric formulas. The incidence of mitral regurgitation is lower if balloon sizes are chosen so that EBDA/BSA is ≤4.0 cm^2/m^2. The single-balloon technique results in a lower incidence of mitral regurgitation but provides less relief of mitral stenosis than the double-balloon technique. Thus, there is an optimal effective balloon dilating area between 3.1 and 4.0 cm^2/m^2 which achieves a maximal mitral valve area with a minimal increase in mitral regurgitation. An echocardiographic score for the mitral valve that can predict the development of severe mitral regurgitation following PMV has also been described [43]. This score takes into account the distribution (even or uneven) of leaflet thickening and calcification, the degree and symmetry of commissural disease, and the severity of subvalvular disease.

Left to right shunt through the created atrial communication occurred in 3–16 % of the patients undergoing PMV. The size of the defect is small as reflected in the pulmonary to systemic flow ratio of <2:1 in the majority of patients. Older age, fluoroscopic evidence of mitral valve calcification, higher echocardiographic score, pre-PMV lower cardiac output, and higher pre-PMV NYHA functional class are the factors that predispose patients to develop left to right shunt post-PMV [49]. Clinical, echocardiographic, surgical, and hemodynamic follow-up of patients with post-PMV left to right shunt demonstrated that the defect closed in approximately 60 %. Persistent left to right shunt at follow-up is small (QP/QS<2:1) and clinically well tolerated. In the series from the Massachusetts General Hospital, there is one patient in whom the atrial shunt remained hemodynamically significant at follow-up. This patient underwent percutaneous transcatheter closure of her atrial defect with a clamshell device. Desideri et al. reported atrial shunting determined by color flow transthoracic echocardiography in 61 % of 57 patients immediately after PMV. The shunt persisted in 30 % of patients at 19±6 (range 9–33) months follow-up [50]. They identified the magnitude of the post-PMV atrial shunt (QP/QS>1.5:1) and use of bifoil balloon (2 balloons on 1 shaft) and smaller post-PMV mitral valve area as independent predictors of the persistence of atrial shunt at long-term follow-up.

Clinical Follow-Up

Long-term follow-up studies after PMV are encouraging [21–23, 25, 26, 28, 34]. Following PMV, the majority of patients have marked clinical improvement and become NYHA classes I or II. The symptomatic, echocardiographic, and hemodynamic improvement produced by PMV persists in intermediate and long-term follow-up. The best long-term results are seen in patients with echocardiographic scores ≤8. When PMV produces a good immediate outcome in this group of patients, restenosis is unlikely to occur at follow-up. Although PMV can result in a good outcome in patients with echocardiographic scores >8, hemodynamic and echocardiographic restenosis is frequently demonstrated at follow-up despite ongoing clinical improvement. Table 26.5 shows long-term follow-up results of patients undergoing PMV at different institutes. We reported an estimated 12-year survival rate of 74 % in a cohort of 879 patients undergoing PMV at the Massachusetts General Hospital (Fig. 26.5). Death at follow-up was directly related to age, post-PMV pulmonary artery pressure, and pre-PMV NYHA functional class IV. In the same group of patients, the 12-year event-free survival (alive and free of mitral valve replacement or repair and redo PMV) was 33 % (Fig. 26.6). Cox regression analysis identified age (risk ratio (R.R.) 1.02; C.I. 1.01–1.03; $p<0.0001$), pre-PMV NYHA functional class IV (R.R. 1.35; C.I. 1.00–1.81; $p=0.05$), prior commissurotomy (R.R. .150; C.I. 1.16–1.92; $p=0.002$), the echocardiographic score (R.R. 1.31; C.I. 1.02–1.67; $p=0.003$), pre-PMV mitral regurgitation ≥2+ (R.R. 1.56; C.I. 1.09–2.22; $p=0.02$), post-PMV mitral regurgitation ≥3+ (R.R. 3.54; C.I. 2.61–4.72; $p<0.0001$), and post-PMV mean pulmonary artery pressure (R.R 1.02; C.I 1.01–1.03; $p<0.0001$) as independent predictors of combined events at long-term follow-up.

Actuarial survival and event-free survival rates throughout the follow-up period were significantly better in patients with echocardiographic scores ≤8. Survival rates were 82 % for patients with echocardiographic score ≤8 and 57 % for patients with score >8 at a follow-up time of 12 years ($p<0.0001$). Event-free survival (38 % vs. 22 %; $p<0.0001$) at 12-year follow-up was also significantly higher for patients with echocardiographic score ≤8. Similar follow-up studies have been reported in other series with the double-balloon technique and with the Inoue technique of PMV [21, 23, 25, 26]. Over 90 % of young patients with pliable valves in sinus rhythm and with no evidence of calcium under fluoroscopy remain free of cardiovascular events at an approximately follow-up of 5 years [17, 22, 34].

Functional deterioration at follow-up is late and related primarily to mitral restenosis [26]. The incidence of restenosis, as assessed by sequential echocardiography, is approximately 40 % after 7 years [25]. Repeat PMV can be proposed if recurrent stenosis leads to symptoms. At the moment, we

Table 26.5 Clinical long-term follow-up after percutaneous mitral valvuloplasty

Author	No. patients	Age (years)	Follow-up	Survival (%)	Event-free survival (%)
Palacios et al.	879	55	12	74	33
Lung et al.	1,024	49	10	85	56
Hernández et al.	561	53	7	95	69
Orrange et al.	132	44	7	83	65
Ben Farhat et al.	30	29	7	100	90
Stefanadis et al.	441	44	9	98	75

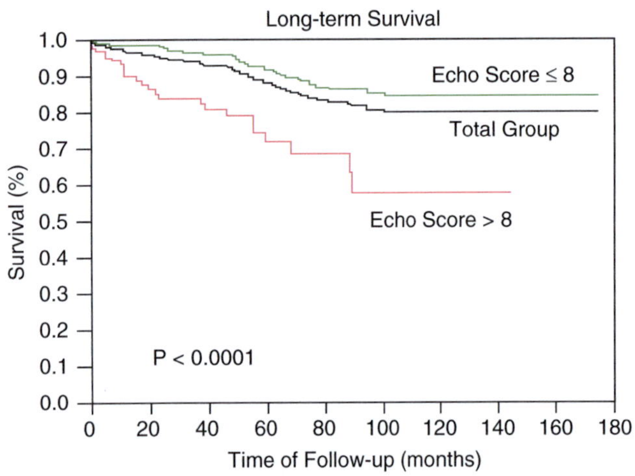

Fig. 26.5 Fifteen-year survival for all patients and for patients with echocardiographic score ≤8 and >8, undergoing percutaneous mitral balloon valvotomy at the Massachusetts General Hospital

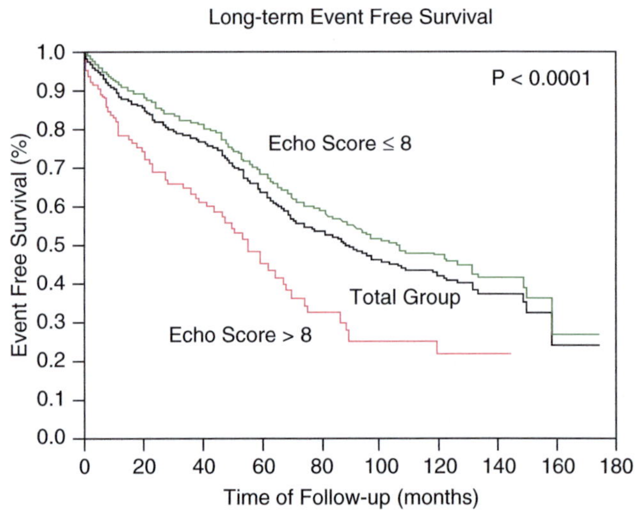

Fig. 26.6 Fifteen-year event-free survival for all patients and for patients with echocardiographic score ≤8 and >8, undergoing percutaneous mitral balloon valvotomy at the Massachusetts General Hospital

have only a small number of series available on redo PMV. They show encouraging results in selected patients with favorable characteristics when restenosis occurs several years after an initially successful procedure and if the predominant mechanism of restenosis is commissural refusion [45].

Follow-Up in the Elderly

Tuzcu et al. reported the outcome of PMV in 99 elderly patients (≥ 65 year) [46]. A successful outcome (valve area ≥1.5 cm² without ≥2+ increase in mitral regurgitation and without left to right shunt of ≥1.5 : 1) was achieved in 46 patients. The best multivariate predictor of success was the combination of echocardiographic score, NYHA functional class, and inverse of mitral valve area. Patients who had an unsuccessful outcome from PMV were in a higher NYHA functional class and had higher echocardiographic scores and smaller mitral valve areas pre-PMV compared to those patients who had a successful outcome. Actuarial survival and combined event-free survival at 3 years were significantly better in the successful group. Mean follow-up was 16 ± 1 months. Actuarial survival (79 ± 7 % vs. 62 ± 10 %; $p = .04$), survival without mitral valve replacement (71 ± 8 % vs. 41 ± 8 %; $p = .002$), and event-free survival (54 ± 12 % vs. 38 ± 8 %; $p = .01$) at 3 years were significantly better in the successful group of 46 patients than the unsuccessful group of 53 patients. Low echocardiographic score was the independent predictor of survival, and the lack of mitral valve calcification was the strongest predictor of event-free survival.

Recently data reported in 96 patients ≥75 years have shown that these patients present a lower pre-PMV mitral valve area (0.8 ± 0.3 vs. 0.9 ± 0.3; $p = 0.005$), a lower post-PMV mitral valve area (1.6 ± 0.6 vs. 1.9 ± 0.7; $p < 0.0001$), and a lower procedural success (51.0 % vs. 71.4 %; $p < 0.0001$) compared with patients <75 years [51]. Patients ≥75 years exhibited a higher inhospital mortality than patients <75 years (3.1 % vs. 0.3 %) with no significant differences in the other procedure-related complications (cardiac tamponade, severe mitral regurgitation, significant left to right shunt, and embolism). Although inhospital mortality was higher, in the majority of these patients, PMV was considered as a palliative treatment. However, technical complications were similar to those more favorable patients aged <75. Survival and event-free survival rates were 60 and 49 % for patients ≥75 years at a follow-up time of 3 years. The echo score is an imperfect predictor of hemodynamic improvement in elderly patients [51, 52].

Unfortunately, no randomized study is available for elderly patients, and a comparison of the results of PMV with those of surgical series is difficult because of the differences in the patients and surgical techniques involved.

Follow-Up of Patients with Calcified Mitral Valves

The presence of fluoroscopically visible calcification on the mitral valve influences the success of PMV. Patients with heavily (≥3 grades) calcified valves under fluoroscopy have a poorer immediate outcome as reflected in a smaller post-PMV mitral valve area and greater post-PMV mitral valve gradient. Immediate outcome is progressively worse as the calcification becomes more severe. The long-term results of percutaneous mitral balloon valvuloplasty are significantly different in calcified and uncalcified groups and in subgroups of the calcified group [53]. The estimated 2-year survival is significantly lower for patients with calcified mitral valves than for those with uncalcified valves (80 % vs. 99 %). The survival curve becomes worse as the severity of valvular calcification becomes more severe. Freedom from mitral valve replacement at 2 years was significantly lower for patients with calcified valves than for those with uncalcified valves (67 % vs. 93 %). Similarly, the estimated event-free survival at 2 years in the calcified group became significantly poorer as the severity of calcification increased. The estimated event-free survival at 2 years was significantly lower for the calcified than for the uncalcified group (63 % vs. 88 %). The actuarial survival curves with freedom from combined events at 2 years in the calcified group became significantly poorer as the severity of calcification increased. These findings are in agreement with several follow-up studies of surgical commissurotomy which demonstrate that patients with calcified mitral valves had a poorer survival compared to those patients with uncalcified valves [54, 55].

Follow-Up of Patients with Previous Surgical Commissurotomy

PMV also has been shown to be a safe procedure in patients with previous surgical mitral commissurotomy [56–61]. Although a good immediate outcome is frequently achieved in these patients, follow-up results are not as favorable as those obtained in patients without previous surgical commissurotomy. Although there is no difference in mortality between patients with or without a history of previous surgical commissurotomy at 4-year follow-up, the number of patients who required mitral valve replacement (26 % vs. 8 %) and/or were in NYHA classes III or IV (35 % vs. 13 %) was significantly higher among those patients with previous commissurotomy. However, when the patients are carefully selected according to the echocardiographic score (≤8), the immediate outcome and the 4-year follow-up results are excellent and similar to those seen in patients without previous surgical commissurotomy.

Follow-Up of Patients with Atrial Fibrillation

We have reported that the presence of atrial fibrillation is associated with inferior immediate and long-term outcome after PMV as reflected in a smaller post-PMV mitral valve area and a lower event-free survival (freedom of death, redo PMV, and mitral valve surgery) at a median follow-up time of 61 months (32 % vs. 61 %; $p<0.0001$) [62]. Analysis of pre-procedural and procedural characteristics revealed that this association is most likely explained by the presence of multiple factors in the atrial fibrillation group that adversely affect the immediate and long-term outcome of PMV. Patients in atrial fibrillation are older and presented more frequently with NYHA class IV, echocardiographic score >8, calcified valves under fluoroscopy, and with history of previous surgical commissurotomy. In the group of patients in atrial fibrillation, we identified severe post-PMV mitral regurgitation (≥ 3+) ($P=0.0001$), echocardiographic score >8 ($p=0.004$), and pre-PMV NYHA class IV ($p=0.046$) as independent predictors of combined events at follow-up. The presence of atrial fibrillation per se should not be the only determinant in the decision process regarding treatment options in a patient with rheumatic mitral stenosis. The presence of an echocardiographic score ≤8 primarily identifies a subgroup of patients in atrial fibrillation in whom percutaneous balloon valvotomy is very likely to be successful and provides good long-term results. Therefore, in this group of patients, PMV should be the procedure of choice.

Follow-Up of Patients with Pulmonary Artery Hypertension

The degree of pulmonary artery hypertension before PMV is inversely related to the immediate and long-term outcome of PMV [28]. Chen et al. [63]. divided 564 patients undergoing PMV at the Massachusetts General Hospital into three groups on the basis of the pulmonary vascular resistance (PVR) obtained at cardiac catheterization immediately prior to PMV: group I with a PVR ≤ 250 dyn sec/cm-5 (normal/mildly elevated resistance) comprised 332 patients (59 %), group II with a PVR between 251 and 400 dyn sec/cm-5 (moderately elevated resistance) comprised 110 patients (19.5 %), and group III with a PVR ≥ 400 dyn sec/cm-5 comprised of 122 patients (21.5 %). Patients in groups I and II were younger and had less severe heart failure symptoms measured by NYHA class and a lower incidence of echocardiographic scores >8, atrial fibrillation, and calcium noted on fluoroscopy than patients in group III. Before and after PMV, patients with higher PVR had a smaller mitral valve area, lower cardiac output, and higher mean pulmonary artery pressure. For groups I, II, and III patients, the immediate success rates for PMV were 68 %, 56 %, and 45 %, respectively. Therefore, patients in the group with severely elevated pulmonary artery resistance before the procedure had lower immediate success rates of PMV. At long-term follow-up, patients with severely elevated pulmonary vascular resistance had a significant lower survival and event-free survival (survival with freedom from mitral valve surgery or NYHA classes III or IV heart failure).

Follow-Up of Patients with Tricuspid Regurgitation

The degree of tricuspid regurgitation before PMV is inversely related to the immediate and long-term outcome of PMV. Sagie et al. divided patients undergoing PMV at the Massachusetts General Hospital into three groups on the basis of the degree of tricuspid regurgitation determined by 2D and color flow Doppler echocardiography before PMV [64]. Patients with severe tricuspid regurgitation before PMV were older and had more severe heart failure symptoms measured by NYHA class and a higher incidence of echocardiographic scores >8, atrial fibrillation, and calcified mitral valves on fluoroscopy than patients with mild or moderate tricuspid regurgitation. Patients with severe tricuspid regurgitation had smaller mitral valve areas before and after PMV than the patients with mild or moderate tricuspid regurgitation. At long-term follow-up, patients with severe tricuspid regurgitation had a significant lower survival and event-free survival (survival with freedom from mitral valve surgery or NYHA classes III or IV heart failure). The degree of tricuspid regurgitation can be diminished when the transmitral pressure gradient is sufficiently relieved with PMV [65].

Follow-Up of the Best Patients for PMV

In patients identified as optimal candidates for PMV, this technique results in excellent immediate and long-term outcome. Optimal candidates for PMV are those patients meeting the following characteristics: (a) age ≤45 years old, (b) normal sinus rhythm, (c) echocardiographic score ≤ 8, (d) no history of previous surgical commissurotomy, and (e) pre-PMV mitral regurgitation ≤1 + Sellers' grade. From 879 consecutive patients undergoing percutaneous mitral balloon valvuloplasty (PMV), we identified 136 patients with optimal pre-procedure characteristics. In these patients, PMV results in an 81 % success rate and a 3.4 % incidence of major inhospital combined events (death and/or MVR). In these patients, PMV results in a 95 % survival and 61 % event-free survival at a 12-year follow-up [28].

Echocardiographic and Hemodynamic Follow-Up

Follow-up studies have shown that the incidence of hemodynamic and echocardiographic restenosis is low after PMV [25, 26, 66, 67]. A study of a group of patients undergoing simultaneous clinical evaluation, 2D Doppler echocardiography, and transseptal catheterization 2 years after PMV reported a 90 % of patients in NYHA classes I and II and 10 % of patients in NYHA class ≥ III [67]. In this study, hemodynamic determination of mitral valve area using the Gorlin equation showed a significant decrease in mitral valve area from 2.0 cm^2 immediately after PMV to 1.6 cm^2 at follow-up. However, there was no significant difference between the echocardiographic mitral valve areas immediately after PMV and at follow-up (1.8 cm^2 and 1.6 cm^2, respectively; p=NS). Although there was a significant difference in the mitral valve area after PMV determined by the Gorlin equation and by 2D echocardiography (2.0 cm^2 vs. 1.8 cm^2), there was no significant difference between the mitral valve area determined by the Gorlin equation and the echocardiographic calculated mitral valve area (1.6 cm^2 for both) at follow-up. The discrepancy between the 2D echocardiographic and Gorlin equation determined post-PMV mitral valve areas is due to the contribution of left to right shunting (undetected by oximetry) across the created interatrial communication which results in both an erroneously high cardiac output and an overestimation of the mitral valve area by the Gorlin equation [68]. Desideri et al. showed no significant differences in mitral valve area (measured by Doppler echocardiography) at 19 ± 6 (range 9–33) months follow-up between the post-PMV and follow-up mitral valve areas. Mitral valve areas were 2.2 ± 0.5 cm^2 and 1.9 ± 0.5 cm^2, respectively [50]. Echocardiographic restenosis (mitral valve area ≤ 1.5 cm^2 with > 50 % reduction of the gain) was estimated in 39 % at 7-year follow-up with the Inoue technique.[25] A mitral area loss ≥0.3 cm^2 was seen in 12 %, 22 %, and 27 % of patients at 3, 5, and 7 years, respectively. Predictors of restenosis included a post-MVA <1.8 cm^2 and an echo score >8.

The Double-Balloon Technique Versus the Inoue Balloon

Today the Inoue approach of PMV is the technique more widely used. There was controversy as to whether the double-balloon or the Inoue technique provided superior immediate and long-term results. We compared the immediate procedural and the long-term clinical outcomes after PMV using the double-balloon technique (n=659) and Inoue technique (n=233) [66]. There were no statistically significant differences in baseline clinical and morphological characteristics between the double-balloon and Inoue patients. Although the post-PMV mitral valve area was larger with the double-balloon technique (1.94 ± 0.72 vs. 1.81 ± 0.58; p=0.01), success rate (71.3 % vs. 69.1 %; p=NS), incidence of ≥3+ mitral regurgitation (9 % vs. 9 %), inhospital complications, and long-term and event-free survival were similar with both techniques. In conclusion, both the Inoue and the double-balloon techniques are equally effective techniques of PMV. The procedure of choice should be performed based on the interventionist experience in the technique.

PMV Versus Surgical Mitral Commissurotomy

Results of surgical closed mitral commissurotomy have demonstrated favorable long-term hemodynamic and symptomatic improvement from this technique. A restenosis rate of 4.2–11.4

per 1,000 patients per year was reported by John et al. in 3,724 patients who underwent surgical closed mitral commissurotomy [69]. Survival after PMV is similar to that reported after surgical mitral commissurotomy. Although freedom from mitral valve replacement and freedom from all events after PMV are lower than reported after surgical commissurotomy, freedom from both mitral valve replacement and all events in patients with echocardiographic scores ≤8 are similar to that reported after surgical mitral commissurotomy [28, 55, 69–76].

Restenosis after both closed and open surgical mitral commissurotomies has been well documented [69–76]. Although surgical closed mitral commissurotomy is uncommonly performed in the United States, it is still used frequently in other countries. Long-term follow-up of 267 patients who underwent surgical transventricular mitral commissurotomy at the Mayo Clinic showed a 79 %, 67 %, and 55 % survival at 10, 15, and 20 years, respectively. Survival with freedom from mitral valve replacement were 57 %, 36 %, and 24 %, respectively [77]. In this study, age, atrial fibrillation, and male gender were independent predictors of death, while mitral valve calcification, cardiomegaly, and mitral regurgitation were independent predictors of repeat mitral valve surgery.

Because of similar patient's selection and mechanism of mitral valve dilatation, similar long-term results should be expected after PMV. Indeed, prospective, randomized trials comparing PMV and surgical closed or open mitral commissurotomy have shown no differences in immediate and 3-year follow-up results between both groups of patients [29–34]. Furthermore, restenosis at 3-year follow-up occurred in 10 and 13 % of the patients treated with mitral balloon valvuloplasty and surgical commissurotomy, respectively [33].

Interpretation of long-term clinical follow-up of patients undergoing percutaneous mitral balloon valvuloplasty as well as their comparison with surgical commissurotomy series is confounded by heterogeneity in patient population. Most surgical series have involved a younger population with optimal mitral valve morphology, pliable with no calcification and no evidence of subvalvular disease. Comparisons were also made at the beginning of PMV. Therefore, surgeons were more experienced than interventional cardiologists. Differences in age and valve morphology may also account for the lower survival and event-free survival of PMV series from United States and Europe [28].

Several studies have compared the immediate and early follow-up results of PMV vs. closed surgical commissurotomy in optimal patients for these techniques. The results of these studies have been controversial showing either superior outcome from PMV or no significant differences between both techniques [29–34]. Patel et al. randomized 45 patients with mitral stenosis and optimal mitral valve morphology to closed surgical commissurotomy and to PMV [29]. They demonstrated a larger increase in mitral valve area with PMV (2.1 ± 0.7 vs. 1.3 ± 0.3 cm^2). Shrivastava et al. compared the results of single-balloon PMV, double-balloon PMV, and closed surgical commissurotomy in three groups of 20 patients each [30]. The mitral valve area post-intervention was larger for the double-balloon technique of PMV. Post-intervention valve areas were 1.9 ± 0.8, 1.5 ± 0.4, and 1.5 ± 0.5 for the double-balloon, the single-balloon, and the closed surgical commissurotomy techniques, respectively. On the other hand, Arora et al. randomized 200 patients with a mean age of 19 ± 7 years and mitral stenosis with optimal mitral valve morphology to PMV and to closed mitral commissurotomy [31]. Both procedures resulted in similar post-intervention mitral valve areas (2.39 ± 0.9 vs. 2.2 ± 0.9 cm^2 for the PMV and the mitral commissurotomy groups, respectively) and no significant differences in event-free survival at a mean follow-up period of 22 ± 6 months. Restenosis documented by echocardiography was low in both groups, 5 % in the PMV group and 4 % in the closed commissurotomy group. Turi et al. randomized 40 patients with severe mitral stenosis to PMV and to closed surgical commissurotomy [32]. The post-intervention mitral valve area at 1 week (1.6 ± 0.6 vs. 1.6 ± 0.7 cm^2) and 8 months (1.6 ± 0.6 vs. 1.8 ± 0.6 cm^2) after the procedures was similar in both groups. Reyes et al. randomized 60 patients with severe mitral stenosis and favorable valvular anatomy to PMV and to surgical commissurotomy [33]. They reported no significant differences in immediate outcome, complications, and 3.5-year follow-up between both groups of patients. Improvement was maintained in both groups, but mitral valve areas at follow-up were larger in the PMV group (2.4 ± 0.6 vs. 1.8 ± 0.4 cm^2). Ben Farhat et al. reported the results of a randomized trial designed to compare the immediate and long-term results of double-balloon PMV vs. those of open and closed surgical mitral commissurotomy in a cohort of patients with severe rheumatic mitral stenosis [34]. This group of patients were from the clinical and morphological point of view optimal candidates for both PMV and surgical commissurotomy (closed or open) procedures. They had a mean age of less than 30 years, absence of mitral valve calcification on fluoroscopy and 2D echocardiography, and an echocardiographic score ≤8 in all patients. Their results demonstrate that the immediate and long-term results of PMV are comparable to those of open mitral commissurotomy and superior to those of closed commissurotomy. The hemodynamic improvement, inhospital complications, and long-term restenosis rate and need for reintervention were superior for the patients treated with either PMV or open commissurotomy than for those treated with closed commissurotomy. The post-intervention mitral valve areas achieved with PMV were similar to the one obtained after open surgical commissurotomy (2.5 ± 0.5 vs. 2.2 ± 0.4 cm^2) but larger than those obtained after closed commissurotomy. These initial changes resulted in an excellent long-term follow-up in the group of patients treated with PMV that was comparable with the open commissurotomy group and superior to the closed commissurotomy group. The inferior results of closed mitral commissurotomy presented by Ben Farhat et al. are in disagreement with previous studies showing no significant differences in immediate and follow-up results between PMV and closed surgical mitral commissurotomy [29–31]. However, the increase in mitral valve area after closed commissurotomy is not uniform and often unsatisfactory. Since open commissurotomy is associated with a thoracotomy, need for cardiopulmonary bypass, higher cost, longer length of hospital stay, and a longer period of convalescence, PMV should be the procedure of choice for the treatment of patients with rheumatic mitral stenosis who are from the clinical and morphological point of view optimal candidates for PMV [35].

PMV in Pregnant Women

Surgical mitral commissurotomy has been performed in pregnant women with severe mitral stenosis. Since the risk of anesthesia and surgery for the mother and the fetus are increased, this operation is reserved for those patients with incapacitating symptoms refractory to medical therapy [78–80]. Under this conditions, PMV can be performed safely after the 20th week of pregnancy with minimal radiation to the fetus [81, 82]. Because of the definite risk in women with severe mitral stenosis of developing symptoms during pregnancy, PMV should be considered when the patient is considering becoming pregnant.

Difference in Outcome Among Women and Men After Percutaneous Mitral Valvuloplasty

We evaluated measures of procedural success and clinical outcome in 1,015 consecutive patients (839 women and 176 men) who underwent PMV. Despite a lower baseline echocardiographic score (7.47 ± 2.15 vs. 8.02 ± 2.18, $P = 0.002$), women were less likely to achieve PMV success (69 % vs. 83 %, adjusted OR 0.44, 95 % CI 0.27–0.74, $P = 0.002$) and had a smaller post-procedural MV area (1.86 ± 0.7 vs. 2.07 ± 0.7 cm^2, $P < 0.001$). Overall procedural and inhospital complication rates did not differ significantly between women and men. However, women were significantly more likely to develop severe MR immediately post-PMV (adjusted OR 2.41, 95 % CI: 1.0–5.83, $P = 0.05$) and to undergo MV surgery (adjusted HR 1.54, 95 % CI: 1.03–2.3, $P = 0.037$) after a median follow-up of 3.1 years. Thus, compared to men, women with rheumatic mitral stenosis who undergo PMV are less likely to have a successful outcome and more likely to require MV surgery on long-term follow-up despite more favorable baseline mitral valve anatomy.

Conclusions

PMV should be the procedure of choice for the treatment of patients with rheumatic mitral stenosis who are, from the clinical and morphological points of view, optimal candidates for PMV. Patients with echocardiographic scores ≤8 have the best results particularly if they are young, are in sinus rhythm, and have no pulmonary hypertension and no evidence of calcification of the mitral valve under fluoroscopy. The immediate and long-term results of PMV in this group of patients are similar to those reported after surgical mitral commissurotomy. Patients with echocardiographic scores >8 have only a 50 % chance to obtain a successful hemodynamic result with PMV, and long-term follow-up results are less good than those from patients with echocardiographic scores ≤8. In patients with echocardiographic scores ≥12, it is unlikely that PMV could produce good immediate or long-term result. They preferably should undergo open-heart surgery. PMV could be performed in these patients if they are non-/high-risk surgical candidates. Finally, much remains to be done in refining indications for patients with few or no symptoms and those with unfavorable anatomy. However, surgical therapy for mitral stenosis should actually be reserved for patients who have ≥2 grades of Sellers' mitral regurgitation by angiography, which can be better treated by mitral valve repair, and for those patients with severe mitral valve thickening and calcification or with significant subvalvular scarring to warrant valve replacement.

Aortic Valvuloplasty

Balloon aortic valvuloplasty (BAV) was first introduced in 1980 as a promising alternative to valve replacement for severe aortic stenosis (AS) treatment, but the early experience showed a limited durability of the therapy due to a high rate of restenosis [71–74]. Therefore, BAV was reserved only to patients who were considered either too old or a high risk for surgical valve replacement because of restenosis, the rate of complications related to the procedure, and the expanded scope of aortic valve surgery [75–79]. However, since the transcatheter aortic valve introduction, the spectrum of patients treated with BAV has increased exponentially, and it is frequently used as a bridge technique before the definitive aortic valve implantation. Moreover, the improved profile of the valvuloplasty balloons with a lower French size and the use of vascular closure techniques have significantly reduced the rate of complications.

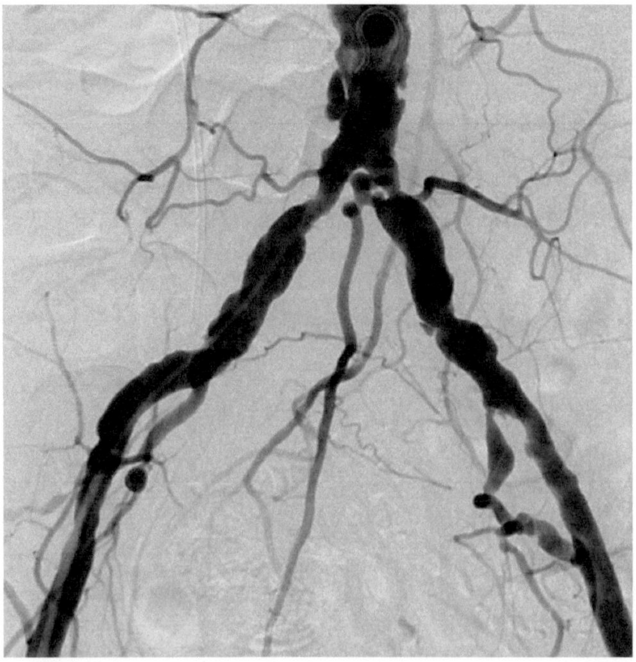

Fig. 26.7 Aortoiliac angiogram using digital subtraction in a balloon aortic valvuloplasty candidate with suspected peripheral arterial disease

Patient Selection and Indications

Symptoms might present several decades later than the onset of degeneration of the aortic valve. When present, initial symptoms tend to be dyspnea on exertion and effort angina, though some patients may present with syncope or heart failure [80]. Once symptoms are detected, the prognosis is poor without intervention: patients are often dead within 5 years of angina, 3 years of syncope, and 2 years of heart failure [81–83]. Surgical valve replacement is currently the standard of care for treatment of symptomatic patients with severe aortic stenosis (class I indication), and the ACC/AHA guidelines limit the BAV use to those patients with hemodynamically unstable severe AS who are at high risk for AVR as bridge to future surgery or for palliation when AVR cannot be performed (class IIb indication) [84]. However, there are other situations where BAV should be also considered.

Children and Young Adults <21 Years

The BAV in this subgroup of patients is durable and with good long-term results. The most common malformation of the aortic valve seen in young patients with AS is the bicuspid valve, and the chances to have a good result with BAV will decrease with an increased age. The severity of the stenosis is measured by the gradient, because many of these patients will be growing and might have a variable area. BAV will be indicated in symptomatic patients or patients with ECG changes and a peak gradient >50 mmHg or asymptomatic patients with a peak gradient >60 mmHg. A gradient reduction of more than 50 % is achieved in around 70 % of the patients [85–88].

Patients with Rheumatic Aortic Valve Stenosis

The mechanism underlying relief of the stenotic lesion with BAV is fracture of calcific deposits within the valve leaflets, stretching of the annulus, and separation of the calcified or fused commissures [89–91]. In patients with rheumatic aortic stenosis, valvuloplasty relieves the stenosis primarily by opening the commissures, and the results might be similar to balloon mitral commissurotomy with acceptable long-term results, and probably better than BAV in senile calcific aortic stenosis.

Bridge to Transcatheter Aortic Valve Implant (TAVI)

This technology is mainly used nowadays on patients with contraindication for surgery (porcelain aorta) or high STS score. The incidence of COPD on these high-risk surgical patients is over 40 % [92], and it might be difficult to ascertain if the shortness of breath is due to the lung and/or heart disease. In these cases, a BAV prior to the TAVI may help to select the patients that might improve the most after the valve implant. Patients with low gradient AS might represent a similar indication of the use of BAV prior to the definitive valve implantation. BAV might be useful to assess if with the relief of the aortic stenosis is followed by improvement in the left ventricular function and then will help to select those patients that might present better outcomes after TAVI.

Procedure

Pre-procedure Evaluation

Because of the severity of the complications related to the balloon valvuloplasty, patients have to be thoroughly evaluated prior to the procedure. The possibility of having complications has to be largely discussed in advance with the patients. The physical exam should focus in the cardiac exam and in the peripheral access. If pulses are reduced, an aortoiliac angiogram should be performed as first step (Fig. 26.7). For those patients with reduced iliofemoral artery caliber, the anterograde approach should be considered. The blood work-up should include coagulation, hemoglobin, and creatinine, and it is worth having a blood cross matching done. We use transthoracic echocardiography (TTE) to quantify the degree of stenosis and to measure the annulus size allowing us to choose the valvuloplasty balloon size.

Vascular Access and Preclosure

To get the arterial access, we use the fluoroscopic approach, placing a hemostat tip at the inferior border of the femoral head under fluoroscopy and puncturing the common femoral artery approximately 1 cm above the location of the hemostat tip. Once the puncture site is decided, mild sedation and local anesthesia are administered. The right common femoral artery and vein are cannulated with a 5 Fr and a 7F sheaths, respectively. A femoral angiogram is performed to assess the position of the sheath, if the puncture is below the femoral bifurcation precludes the use of that puncture site to passage of the larger valvuloplasty sheath. At this point, an aortoiliac angiogram should be done placing a 5F pigtail through the sheath to assess the contralateral femoral bifurcation. The angiogram can be used in reference to get access on the left femoral artery. If the puncture site is adequate and there is no significant stenosis of the common femoral, preclosure with two suture systems can be performed. Advancing a Wholey wire, the 5F sheath is removed and the first Perclose device is placed; before removing it completely, the wire is readvanced through the device (hole pointed by a small arrow). The second device is advanced then and same maneuver is done with the wire preserving the femoral access. The devices should be positioned keeping a 90° angle between the two deployment sites. Finally, a 10–14F sheath is placed over the wire depending on the valvuloplasty balloon size and manufacturer.

Assessment of Aortic Stenosis Severity and Coronary Arteries

A 7F Swan–Ganz catheter is advanced from the femoral vein, and baseline right-sided pressures are recorded. Cardiac output measurements using either thermodilution or the Fick principle should wait until the aortic valve has been crossed to reduce the error in calculation of aortic valve area. Coronary angiography is performed at this point to assess concomitant coronary artery disease; if any significant stenosis is found, coronary stenting should be done before the BAV. Aortic angiography is performed with the pigtail placed above the aortic valve in the LAO cranial projection to assess the degree of aortic regurgitation. BAV should be avoided in patients with aortic regurgitation ≥grade 2.

To cross the valve, we use a 6 Fr Amplatz catheter and a straight 0.035 in. guide wire (Fig. 26.8a). We prefer the Judkins right or a multipurpose if the aortic root is more horizontal. The straight AP projection or slight left cranial helps to identify the right and left cusps. The Amplatz catheter should be with the tip pointed at the orifice between the left and right cusps; advance the straight wire 2 in. out of the catheter and rotate the catheter clockwise. When the catheter and the wire are whipped by the flow, advance the wire and the catheter altogether across the valve. Once the valve has been crossed, the wire position is confirmed in the RAO projection, and the crossing catheter is advanced into the left ventricle (Fig. 26.8b). Exchange the AL catheter for a double-lumen pigtail using an extra stiff wire. Place a large curve on the end of the wire to increase the stability of the wire in the left ventricle and to decrease the risks of ventricular perforation. The transvalvular gradient can be obtained with the double-lumen pigtail, and cardiac output should be measured as well to assess the aortic valve area.

Retrograde Balloon Valvuloplasty

The Amplatz extra stiff 0.035" wire is readvanced into the left ventricle keeping the large curve (Fig. 26.8c). A temporary pacing wire is placed for rapid pacing during the valvuloplasty. The rapid pacing will help reduce the stroke volume temporarily and will help to position and stabilize better the valvuloplasty balloon. Choose a balloon with a 1:1 annulus to balloon ratio. There are several valvuloplasty balloon catheters available, most of them go up to 25 mm and are compatible with a 12F sheath. The 4 cm length balloons are preferred to increase the stability during the inflation, but in those patients with small ventricle, 3 cm balloons should be considered to reduce the risk of temporary AV block.

One major challenge during the BAV is maintaining the position of the balloon stable during the inflation. Choosing longer balloons and using the rapid pacing are two maneuvers that will help to keep the balloon stable, but coordination between the two operators is needed. While one of the operators positions the balloon and holds it altogether with the wire, the other operator inflates the balloon quickly until the waist in the balloon disappears completely (Fig. 26.8d). If the balloon moves during the inflation, deflate it partially and reposition it again. Some groups connect a smaller syringe to the sidearm with a stopcock to boost the balloon. This maneuver increases the risk of balloon rupture, and in some occasions, it is not possible to remove it through the sheath. When this happens, both the balloon and the sheath have to be pulled altogether. If this does not work, it might be because the balloon has ruptured horizontally, and on these cases, the tip of the balloon has to be snared and removed from the opposite groin. Second and third inflations can be attempted if the patient appears to tolerate the consecutive inflations. Once the balloon is fully inflated, it has to be deflated as rapidly as possible. Diluting the contrast with saline will make the inflations and deflations easier and faster; any dilution over 1:5 should be enough to keep a good radiopacity to visualize the balloon.

After the two or three fully balloon inflations, the balloon is removed keeping the wire inside the left ventricle. Doing a counter clockwise movement at the same time that we pull out the balloon will avoid sticking the balloon on the sheath. The double-lumen pigtail is placed back in the left ventricle and the gradient and valve area are measured again. In most

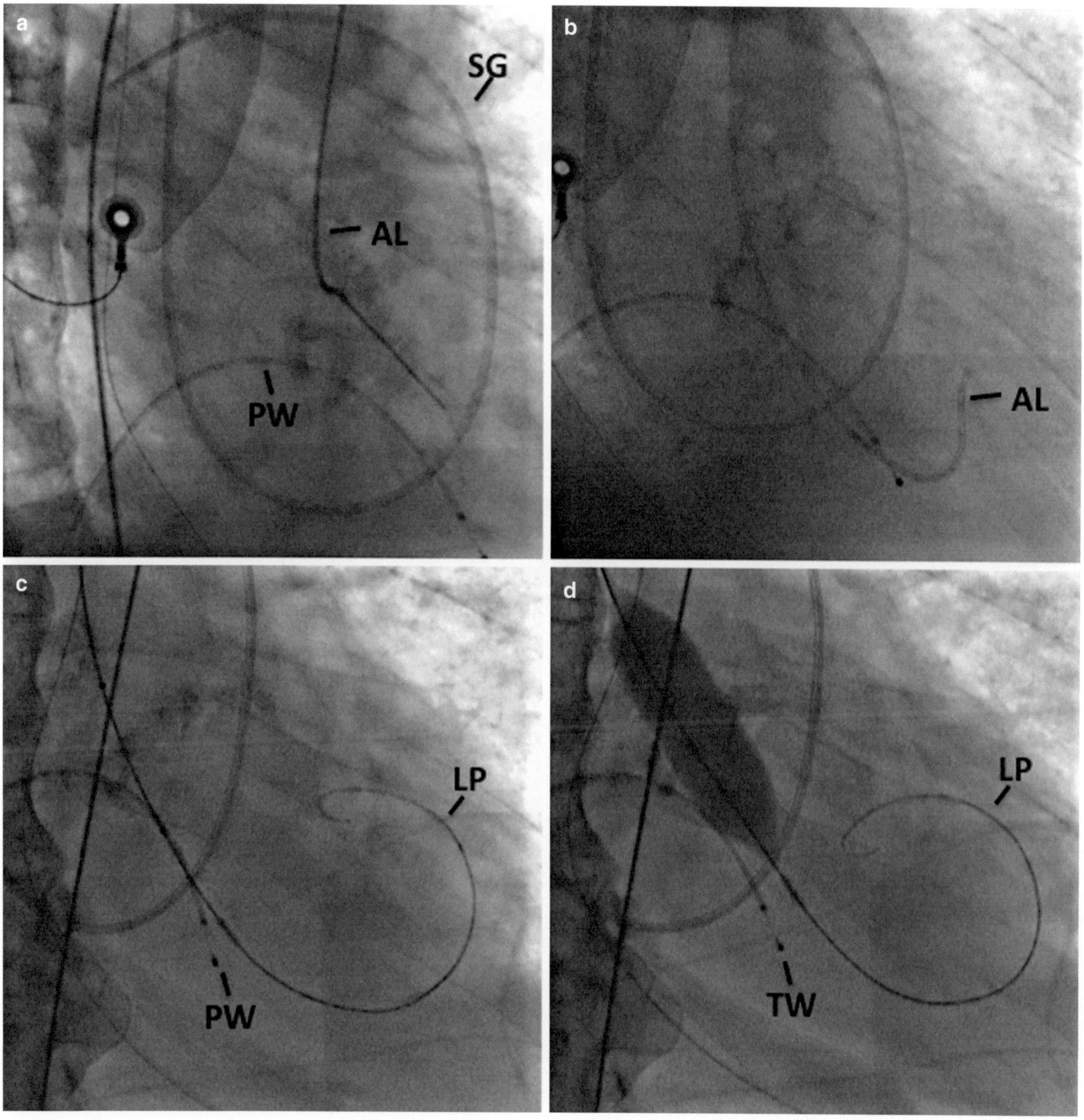

Fig. 26.8 Steps of retrograde balloon aortic valvuloplasty. (**a**) The stenotic aortic valve is crossed using a 6 Fr Amplatz left catheter and a straight 0.035 in. guide wire. (**b**) The Amplatz left catheter is then advanced into the left ventricle and the wire removed. Ideally, the catheter should be curved along the left ventricular apex. (**c**) An Amplatz extra stiff 0.035" wire with a generous loop (*LP*) is then used to exchange the Amplatz left catheter for a double-lumen pigtail catheter and then for the valvuloplasty balloon. (**d**) The balloon is then inflated during rapid pacing (*AL* Amplatz left catheter, *PW* temporary pacing wire, *SG* Swan–Ganz catheter)

of the cases, the valve area increases 0.2–0.4 cm^2. If no increase is observed in the valve area, the valvuloplasty can be repeated increasing the balloon diameter by 2 mm. The aortic regurgitation can be assessed before increasing the size of the balloon, but doing that we will have to remove the wire in the left ventricle, and we will need to cross the valve again. In our center, we evaluate the aortic diastolic pressure, and if no significant drop is observed, we go up with a larger balloon without doing an aortography.

At the completion of the procedure, the arterial sheath is removed. If preclosure with a suture device has been placed, a wire should be passed back into the sheath and the initial knots tied over the wire as the sheath is withdrawn, so that if hemostasis is not successful, a new Perclose can be advanced.

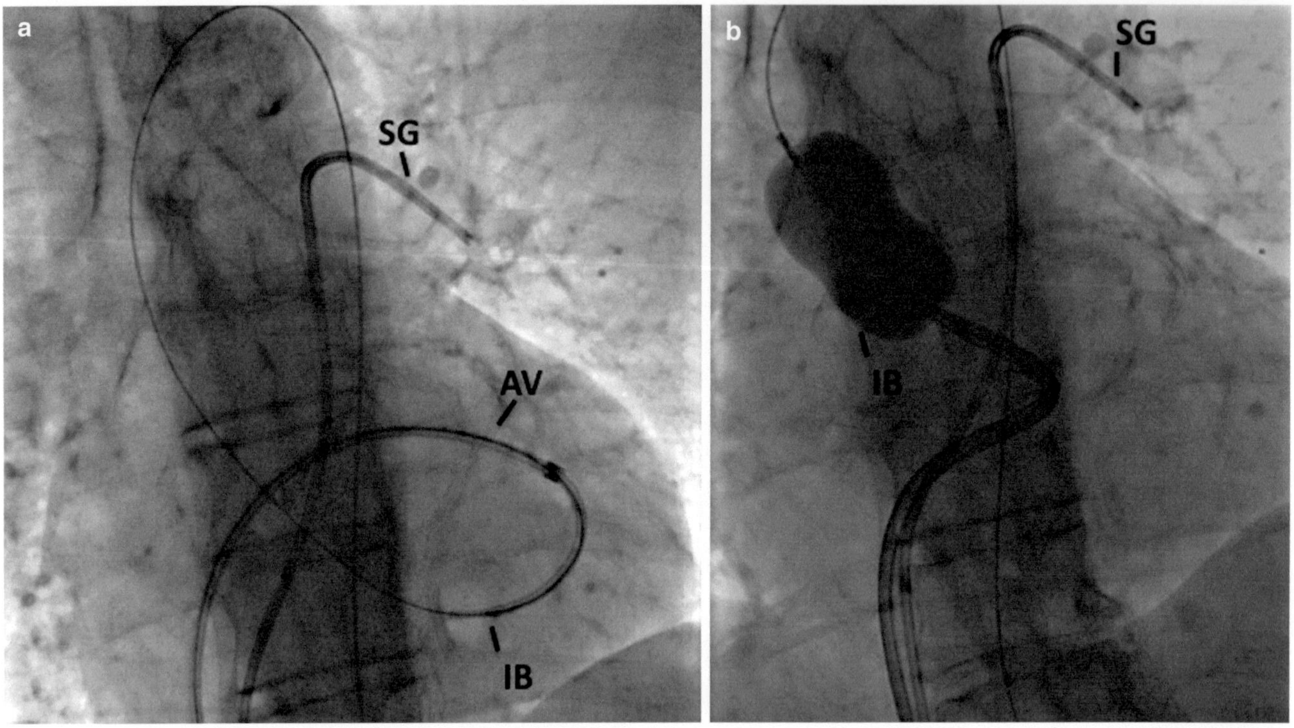

Fig. 26.9 Anterograde balloon aortic valvuloplasty. Fluoroscopic images demonstrating stages of anterograde balloon aortic valvuloplasty. (**a**) A Mullins sheath is advanced via transseptal puncture into the left ventricle. A wire is then advanced into the descending aorta and snared from the femoral artery. In order to avoid injury to the mitral valve, a large arteriovenous loop is created within the left ventricle. An Inoue balloon catheter is then advanced while partially inflated through the left ventricle and across the aortic valve. (**b**) Finally, balloon aortic valvuloplasty is performed while pulling the Inoue balloon catheter against the aortic valve (*AV* arteriovenous loop, *IB* Inoue balloon catheter, *SG* Swan–Ganz catheter)

If this does not work, the sheath can be replaced and pulled later depending on the ACT. If the preclosure technique has not been used, the sheath is removed manually and prolonged compression is typically necessary.

Antegrade Aortic Valuloplasty

If arterial access is not possible, the aortic valve can be dilated via the antegrade route. This method is more challenging and requires a higher grade of experience because of the potential damage of the mitral valve. In this approach, a transseptal puncture is performed and a wire is looped in the left ventricle and advanced across the aortic valve. The wire is snared in the descending aorta with a gooseneck snare advanced through the femoral artery. An arteriovenous loop is created that will allow advancing the valvuloplasty balloon through the septum and position it across the aortic valve. The main advantage in this technique is the reduction of the French size in the arterial site, and the main limitation is the complex approach required including a transseptal puncture and the creation of the arteriovenous loop.

Cannulate the right common femoral artery and vein with a 5 Fr and an 8F sheaths, respectively. After the transseptal puncture, the Mullins sheath is placed in the left atrium. Advance a balloon-wedge catheter or a floppy multipurpose catheter through the Mullins sheath in the left ventricle and try to loop it in the apex pointing the tip of the catheter toward the aortic valve. A 0.032" extra stiff wire is advanced then, and most of the times, it will cross the valve easily. In some rare occasions, the catheter will need to be advanced further to give more support to the wire. In the case that we are using a balloon-wedge catheter, we can take advantage of the flow to position it below the valve; if we slightly deflate, it we will be able to cross the valve directly with the catheter. Advance the wire into the descending aorta and with a 15 mm gooseneck snare, capture it and exteriorize the wire through the arterial femoral sheath. The venous sheath is upgraded to a 14F sheath. Once the arteriovenous loop has been created (Fig. 26.9a), we have to decide if we are using an Inoue balloon or a conventional balloon. The main advantages of the first are (1) that it is going to be easier to loop it into the ventricle and advance it across the aortic valve, (2) the inflation–deflation of the balloon is much more rapid, and (3) a larger final aortic valve area might be obtained [93]. However, the shaft of the Inoue balloon is stiffer than the conventional balloon, and it is difficult to keep a wide loop during the inflations producing a more severe mitral regurgitation due

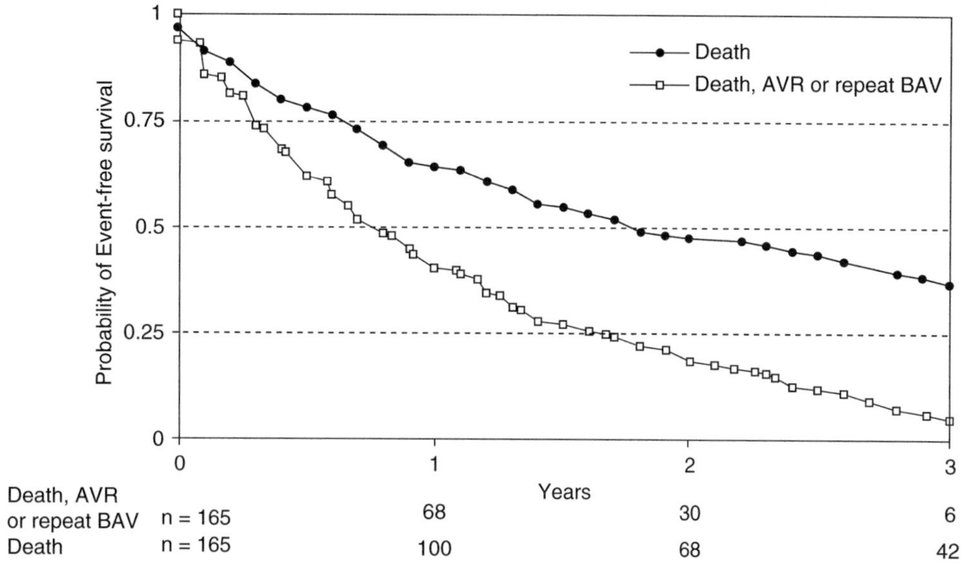

Fig. 26.10 Actuarial and event-free survival after balloon aortic valvuloplasty illustrating the probability of actuarial and event-free survival from the date of initial balloon aortic valvuloplasty. Events are defined as death, aortic valve replacement (*AVR*), or a second balloon aortic valvuloplasty (repeat *BAV*) (From Lieberman et al. [95], with permission)

to a tenting of the valve with the shaft (Fig. 26.9b). The conventional balloons have a more complicated navigability, but once positioned across the valve, it is easier to open the loop advancing the wire and thus, reducing the degree of mitral regurgitation.

After a couple of inflations, the balloon is removed keeping the arteriovenous loop in place. Advancing the Mullins sheath in the left ventricle, we can measure the gradient and decide if we need to increase the diameter of the balloon or to stop the procedure at this point.

Post-catheterization Orders

After the valvuloplasty, patients have to be closely followed. Most of the patients are really fragile patients that might destabilize easily with any complication. Explore the pulses and groins during the following hours to the intervention to check for possible embolic events or hematomas, respectively. In some cases, patients fall into heart failure after the procedure, and the diuretic dose has to be increased. We routinely check the creatinine and hematocrit at 6 and 12 h after the procedure and perform a new TTE in the 24 h after the procedure to reassess the results of the valvuloplasty.

Results

The long-term results of the BAV suggest that there is no increase in the survival of the patients treated with valvuloplasty [94–96] (Fig. 26.10). Moreover, the procedure has been associated with a high rate of restenosis and procedural complications. For these reasons, the aortic valvuloplasty has been reserved for palliative use during a long time. However, the improvement in the balloon catheters with lower profile, the use of vascular closure techniques, and the introduction of the transcatheter valves have got back this technique, and the number of BAV has increased exponentially in the last years.

The BAV improves the hemodynamics of severe aortic stenosis to a modest degree. The average valve area increases from 0.5 to 0.8 cm^2, peak-to-peak systolic pressure gradients decrease 30–50 %, and small improvements in the left ventricular end-diastolic pressure, pulmonary artery pressure, and cardiac output are noted [72]. These results might improve even more when the anterograde approach is used.

Complications

Brady- and Tachyarrhythmia

The assessment of baseline EKG prior to the procedure is important; the patients with an underlying defect of the conduction system such as preexisting left or right bundle branch block or atrioventricular (AV) block are more susceptible to developing advanced atrioventricular block. Inflation of the balloon catheter across the aortic valve can disturb the electrical conduction system by direct trauma, causing intraventricular conduction defect or bundle branch block. In the majority of cases, this is a transient disorder with recovery within 48 h. Since a temporary wire is placed before the valvuloplasty for the rapid pacing, we keep it after the procedure in the cases that the conduction defect is persistent.

Ventricular arrhythmias are frequent during the wire and balloon manipulation inside the left ventricle. A simple reposition of the wire or releasing the tension might be enough to stop these arrhythmias. In rare occasions, patients might develop a sustained ventricular tachycardia or even fibrillation; for this reason, the defibrillator patches should be positioned prophylactically.

Vascular Injury

As the vascular access is performed on frail patients of advanced age, whose arteries may have significant atherosclerosis, there is always a risk of inadvertent trauma of a vessel, resulting in hematoma formation, retroperitoneal bleeding, vascular perforation, dissection, or atheroembolization. Moreover, these major vascular complications are associated with increased mortality and morbidity; therefore, an adequate arterial access in these patients is essential. Peripheral angioplasty balloons from 7 to 10 mm should be available in the room, if a perforation occurs a fast actuation might be lifesaving.

Vascular surgery has been required in 5 % of the patients, but the introduction of the suture closure techniques has reduced dramatically the need for surgery and blood transfusion [97, 98].

Massive Aortic Regurgitation

Massive aortic regurgitation after BAV can be a fatal complication. In patients with small stature or heavily calcified valves, it is recommended to dilate the valve in a stepwise fashion from the small-sized to the larger-sized balloon. If massive regurgitation occurs and the patient is hemodynamically stable, urgent surgery or TAVI has to be considered. In stable patients, the valve replacement procedure can be postponed and done electively.

Ventricular Perforation and Tamponade

Cardiac tamponade has been reported in about 1 % of the PAVs. The perforation might be due to the stiff wire placed in the left ventricle or due to an aggressive advancement of the balloon across the valve. To avoid this complication, it is important to keep a large loop on the tip of the wire all the time and have the wire controlled all along the procedure. Moreover, it is important to confirm the pressure drop during the rapid pacing; otherwise, the balloon might melon seed and perforate the ventricle kinking the wire. Performance of pericardiocentesis is a requisite skill for these procedures.

Embolic Events

The occurrence of clinically apparent cerebral events is below 2 %. Patients should be treated with 70 IU/Kg of heparin at the beginning of the procedure. Aggressive crossing technique of the valve should be avoided, and the wire and the catheter have to be retrieved and flushed every 3 min if the valve is difficult to cross. Neurologic symptoms might present due to prolonged hypotension, particularly in patients with cerebrovascular disease. Short balloon inflation–deflation and hemodynamic support with inotropic drugs are highly recommended. The development of neurologic changes should prompt urgent imaging and consultation with a neurologist.

Death

Death in the hospital occurs in 5–8 % of patients; 1 % will expire in the catheterization laboratory. The majority of these deaths occur as the result of fatal complication of the procedure (arrhythmia, rupture of the aorta, ventricle perforation) or due to a progressive heart failure and cardiogenic shock in patients with severely depressed left ventricular function.

References

1. Inoue K, Owaki T, Nakamura T, Kitamura F, Miyamoto N. Clinical application of transvenous mitral commissurotomy by a new balloon catheter. J Thorac Cardiovasc Surg. 1984;87:394–402.
2. Lock JE, Kalilullah M, Shrivastava S, Bahl V, Keane JF. Percutaneous catheter commissurotomy in rheumatic mitral stenosis. N Engl J Med. 1985;313:1515–18.
3. Al Zaibag M, Ribeiro PA, Al Kassab SA, Al Fagig MR. Percutaneous double balloon mitral valvotomy for rheumatic mitral stenosis. Lancet. 1986;1:757–61.
4. Palacios I, Block PC, Brandi S, Blanco P, Casal H, Pulido JI, Munoz S, D'Empaire G, Ortega MA, Jacobs M, Vlahakes G. Percutaneous balloon valvotomy for patients with severe mitral stenosis. Circulation. 1987;75:778–84.
5. Mc Kay CR, Kawanishi DT, Rahimtoola SH. Catheter balloon valvuloplasty of the mitral valve in adults using a double balloon technique. Early hemodynamic results. JAMA. 1987;257:1753–61.
6. Cohen DJ, Kuntz RE, Gordon SPF, Piana RN, Safian RD, McKay RG, Baim DS, Grossman W, Diver DJ. Predictors of long-term outcome after percutaneous mitral valvuloplasty. N Engl J Med. 1991;327:1329–35.
7. Arora R, Kalra GS, Murty GS, Trehan V, Jolly N, Mohan JC, Sethi KK, Nigam M, Khalilullah M. Percutaneous transatrial mitral commissurotomy: immediate and intermediate results. J Am Coll Cardiol. 1994;23:1327–32.
8. Chen CR, Cheng TO. Percutaneous balloon mitral valvuloplasty by the Inoue technique: a multicenter study of 4832 patients in China. Am Heart J. 1995;129:1197–203.
9. Dean LS, Mickel M, Bonan R, Holmes Jr DR, O'Neill WW, Palacios IF, Rahimtoola S, Slater JN, Davis K, Kennedy JW. Four-year follow-up of patients undergoing percutaneous balloon mitral commissurotomy. A report from the National Heart, Lung, and Blood Institute Balloon Valvuloplasty Registry. J Am Coll Cardiol. 1996;28:1452–7.
10. Orrange SE, Kawanishi DT, Lopez BM, Curry SM, Rahimtoola SH. Actuarial outcome after catheter balloon commissurotomy in patients with mitral stenosis. Circulation. 1997;97:245–50.
11. Chen CR, Cheng TO, Chen JY, Huang YG, Huang T, Zhang B. Long-term results of percutaneous balloon mitral valvuloplasty for mitral stenosis: a follow-up study to 11 years in 202 patients. Cathet Cardiovasc Diagn. 1998;43:132–9.
12. Stefanadis CI, Stratos CG, Lambrou SG, Bahl VK, Cokkinos DV, Voudris VA, Foussas SG, Tsioufis CP, Toutouzas PK. Retrograde nontransseptal balloon mitral valvuloplasty: immediate results and intermediate long-term outcome in 441 cases–a multicenter experience. J Am Coll Cardiol. 1998;32:1009–16.
13. Cribier A, Eltchaninoff H, Koning R, Rath PC, Arora R, Imam A, El-Sayed M, Dani S, Derumeaux G, Benichou J, Tron C, Janorkar S, Pontier G, Letac B. Percutaneous mechanical mitral commissurotomy with a newly designed metallic valvulotome: immediate results of the initial experience in 153 patients. Circulation. 1999;99:793–9.

14. Hernandez R, Banuelos C, Alfonso F, Goicolea J, Fernandez-Ortiz A, Escaned J, Azcona L, Almeria C, Macaya C. Long-term clinical and echocardiographic follow-up after percutaneous mitral valvuloplasty with the Inoue balloon. Circulation. 1999;99:1580–6.
15. Iung B, Garbarz E, Michaud P, Helou S, Farah B, Berdah P, Michel PL, Cormier B, Vahanian A. Late results of percutaneous mitral commissurotomy in a series of 1024 patients: analysis of late clinical deterioration: frequency, anatomic findings and predictive factors. Circulation. 1999;99:3272–8.
16. Cribier A, Eltchaninoff H, Carlot R, et al. Percutaneous mechanical mitral commissurotomy with the metallic valvulotome: detailed technical aspects and overview of the results of the multicenter registry in 882 patients. J Interv Cardiol. 2000;13:255–62.
17. Palacios IF, Sanchez PL, Harrell LC, Weyman AE, Block PC. Which patients benefit from percutaneous mitral balloon valvuloplasty? Prevalvuloplasty and postvalvuloplasty variables that predict long-term outcome. Circulation. 2002;105:1465–71.
18. Patel JJ, Shama D, Mitha AS, Blyth D, Hassen F, Le Roux BT, Chetty S. Balloon valvuloplasty versus closed commissurotomy for pliable mitral stenosis: a prospective hemodynamic study. J Am Coll Cardiol. 1991;18:1318–22.
19. Shrivastava S, Mathur A, Dev V, Saxena A, Venugopal P, Sampath Kumar A. A comparison of immediate hemodynamic response of closed mitral commissurotomy, single-balloon, and double-balloon mitral valvuloplasty in rheumatic mitral stenosis. J Thorac Cardiovasc Surg. 1992;104:1264–7.
20. Arora R, Nair M, Kalra GS, Nigam M, Khalilullah M. Immediate and long-term results of balloon and surgical closed mitral valvotomy: a randomized comparative study. Am Heart J. 1993;125:1091–4.
21. Turi ZG, Reyes VP, Raju BS, Raju AR, Kumar DN, Rajagopal P, Sathyanarayana PV, Rao DP, Srinath K, Peters P, et al. Percutaneous balloon versus surgical closed commissurotomy for mitral stenosis: a prospective, randomized trial. Circulation. 1991;83:1179–85.
22. Reyes VP, Raju BS, Wynne J, Stephenson LW, Raju R, Fromm BS, Rajagopal P, Mehta P, Singh S, Rao DP, et al. Percutaneous balloon valvuloplasty compared with open surgical commissurotomy for mitral stenosis. N Engl J Med. 1994;331:961–7.
23. Ben Farhat M, Ayari M, Maatouk F, Betbout F, Gamra H, Jarra M, Tiss M, Hammami S, Thaalbi R, Addad F. Percutaneous balloon versus surgical closed and open mitral commissurotomy: seven-year follow-up results of a randomized trial. Circulation. 1998;97:245–50.
24. Vahanian A, Palacios IF. Percutaneous approaches to valvular disease. Circulation. 2004;109:1572–9.
25. Rd S, Levy MJ, Amplatz K, Lillehei CW. Left retrograde cardioangiography in acquired cardiac disease. Am J Cardiol. 1964;14:437–47.
26. Babic UU, Pejcic P, Djurisic Z, Vucinic M, Grujicic SM. Percutaneous transarterial balloon valvuloplasty for mitral valve stenosis. Am J Cardiol. 1986;57:1101–4.
27. Stefanadis C, Stratos C, Pitsavos C, Kallikazaros I, Triposkiadis F, Trikas A, Vlachopoulos C, Gavaliatsis I, Toutouzas P. Retrograde nontransseptal balloon mitral valvuloplasty. Immediate results and long term follow-up. Circulation. 1992;85:1760–7.
28. Mc Kay RG, Lock JE, Safian RD, Come PC, Diver DJ, Baim DS, Berman AD, Warren SE, MAndell VE, Rotal HD, Grossman W. Balloon dilatation of mitral stenosis in adults patients: postmortem and percutaneous mitral valvuloplasty studies. J Am Coll Cardiol. 1987;9:723–31.
29. Acar C, Jebara VA, Grare P, Chachques JC, Dervanian P, Vahanian A, Carpentier A. Traumatic mitral insufficiency following percutaneous mitral dilatation: anatomic lesions and surgical implications. Eur J Cardiothorac Surg. 1992;6:660–4.
30. Herrmann HC, Lima JA, Feldman T, Chisholm R, Isner J, O'Neill W, Ramaswamy K. Mechanisms and outcome of severe mitral regurgitation after Inoue balloon valvuloplasty. J Am Coll Cardiol. 1993;27:783–9.
31. Wilkins GT, Weyman AE, Abascal VM, Block PC, Palacios IF. Percutaneous balloon dilatation of the mitral valve: an analysis of echocardiographic variables related to outcome and the mechanism of dilatation. Br Heart J. 1988;60:229–308.
32. Padial LR, Freitas N, Sagie A, Newell JB, Weyman AE, Levine RA, Palacios IF. Echocardiography can predict which patients will develop severe mitral regurgitation after percutaneous mitral valvulotomy. J Am Coll Cardiol. 1996;27:1225–31.
33. Abascal VM, O'Shea JP, Wilkins GT, Palacios IF, Thomas JD, Rosas E, Newell JB, Block PC, Weyman AE. Prediction of successful outcome in 130 patients undergoing percutaneous balloon mitral valvotomy. Circulation. 1990;82:448–56.
34. Herrman HC, Wilkins GT, Abascal VM, Weyman AE, Block PC, Palacios IF. Percutaneous balloon mitral valvotomy for patients with mitral stenosis: analysis of factors influencing early results. J Thorac Cardiovasc Surg. 1988;96:33–8.
35. Tuzcu EM, Block PC, Griffin BP, Newell JB, Palacios IF. Immediate and long term outcome of percutaneous mitral valvotomy in patients 65 years and older. Circulation. 1992;85:963–71.
36. Abascal VM, Wilkins GT, Choong CY, Block PC, Palacios IF, Weyman AE. Mitral regurgitation after percutaneous mitral valvuloplasty in adults: evaluation by pulsed Doppler echocardiography. J Am Coll Cardiol. 1988;2:257–63.
37. Roth RB, Block PC, Palacios IF. Predictors of increased mitral regurgitation after percutaneous mitral balloon valvotomy. Cathet Cardiovasc Diagn. 1990;20:17–21.
38. Casale P, Block PC, O'Shea JP, Palacios IF. Atrial septal defect after percutaneous mitral balloon valvuloplasty: immediate results and follow-up. J Am Coll Cardiol. 1990;15:1300–4.
39. Desideri A, Vanderperren O, Serra A, Barraud P, Petritclerc R, Lesperance J, Dyrda I, Crepeaau J, Bonan R. Long term (9 to 33 months) echocardiographic follow-up after successful percutaneous mitral commissurotomy. Am J Cardiol. 1992;69: 1602–6.
40. Sanchez PL, Rodríguez-Alemparte M, Inglessis I, Palacios IF. The impact of age in the immediate and long-term outcomes of percutaneous mitral balloon valvuloplasty. J Interv Cardiol. 2005 Aug;18(4):217–25.
41. Sutaria N, Elder AT, Shaw TR. Long term outcome of percutaneous mitral balloon valvotomy in patients aged 70 and over. Heart. 2000;83:433–8.
42. Tuzcu EM, Block PC, Griffin B, Dinsmore R, Newell JB, Palacios IF. Percutaneous mitral balloon valvotomy in patients with calcific mitral stenosis: immediate and long term outcome. J Am Coll Cardiol. 1994;23:1604–9.
43. Williams JA, Littmann D, Warren R. Experience with the surgical treatment of mitral stenosis. N Engl J Med. 1958;258:623–30.
44. Scannell JG, Burke JF, Saidi F, Turner JD. Five-year follow-up study of closed mitral valvotomy. J Thorac Cardiovasc Surg. 1960;40:723–30.
45. Rediker DE, Block PC, Abascal VM, Palacios IF. Mitral balloon valvuloplasty for mitral restenosis after surgical commissurotomy. J Am Coll Cardiol. 1988;2:252–6.
46. Medina A, Suarez De Lezo J, Hernandez E, Pan M, Romero M, Melian F, Sancho M, Bethencourt A, Vivancos R, Jimenez F, et al. Balloon valvuloplasty for mitral restenosis after previous surgery. A comparative study. Am Heart J. 1990;120:568–71.
47. Davidson CJ, Bashore TM, Mickel M, Davis K. Balloon mitral commissurotomy after previous surgical commissurotomy. The National Heart, Lung, and Blood Institute Balloon Valvuloplasty Registry participants. Circulation. 1992;86:91–9.
48. Jang IK, Block PC, Newell JB, Tuzcu EM, Palacios IF. Percutaneous mitral balloon valvotomy for recurrent mitral stenosis after surgical commissurotomy. Am J Cardiol. 1995;75:601–5.

49. Lau KW, Ding ZP, Gao W, Koh TH, Johan A. Percutaneous balloon mitral valvuloplasty in patients with mitral restenosis after previous surgical commissurotomy. A matched comparative study. Eur Heart J. 1996;17:1367–72.
50. Eltchaninoff H, Tron C, Cribier A. Effectiveness of percutaneous mechanical mitral commissurotomy using the metallic commissurotomy in patients with restenosis after balloon or previous surgical commissurotomy. Am J Cardiol. 2003;91:425–8.
51. Leon MN, Harrell LC, Simosa HF, Mahdi NA, Pathan A, Lopez-Cuellar J, Inglessis I, Moreno PR, Palacios IF. Mitral balloon valvotomy for patients with mitral stenosis in atrial fibrillation: immediate and long-term results. J Am Coll Cardiol. 1999;34:1145–52.
52. Chen MH, Semigran M, Schwammenthal E, Harrell L, Palacios IF. Impact of pulmonary resistance on short and long term outcome after percutaneous mitral valvuloplasty. Circulation. 1993; (Suppl I):1825.
53. Sagie A, Schwammenthal E, Newell JB, Harrell L, Weyman AE, Levine RA, Palacios IF. Significant tricuspid regurgitation is a marker for adverse outcome in patients undergoing mitral balloon valvotomy. J Am Coll Cardiol. 1994;24:696–702.
54. Song JM, Kang DH, Song JK, Jeong YH, Lee CW, Hong MK, Kim JJ, Park SW, Park SJ. Outcome of significant functional tricuspid regurgitation after percutaneous mitral valvuloplasty. Am Heart J. 2003;145:371–6.
55. Sanchez PL, Harrell LC, Salas RE, Palacios IF. Learning curve of the Inoue technique of percutaneous mitral balloon valvuloplasty. Am J Cardiol. 2001;88:662–7.
56. Block PC, Palacios IF, Block EH, Tuzcu EM, Griffin B. Late (two year) follow-up after percutaneous mitral balloon valvotomy. Am J Cardiol. 1992;69:537–41.
57. Petrossian GA, Tuzcu EM, Ziskind AA, Block PC, Palacios IF. Atrial septal occlusion improves the accuracy of mitral valve area determination following percutaneous mitral balloon valvotomy. Cathet Cardiovasc Diagn. 1991;22:21–4.
58. John S, Bashi VV, Jairaj PS, et al. Closed mitral valvotomy: early results and long term follow up of 3724 patients. Circulation. 1983;68:891–6.
59. Ellis LR, Harken DE, Black H. A clinical study of 1,000 consecutive cases of mitral stenosis two to nine years after mitral valvuloplasty. Circulation. 1959;19:803–20.
60. Elis FH, Kirklin JW, Parker RL, Burchell HB, Wood EH. Mitral commissurotomy: an overall appraisal of clinical and hemodynamic results. Arch Intern Med. 1954;94:774–84.
61. Hoeksema TD, Wallace RB, Kirklin JW. Closed mitral commissurotomy. Am J Cardiol. 1966;17:825–8.
62. Kirklin JW. Percutaneous balloon versus surgical closed commissurotomy for mitral stenosis. Circulation. 1991;83:1450–1.
63. Higgs LM, Glancy DL, O'Brien KP, Epstein SE, Morrow AG. Mitral restenosis: an uncommon cause of recurrent symptoms following mitral commissurotomy. Am J Cardiol. 1970;26: 34–7.
64. Glover RP, Davila JC, O'Neil TJE, Janton OH. Does mitral stenosis recur after commissurotomy? Circulation. 1955;11:14–28.
65. Hickey MSJ, Blackstone EH, Kirklin JW, Dean LS. Outcome probabilities and life history after surgical mitral commissurotomy: Implications for balloon commissurotomy. J Am Coll Cardiol. 1991;17:29–42.
66. Rihal CS, Schaff HV, Frye RL, Bailey KR, Hammes LN, Holmes Jr DR. Long-term follow-up of patients undergoing closed transventricular mitral commissurotomy: a useful surrogate for percutaneous balloon mitral valvuloplasty. J Am Coll Cardiol. 1992;20:781–6.
67. Bernal JM, Miralles PJ. Cardiac surgery with cardiopulmonary bypass during pregnancy. Obstet Gynecol Surg. 1998;41(1):1–6.
68. Vosloo S, Reichart B. The feasibility of closed mitral valvotomy in pregnancy. J Thorac Cardiovasc Surg. 1987;93:675.
69. Palacios IF, Block PC, Wilkins GT, Rediker DE, Daggett WM. Percutaneous mitral balloon valvotomy during pregnancy in patients with severe mitral stenosis. Cathet Cardiovasc Diagn. 1988;15:109–11.
70. Mangione JA, Zuliani MF, Del Castillo JM, Nogueira EA, Arie S. Percutaneous double balloon mitral valvuloplasty in pregnant women. Am J Cardiol. 1989;64:99–102.
71. Safian RD, Berman AD, Diver DJ, McKay LL, Come PC, Riley MF, Warren SE, Cunningham MJ, Wyman RM, Weinstein JS, et al. Balloon aortic valvuloplasty in 170 consecutive patients. N Engl J Med. 1988;319(3):125–30.
72. Otto CM, Mickel MC, Kennedy JW, Alderman EL, Bashore TM, Block PC, Brinker JA, Diver D, Ferguson J, Holmes Jr DR, et al. Three-year outcome after balloon aortic valvuloplasty. Insights into prognosis of valvular aortic stenosis. Circulation. 1994;89(2):642–50.
73. Kuntz RE, Tosteson AN, Berman AD, Goldman L, Gordon PC, Leonard BM, McKay RG, Diver DJ, Safian RD. Predictors of event-free survival after balloon aortic valvuloplasty. N Engl J Med. 1991;325(1):17–23.
74. O'Neill WW. Predictors of long-term survival after percutaneous aortic valvuloplasty: report of the Mansfield Scientific Balloon Aortic Valvuloplasty Registry. J Am Coll Cardiol. 1991;17(1):193–8.
75. Culliford AT, Galloway AC, Colvin SB, Grossi EA, Baumann FG, Esposito R, Ribakove GH, Spencer FC. Aortic valve replacement for aortic stenosis in persons aged 80 years and over. Am J Cardiol. 1991;67(15):1256–60.
76. Lytle BW, Cosgrove DM, Taylor PC, Goormastic M, Stewart RW, Golding LA, Gill CC, Loop FD. Primary isolated aortic valve replacement. Early and late results. J Thorac Cardiovasc Surg. 1989;97(5):675–94.
77. Pereira JJ, Lauer MS, Bashir M, Afridi I, Blackstone EH, Stewart WJ, McCarthy PM, Thomas JD, Asher CR. Survival after aortic valve replacement for severe aortic stenosis with low transvalvular gradients and severe left ventricular dysfunction. J Am Coll Cardiol. 2002;39(8):1356–63.
78. Rothenburger M, Drebber K, Tjan TD, Schmidt C, Schmid C, Wichter T, Scheld HH, Deiwick M. Aortic valve replacement for aortic regurgitation and stenosis, in patients with severe left ventricular dysfunction. Eur J Cardiothorac Surg. 2003;23(5):703–9. discussion 709.
79. Sharony R, Grossi EA, Saunders PC, Schwartz CF, Ciuffo GB, Baumann FG, Delianides J, Applebaum RM, Ribakove GH. Culliford AT and others. Aortic valve replacement in patients with impaired ventricular function. Ann Thorac Surg. 2003;75(6): 1808–14.
80. Kennedy KD, Nishimura RA, Holmes Jr DR, Bailey KR. Natural history of moderate aortic stenosis. J Am Coll Cardiol. 1991;17(2): 313–19.
81. Selzer A. Changing aspects of the natural history of valvular aortic stenosis. N Engl J Med. 1987;317(2):91–8.
82. Frank S, Johnson A, Ross Jr J. Natural history of valvular aortic stenosis. Br Heart J. 1973;35(1):41–6.
83. Ross Jr J, Braunwald E. Aortic stenosis. Circulation. 1968; 38(1 Suppl):61–7.
84. Bonow RO, Carabello BA, Chatterjee K, de Leon AC Jr, Faxon DP, Freed MD, Gaasch WH, Lytle BW, Nishimura RA, O'Gara PT, et al. 2008 Focused update incorporated into the ACC/AHA 2006 guidelines for the management of patients with valvular heart disease: a report of the American College of Cardiology/American Heart Association Task Force on Practice Guidelines (Writing Committee to Revise the 1998 Guidelines for the Management of Patients With Valvular Heart Disease): endorsed by the Society of Cardiovascular Anesthesiologists, Society for Cardiovascular Angiography and Interventions, and Society of Thoracic Surgeons. Circulation. 2008;118(15):e523-661.

85. Huhta JC, Carpenter Jr RJ, Moise Jr KJ, Deter RL, Ott DA, McNamara DG. Prenatal diagnosis and postnatal management of critical aortic stenosis. Circulation. 1987;75(3):573–6.
86. Pass RH, Hellenbrand WE. Catheter intervention for critical aortic stenosis in the neonate. Catheter Cardiovasc Interv. 2002;55(1): 88–92.
87. Rao PS, Jureidini SB. Transumbilical venous, anterograde, snare-assisted balloon aortic valvuloplasty in a neonate with critical aortic stenosis. Cathet Cardiovasc Diagn. 1998;45(2):144–8.
88. Beekman RH, Rocchini AP, Andes A. Balloon valvuloplasty for critical aortic stenosis in the newborn: influence of new catheter technology. J Am Coll Cardiol. 1991;17(5):1172–6.
89. McKay RG, Safian RD, Lock JE, Mandell VS, Thurer RL, Schnitt SJ, Grossman W. Balloon dilatation of calcific aortic stenosis in elderly patients: postmortem, intraoperative, and percutaneous valvuloplasty studies. Circulation. 1986;74(1):119–25.
90. Safian RD, Mandell VS, Thurer RE, Hutchins GM, Schnitt SJ, Grossman W, McKay RG. Postmortem and intraoperative balloon valvuloplasty of calcific aortic stenosis in elderly patients: mechanisms of successful dilation. J Am Coll Cardiol. 1987;9(3): 655–60.
91. Isner JM, Samuels DA, Slovenkai GA, Halaburka KR, Hougen TJ, Desnoyers MR, Fields CD, Salem DN. Mechanism of aortic balloon valvuloplasty: fracture of valvular calcific deposits. Ann Intern Med. 1988;108(3):377–80.
92. Smith CR, Leon MB, Mack MJ, Miller DC, Moses JW, Svensson LG, Tuzcu EM, Webb JG, Fontana GP, Makkar RR, et al. Transcatheter versus surgical aortic-valve replacement in high-risk patients. N Engl J Med. 2011;364(23):2187–98.
93. Eisenhauer AC, Hadjipetrou P, Piemonte TC. Balloon aortic valvuloplasty revisited: the role of the Inoue balloon and transseptal antegrade approach. Catheter Cardiovasc Interv. 2000;50(4):484–91.
94. Eltchaninoff H, Cribier A, Tron C, Anselme F, Koning R, Soyer R, Letac B. Balloon aortic valvuloplasty in elderly patients at high risk for surgery, or inoperable. Immediate and mid-term results. Eur Heart J. 1995;16(8):1079–84.
95. Lieberman EB, Bashore TM, Hermiller JB, Wilson JS, Pieper KS, Keeler GP, Pierce CH, Kisslo KB, Harrison JK, Davidson CJ. Balloon aortic valvuloplasty in adults: failure of procedure to improve long-term survival. J Am Coll Cardiol. 1995;26(6):1522–8.
96. Kastrup J, Wennevold A, Thuesen L, Nielsen TT, Kassis E, Fritz-Hansen P, Thayssen P. Short- and long-term survival after aortic balloon valvuloplasty for calcified aortic stenosis in 137 elderly patients. Dan Med Bull. 1994;41(3):362–5.
97. Mylonas I, Sakata Y, Salinger M, Sanborn TA, Feldman T. The use of percutaneous suture-mediated closure for the management of 14 French femoral venous access. J Invasive Cardiol. 2006;18(7):299–302.
98. Solomon LW, Fusman B, Jolly N, Kim A, Feldman T. Percutaneous suture closure for management of large French size arterial puncture in aortic valvuloplasty. J Invasive Cardiol. 2001;13(8):592–6.

Transcatheter Aortic Valve Therapy

27

Anita Asgar and Raoul Bonan

Therapy of aortic stenosis, once the exclusive realm of cardiac surgery, has undergone major paradigm shifts in the past 10 years with the development, proof of concept, and completion of randomized controlled trials of transcatheter valve therapy. In fact, prior to 2002 the treatment of elderly high-risk individuals with aortic stenosis was limited to medical therapy with the option of palliative aortic valvuloplasty. Exhaustive work continues in the field to determine suitable patients and optimal valve sizing as well as to further our understanding of the long-term role of this technology in lower-risk patients. This chapter aims to provide a practical overview of this technology with an emphasis on understanding the basic anatomy for transcatheter intervention, optimizing patient selection and procedural tips and tricks, and a summary of the current scientific evidence.

Anatomy of the Aortic Valve

A rudimentary understanding of the anatomy of the aortic valve has long been sufficient for the diagnosis and management of aortic stenosis however; the advent of transcatheter therapy has necessitated a deeper grasp of anatomy and anatomic relationships to safely perform the procedure.

The aortic valve is, in the majority of cases, a trileaflet valve. The valve leaflets are composed of fibrous tissue lined on both the aortic and ventricular surfaces with endothelial tissue. The valve leaflets are attached basally to the ventricular myocardium and throughout their length to the aortic root. The aorta, valve leaflets, and ventricle form a series of rings as described by Piazza et al. which lie between the sinotubular junction and the basal attachment of the valve leaflets [1].

The first true ring is that formed by the sinotubular junction of the aorta. The second is comprised of the ventriculoarterial junction. The valve leaflets extend toward the ventricle from the sinotubular junction, cross the ventriculoarterial junction, and then insert into the ventricular myocardium at what is described as the basal attachment point. At this level, the leaflet insertion creates a virtual ring.

The importance of this description is in understanding the location of the "aortic annulus" (Fig. 27.1). In fact, there is no true annulus of the aortic valve; however, evaluation of the annulus is required for selection of a transcatheter valve. For practical purposes, the measurement used and described is the measurement made at the basal attachment of the valve leaflets, the so-called virtual ring. Appropriate assessment of this region by transthoracic echo must measure from sinus to

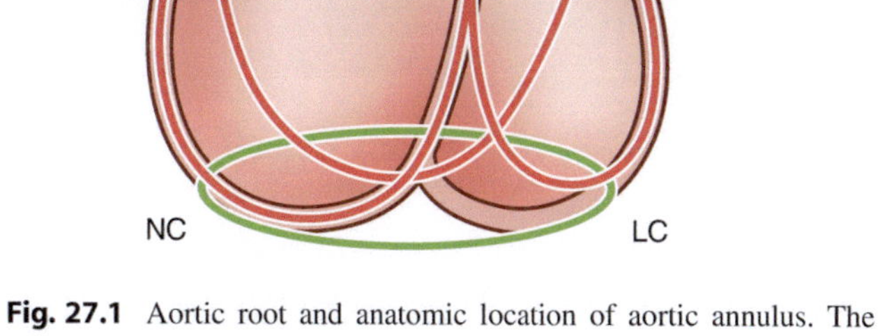

Fig. 27.1 Aortic root and anatomic location of aortic annulus. The *three red rings* represent the aortic valve cusps, with the *green circle* placed at the nadir of the aortic cusps denoting the annular plane (*LC* left coronary cusp, *NC* noncoronary cusp)

A. Asgar, MD, FRCPC (✉)
Transcatheter Valve Therapy Clinic,
Institut de Cardiologie de Montreal, Montreal, QC, Canada
e-mail: anita.asgar@gmail.com

R. Bonan, MD, FACC
Department of Medicine,
Montreal Heart Institute, Montreal, QC, Canada

C.A. Thompson (ed.), *Textbook of Cardiovascular Intervention*,
DOI 10.1007/978-1-4471-4528-8_27, © Springer-Verlag London 2014

commissure to avoid off-axis measurements that underestimate the "annular" dimensions (Fig. 27.2).

In addition to being aware of the anatomy of the aortic valve, it is imperative to understand the relationship of the valve to the surrounding structures: in particular, the coronary arteries, sinuses of valsalva, membranous septum, and mitral valve.

The coronary arteries are located in the anteriorly located right and left sinuses of Valsalva. During transcatheter valve procedures, the location of the coronary arteries is of vital importance in order to minimize the risk of coronary obstruction by the native valve during deployment of the bioprosthetic valve. A study of individuals with aortic stenosis undergoing multi-slice computed tomography (CT) demonstrated that the mean distance from the level of the basal attachment point of the aortic valve leaflets to the ostium of the left coronary and right coronary artery was 14.4 ± 2.9 mm and 17.2 ± 3.3 mm, respectively [2]. Current recommendations for minimum distance to the coronary arteries are 14 mm to prevent coronary obstruction. Measurement of coronary artery distance from the valve is only part of the story of coronary obstruction, another important factor being the width of the sinuses of Valsalva. Care must be taken to ensure that there is adequate room for displacement of the native leaflets prior to TAVR. This may be assessed by angiography or multi-slice CT or even during balloon valvuloplasty in case of contradictory results.

The final anatomic considerations include the relationship between the aortic valve and mitral valve and the conduction system. The mitral valve is in fibrous continuity with the aortic valve and is located posterior to the aorta with the anterior mitral leaflet lying in close proximity to the left ventricular outflow tract. Suboptimal positioning of the transcatheter valve prosthesis low in the left ventricular outflow tract could impinge on the movement and function of the anterior mitral leaflet. Location of the conduction system is another important concern in light of relatively high rates of pacemaker post-TAVR that are not fully understood. In fact, the atrioventricular node is located near the membranous septum of the left ventricle and therefore is neighboring the aortic valve. This relationship likely explains the rates of pacemaker implantation following aortic valve surgery. Therefore, it is not unreasonable to assume that implantation of a transcatheter valve in this region could also impact the development of conduction system abnormalities. Multiple theories exist regarding contribution to development of new conduction system disturbances including the depth of prosthesis implant. A retrospective study of 70 patients undergoing TAVR identified depth of implant and preexisting right bundle branch block as potential risk factors for permanent pacemaker implantation [3]. Other theories include the volume of calcification of the device landing zone which may create a mass effect or pressure on the conduction system in that region post device deployment [4].

Patient Selection

At present, transcatheter valve therapy, with the Edwards SAPIEN THV, has been approved by the Food and Drug Administration (FDA) for the treatment of aortic stenosis in high-risk patients, those who are not eligible for open-heart surgery for replacement of their aortic valve and have a "calcified aortic annulus (calcium buildup in the fibrous ring of the aortic heart valve)." It is also advised

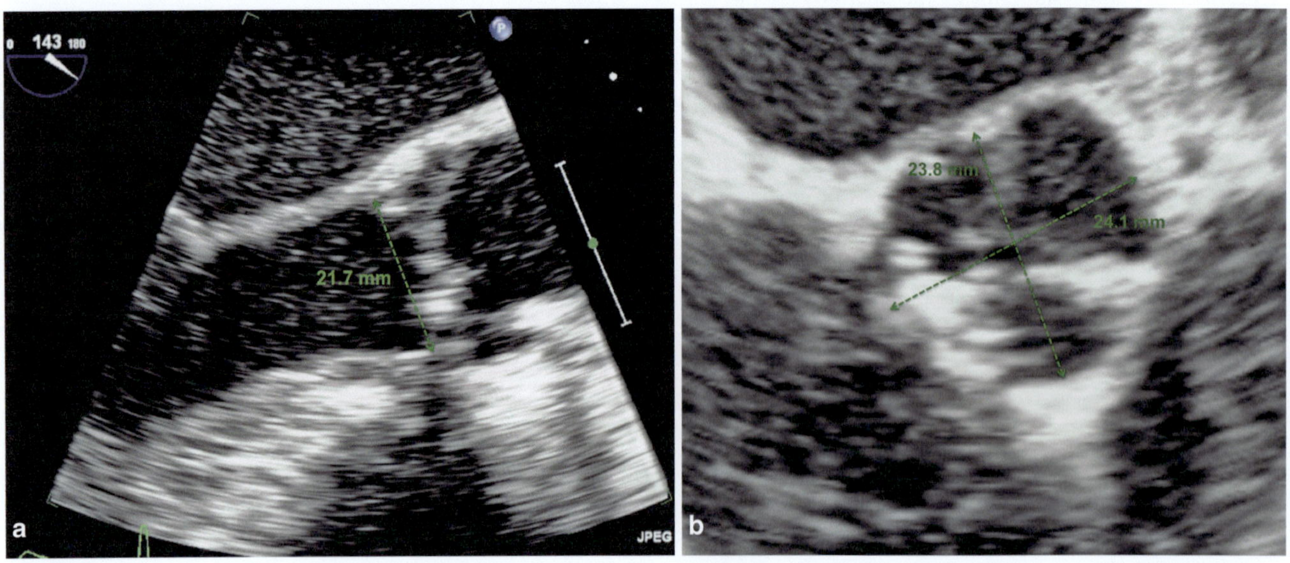

Fig. 27.2 (**a** and **b**) Transthoracic echocardiographic images of the annulus measurement from sinus to commissure

that a heart surgeon should be involved in determining if the SAPIEN THV is an appropriate treatment for the patient [5].

In practical terms, high-risk patients are those in whom the surgical risk is felt to be prohibitive. These patients are those defined in PARTNER A [6], patients at high risk for operative complications or death on the basis of coexisting conditions that were associated with a risk of death of at least 15 % by 30 days after the procedure or Society of Thoracic Surgeons (STS) Score of at least 10 %. The STS Score is a risk prediction model based on an algorithm that utilizes coexisting illnesses to predict the risk of mortality following surgical intervention. There is however a fine and poorly defined line between high risk due to comorbidities and too sick due to comorbidities. Differentiating between the two is the focus of ongoing investigation into identifying markers of frailty that may help aid the decision-making process. Gait speed is one such marker of morbidity, disability, and survival in older patients and has been shown to predict mortality and length of stay in patients undergoing cardiac surgery [7]. Recent work into the assessment of frailty using gait speed in patients undergoing evaluation for transcatheter aortic valve implantation demonstrated a high prevalence of slow gait speed in these patients. Furthermore, this marker of frailty was not accurately predicted by traditional methods of patient risk assessment [8]. For the time being, it is important to realize the limitations of conventional risk assessment tools and perhaps incorporate new markers of frailty in the overall patient evaluation. The ideal candidate is likely the elderly patient with multiple comorbidities but yet a reasonable quality of life that is expected to improve following intervention.

Once a patient is confirmed to be a high-risk surgical candidate, further investigations are required to establish the anatomic suitability of the patient for intervention. This requires careful investigation with echocardiography, coronary angiography, and evaluation of vascular access most commonly performed using multi-slice computed tomography (CT).

Echocardiographic Evaluation

Echocardiographic evaluation of aortic stenosis prior to TAVR involves confirmation of the presence of severe aortic stenosis as well as an assessment of left ventricular function and the existence of other associated valvular abnormalities such as mitral regurgitation that may have an impact during the procedure. In addition, the aortic annulus is evaluated by echo. As described previously, the annular dimension as estimated by echo must be done carefully to avoid underestimation from oblique measurements. This is best done in the parasternal long-axis view and by measuring from commissure to sinus rather than obliquely from sinus to sinus (Fig. 27.2). The assessment of pulmonary hypertension provides additional information of patient risk.

Coronary Angiography

Coronary angiography is an essential part of the assessment process for TAVR. The key role is to establish the presence of coronary artery disease and evaluate coronary artery grafts if present. The decision to intervene on existing coronary disease is debatable, and many experts suggest only intervening in the presence of prognostic lesions or in symptomatic patients. The presence of coronary artery disease appears to be associated with a worse prognosis. Data from a recent review of feasibility study data demonstrated that previous coronary artery bypass grafting (CABG) or percutaneous coronary intervention (PCI) was associated with a tenfold higher mortality at 30 days and a twofold higher mortality at any time following TAVI [9]. In addition to coronary evaluation, invasive angiography can be used to verify the measurements of the peripheral vessels and aorta using a marker pigtail.

Multi-slice CT

Computed tomography (CT) has become an almost essential component of patient evaluation pre-TAVR. This one technique can provide invaluable information on annular geometry and measurements and aortic dimensions as well as assess iliofemoral access, including tortuosity and calcification (Fig. 27.3).

The aortic annulus is a complex structure as previously described. Reconstruction of CT data allows an understanding of the oval geometry of the annulus and provides both the minimum and maximum diameters. In fact, in comparison with TTE, CT has been found to be more accurate in assessment of oval annuli and closely approximates results obtained from intraoperative TEE [10, 11]. In addition, CT enables accurate measurement of the height of the coronary artery ostia in relation to the annulus, which is crucial in minimizing risks of coronary artery obstruction. Aortic root measurements can also be easily obtained and are of particular importance for implantation of the Medtronic CoreValve, which is contraindicated in a very dilated ascending aorta (>45 mm).

Finally, thorough evaluation of the peripheral vasculature is best obtained using CT that permits visualization of the burden and distribution of calcium in the vessels as well as allowing reconstruction demonstrating the tortuosity of the vessels. In addition, CT can identify other high-risk features including dissections and complex atheroma in the aorta [12].

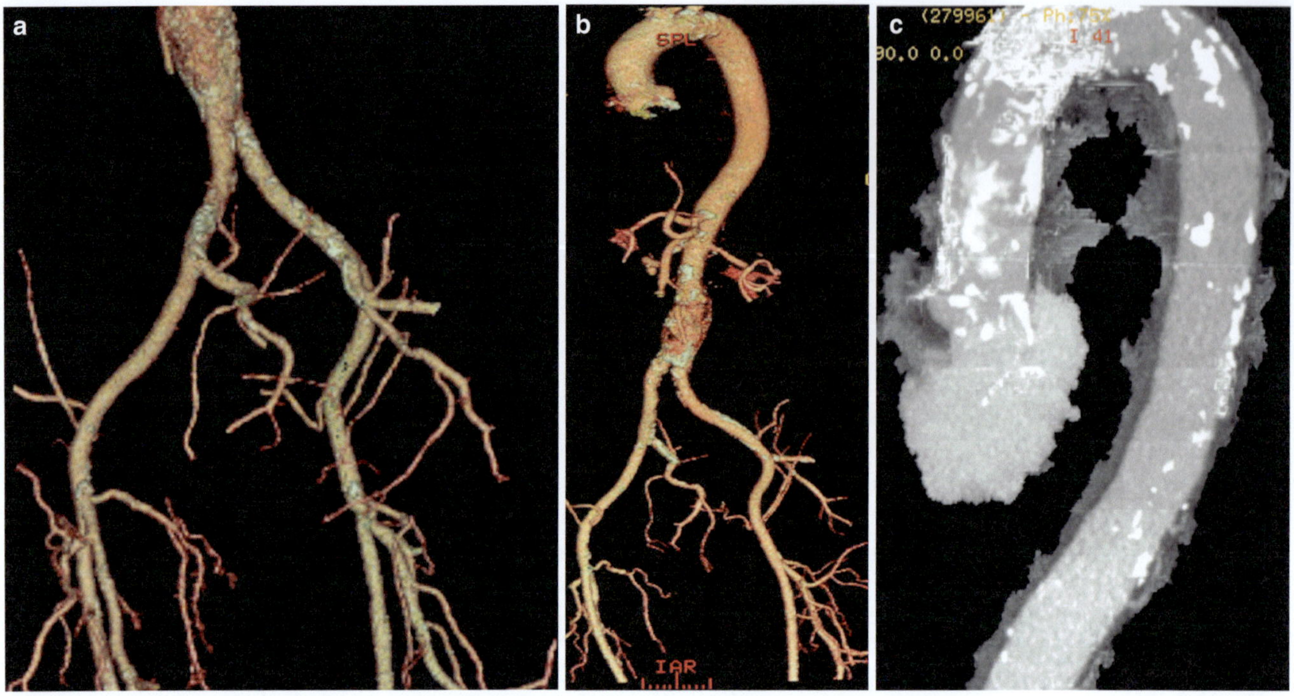

Fig. 27.3 (**a**) CT image of the iliac and femoral vessels demonstrating calcification and tortuosity. (**b**) Volume rendered CT image of the aorta and peripheral vessels. (**c**) CT image of the aorta demonstrating calcification in the ascending and transverse segments

Balloon-Expandable Prosthesis: Edwards SAPIEN THV

The Edwards SAPIEN THV (Edwards LifeSciences) is a balloon-expandable transcatheter aortic valve (Fig. 27.4). The valve consists of a bovine trileaflet pericardial valve housed within a stainless steel stent (cobalt chromium in the case of the SAPIEN XT). A pericardial skirt to prevent paravalvular leaks at the annular level covers a portion of the stent. The device is deployed retrogradely via the aorta by balloon expansion during rapid ventricular pacing. The device is available in three sizes, 23, 26, and 29 mm, which can only be used via the transapical route. These valves can treat a native annulus of between 18 and 26 mm. The femoral delivery catheter, referred to as the RetroFlex 3, has an internal diameter of either 22 or 24French requiring a femoral access of a minimum of 8 mm. The newer generation devices (SAPIEN XT) available outside the United States have an internal diameter of 16 or 18French [13].

Self-Expanding Aortic Prosthesis: Medtronic CoreValve

The Medtronic CoreValve Revalving System consists of three components: CoreValve bioprosthesis, the delivery catheter, and the disposable loading system.

The CoreValve bioprosthesis is a porcine pericardial valve sutured into a self-expandable nitinol frame. The nitinol frame is made of laser cut nitinol with diamond cells and a distinct funnel-like shape that measures between 53 and 55 mm in length. The frame has three distinct regions of radial force at the distal, mid, and outflow portion of the device. The distal portion of the device has high radial force to maintain intra-annular anchoring and is covered with a pericardial skirt to minimize paravalvular aortic regurgitation. The mid portion is constrained at the level of the porcine pericardial leaflets and is designed to avoid impingement of the coronary arteries while providing supra-annular leaflet function. The outflow portion of the prosthesis has low radial force and provides a means of orienting the device in the ascending aorta (Fig. 27.5). The valve leaflets are composed of six separate segments of porcine pericardium that are sutured to the frame in a supra-annular position. The supra-annular position reduces leaflet stress and optimizes leaflet motion [14]. In addition, it ensures optimal valve function despite inadequate frame expansion as described by Jilaihawi et al. [15]. The valve is currently available in three sizes, all of which utilize the same 18French delivery catheter: 26, 29, and 31 mm to treat aortic annuli between 20 and 29 mm.

TAVR Procedure: A Step-by-Step Guide

There are two currently available devices for TAVR, the Edwards SAPEIN THV and the Medtronic CoreValve (Figs. 27.6 and 27.7). The two devices differ in their means of deployment and the specifics for each will be discussed in

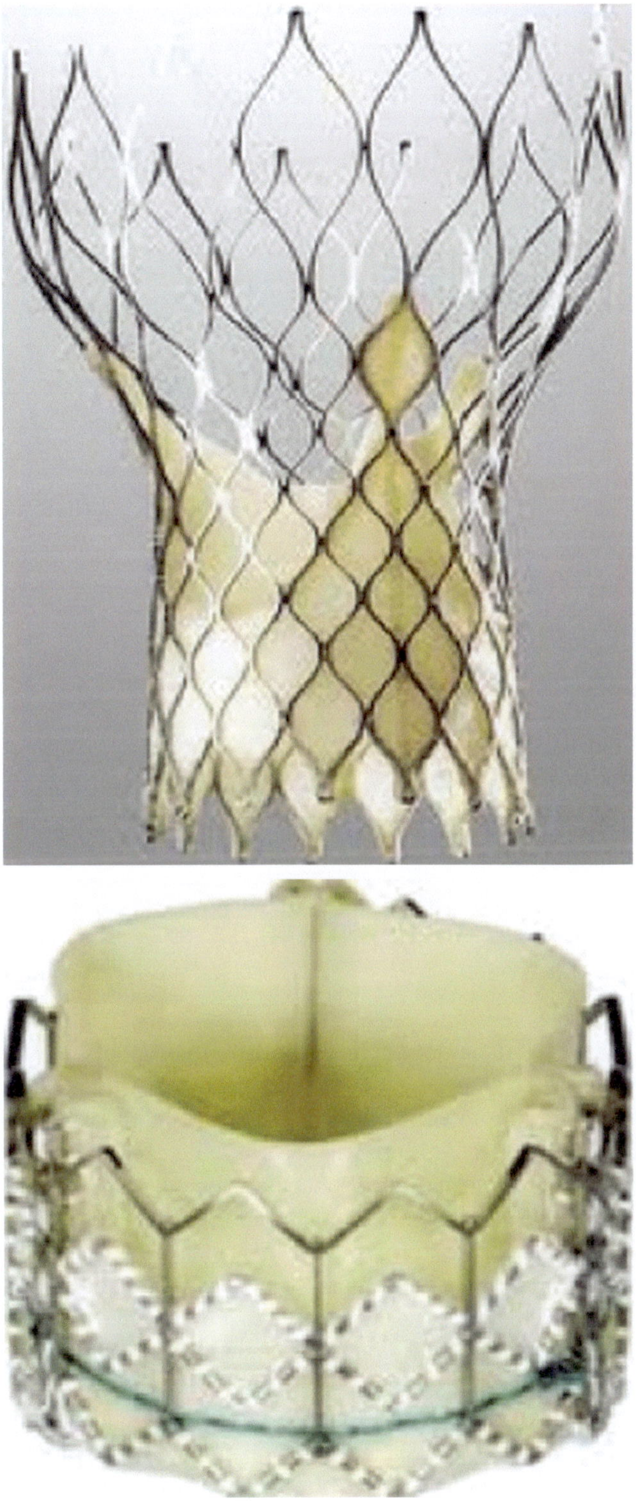

Fig. 27.4 Medtronic CoreValve (*left*) and Edwards SAPIEN (*right*) THV

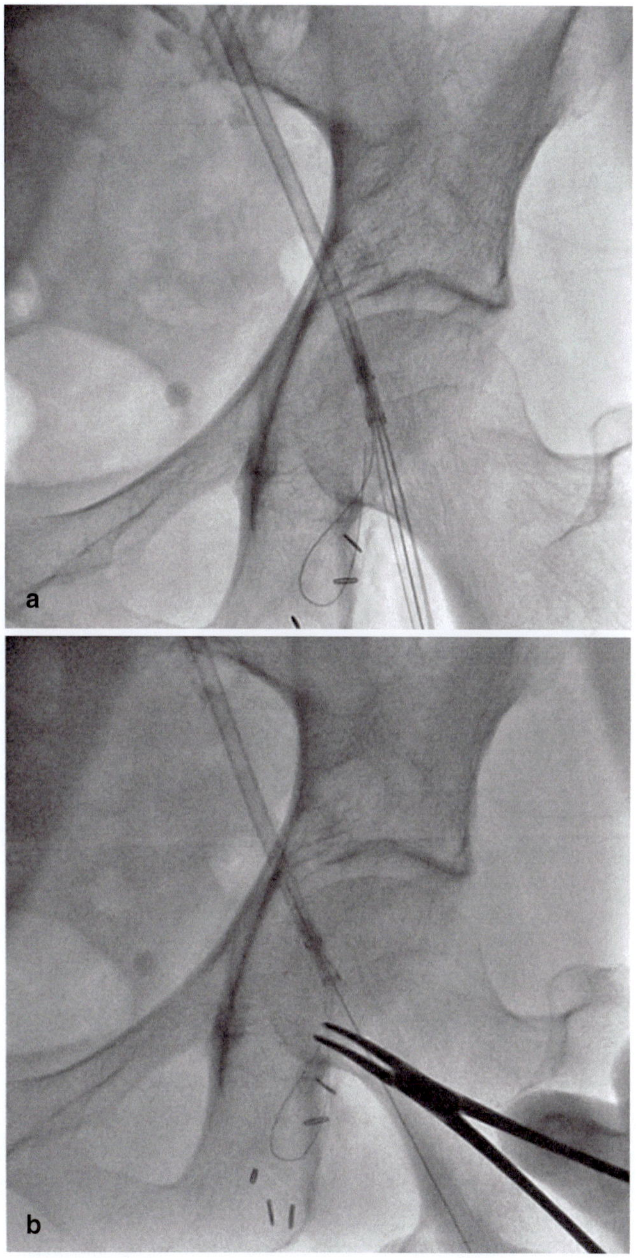

Fig. 27.5 (**a** and **b**) Outflow portion of the CoreValve prosthesis has low radial force and provides a means of orienting the device in the ascending aorta

more detail following this section which deals with basic steps of the procedure with tips and tricks discussed along the way.

The TAVI procedure can be divided up into three stages: vascular access, aortic valvuloplasty and valve implantation, and vascular access closure.

Vascular Access

Femoral vascular access is the predominant route for the majority of TAVI procedures worldwide. Initial experience with both technologies focused on surgical cutdown and closure for TAVR, but this has rapidly progressed to a completely percutaneous procedure with the introduction of the 18French systems and expandable sheaths. The cornerstone of successful management of vascular access begins with the puncture site selection. Angiographic and CT imaging pre-procedure provides an overview of vessel calcification and

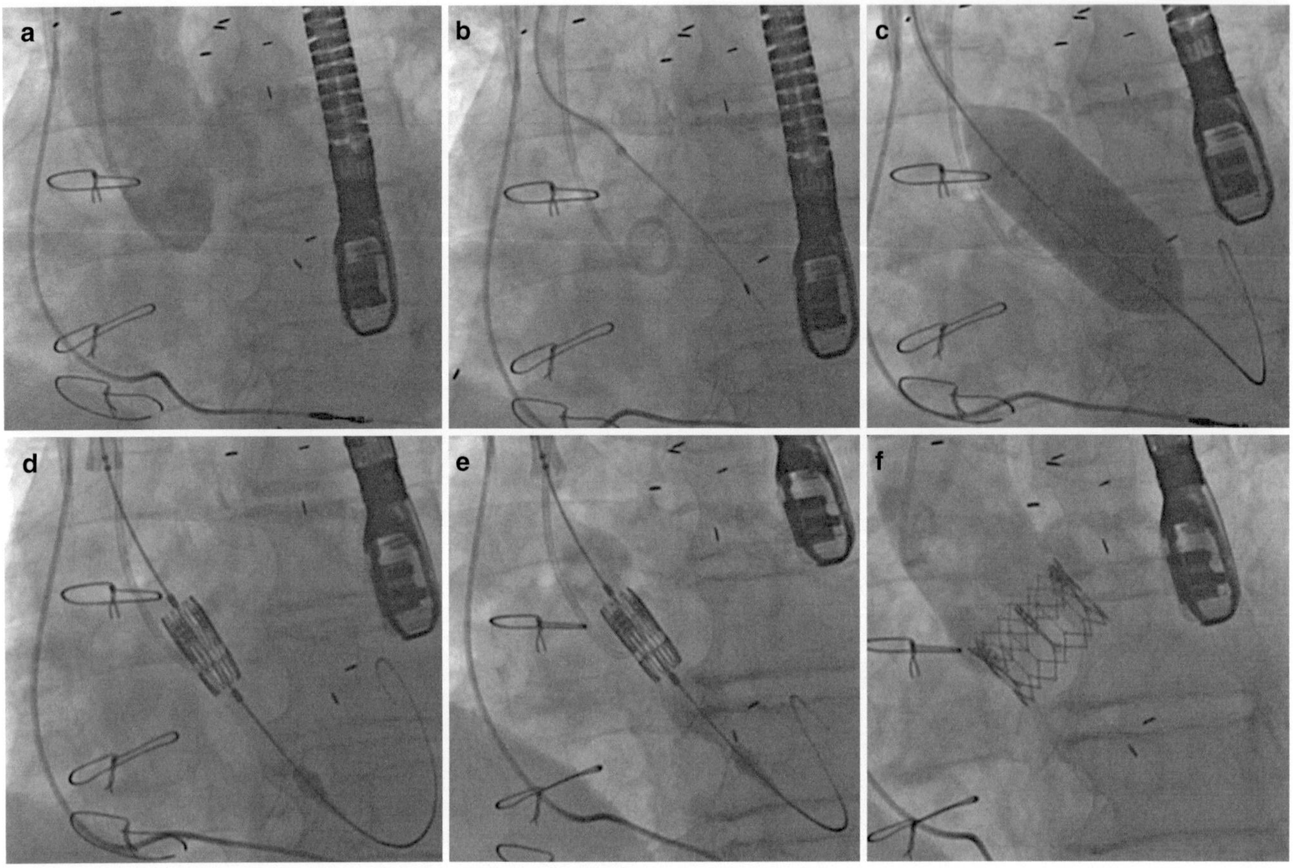

Fig. 27.6 (**a**) Aortogram pre-TAVI. (**b**) Crossing the aortic valve using an AL1 catheter and straight-tipped wire. (**c**) Aortic valvuloplasty. (**d**) Positioning of the Edwards SAPIEN valve. (**e**) Balloon inflation of the Edwards SAPIEN valve. (**f**) Final angiographic result

tortuosity, which should be taken into consideration to select a puncture site above the femoral bifurcation. We recommended puncturing the contralateral side and then performing an angiogram via a pigtail inserted antegradely into the common femoral artery on the puncture side. Alternatively, the use of ultrasound-guided puncture may be of additional benefit to ensure placement above the bifurcation and avoid regions of heavily calcified plaque. The actual puncture may be performed with a standard needle or micropuncture needle, followed by introduction of a 5 or 6F sheath. In obese patients, it may be prudent to perform the puncture with a more vertical angle to minimize the distance between the puncture and vessel wall.

Once angiography confirms placement of the sheath above the bifurcation, the access is prepared for pre-closure using either a Prostar device or two Perclose ProGlide vascular closure systems (Abbott Vascular, Redwood, CA). Regardless of the closure device chosen, there are a few important technical considerations. Firstly, the skin tract must be opened sufficiently to allow the device to advance freely down to the vessel wall and permit movement of the suture knot without being stuck in the subcutaneous tissue. In the case of the Prostar, it is important to ensure free movement of the sutures and keep the sutures moist throughout the procedure to facilitate knot tying and sliding at sheath removal. Second, it is prudent to perform fluoroscopy during needle deployment to ensure that the needles have penetrated the vessel wall without becoming stuck in an area of plaque or calcium. If the needles do become stuck and cannot be fully withdrawn (picture), they will have to be re-advanced forward and the device changed. At that point it may be wise to consider use of the contralateral side or surgical closure following the procedure.

Successful pre-closure of the vessel is followed by vessel dilation and sheath insertion. In smaller anatomy, successive vessel dilation followed by sheath insertion is recommended. Additional strategies for small vessel size include use of a lubricant such as Rotaglide to facilitate sheath insertion or the use of an expandable sheath such as the SoloPath (Terumo Medical) or Edwards eSheath (Edwards LifeSciences). Both of these devices enter the vessel in a smaller French size, and in the case of the SoloPath, the balloon dilator is inflated to expand the sheath from 12 to 19Fr. For tortuous anatomy advancing

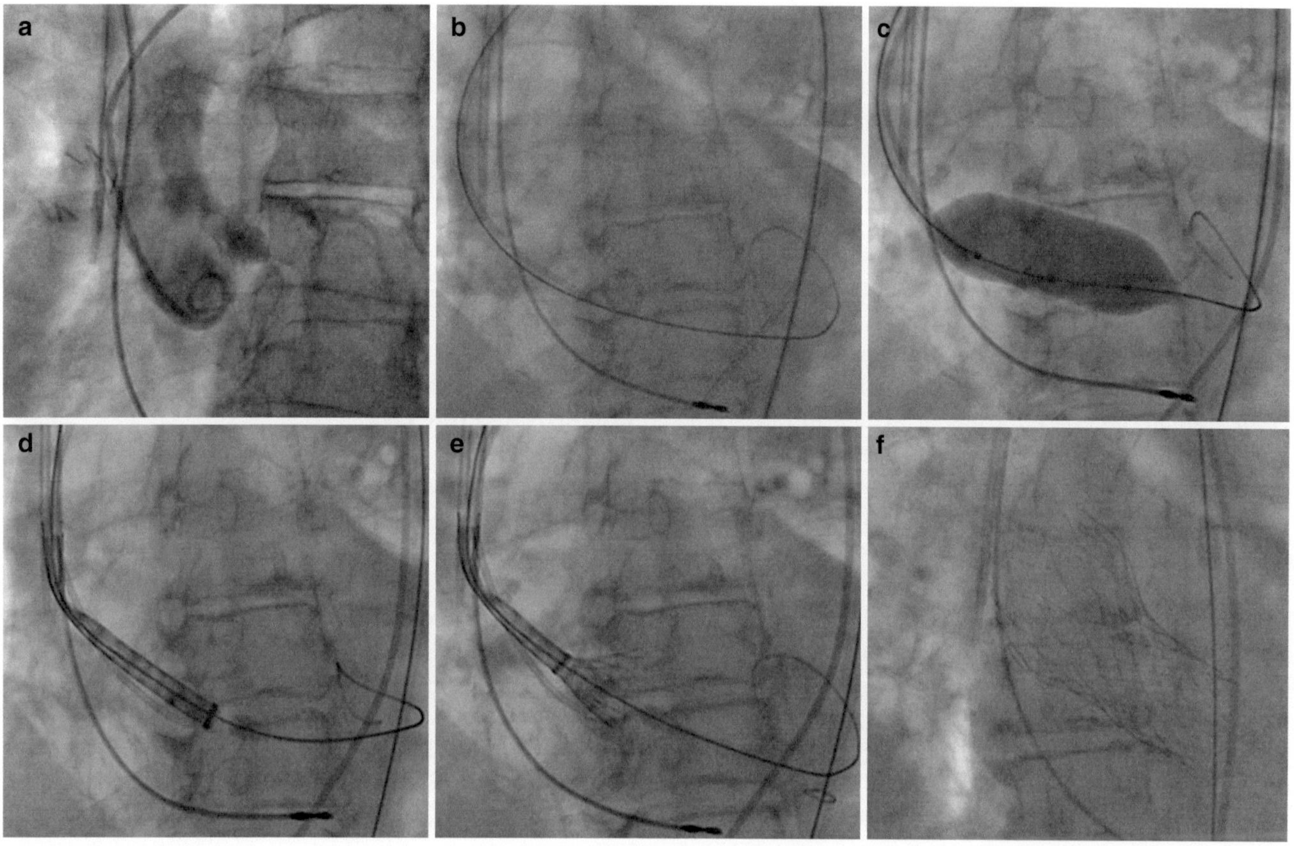

Fig. 27.7 Deployment of the Medtronic CoreValve. (**a**) Initial aortogram. (**b**) Positioning of the superstiff wire for valve deployment. (**c**) Aortic valvuloplasty. (**d**) Positioning of the Medtronic CoreValve. (**e**) Initial stages of the valve deployment. (**f**) Final result of the Medtronic CoreValve

the sheath into the aorta may be challenging and a stiff wire is recommended to aid passage of the sheath without kinking of the wire.

Aortic Valvuloplasty and Valve Implantation

Placement of the large sheath in the aorta is then followed by crossing of the aortic valve and placement of the stiff wire in the ventricle to perform the aortic valvuloplasty. Aortography prior to the procedure is helpful to establish the working and implantation view for valve implantation and valve crossing. The goal is to find the angulation that has all three cusps of the valve in the same plane and is therefore perpendicular to the valve annulus. This can be achieved by performing orthogonal aortograms or by using reconstructed CT data to provide the optimal angulation [12].

Crossing the stenosed aortic valve is best accomplished using an Amplatz left (AL1) coronary catheter and a soft straight-tipped wire. Ideally to avoid embolization of valve material, the wire should be advanced gently in the direction of the jet ejected, which is often eccentric. Care must be taken to not be too aggressive as leaflet perforation by the wire can occur and result in complications if the valvuloplasty is performed through a leaflet perforation.

Once the valve has been crossed, the left ventricular end-diastolic pressure is recorded to establish a hemodynamic baseline and the stiff curved wire is advanced into the ventricle. The curved wire is prepared prior to crossing the valve to ensure that the transition zone of the wire is safely curved away from the apex of the ventricle to avoid perforations once the wire is advanced. The wire should be advanced distally into the ventricle to provide optimal stability for valve implantation.

Aortic valvuloplasty is performed using a compliant balloon, the sizing based on the annular assessment performed by echocardiography and CT scan. Valvuloplasty is most commonly performed with rapid ventricular pacing to minimize balloon movement during inflation. This is not obligatory; however, it is commonly performed. Of particular importance is the complete deflation of the balloon prior to cessation of pacing to prevent excessive balloon motion. We generally use a 20 mm balloon for small valves and a 22 mm balloon for the larger valves. The goal of the annuloplasty is to open the stenotic valve without causing significant aortic insufficiency that could potentially destabilize the patient.

In the case of hemodynamic deterioration post-valvuloplasty, it is important to have the valve prepared and ready for implantation immediately following the valvuloplasty.

Edwards SAPIEN THV

The Edwards valve is a balloon-expandable valve and as such is deployed instantly with balloon inflation. The valve is crimped onto the delivery balloon and then advanced into the aorta. The valve is positioned to maintain 50 % above and below the level of the annulus. Rapid ventricular pacing is an absolute necessity for this procedure to lower blood pressure and the force of cardiac ejection, which may otherwise result in valve embolization. If post-dilation of the valve is required, it is ideally done with the deployment balloon.

Self-Expanding Medtronic CoreValve

Deployment of the self-expanding Medtronic CoreValve is performed slowly by gradually withdrawing the sheath covering the valve. During the deployment, the position of the valve can be adjusted to obtain an optimal position at approximately 4–6 mm below the level of the annulus. Once the valve has been deployed to one-third, the native valve is blocked and deployment must be more rapid to two-thirds, to allow the prosthetic valve to function. Faster cardiac pacing (heart rate 100–120) can be used during this phase to minimize valve movement. At this point, the remainder of valve deployment can progress slowly until confirmation of complete prosthesis release from the delivery catheter.

Evaluation of the hemodynamic result post-TAVR involves reassessment of left ventricular end-diastolic pressures and aortic valve gradient. Indications for further intervention, such as post-dilation, would include hemodynamically significant aortic insufficiency. In such cases the mechanism of the aortic insufficiency would dictate the next appropriate step: under-expansion of the device would require post-dilation of the valve, whereas improper valve placement may require snaring of the valve or a second implant.

Vascular Access Closure

A successful valve implant is not the end of the procedure as vessel closure remains. Results from randomized controlled trials and registries have demonstrated that vascular access complications and bleeding are independently associated with an increased mortality [6]. Angiograms should be performed as the sheath is withdrawn into the iliac artery to confirm vessel integrity and rule out dissection or rupture. We recommend placing a wire and sheath across the iliac bifurcation from the contralateral side to enable balloon occlusion of the vessel in the case of bleeding from vessel closure failure or other complications. This technique has been described as the crossover balloon technique by some groups and is associated with fewer vascular complications [16].

Evidence for Transcatheter Aortic Valve Implantation

Balloon-Expandable Technology: Edwards SAPIEN THV

The Edwards SAPIEN THV is the transcatheter aortic valve to have been studied in a randomized controlled trial, Placement of AoRTic TraNscathetER Valve, PARTNER A and B. These trials examined the effectiveness of transcatheter valve therapy with the SAPIEN valve in high-risk surgical patients vs. standard surgical aortic valve replacement (Cohort A, PARTNER A) and in patients considered to be inoperable vs. medical therapy (Cohort B, PARTNER B).

PARTNER B was reported first in 2010. This trial randomized 358 inoperable patients to standard medical therapy including balloon aortic valvuloplasty or transcatheter valve therapy with the Edwards SAPIEN valve via transfemoral access. The primary end point was the rate of death from any cause over the duration of the trial. All patients were followed for at least 1 year, and crossover from the standard-therapy group to the TAVI group was not permitted. At 1-year follow-up, TAVI significantly reduced death from any cause in this inoperable patient group to 30.7 % vs. 50.7 % ($p<0.001$) in the medical arm, despite the fact that 83 % of patients in the medical treatment arm also underwent balloon valvuloplasty. In addition, this trial demonstrated the high mortality of aortic stenosis in the inoperable cohort, which was 50 % at 1 year [13]. TAVI was also associated with a significant increase in vascular complications, 16.2 % vs. 1.1 % ($p<0.001$), and a nonsignificant increase in the incidence of major strokes, 5.0 % vs. 1.1 %, $P=0.06$. Overall, this trial was felt to be overwhelmingly positive in favor of TAVI for the treatment of symptomatic severe AS in inoperable patients. Subsequent 2-year follow-up demonstrated a slight catch-up phenomenon with an increase in mortality to 43.3 % in the TAVI group vs. 68.0 % in the medical treatment group, $p<0.001$; however, the difference remained significant. In addition, rates of rehospitalization were lower in the TAVI group. One of the important observations in the 2-year follow-up was that despite a continued benefit of TAVI over medical therapy, the presence of significant comorbidities does attenuate the benefit of TAVI in this cohort of patients [17].

PARTNER A randomized 699 high-risk surgical patients to either TAVI via transfemoral or transapical route or standard surgical aortic valve replacement (AVR). The primary end point of the trial was non-inferiority of TAVI to surgical AVR in the rate of death from any cause at 1 year in the intention-to-treat population. In the transcatheter group, 244 patients were assigned to undergo transfemoral placement, and 104 were assigned to undergo transapical placement on the basis of the presence of significant peripheral vascular disease. A total of 351 patients were assigned to undergo surgical valve replacement. The rates of death from any cause were 3.4 % in the TAVI group and 6.5 % in the surgical group at 30 days ($P=0.07$) and 24.2 % and 26.8 %, respectively, at 1 year ($P=0.44$). This reduction of 2.6 percentage points in the TAVI group met the predefined non-inferiority end point $P=0.001$. TAVI was however associated with higher rates of major stroke at 30 days (3.8 % vs. 2.1 %, $P=0.20$); however, this was not significant. Major vascular complications were significantly more frequent with transcatheter replacement (11.0 % vs. 3.2 %, $P<0.001$); adverse events that were more frequent after surgical replacement included major bleeding (9.3 % vs. 19.5 %, $P<0.001$) and new-onset atrial fibrillation (8.6 % vs. 16.0 %, $P=0.006$) [6].

At 2-year follow-up, the rates of death from any cause were similar in the TAVR and surgery groups, and there was no significant difference in stroke between the two groups. Of note, paravalvular aortic regurgitation was more frequent with TAVI and was associated with higher late mortality [18]. In conclusion, in high-risk surgical patients with aortic stenosis, TAVI is a reasonable treatment alternative.

Clinical Evidence for Self-Expanding Technology: Medtronic CoreValve

In May 2007 the CoreValve Revalving System received CE Mark approval and the technology became available for the treatment of high-risk aortic stenosis patients in Europe. Since that time, over 12,000 implants have been performed worldwide. Such widespread adoption of the technology has resulted in increased operator experience, higher procedural success, and the recognition of new challenges.

Cardiac conduction system abnormalities are not uncommon in patients with aortic valve stenosis, and surgical aortic valve replacement has been associated with the requirement of a permanent pacemaker in 3–8 % of patients, in part due to the proximity of the conduction system to the aortic valve. Initial case reports had highlighted an increased incidence of conduction anomalies post-TAVI, and this was further described by a retrospective study that demonstrated a possible link between positioning of the Medtronic CoreValve and the incidence of left bundle branch block (LBBB) and subsequent pacemakers [19]. The exact mechanism of conduction system anomalies is unclear but there are numerous theories. Given the proximity of the atrioventricular node and left bundle to the aortic valve and left ventricular outflow tract, the depth of prosthesis implant may have an effect. A retrospective study of 70 patients undergoing TAVI identified depth of implant and preexisting right bundle branch block as potential risk factors for permanent pacemaker implantation [3]. Other theories include the volume of calcification of the device landing zone which may create a mass effect or pressure on the conduction system in that region post device deployment [4]. Interestingly, other work has demonstrated that LBBB often develops post-balloon valvuloplasty suggesting perhaps a traumatic etiology that occurs prior to valve implantation that may be related to oversizing of the balloon with respect to the aortic annulus [20]. Although plausible this does not explain the relatively lower incidence of permanent pacemakers required in those patients receiving the Edwards device which is balloon-expandable and requires a minimum of two balloon dilation rather than one.

Two-year follow-up data from the third-generation safety and efficacy trial were published in 2011. These data included 126 patients treated with the 18French CoreValve Revalving System from 2006 to 2008 in Europe and Canada. Procedural success was modest, 83 %; however, this was relatively early in the overall experience with the technology, and 30-day mortality was 15.2 %. At 2-year follow-up, all-cause mortality was 38.1 % and permanent pacemakers were required in 26.2 % of patients for atrioventricular conduction abnormalities. There was no evidence of deterioration in the hemodynamic result during the 2-year follow-up, and improvements in functional class were also maintained. Importantly, this study illustrated the durability of the transcatheter Medtronic CoreValve at a minimum of 2 years [21].

The largest published series of patients treated with the third-generation CoreValve Revalving System, an Italian multicenter study, had high rates of procedural success with low procedural mortality, 98 % and 0.9 %, respectively, in this high-risk elderly population. This series identified factors predictive of mortality including conversion to open-heart surgery, cardiac tamponade, major access complications, and low ejection fraction. Of note the highest mortality was observed within the first 2 weeks following the procedure, often related to procedural complications. Mortality continued at a steady rate in this population of 0.9 % per month during the first year as a result of patient comorbidities, for a 1-year mortality rate of 15 %. The rates of vascular access complications were low, 2 %, and the need for a permanent pacemaker was 17.4 % at 30 days [22]. At present, the Medtronic CoreValve is being studied in a randomized controlled trial in the United States, with the results likely to be available at the end of 2013.

Summary

In ten short years, transcatheter aortic valve implantation has moved from first-in-man to completion of randomized controlled trials. This technology now enables the treatment of patients once felt to be inoperable and has been demonstrated to be an alternative for those at high surgical risk. Despite the advances made, much remains to be learned in regard to patient selection to optimize benefit, optimal device, and annular sizing and the long-term clinical outcomes. For the interventional cardiologist and surgeon, this therapy offers an opportunity to collaborate through systematic evaluation, procedure planning, and execution, to ensure optimal patient outcomes.

References

1. Piazza N, et al. Early and persistent intraventricular conduction abnormalities and requirements for pacemaking after percutaneous replacement of the aortic valve. JACC Cardiovasc Interv. 2008;1(3):310–16.
2. Tops LF, Wood DA, Delgado V, Schuijf JD, Mayo JR, Pasupati S, et al. Noninvasive evaluation of the aortic root with multislice computed tomography implications for transcatheter aortic valve replacement. JACC Cardiovasc Imaging. 2008;1(3):321–30. doi:10.1016/j.jcmg.2007.12.006.
3. Fraccaro C, et al. Incidence, predictors, and outcome of conduction disorders after transcatheter self-expandable aortic valve implantation. Am J Cardiol. 2011;107(5):747–54.
4. Latsios G, et al. "Device landing zone" calcification, assessed by MSCT, as a predictive factor for pacemaker implantation after TAVI. Catheter Cardiovasc Interv. 2010;76(3):431–9.
5. FDA press release, November 2011
6. Smith CR, Leon MB, Mack MJ, Miller DC, Moses JW, Svensson LG, et al. Transcatheter versus surgical aortic-valve replacement in high-risk patients. N Engl J Med. 2011;364(23):2187–98. doi:10.1056/NEJMoa1103510.
7. Afilalo J, Eisenberg MJ, Morin JF, Bergman H, Monette J, Noiseux N, et al. Gait speed as an incremental predictor of mortality and major morbidity in elderly patients undergoing cardiac surgery. J Am Coll Cardiol. 2010;56(20):1668–76. doi:10.1016/j.jacc.2010.06.039.
8. Green P, Woglom AE, Genereux P, Maurer MS, Kirtane AJ, Hawkey M, et al. Gait speed and dependence in activities of daily living in older adults with severe aortic stenosis. Clin Cardiol. 2012. doi:10.1002/clc.21974.
9. Dewey TM, Brown DL, Herbert MA, Culica D, Smith CR, Leon MB, et al. Effect of concomitant coronary artery disease on procedural and late outcomes of transcatheter aortic valve implantation. Ann Thorac Surg. 2010;89(3):758–67. doi:10.1016/j.athoracsur.2009.12.033. discussion 767.
10. Buzzatti N, Maisano F, Latib A, Cioni M, Taramasso M, Mussardo M, et al. Computed tomography-based evaluation of aortic annulus, prosthesis size and impact on early residual aortic regurgitation after transcatheter aortic valve implantation. Eur J Cardiothorac Surg. 2012. doi:10.1093/ejcts/ezs155.
11. Kempfert J, Van Linden A, Lehmkuhl L, Rastan AJ, Holzhey D, Blumenstein J, et al. Aortic annulus sizing: echocardiographic vs. computed tomography derived measurements in comparison with direct surgical sizing. Eur J Cardiothorac Surg. 2012. doi:10.1093/ejcts/ezs064.
12. Leipsic J, Gurvitch R, Labounty TM, Min JK, Wood D, Johnson M, et al. Multidetector computed tomography in transcatheter aortic valve implantation. JACC Cardiovasc Imaging. 2011;4(4):416–29. doi:10.1016/j.jcmg.2011.01.014.
13. Leon MB, Kodali S, Williams M, Oz M, Smith C, Stewart A, et al. Transcatheter aortic valve replacement in patients with critical aortic stenosis: rationale, device descriptions, early clinical experiences, and perspectives. Semin Thorac Cardiovasc Surg. 2006;18(2):165–74. doi:10.1053/j.semtcvs.2006.08.002.
14. Grube E, et al. First report on a human percutaneous transluminal implantation of a self-expanding valve prosthesis for interventional treatment of aortic valve stenosis. Catheter Cardiovasc Interv. 2005;66(4):465–9.
15. Jilaihawi H, Asgar A, Bonan R. Good outcome and valve function despite Medtronic-CoreValve underexpansion. Catheter Cardiovasc Interv. 2010;76(7):1022–5.
16. Genereux P, Kodali S, Leon MB, Smith CR, Ben-Gal Y, Kirtane AJ, et al. Clinical outcomes using a new crossover balloon occlusion technique for percutaneous closure after transfemoral aortic valve implantation. JACC Cardiovasc Interv. 2011;4(8):861–7. doi:10.1016/j.jcin.2011.05.019.
17. Makkar RR, Fontana GP, Jilaihawi H, Kapadia S, Pichard AD, Douglas PS, et al. Transcatheter aortic-valve replacement for inoperable severe aortic stenosis. N Engl J Med. 2012;366(18):1696–704. doi:10.1056/NEJMoa1202277.
18. Kodali SK, Williams MR, Smith CR, Svensson LG, Webb JG, Makkar RR, et al. Two-year outcomes after transcatheter or surgical aortic-valve replacement. N Engl J Med. 2012;366(18):1686–95. doi:10.1056/NEJMoa1200384.
19. Piazza N, de Jaegere P, Schultz C, Becker AE, Serruys PW, Anderson RH. Anatomy of the aortic valvar complex and its implications for transcatheter implantation of the aortic valve. Circ Cardiovas Interv. 2008;1:74–81.
20. Nuis RJ, et al. Timing and potential mechanisms of new conduction abnormalities during the implantation of the Medtronic CoreValve System in patients with aortic stenosis. Eur Heart J. 2011;32(16):2067–74.
21. Buellesfeld L, et al. 2-year follow-up of patients undergoing transcatheter aortic valve implantation using a self-expanding valve prosthesis. J Am Coll Cardiol. 2011;57(16):1650–7.
22. Tamburino C, et al. Incidence and predictors of early and late mortality after transcatheter aortic valve implantation in 663 patients with severe aortic stenosis. Circulation. 2011;123(3):299–308.

Percutaneous Management of Mitral Regurgitation

28

Jason H. Rogers and John M. Lasala

Proper function of the mitral valve (MV) requires the structural integrity of and delicate interplay between individual components of the "mitral apparatus" (Fig. 28.1). Adequate mitral leaflet mobility during diastole and coaptation during systole are related to proper function of the mitral annulus, chordae tendineae, papillary muscles, left ventricle, and left atrium. Clinical pathology of the apparatus can result in either mitral stenosis or mitral regurgitation. Mitral stenosis can be treated medically, with percutaneous balloon valvuloplasty or with surgery. This topic is covered in a separate chapter in this book. Mitral regurgitation (MR) is an important and often under-recognized entity in which blood regurgitates into the left atrium from the left ventricle during systole. Surgical MV replacement can be performed, making use of numerous repair techniques. Published guidelines have established indications for surgical MV correction, generally for patients with symptoms, evidence of LV enlargement or systolic dysfunction, or atrial fibrillation [1, 2]. These guidelines have annually resulted in approximately 40,000 mitral valve operations in the United States and a comparable number in Europe [3]. However, an unmet clinical need exists for a large population of patients with congestive heart failure-associated MR, with comorbidities, or with high surgical risk who do not currently undergo surgery because of a failure to refer due to perceived excessive surgical morbidity and mortality [4, 5]. Because MR reduction in these patients can improve quality of life and result in favorable LV remodeling, percutaneous approaches for treating MR have been developed extensively in the last decade. We herein describe existing and emerging therapies that are rapidly assuming importance as therapeutic options for patients with MR.

J.H. Rogers, MD (✉)
Division of Cardiovascular Medicine,
UC Davis Medical Center,
4860 Y Street, Suite 2820, Sacramento,
CA 95817, USA
e-mail: jason.rogers@ucdmc.ucdavis.edu

J.M. Lasala, MD, PhD
Interventional Cardiology,
Cardiac Catheterization Laboratory,
Washington University School of Medicine,
One Barnes-Jewish Hospital,
St. Louis, MO 63110, USA

Mitral Regurgitation: Etiology, Prevalence, and Clinical Background

The etiologies of MR are multiple and have been described by Carpentier, Barlow, and others (Fig. 28.2) [6–8]. Degenerative mitral regurgitation (DMR, Carpentier Type II dysfunction) is the result of structurally abnormal leaflets or chordae and occurs in fibroelastic deficiency with leaflet prolapse, myxomatous leaflet degeneration, or Barlow's disease with diffuse excess tissue and chordal elongation. The 10-year natural history of severe MR due to a flail posterior leaflet is known, with 90 % of patients expiring or requiring an MV operation [9]. Surgical MV repair has traditionally been the preferred treatment for degenerative MR, since it affords improved postoperative outcomes and survival when compared to MV replacement [10]. Surgical intervention for degenerative MR consists of multiple techniques including leaflet repair with resection, chordal transfer, use of polytetrafluoroethylene neochordae, and prosthetic ring or band annuloplasty [11].

Functional MR (FMR, Carpentier Type I, or IIIb) is a direct consequence of underlying left ventricular dysfunction and annular dilation, which secondarily impairs the coaptation of otherwise structurally normal leaflets. Surgical correction of FMR has been shown to improve functional class and left ventricular remodeling [12], but a survival benefit has yet to be shown [13]. Additionally, even with current surgical annuloplasty techniques, up to one-third of treated patients have moderate or greater MR recur within 1 year of surgery [14–16]. Preoperative predictors of recurrent MR

C.A. Thompson (ed.), *Textbook of Cardiovascular Intervention*,
DOI 10.1007/978-1-4471-4528-8_28, © Springer-Verlag London 2014

Fig. 28.1 The mitral valve apparatus

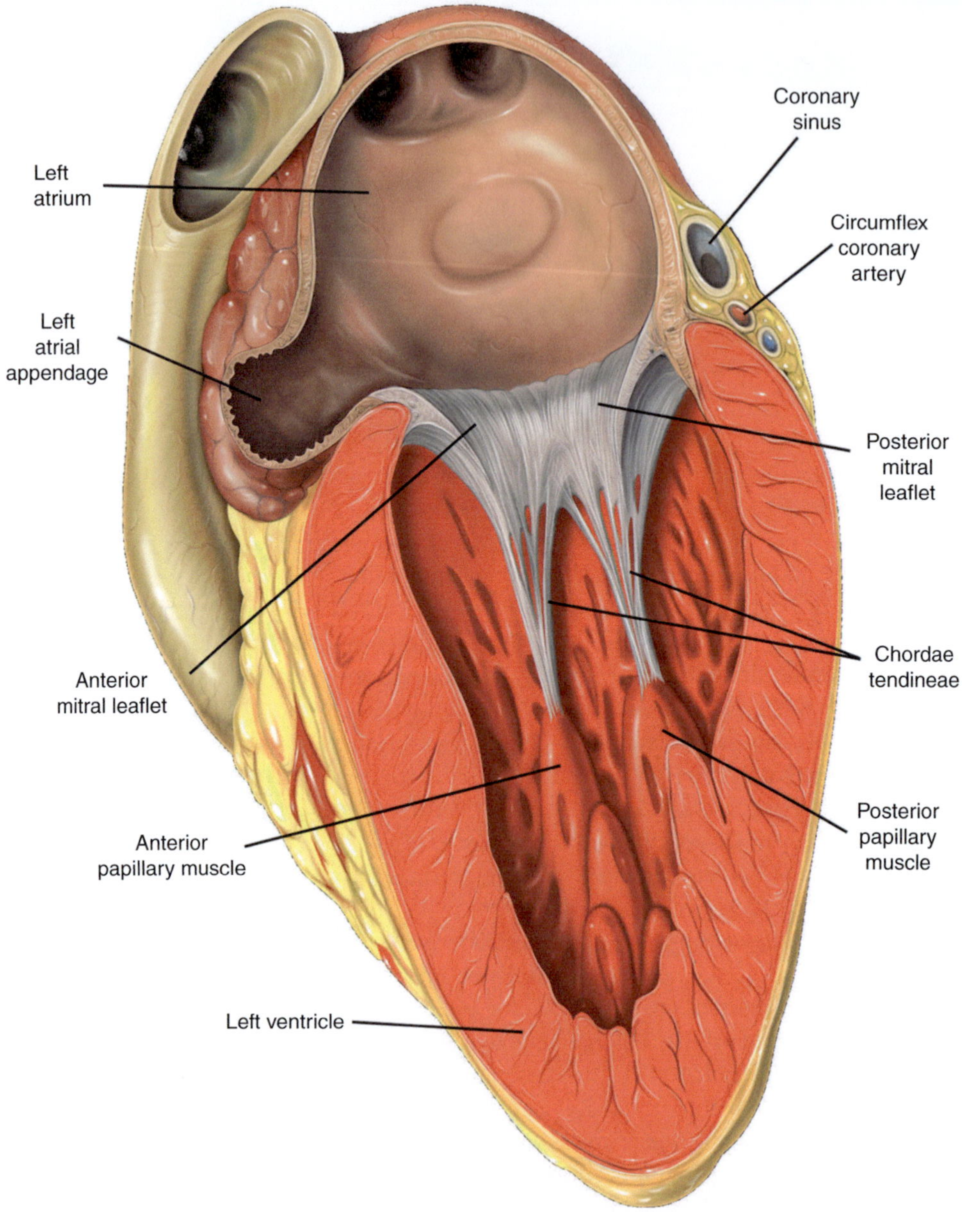

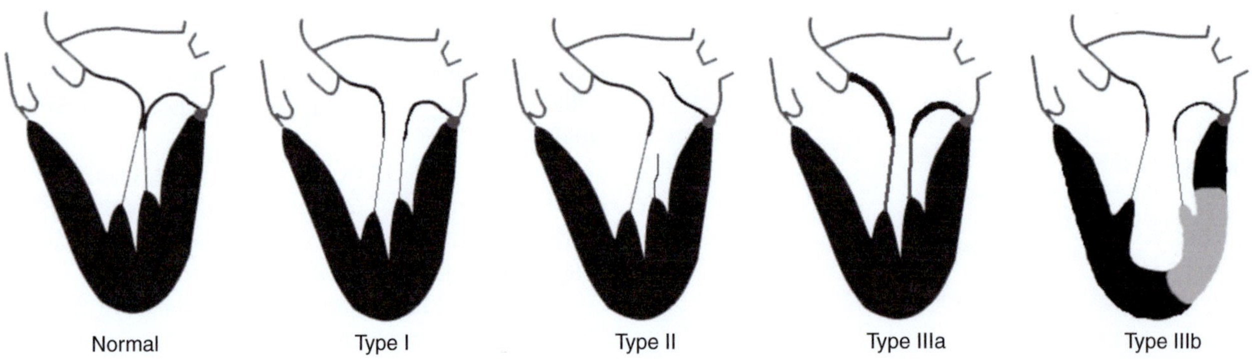

Fig. 28.2 The Carpentier classification of mitral valve regurgitation. These represent the basic mechanistic etiologies for mitral regurgitation. More than one type can coexist in a given individual. Shown at left is the normal mitral valve apparatus. *Type I*: normal leaflet motion with annular dilation; *Type II*: increased leaflet motion (leaflet prolapse or flail); *Type IIIa*: restricted leaflet motion in systole and diastole, usually associated with leaflet and subvalvular thickening (rheumatic); *Type IIIb*: restricted leaflet motion in systole, often seen in ischemic cardiomyopathy with history of infarct (light region in left ventricle) (From Feldman et al. [68], Chap. 1, p 3 with permission)

Table 28.1 Percutaneous therapies for mitral valve regurgitation

Target of therapy	Device name (manufacturer)	Mechanism of action
Leaflet repair	MitraClip (Abbott)	Clip-based edge-to-edge repair
	Percu-Pro (Cardiosolutions)	Regurgitant orifice space occupying
	Mobius (Edwards)	Suture-based edge-to-edge repair
Chordal implant	NeoChord (NeoChord)	Synthetic chordae tendineae
Indirect annuloplasty	Carillon (Cardiac Dimensions)	Coronary sinus reshaping
	Monarc (Edwards)	Coronary sinus reshaping
	PTMA device (Viacor)	Coronary sinus reshaping
	Mitral cerclage (NIH)	Coronary sinus—right atrial encircling
	PS3 System (MVRx)	Transatrial coronary sinus— atrial septal shortening
Direct annuloplasty	Mitralign (Mitralign)	2×2 plicating anchors through posterior annulus
	AccuCinch (Guided Delivery Systems)	Plicating anchors in ventricular side of mitral annulus
	Cardioband (Valtech)	Plicating anchors on atrial side of mitral annulus
	QuantumCor (QuantumCor)	Radio-frequency energy shrinking annular collagen
	Millipede (Millipede)	Semirigid circumferential annular ring
Left ventricular reshaping	iCoapsys (Edwards)	Transventricular reshaping
	BACE (Mardil)	External basal myocardial reshaping
Mitral valve replacement	Endovalve-Herrmann (Endovalve)	Valve replacement
	CardiAQ (CardiAQ)	Valve replacement
	Tiara (Neovasc)	Valve replacement

and poor outcomes after restrictive annuloplasty for FMR include LV end-diastolic diameter >65 mm [17], posterior leaflet angle ≥45° [18], and MV coaptation depth ≥11 mm [19]. It is estimated that as many as 500,000 people in North America alone have clinically significant congestive heart failure-associated MR, many of whom are currently not offered mitral valve intervention. Since even asymptomatic patients with severe MR have higher 5-year rates of death, heart failure, and atrial fibrillation, consideration of valve repair is clinically warranted in these patients. Until the advent of percutaneous mitral valve procedures, surgical mitral valve repair or replacement had been the sole option for treating MR.

Categories of Percutaneous Approaches to Mitral Regurgitation

Since mitral valve function depends on the coordinated interaction of the "mitral apparatus," surgical therapies have been developed to address all of the individual derangements of the annulus, leaflets, chordae tendineae, and left ventricle. In cases where repair is not possible, mitral valve replacement can be performed. Percutaneous approaches have broadly mimicked surgical approaches, although several novel approaches have been developed. These technologies have been categorized as those acting on or involving the leaflets, annulus, chordal implants, LV remodeling techniques, and percutaneous mitral valve replacement (Table 28.1) [20].

Leaflet Repair

MitraClip Therapy

MitraClip therapy has become an important therapeutic option for patients with mitral regurgitation, and important investigations centered upon this therapy have given credence and momentum to the entire field of percutaneous mitral valve repair [21]. MitraClip therapy is based on the surgical edge-to-edge repair first described by Alfieri [22]. The surgical technique involves the use of suture to convert a regurgitant mitral orifice into a competent double-orifice valve. The inspiration for this technique came from observing the morphology of a congenital double-orifice mitral valve. The MitraClip device consists of a percutaneously delivered MRI-compatible cobalt chromium implant with two arms and two grippers used to grasp the opposing free edges of the anterior and posterior leaflet in order to improve leaflet coaptation and generate a double-orifice valve. Each MitraClip arm is 4 mm wide and 8 mm long and is covered with a polyester fabric to promote tissue ingrowth.

The MitraClip procedure is performed in a standard cardiac catheterization laboratory and requires a multidisciplinary team, including 1–2 interventional cardiologists, an echocardiographer, and an anesthesiologist. The procedure is performed under general anesthesia for patient comfort and to allow breath holding and to avoid patient movement during the delicate grasping steps. However, it is feasible to perform the procedure under conscious sedation [23]. The device is delivered from the femoral vein by a transseptal route using a steerable guide catheter (24 Fr proximally and

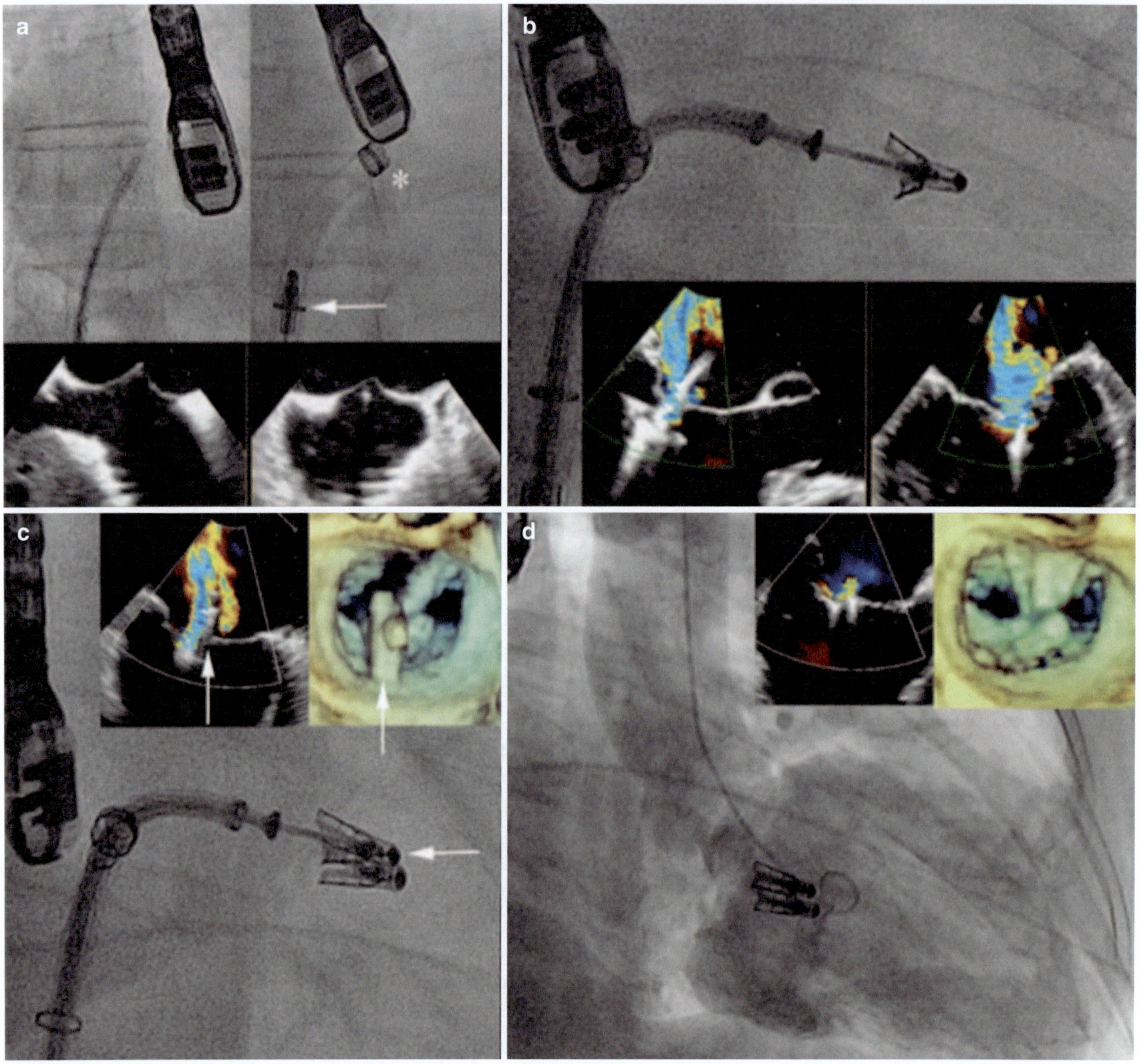

Fig. 28.3 MitraClip procedure. Although echocardiography (2-D and 3-D TEE) is the predominant modality for imaging and guiding the MitraClip procedure, fluoroscopy also provides important information. (**a**) Transseptal puncture is performed using standard technique under biplane TEE guidance to ensure adequate height above the mitral valve plane. The guiding catheter (*asterisk*) is then placed into the left atrium over a wire, through which the MitraClip (*arrow*) is delivered. (**b**) The MitraClip is positioned within the regurgitant jet using orthogonal TEE views before grasping the leaflets. (**c**) In this case, there was a residual regurgitant jet lateral to the first MitraClip; therefore, a second MitraClip (*arrow*) was positioned and deployed. (**d**) Two adjacent MitraClips in place after deployment with generation of a double-orifice valve with trace residual regurgitation

22 Fr at the interatrial septum), through which the steerable clip delivery system (CDS) with the MitraClip attached at the distal end is delivered. The MitraClip is steered and advanced under echocardiographic and fluoroscopic guidance into the left ventricle at the point of maximal regurgitation and withdrawn with the arms opened to allow capture of both leaflets with the grippers and arms. Once secure leaflet capture is confirmed, the MitraClip can then be tightened to improve coaptation and reduce MR further. If the desired result is achieved, the MitraClip is released from the catheter (Fig. 28.3). If the grasp is suboptimal, the clip can be reopened, the leaflets released, and the grasping procedure repeated. The procedure is performed with heparin for anticoagulation. After implantation, aspirin (325 mg) is given for 6 months and clopidogrel (75 mg) for 30 days. SBE prophylaxis is generally recommended for 6 months after the

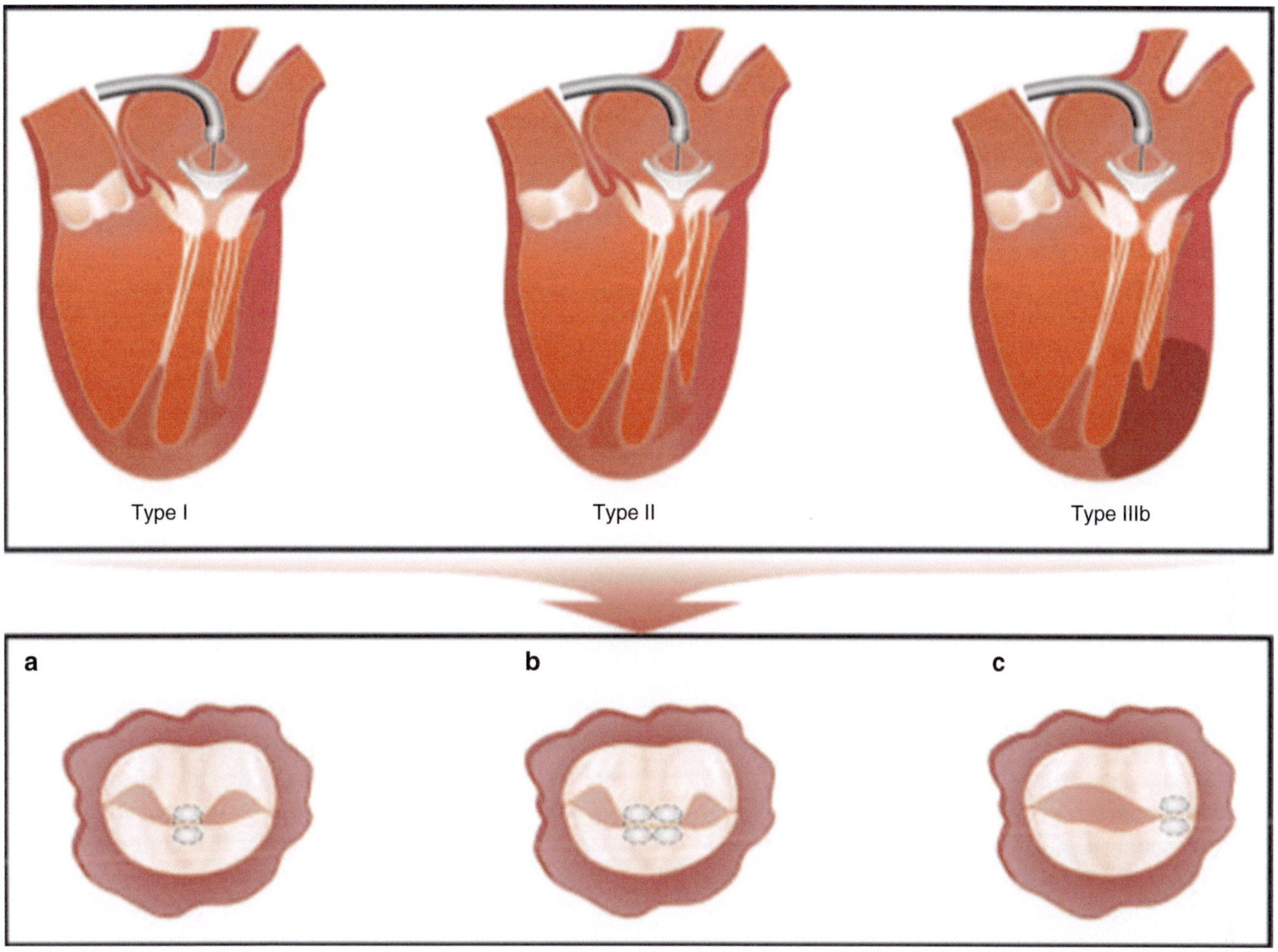

Fig. 28.4 Multiple pathologies are treatable with MitraClip therapy. The *top panel* shows multiple Carpentier-type etiologies of MR that can be treated with MitraClip therapy. *Lower panel* illustrates the final common pathway for MitraClip therapy, which consists of generating a double-orifice valve. One or more MitraClips can be placed centrally (**a**, **b**). For lateral or commissural jets, a MitraClip can be placed in the para-commissural region with a resultant single orifice (**c**) (From Rogers and Franzen [21], with permission)

procedure. The only limitation to the number of MitraClips implanted from a safety standpoint is the development of mitral stenosis. It has been shown that MitraClip repair with one or two clips using the EVEREST inclusion criteria of a baseline MVA ≥ 4.0 cm^2 does not result in significant mitral stenosis [24]. MitraClip therapy results in an acute post-procedural improvement in forward stroke volume and cardiac output, while decreasing LV end-diastolic pressure and end-diastolic volume [25]. MitraClip therapy is intended for the treatment of MR that has a primarily central origin (A2/P2 interface), based on the original surgical technique described by Alfieri. The MitraClip has been applied successfully to a wide spectrum of degenerative (anterior, posterior, and bileaflet prolapse) and functional pathologies with central regurgitant jets. Regardless of regurgitation etiology, the final common objective of MitraClip implantation is the generation of a double-orifice valve. Off-label use to treat lateral regurgitant jets has been described (Fig. 28.4).

EVEREST Trials

The North American EVEREST (Endovascular Valve Edge-to-Edge Repair Study) trials represent the safety and feasibility (EVEREST I) and pivotal (EVEREST II) MitraClip trials, which established the initial algorithms for clinical and echocardiographic patient selection and the procedural protocols and utilized echocardiographic core-lab follow-up.

The EVEREST I safety and feasibility trial enrolled 55 subjects and was reported with an additional 52 patients treated in the pre-randomization start-up (roll-in) phase of the EVEREST II pivotal trial [26]. Patients were selected if they were candidates for MV surgery, met major ACC/AHA indications for MV surgery, and had very specific echocardiographic criteria including a primary central regurgitant jet associated with the A2/P2 segments, a leaflet coaptation length ≥ 2 mm, a coaptation depth ≤ 11 mm, a flail gap <10 mm, and a flail width <15 mm. Key exclusion criteria included LVEF ≤25 %, LV end-systolic dimension >55 mm, mitral valve orifice area <4 cm^2, or recent myocardial infarction. Of the 107 patients who underwent the MitraClip procedure in this early clinical experience, 70 (74 %) achieved acute procedural success (APS), defined as a post-procedure reduction of MR to ≤2+. Of subjects who did not achieve APS, 17 (16 %) had MitraClip implantation with acute MR grade >2+, and 11 (10 %) had no MitraClip implanted with post-procedure MR>2+. At 12 months, not including crossover to surgery, 50 of 76 APS patients (66 %) had echocardiographic follow-up and continued with MR ≤ 2+. A total of 32 patients underwent MV surgery after a clip procedure, and when repair was planned, 84 % were successfully repaired. Freedom from death at up to 3 years follow-up was 90.1 %, and freedom from surgery was 76.3 %. The majority of patients included had degenerative MR (79 %), but patients with functional MR (21 %) had similar acute results and durability.

The landmark EVEREST II trial was the first randomized trial of a percutaneous mitral repair device measured against conventional surgical therapy and also represents the first echocardiographic core-lab adjudicated follow-up after surgical mitral valve repair [27]. This trial randomized 279 patients with 3–4+ MR amenable to surgical repair prospectively to receive either MitraClip therapy ($n=184$) or conventional surgical repair or replacement ($n=95$) in a 2:1 ratio. The primary safety endpoint was any major adverse event (MAE) at 30 days. Prespecified MAEs were death, major stroke, reoperation of mitral valve, urgent/emergent CV surgery, myocardial infarction, renal failure, deep wound infection, ventilation >48 h, new onset permanent atrial fibrillation, septicemia, GI complication requiring surgery, or transfusion ≥2 units. The composite primary efficacy endpoint was defined as 12-month-freedom death, new surgery for mitral valve dysfunction, or MR > 2+. The intention-to-treat 30-day MAE rate was lower in the MitraClip group when compared to the surgery group (15 % vs. 48 %, superiority $P<0.001$). The MAE difference was driven largely by transfusion requirements in the surgical arm; however, in response to this criticism, a modified MAE analysis which defined major bleeding as transfusion ≥4 units or requiring surgical intervention still demonstrated a lower MAE rate in the MitraClip group (5.0 % vs. 30.9 %, $P<0.0001$) [28]. Primary clinical efficacy at 12 months by intention to treat was achieved in 55 % of the MitraClip device patients and 73 % of the surgery group (non-inferiority $P=0.007$). After 2-year follow-up, primary clinical efficacy was preserved in 52 % of the percutaneous-repair group and 66 % in the surgery group ($P=0.04$, non-inferiority). There was no need for emergency surgery in any patient treated with MitraClip therapy. It is important to emphasize that the EVEREST II trial examined the safety and efficacy of MitraClip therapy as an initial strategy in the treatment of patients with MR. Not every MitraClip procedure was successful in reducing MR, but of these failures in reaching acute procedural success, the majority went on to have successful subsequent mitral valve surgery. Both the MitraClip and surgically treated subjects had favorable LV remodeling and improvements in quality of life at 12 months. A non-prespecified subgroup analysis showed that for subjects with age ≥70 years, functional MR, and LVEF <60 %, surgery was not superior to percutaneous treatment with regard to efficacy. Concomitant with the EVEREST II trial, a single-arm "high risk registry" (HRR) enrolled 78 patients with primarily FMR and an STS or surgeon-estimated surgical procedural mortality risk of ≥12 %. The HRR demonstrated superior safety compared to the estimated surgical risk, as well as favorable LV remodeling and improved symptoms in most patients.

It is desirable that subsequent surgical options for MV repair are preserved after MitraClip implantation. This is most important in low surgical risk patients with degenerative MR. However, it is debatable whether mitral valve repair after a failed MitraClip procedure in functional mitral regurgitation should even be attempted, as a mortality difference has not been shown between repair and replacement in patients with ischemic MR up to 6 years after surgery [29]. Nonetheless, it has been shown that surgical repair can be performed in many subjects successfully after MitraClip therapy, with successful repair having been reported up to 5 years after implantation [30, 31]. It is clear that not every patient will be able to have successful surgical repair after MitraClip therapy, and it is very likely that fibrosis over time will hinder successful clip removal without injuring the leaflets. The degree to which this limitation will be clinically significant requires further study. The presence of anterior/bileaflet flail or prolapse has been shown to be a significant predictor of the need for MV replacement. However, surgeon experience (defined as the number of surgeries performed annually), duration of implant, or an operative note of valve injury or difficulty removing the device did not have an impact on whether a repair or replacement was performed [32].

European Registry Results

In March 2008, the MitraClip received CE-mark approval. Since then, the majority of MitraClip implants have been performed in Europe. In addition, the clinical characteristics of European patients are different from those enrolled in the EVEREST trials, as the relatively limiting mitral leaflet anatomic criteria were not consistently observed. The two largest reports to date on the European MitraClip experience emanate from a single center in Germany [33] and two centers in Italy [34], for a total of 82 patients. Both centers reported favorable acute and short-term outcomes in patients at high risk for surgery with primarily FMR and low ejection fractions. Data from the EVEREST trials and European registries are summarized in Table 28.2.

Table 28.2 Comparative summary of major MitraClip clinical trials

	% (Per)	EVEREST/N on EVEREST eligibility	Degenerative/ Functional ecology	Age, Mean	Baseline LVEF %	STS Score/Logistic EuroSCORE, Mean	Baseline NYHA II/IV, %	Follow-up NYHA II/IV, %	Mean MR grade at baseline	MR ≤2+ at follow-up	Echocardio-graphic Core Lab	Procedural mortality/In hospital death
EVEREST and EVEREST II Roll-In Registry (USA), Feldman et al.	107	100 %/0 %	79 %/21 %	71	62	NR/NR	46 %	8 % (at 12 months)	3.3	74 % (discharge)/ 66 % (12 months)	Yes	0(0 %)/1(0.9 %)
EVEREST II Randomized Trail (USA), Feldman et al.	184	100 %/0 %	73 %/27 %	67	60	NR/NR	52 %	2 %	3.2	79 % (12 months)	Yes	0(0 %)/2 (1 %) @ 30 days
German Experience Franzen et al.	51	31 %/69 %	31 %/69 %	73	36	16/28	98 %	33 % (at discharge)	3.6	94 % (at discharge)	No	0(0 %)/ 0(0 %)
Italian Experience Tamburino et al.	51	100 %/0 %	42 %/58 %	71	42	10.3/14.3	87 %	0 % (at 30 days)	3.9	97 % (30 days)	No	0(0 %)/NR

From Rogers and Franzen [21], with permission
NR not reported

In the German experience, MitraClip therapy was used in 51 patients with ≥3 + MR who were at high risk for mitral valve surgery based on a logistic EuroSCORE >20, an STS score >12, or by other clinical factors which the team felt conferred a high surgical risk. Patients in this series had worse LV function and more adverse valve morphology than those enrolled in the EVEREST trials. Specifically, 35 patients (69 %) had LV or leaflet characteristics that would have excluded them from enrollment in the EVEREST trials. Despite these adverse characteristics, acute outcomes were favorable, with reduction in MR severity two or more grades in 65 % of subjects and no clinically significant mitral stenosis, procedure-related major adverse events, or inhospital mortality. Longer-term outcomes from this cohort have not been reported, and therefore effects on prognosis and durability of left ventricular remodeling and MR reduction remain unanswered.

In two Italian centers, 31 subjects who were high risk for surgery underwent MitraClip therapy. Although clinical and anatomic leaflet criteria were similar to the EVEREST trials, there was no exclusion for very low LV ejection fraction or severe LV enlargement. Acute device success was observed in 97 % of patients, with sustained MR reduction and favorable LV remodeling seen at 30 days. The higher acute success rates in this series as compared to the EVEREST trials may reflect the lack of a blinded core lab, a different patient population, more liberal use of two clips, and an accelerated procedural learning curve as a result of prior experience in North America. Longer-term efficacy and durability in this initial cohort has not yet been reported. Hopefully the ongoing North American REALISM registry will validate these outcomes.

MitraClip Future Directions

The MitraClip has emerged as an important therapeutic option for patients with mitral regurgitation. The device has excellent safety; acute outcomes are favorable, and for those patients with acute procedural success, midterm durability (up to 2 years) is reasonable. For patients at low surgical risk with degenerative MR, surgical mitral valve repair has set a high standard, with a 10-year freedom from reoperation of up to 97 % [35]. Based on adoption patterns in Europe, recent utilization trends in North America, and subgroup analyses from the EVEREST II trial, it would appear that patients who are older, at higher risk for surgical therapy, or with functional MR and depressed ejection fractions will constitute the initial target population for MitraClip therapy. Since functional MR is primarily a ventricular problem, it remains to be seen whether a pure leaflet intervention will have durable efficacy or will be superior to best medical therapy with cardiac resynchronization therapy. If so, a very large population of patients could benefit. The potential importance of concomitant annuloplasty as an adjunct to MitraClip remains unanswered. Failure to perform annuloplasty at the time of surgical degenerative leaflet repair has been shown to adversely affect repair durability [36–38]. Future iterations of the MitraClip may simplify leaflet insertion and grasping. 3-D transesophageal echocardiography (TEE), which was not widely available at the outset of the MitraClip experience, has been shown to lessen procedure times and improve visualization [39].

Other Leaflet Repair Technologies

The Mobius device (Edwards Lifesciences, Irvine, California) uses an innovative transseptal catheter with suction capability to grasp the leaflets and deliver suture to create a double-orifice valve. The procedure was performed successfully on 15 patients in 4 international centers with acute reduction of MR by ≥1 grade in 9 patients and sustained improvement in 6 patients at 30 days. Due to the limited clinical benefit and lack of durability, human clinical development was abandoned [40]. However, if in the future the technical aspects of suture delivery can be improved, the procedure may yet have utility.

The Cardiosolutions Percu-Pro™ System (Cardiosolutions Inc., Stoughton, MA) is a percutaneously delivered polyurethane-silicone polymer "Mitra-Spacer."

This is a balloon-shaped spacer that occupies the regurgitant mitral orifice and is anchored to the left ventricular apex (Fig. 28.5). Animal studies have shown that the device is nonthrombotic with minimal inflammatory response. Human implants are planned.

Chordal Implantation

NeoChord

The NeoChord device is a beating-heart, sternal-sparing, transapical approach to implantation of artificial chordae tendineae in patients with leaflet prolapse or flail (Fig. 28.6). The LV apex is exposed via a left lateral mini-thoracotomy. The procedure is guided by TEE, and a catheter is used to grasp the leaflets and attach artificial chordae that are anchored to the LV apex. The system utilizes a unique fiberoptic feedback system to ensure the target leaflet is appropriately centered in the jaws of the device. In addition to being minimally invasive, the beating-heart aspect of the procedure allows the operator to assess real-time reduction in MR by varying chord tension. The European TACT Trial (Transapical Artificial Chordae Tendineae) is underway and targets subjects with severe degenerative mitral regurgitation.

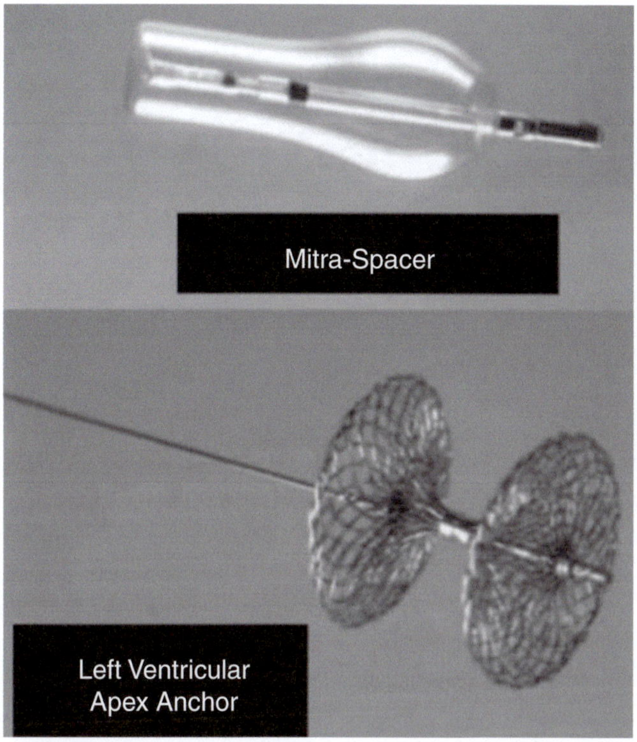

Fig. 28.5 The Percu-Pro system. The space occupying Mitra-Spacer balloon acts as a "buoy" filling the mitral regurgitant orifice and is anchored by a tether to the left ventricular apex

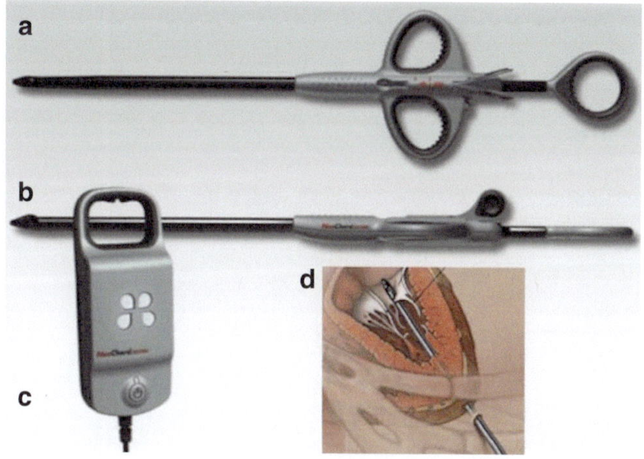

Fig. 28.6 NeoChord device. The NeoChord device is delivered from a transapical approach and consists of a catheter to grasp the leaflet (**a**), an exchangeable cartridge containing ePTFE suture (**b**), and an integrated fiber-optic display to verify leaflet capture (**c**). *Panel* (**d**) shows the system in use

Annular Shape Change Approaches

Surgical annuloplasty is an effective stand-alone treatment for functional MR and is an important adjunct to leaflet repair procedures for degenerative mitral regurgitation. Percutaneous techniques have been developed to mimic surgical annuloplasty. Most approaches have attempted to reshape the annulus "indirectly" by reshaping the coronary sinus. Other techniques employ more "direct" annuloplasty by attaching a series of anchors near or on the annulus which can be drawn together (plicated) with suture, with the goal of reducing the mitral annular circumference and the septal-lateral dimension. Finally, technology is under development to completely replicate a surgical annuloplasty with a semi-rigid implantable circumferential annular ring.

Indirect Annuloplasty

The coronary sinus (CS) travels in close proximity to the mitral annulus (Fig. 28.7). The CS travels 5–10 mm superior and diagonally to the plane of the mitral annulus [41] and is typically connected to the mitral annulus by nonfibrous atrial myocardium. Any conformational change in the CS must be transmitted through this sinoannular tissue, which attenuates any applied force, and may remodel and redilate over time resulting in compromised durability. Several devices have been developed which can be placed within the CS. By tensioning these systems by various means, the circumference of the mitral annulus can be decreased with some reduction in the septal-lateral dimension and reduction in MR. Although these devices can be deployed with relative ease, there remain significant limitations including the lack of robust and reproducible efficacy and the risk of coronary artery compression. A coronary artery (usually the circumflex) has been shown to travel between the CS and mitral annulus in up to 68 % of cases [42]. This relationship puts the circumflex coronary artery at risk for compression during CS device placement.

Cardiac Dimensions Carillon Device

The Carillon Mitral Contour System (Cardiac Dimensions, Inc., Kirkland, WA) consists of a pair of helical self-expanding nitinol distal and proximal anchors connected by a nitinol bridge. The device is placed percutaneously in the coronary sinus from a right internal jugular vein approach and can be retrieved acutely if positioning or MR reduction is not favorable. The bridge can be shortened after the anchors are deployed in order to plicate posterior annular tissue and create movement of the posterior annulus anteriorly and reduce the septal-lateral dimension (Fig. 28.8).

The AMADEUS trial was the first investigation into the potential role of a percutaneous CS-based intervention to reduce functional mitral regurgitation (FMR) in patients with heart failure [43], and, on the basis of the findings, the Carillon device was granted CE-mark approval in 2009.

In the AMADEUS trial, 48 symptomatic patients with dilated cardiomyopathy, at least moderate FMR, and an ejection fraction <40 % were enrolled. Thirty patients had successful device implantation with the primary safety endpoint—a composite of death, myocardial infarction, or device-related complication—evaluated at 30 days. Echocardiographic FMR grade and functional indices

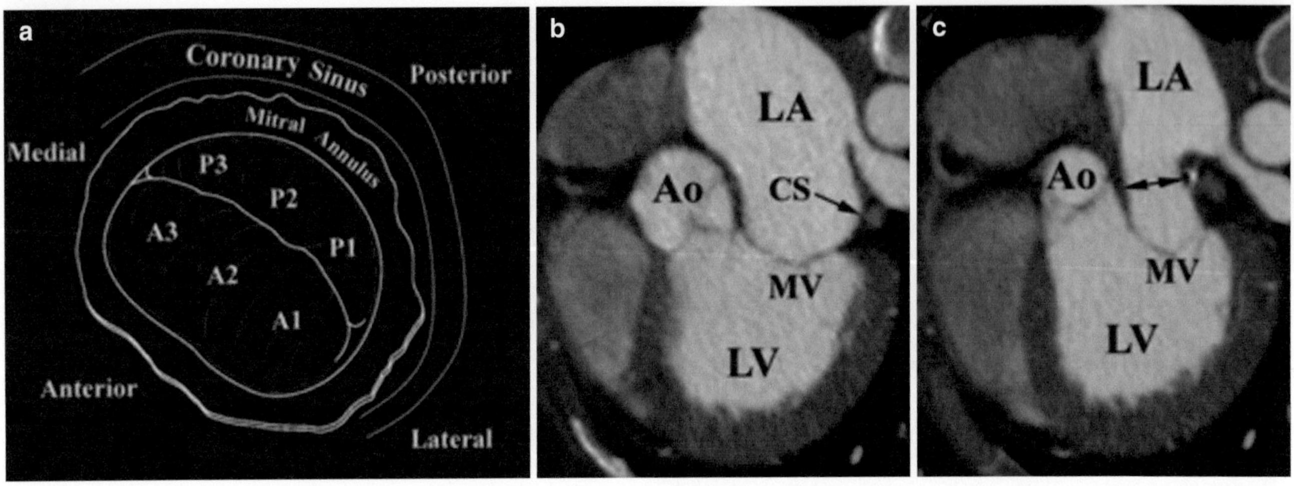

Fig. 28.7 Indirect mitral annuloplasty using the coronary sinus. (**a**) The coronary sinus (*CS*) encircles the posterior mitral annulus. (**b**) CT scan of subject with functional MR showing relationship of CS (*arrow*) to the mitral valve. Note that they are not coplanar. (**c**) Movement of the CS with device results in narrowing of the left atrial lumen above the mitral valve (*double-headed arrow*), with secondary indirect decrease in the mitral annulus diameter. *CS* coronary sinus, *LV* left ventricle, *LA* left atrium, *AO* aorta, *MV* mitral valve

(NYHA functional class, Kansas City Cardiomyopathy Questionnaire, and 6-min walk test) were assessed at baseline, 1 month, and 6 months. Of the 48 patients enrolled in the trial, 6 (13 %) experienced a major adverse event within 30 days; one of these six patients died, with the remaining events consisting of either clinically silent myocardial infarction or coronary sinus dissection and/or perforation. The causes for coronary sinus injury were procedural, taking place early in the trial, and changes were made in technique for subsequent implants. Coronary arteries were crossed in 36 of 43 (84 %) implant attempts. When coronary compromise was identified, the Carillon device could be safely removed prior to implantation. There was a 22–32 % reduction in mitral regurgitation grade at 6 months by a composite of four echocardiographic parameters used, with no significant erosion in 30-day mitral regurgitation values at 6 months. Although quality of life and functional indices all improved in follow-up, there was no significant change in left ventricular size or left ventricular ejection fraction at 6 months. Additionally, the anteroposterior mitral annular diameter decreased from an average of 42.0 mm at baseline to only 37.8 mm at 6-month follow-up—representing a relatively small 10 % diameter reduction—and never attained a correction back to normal. The AMADEUS trial was important evidence that a CS-based device could be used safely to reduce MR and improve quality of life in patients with FMR.

The findings in the AMADEUS trial were strengthened by the more recently reported prospective nonrandomized TITAN trial, in which 53 patients with symptomatic FMR were enrolled for device therapy. Thirty six patients (68 %) underwent successful device implantation, whereas 17 were not implanted due to insufficient MR reduction or transient coronary compromise. Device therapy showed significant reduction in MR grade, favorable LV remodeling, and improved quality of life when compared to the control group of non-implanted subjects. There were several clinically silent wireform fractures seen in this trial. A newer Carillon mXE2 device has recently been introduced and will be used in future trials. Pre-procedure computed tomography scanning has been used in the Carillon studies and can provide some useful anatomic information for planning the procedure, but has not reliably been able to predict efficacy or coronary artery compression.

Edwards Monarc Device

The Monarc device (Edwards Lifesciences, Irvine, CA) has a distal self-expanding anchor, a middle spring-like "bridge," and a proximal self-expanding anchor. The distal anchor is placed near the anterior interventricular vein and the proximal anchor near the ostium of the CS. The bridge has shape memory properties that result in shortening forces at body temperature after dissipation of a dissolvable element in the center of the device. This device is unique in that acute MR reduction is not observed, but rather occurs after a 3- to 6-week period after the spacer material dissolves and results in device shortening. This delayed-shortening property raises a concern for late coronary artery compression. A pilot study in humans with the first-generation Viking device showed some improvement in chronic MR, but 1 out of the 5 patients could not have the device successfully implanted, and 3 of the 4 who did had evidence of bridge separation or fracture during follow-up [44]. A second-generation device (Monarc device) correcting these problems was then studied in the prospective nonrandomized EVOLUTION I and II trials (Clinical Evaluation of the Edwards Lifesciences Percutaneous Mitral Annuloplasty System for The Treatment of Mitral Regurgitation). The EVOLUTION I trial of functional MR demonstrated implantation success in 82 % (59 of

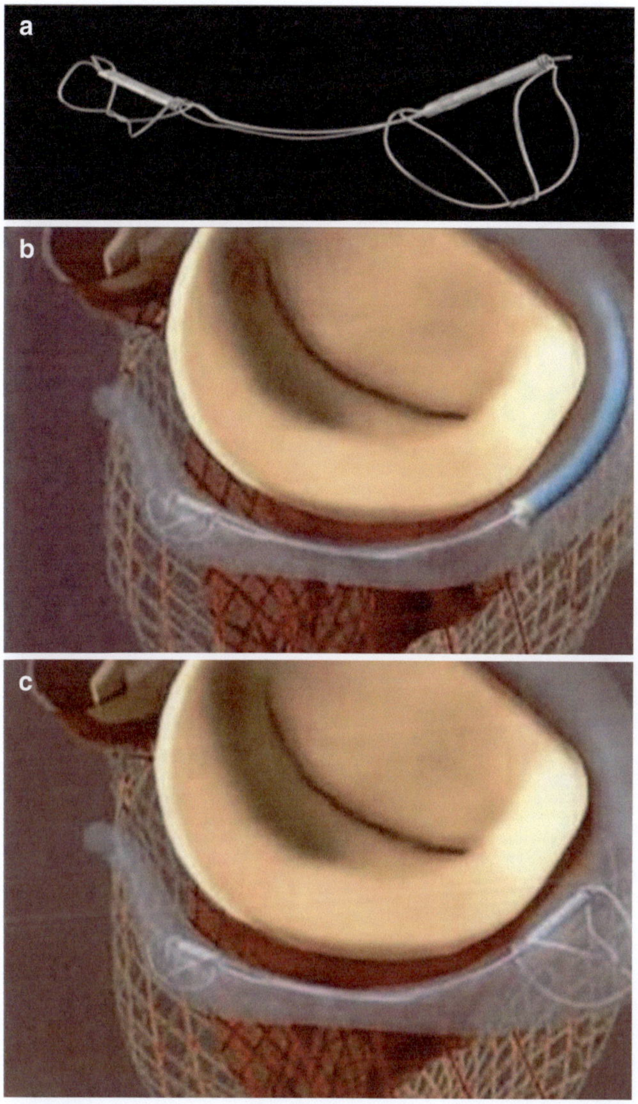

Fig. 28.8 Cardiac dimensions Carillon device. (**a**) The Carillon device. The distal anchor is smaller and deployed first (**b**), traction applied, followed by proximal anchor deployment (**c**) (From Feldman et al. [68], Chap. 1, p 7 with permission)

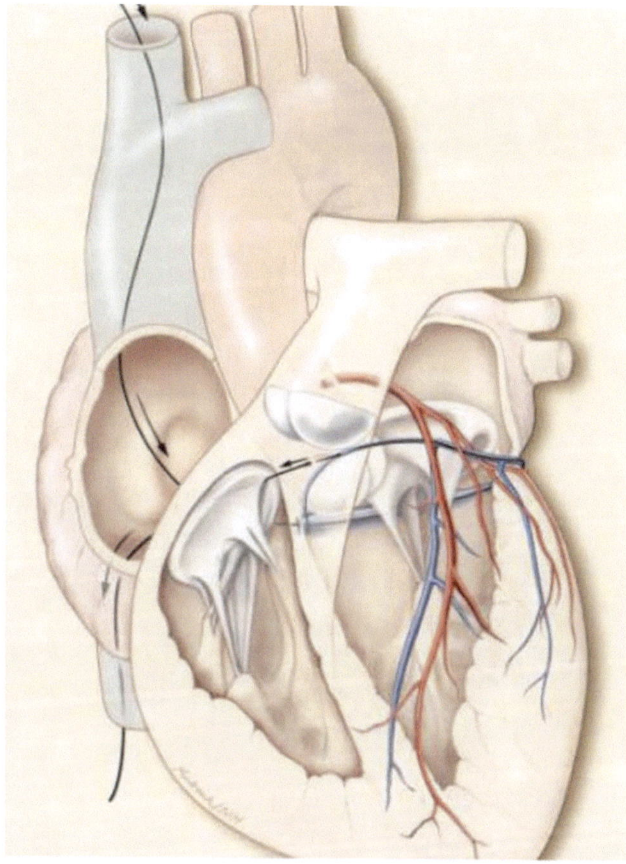

Fig. 28.9 Cerclage annuloplasty. The mitral valve is encircled by a guidewire which can be tensioned to reduce the mitral annular circumference and diameter

72 patients), with 13 failures (18 %) due to tortuous anatomy or inappropriate CS dimensions. Two myocardial infarctions occurred due to coronary artery compression. Event-free survival was 91 % at 30 days and 82 % at 1 year. MR reduction $\geq$ 1 grade was seen in 50 % of subjects at 12 months [45]. Despite encouraging initial clinical results, the MONARC program is no longer undergoing active investigation.

Viacor PTMA Device

The Viacor percutaneous transvenous mitral annuloplasty (PTMA) device (Viacor, Inc., Wilmington, Massachusetts) uses a coronary sinus catheter containing up to three nitinol rods of varying length and stiffness that exert an anterior displacement force. The safety and feasibility of this device was reported for 19 subjects who underwent temporary "diagnostic device" implantation to assess acute MR reduction. The device was successfully implanted in nine subjects. Four of the implants were subsequently removed because of device migration and/or diminished efficacy. There were no procedure or device-related major adverse events with permanent sequelae observed in any of the diagnostic or implant patients. In conclusion, although it was feasible to implant this device in humans, further device development has been abandoned due to limited MR reduction and technical issues [46].

Other Coronary Sinus-Based Devices

Cerclage annuloplasty (Fig. 28.9) is an investigational technique which uses magnetic resonance imaging fused with fluoroscopy to pass a wire from the right atrium, through the coronary sinus, thereby allowing it to reenter the right atrium by traversing a short segment of the basal septal myocardium. In this way it encircles the annulus. By tensioning the guidewire in a porcine model of ischemic cardiomyopathy, mitral annular size and MR grade can be decreased. A small nitinol tube has been developed to prevent guidewire coronary artery compression by acting as a miniature arch over the artery [47].

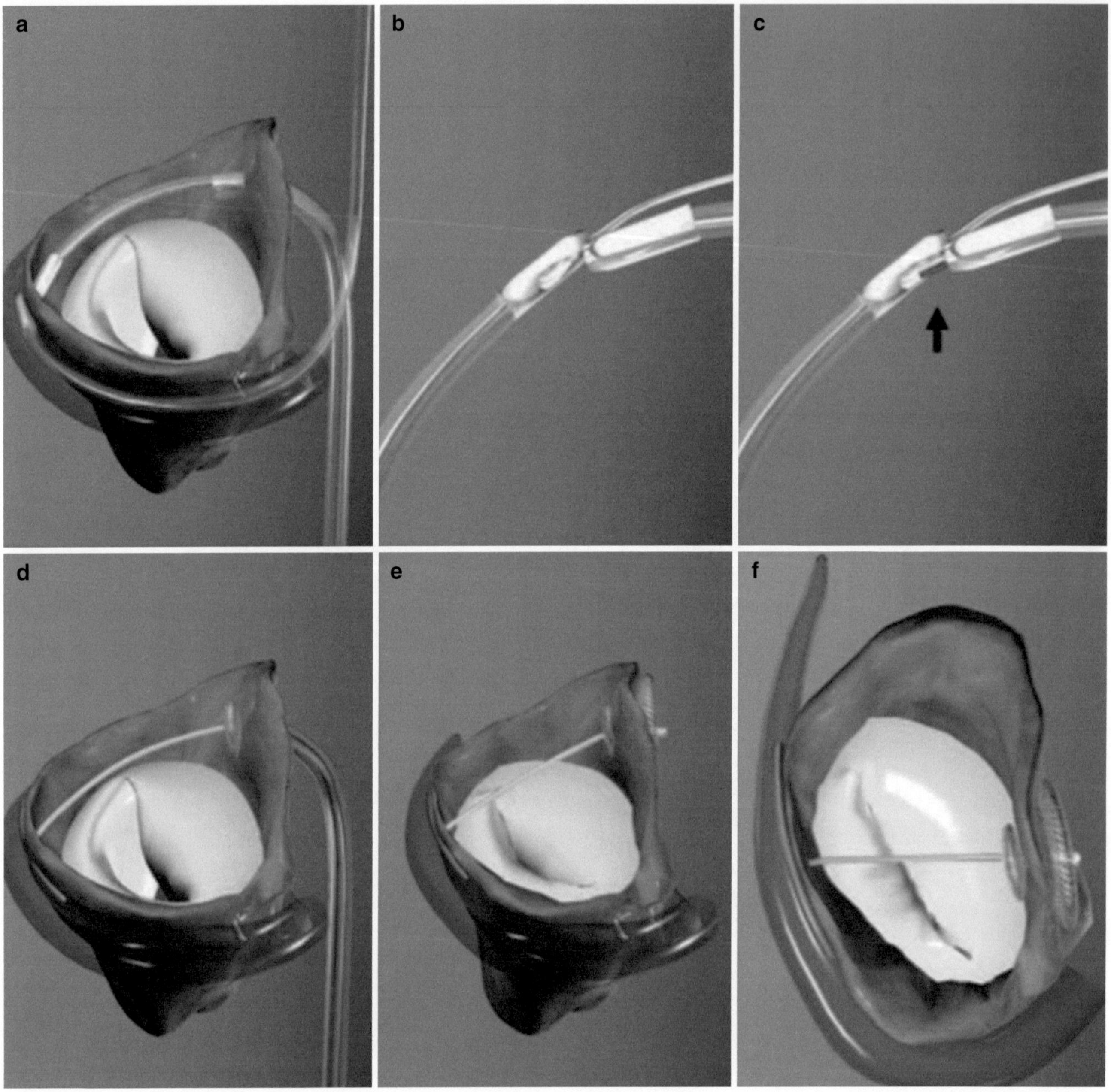

Fig. 28.10 Percutaneous septal sinus shortening (PS3) procedure. (**a**) Magnet- tipped catheters are placed in the coronary sinus and left atrium and "linked" together behind the P2 scallop of the posterior mitral leaflet. (**b**) Close-up of magnetically linked catheters. (**c**) Crossing catheter (*arrow*) is used to safely cross from the left atrium into the coronary sinus, which allows passage of a guidewire. (**d**) The PS3 system in place before tensioning with an anchor in the coronary sinus and an anchor on the interatrial septum. (**e**) Tensioning and locking the suture which connects the two anchors results in reduction of functional MR. (**f**) Superior view of the PS3 system showing remodeling of the mitral annulus and improved leaflet coaptation

The Percutaneous Septal Sinus Shortening System (PS^3 System, MVRx, Belmont, CA) uses magnetic catheters in order to allow accurate placement of a "bridge" which connects anchors in the coronary sinus and the interatrial septum (Fig. 28.10). Once this connection is made between the CS and the interatrial septum, tension can be applied to the bridge element, effectively shortening the septal-lateral (SL) dimension. Using an ovine model, the investigators found that device implantation with an average 24 % SL diameter reduction resulted in acute and chronic MR reduction [48]. Since this approach had shown early promise, temporary devices were implanted in a first-in-human study, confirming efficacy and significantly reducing MR [49]. Further human studies are planned.

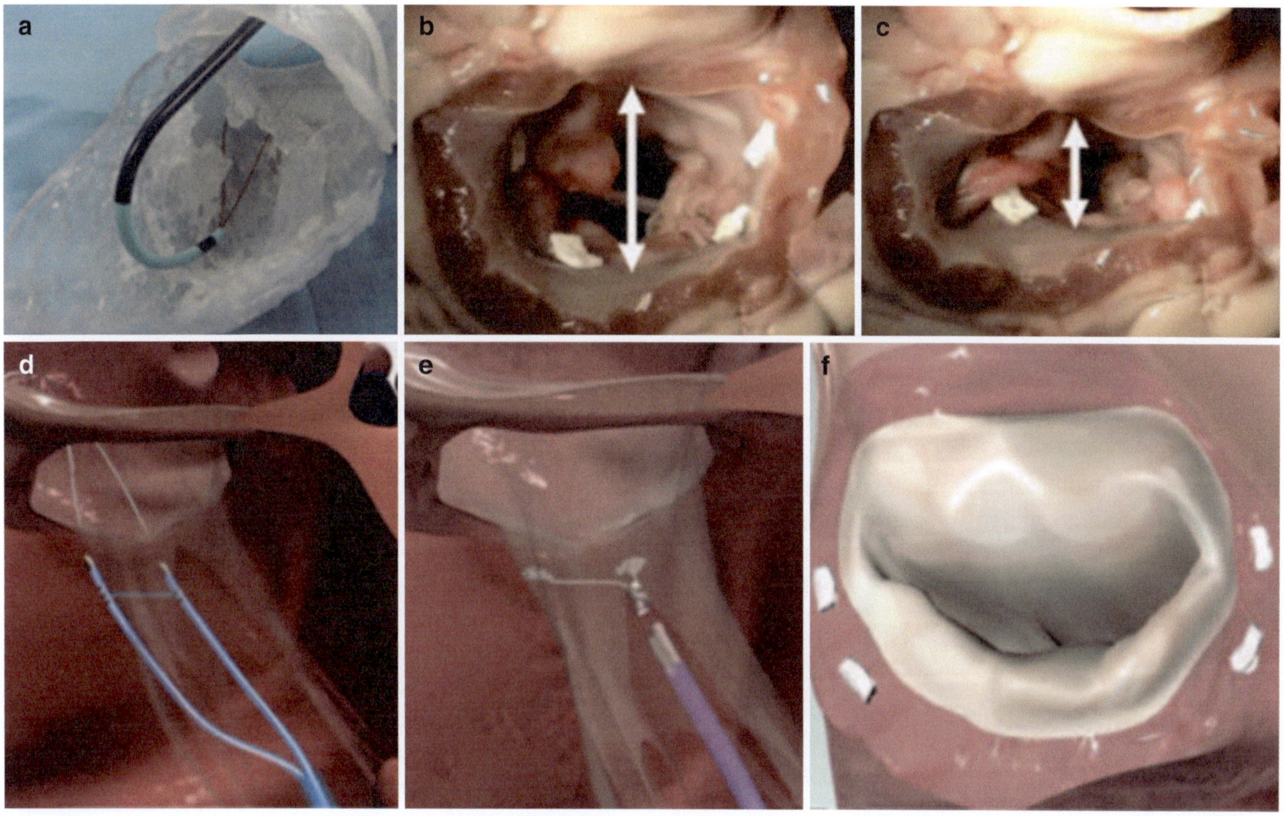

Fig. 28.11 Mitralign annuloplasty system. (**a**) Model demonstrating deflectable catheter which allows passage of the "bident"-crossing wires through the mitral annulus from the left ventricle to the left atrium. (**b**) Paired pledgeted sutures are placed on opposite sides of the posterior annulus and then tensioned (**c**) to reduce the septal-lateral diameter (*arrow*) and improve leaflet coaptation. (**d**) Bident wires are passed across the annulus. (**e**) The anchor suture is pulled together and locked. (**f**) Final appearance of 2×2 annular plication (Figures (d), (e), and (f) from Feldman et al. [68], Chap. 1, p 8 with permission)

Direct Annuloplasty

Surgical closed-ring mitral annuloplasty is currently considered the surgical gold standard for the treatment of functional mitral regurgitation, with predictable and durable reductions in mitral annular circumference and the septal-lateral diameter. Prior to the advent of open and closed rigid rings, suture-based annuloplasty based on the prior work by Paneth and Burr had been used [50]. This technique has been shown to reduce the septal-lateral diameter in patients undergoing adjunctive annuloplasty in the setting of degenerative leaflet repair or for repair of functional mitral regurgitation [51, 52]. However, the durability of suture-based or nonrigid annuloplasty has been shown to be inferior to rigid mitral annular rings, with progression in mitral annular dimensions over time [16, 51]. Nonetheless, given the ability to achieve suture-based annuloplasty through percutaneous approaches, several percutaneous approaches have been developed. Other novel approaches include the application of radio-frequency energy and the development of a percutaneously delivered semirigid circumferential mitral annuloplasty ring.

Mitralign Percutaneous Annuloplasty System

The Mitralign Percutaneous Annuloplasty System (Mitralign, Inc., Tewksbury, MA) is based on surgical suture annuloplasty of the mitral valve. The Mitralign procedure involves a left ventricular approach through retrograde femoral arterial access. A deflectable catheter is placed under the posterior mitral leaflet, adjacent to the annular tissue beneath the valve. The procedure is performed under fluoroscopic and echocardiographic guidance. A specially designed catheter carries two crossing wires (the "bident") that are passed from the ventricular aspect of the annulus into the left atrium using a brief application of radio-frequency energy. These wires then serve as the guides over which two sets of paired anchors are placed through the posterior annulus of the mitral valve. These anchors are plicated together, resulting in segmental posterior annuloplasty and reduction in mitral regurgitation (Fig. 28.11). This technology is undergoing safety and feasibility testing in Europe and South America.

Guided Delivery Systems AccuCinch System

The AccuCinch system (Guided Delivery Systems, Santa Clara, CA), which is also based on the suture annuloplasty method, is focused on correction of annular dilation. This procedure uses a retrograde femoral arterial approach to gain access to the ventricular aspect of the mitral annulus. A proprietary catheter is placed under the posterior mitral leaflet, adjacent to the annular tissue beneath the valve. Using this catheter, 9–12 anchors can be placed from the anterior to posterior commissures along the posterior mitral annulus. The anchors are then connected by a suture element and plicated to provide reductions in the mitral annular circumference and mitral regurgitation. It has also been described that this technique could be used to plicate the posterior wall of the left ventricle to improve ventricular geometry and potentially reduce functional MR. Chronic surgical implants in humans have been completed, and percutaneous human implants are being performed.

The QuantumCor System

The QuantumCor System (QuantumCor, Bothell, WA) is based on the concept of thermal remodeling of collagen. Since the mitral valve annulus has significant collagen content, catheter-based application of radio-frequency (RF) energy at subablative temperatures to the mitral annulus will heat and contract the collagen fibers, thereby reducing mitral annular circumference. This technology has been proven to reduce mitral annular dimensions and mitral regurgitation in an animal model [53]. Histologic follow-up showed that the lesions generated did not compromise the structural integrity of the atrium or mitral leaflets. The energy is applied circumferentially to the mitral annulus using a proprietary catheter that is used to apply RF energy. The favorable aspects of this technology are that no material is left behind and that repeat applications can be applied. Therapy in humans has not yet been reported.

Supra-annular Rings

The Millipede system (Millipede, Inc., Minneapolis, MN) is a device in preclinical development which attempts to mimic a surgical circumferential and rigid annuloplasty. This consists of the placement of a novel expandable annular ring with an innovative attachment system via either minimally invasive surgical or percutaneous methods to restore the native mitral annular shape and diameter. The device could be used to treat functional MR or as an adjunct to leaflet repair technologies.

The Cardioband (Valtech Ltd., Or Yehuda, Israel), allows a series of anchors to be placed percutaneously into the left atrial aspect of the mitral annulus. These anchors are connected by a sleeve which can be tensioned, resulting in reduction of the mitral annular circumference. Early human experience has been promising.

Ventricular Reshaping Technologies

The iCoapsys system (Edwards, Irvine, CA) is a novel method of reshaping the left ventricle by means of a percutaneously placed system. The procedure is based on the surgically placed Coapsys system which has been shown to result in sustained reduction in mitral regurgitation at 1 year [54]. Under fluoroscopic and echocardiographic guidance, intrapericardial-anchoring devices are placed on the epicardial ventricular surfaces in an anterior-posterior configuration and are connected by a tethering or anchoring suture that passes horizontally through the left ventricle. By applying tension to the anchoring suture, the geometry of the ventricle is changed (Fig. 28.12). Likewise, the mitral annular diameter is decreased, resulting in improved leaflet coaptation. After several human implants, further development of the device was terminated due to device complexity and other technical issues. Nonetheless, the device was important in validating the concept that FMR is a ventricular disease, and that by remodeling the LV, MR reduction can be observed.

The BACE device (Basal Annuloplasty of the Cardia Externally, Mardil Inc., Morrisville, North Carolina) requires a mini-thoracotomy and is implanted on a beating heart. A silicone band with inflatable chambers is placed around the atrioventricular groove. This reportedly can result in reshaping of the mitral annulus with improved leaflet coaptation.

Percutaneous Mitral Valve Replacement

Although surgical mitral valve repair is generally preferable to replacement for degenerative MR, developing transcatheter mitral valve replacement therapies is important for several reasons. First, some complex mitral valve pathologies will not be amenable to percutaneous repair or will require combinations of percutaneous technologies which may not be feasible. Percutaneous valve replacement may result in superior reduction of MR compared to repair, and this may be of particular importance if the goal of a procedure is to attain "zero MR." For patients with FMR, replacement may be an attractive option, as there is no mortality difference between repair and replacement in patients with ischemic MR up to 6 years after surgery [29]. However, multiple challenges exist. Secure anchoring and attachment of percutaneous valves will be very important, as paravalvular leaks will

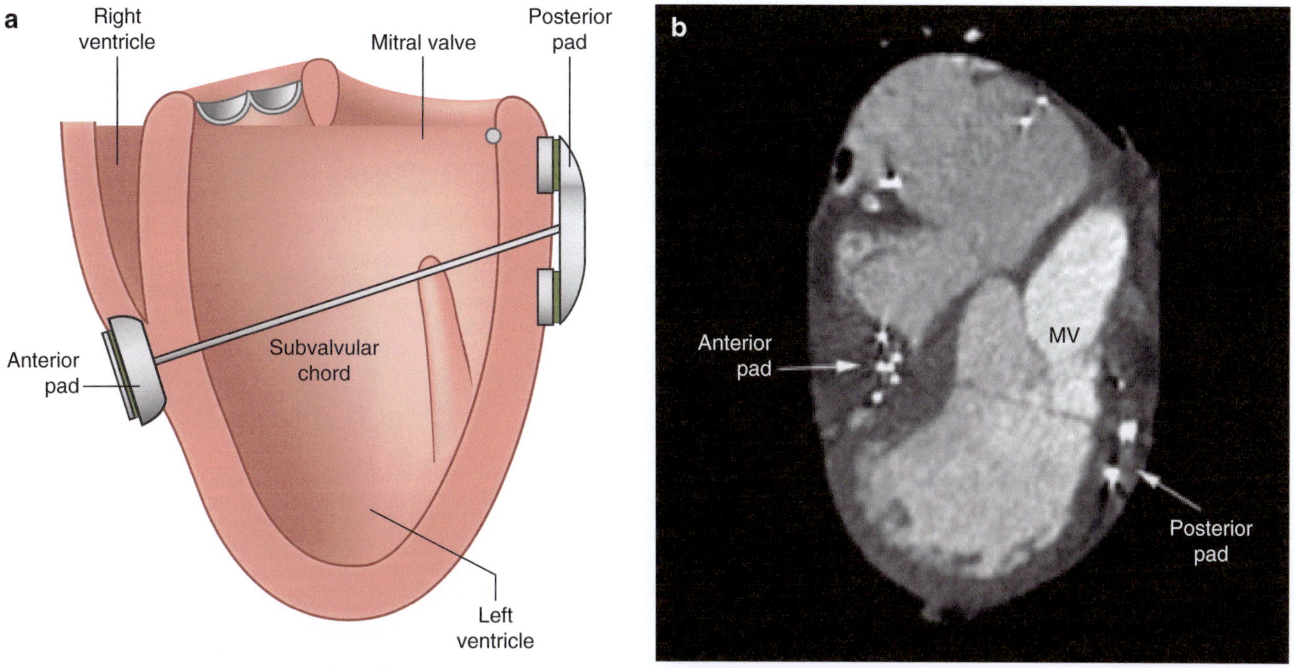

Fig. 28.12 iCoapsys system. Components of the iCoapsys system are shown (**a**), as well as CT scan imaging of the device spanning the left ventricle after implantation (**b**)

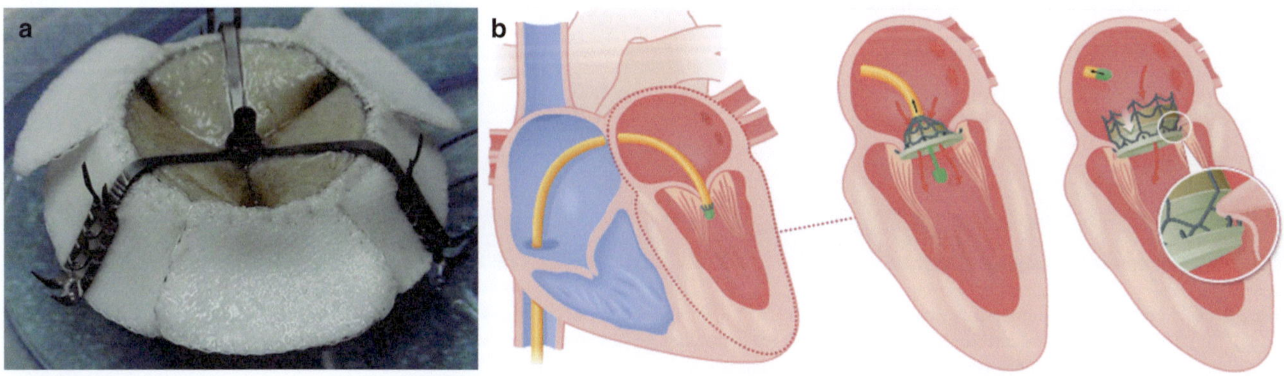

Fig. 28.13 Percutaneous Mitral Valve Replacements. (**a**) The Endovalve-Herrmann prosthesis, shown also in collapsed form (inset). (**b**) Schematic of delivery of CardiAQ prosthesis via transseptal route with self-expanding frame. from Feldman et al. [68], Chap. 1, p 10 with permission

likely not be well tolerated. In addition, patients with FMR will generally have large mitral annular diameters, and developing devices which expand to fill these large diameters will be necessary.

The Endovalve-Herrmann Mitral Valve (Endovalve, Inc., Princeton, NJ) is a foldable nitinol valve in preclinical development with a sealing skirt that attaches to the mitral valve apparatus. It is fully valve sparing and repositionable before release. The CardiAQ prosthesis (CardiAQ Valve Technologies, Winchester, MA), which is also in preclinical development, is delivered by a transseptal approach. The valve is attached to a self-expanding nitinol frame which centers itself on the mitral annulus (Fig. 28.13).

Percutaneous Closure of Mitral Paravalvular Leaks

Surgical mitral valve replacement requires suture-mediated attachment of a bioprosthetic or mechanical mitral valve to the native mitral annulus. Mitral paravalvular leak (PVL) occurs when there is a physical separation between the prosthetic valve sewing ring and the native annulus. The etiologies of PVLs are multiple and may be related to technical issues at the time of surgery, subsequent endocarditis with erosion, or native annular calcium which does not allow secure suture attachment [55–57]. Although mitral PVLs have been reported to be a relatively rare occurrence, their

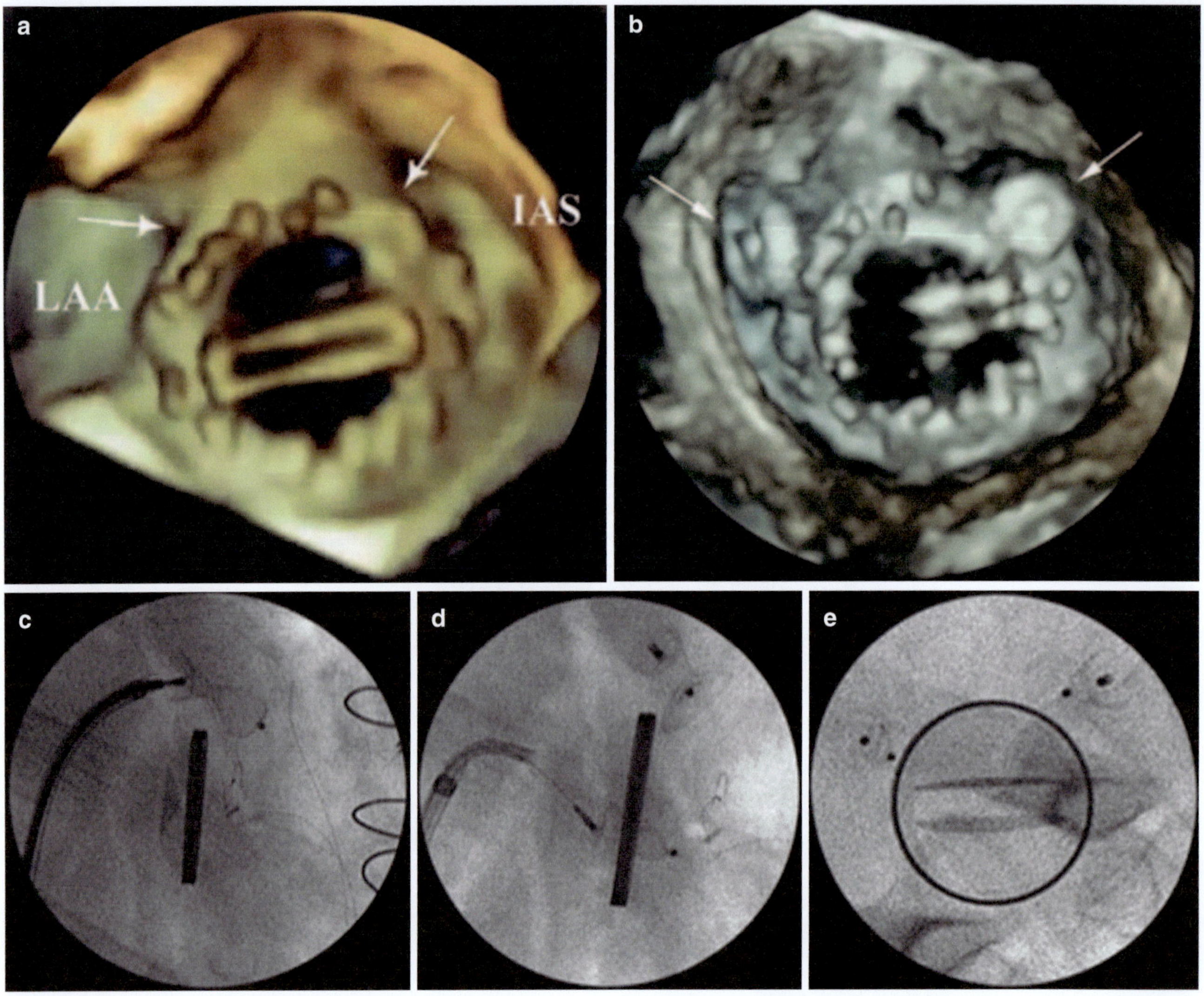

Fig. 28.14 Percutaneous mitral paravalvular leak closure. (**a**) 3-dimensional transesophageal echocardiographic (TEE) images showing mechanical mitral valve with pre-procedure lateral and medial paravalvular leak (PVL) defects (*arrows*) near the left atrial appendage (LAA) and interatrial septum (IAS). (**b**) Post-procedure 3-D TEE showing occluder devices in position with no interference of mechanical leaflet function. (**c**) RAO fluoroscopy of lateral PVL occluder being placed. (**d**) RAO fluoroscopy of medial PVL occluder being placed. (**e**) Final LAO caudal fluoroscopic view of mitral valve with both occluders in place

true prevalence may be higher since PVLs may not be detected if they are asymptomatic and since they are often not easily localized with routine transthoracic echocardiography [58]. Although most smaller defects are clinically asymptomatic and do not require intervention, clinically significant larger mitral PVLs can result in anemia due to hemolysis or congestive heart failure due to elevated left atrial pressures [59]. Reoperations for mitral PVLs carry significant morbidity and mortality and may not guarantee absence of recurrent PVLs since the quality of the native annular tissue is often suboptimal to begin with [60].

Formal society guidelines for percutaneous repair of mitral PVLs have not yet been published, but the procedure has evolved over the last decade and is increasingly applied in current practice. Clinical success rates have been reported in the range of ~60–90 %, but with a need for re-intervention in up to 40 % of cases [59, 61, 62]. Percutaneous PVL closures are challenging structural interventional procedures and, like other percutaneous therapies for mitral regurgitation, require an advanced understanding of anatomy, skilled ultrasound guidance (preferably with 3-D TEE), and a complete inventory of structural heart-related equipment including wires, specialty guides, and various occluders. Since one often encounters unexpected challenges during the procedure, the ability to adapt and innovate intraprocedurally is critical for success.

The procedure is performed under general anesthesia for patient comfort and to allow often lengthy TEE imaging to guide therapy. Localization and adequate visualization of the defect by 3-D TEE is preferred [63, 64]. The basic approach for closing PVLs consists of wiring the defect (antegrade transseptal or retrograde from a transaortic or transapical approach), establishing a stable guide position through the defect and then delivering an occluder successfully to reduce the regurgitant flow without impinging on important adjacent structures such as the prosthetic valve leaflets. Fluoroscopic views of the mitral annulus which are helpful are the RAO (side view) and LAO caudal (en face) views. Heparin is typically given for intraprocedural anticoagulation due to lengthy dwell times in the left atrium. Attention must be paid to device position as both mechanical and bioprosthetic valve dysfunction and erosion have been described as complications of the procedure [65, 66].

Since there are no specifically approved occluder devices for the treatment of mitral PVLs, "off-label" application of numerous occluder devices has been reported, including the Amplatzer septal occluder, patent ductus arteriosus occluder, muscular VSD occluder, and the Amplatzer Vascular Plugs I, II, III and IV [62]. An inherent limitation of all of these devices (with the exception of the Amplatzer Vascular Plug III) is that they are cylindrical in cross section, whereas the PVL tracts are often slit-like, crescent- or oval-shaped, and may have a serpiginous tunnel with alternating horizontal and vertical sections. There may be multiple discrete PVLs in the same patient, and the defects may also be quite wide. For wide defects, two smaller adjacently deployed occluders (through two adjacent delivery guides) may be required for adequate closure. The Amplatzer Vascular Plug III is a unique occluder that has a rectangular cross section and may therefore be more ideally suited for closure of crescentic paravalvular leaks. Despite this unique shape, it is not always possible to reliably orient the device so that it aligns with the defect. An initial report using this device is encouraging, but larger studies are needed to confirm efficacy [67]. In general, percutaneous repair should not be attempted in the event of regurgitant arcs greater than 90°, active endocarditis, or an unstable "rocking" valve. Hemolysis may occur after successfully reducing MR for treatment of heart failure symptoms. The etiology of hemolysis is multifactorial and includes unfavorable regurgitant tract morphology, increased jet velocities after device placement, and inherent red blood cell fragility. Hemolysis should initially be treated with supportive therapy such as red cell transfusions and erythropoietin and may take up to several months to abate as the device endothelializes and as the regurgitant tract morphology changes over time.

Post-procedure, patients must be followed with serial echocardiography to ensure durability of therapy and to document the absence of device migration over time. Antiplatelet therapy is given post-procedure and usually consists of aspirin and clopidogrel. With proper planning and patient selection, the majority of defects can be at least partially closed with currently available occludes. A case example of dual mitral paravalvular leak closure is shown in Fig. 28.14.

Conclusion

Interventional cardiology has seen the advent of a new era in the transcatheter management of mitral valve disease. The challenges for all these devices will be to demonstrate safety and either equivalent or superior efficacy in comparison to traditional management strategies, whether medical or surgical. We must strive to properly select patients for these new therapies and to develop effective technologies [51] to treat populations at high risk for surgery. Patience, collaboration, and vision are needed to fully develop these strategies.

References

1. Bonow RO, Carabello BA, Chatterjee K, et al. 2008 Focused update incorporated into the ACC/AHA 2006 guidelines for the management of patients with valvular heart disease: a report of the American College of Cardiology/American Heart Association Task Force on Practice Guidelines (Writing Committee to Revise the 1998 Guidelines for the Management of Patients With Valvular Heart Disease): endorsed by the Society of Cardiovascular Anesthesiologists, Society for Cardiovascular Angiography and Interventions, and Society of Thoracic Surgeons. Circulation. 2008;118(15):e523–661.
2. Vahanian A, Baumgartner H, Bax J, et al. Guidelines on the management of valvular heart disease: The Task Force on the Management of Valvular Heart Disease of the European Society of Cardiology. Eur Heart J. 2007;28(2):230–68.
3. Gammie JS, O'Brien SM, Griffith BP, Ferguson TB, Peterson ED. Influence of hospital procedural volume on care process and mortality for patients undergoing elective surgery for mitral regurgitation. Circulation. 2007;115(7):881–7.
4. Mirabel M, Iung B, Baron G, et al. What are the characteristics of patients with severe, symptomatic, mitral regurgitation who are denied surgery? Eur Heart J. 2007;28(11):1358–65.
5. O'Brien SM, Shahian DM, Filardo G, et al. The Society of Thoracic Surgeons 2008 cardiac surgery risk models: Part 2–isolated valve surgery. Ann Thorac Surg. 2009;88(1 Suppl):S23–42.
6. Carpentier A. Cardiac valve surgery–the "French correction". J Thorac Cardiovasc Surg. 1983;86(3):323–37.
7. Adams DH, Rosenhek R, Falk V. Degenerative mitral valve regurgitation: best practice revolution. Eur Heart J. 2010;31(16): 1958–66.
8. Barlow JB, Pocock WA. The significance of late systolic murmurs and mid-late systolic clicks. Md State Med J. 1963;12:76–7.
9. Ling LH, Enriquez-Sarano M, Seward JB, et al. Clinical outcome of mitral regurgitation due to flail leaflet. N Engl J Med. 1996;335(19):1417–23.
10. Enriquez-Sarano M, Schaff HV, Orszulak TA, Tajik AJ, Bailey KR, Frye RL. Valve repair improves the outcome of surgery for mitral regurgitation. A multivariate analysis. Circulation. 1995;91(4): 1022–8.

11. Seeburger J, Falk V, Borger MA, et al. Chordae replacement versus resection for repair of isolated posterior mitral leaflet prolapse: a egalite. Ann Thorac Surg. 2009;87(6):1715–20.
12. Bax JJ, Braun J, Somer ST, et al. Restrictive annuloplasty and coronary revascularization in ischemic mitral regurgitation results in reverse left ventricular remodeling. Circulation. 2004;110(11 Suppl 1):II103–8.
13. Wu AH, Aaronson KD, Bolling SF, Pagani FD, Welch K, Koelling TM. Impact of mitral valve annuloplasty on mortality risk in patients with mitral regurgitation and left ventricular systolic dysfunction. J Am Coll Cardiol. 2005;45(3):381–7.
14. Hung J, Papakostas L, Tahta SA, et al. Mechanism of recurrent ischemic mitral regurgitation after annuloplasty: continued LV remodeling as a moving target. Circulation. 2004;110(11 Suppl 1):II85–90.
15. Marwick TH. Restrictive annuloplasty for ischemic mitral regurgitation: too little or too much? J Am Coll Cardiol. 2008; 51(17):1702–3.
16. McGee EC, Gillinov AM, Blackstone EH, et al. Recurrent mitral regurgitation after annuloplasty for functional ischemic mitral regurgitation. J Thorac Cardiovasc Surg. 2004;128(6):916–24.
17. Braun J, van de Veire NR, Klautz RJ, et al. Restrictive mitral annuloplasty cures ischemic mitral regurgitation and heart failure. Ann Thorac Surg. 2008;85(2):430–6. discussion 436–437.
18. Magne J, Pibarot P, Dagenais F, Hachicha Z, Dumesnil JG, Senechal M. Preoperative posterior leaflet angle accurately predicts outcome after restrictive mitral valve annuloplasty for ischemic mitral regurgitation. Circulation. 2007;115(6):782–91.
19. Calafiore AM, Gallina S, Di Mauro M, et al. Mitral valve procedure in dilated cardiomyopathy: repair or replacement? Ann Thorac Surg. 2001;71(4):1146–52. discussion 1152–1143.
20. Chiam PT, Ruiz CE. Percutaneous transcatheter mitral valve repair: a classification of the technology. JACC Cardiovasc Interv. 2011; 4(1):1–13.
21. Rogers JH, Franzen O. Percutaneous edge-to-edge MitraClip therapy in the management of mitral regurgitation. Eur Heart J. 2011;32(19):2350–7.
22. Alfieri O, Maisano F, De Bonis M, et al. The double-orifice technique in mitral valve repair: a simple solution for complex problems. J Thorac Cardiovasc Surg. 2001;122(4):674–81.
23. Ussia GP, Barbanti M, Tamburino C. Feasibility of percutaneous transcatheter mitral valve repair with the MitraClip system using conscious sedation. Catheter Cardiovasc Interv. 2010;75(7):1137–40.
24. Herrmann HC, Kar S, Siegel R, et al. Effect of percutaneous mitral repair with the MitraClip device on mitral valve area and gradient. EuroIntervention. 2009;4(4):437–42.
25. Siegel RJ, Biner S, Rafique AM, et al. The acute hemodynamic effects of MitraClip therapy. J Am Coll Cardiol. 2011;57(16):1658–65.
26. Feldman T, Kar S, Rinaldi M, et al. Percutaneous mitral repair with the MitraClip system: safety and midterm durability in the initial EVEREST (Endovascular Valve Edge-to-Edge REpair Study) Cohort. J Am Coll Cardiol. 2009;54(8):686–94.
27. Feldman T, Foster E, Glower DG, et al. Percutaneous repair or surgery for mitral regurgitation. N Engl J Med. 2011;364:1395–406.
28. Feldman T, Mauri L, Kar S, et al. EVEREST II randomized clinical trial: a critical assessment of the safety data in patients treated with the MitraClip. J Am Coll Cardiol. 2010;56(13, Supplement 1):B23.
29. Magne J, Girerd N, Senechal M, et al. Mitral repair versus replacement for ischemic mitral regurgitation: comparison of short-term and long-term survival. Circulation. 2009;120(11 Suppl):S104–11.
30. Argenziano M, Skipper E, Heimansohn D, et al. Surgical revision after percutaneous mitral repair with the MitraClip device. Ann Thorac Surg. 2010;89(1):72–80. discussion p 80.
31. Rogers JH, Yeo KK, Carroll JD, et al. Late surgical mitral valve repair after percutaneous repair with the MitraClip system. J Card Surg. 2009;24(6):677–81.
32. Glower D, Young JN, Alexander J, et al. EVEREST II randomized clinical trial: a critical assessment of anatomical predictors of de novo mitral valve replacement or following the MitraClip procedure. J Am Coll Cardiol. 2010;56(13, Supplement 1):B25.
33. Franzen O, Baldus S, Rudolph V, et al. Acute outcomes of MitraClip therapy for mitral regurgitation in high-surgical-risk patients: emphasis on adverse valve morphology and severe left ventricular dysfunction. Eur Heart J. 2010;31(11):1373–81.
34. Tamburino C, Ussia GP, Maisano F, et al. Percutaneous mitral valve repair with the MitraClip system: acute results from a real world setting. Eur Heart J. 2010;31(11):1382–9.
35. Johnston DR, Gillinov AM, Blackstone EH, et al. Surgical repair of posterior mitral valve prolapse: implications for guidelines and percutaneous repair. Ann Thorac Surg. 2010;89(5):1385–94.
36. Flameng W, Herijgers P, Bogaerts K. Recurrence of mitral valve regurgitation after mitral valve repair in degenerative valve disease. Circulation. 2003;107(12):1609–13.
37. Gillinov AM, Cosgrove DM, Blackstone EH, et al. Durability of mitral valve repair for degenerative disease. J Thorac Cardiovasc Surg. 1998;116(5):734–43.
38. DiBardino DJ, ElBardissi AW, McClure RS, Razo-Vasquez OA, Kelly NE, Cohn LH. Four decades of experience with mitral valve repair: analysis of differential indications, technical evolution, and long-term outcome. J Thorac Cardiovasc Surg. 2010;139(1):76–83. discussion 83–74.
39. Biner S, Perk G, Kar S, et al. Utility of combined two-dimensional and three-dimensional transesophageal imaging for catheter-based mitral valve clip repair of mitral regurgitation. J Am Soc Echocardiogr. 2011;24(6):611–17.
40. Webb JG, Maisano F, Vahanian A, et al. Percutaneous suture edge-to-edge repair of the mitral valve. EuroIntervention. 2009; 5(1):86–9.
41. Maselli D, Guarracino F, Chiaramonti F, Mangia F, Borelli G, Minzioni G. Percutaneous mitral annuloplasty: an anatomic study of human coronary sinus and its relation with mitral valve annulus and coronary arteries. Circulation. 2006;114(5):377–80.
42. Tops LF, Van de Veire NR, Schuijf JD, et al. Noninvasive evaluation of coronary sinus anatomy and its relation to the mitral valve annulus: implications for percutaneous mitral annuloplasty. Circulation. 2007;115(11):1426–32.
43. Schofer J, Siminiak T, Haude M, et al. Percutaneous mitral annuloplasty for functional mitral regurgitation: results of the CARILLON Mitral Annuloplasty Device European Union Study. Circulation. 2009;120(4):326–33.
44. Webb JG, Harnek J, Munt BI, et al. Percutaneous transvenous mitral annuloplasty: initial human experience with device implantation in the coronary sinus. Circulation. 2006;113(6):851–5.
45. Harnek J, Webb JG, Kuck KH, et al. Transcatheter implantation of the MONARC coronary sinus device for mitral regurgitation: 1-year results from the EVOLUTION phase I study (Clinical Evaluation of the Edwards Lifesciences Percutaneous Mitral Annuloplasty System for the Treatment of Mitral Regurgitation). JACC Cardiovasc Interv. 2011;4(1):115–22.
46. Sack S, Kahlert P, Bilodeau L, et al. Percutaneous transvenous mitral annuloplasty: initial human experience with a novel coronary sinus implant device. Circ Cardiovasc Interv. 2009;2(4):277–84.
47. Kim JH, Kocaturk O, Ozturk C, et al. Mitral cerclage annuloplasty, a novel transcatheter treatment for secondary mitral valve regurgitation: initial results in swine. J Am Coll Cardiol. 2009;54(7):638–51.
48. Rogers JH, Macoviak JA, Rahdert DA, Takeda PA, Palacios IF, Low RI. Percutaneous septal sinus shortening. A novel procedure for the treatment of functional mitral regurgitation. Circulation. 2006;113(19):2329–34.
49. Palacios IF, Condado JA, Brandi S, et al. Safety and feasibility of acute percutaneous septal sinus shortening: first-in-human experience. Catheter Cardiovasc Interv. 2007;69(4):513–18.

50. Burr LH, Krayenbuhl C, Sutton MS. The mitral plication suture: a new technique of mitral valve repair. J Thorac Cardiovasc Surg. 1977;73(4):589–95.
51. Aybek T, Risteski P, Miskovic A, et al. Seven years' experience with suture annuloplasty for mitral valve repair. J Thorac Cardiovasc Surg. 2006;131(1):99–106.
52. Nagy ZL, Bodi A, Vaszily M, Szerafin T, Horvath A, Peterffy A. Five-year experience with a suture annuloplasty for mitral valve repair. Scand Cardiovasc J. 2000;34(5):528–32.
53. Heuser RR, Witzel T, Dickens D, Takeda PA. Percutaneous treatment for mitral regurgitation: the QuantumCor system. J Interv Cardiol. 2008;21(2):178–82.
54. Mishra YK, Mittal S, Jaguri P, Trehan N. Coapsys mitral annuloplasty for chronic functional ischemic mitral regurgitation: 1-year results. Ann Thorac Surg. 2006;81(1):42–6.
55. Miller DL, Morris JJ, Schaff HV, Mullany CJ, Nishimura RA, Orszulak TA. Reoperation for aortic valve periprosthetic leakage: identification of patients at risk and results of operation. J Heart Valve Dis. 1995;4(2):160–5.
56. Rallidis LS, Moyssakis IE, Ikonomidis I, Nihoyannopoulos P. Natural history of early aortic paraprosthetic regurgitation: a five-year follow-up. Am Heart J. 1999;138(2 Pt 1):351–7.
57. Schoen FJ, Levy RJ. Pathology of substitute heart valves: new concepts and developments. J Card Surg. 1994;9(2 Suppl):222–7.
58. Jindani A, Neville EM, Venn G, Williams BT. Paraprosthetic leak: a complication of cardiac valve replacement. J Cardiovasc Surg (Torino). 1991;32(4):503–8.
59. Pate GE, Al Zubaidi A, Chandavimol M, Thompson CR, Munt BI, Webb JG. Percutaneous closure of prosthetic paravalvular leaks: case series and review. Catheter Cardiovasc Interv. 2006;68(4):528–33.
60. Echevarria JR, Bernal JM, Rabasa JM, Morales D, Revilla Y, Revuelta JM. Reoperation for bioprosthetic valve dysfunction. A decade of clinical experience. Eur J Cardiothorac Surg. 1991; 5(10):523–6. discussion 527.
61. Sorajja P, Cabalka AK, Hagler DJ, et al. Successful percutaneous repair of perivalvular prosthetic regurgitation. Catheter Cardiovasc Interv. 2007;70(6):815–23.
62. Kim MS, Casserly IP, Garcia JA, Klein AJ, Salcedo EE, Carroll JD. Percutaneous transcatheter closure of prosthetic mitral paravalvular leaks: are we there yet? JACC Cardiovasc Interv. 2009;2(2): 81–90.
63. Johri AM, Yared K, Durst R, et al. Three-dimensional echocardiography-guided repair of severe paravalvular regurgitation in a bioprosthetic and mechanical mitral valve. Eur J Echocardiogr. 2009;10(4):572–5.
64. Singh P, Manda J, Hsiung MC, et al. Live/real time three-dimensional transesophageal echocardiographic evaluation of mitral and aortic valve prosthetic paravalvular regurgitation. Echocardiography. 2009;26(8):980–7.
65. Mandegar MH, Roshanali F. Prosthetic valve malfunction after Amplatzer closure of paravalvular leak. Ann Thorac Surg. 2011;91(2):614.
66. Rogers JH, Morris AS, Takeda PA, Low RI. Bioprosthetic leaflet erosion after percutaneous mitral paravalvular leak closure. JACC Cardiovasc Interv. 2010;3:122–3.
67. Nietlispach F, Johnson M, Moss RR, et al. Transcatheter closure of paravalvular defects using a purpose-specific occluder. JACC Cardiovasc Interv. 2010;3(7):759–65.
68. Feldman T et al. Atlas of percutaneous edge-to-edge mitral valve repair. New York: Springer; 2013.

Upper Extremity Interventions

29

Tracy Huynh and Carlos Mena-Hurtado

Upper extremity interventions account for 15 % of all symptomatic, extracranial cerebrovascular disease. Brachiocephalic/innominate and subclavian artery lesions account for the majority of upper extremity endovascular procedures with atherosclerotic occlusive disease as the principle etiology. Subclavian stenosis most frequently involves the ostial and/or proximal segment of the subclavian artery. The left subclavian artery is more frequently involved than the right [1].

Symptomatic subclavian and brachiocephalic stenotic lesions have historically been treated with open surgical revascularization. Technological advances and the evolution of endovascular therapies over the past decade have made percutaneous revascularization a feasible and safe alternative to surgery. High technical success rates (95 %) [2] and durable long-term primary and secondary patency rates approaching 80–95 % [2] have led to a paradigm shift in the way these lesions are now treated.

Surgical revascularization has been the standard of care for symptomatic subclavian/innominate artery obstruction. Although the technical success rate of surgery is high, there is a risk of major complications including stroke in 0.5–5 %, perioperative death (2–3 %), myocardial infarction, and an overall complication rate of 13–19 % based on older registries [3]. Catheter-based endovascular therapies reduce the morbidity and mortality associated with surgery. Patel et al. reported technical success rate with endovascular revascularization of 99.4 % (174/177) for stenotic lesions and 90.5 % for occlusions (19/21) [4]. Primary patency was reported to be 83 % and secondary patency 96 % [8].

T. Huynh, MD (✉)
Interventional Cardiology,
Yale-New Haven Hospital, New Haven, CT, USA
e-mail: tnhuynh@mednet.ucla.edu

C. Mena-Hurtado, MD
Coronary and Peripheral Interventions,
Department of Medicine, Yale New Haven Hospital,
Yale University, Fitkin Memorial Pavilion,
789 Howard Ave, 3rd Fl., New Haven, CT 06519, USA

Advantages to endovascular approach include lower morbidity and mortality with a shorter length of stay, use of conscious sedation obviating the need for general anesthesia, and lower risk of cranial nerve injury, myocardial infarction, wound infection, death, and stroke. Overall morbidity in open surgical repair versus endovascular repair (6–28 % vs. 2–11 %) and mortality (0–2.2 % vs. 0–1 %) is higher [5]. Taken as a whole, this has contributed to endovascular revascularization supplanting surgery as the initial treatment of subclavian or innominate artery stenosis.

Anatomy

The subclavian artery arises from the bifurcation of the brachiocephalic artery on the right and directly from the aortic arch on the left (Fig. 29.1). In 0.5 % of patients,

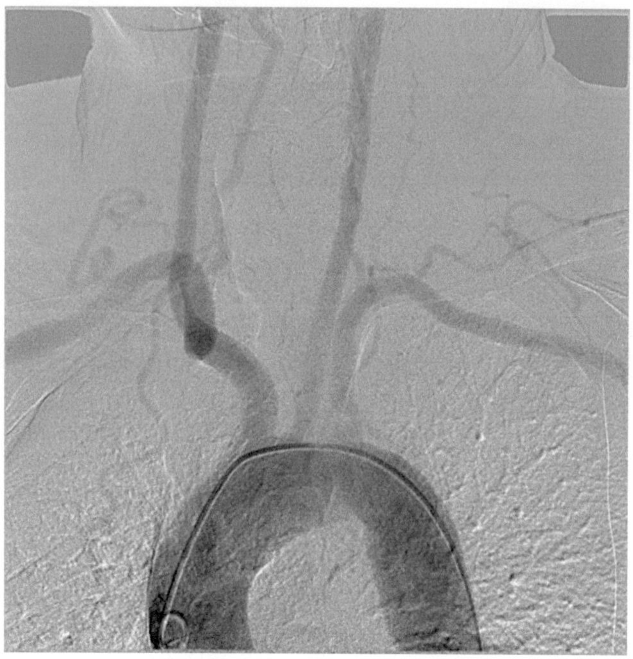

Fig. 29.1 Normal aortic arch

C.A. Thompson (ed.), *Textbook of Cardiovascular Intervention*,
DOI 10.1007/978-1-4471-4528-8_29, © Springer-Verlag London 2014

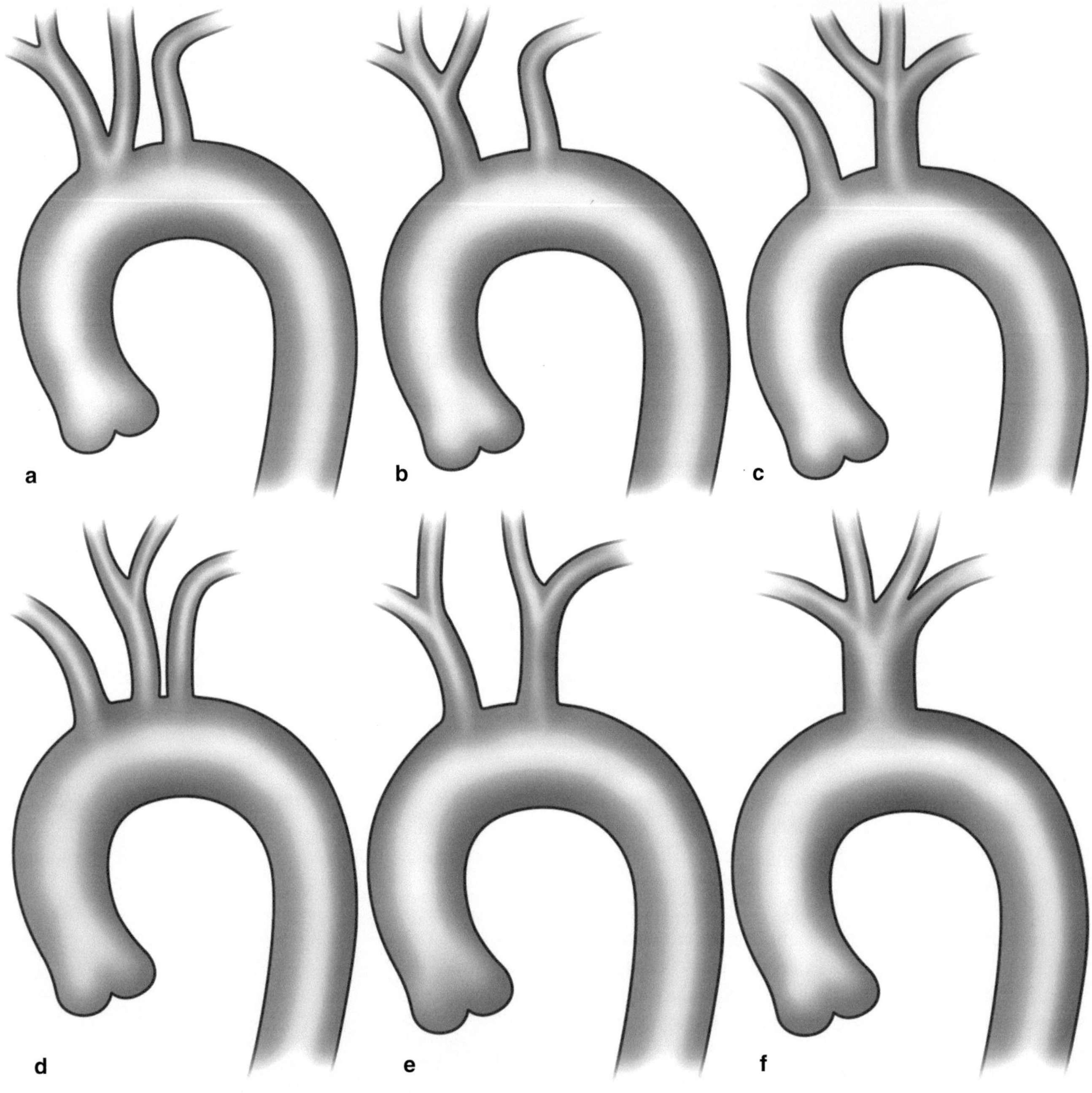

Fig. 29.2 Aortic arch variants - (**a**) common trunk of brachiocephalic trunk and right common carotid artery (bovine arch), (**b**) left common carotid artery arising from brachiocephalic trunk, (**c**) right and left common carotid arising from left subclavian artery, (**d**) right and left carotid arteries arising from common aortic trunk, (**e**) left common carotid artery arising from left subclavian artery, and (**f**) common trunk for subclavian and carotid arteries

the right subclavian artery arises anomalously from its own origin as the terminal vessel of the descending aorta. The left subclavian artery may arise anomalously from the innominate artery in 10 % of patients (bovine arch). Other variants exist, such as a common origin of the innominate and left subclavian artery and the origination of the left vertebral artery directly from the aortic arch (Fig. 29.2).

The most important branches of the subclavian artery arise from the proximal segment of the artery (the vertebral and the internal mammary branches of the subclavian artery). These branches supply the posterior cerebral circulation (vertebral) and anterior chest wall (internal mammary artery). In 5 % of patients, the left vertebral artery arises directly from the aortic arch between the left subclavian artery and left common carotid artery. The subclavian artery is divided into three parts: proximal (ostium to origin of vertebral artery), middle (segment including vertebral and IMA), and distal (segment beyond IA to lateral border of pectoralis minor).

At the lateral margin of the first rib, the subclavian artery becomes the axillary artery. The axillary artery gives off the anterior and posterior circumflex humeral branches before continuing on as the brachial artery at the distal aspect of the humerus. In the forearm, the brachial artery supplies the deep brachial branch that runs posteriorly and the superior and inferior ulnar collateral arteries. At the elbow, the brachial artery gives rise to the radial and the ulnar arteries.

The ulnar artery is usually the larger of the two branches in the forearm, and it gives rise to the anterior and posterior ulnar recurrent arteries supplying collateral flow to the elbow before giving rise to the common interosseous artery in the antecubital fossa. The ulnar artery then descends along the medial aspect of the forearm. The radial artery gives off a recurrent radial branch before traversing the lateral aspect of the forearm. In some cases, the radial artery may originate high from the axillary (1–3 % cases) or upper brachial artery (15–20 % cases) [4].

In the hand, the ulnar artery supplies the superficial palmar arch, while the radial artery supplies the deep palmar arch (Fig. 29.3). In 10 % of cases, the anterior interosseous or median artery supplies the deep palmar arch. The princeps pollicis and radialis indicis arteries arise from the radial artery and supply the thumb and index finger. The superficial palmar arch gives off three or four common palmar digital arteries, and the deep palmar arch gives off the palmar metacarpal arteries. At the bases of the proximal phalanges, adjacent metacarpal vessels from each arch join and divide into the proper digital arteries to supply the fingers.

Patient Selection

As with all endovascular procedures, careful patient selection is crucial to maximizing patient safety and procedural success rates while minimizing the risk of complications. This requires careful planning and a fundamental knowledge of normal and abnormal vascular anatomy in addition to details of each patient's history, physical examination, and noninvasive test results. An understanding of the technical nuances, safety, indications, and potential complications is essential before undertaking a peripheral intervention.

In general, endovascular revascularization is reserved for patients with symptomatic subclavian or brachiocephalic disease. However, most patients with subclavian or brachiocephalic artery disease are asymptomatic due to the

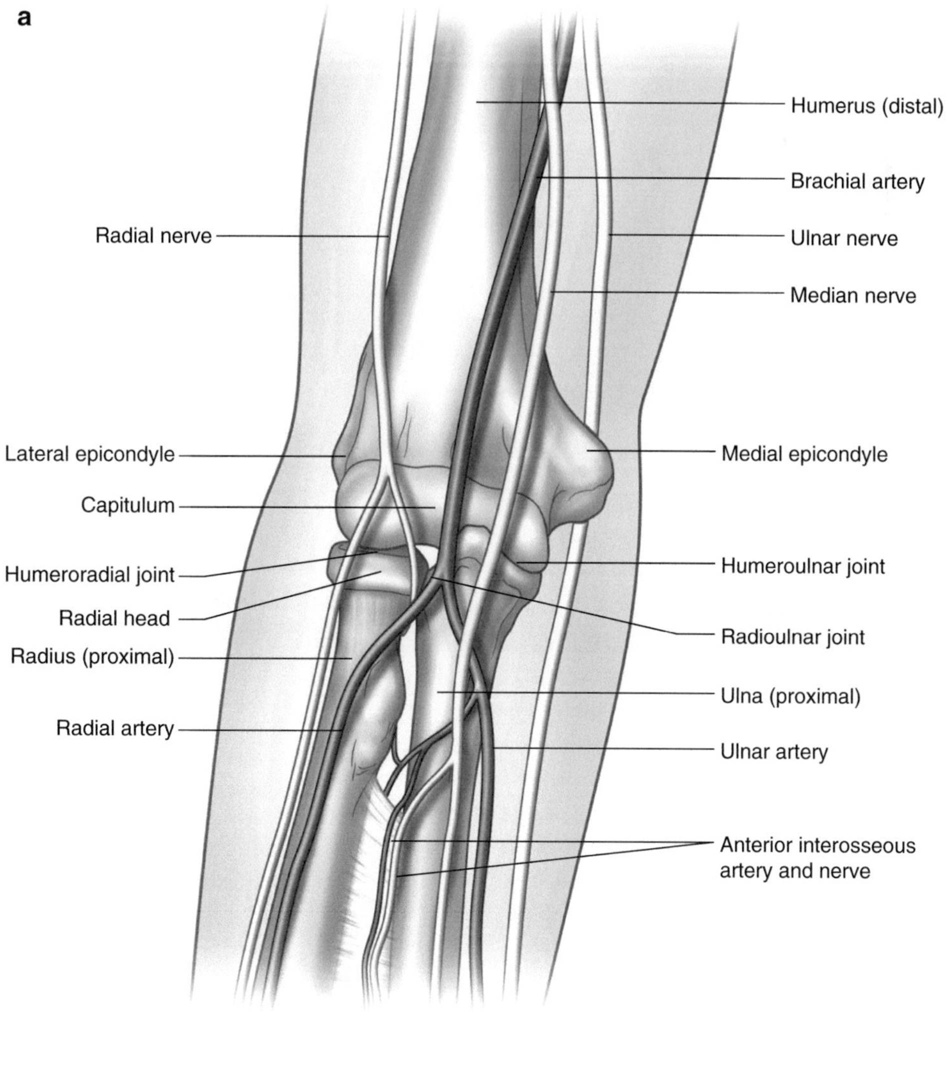

Fig. 29.3 (**a** and **b**) Brachial and hand circulation

Fig. 29.3 (continued)

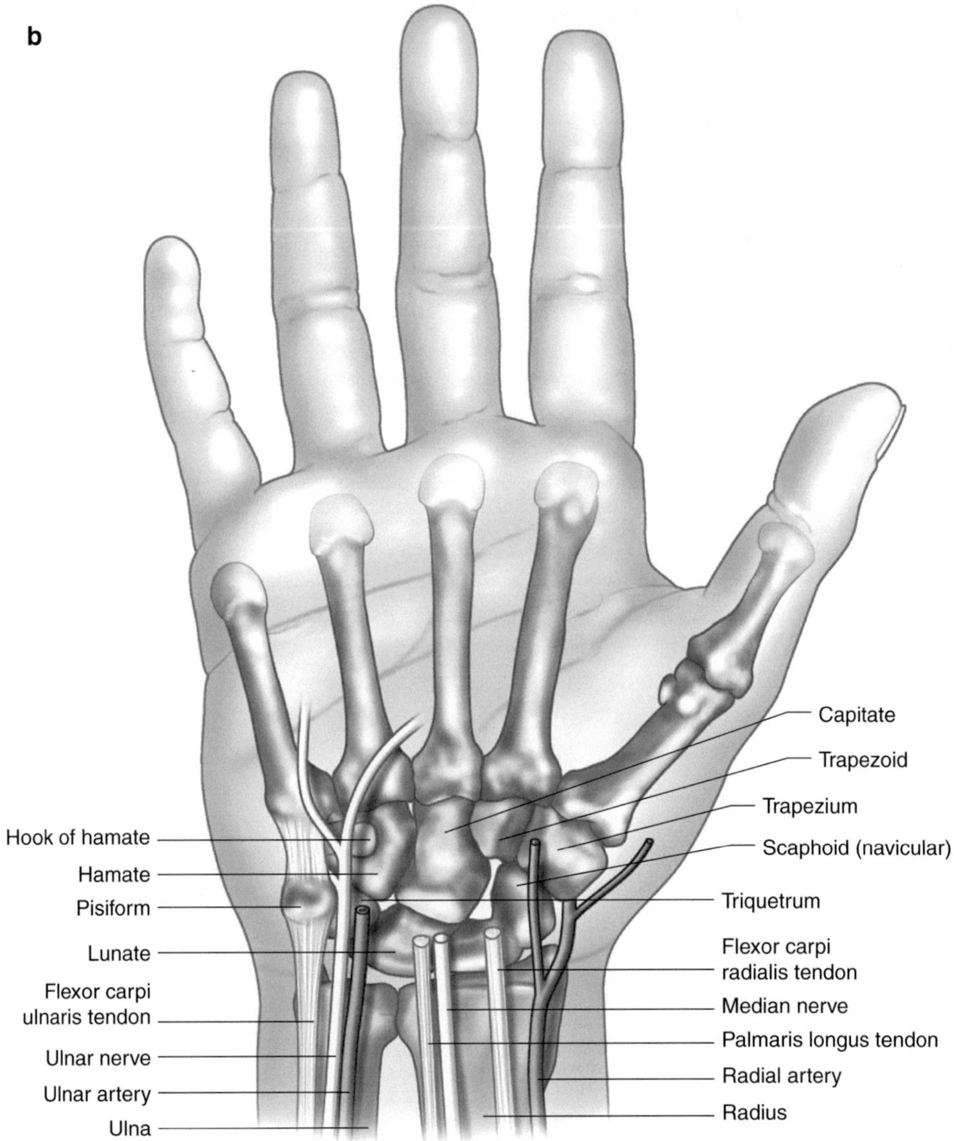

slow development of atherosclerosis over time and the rich network of collateral flow that develops. These lesions are usually detected incidentally by the finding of asymmetric arm blood pressures difference of >15 mmHg or on noninvasive imaging performed for another indication. Arm pain, fatigue, ache, heaviness, or numbness with exertion may be misdiagnosed as arthritis, a pinched nerve, or other neuromusculoskeletal disorders. Evidence of distal thromboembolism, acute upper extremity limb ischemia, or chronic ischemic symptom (ischemic rest pain or digital ulceration) is a sign of upper extremity stenosis or occlusion. Symptoms such as dizziness, diplopia, nystagmus, ataxia, vertigo, drop attacks, or syncope may be due to compromise of the posterior cerebral circulation as a result of significant subclavian steal syndrome (SSS) with retrograde vertebral flow in the setting of significant subclavian stenosis (Table 29.1).

Table 29.1 Indications for upper extremity intervention

Indication
Upper extremity claudication
Vertebrobasilar insufficiency
Ischemia or ulceration due to distal embolization
Subclavian steal syndrome (SSS):
Coronary-subclavian steal symptoms
Vertebral-subclavian steal symptoms
Preemptive protection of coronary artery bypass graft (IMA)
Protection of axillofemoral bypass or lower extremity claudication with axillofemoral graft
Protection of axillo-axillo bypass graft
Protection of arterio-venous fistula
Preemptive left subclavian stenting prior to thoracic endovascular aortic repair (TEVAR) [9]

From Aiello and Morrissey [5], with permission

In patients with prior bypass surgery, angina or ischemia due to compromised flow through the IMA bypass graft may occur due to subclavian stenosis or brachiocephalic stenosis on the right.

The major contraindication to subclavian/brachiocephalic intervention is the presence of an acute thrombus. Embolization to the vertebral artery or right internal carotid artery during subclavian or brachiocephalic artery intervention is an important complication. With thrombotic lesions, we recommend treatment with either thrombolytics or anticoagulation for 4 weeks prior to intervention. The use of embolic protection devices should also be considered. Patients with long occlusions (>5 cm) combined with severe calcification and occlusions in proximity of the vertebral artery ostium and patients with arteritis should be considered for surgical revascularization.

The major risk of upper extremity interventions is the risk of distal embolization; however, this risk is low and generally less than 1 % in most series. [4] Access site complications are another common complication with a rate of up to 5 % in some series. The major risk for access site complication is brachial access due to difficulty to control hemostasis, hematoma, thrombosis, fistula formation, and pseudoaneurysm. Stent migration has also been reported, possibly due to stent malapposition. The rate of stent restenosis is less than 10–15 % and comparable to surgical failure rates [2]. Other complications related to access site including groin infection and nerve injury.

Upper Extremity Angiography

An arch aortogram should be performed first in a left anterior oblique (LAO) 45° projection using an angled pigtail catheter positioned approximately 3–4 cm above the aortic root. This is done using a power injection on the digital subtraction angiography (DSA) mode using 40 ml of contrast at 20 ml/s at 900 psi. Raising the table and minimizing the distance between the patient and image intensifier will allow one to maximize the field of view. Delineation of the origin of the subclavian artery and its relation to the stenotic area and the vertebral and internal mammary arteries is crucial. Careful attention should be paid to arch angulation, anomalous circulation and great vessel takeoff, tortuosity involving the brachiocephalic or proximal subclavian arteries, or the presence of a type II or III aortic arch. This will assist in determining whether a long sheath or guide catheter system should be used to engage the branch vessels and influence the choice of equipment selected. Iodixanol (Visipaque), an iso-osmolar nonionic contrast agent, is the preferred contrast agent for use in peripheral angiography as it is readily tolerated and does not burn.

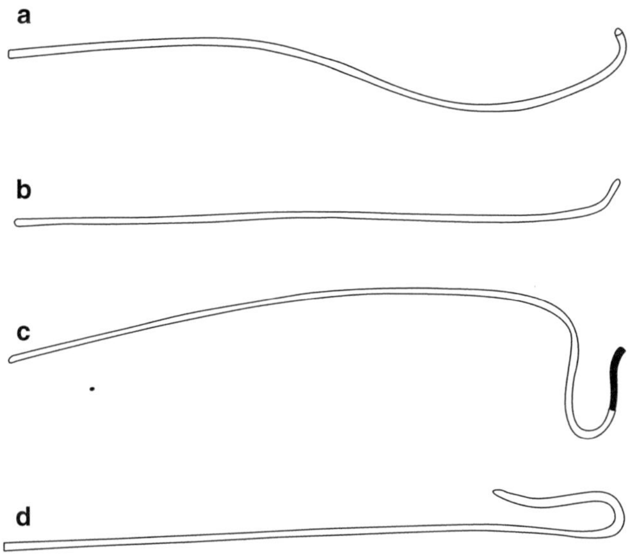

Fig. 29.4 Diagnostic catheters that are used in carotid angiography and stenting. (**a**) The most commonly used catheter is the JR4. (**b**) The angled glide catheter can be used in simple arches. (**c**) The Vitek and (**d**) Simmons are the reverse-angled catheters that are used in difficult arches

Appropriate catheter selection is vital in successful engagement of the lesion and peripheral intervention. Using the arch aortogram as a roadmap, selective engagement of the brachiocephalic artery and left subclavian artery can be achieved using a multitude of catheters (JR 4, Multipurpose, Berenstein, angled glide) in the LAO 45° projection. For most patients, selective engagement of the arch vessels can be achieved using a 5 Fr JR 4 or angled glide catheter. In patients with type III arches, alternative catheters such as Vitek, Simmons, Headhunter-1 catheters may be used with careful handling (Fig. 29.4). The Vitek catheter is brought into the descending artery over a 0.035″ wire. After the wire is removed, the catheter is then advanced and rotated in a clockwise direction and advanced to engage the arch vessels. To disengage, the catheter is rotated counterclockwise and withdrawn. After successful engagement of the brachiocephalic or subclavian artery, selective angiography should be performed in multiple views using DSA. The bifurcation of the brachiocephalic and right subclavian artery is best delineated in a right anterior oblique (RAO) projection. The origin of the right vertebral and right internal mammary artery (RIMA) is best laid out in the LAO projection. For the left subclavian artery, the origin of the left vertebral artery and LIMA is best visualized in the RAO projection, while the bifurcation of the left subclavian artery and common carotid artery is best delineated in an LAO projection. In patients suspected of having thoracic outlet syndrome, angiography should be performed in the posterior-anterior (PA) position with the arm in neutral position and then repeated with the arm abducted and externally rotated.

Selective angiography of the axillary or brachial arteries requires advancement of a diagnostic catheter into the distal subclavian artery. We recommend the use of a soft-tipped 0.035 wire such as a Versacore, Wholey, Magic Torque, or Bentson wire. A JR 4, Berenstein, or angled glide catheter is used to perform selective angiography. Vitek or Simmons catheters should be exchanged out for one of these catheters as they are less likely to cause vascular trauma.

Adequate angiography of the forearm and fingers requires advancement of the diagnostic catheter into the distal brachial artery. We recommend liberal use of vasodilators such as nitroglycerin and calcium channel blockers. The fingers and thumb should be abducted. The use of a warm compress may help with vasodilation. In general, a posterior-anterior (PA) projection provides adequate delineation of these vessels.

Subclavian and Brachiocephalic Artery Intervention

After selective upper extremity angiography is performed, selective engagement of the subclavian or innominate artery is achieved using either a short sheath and diagnostic catheter or a long sheath.

Choice of Access Site

The choice of access site for upper extremity intervention is strongly influenced by the severity of the obstruction. A long sheath may be delivered selectively into the branch vessels. Most subclavian stenosis can be approached from the femoral artery with high success rates. Femoral access is the preferred approach for its simplicity, allowing visualization of the ostium of the vessel. In addition, it is associated with fewer access site complications when performing upper extremity interventions and permits for delivery of larger sheaths. For complete occlusions or ostial lesions, access via the ipsilateral radial or brachial artery is preferred as this provides superior guide catheter and wire support. Brachial site access, however, is associated with higher access site complications, with up to 5 % rate of brachial artery thrombosis when using 7 Fr sheaths [6, 7].

From the femoral approach, we selectively engage the origin of the subclavian artery using a 5 Fr diagnostic catheter, advance a 0.035″ stiff guidewire (Glide Advantage, Rosen, TAD) across the lesion, and then deliver a 6–8 Fr 90 cm long sheath (destination or shuttle sheath) over the guide catheter and position it at the subclavian ostium using a telescoping technique (Fig. 29.5). For tortuous or high-grade aorto-iliac disease, access via the radial or brachial artery may be preferred.

Pharmacology

All patients are pretreated with aspirin 325 mg and a thienopyridine (generally clopidogrel 600 mg) prior to the procedure. Systemic anticoagulation is then administered, either with unfractionated heparin after a bolus of 70 units/

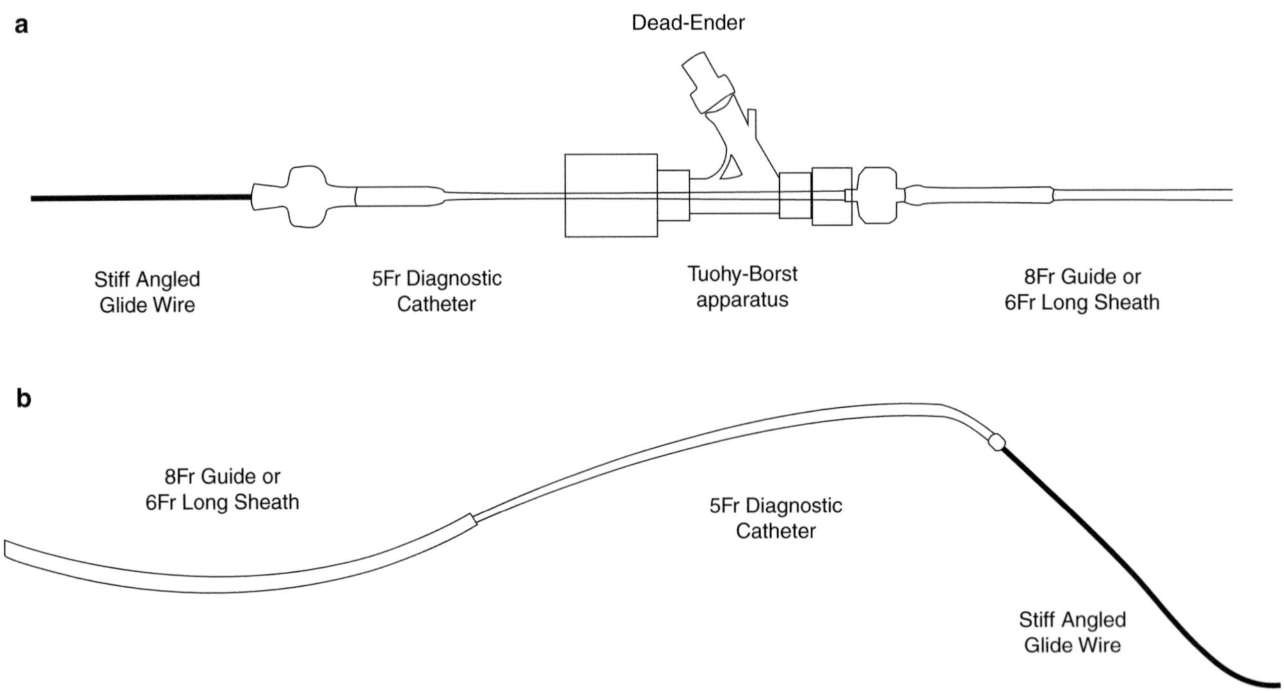

Fig. 29.5 The "telescoping technique." (**a**) The *back end* consists of a 5F diagnostic catheter "telescoped" through a Tuohy-Borst apparatus and an 8F guide/6F long sheath. (**b**) The *top end* of this system with a stiff angled glidewire (From MacDonald and Stansby [10], Ch. 12, with permission)

kg to achieve an activated clotting time (ACT) of 250–300 s or with bivalirudin in patients with contraindications to heparin.

Balloon Angioplasty

Stenotic lesions can be crossed with multiple wires (0.014, 0.018, and 0.035). For occlusions, an angled glidewire and catheter are generally preferred. Most balloons fit over a 0.035″ wire and several are deliverable over a 0.018″ wire. The risk of dissection can be minimized using a conservative approach to balloon sizing, using a balloon diameter 70 % of the estimated vessel diameter or 2 sizes smaller to minimize risk of dissection. For most subclavian vessels, this is 5–7 mm. Intravascular ultrasound may also be helpful in vessel sizing. With the excellent results achieved with stenting, stand-alone balloon angioplasty is rarely performed nowadays.

Stenting

Subclavian lesions proximal to the vertebral artery are treated using balloon-expandable stents to allow for accurate stent deployment with respect to the aortic arch and vertebral artery (Fig. 29.6). These stents provide the strong radial force required in this area. Self-expanding stents can be used for longer lesions or in the mid and distal subclavian arteries beyond the vertebral artery. In general, most subclavian arteries are 6–8 mm in diameter. For ostial lesions, we prefer balloon-expandable stents for accurate stent deployment, being careful not to impinge on the IMA or vertebral arteries. The stent should extend a few millimeters into the aorta and the stent flared with post-dilation. Stent deployment involving the ostium should be performed in multiple orthogonal views. In general, we recommend a diameter equivalent to that of the reference vessel when using balloon-expandable stents and selection of a stent with a diameter 1 mm larger than that of the reference vessel for self-expanding stents.

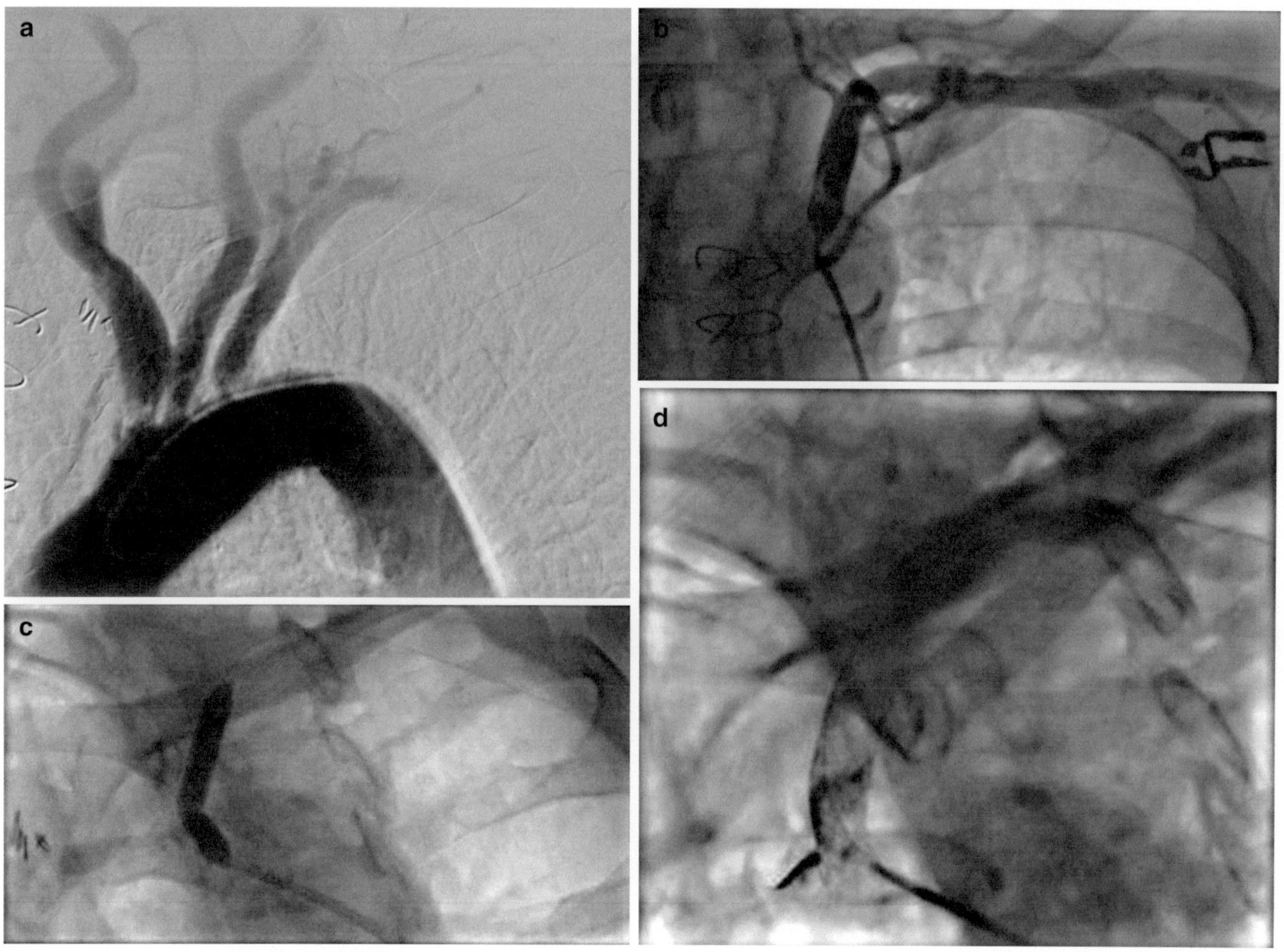

Fig. 29.6 Patient with coronary-subclavian steal, CABG, and anterior ischemia. (**a**) Scout image demonstrating left subclavian artery stenosis. (**b**) Selective angiography demonstrating high-grade left subclavian stenosis. (**c**) Demonstration of adequate stent placement extending into aorta. (**d**) Final result

For occlusive lesions, additional access using the radial or brachial artery is required (Fig. 29.7). In general, a 6 Fr 23–55 mm length sheath is used from the ipsilateral upper extremity. These lesions are generally crossed with an angled glidewire and catheter. Sometimes, a stiff 0.014″ wire (Confianza, Miracle Bros 6 g) may be successful in crossing the lesion. Finding the true lumen at the ostium of the subclavian artery is crucial as dissection into the aorta may compromise flow to other arch vessels. The use of intravascular ultrasound may be helpful in confirming

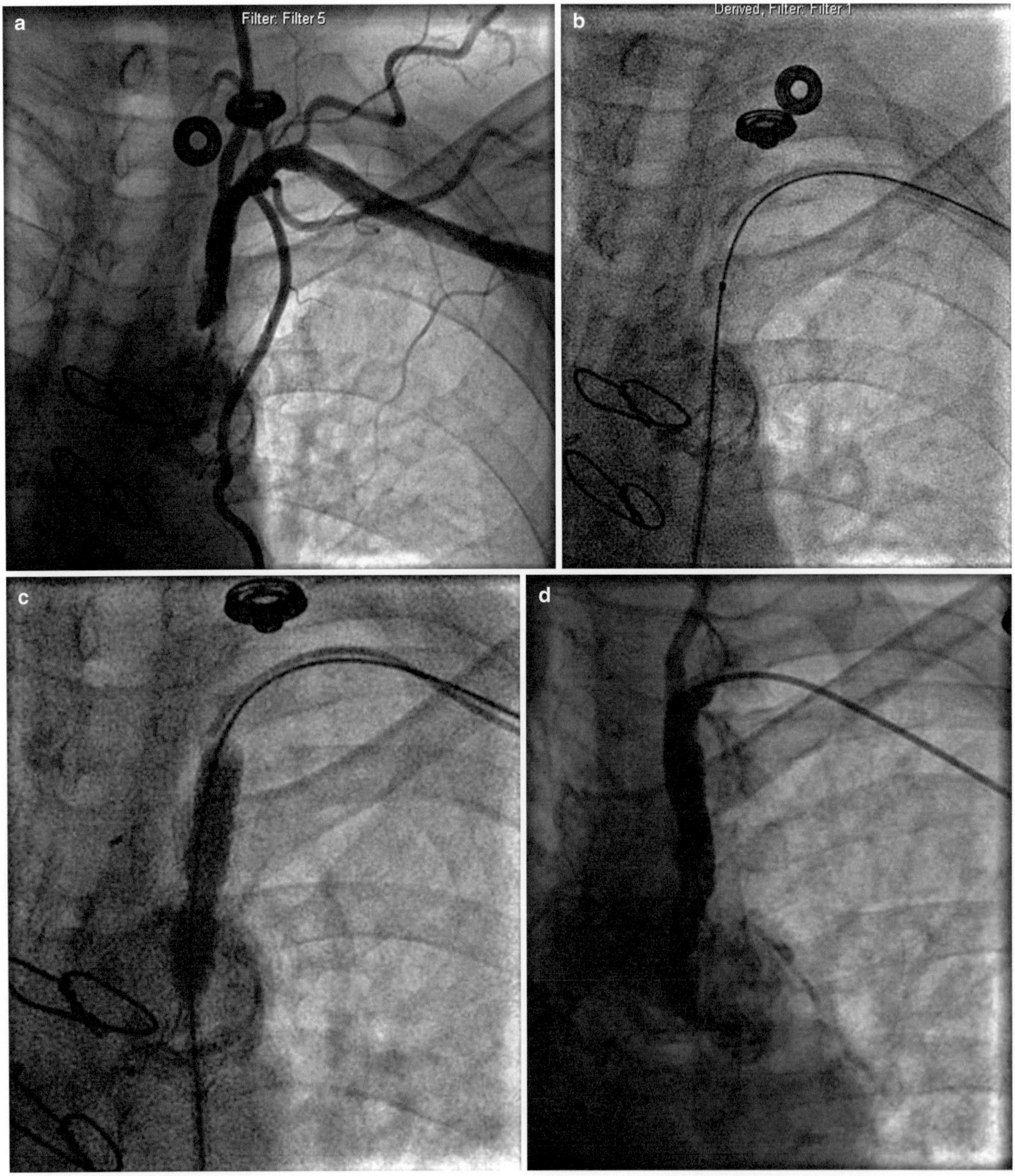

Fig. 29.7 (**a**–**d**) Patient with occlusive lesion requiring brachial access

true lumen position. Success rates for stenting of occlusions are lower than for stenotic lesions (80–90 %) and are dependent on operator experience. Technical success rate is defined as ≤30 % residual stenosis, blood pressure difference ≤10 mmHg, and pressure gradient across the lesion <5 mmHg. Risk factors for in-stent restenosis include the use of more than one stent, smaller stent diameter, and residual blood pressure difference post intervention [8].

For brachiocephalic intervention, there is a higher risk of embolization. In this case, the use of an embolic protection device (EPD) should be considered although its use remains controversial. There are many available, with distal filter protection devices placed in the internal carotid artery being most common. All EPDs require additional right brachial artery access. In general, an IM catheter is delivered from the brachial artery and a filter is deployed in the internal carotid artery. The brachiocephalic lesion is crossed antegrade from the aorta and a wire is delivered into the external carotid artery. Balloon angioplasty and stenting is performed similar to subclavian intervention.

Post-procedural Management

In general, most patients tolerate the procedure well and are able to be discharged the following day. Patients should be maintained on dual antiplatelet therapy with aspirin and a thienopyridine for a minimum of 1 month and then single antiplatelet therapy indefinitely. Prior to discharge, blood pressure recordings in both arms should be documented. During follow-up, patients should be assessed for recurrence of symptoms. Duplex ultrasound may be performed if clinical suspicion arises of restenosis. In general, early detection of stenosis before progression to occlusion is important in maintaining secondary patency rates above 90–95 %.

References

1. Shadman R, Criqui MH, Bundens WP, et al. Subclavian artery stenosis: prevalence, risk factors, and association with cardiovascular diseases. J Am Coll Cardiol. 2004;44:618–23.
2. Patel SN, White CJ, Collins TJ, et al. Catheter-Based Treatment of the Subclavian and Innominate Arteries. Cathet Cardiovasc Interv. 2008;71:963–8.
3. Palchik E, Bakken AM, Wolford HY, et al. Subclavian artery revascularization: an outcome analysis based on mode of therapy and presenting symptoms. Ann Vasc Surg. 2008;22(1):70–8.
4. Capers IV Q, Phillips J. Advances in percutaneous therapy for upper extremity arterial disease. Cardiol Clin. 2011;29:351–61.
5. Aiello F, Morrissey NJ. Open and endovascular management of subclavian and innominate arterial pathology. Semin Vasc Surg. 2011;24:31–5.
6. Sullivan TM, Gray BH, Bacharach JM, et al. Angioplasty and primary stenting of the subclavian, innominate and common carotid arteries in 83 patients. J Vasc Surg. 1998;25:1059–65.
7. Rodriquez-Lpez JA, Werner A, Martinez R, et al. Stenting for atherosclerotic occlusive disease of the subclavian artery. Ann Vasc Surg. 1999;13:254–60.
8. Przewlocki T, Kablak-Ziembicka A, Pieniazek P, et al. Determinants of immediate and long-term results of subclavian and innominate artery angioplasty. Cathet Cardiovasc Interv. 2006;67:519–26.
9. Matsumara JS, Rizvi AZ. Left subclavian artery revascularization: Society for Vascular Surgery Practice Guidelines. J Vasc Surg. 2010;52:65S–70.
10. MacDonald S, Stansby G. Practical carotid stenting. New York: Springer; 2009.

30 Percutaneous Management of Lower Extremity Arterial Disease: Patient Selection, Techniques, and Technologies

Subhash Banerjee and Kimberly Brayton

Peripheral arterial disease (PAD) involving lower extremity arterial vessels is a common manifestation of generalized atherosclerosis that affects a large proportion of the adult population worldwide [1]. Though intermittent claudication and critical limb ischemia are recognized presentations of lower extremity PAD, it is important to point out that a large number of patients present with subclinical forms of PAD and are asymptomatic. In fact, the presence of symptomatic expression of lower extremity PAD defines a small subset of the total population with the disease; it is estimated that out of nearly eight million men and women with PAD in the United States, 20–50 % are asymptomatic [2].

Management of symptomatic PAD is multidisciplinary and is most effective when it involves a closely coordinated approach between primary care providers, interventional cardiologists, radiologists, and vascular surgeons [3]. Significant technological strides made in the area of endovascular therapy, together with a marked increase in endovascular training, have led to a remarkable improvement in endovascular capabilities and procedural volumes around the globe. Endovascular procedures are also favored given the increased risk of adverse cardiovascular events associated with vascular surgical procedures in patients with PAD [4]. Ultimately, the decision to pursue endovascular therapy versus surgical revascularization is individualized and depends on patient characteristics as well as lesion characteristics. The most widely used system of lesion classification in peripheral artery disease is set forth in the TransAtlantic Inter-Society Consensus (TASC) documents, shown for aortoiliac disease in Fig. 30.1 and for femoropopliteal disease in Fig. 30.2. The rest of the chapter offers an overview of the indications for endovascular management, as well as an introduction to the endovascular techniques and technologies applied in current practice.

S. Banerjee, MD (✉) • K. Brayton, MD
Division of Cardiology,
VA North Texas Healthcare System, Dallas, TX, USA

UT Southwestern Medical School, Dallas, TX, USA
e-mail: subhash.banerjee@va.gov

Patient and Lesion Selection for Endovascular Management of Claudication

The therapeutic goal of endovascular treatment in patients with claudication is improving quality of life. Endovascular procedures are primarily indicated for claudicants who have an inadequate response to exercise or pharmacological therapy. Clinical outcomes are most durable for TASC type A iliac and femoropopliteal arterial lesions [6]. This is a class I indication in the American College of Cardiology (ACC)/American Heart Association (AHA) guidelines for the management of patients with peripheral arterial disease [6]. Note that the guideline-based support for endovascular intervention for the management of claudication is limited to suprapopliteal lesions – there is no routine indication for infrapopliteal percutaneous interventions for claudication.

Translesional pressure gradients (with and without vasodilation) should be obtained for the evaluation of lesions of intermediate (50–70 % diameter) angiographic severity. However, catheter-derived pressure gradient measurements across vascular lesions may lead to overestimation of the physiologic significance of these lesions and thus to inappropriate intervention. Instead, use of a pressure wire for hemodynamic interrogation may be a better tool for the assessment of the hemodynamic significance of a peripheral vascular lesion [7]. A study from our group reported the association between an invasive hemodynamic measure (translesional gradient), patient symptom status (assessed by a walking impairment questionnaire), and a noninvasive measure of ankle-brachial index in the infrainguinal arterial distribution. A translesional gradient ≥11 mmHg (assessed with a 0.014″ pressure wire) after 100 μg of intra-arterial adenosine was 100 % specific, reasonably sensitive (sensitivity 71.43 %), and provided

C.A. Thompson (ed.), *Textbook of Cardiovascular Intervention*,
DOI 10.1007/978-1-4471-4528-8_30, © Springer-Verlag London 2014

Type A lesions

- Unilateral or bilateral stenoses of CIA
- Unilateral or bilateral single short (≤3 cm) stenosis of EIA

Type B lesions

- Short (≤3cm) stenosis of infrarena aorta
- Unilateral CIA occlusion
- Single or multiple stenosis totaling 3–10 cm involving the EIA not extending into the CFA
- Unilateral EIA occlusion not involving the origins of internal iliac or CFA

Type C lesions

- Bilateral CIA occlusions
- Bilateral EIA stenoses 3–10 cm long not extending into the CFA
- Unilteral EIA stenosis extending into the CFA
- Unilateral EIA occlusion that involving the origins of internal iliac or CFA
- Heavily calcified unilateral EIA occlusion with or without involvement of origins of internal iliac and/or CFA

Type D lesions

- Infra-renal aortoiliac occlusion
- Diffuse disease involving the aorta and both iliac arteries requiring treatment
- Diffuse multiple stenoses involving the unilateral CIA, EIA, and CFA
- Unilateral occlusions of both CIA and EIA
- Bilateral occlusion of EIA
- Illiac stenoses in patients with AAA requiring treatment and not amenable to endograft placement or other lesions requiring open aortic or iliac surgery

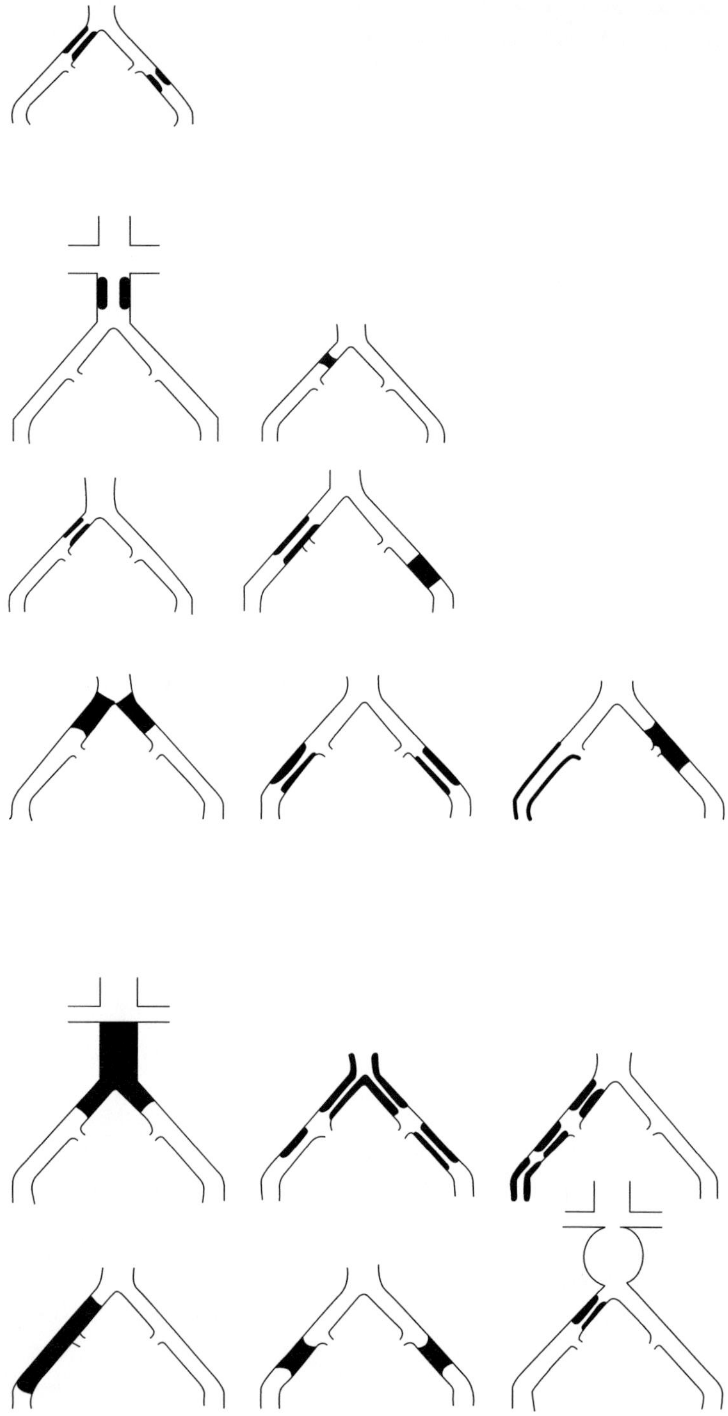

Fig. 30.1 TASC classification of aortoiliac disease (From Norgren et al. [5], with permission)

the greatest discriminating ability to diagnose symptomatic PAD. Assessment of lower extremity hyperemic translesional gradients could have several important applications in daily clinical practice. It could allow the determination of the functional severity of arterial lesions in patients who undergo angiography for PAD symptoms, potentially target treatment of such lesions, and assess response to endovascular treatment [8].

There is ample evidence for the durability of stents as a primary therapy for common iliac and external iliac lesions, with particularly robust data for common iliac stenting. Stents may be provisionally used in all iliac artery distributions for suboptimal or failed balloon angioplasty (PTA).

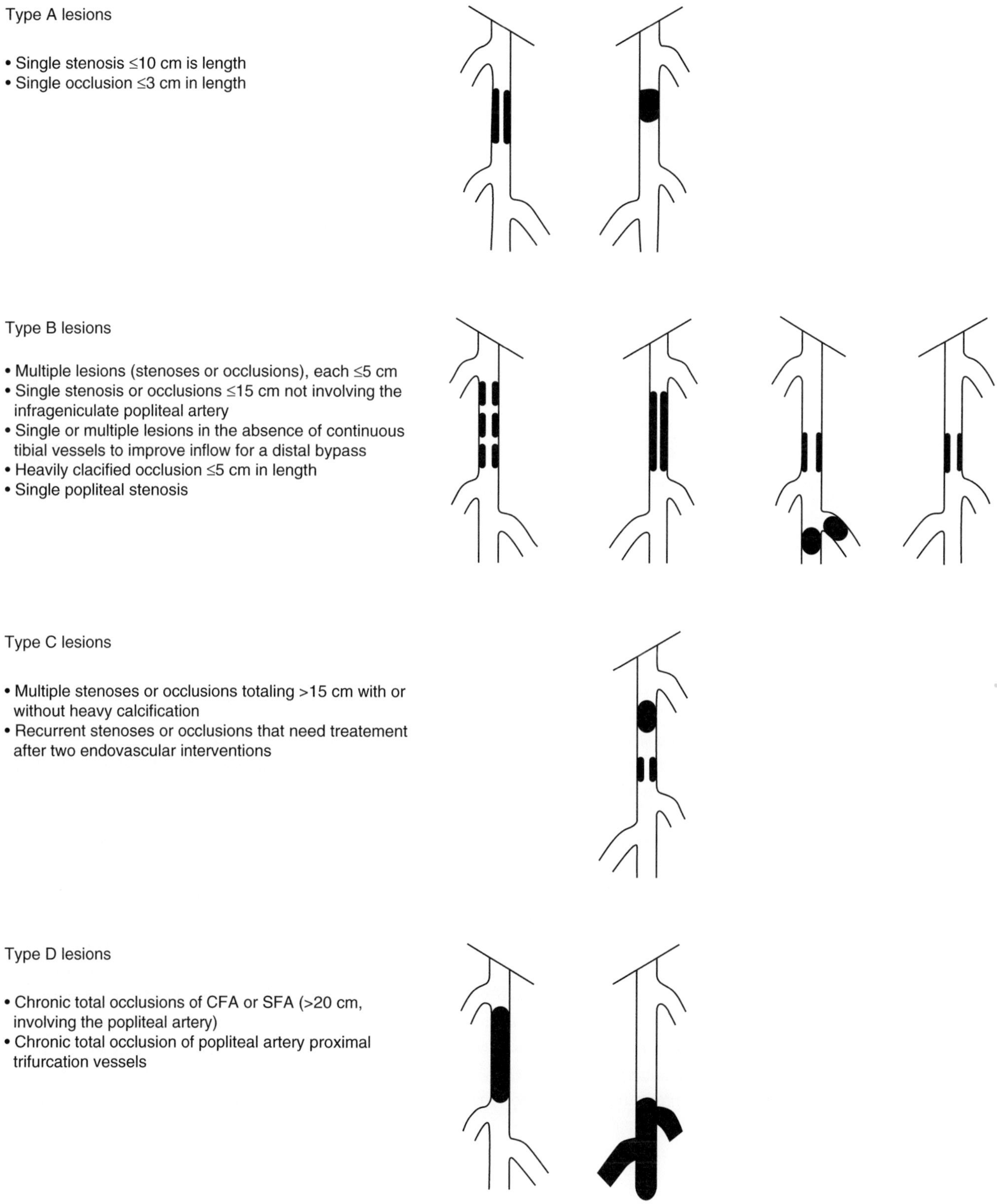

Fig. 30.2 TASC classification of femoropopliteal disease (From Norgren et al. [5], with permission)

Failed iliac PTA is generally defined as a persistent translesional gradient, residual diameter stenosis greater than 50 %, or flow-limiting dissection [9].

The effectiveness of stents, atherectomy, cutting balloons, and lasers for the treatment of femoral-popliteal arterial lesions is not well established. In fact, there is a notable absence of

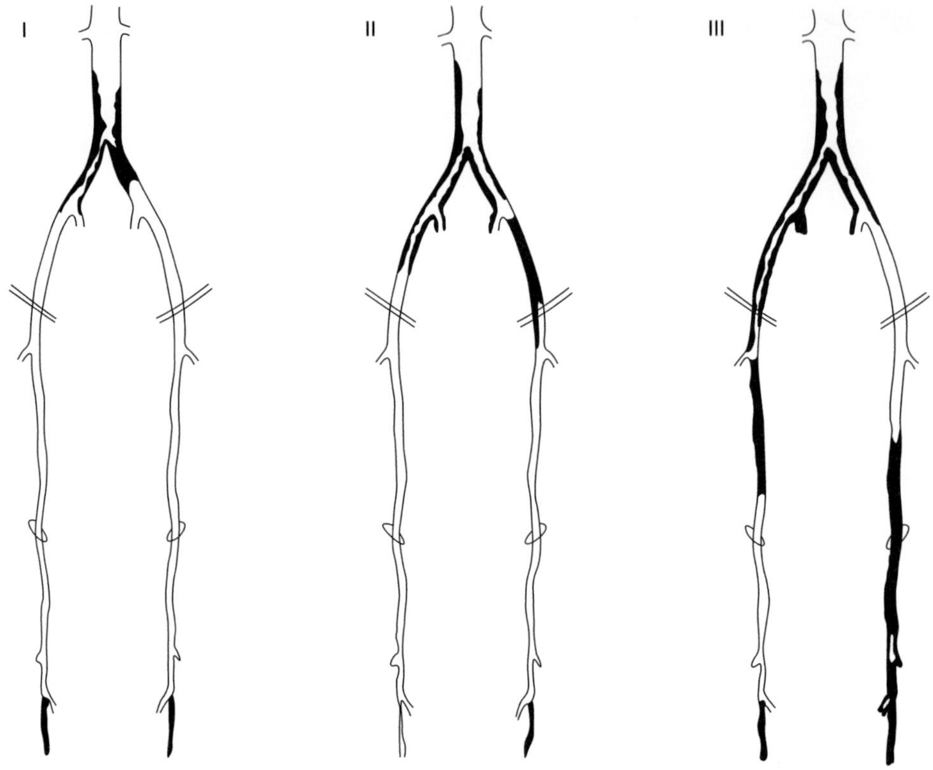

Fig. 30.3 Distribution of aortoiliac occlusive disease

guideline support, favorable case studies, or even single-arm registries. However, many of these devices have nonetheless become standard during endovascular interventions [6, 10].

Finally, some lesions are best approached as a hybrid procedure with both endovascular and surgical therapies. Suprainguinal iliac artery atherosclerosis often involves the distal aorta and may extend across the inguinal ligament into the common femoral artery. Therefore, it is not uncommon to view iliac artery disease as an aortoiliac process. Figure 30.3 illustrates some common patterns of aortoiliac disease. Extension of this disease process below the inguinal ligament constitutes a major obstacle to endovascular therapy, and the presence of occlusive disease may complicate infra-inguinal surgical reconstruction, given the lack of suitable inflow. Given these challenges, some patients with aortoiliac occlusive disease with infrainguinal extension may be managed using hybrid procedures. An example of such a hybrid procedure would involve stenting of the iliac arteries into the common femoral artery, with direct repair of the common femoral by endarterectomy with or without path angioplasty or an interposition graft [11].

Patient and Lesion Selection for Endovascular Management of Critical Limb Ischemia

Critical limb ischemia (CLI) is defined by the presence of rest pain, ulcers, or tissue loss attributed to arterial occlusive disease and is associated with great morbidity and mortality. Acute critical limb ischemia refers to patients in whom CLI symptoms have been present for <14 days, whereas symptoms persisting beyond 14 days are referred to as chronic critical limb ischemia.

Therapeutic goals of endovascular treatment of patients with CLI include relieving ischemic pain, healing ulcers, preventing major amputation, improving quality of life, and increasing survival [12]. Findings of the BASIL trial show that patients with severe limb ischemia, with a life expectancy of >2 years, and with a usable vein may derive greater benefit from bypass surgery because of the long-term patency of the saphenous vein. However, in the subset of patients with life expectancy of <2 years or those without an adequate vein, endovascular intervention should be considered as results of prosthetic bypass show poor durability in infrainguinal lesions [13]. It is important to note that given the diverse presentations and anatomic variations of PAD in patients with CLI, endovascular treatment should be undertaken exclusively by highly skilled and experienced physicians or groups of specialists.

In patients presenting with CLI with combined inflow (aortoiliac) and outflow (iliofemoral or femoropopliteal) disease, endovascular treatment should first be directed to inflow lesions [14]. However, restoration of pulsatile flow to the foot is generally needed for the healing of ischemic ulcers or gangrene. Therefore, if ischemic ulcers, gangrene, or infection persist after treatment of inflow disease and the ABI is below 0.8, an outflow vessel intervention should be performed [14].

Traditionally, procedural success of an endovascular intervention in CLI has been defined as <30 % residual diameter stenosis of critical inflow vessels and straight-line outflow in at least one infrapopliteal vessel to the pedal arch [15]. However, this definition fails to require targeted revascularization of ischemic tissue, and likely for this reason, nontargeted below-the-knee vessel interventions often lead to unsatisfactory clinical outcomes. Targeted therapy is possible using an angiosome-based approach, which provides a three-dimensional view of the tissue territories supplied by source arteries and has been used by general surgeons and plastic surgeons for limb and tissue salvage [16]. In a study comparing an angiosome-guided direct approach to CLI intervention compared to an indirect approach not angiosome guided, the limb salvage rate was significantly higher in the direct group than in the indirect group (86 % vs. 69 %, $p=.03$ at 1 year; 82 % vs. 64 %, $p=.029$ at 2 years; 82 % vs. 64 %, $p=.029$ at 3 years; and 82 % vs. 64 %, $p=.029$ at 4 years) [17].

Acute critical limb ischemia is a clinical emergency requiring rapid evaluation and treatment. Treatment begins with immediate anticoagulation with unfractionated heparin. Based on the results of several randomized trials, there is no clear superiority for endovascular management versus surgery on 30-day limb salvage or mortality, though surgery is used more often in practice [18]. Endovascular management options include catheter-based thrombolysis or thrombectomy [19].

Endovascular Intervention of Iliac Arteries

Surgical aortobifemoral bypass for iliac artery PAD has excellent 1-, 3-, and 5-year patency rates, and all iliac procedures, including endovascular interventions, are benchmarked against it. However, where outcomes between endovascular procedures and surgery are similar, endovascular procedures are favored due to the lower morbidity associated with minimally invasive approaches. The TASC guidelines specify that endovascular therapy is the treatment of choice for TASC A lesions and surgery the treatment of choice for TASC D lesions. They are less clear as to the optimal management of TASC B and C lesions, stating that in general endovascular treatment is preferred for type B lesions and surgery preferred for good-risk patients with type C lesions, but this is with the caveat that it should be an individualized choice for these lesions taking into account comorbidities and patient preferences [5]. It is worth noting that the guidelines might be lagging behind contemporary practice, with endovascular therapies increasing being chosen even in TASC type C and D lesions with good results.

Acute procedural success of PTA of iliac stenoses is >90 % overall. It is 100 % for focal iliac lesions and 80 % for long lesions and occlusions. While considering the management of iliac artery disease, it is critical to carefully evaluate the distribution and severity of atherosclerotic disease. Five-year patency rates of PTA for iliac lesions are between 70 and 72 % [20], and Murphy et al. reported an 8-year primary patency rate of 74 % with iliac artery stenting [21].

The Dutch Iliac Stent Trial compared routine iliac artery stenting to PTA with a provisional stent approach [22]. However, there was a high crossover rate with nearly half (43 %) of the patients randomized to PTA requiring stenting for a suboptimal result during the primary procedure. Re-intervention rates were similar in both arms at 2 (7 % PTA and 4 % stenting) [22] and 5 years (18 % PTA and 20 % stenting) [23]. There were no differences in iliac patency, ankle-brachial index (ABI), or quality of life between the two groups. A 2,116 patient meta-analysis comparing iliac artery PTA and stenting in claudicants and CLI reported a higher technical success rate with stenting; however, 30-day mortality was similar [9]. The 4-year primary patency rates were 65 % (PTA) and 77 % (stent) for stenoses and 54 % (PTA) versus 61 % (stent) for occlusion, with the inclusion of all reported technical failures.

Endovascular treatment of aortoiliac bifurcation lesions is not feasible with PTA but can be performed with high technical success with implantation of "kissing" stents, with 78 and 98 % 3-year primary and secondary patency rates [24]. High primary and secondary patency rates of 79 and 87 % at 1 year and 69 and 81 % at 3 years, respectively, have also been reported for stenting of iliac artery chronic total occlusions [25].

There are three types of stents typically used in peripheral interventions: uncovered balloon-expandable, covered balloon-expandable, and self-expanding stents. The type of stent chosen for a particular intervention is often determined by lesion location as well as lesion characteristics. There are no head-to-head studies of balloon-expandable versus self-expanding stents in the iliac distribution; however, there are studies comparing various covered versus bare-metal stent types, as discussed in more detail below.

Generally, in aortoiliac interventions, uncovered balloon-expandable stents are preferred over self-expanding stents. This is true for several reasons. Balloon-expandable stents have better radial strength, which is useful in heavily calcified lesions. Also, balloon-expandable stents have minimal foreshortening and allow for precise stent placement, which make them particularly suitable for stenting into the aorta using the kissing stent technique. The 2-year results of the MELODIE trial reported the safety and effectiveness of the balloon-expandable Express LD Vascular stent for the treatment of atherosclerotic iliac artery disease [26]. Primary patency was 92.1 % at 6 months and 87.8 % at 2 years. The rate of major adverse events (MAE) was 6.3 % at 6 months and 10.2 % at 2 years. Of the three event types included in the definition of MAE, only target lesion revascularization occurred, and 2-year ABI remained significantly improved compared to baseline (0.85 vs. 0.63, $p<0.0001$). Most iliac stents studied are made up of stainless steel; however, the Assurant balloon-expandable cobalt stent has received Food and Drug Administration (FDA) approval for iliac artery implantation. The ACTIVE trial

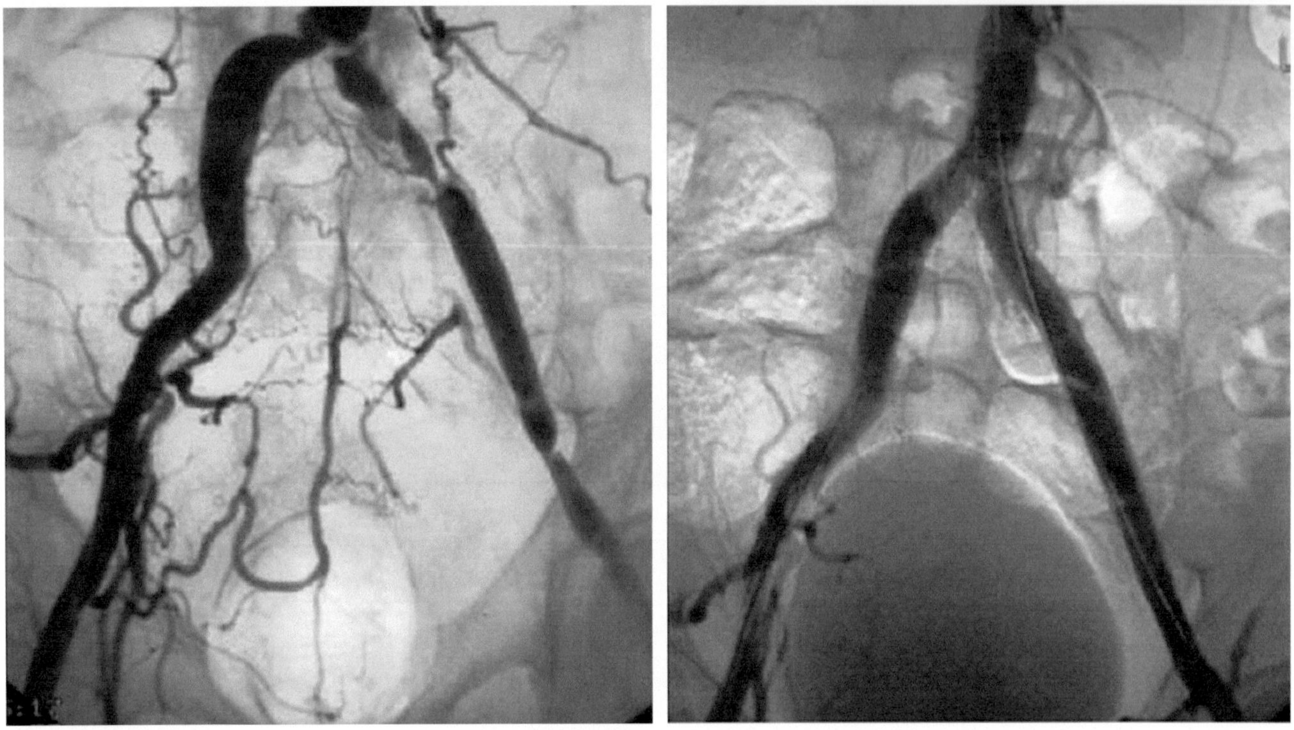

Fig. 30.4 Successful endovascular treatment of the left common iliac artery

(unpublished; ClinicalTrials.gov Identifier: NCT00753337) reported a rate of 0.8 % for major adverse events, target lesion revascularization (TLR) and target vessel revascularization (TVR). In addition, the device also achieved a 99.2 % primary patency rate through 9 months of follow-up.

Covered balloon-mounted stents are generally reserved for complications or lesions with features which suggest high risk for embolization, i.e., eccentric ulcers or exophytic calcifications. A recent trial, COBEST (Covered Versus Balloon Expandable Stent Trial), of 125 patients with severe aortoiliac disease demonstrated that in the overall cohort, lesions treated with a covered stent were significantly more likely to remain free from binary restenosis than those that were treated with a bare-metal stent (hazard ratio [HR], 0.35; 95 % confidence interval (CI), 0.15–0.82; $p=.02$). Subgroup analyses demonstrated that covered and bare-metal stents produced similar and acceptable results for TASC B lesions; however, covered stents performed better for TASC C and D lesions in terms of long-term patency and clinical outcomes [27].

Self-expanding stents provide greater flexibility and are best suited for external iliac and more downstream lesions. A study comparing outcomes of two self-expanding stents for the treatment of iliac artery lesions reported 1-year primary patency rates of 94.7 and 91.1 % (not significant), respectively, with similar complication and symptomatic improvement rates regardless of the type of stent [28].

In conclusion, for type A iliac lesions, endovascular therapy is appropriate. For type D, surgery is most appropriate. For classes B and C, neither approach is clearly superior to the other, but endovascular therapy is more commonly used for class B and surgery more common for class C. Factors negatively affecting the patency of endovascular iliac interventions include poor quality of runoff vessels, severe limb ischemia, and long length of diseased segments. Female gender has also been suggested to decrease patency of external iliac artery stents [29].

Most iliac artery interventions are performed using common femoral access. During aortoiliac interventions careful analysis of the distal aorta and iliac vessel angiograms should be performed. Accessory renal arteries are found in approximately 15 % of patients and may arise from a variety of locations, such as the distal infrarenal abdominal aorta. Failure to recognize this variant during aortoiliac interventions could result in jailing and possibly occluding the renal artery, which could lead to ischemic renal injury. Using a wide (>12-in. diameter) image intensifier and digital subtraction angiography could aid in the recognition of this arterial variant. Transradial or brachial artery access for iliac interventions is feasible and is associated with lower periprocedural bleeding complications. These accesses are best suited for crossing flush occlusions of the proximal common iliac arterial segments, in patients with common femoral artery disease or patients with infrainguinal grafts [30]. Figure 30.4 demonstrates a case of successful endovascular treatment of a left common iliac artery through radial artery access.

Approximately one-third of obstructive lesions in peripheral arterial occlusive disease affect the aortoiliac segment. One of the main challenges when treating completely occluded iliac arteries is crossing the occluded segment safely. Retrograde, crossover, and brachial access individually or dual access is often required for endovascular treatment of iliac total occlusions. A primary guide wire (0.035″) generally with a support catheter can be used; however, blunt microdissection techniques (Frontrunner® and CrossBoss®) are becoming the more popular approach. Subintimal entry of the guide wire may occur during recanalization of an aortoiliac occlusion. Though experience with specific reentry devices in the iliac arteries is limited, the Pioneer system may be preferable because of its intravascular ultrasound-based orientation that may facilitate positioning of the device and reentry into the true lumen of the distal aorta [31].

Endovascular Intervention of Infrainguinal Vessels

The primary reason for the selection and ultimately exponential growth in infrainguinal endovascular procedures is to avoid the morbidity and mortality associated with open surgical reconstructions. Especially for lesions <10 mm in length, PTA of infrainguinal arterial vessels may be the preferred option [32]. The gap between the findings of the revised TASC document and contemporary endovascular practice worldwide is nowhere as wide as for the femoropopliteal and below-the-knee (BTK) interventions. This is primarily due to recent advancements in device development and advances in technical approach, all of which have increased success of endovascular treatment of complex femoropopliteal and chronic total occlusions to rates >85 %. The newer devices include hydrophilic guide wires, microdissection, and reentry catheters [32]. Therapeutic effectiveness of an endovascular approach to infrainguinal disease is dependent on the complexity of the underlying disease and clinical presentation of the patient. The immediate technical success and short- and intermediate-term patency rates achieved with the traditional endovascular modalities have been promising, with overall immediate technical and clinical success rate of PTA of femoropopliteal artery stenoses in all series exceeding 95 % [33]. However, long-term patency rates in the treatment of femoropopliteal disease have proved disappointing. The usefulness of conventional angioplasty is limited by elastic recoil, flow-limiting dissection, and high restenosis rates. The efficacy of stents has been limited by high restenosis and stent fracture rates.

In a balloon angioplasty performance analysis performed by Rocha-Singh et al., 12-month duplex ultrasound-derived patency was established to be low, at 33 % [34]. In a meta-analysis of balloon angioplasty and stent implantation studies for occlusive femoropopliteal PAD, Mwipatayi et al. reported a 45–84.2 % and a 25–77.2 % 1-year and 2-year primary patency rates following balloon angioplasty, compared to a 63–90 % 1-year and 46–87 % 2-year primary patency rates in the stent implantation group [27]. Based on these findings, the investigators concluded that stent placement for femoropopliteal occlusive disease does not increase the patency rate when compared with angioplasty alone at 1 year. Kasapis et al. in a meta-analysis of 10 randomized controlled trials compared routine stent implantation to PTA for femoropopliteal artery disease in 724 limbs treated with stents and in 718 limbs treated with balloon angioplasty and provisional stent strategy [35]. The follow-up period was 9–24 months, mean lesion length 45.8 mm in the stent and 43.3 mm in the provisional stent groups, respectively. Immediate technical failure was significantly higher in the balloon angioplasty with provisional stent group than in the stent group (17.1 % vs. 5.9 %, relative risk (RR) = 0.28, 95 % CI 0.15–0.54, $p = 0.001$). There was a trend for lower restenosis in the stent group, 37.6 % versus 45.3 % in provisional stent group (RR 0.85, 95 % CI 0.69–1.06, $p = 0.146$). There was no difference in the need for target vessel revascularization (20 % in-stent group vs. 20.2 % in provisional stent group, RR 0.98, 95 % CI 0.78–1.23, $p = 0.89$). These data do not support use of routine stenting as the primary endovascular treatment for short SFA lesions. A meta-regression analysis in the study from Kasapis et al. suggested that stenting may be beneficial for longer lesions [35, 36]. Despite methodological robustness, these findings were limited by the study's inability to account for the wide variability of endovascular techniques and technologies used, limiting the practical relevance of such data. Data from more recent randomized clinical trials are also not conclusive. In the Femoral Artery Stenting Trial (FAST), Krankengerg et al. reported 1-year binary restenosis rates of 38.6 and 31.7 % with balloon angioplasty and nitinol stents implants in the SFA, respectively [36]. These findings are in contrast to another randomized study performed by Schillinger et al. who observed a 12-month binary restenosis rate of 36.7 % in their SFA nitinol stent group patients, compared to 63.5 % in the balloon angioplasty group. It is important to mention that the mean lesion length was approximately 45 mm in FAST and 101 mm in the study by Schillinger et al [37, 38]. Moreover, in FAST, significantly fewer chronic total occlusions of the SFA were included in the balloon angioplasty arm compared to the stent arm, and stenting with nitinol self-expanding stents showed a 15 % lower restenosis rate in diabetic subjects. The findings from the Randomized Study Comparing the Edwards Self-Expanding Lifestent versus Angioplasty-alone In Lesions Involving the SFA and/or Proximal Popliteal Artery (RESILIENT) trial also show that angioplasty is effective for certain types of lesions, particularly those under 5 cm in length [38].

The subset of PAD patients with diabetes deserves special attention. Patients with diabetes have significantly more diffuse and angiographically more severe PAD. An observational study of 65 consecutive patients who underwent long-segment (≥10 cm) SFA stenting found that 40 % of patients developed in-stent restenosis during the median 8-month follow-up. Cumulative freedom from restenosis at 6 and 12 months was 79 and 54 %, respectively, for the overall cohort. However, in diabetics, the 6- and 12-month freedom from restenosis was 68 and 22 %, respectively, compared to nondiabetics, with rates of 84 and 71 %, at the same time periods (adjusted HR of 3.8, $p=0.01$) [39]. This observation of high restenosis rates in patients with diabetes mellitus, especially after long-segment femoropopliteal stenting using self-expanding nitinol stents, has been confirmed by other studies and remains a challenging clinical problem. Despite these observations, SFA stenting remains highly prevalent in patients with diabetes mellitus, given the dismal (<30 %) 1-year patency rates following balloon angioplasty of long segments of stenosed or occluded SFAs.

Endovascular Intervention of Popliteal and Infrapopliteal Vessels

The management of popliteal and infrapopliteal arterial disease is challenging, and surgery remains the gold standard for treating infrapopliteal disease. The majority of patients with symptomatic PAD of the popliteal and infrapopliteal arteries have multilevel disease with atherosclerosis in the aortoiliac and femoropopliteal segments as well, with a minority of patients with symptomatic disease from isolated popliteal or infrapopliteal PAD [5, 40]. The anatomic challenges of intervening on the small and often heavily calcified tibial and pedal arteries have led to the generally inferior results of infrapopliteal revascularization compared to revascularization of larger proximal arterial segments, and consequently, intervention in patients with infrapopliteal PAD is generally reserved for patients with CLI, as these patients have the highest risk of limb loss and death [41].

If endovascular treatment of an infrapopliteal lesion is ultimately decided upon, evaluation and treatment of proximal lesions (aortoiliac or femoropopliteal) is usually necessary for successful treatment of lesions at or below the knee [42]. The mainstay of infrapopliteal intervention has been angioplasty, with stenting reserved for flow-limiting dissections in patients with CLI. A meta-analysis of infrapopliteal angioplasty for chronic critical limb ischemia combined data from 30 trials and found a pooled estimate of success of 89.0 % ± 2.2 % for immediate technical result. Results at 1 and 36 months were 77.4 % ± 4.1 % and 48.6 % ± 8.0 % for primary patency, 93.4 % ± 2.3 % and 82.4 % ± 3.4 % for limb salvage, and 98.3 % ± 0.7 % and 68.4 % ± 5.5 % for patient survival. The authors concluded that the technical success rate and durability of results were inferior to surgery outcomes, but the limb salvage rates were equivalent, supporting a potential role for angioplasty as an alternative to surgery [43].

Data comparing angioplasty to stenting (BMS or DES) are limited, though several trials involving BMS, DES, and drug-coated balloons (DCB) are currently underway [44]. Randon et al. compared PTA to PTA plus placement of a single bare metal in 38 limbs of 35 patients with CLI (Rutherford class 4–6) and a >70 % stenosis of a tibial vessel. The mean length of angioplasty was 3.9 cm (range, 2–10 cm), and the mean stent length was 2.15 cm (range, 1.2–4 cm). There was no significant difference in 12-month primary patency rates (66 % PTA vs. 56 % PTA + BMS), secondary patency rates (79.5 % vs. 64 %), limb salvage rates (90 % vs. 91.7 %), or survival rates (69.3 % vs. 74.1 %) [45]. In 2011, Rastan et al. published a randomized multicenter trial of BMS versus sirolimus-eluting stents in 161 patients with >70 % stenosis of a tibial artery and target lesion length <4.5 cm. Of the study patients, 86 (53 %) had intermittent claudication (Rutherford class 2 or 3) and 75 (47 %) had CLI (Rutherford class 4 or 5). The primary outcome was binary restenosis at 12 months. Although the authors reported a significant difference in 12-month in-stent restenosis rates (44.4 % BMS vs. 19.4 % DES, $p=0.004$), only results for the 77.6 % of patients completing the 12-month follow-up were reported, rather than the results of a right-censored Kaplan-Meier survival analysis. A Kaplan-Meier survival analysis for the composite end point of "event-free survival" (freedom from death, minor or major amputation or target lesion revascularization) showed no difference between the groups [46]. We look forward to the completion of the trials in progress to better clarify the appropriate roles of angioplasty, BMS, and DES in popliteal and infrapopliteal endovascular procedures.

Cryoplasty

Cryoplasty induces smooth muscle cell (SMC) apoptosis while limiting cell necrosis, and it has been hypothesized that this may reduce ISR and has been thought to hold particular promise for diabetic patients who tend to have more aggressive and severe disease and who have an accelerated and exuberant SMC proliferative response to vascular injury [47]. Endovascular treatment of such extensive PAD frequently requires nitinol stent implants and may benefit from application of cryoplasty as an adjunctive post-dilation strategy to lower restenosis and repeat revascularization rates from current levels of >50 %.

In one of the most recent studies of cryoplasty, the authors retrospectively analyzed data from the angiograms and

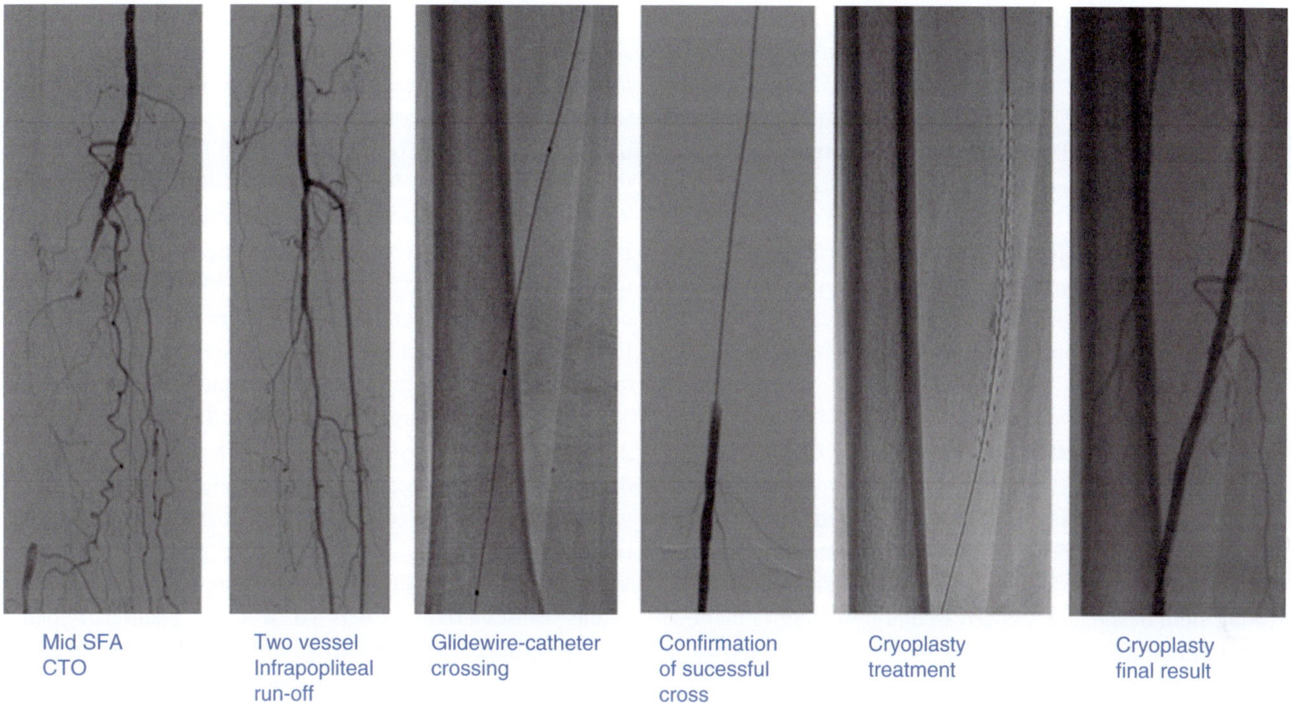

Fig. 30.5 Successful intervention of a mid-SFA CTO using cryoplasty. *CTO* Chronic total occlusion

medical records of unselected nonrandom patients from a single center who underwent cryoplasty for PAD from January 2004 through November 2006. The study population comprised 99 patients who received treatment for 132 atherosclerotic lesions, including 62 lesions in the SFA, 28 in the popliteal artery, and 25 in arteries below the knee. Mean lesion length was 39 ± 15.9 mm. Periprocedural success was achieved in 98.5 % of the interventions. Dissections occurred in 12.2 % of patients treated successfully without bailout stenting or additional balloon inflations. At 6 months, re-intervention was required for 42 % of patients. Mean ankle-brachial indices improved significantly after treatment ($p<0.0001$) [48]. However, the intermediate-term efficacy was compromised by dissections and frequent need for re-intervention.

It may be useful to consider the application of cryoplasty in particular anatomic locations. In the SFA, cryoplasty can be applied through the PolarCath® balloon dilation system, in which a double-layered balloon inflated with nitrous oxide instead of saline and delivers cryotherapy precisely at −10 °C to the arterial wall [49]. It is important to indicate that studies comparing PolarCath® cryoplasty to balloon angioplasty have reported mixed results, with some showing improved patency rates and others increased restenosis, including two trials demonstrating lower patency in a diabetic population. These studies have all been single or multicenter observational experiences, they have generally not used cryotherapy as an adjunct to stent-based therapy in a diabetic patient population, and they have not used cryotherapy in high-risk lesions. In fact, the recently presented COBRA trial (Cryoplasty or Conventional Balloon Post-dilation of Nitinol Stents for Revascularization of Peripheral Arterial Segments) is the first such trial to demonstrate that delivery of cryotherapy in addition to a vascular scaffold can be used to treat complex SFA disease and reduce in-stent restenosis. Figure 30.5 shows successful intervention of a mid-SFA chronic total occlusion using cryoplasty.

Laird et al. in a prospective, multicenter trial that evaluated the efficacy of cryoplasty for femoropopliteal disease reported a clinical patency in this group of 82.2 % and a primary patency determined by duplex ultrasound of 70.1 % at 9 months [50]. In a long-term (3-year) observational study from Diaz et al. of cryoplasty for femoropopliteal PAD, the reported patency rates at 6 months and at 1, 2, and 3 years of follow-up were 71.5, 61.2, 60, and 56 %, respectively [48]. Jahnke et al. evaluated the safety and efficacy of cryoplasty versus conventional angioplasty for focal popliteal arterial occlusive disease in a single-center randomized trial and reported 9-month patency rate of 79 % with cryoplasty compared to 67 % with conventional balloon angioplasty [51]. There was a trend toward higher patency after cryoplasty, but differences were not statistically significant and results of longer-term follow-up are awaited. In an earlier observational study from our group, cryoplasty alone was superior to cryoplasty with adjunctive, bailout stent placement [52].

The below-the-knee chill or BTK-CHILL trial prospectively examined the use of primary cryoplasty for BTK occlusive disease in patients with critical limb ischemia (CLI). At 1 year, 21 % of patients underwent target limb revascularization [53]. Rates of major amputation and death at 1 year were 0 % and 0 % for patients with initial Rutherford category 4; 11.4 and 0 %, respectively, for initial category 5; and 40.0 and 31.8 % for initial category 6. The authors concluded that cryoplasty therapy is a safe and effective method of treating infrapopliteal disease, providing excellent results and a high rate of limb salvage in patients with CLI.

Drug-Eluting Stents and Balloons

In October 2011, the FDA Circulatory System Devices Panel of the Medical Devices Advisory Committee voted unanimously to approve the Zilver PTX (Cook Medical) paclitaxel-eluting stent designed for endovascular treatment of de novo or re-stenotic above-the-knee lesions in femoral arteries in patients with symptomatic peripheral arterial disease (PAD). The self-expanding nitinol Zilver PTX stent is polymer free and is coated on its outer surface with paclitaxel (dose density of 3 mcg/mm^2). This device will be the first-ever paclitaxel-eluting stent available in the USA for the treatment of symptomatic PAD. The paclitaxel-coated Zilver PTX stent prospective multicenter randomized trial of bare-metal versus paclitaxel-eluting nitinol stents for SFA disease had two randomization protocols. Patients were initially randomized to treatment with either PTA or the Zilver PTX paclitaxel-eluting peripheral stent. Those who had >30 % residual stenosis or a >5-mmHg pressure gradient following 2–3 min of PTA balloon inflation ("suboptimal PTA") were again randomized to a provisional bare-metal Zilver stent or the Zilver PTX. After 1 year, 83.1 % of the stented segments treated with Zilver PTX were patent, compared with 32.8 % in the PTA-treated patients ($p<0.01$). Zilver PTX still performed much better than optimal PTA, 83.1 % compared with 65.3 % ($p<0.01$). In the provisional stenting group the 12-month patency rate was 89.9 % in the Zilver PTX-treated patients compared with 73 % for the bare-metal-stent-treated patients ($p=0.01$). The patency rate for the Zilver PTX-treated patients was also significantly better ($p<0.01$) than the optimal PTA and provisional bare-metal stent groups combined ("standard-of-care" group). The 12-month patency rate for this combined group was 67 %. Stent fractures were rare, only 0.9 % at 12 months. It is important to point out that the average lesion length was 66 mm, and nearly 50 % of included patients were diabetic [54].

While drug-eluting stents seem to show promise for peripheral lesions, they have attendant risks of stent fracture as well as in-stent restenosis. This has prompted interest in non-stent-based local drug delivery systems, especially drug-eluting balloons. Results of several preclinical in vitro and animal studies suggested that short-term exposure of injured arteries to paclitaxel eluted from regular PTA balloons might be sufficient to reduce late lumen loss and restenosis rates [55–57]. The German THUNDER (Local Taxane with Short Exposure for Reduction of Restenosis in Distal Arteries) trial studied the effect of paclitaxel on restenosis following angioplasty of stenotic or occluded femoropopliteal arteries using paclitaxel-coated angioplasty balloons compared with conventional PTA. One hundred and fifty-four patients were randomized. At 6 months, the paclitaxel-coated balloon had significantly less restenosis and lower 6-, 12-, and 24-month target lesion revascularization rates. The primary end point of mean late lumen loss was evaluated in 83 patients who underwent angiographic follow-up, and it was significantly lower in the group treated with paclitaxel-coated balloons compared to the control group (0.4 ± 1.2 mm vs. 1.7 ± 1.8 mm, $p<0.001$). The 12-month rate of target lesion revascularization was 10 % in the paclitaxel-coated balloon group, compared with 48 % in the control group ($p<0.001$). Even at 24 months, the rate of additional revascularization remained significantly less for the paclitaxel balloon group ($p<0.001$) [58]. The results of the Thunder trial were confirmed by the FemPac pilot trial, in which 87 patients with femoropopliteal artery occlusion or stenosis were randomly assigned to treatment with either standard balloon angioplasty or the paclitaxel-coated balloon. At 6-month follow-up, patients treated with the paclitaxel-coated balloon had significantly reduced late lumen loss compared to the control group ($p=0.031$). The number of TLR was significantly lower in the paclitaxel-coated balloon group than in control subjects ($p=0.002$), and the difference in TLR between both treatment groups was maintained 18–24 months post-intervention. Furthermore, patients in the coated balloon group also had improvement in Rutherford class ($p=0.045$), but no difference in improvement of ankle-brachial index was found [59]. Studies of other paclitaxel-coated balloon systems are ongoing [60]. Taken together, the existing preclinical and clinical studies indicate that short-term exposure of injured peripheral arteries to paclitaxel may be sufficient to inhibit restenosis and specifically suggest an important role for drug-eluting balloons in endovascular therapy for PAD.

Biodegradable Stents

As previously mentioned, stent-based therapies in peripheral arterial interventions are associated with significant long-term complications including in-stent restenosis and stent fracture. Biodegradable stents (made of either a polymeric substrate or of corrodible metals) offer a semipermanent alternative to typical drug-eluting stents that may, in theory, circumvent many of the immunologic and inflammatory response issues seen with long-term stent failure in peripheral applications [61]. The majority of studies with biodegradable stents to date have been in coronary artery interventions; however, there have been a few trials of peripheral vascular applications. The Perseus trial was a nonrandomized, single-center trial evaluating the Igaki-Tamai polymeric stent in 45 patients with significant superficial femoral artery lesions. They reported a 100 % technical success rate with no recurrent stenosis at 6 months and a 30 % restenosis rate (defined as >50 % recurrent occlusion) at 6 months [62]. An absorbable magnesium alloy stent was tested in 20 patients with infrapopliteal lesions causing critical limb ischemia (Rutherford class IV/V). The primary clinical patency rate of the stent was 89.5 % at 3 months, and a limb salvage rate of 94.7 % at 1 year was reported [63, 64]. These results are interesting but far from definitive. One specific concern that has been voiced regards whether biodegradable stents have sufficient radial strength for use in femoropopliteal lesions [65]. Ultimately these preliminary studies must be followed by large, randomized trials before the use of biodegradable stents can be widely adopted in peripheral vascular procedures.

References

1. Criqui MH, Denenberg JO, Langer RD, Fronek A. The epidemiology of peripheral arterial disease: importance of identifying the population at risk. Vasc Med. 1997;2:221–6.
2. McDermott MM, Fried L, Simonsick E, Ling S, Guralnik JM. Asymptomatic peripheral arterial disease is independently associated with impaired lower extremity functioning: the women's health and aging study. Circulation. 2000;101:1007–12.
3. Hallett JW, Rooke TW, Koch M. The Mayo Vascular Center experience. Cardiovasc Surg. 1998;6:333–6.
4. O'Brien G, Martin Z, Haider N, et al. An analysis of vascular surgery in elderly patients to determine whether age affects treatment strategy. Ir J Med Sci. 2012;181(1):73–6.
5. Norgren L, Hiatt WR, Dormandy JA, et al. Inter-society consensus for the management of peripheral arterial disease. Int Angiol. 2007;26:81–157.
6. Hirsch AT, Haskal ZJ, Hertzer NR, et al. ACC/AHA 2005 guidelines for the management of patients with peripheral arterial disease (lower extremity, renal, mesenteric, and abdominal aortic): executive summary a collaborative report from the American Association for Vascular Surgery/Society for Vascular Surgery, Society for Cardiovascular Angiography and Interventions, Society for Vascular Medicine and Biology, Society of Interventional Radiology, and the ACC/AHA Task Force on Practice Guidelines (Writing Committee to Develop Guidelines for the Management of Patients With Peripheral Arterial Disease) endorsed by the American Association of Cardiovascular and Pulmonary Rehabilitation; National Heart, Lung, and Blood Institute; Society for Vascular Nursing; TransAtlantic Inter-Society Consensus; and Vascular Disease Foundation. J Am Coll Cardiol. 2006;47: 1239–312.
7. Garcia LA, Carrozza Jr JP. Physiologic evaluation of translesion pressure gradients in peripheral arteries: comparison of pressure wire and catheter-derived measurements. J Interv Cardiol. 2007;20:63–5.
8. Banerjee S, Badhey N, Lichtenwalter C, Varghese C, Brilakis ES. Relationship of walking impairment and ankle-brachial index assessments with peripheral arterial translesional pressure gradients. J Invasive Cardiol. 2011;23:352–6.
9. Bosch JL, Hunink MG. Meta-analysis of the results of percutaneous transluminal angioplasty and stent placement for aortoiliac occlusive disease. Radiology. 1997;204:87–96.
10. Ramaiah V, Gammon R, Kiesz S, et al. Midterm outcomes from the TALON Registry: treating peripherals with SilverHawk: outcomes collection. J Endovasc Ther. 2006;13:592–602.
11. Sharafuddin MJ, Kresowik TF, Hoballah JJ, Nicholson RM, Sharp WJ. Combined direct repair and inline inflow stenting in the management of aortoiliac disease extending into the common femoral artery. Vasc Endovascular Surg. 2011;45:274–82.
12. Zeller T, Sixt S, Rastan A. New techniques for endovascular treatment of peripheral artery disease with focus on chronic critical limb ischemia. Vasa. 2009;38:3–12.
13. Bradbury AW, Adam DJ, Bell J, et al. Bypass versus Angioplasty in Severe Ischaemia of the Leg (BASIL) trial: Analysis of amputation free and overall survival by treatment received. J Vasc Surg. 2010;51:18S–31.
14. Bernstein EF, Rhodes GA, Stuart SH, Coel MN, Fronek A. Toe pulse reappearance time in prediction of aortofemoral bypass success. Ann Surg. 1981;193:201–5.
15. Dorros G, Jaff MR, Dorros AM, Mathiak LM, He T. Tibioperoneal (outflow lesion) angioplasty can be used as primary treatment in 235 patients with critical limb ischemia: five-year follow-up. Circulation. 2001;104:2057–62.
16. Taylor GI, Palmer JH. The vascular territories (angiosomes) of the body: experimental study and clinical applications. Br J Plast Surg. 1987;40:113–41.
17. Iida O, Nanto S, Uematsu M, et al. Importance of the angiosome concept for endovascular therapy in patients with critical limb ischemia. Catheter Cardiovasc Interv. 2010;75:830–6.
18. Berridge DC, Kessel D, Robertson I. Surgery versus thrombolysis for acute limb ischaemia: initial management. Cochrane Database Syst Rev. 2002;2002:CD002784.
19. Silva JA, Ramee SR, Collins TJ, et al. Rheolytic thrombectomy in the treatment of acute limb-threatening ischemia: immediate results and six-month follow-up of the multicenter AngioJet registry. Possis Peripheral AngioJet Study AngioJet Investigators. Cathet Cardiovasc Diagn. 1998;45:386–93.
20. Becker GJ, Katzen BT, Dake MD. Noncoronary angioplasty. Radiology. 1989;170:921–40.
21. Murphy TP, Ariaratnam NS, Carney Jr WI, et al. Aortoiliac insufficiency: long-term experience with stent placement for treatment. Radiology. 2004;231:243–9.
22. Tetteroo E, van der Graaf Y, Bosch JL, et al. Randomised comparison of primary stent placement versus primary angioplasty followed by selective stent placement in patients with iliac-artery occlusive disease. Dutch Iliac Stent Trial Study Group. Lancet. 1998;351:1153–9.
23. Klein WM, van der Graaf Y, Seegers J, Moll FL, Mali WP. Long-term cardiovascular morbidity, mortality, and reintervention after endovascular treatment in patients with iliac artery disease: The Dutch Iliac Stent Trial Study. Radiology. 2004;232:491–8.
24. Haulon S, Mounier-Vehier C, Gaxotte V, et al. Percutaneous reconstruction of the aortoiliac bifurcation with the "kissing stents" technique: long-term follow-up in 106 patients. J Endovasc Ther. 2002;9:363–8.
25. Uher P, Nyman U, Lindh M, Lindblad B, Ivancev K. Long-term results of stenting for chronic iliac artery occlusion. J Endovasc Ther. 2002;9:67–75.
26. Stockx L, Poncyljusz W, Krzanowski M, Schroe H, Allocco DJ, Dawkins KD. Express LD vascular stent in the treatment of iliac artery lesions: 24-month results from the MELODIE trial. J Endovasc Ther. 2010;17:633–41.

27. Mwipatayi BP, Thomas S, Wong J, et al. A comparison of covered vs bare expandable stents for the treatment of aortoiliac occlusive disease. J Vasc Surg. 2011;54:1561–70e1.
28. Ponec D, Jaff MR, Swischuk J, et al. The Nitinol SMART stent vs Wallstent for suboptimal iliac artery angioplasty: CRISP-US trial results. J Vasc Interv Radiol. 2004;15:911–8.
29. Timaran CH, Ohki T, Gargiulo 3rd NJ, et al. Iliac artery stenting in patients with poor distal runoff: influence of concomitant infrainguinal arterial reconstruction. J Vasc Surg. 2003;38:479–84. discussion 84–5.
30. Korabathina R, Yadav SS, Coppola JT, Staniloae CS. Transradial approach to lower extremity interventions. Vasc Health Risk Manag. 2010;6:503–9.
31. Etezadi V, Benenati JF, Patel PJ, Patel RS, Powell A, Katzen BT. The reentry catheter: a second chance for endoluminal reentry at difficult lower extremity subintimal arterial recanalizations. J Vasc Interv Radiol. 2010;21:730–4.
32. Muradin GS, Bosch JL, Stijnen T, Hunink MG. Balloon dilation and stent implantation for treatment of femoropopliteal arterial disease: meta-analysis. Radiology. 2001;221:137–45.
33. Han DK, Shah TR, Ellozy SH, Vouyouka AG, Marin ML, Faries PL. The success of endovascular therapy for all TransAtlantic Society Consensus graded femoropopliteal lesions. Ann Vasc Surg. 2011;25:15–24.
34. Rocha-Singh KJ, Jaff MR, Crabtree TR, Bloch DA, Ansel G. Performance goals and endpoint assessments for clinical trials of femoropopliteal bare nitinol stents in patients with symptomatic peripheral arterial disease. Catheter Cardiovasc Interv. 2007;69:910–9.
35. Kasapis C, Henke PK, Chetcuti SJ, et al. Routine stent implantation vs. percutaneous transluminal angioplasty in femoropopliteal artery disease: a meta-analysis of randomized controlled trials. Eur Heart J. 2009;30:44–55.
36. Krankenberg H, Schluter M, Steinkamp HJ, et al. Nitinol stent implantation versus percutaneous transluminal angioplasty in superficial femoral artery lesions up to 10 cm in length: the femoral artery stenting trial (FAST). Circulation. 2007;116:285–92.
37. Schillinger M, Sabeti S, Loewe C, et al. Balloon angioplasty versus implantation of nitinol stents in the superficial femoral artery. N Engl J Med. 2006;354:1879–88.
38. Laird JR, Katzen BT, Scheinert D, et al. Nitinol stent implantation versus balloon angioplasty for lesions in the superficial femoral artery and proximal popliteal artery: twelve-month results from the RESILIENT randomized trial. Circ Cardiovasc Interv. 2010;3: 267–76.
39. Sabeti S, Mlekusch W, Amighi J, Minar E, Schillinger M. Primary patency of long-segment self-expanding nitinol stents in the femoropopliteal arteries. J Endovasc Ther. 2005;12:6–12.
40. Gray BH, Grant AA, Kalbaugh CA, et al. The impact of isolated tibial disease on outcomes in the critical limb ischemic population. Ann Vasc Surg. 2010;24:349–59.
41. Hirsch AT, Haskal ZJ, Hertzer NR, et al. ACC/AHA 2005 Practice Guidelines for the management of patients with peripheral arterial disease (lower extremity, renal, mesenteric, and abdominal aortic): a collaborative report from the American Association for Vascular Surgery/Society for Vascular Surgery, Society for Cardiovascular Angiography and Interventions, Society for Vascular Medicine and Biology, Society of Interventional Radiology, and the ACC/AHA Task Force on Practice Guidelines (Writing Committee to Develop Guidelines for the Management of Patients With Peripheral Arterial Disease): endorsed by the American Association of Cardiovascular and Pulmonary Rehabilitation; National Heart, Lung, and Blood Institute; Society for Vascular Nursing; TransAtlantic Inter-Society Consensus; and Vascular Disease Foundation. Circulation. 2006;113:e463–654.
42. Sadek M, Ellozy SH, Turnbull IC, Lookstein RA, Marin ML, Faries PL. Improved outcomes are associated with multilevel endovascular intervention involving the tibial vessels compared with isolated tibial intervention. J Vasc Surg. 2009;49:638–43. discussion 43–4.
43. Romiti M, Albers M, Brochado-Neto FC, Durazzo AE, Pereira CA, De Luccia N. Meta-analysis of infrapopliteal angioplasty for chronic critical limb ischemia. J Vasc Surg. 2008;47:975–81.
44. Gasper WJ, Runge SJ, Owens CD. Management of infrapopliteal peripheral arterial occlusive disease. Curr Treat Options Cardiovasc Med. 2012;14(2):136–48.
45. Randon C, Jacobs B, De Ryck F, Vermassen F. Angioplasty or primary stenting for infrapopliteal lesions: results of a prospective randomized trial. Cardiovasc Intervent Radiol. 2010;33:260–9.
46. Rastan A, Tepe G, Krankenberg H, et al. Sirolimus-eluting stents vs. bare-metal stents for treatment of focal lesions in infrapopliteal arteries: a double-blind, multi-centre, randomized clinical trial. Eur Heart J. 2011;32:2274–81.
47. Jude EB, Oyibo SO, Chalmers N, Boulton AJ. Peripheral arterial disease in diabetic and nondiabetic patients: a comparison of severity and outcome. Diabetes Care. 2001;24:1433–7.
48. Diaz ML, Urtasun F, Barberena J, Aranzadi C, Guillen-Grima F, Bilbao JI. Cryoplasty versus conventional angioplasty in femoropopliteal arterial recanalization: 3-year analysis of reintervention-free survival by treatment received. Cardiovasc Intervent Radiol. 2011;34:911–7.
49. Karthik S, Kessel DO. Cryoplasty–where is the evidence? Acta Chir Belg. 2007;107:500–3.
50. Laird J, Jaff MR, Biamino G, et al. Cryoplasty for the treatment of femoropopliteal arterial disease: results of a prospective, multicenter registry. J Vasc Interv Radiol. 2005;16:1067–73.
51. Jahnke T. Cryoplasty for the treatment of femoropopliteal arterial disease: will freezing solve the problem of cold feet? J Vasc Interv Radiol. 2005;16:1051–4.
52. Banerjee S, Brilakis ES, Das TS, Lichtenwalter CS. Treatment of complex superficial femoral artery lesions with PolarCath cryoplasty. Am J Cardiol. 2009;104:447–9.
53. Das T, McNamara T, Gray B, et al. Cryoplasty therapy for limb salvage in patients with critical limb ischemia. J Endovasc Ther. 2007;14:753–62.
54. Dake MD, Ansel GM, Jaff MR, et al. Paclitaxel-eluting stents show superiority to balloon angioplasty and bare metal stents in femoropopliteal disease: twelve-month Zilver PTX randomized study results. Circ Cardiovasc Interv. 2011;4:495–504.
55. Scheller B, Speck U, Romeike B, et al. Contrast media as carriers for local drug delivery. Successful inhibition of neointimal proliferation in the porcine coronary stent model. Eur Heart J. 2003;24:1462–7.
56. Scheller B, Speck U, Abramjuk C, Bernhardt U, Bohm M, Nickenig G. Paclitaxel balloon coating, a novel method for prevention and therapy of restenosis. Circulation. 2004;110:810–4.
57. Albrecht T, Speck U, Baier C, Wolf KJ, Bohm M, Scheller B. Reduction of stenosis due to intimal hyperplasia after stent supported angioplasty of peripheral arteries by local administration of paclitaxel in swine. Invest Radiol. 2007;42:579–85.
58. Tepe G, Zeller T, Albrecht T, et al. Local delivery of paclitaxel to inhibit restenosis during angioplasty of the leg. N Engl J Med. 2008;358:689–99.
59. Werk M, Langner S, Reinkensmeier B, et al. Inhibition of restenosis in femoropopliteal arteries: paclitaxel-coated versus uncoated balloon: femoral paclitaxel randomized pilot trial. Circulation. 2008;118:1358–65.
60. Tepe G, Schmitmeier S, Speck U, Schnorr B, Kelsch B, Scheller B. Advances on drug-coated balloons. J Cardiovasc Surg. 2010;51: 125–43.
61. Brown DA, Lee EW, Loh CT, Kee ST. A new wave in treatment of vascular occlusive disease: biodegradable stents–clinical experience and scientific principles. J Vasc Interv Radiol. 2009;20:315–24. quiz 25.

62. Biamino G, Schmidt A, Scheinert D. Treatment of SFA lesions with PLLA biodegradable stents: results of the PERSEUS study. J Endovasc Ther. 2005;12:I5.
63. Peeters P, Bosiers M, Verbist J, Deloose K, Heublein B. Preliminary results after application of absorbable metal stents in patients with critical limb ischemia. J Endovasc Ther. 2005;12:1–5.
64. Bosiers M, Deloose K, Verbist J, Peeters P. First clinical application of absorbable metal stents in the treatment of critical limb ischemia: 12-month results. Vasc Dis Manage. 2006;2:86–91.
65. Schillinger M, Minar E. Past, present and future of femoropopliteal stenting. J Endovasc Ther. 2009;16 Suppl 1:I147–52.

Application of Advanced Technologies for the Treatment of Lower Extremity Arterial Disease

31

Faisal Hasan

Lower extremity peripheral arterial occlusive disease poses a unique challenge to traditional angioplasty-based endovascular therapies. Factors that negatively affect the long-term results of percutaneous intervention include the length of the diseased segment, the presence of total occlusion, diabetes mellitus, poor distal runoff, and critical limb ischemia as the clinical presentation [1, 2]. Chronic total occlusion may be present in up to 40 % of patients undergoing treatment for symptomatic peripheral arterial disease, and procedural success rates have historically been lower in the setting of chronic total occlusion [2, 3]. These challenges have spawned the development of a host of new technologies in an attempt to improve the safety and effectiveness of percutaneous revascularization for lower extremity peripheral arterial disease.

Intraluminal Recanalization Devices

Treatment of chronic total occlusions is challenging and often leads to prolonged procedure time, increased operator and patient radiation exposure, higher contrast load, and periprocedural complications including perforation, dissection, loss of collaterals, and creation of an arteriovenous fistula [2–6]. Multiple methods have been developed for chronic total occlusions. Subintimal angioplasty, one of the most widely used techniques, was first described by Bolia et al. in a case in which an inadvertent subintimal channel of a totally occluded popliteal artery was dilated and subsequently found to maintain its patency for 9 years [4]. This approach has been used in thousands of procedures worldwide. However, this technique is known to have significant limitations. The success of the subintimal angioplasty technique in totally occluded vessels is influenced not only by the length of the occlusion, severity of plaque calcification, and diffuse disease of the distal target but also technical experience.

The increasingly complex nature of peripheral vascular disease is a major limitation to this technique. Long lesion lengths and calcification of CTOs prevent crossing or reentry into the true lumen. The subintimal dissection approach also limits the use of newer atherectomy devices. Lastly, the entry and reentry of the occlusion with the subintimal wire approach has been plagued with considerable periadventitial hematomas and/or vessel perforations [5–11]. Thus, methods that successfully gain access across CTOs of lower extremity vessels through central lumen crossing and limit the creation of subintimal dissection planes can potentially prevent some of the drawbacks of the subintimal dissection method. Maintaining an intraluminal course also increases available treatment options with a wide array of atherectomy devices now available.

FRONTRUNNER

The FRONTRUNNER device (Cordis) consists of a handle assembly and integrated catheter rotator, a proximal braided and distal shapeable shaft, and a distal microdissection tip composed of bilateral hinged pieces. It has a hydrophilic coating along the entire catheter length to facilitate CTO crossing. It works on the principle of controlled blunt microdissection using a pair of miniature hinged jaws that can be actuated from the catheter handle. The crossing profile is 0.039 in. with the jaws closed, reaches a maximum diameter of 2.3 mm with the jaws open, and is available in 90- and 140-cm lengths (Figs. 31.1a, b and 31.2a, b). The device is particularly useful in crossing the proximal and distal caps of chronic total occlusions. The jaws of the FRONTRUNNER can be used to create a microchannel, through which the device can then be advanced. The device does not have a guidewire lumen, and once a lesion is crossed, a dedicated MicroGuide catheter is advanced over the FRONTRUNNER

F. Hasan, MD, FACC
Section of Cardiovascular Medicine,
Yale University School of Medicine, New Haven, CT, USA
e-mail: faisal.hasan@yale.edu

C.A. Thompson (ed.), *Textbook of Cardiovascular Intervention*,
DOI 10.1007/978-1-4471-4528-8_31,

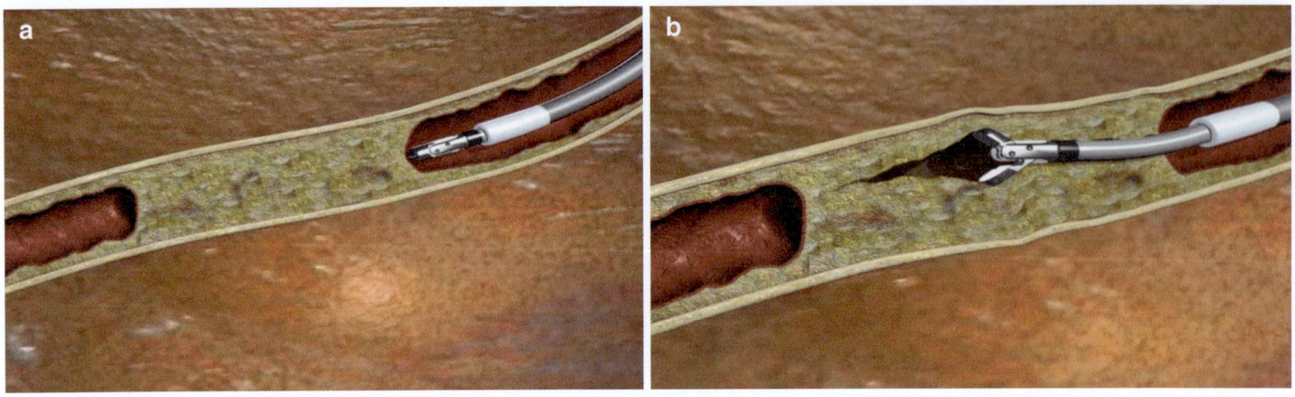

Fig. 31.1 (**a**) FRONTRUNNER XP Catheter engaging a peripheral chronic total occlusion lesion (**b**) FRONTRUNNER XP blunt microdissection within chronic total occlusion segment

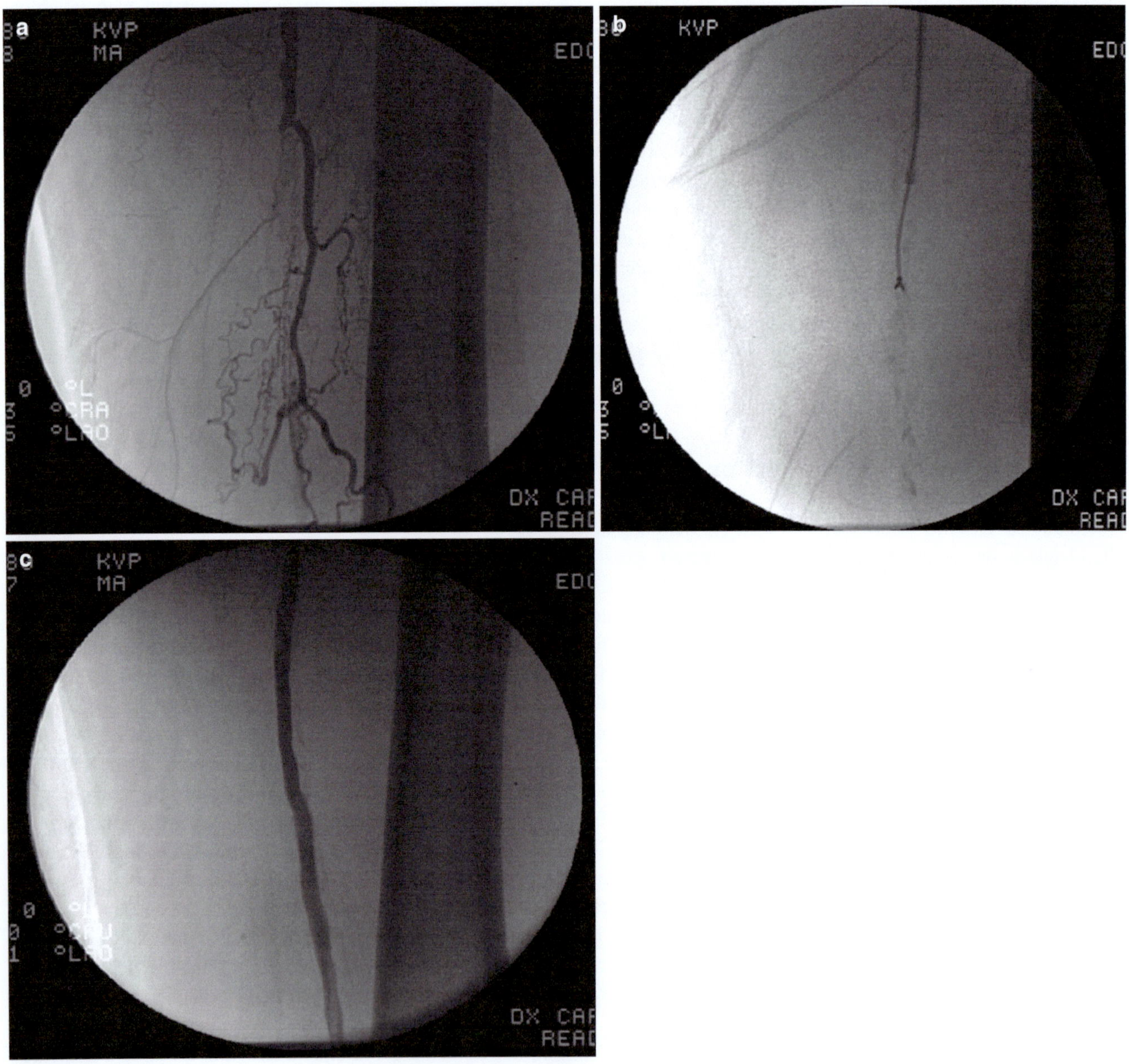

Fig. 31.2 (**a**) Chronic total occlusion of superficial femoral artery. (**b**) FRONTRUNNER XP blunt microdissection within chronic total occlusion. (**c**) Final post stent angiogram

catheter to its tip, and the catheter is then withdrawn. A guidewire can then be placed through the MicroGuide over which further therapies such as balloons, stents, and atherectomy devices may be delivered. The device has been reported to be safe and feasible, with a 91 % success rate in treating pelvic and lower limb chronic total occlusions in a series of 36 patients with 44 symptomatic chronic total occlusions that had failed conventional percutaneous revascularization [12].

CROSSER Catheter

The CROSSER chronic total occlusion recanalization system (Bard Peripheral Vascular) is an innovative device that uses high-frequency mechanical vibrations (20,000 cycles per second to a depth of 20 μm) propagated through a nitinol core wire to a stainless steel tip (Fig. 31.3). The system is comprised of an electronic CROSSER generator, foot switch, high-frequency transducer, the FlowMate Injector, and CROSSER catheter. The generator applies AC current to the piezoelectric crystals in the transducer, which then converts, amplifies, and transmits this energy to the catheter tip. The vibrational mechanical impact and cavitational effects result in penetration of the occluded artery. The catheter is mounted on a standard 0.014-in. guidewire and is compatible with a 5F guiding catheter.

For the typical procedure with an over-the-wire catheter, a 0.014 guidewire is advanced to the proximal cap of the chronic total occlusion. The CROSSER is then passed over the guidewire until it comes in contact with the proximal cap. The guidewire is withdrawn and the device is activated with the foot pedal and slowly advanced into the occlusion. Gentle forward pressure is applied to cross the lesion, allowing the device to find its way. Once crossing of the lesion is confirmed by angiography, the guidewire is advanced into the distal lumen. Use of chilled saline for irrigation is essential to avoid excessive heating of the device. Guidewires with polymer-coated distal ends should not be used.

The basis for infrainguinal approval of the CROSSER device was the PATRIOT trial [13]. In this study, a technical success rate of 84 % was achieved in crossing peripheral CTOs. The average occlusion length was 117.5 mm, and 75 % of the lesions were moderate to severely calcified. Available case series demonstrated a success rate of 41–75 % in peripheral interventions with the CROSSER device [14, 15].

The TruePath Crossing Device

The TruePath device (Boston Scientific Corporation, Natick, MA) is designed to penetrate hard or calcified occlusions and create microdissection in CTOs to facilitate access to the distal true lumen (Fig. 31.4). It is a 0.018-in. wire with a diamond-coated tip that rotates at 13,000 rpm. A support catheter is used to advance the TruePath to the lesion. The device is then activated and advanced across the lesion. It has a built-in safety mechanism with audible and visual alerts if excessive resistance is encountered. The working length is 165 cm, which can be extended to 300 cm to allow for catheter exchanges. The tip may be bent up to 15° for added steerability. A support catheter is mandatory when using the

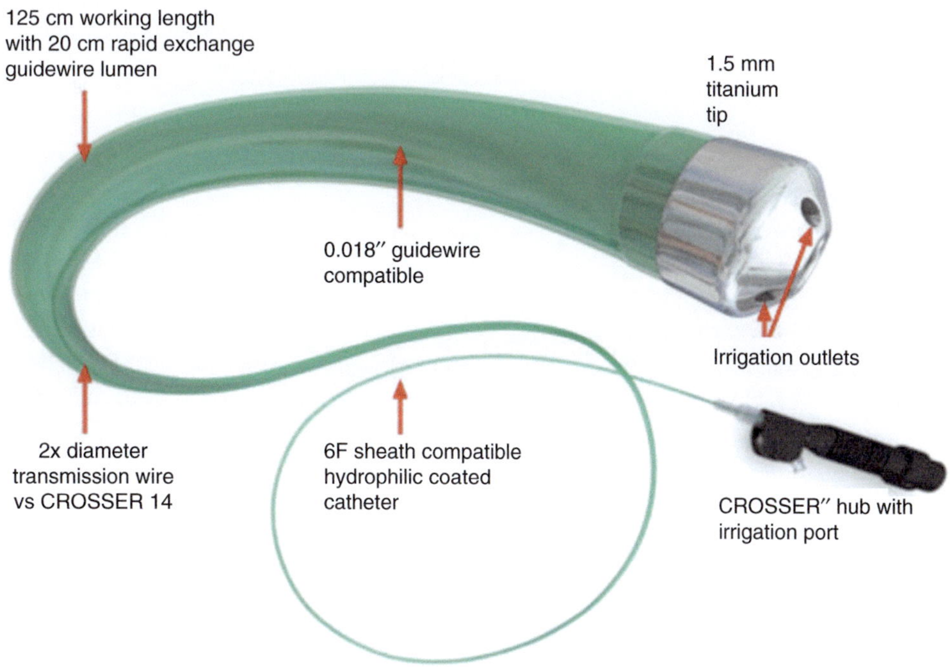

Fig. 31.3 (**a** and **b**) CROSSER chronic total occlusion recanalization system (©2012 C. R. Bard, Inc. Used with permission)

Fig. 31.3 (continued)

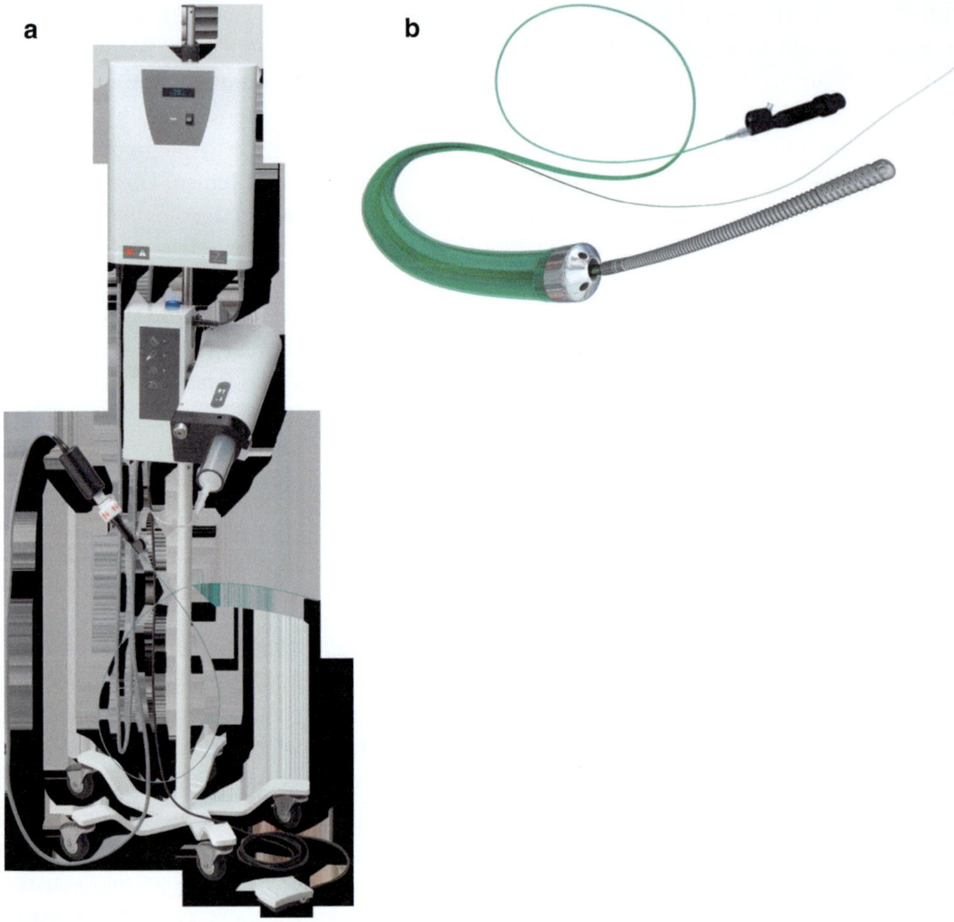

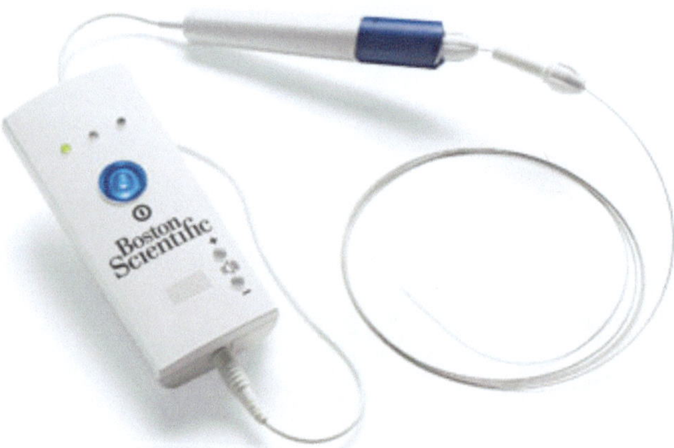

Fig. 31.4 TruePath catheter (Courtesy of Boston Scientific Corporation, Natick, MA)

TruePath device. A preshaped support catheter is preferred with this device. For added support, the device tip should not be extended 1 cm beyond the support catheter. Shaping the device tip may help with steerability through complex occlusions. Gentle forward pressure and slow device advancement is recommended.

TruePath was originally evaluated in the investigational device exemption ReOpen study in which a technical success rate of 80 % and primary safety end point rate of 98.8 % was achieved. The mean lesion length was 166 mm, the fluoroscopy time was 29 min, and the device activation time was 8.2 min.

Avinger Devices

The Wildcat, Kittycat, and Ocelot devices (Avinger, Inc., Redwood City, CA) utilize a corkscrew action to traverse CTOs. The Wildcat is a 0.035-in. catheter with a hydrophilic coating that facilitates tracking through complex lesions in the SFA. The rotatable tip assumes both passive (wedges in) and active (wedges out) configurations. The tip is initially advanced to the lesion and rotated in the passive mode. For more fibro-calcified lesions, the active mode may be used to traverse the CTO. The tip may be rotated manually or with a handheld motorized unit called the juicebox. The 0.014-in. versions of this device (Kittycat and Kittycat 2) provide smaller crossing profiles and longer working lengths for tight above-the-knee lesions or tibial vessels. The Ocelot device (Avinger, Inc.)

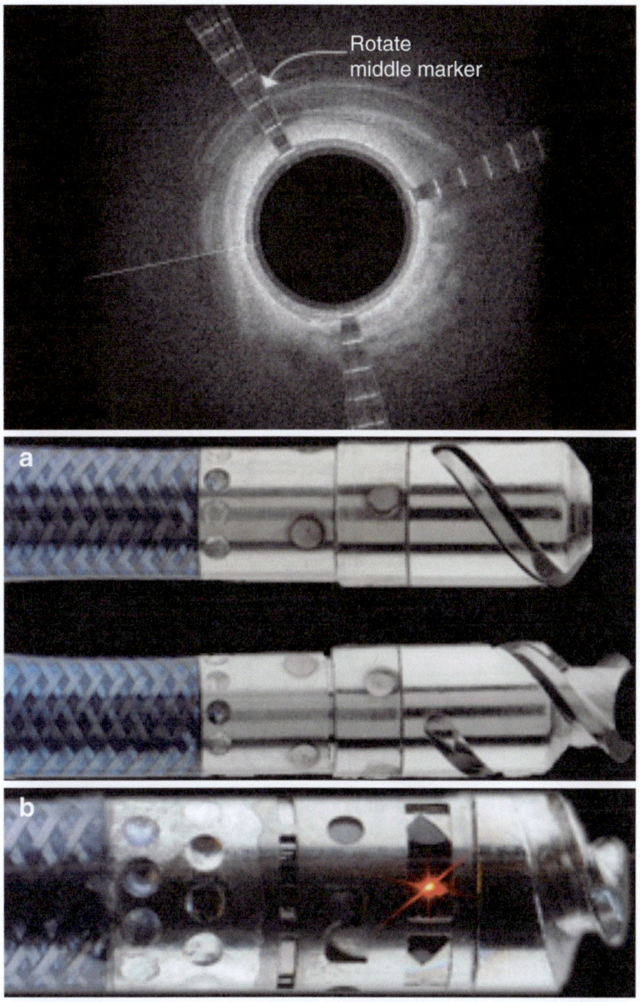

Fig. 31.5 (**a**) Ocelot device and (**b**) Optical coherence tomography orientation system (Courtesy of Avinger, Redwood City, CA)

is the latest addition to this family that incorporates real-time optical coherence tomography built into the catheter to guide intraluminal crossing (Fig. 31.5). The catheter tip may be rotated clockwise, counterclockwise, or a combination of the two with a gentle forward pressure. Counterclockwise rotation is less aggressive and should generally be tried first. The device should not be rotated in one direction for prolonged periods of time. Passive mode may be effective in softer occlusions and can be attempted before active mode. The active mode is more effective in fibrocalcific lesions. If significant resistance is encountered at the proximal or distal cap, only gentle forward pressure should be applied, allowing the device wedges to do the work. If the catheter becomes subintimal, it is withdrawn and additional attempts are made to reenter the true lumen or the tip of the catheter is deflected.

Wildcat was evaluated in the CONNECT (Chronic Total Occlusion Crossing With the Wildcat Catheter) trial in which the technical success rate of crossing CTOs was 89.3 %, with

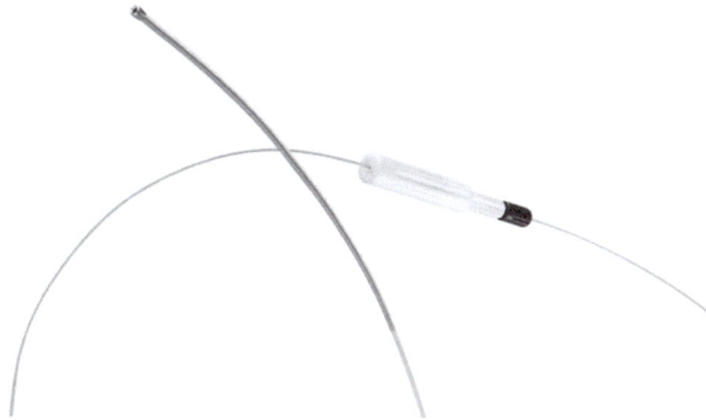

Fig. 31.6 Viance CTO Crossing Catheter (Covidien) – this catheter has a rounded tip which facilitates crossing via rapid rotation from external torque system

a primary safety rate of >95 %. The average lesion length was 174 mm, and approximately half of the lesions were moderately calcified.

Viance and Enteer Peripheral CTO Crossing and Reentry Devices

This is a novel peripheral CTO crossing system (Covidien) and has yet to be approved by the US Food and Drug Administration for peripheral vascular use (Figs. 31.6 and 31.7). The system is based on a coronary system called the CrossBoss and Stingray devices. It is composed of a crossing catheter that facilitates recanalization of the lesion and a reentry device to facilitate access to the distal true lumen, in case of subintimal tracking. The crossing catheter has a working length of 150 cm and tracks over a 0.014-in. guidewire. It has a coiled shaft and an atraumatic distal tip to prevent vessel exit. Using a torque device, the catheter is rapidly spun in either direction to facilitate advancement through the lesion. If the crossing catheter enters the subintimal plane, the reentry device is used to access the distal true lumen. This is the only reentry device designed for below-the-knee use. The reentry system consists of an orienting balloon catheter and a reentry guidewire. The balloon catheter has a 150-cm shaft length and is 0.018-in. wire compatible. The balloon is available in two sizes (3.75 × 20 mm and 2.75 × 20 mm) to facilitate reentry both above and below the knee. The balloon has a flat shape, which is designed to self-orient one of two 180° offset exit ports toward the vessel true lumen upon low-pressure inflation.

The location of the true lumen is determined with fluoroscopic guidance. When the balloon is at the desired reentry location, the primary guidewire is removed, and the barbed reentry guidewire is introduced. The 0.014-in. reentry guidewire has an angled tip that is designed to be introduced

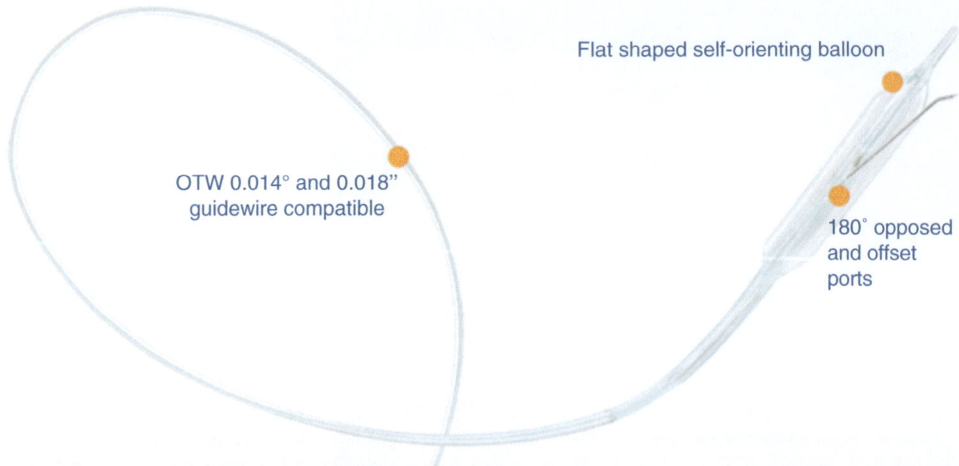

Fig. 31.7 Enteer balloon orientation catheter for lumen reentry – offset sideports consistently orient for true-lumen access (Courtesy of Covidien, Mansfield, MA)

through the appropriate exit port. Once the reentry wire is in the true lumen, the reentry balloon is removed followed by wire exchange and intervention.

Atherectomy Devices

PAD is a progressive chronic disease that requires a continuum of treatment, where few patients are treated once. Treatments that restore blood flow without reducing the ability to treat the vessel in the future are better suited for PAD. Atherectomy is seen by many as an ideal therapy for PAD because it can restore flow while removing the plaque burden and does not leave behind a permanent obstacle to future treatments such as a stent. There are currently four atherectomy systems approved in the United States.

Laser Atherectomy

Continuous-wave, hot-tipped lasers were evaluated and abandoned for peripheral arterial use in the late 1980s because of high complication rates caused by thermal damage to surrounding tissue [16]. In contrast, excimer laser-assisted angioplasty of the leg arteries has been practiced commercially in Europe since 1994. The Turbo Elite and Turbo-Tandem (Spectranetics) are commercially available excimer laser devices indicated for atherectomy of infrainguinal arteries (Fig. 31.8). These devices use flexible fiber-optic catheters to deliver intense bursts of ultraviolet energy in short pulse durations. The advantage of ultraviolet light lies in its short penetration depth and in its ability to break molecular bonds directly by a photochemical rather than thermal process. The excimer laser catheter removes a tissue layer of 10 μm with each pulse of energy. Tissue is ablated only on contact, without a consequent rise in temperature to surrounding tissue. Current data also suggests that ultraviolet light ablates thrombus and inhibits platelet aggregation [17].

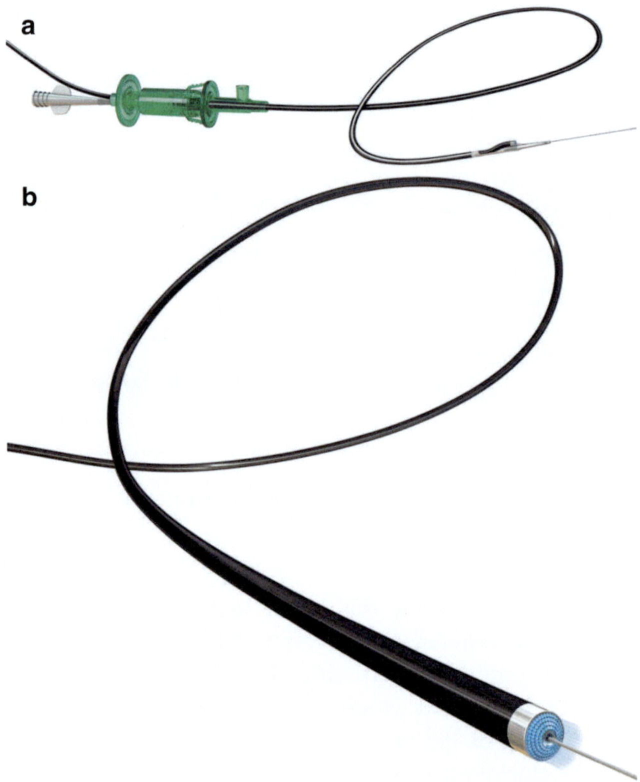

Fig. 31.8 (**a**) Turbo Tandem Laser Guide Catheter (**b**) Turbo Elite Laser Ablation Catheter. Concentric laser atherectomy (Courtesy of Spectranetics, Corp., Colorado Springs, CO)

Potential advantages of laser atherectomy include the ability to treat long occlusions and complex disease effectively, thereby providing a better angiographic result with less distal embolization and less need for stenting. The excimer laser can also be used to facilitate crossing of chronic total occlusions using a technique in which the guidewire is advanced just proximal to the lesion and the excimer laser catheter is brought into contact with the occlusion (Fig. 31.8). The laser catheter is gently advanced ahead and activated for 5–10 s in an attempt to penetrate the fibrous cap. The guidewire is then used to probe the lesion to find a channel. If a channel cannot be found, the laser is reactivated, and the above technique is repeated. Scheinert and colleagues analyzed the results of 411 consecutive excimer laser-assisted recanalization procedures for long SFA occlusions (mean occlusion length, 19.4 cm) in 318 patients. Despite the treatment of long occlusions, the technical success rate was high (90.5 %). Bailout stenting was needed in only 7.3 % of cases. Other complications were infrequent and included acute reocclusion (1 %), perforation (2.2 %), and distal embolization (3.9 %). The primary patency rate at 1 year was disappointing; however, with careful surveillance and early reintervention, a secondary patency rate of 75.1 % at 1 year was achieved after treatment of these long SFA occlusions [18].

Excimer laser-assisted intervention also has been evaluated for the treatment of complex occlusive disease in patients presenting with critical limb ischemia. In the Laser Angioplasty for Critical Limb Ischemia (LACI) trial, 145 patients (155 critically ischemic limbs) were treated with excimer laser-assisted intervention at 15 sites in the United States and Germany. All patients were poor candidates for surgical revascularization because of diffuse distal disease, with poor targets for bypass, the absence of venous conduit, or significant medical or cardiac comorbidities placing the patient at high risk for complications from surgery. A total of 423 lesions were treated in the SFA (41 %), popliteal (15 %), and infrapopliteal (41 %) arteries. The majority of patients (70 %) had a combination of stenoses and occlusions, and the mean treatment length was 16 cm. Despite these unfavorable lesion and patient characteristics, an excellent limb salvage rate of 93 % was achieved at 6 months [19]. There have been numerous improvements in laser catheter technology over the years making it an excellent option for treating long and complex infrainguinal occlusions.

Excisional Atherectomy

The TurboHawk and SilverHawk Plaque Excision System (Covidien) are forward-cutting atherectomy devices. When the catheter is activated and manually advanced through a lesion, a high-speed cutting blade excises a ribbon of plaque that is collected into the catheter nose cone (Fig. 31.9). Multiple catheter passes are made through the lesion, during which the blade is redirected sequentially toward all quadrants of the vessel lumen. The SilverHawk catheter now comes in seven different sizes to allow treatment of femoral, popliteal, tibial, and even pedal vessels. Two of the catheters have extra-large nosecones for greater plaque capacity, whereas the MS catheter has a slightly lower-profile blade that was designed for greater efficacy in calcified lesions. Some of the catheters feature a design modification that allows easier flushing of the nosecone.

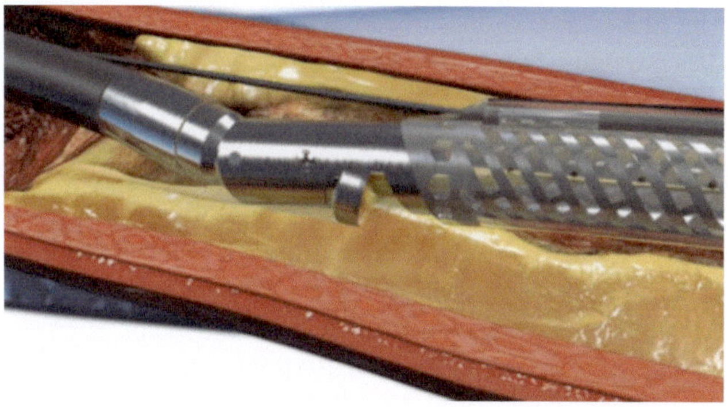

Fig. 31.9 TurboHawk and SilverHawk (Covidien) atherectomy systems

Several single-center experiences with the SilverHawk have been published. Zeller and colleagues [20] have published their experience with femoropopliteal excisional atherectomy. They treated 131 lesions in 100 limbs in 84 patients presenting with Rutherford category 2–5 ischemia. Forty-five lesions were de novo (group 1; 34 %), 43 lesions were native vessel restenosis (group 2; 33 %), and 43 lesions were in-stent restenosis (group 3; 33 %). The technical success rate was 86 % for atherectomy alone and 100 % after adjunctive therapies. Primary patency, defined as freedom from 50 % restenosis by duplex ultrasound at 18 months, was 73 %, 42 %, and 49 % in the three groups, respectively. The secondary patency rates at 18 months were 89 %, 67 %, and 79 %, respectively. The authors concluded that long-term technical and clinical results after atherectomy of femoropopliteal lesions are in favor of de novo lesions compared with restenotic lesions [20]. Kandzari and colleagues [21] also evaluated SilverHawk atherectomy for patients presenting with critical limb ischemia (Rutherford category 5–6). A total of 76 limbs were treated in 69 patients at seven centers in the United States. Approximately 40 % of the lesions treated were in the infrapopliteal vessels. Procedural success was achieved in 99 % of cases. Complications were infrequent, and target-lesion revascularization occurred in only 4 % of cases. Limb salvage (avoidance of major amputation) was achieved in 87 % of patients at 6 months [21].

Rotational Atherectomy

This resurgence in interest in atherectomy devices for peripheral vascular use has led to the development of two new rotational atherectomy systems. The Jetstream Navitus atherectomy device (Bayer Healthcare) has expandable, rotating scraping blades ("flutes") with ports between the flutes that allow flushing and aspiration of plaque material or thrombus. The device has a front-facing differential cutting tip driven by an external drive pod and continuous active aspiration. It is effective in different lesion morphologies.

The blades next to the tip can expand to a larger diameter thus providing two cutting diameters in one device.

The Diamondback Stealth Orbital Atherectomy System (Cardiovascular Systems, St Paul, Minn) is a high-speed rotational atherectomy system that incorporates an eccentric, diamond-coated abrasive crown. Crowns are available in 1.25-, 1.5-, and 2-mm sizes. When rotated at high speeds, the abrasive crown moves in an orbital path within the artery, potentially creating a lumen larger than the diameter of the crown while generating only small particles that pass through the capillary circulation. An 0.014 Viper wire guidewire is used with the device.

True-Lumen Reentry Catheters

Multiple technologies are now available to allow passage of a guidewire beyond an occlusion or stenosis, but this is often in a subintimal fashion. Reentering the true lumen with conventional guidewires is often a lengthy and unsuccessful venture. Three devices are currently available that facilitate true-lumen reentry, the Enteer reentry system, the OUTBACK LTD reentry catheter, and the Pioneer reentry catheter. In addition to ensuring a high success rate in reentering the true lumen, these devices may reduce the chance of vessel perforation and procedure times.

OUTBACK LTD Reentry Catheter

The OUTBACK LTD reentry catheter (Cordis) is a 6-Fr sheath compatible, 120 cm in length with a single 0.014-in. wire lumen. The catheter consists of a deployment handle mounted to a rotating hemostasis valve, which is attached to the proximal catheter shaft. At the distal end of the catheter is a 22-gauge reentry needle. A 0.014 in. wire is advanced in the subintimal space adjacent to the reentry point. The device is passed over this wire into the subintimal space to the desired reentry location. The catheter is then oriented under fluoroscopy by means of distal "L" and "T" markers at the end of the catheter and the needle is aligned with the true lumen. The wire is then partially withdrawn, and the needle is advanced into the true lumen by moving the deployment slide forward. The wire can then be advanced into the true lumen, and conventional therapies can be delivered.

The OUTBACK catheter was first evaluated in a series of 36 patients with peripheral (primarily iliac and femoral) chronic total occlusions initially approached with percutaneous controlled blunt microdissection. Of all successful cases, 35 % (14 of 40) required true-lumen reentry, which was successfully achieved with this device [12]. In another series of 100 consecutive endovascular occlusions in which the distal true lumen could not be reentered, there was a reported 95 % clinical success rate in reentering the true lumen with available reentry catheters and successfully completing the intervention [22].

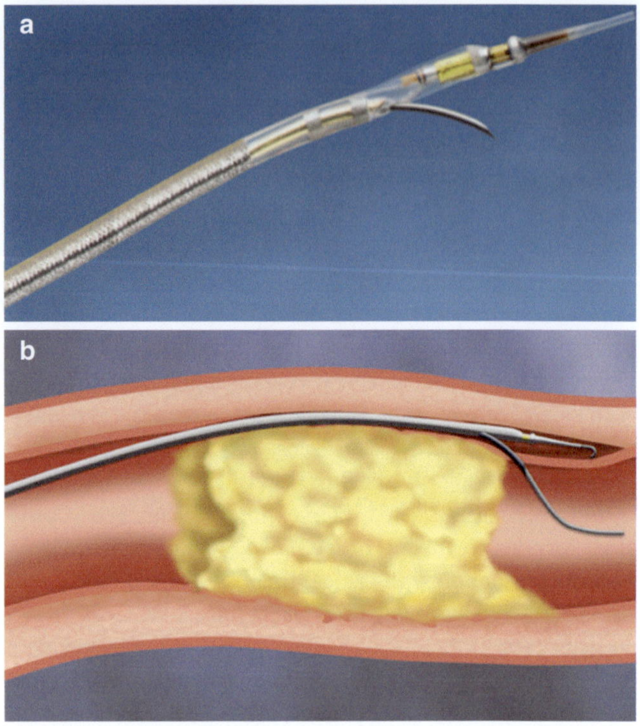

Fig. 31.10 (**a**) Pioneer Reentry Catheter (Medtronic, Inc.) – can be directed over the true lumen by distal rapid exchange port. A reentry needle can puncture the true lumen with real-time phased-array ultrasound guidance and wire access then subsequently obtained in the distal true lumen. (**b**) Pioneer Reentry Catheter (Medtronic, Inc.) – schematic of IVUS – guided needle puncture and lumen wiring

Pioneer Catheter

The Pioneer catheter (Medtronic) is another device designed to assist true-lumen reentry (Fig. 31.10). This catheter incorporates a distal 25-gauge nitinol reentry needle with an integrated 64-element phased-array intravascular ultrasound transducer to allow directed ultrasound-guided reentry into the true lumen. The basic principle is the same as the OUTBACK catheter with the added advantage of IVUS guidance. This catheter is 120-cm long, accommodates two 0.014-in. guidewires (one to track the device and one for the reentry needle), and is compatible with a 7F sheath. The subintimal wire is advanced to the reentry position and the device is brought into the subintimal tract over the wire. Under intravascular ultrasound imaging, color flow is identified in the true lumen. The catheter is rotated to position the true lumen at the "12 o'clock" position, after which the needle is advanced and the true lumen is wired. The distance of needle travel is adjustable from the handle. The Pioneer catheter is then removed and intervention performed over the wire. Prior studies have shown the Pioneer catheter to be safe and effective in true-lumen reentry, with low recanalization times for endovascular chronic total occlusions [23–25].

In summary, the arrival of CTO, plaque debulking, and true lumen reentry devices as enablers for the treatment of lower extremity atherosclerotic disease has opened a new door of hope for thousands of patients who were previously reliant on higher-risk surgical therapy or without options.

References

1. Johnston KW. Femoral and popliteal arteries: reanalysis of results of balloon angioplasty. Radiology. 1992;183:767–71.
2. Capek P, McLean GK, Berkowitz HD. Femoropopliteal angioplasty: factors influencing long-term success. Circulation. 1991; 83(Suppl I):170–80.
3. Morgenstern BR, Getrajdman GI, Laffey KJ, Bixon R, Martin EC. Total occlusions of the femoropopliteal artery: high technical success rate of conventional balloon angioplasty. Radiology. 1989; 172(pt 2):937–40.
4. Bolia A, Miles KA, Brennan J, et al. Percutaneous transluminal angioplasty of occlusions of the femoral and popliteal arteries by subintimal dissection. Cardiovasc Intervent Radiol. 1990;13:357–63.
5. Shaw MB, DeNunzio M, Hinwood D, et al. The results of subintimal angioplasty in a district general hospital. Eur J Vasc Endovasc Surg. 2002;24:524–7.
6. Horesh L. Subintimal angioplasty for the management of chronic total occlusions. Endovasc Today. 2005;4:31–6.
7. Vraux H, Hammer F, Verhelst R, et al. Subintimal angioplasty of tibial vessel occlusions in the treatment of critical limb ischemia: mid-term results. Eur J Vasc Endovasc Surg. 2000;20:441–6.
8. Tisi PV, Mirnezami A, Baker S, et al. Role of subintimal angioplasty in the treatment of chronic lower limb ischemia. Eur J Vasc Endovasc Surg. 2002;24:417–22.
9. McCarthy RJ, Neary W, Roobottom C, et al. Short-term results of femoropopliteal subin- timal angioplasty. Br J Surg. 2000;87: 1361–5.
10. Joye JD. Optimizing acute success in lower extremity chronic total occlusions. Endovasc Today. 2003;2:51–4.
11. Lipsitz EC, Ohki T, Veith FJ, et al. Does subintimal angioplasty have a role in the treat- ment of severe lower extremity ischemia? J Vasc Surg. 2003;37:386–91.
12. Mossop PJ, Amukotuwa SA, Whitbourn RJ. Controlled blunt microdis- section for percutaneous recanalization of lower limb arterial chronic total occlusions: a single center experience. Catheter Cardiovasc Interv. 2006;68:304–10.
13. PATRIOT evaluates FlowCardia's Crosser to mediate CTO recanalization. Endovascular Today. http://www.evtoday.com/eNews/eNews102909.htm. Accessed 23 Dec 2009.
14. Khalid MR, Khalid FR, Farooqui FA, et al. A novel catheter in patients with peripheral chronic total occlusions: a single center experience. Catheter Cardiovasc Interv. 2010;76:735–9.
15. Tiroch K, Cannon L, Reisman M, et al. High-frequency vibration for the recanalization of guidewire refractory chronic total coronary occlusions. Catheter Cardiovasc Interv. 2008;72: 771–80.
16. Wollenek G, Laufer G. Comparative study of different laser systems with special regard to angioplasty. Thorac Cardiovasc Surg. 1988;36 Suppl 2:126–32.
17. Lawrence JB, Prevosti LG, Kramer WS, Smith PD, Bonner RF, Lu DY, Leon MB. Pulsed laser and thermal ablation of atherosclerotic plaque: morphometrically defined surface thrombogenicity in studies using an annular perfusion chamber. J Am Coll Cardiol. 1992;19:1091–100.
18. Scheinert D, Laird Jr JR, Schroder M, Steinkamp H, Balzer JO, Biamino G. Excimer laser-assisted recanalization of long, chronic superficial femoral artery occlusions. J Endovasc Ther. 2001;8: 156–66.
19. Laird JR, Zeller T, Gray BH, Scheinert D, Vranic M, Reiser C, Biamino G. Limb salvage following laser-assisted angioplasty for critical limb ischemia: results of the LACI multicenter trial. J Endovasc Ther. 2006;13:1–11.
20. Zeller T, Rastan A, Sixt S, Schwarzwalder U, Schwarz T, Frank U, Burgelin K, Muller C, Rothenpieler U, Flugel PC, Tepe G, Neumann FJ. Long-term results after directional atherectomy of femoro-popliteal lesions. J Am Coll Cardiol. 2006;48:1573–8.
21. Kandzari DE, Kiesz RS, Allie D, Walker C, Fail P, Ramaiah VG, Cardenas J, Vale J, Chopra A, Gammon RS. Procedural and clinical outcomes with catheter-based plaque excision in critical limb ischemia. J Endovasc Ther. 2006;13:12–22.
22. Joye JD, Serry R, St. Goar FG, Zetterlund P. Clinical success in 100 consecutive endovascular occlusion cases using re-entry catheters for failed sub-intimal approach. J Am Coll Cardiol. 2006;47 Suppl 2:31B. Abstract.
23. Saket RR, Razavi MK, Padidar A, Kee ST, Sze DY, Dake MD. Novel intravascular ultrasound-guided method to create transintimal arterial communications: initial experience in peripheral occlusive disease and aortic dissection. J Endovasc Ther. 2004;11: 274–80.
24. Saketkhoo RR, Razavi MK, Padidar A, Kee ST, Sze DY, Dake MD. Percutaneous bypass: subintimal recanalization of peripheral occlusive disease with IVUS guided luminal re-entry. Tech Vasc Interv Radiol. 2004;7:23–7.
25. Javed U, Laird JR. Specialty crossing devices: understanding the learning curve. Endovascular Today. http://www.bmctoday.net/evtoday/2012/05/article.asp?f=specialty-crossing-devices-understanding-the-learning-curve. Accessed May 2012.

Percutaneous Management of Renovascular Diseases

32

R. Kevin Rogers and Joseph M. Garasic

Dr. Andreas Gruntzig published the first account of performing renal artery angioplasty in 1978 [1]. In 1983, Dr. Thomas Sos reported favorable outcomes at nearly 2 years following angioplasty in 89 patients with renal artery stenosis due to either atherosclerosis or fibromuscular dysplasia [1]. Subsequently, with improved technology – notably, endovascular stents – endovascular treatment has emerged as the preferred revascularization modality for renal artery stenosis.

Renal artery stenosis is the most common renovascular disease treated percutaneously. Atherosclerosis accounts for 90 % of renal artery stenosis [2, 3]. Several epidemiologic features of atherosclerotic renal artery stenosis – its prevalence, natural history, and association with adverse outcomes – set the stage for interest in the percutaneous revascularization of this disease:

Atherosclerotic Renal Artery Stenosis Is Prevalent

The prevalence of atherosclerotic renal artery stenosis has been described in population-based, autopsy, and referred populations and has been summarized in multiple reviews [2–5]. The prevalence is highest among patients with known atherosclerotic disease. For example, in 319 patients undergoing catheter-based angiography for aortic or peripheral atherosclerotic disease, >50 % stenosis of a renal artery was found in 38 % patients [6]. The prevalence remains high for patients suspected to have coronary artery disease. In over 20,000 patients referred for coronary angiography across seven studies, the prevalence of >50 % renal artery stenosis by angiography ranged from 6.3 to 23 % [2, 5]. In the general population, the prevalence is lower but not insignificant. That is, in a study of 834 Medicare patients with a mean age of 77 years, nearly 7 % had a renal artery stenosis of >60 % by screening duplex ultrasonography [4].

Atherosclerotic Renal Artery Stenosis Is Progressive

Multiple retrospective and prospective natural history studies have described the course of renal artery stenosis as progressive [2, 7–13]. By serial angiographic assessment of stenoses in early studies and by duplex ultrasonographic evaluation in later studies, 30–70 % of patients had progression of renal artery stenoses. These rates varied depending on the length of follow-up and how stenoses were defined. Progression to occlusion was more common in more severe stenoses [12, 13]. It should be noted that the enrollment for many, if not all, of these studies predated contemporary medical therapy. Thus, atherosclerotic disease of the renal arteries may have a different natural history than was once thought. This observation may partially explain the lower than expected event rates in trials of medical therapy for atherosclerotic renal artery stenosis. Nonetheless, the early reported natural history of atherosclerotic renal artery disease increased interest in the perceived need for revascularization.

Atherosclerotic Renal Artery disease Is Associated with Adverse Outcomes

An incidental renal artery stenosis >50 % by screening angiography was found to be an independent predictor of all-cause mortality in patients referred for coronary angiography [4]. Not only does atherosclerotic renal artery stenosis predict mortality; it does so in a dose-dependent relationship. In nearly 4,000 patients undergoing screening abdominal aortography, 4-year survival was 90 % for those with no renal artery stenosis, compared to ~70 % for those with a renal artery stenosis of 50–95 and 48 % for those with a renal artery stenosis of >95 % [14].

R.K. Rogers, MD, MSc • J.M. Garasic, MD (✉)
Division of Cardiology, Massachusetts General Hospital, GRB-8-821, Boston, MA 02114, USA
e-mail: jgarasic@partners.org

C.A. Thompson (ed.), *Textbook of Cardiovascular Intervention*,
DOI 10.1007/978-1-4471-4528-8_32, © Springer-Verlag London 2014

In summary, the high prevalence, progressive natural history, and association with adverse outcomes of atherosclerotic renal artery stenosis fueled initial enthusiasm for renal artery revascularization. This excitement was bolstered by technical success rates of 95–100 % for renal artery stenting from observational studies [5, 10, 15–22]. Accordingly, percutaneous renal revascularization procedures increased from 8,000 to 35,000 yearly from 1996 through 2005 in the United States according to Medicare claims [23]. Clinical success rates reported in observational studies have also been favorable but not as impressive as angiographic success. On average, hypertensive patients who undergo renal artery stenting enjoy improvement in blood pressure control in 50–70 % of cases, but cure in <10–20 % [2, 3, 24]. Similarly, improvement or stabilization in renal function is achieved in approximately 70–80 % of reported cases, with deterioration in renal function in the remainder of patients and rare progression to end-stage renal disease [3, 5].

However, results from subsequent randomized trials of percutaneous revascularization compared to medical therapy have raised doubts among many regarding the benefits of stenting for atherosclerotic renal artery stenosis. Despite methodologic flaws and limited generalizability to patients with severe disease, these trials have rightfully illustrated the importance of patient selection for renal artery revascularization to achieve favorable outcomes. This evidence has also highlighted the importance of further attention to detail regarding the optimal techniques for percutaneous renal revascularization (e.g., distal embolic protection). Thus, vascular specialists require both exemplary clinical and technical expertise for patient evaluation and selection for *therapeutic* revascularization of this disease.

This chapter provides the fundamental knowledge base for the interventionalist treating atherosclerotic renal artery disease, including its diagnostic evaluation, a critical summary of randomized trials of percutaneous revascularization versus medical therapy, and endovascular techniques for assessing and treating renal artery lesions. In addition, the clinical and endovascular approach to renal fibromuscular dysplasia, the second most common cause of renal artery stenosis, is summarized, and an overview of transplant renal artery stenosis is provided. Finally, the role of endovascular therapy for acute renovascular disorders is introduced.

Pertinent Anatomy and Pathophysiology

Renal Vascular Anatomy for the Interventionalist

The renal arteries arise from the aorta at the level of the 1st–2nd lumbar vertebra, just below the takeoff of the superior mesenteric artery [25]. The right renal artery typically has a somewhat anterior takeoff that is slightly superior to the left renal artery, which arises slightly posteriorly. Thus, some left anterior oblique angulation (10–15°) is often optimal for imaging the origin of the renal arteries.

The renal arteries branch into segmental, lobar, interlobar, arcuate, and interlobular arteries. Veins parallel these arteries, eventually draining into the inferior vena cava. In a majority of cases (55 %), single renal arteries are present bilaterally. However, a number of variations are commonly seen including early branching segmental arteries (14 %), dual renal arteries supplying a single kidney (8 %), and an accessory renal artery (7 %) (Fig. 32.1) [24]. The caliber of a renal artery depends in large part on the presence of accessory renal arteries. A single renal artery is typically 5–7 mm in diameter, whereas dual renal arteries or an accessory renal artery would be smaller.

Potential sources of collateral supply in the event of renal arterial occlusion include intercostal, lumbar, internal iliac, and adrenal arteries [26]. These anastomotic pathways occur at the level of perforating capsular arterioles. However, the renal artery is functionally an "end artery," and though these collaterals may preserve viability in the short term in the event of acute renal artery occlusion, they are insufficient to prevent progressive loss of renal mass in the setting of chronic occlusive disease [27]. In contrast, collateral venous pathways are likely to provide adequate outflow to maintain viability in the event of a chronic renal vein occlusion [28].

Pathophysiology of Renal Artery Stenosis

Renal artery stenosis can cause hypertension, renal dysfunction, and cardiopulmonary disturbance syndromes (Fig. 32.2).

The mechanism of hypertension in renal artery stenosis is thought to be related to activation of the renin-angiotensin axis. Decreased renal perfusion pressure distal to the culprit stenosis leads to elevation in serum renin levels. Elevated renin results in increased angiotensin II production. The outcome is vasoconstriction, decreased sodium excretion in the affected kidney, and activation of the sympathetic nervous system. If the stenosis is unilateral, vasoconstriction is thought to be the primary mechanism of hypertension. If the stenosis is bilateral, sodium and volume retention is the primary cause of hypertension [3, 30]. Similarly, volume retention can lead to pulmonary edema, and uncontrolled hypertension can exacerbate symptoms from obstructive coronary artery disease.

The mechanistic link between renal artery stenosis, ischemic injury to the kidney, and renal dysfunction is less clear, partly because the kidney requires only 10 % of the oxygen delivered under normal circumstances [30]. That is, renal excretory dysfunction in the setting of renal artery stenosis may not be due to ischemia, per se. The deleterious effect of concomitant hypertension may have a more prominent role

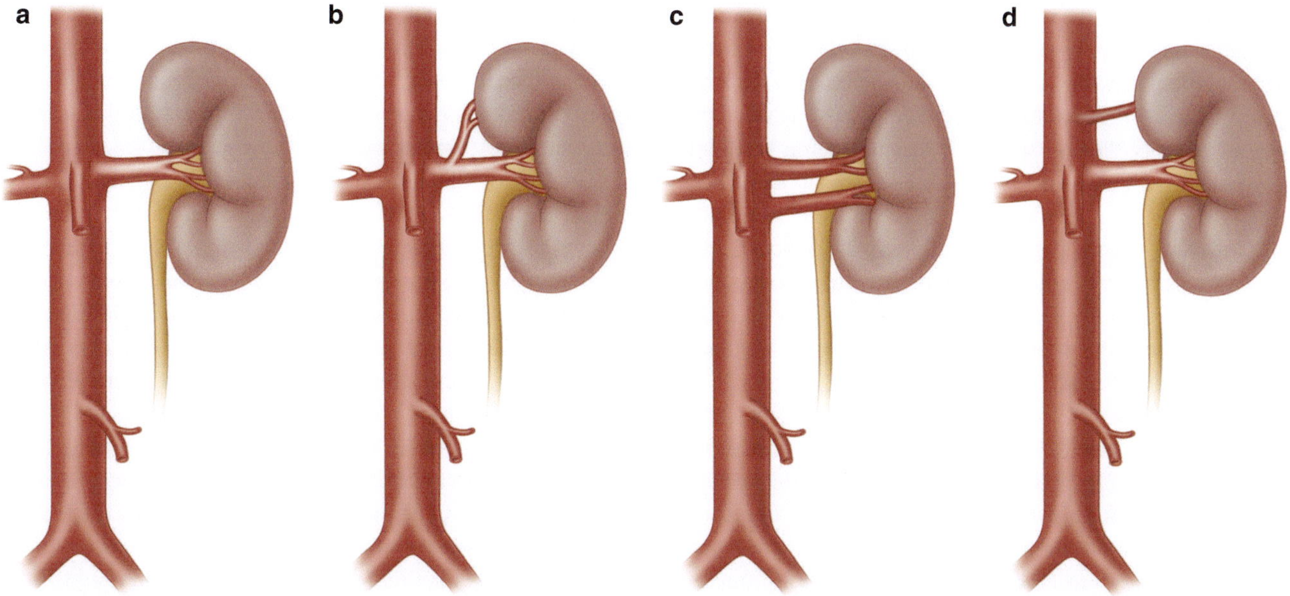

Fig. 32.1 Anatomic variants of renal arteries. (**a**) In a majority of cases (55 %), single renal arteries are present bilaterally. Other variants include (**b**) early branching segmental arteries (14 %), (**c**) dual renal arteries supplying a single kidney (8 %), and (**d**) an accessory renal artery (7 %) (From Safian and Madder [24] with permission)

Fig. 32.2 Pathophysiology of renal artery stenosis (From Fernando and Garasic [29] with permission)

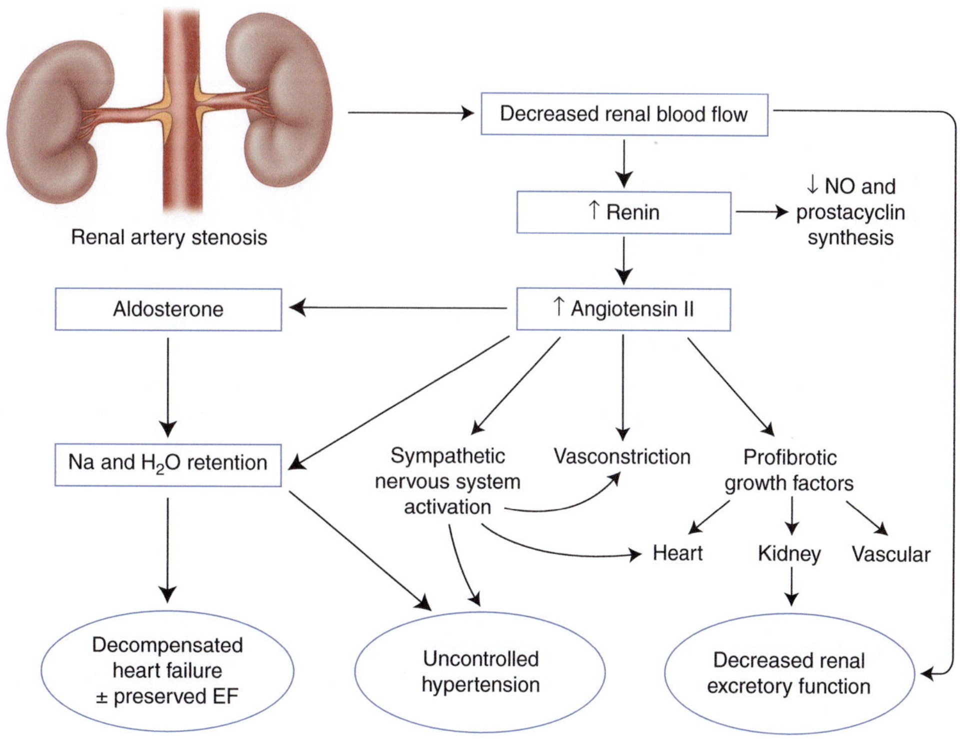

than actual ischemia. Profibrotic mediators induced by angiotensin II – such as transforming growth factor beta, nuclear factor–kB, and platelet-derived growth factor – may also be responsible for renal injury [31–34]. Finally, local atheroembolic events from the culprit renal artery stenosis to the renal parenchyma may contribute [35].

Renal Translesional Hemodynamics

As for lesion assessment in the coronary circulation, the concept of translesional hemodynamic assessment is becoming an increasingly important aspect of renal artery intervention for many of the same reasons [36]. The correlation of angiographic stenosis with the actual physiologic severity of a renal artery stenosis is limited [36–38]. Therefore, translesional hemodynamic assessment is attractive. However, simply measuring a pressure gradient across a stenosis is not necessarily "lesion specific"; that is, such a gradient is dependent on the aortic pressure, the size of the catheter across the lesion, the downstream renal microvasculature, and the renal venous pressure in addition to the actual severity of the stenosis [36]. To circumvent these confounding issues, *hyperemic translesional gradients* and the *fractional flow reserve* can be employed, which requires understanding of the concept of *renal flow reserve*.

The *renal flow reserve* is the proportional increase in renal blood flow in a state of hyperemia compared to baseline in a normal kidney [39]. The renal flow reserve reflects the capacity of overall blood flow to a kidney to increase in response to vasodilatation of the renal microvasculature. In a normal kidney, the flow reserve approaches two with maximal hyperemia [40]. In a stenotic renal artery with normal or diseased parenchymal vessels, the flow reserve is less than in a normal kidney [39]. The lack of vasoreactivity of the renal microvasculature in the post-stenotic kidney may reflect maximal vasodilatation or irreversible microvascular disease. Following revascularization of the post-stenotic kidney with normal parenchymal vessels, the flow reserve increases to supranormal values, indicating lack of maximal vasodilatation of the renal microvasculature at rest and lack of irreversible renal microvascular disease [39]. In contrast, in the stenotic renal artery with abnormal parenchymal vessels, the flow reserve should remain abnormal following revascularization, indicating irreversible microvascular disease.

If the renal artery diameter remains constant, then the renal flow reserve is equal to the hyperemic average peak velocity divided by the baseline average peak velocity. Invasive measurement of flow velocities requires a Doppler wire, which is not widely available. Thus, *fractional flow reserve* is often used as a surrogate for direct measurement of flow velocities, when assessing the effects of a stenosis on flow reserve.

Renal fractional flow reserve is defined as the maximal renal blood flow through a stenotic renal artery divided by the maximal flow in the artery without a stenosis [36]. Maximal renal blood flow in a stenotic artery is equal to the difference of the hyperemic pressure distal to the stenosis and the mean central venous pressure divided by the renal arteriolar resistance. Similarly, the maximal renal blood flow in the absence of a stenosis is equal to the difference of the mean aortic pressure and the mean central venous pressure divided by the renal arteriolar resistance [36]. Under maximal hyperemia, the renal resistance is assumed to be constant and negligible. The central venous pressure is typically near 0 mmHg and negligible. In such conditions, the fractional flow reserve can be calculated with the ratio of the hyperemic pressure distal to the stenosis divided by the mean aortic pressure [41]. However, this assumption is not the case in patients with decompensated heart failure in which disregarding the elevated central venous pressure will result in a falsely elevated (less severe) estimated fractional flow reserve [41].

Because of the limited flow reserve of the renal circulation, particularly in the presence of renal artery stenosis, it may be more appropriate to simply measure *hyperemic translesional pressure gradients* [38]. In the post-stenotic kidney, the efferent arterioles constrict to maintain filtration pressure, which increases the pressure distal to the stenosis. Thus, a significant translesional pressure gradient may be masked at baseline. To remove this confounder, an arteriolar vasodilator specific to the kidney can be administered. Medications that are used to dilate the renal microvasculature and induce hyperemia include papaverine, dopamine, fenoldopam, and isosorbide dinitrate. Dopamine is thought to best achieve maximal hyperemia in the kidney [40]. In contrast, isosorbide dinitrate preferentially vasodilates the main renal arteries and thus does not establish a state of complete hyperemia.

In summary, the clinical implications of assessing hyperemic translesional gradients are multifold. First, removing the effects of efferent arteriolar vasoconstriction is necessary to more accurately assess the hemodynamic significance of a proximal renal artery stenosis [40]. Second, return of vasoreactivity of the renal microvasculature following revascularization may be a surrogate for viability of the kidney and/or reversibility of the clinical syndrome caused by the renal artery stenosis [40, 42].

Clinical Approach to Renal Vascular Diseases

By far, the most common renal vascular disease is renal artery stenosis. Atherosclerosis accounts for >90 % of renal artery stenosis, while fibromuscular dysplasia is the second most common cause (Table 32.1). Transplant renal artery stenosis is a rare, yet emerging, entity. Acute renal vascular disorders are a much less common category of renovascular disease.

Atherosclerotic Renal Artery Stenosis

Presentation

Atherosclerotic renal artery stenosis can cause hypertension, renal excretory dysfunction, and cardiopulmonary disturbance syndromes. A patient with hypertension and renal artery stenosis may have essential hypertension, hypertension due to the renal artery stenosis (*i.e.*, "renovascular hypertension"), or both. Likewise, a patient with renal ischemia may have excretory dysfunction of the post-stenotic

Table 32.1 Comparison of renal artery stenosis due to atherosclerosis or fibromuscular dysplasia

	Atherosclerosis	Fibromuscular dysplasia
Typical clinical syndrome	Renal dysfunction	Hypertension
Typical demographic	Older patients with multiple risk factors or evidence of atherosclerosis	Younger females
Imaging characteristics	Ostial or proximal stenoses, often calcified	Middle/distal stenoses "Beads-on-a-string" of medial fibroplasia Smooth or napkin-ring stenoses or redundancy if intimal fibroplasia
Diagnostic invasive approach	Translesion hemodynamic assessment encouraged	Translesion pressure gradient and IVUS extremely important for medial fibroplasia
Therapeutic invasive approach	Stenting recommended	Angioplasty usually sufficient
Outcomes	Cure/improvement 50–70 %	Cure/improvement 70–90+%

Abbreviations: *IVUS* intravascular ultrasound

kidney; however, disease of the parenchyma may be due to ischemia (*i.e.*, "ischemic nephropathy"), hypertension (*i.e.*, "hypertensive nephropathy"), diabetes (*i.e.*, "diabetic nephropathy"), or other causes [24].

Hypertension is commonly found in patients with renal artery stenosis. Several clinical features classically distinguish hypertension due to renal artery stenosis from essential hypertension. The age of onset is typically either younger or older than that for essential hypertension. If a patient presents with hypertension under the age of 30 years, then renal artery stenosis – particularly, due to fibromuscular dysplasia – should be considered. A late presentation (>55 years) is also suggestive of a secondary cause such as renal artery stenosis. Older patients will also often have known atherosclerosis of other arterial beds. Hypertension due to renal artery stenosis may be refractory to multiple medications, be rapidly progressive, or be malignant with evidence of end organ damage [2].

Renal ischemia is another manifestation of renal artery stenosis that may occur with or without renovascular hypertension. Excretory dysfunction is difficult to detect by serum creatinine unless there is bilateral renal artery ischemia or ischemia of a solitary kidney. Several clinical features can help distinguish excretory dysfunction from renal ischemia from other causes of renal dysfunction, a difficult task for the clinician. A rapid increase in serum creatinine following the initiation of angiotensin-converting enzymes is suggestive of bilateral renal artery stenosis. Alternative causes of renal dysfunction – hypertension, diabetes, intrinsic renal disease, or post-obstructive causes – should be absent, though this is not always the case. Proteinuria is common to many forms of nephropathy, including ischemic nephropathy, but the urinary sediment should be acellular in the presence of renal ischemia [43]. If an elevated serum creatinine exists in the presence of unilateral renal artery stenosis, the diagnosis of clinically significant renal artery stenosis should be questioned as a normally functioning single kidney is adequate to maintain normal serum creatinine levels [3].

Cardiopulmonary syndromes include decompensated heart failure, classically manifested by "flash pulmonary edema," and unstable angina. Cardiopulmonary syndromes are often seen in association with uncontrolled hypertension and/or renal dysfunction. Clinically significant renal artery stenosis should be expected in the setting of decompensated heart failure in the absence of left ventricular or valvular dysfunction [4].

Diagnostic Testing

Diagnostic evaluation must go beyond simple demonstration of an anatomically severe renal artery stenosis. Rather, to optimally select which patients might benefit from revascularization, the clinician should seek information regarding the physiologic severity of a lesion, parenchymal disease of the post-stenotic kidney, and the cause-effect relationship of a stenosis to a particular clinical syndrome. Granted, it is challenging to demonstrate these features in every case, but this approach is useful in guiding the evaluation of patients with renal artery stenosis. The lack of such an approach has likely contributed to the inability of prior randomized trials to show a benefit of renal artery revascularization over medical therapy alone.

Serologic Studies

Serum creatinine is perhaps the most commonly used test to assess for nephropathy of any cause. However, serum creatinine levels do not become elevated until more than 50 % of renal mass is lost [24].

Baseline serum creatinine and estimated glomerular filtration rate have been an inconsistent predictor of clinical improvement following renal artery stenting, often due to lack of strong competing predictor variables adjusted for in various prediction models [44–49]. However, the rate of decline of renal dysfunction (expressed by slope of 1/serum creatinine over time) prior to revascularization may be a predictor of improvement following revascularization, with a steeper rate of decline indicating a higher chance of improvement in renal function as compared to stable, longstanding excretory dysfunction [45, 49]. It may be that actively declining renal function is a surrogate for residual viability.

Other noninvasively collected serologic studies that have been studied in the diagnostic evaluation of renal artery stenosis include *plasma renin activity* and *B-type natriuretic peptide*. Plasma renin activity (measured before and/or after administration of captopril) has poor diagnostic characteristics for the detection of physiologically significant renal artery stenosis and is not recommended (class III) by the American Heart Association in the evaluation of renal artery stenosis [2]. On the other hand, B-type natriuretic peptide is more promising. This hormone may predict improvement in hypertension following renal artery revascularization. In a small cohort of patients ($n=27$) with refractory hypertension and atherosclerotic renal artery stenosis, 17 of 22 patients with a BNP level greater than 80 pg/mL prior to renal artery stenting were shown to have improvement in hypertension (<140/90 mmHg or decrease in DBP by 15 mmHg on same or fewer antihypertensives) at a mean follow-up of 3.5 ± 1.3 months [50]. In contrast, 0 of five patients with a BNP<=80 pg/mL had improvement in hypertension post-stenting. Of note, these results do not generalize to patients with renal excretory dysfunction due to renal artery stenosis or cardiopulmonary disturbance syndromes as exclusion criteria for this study included serum creatinine>=2 mg/dL and decompensated heart failure. Also, the optimal BNP cutoff for this indication should be validated in other study populations. The interpretation of early results from the Hercules (Herculink Elite Renal Stent to Treat Renal Artery Stenosis) study has been pessimistic regarding the predictive ability of BNP for improvement in hypertension following revascularization.

Urine Studies

Proteinuria is a nonspecific marker of nephropathy of multiple causes, including ischemic nephropathy [43]. The degree of proteinuria may have predictive ability regarding improvement in renal function following revascularization for renal artery stenosis. In a retrospective study of 83 patients with renal dysfunction who had undergone percutaneous renal artery revascularization, the presence of >0.6 g/day of urinary protein had an odds ratio of 6.4 (95 % CI 1.4–27.6) for lack of improvement in renal function following revascularization at a mean follow-up of 22 months [51]. Thus, higher degrees of proteinuria may predict less residual renal function to be salvaged by revascularization.

The *urinary sediment* should be bland in patients with ischemic nephropathy. The presence of cellular casts, for example, is suggestive of an alternative, or additional, cause of nephropathy.

Noninvasive Imaging

Duplex ultrasonography is an excellent initial imaging study in the evaluation of renal artery stenosis. It can provide anatomic information on lesion severity (2-D imaging), physiologic information on lesion severity (color and spectral Doppler and velocity measurements), and insight into parenchymal disease (renal resistive index and renal size). Though not universally adopted by vascular laboratories, a peak systolic velocity >200 cm/s and a renal artery/aortic peak systolic velocity ratio of 3.5 is generally consistent with a physiologically significant stenosis. Limitations of duplex ultrasonography include a high degree of expertise needed by the ultrasonographer and inability to attain high quality images due to patient habitus or bowel gas.

Exclusion criteria for many studies of renal artery revascularization have included a renal size <7 cm, assuming this finding is a surrogate for non-viability of the post-stenotic kidney. A normal-sized kidney is >/=10 cm and is reassuring that residual renal function is present. In a prospective cohort study of 215 patients who had undergone renal artery stenting for uncontrolled hypertension, a renal parenchymal/pelvic ratio was an independent predictor of improvement in mean blood pressure 1 year after the intervention [48].

The renal resistive index is defined by the formula 1 – (EDV/PSV). Values >0.80 are considered abnormal and representative of small vessel renovascular disease. This parameter can be a useful prognosticator if interpreted correctly in the context of a particular patient's clinical circumstances. In a prospective cohort study of 138 patients who had undergone renal artery revascularization, a renal resistive index >=0.80 was a strong independent predictor of lack of improvement in renal function following revascularization. Conversely, an index <0.80 was a strong independent predictor of improvement in both renal function and hypertension [52]. Of note, if a segment distal to a critical stenosis is insonated, the RRI will be normal (due to a *parvus et tardus* waveform) but is not necessarily indicative of lack of parenchymal vascular disease. Thus, the renal resistive index is more useful as a prognostic test than as a diagnostic study for renal artery stenosis.

Computed tomographic angiography and *magnetic resonance angiography* are considered to be accurate diagnostic tests for characterizing the anatomic severity of the typical ostial of proximal renal artery stenosis found in atherosclerotic disease [53]). In a meta-analysis of 25 studies encompassing 998 patients, gadolinium-enhanced magnetic resonance angiography had a sensitivity of 97 % (95 % CI: 93±98 %) and specificity of 93 % (95 % CI: 91±95 %) for severe renal artery stenosis in general with catheter-based angiography as the gold standard [54]. Additional advantages and limitations of CT and MR angiography are listed in Table 32.2.

Table 32.2 Comparison of imaging modalities for renal artery stenosis

Modality	Pros	Cons
Doppler ultrasonography	Inexpensive Noninvasive No radiation exposure No contrast use Able to obtain functional information	Highly operator dependent Limited visibility in obese patients Challenging in transplant renal artery stenosis
CT angiography	Good characterization of aorta and proximal large vessel stenoses	Radiation exposure Use of contrast Limited visibility in presence of severe calcification Can be difficult to see mid/distal renal arteries (FMD, dissection)
MRA	Good characterization of aorta and proximal large vessel stenoses No radiation exposure	Expensive Can be difficult to see mid/distal renal arteries (FMD, dissection) High false-positive rate
Scintigraphy	Physiologic information on stenosis severity Information on excretory function	Poor diagnostic characteristics in presence of bilateral renal artery stenosis, renal artery stenosis to a solitary kidney, and global nephropathy of any cause
Invasive angiography	Superior anatomic definition of stenoses Hemodynamic assessment	Risk of vascular complications Radiation exposure Use of contrast (less than CT angiography)

Abbreviations: *CT* computed tomographic, *FMD* fibromuscular dysplasia, *MRA* magnetic resonance angiography

Renal scintigraphy is another noninvasive imaging modality for the evaluation of renal artery stenosis. This test involves intravenous administration of a technetium 99 m-labeled compound to a patient followed by imaging to assess the time to maximum activity of a tracer in the kidney. Additionally, the symmetry of tracer uptake between kidneys, the retention of tracer in the renal cortex, and the effect of captopril on these same parameters on repeat imaging following the administration of oral captopril is determined. This study provides information about size, perfusion, and excretory function. Delayed uptake and decreased uptake compared to contralateral kidney are suggestive of renal ischemia. Cortical retention of tracer is indicative of nephropathy in general. The diagnostic characteristics of this modality for physiologically significant renal artery stenosis is poor in the setting of bilateral renal artery stenosis, renal artery stenosis to a solitary kidney, and global nephropathy of any cause [2]. However, abnormal unilateral function, defined by a ratio of <=0.45 of estimated blood flow to the affected kidney/total bilateral renal blood flow, has been shown to be an independent predictor of improvement in hypertension or renal function in a prospective cohort study of 40 patients who underwent renal artery stenting for uncontrolled hypertension or renal dysfunction [55]. Likely, lateralization of perfusion on a renal scintigram is a surrogate for a hemodynamically significant stenosis.

Catheter-Based Evaluation

Catheter-based angiography is considered the gold standard technique for characterizing the anatomic severity of a renal artery stenosis (Fig. 32.3a). This modality is typically not the 1st-line imaging test for atherosclerotic renal artery stenosis due to the small but real risk of vascular complications. However, it should be mentioned that less contrast is required for diagnostic catheter-based angiography (<20–25 cc for abdominal aortography; <10 cc for each renal artery) compared to CT angiography (>85 cc iodinated contrast) [53]. The technique of catheter-based angiography is discussed later in the chapter.

Measurement of translesional pressure gradients provides important diagnostic information as angiographic evaluation alone is thought to be an inaccurate measure of lesion severity [36, 41, 56, 57] (Fig. 32.3b). With a flow wire or small caliber catheter, systolic and mean translesional pressures can be measured at rest. With a flow wire, a hyperemic translesional systolic and mean gradient as well as a fractional flow reserve can be measured after the administration of a renal vasodilator. In a prospective study of 17 patients with medically refractory hypertension, 86 % of those with a FFR<0.8 after intra-arterial administration of papaverine had improvement in hypertension at 90 days following renal artery stenting. In contrast, only 30 % of those with a hyperemic FFR>0.8 experienced improved blood pressure control [36]. In another prospective study of 62 patients with unilateral renal artery stenosis 50–90 % by qualitative angiography, among multiple hemodynamic, angiographic, and IVUS variables, a hyperemic systolic gradient measured by a flow wire was the only independent predictor of clinical improvement in hypertension at 12 months following renal artery stenting. In this study, 84 % of those with a hyperemic systolic gradient >=21 mmHg showed improvement in blood pressure control compared to 36 % for those with a hyperemic systolic gradient <21 mmHg [38]. Similar findings

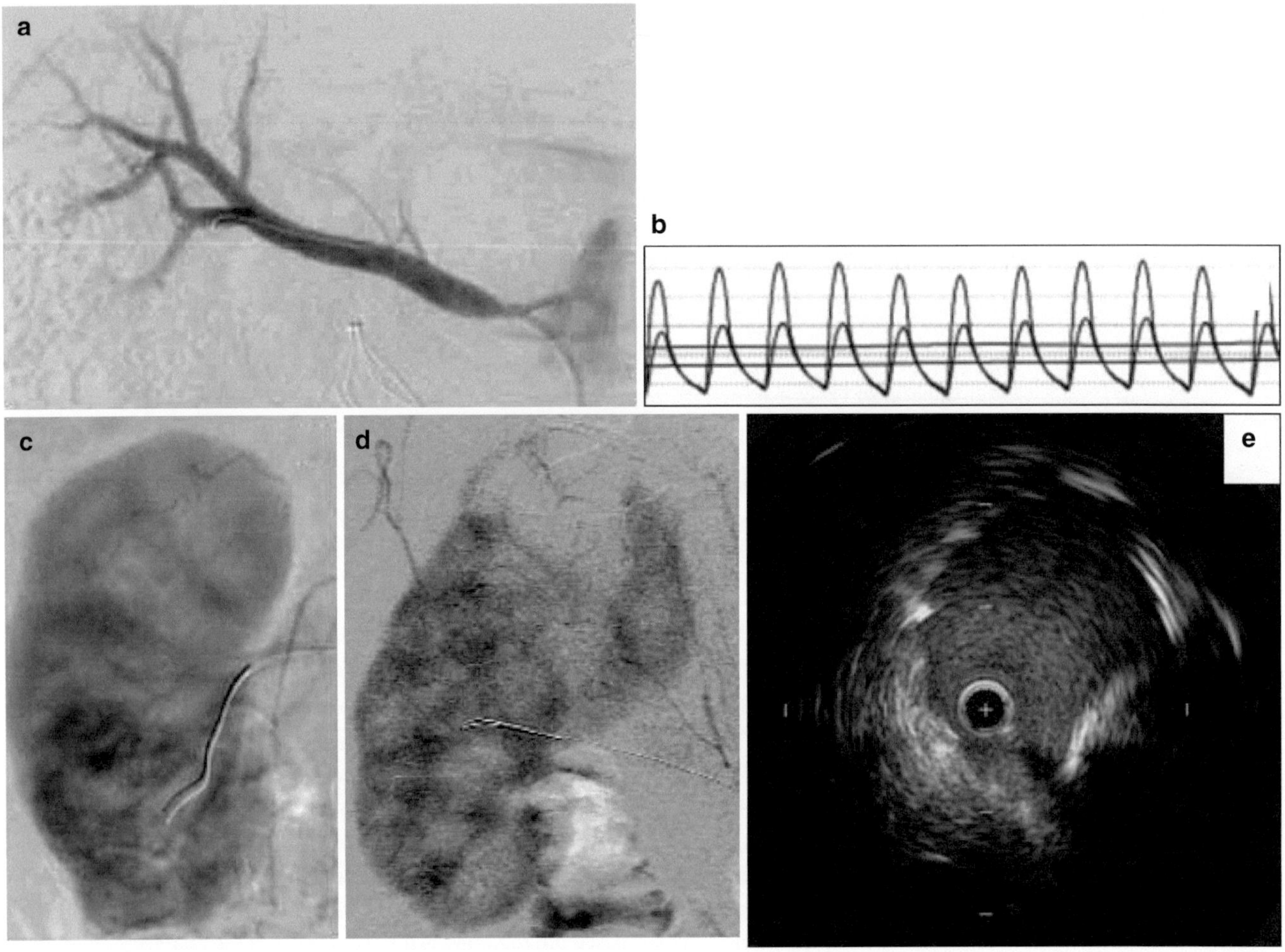

Fig. 32.3 Catheter-based assessment of renal artery stenosis. (**a**) Selective right renal angiogram demonstrating the typical ostial location of an atherosclerotic renal artery stenosis. (**b**) Translesional hemodynamic measurements obtained from a 0.014-in. flow wire in a different patient. After intrarenal administration of 40 mg of papaverine, the FFR was 0.6 and the hyperemic systolic gradient was 40 mmHg. (**c**) Normal nephrogram. (**d**) Nephrogram indicating abnormal perfusion of the upper pole of the kidney. (**e**) IVUS showing underdeployed renal artery stent that was subsequently post-dilated

were demonstrated in a prospective study of 53 patients with unilateral renal artery stenosis and refractory hypertension in which a dopamine-induced hyperemic mean gradient was the strongest predictor, among other translesional hemodynamic variables, of improvement in hypertension after renal artery stenting [37]). In this study, a dopamine-induced hyperemic mean gradient had an area under the receiver operator characteristic curve of 0.77 (95 % CI 0.64–0.90) for improvement in hypertension 3 months following stenting. The optimal cutoff value was 20 mmHg.

The predictive ability of hyperemic gradients likely reflects more accurate assessment of lesion severity by removing the effects of downstream resistance that confounds lesion assessment at rest. Furthermore, response in the parenchymal vessels to a vasodilator may represent reversibility of disease and viability of the kidney. The technique of obtaining translesional pressure gradients is discussed later in the chapter [40, 42].

Renal vein renin sampling via a catheter selectively placed in the renal veins has been described in the assessment of renal artery stenosis. In a prospective study of 50 patients with refractory hypertension and unilateral renal artery stenosis, a ratio of <1.5 of the plasma renin activity from the renal vein of the post-stenotic kidney to the plasma renin activity from the renal vein of the contralateral kidney was an independent predictor of failure to improve hypertension following revascularization [58]. Such lateralization of renal vein renin levels may be a surrogate for an ipsilateral, physiologically significant renal artery stenosis. Thus, it is unclear if this modality would have practical, incremental information to translesional hemodynamic data. Clinical utility is also limited if results of the renin assay cannot be obtained in "real time." The role of renal vein renin sampling may be more useful in guiding the decision to perform nephrectomy of a post-stenotic atrophic kidney in a patient with refractory hypertension [2].

Table 32.3 2005 ACC/AHA guidelines for renal artery revascularization

Class of indication	Level of evidence	Indication
I	B	Hemodynamically significant RAS with recurrent, unexplained HF, or sudden unexplained pulmonary edema
IIa	B	RAS with either (a) accelerated, resistant, or malignant hypertension, (b) hypertension with unilateral small kidney, and (c) hypertension with medical intolerance
IIa	B	CKD with bilateral RAS or RAS to solitary kidney
IIa	B	RAS and unstable angina
IIb	C	Asymptomatic bilateral RAS or solitary viable kidney with hemodynamically significant RAS
IIb	C	Asymptomatic unilateral hemodynamically significant RAS in a viable kidney
IIb	C	RAS and CKD with unilateral RAS with two kidneys present

From Hirsch et al. [2]

Abbreviations: *ACC* American College of Cardiology, *AHA* American Heart Association, *RAS* renal artery stenosis, *HF* decompensated heart failure; *CKD* chronic kidney disease

The *nephrogram* (cineangiographic visualization of contrast uptake into the renal parenchyma) can provide information on the extent of parenchymal disease and may be predictive of outcomes following revascularization (Fig. 32.3c, d). In a retrospective study of 24 hypertensive patients with unilateral renal artery stenosis and 17 controls, Mahmud et al. analyzed the ability of two aspects of the nephrogram to predict outcomes following renal artery stenting. The authors showed that improvement in *renal frame count* (number of frames required for contrast to reach the distal parenchyma) and *renal blush grade* (objective score of intensity of parenchymal opacification by contrast) after renal artery stenting predicted better blood pressure control post-intervention [59]. Of note, to determine renal frame count as defined in this study would require image acquisition at 30 frames/s, which is faster than that typically used for digital subtraction angiography. It will be interesting if related future research determines whether any pre-interventional features of the nephrogram are also predictive.

Intravascular ultrasound (IVUS) has been described for renal artery stenting [38, 60] (Fig. 32.3e). The predictive characteristics of IVUS for improvement in blood pressure were studied in 62 patients undergoing renal artery revascularization [38]. The minimum luminal area had an area under the receiver operator characteristic curve of 0.86 (95 % CI 0.76–0.95), indicating excellent predictive value for improvement at 12 months following revascularization. The optimal cut point for the minimum luminal area was 7.8 mm^2, which had 79 % predictive accuracy. IVUS may improve technical results, as well. In a retrospective study of 131 patients undergoing IVUS-guided renal artery stenting, IVUS identified 22 (14 %) cases of stent malapposition or underexpansion, 8 (5 %) dissections and 6 (4 %) in geographic miss of the ostium [38, 60]. These findings were not apparent on angiography.

Management

All patients with atherosclerotic renal artery stenosis should receive appropriate medical therapy for atherosclerosis including antiplatelet therapy, HMG CoA reductase inhibitors (statins), and blood pressure control in addition to counseling for smoking cessation and lifestyle modifications. The challenging clinical decision making for renal artery stenosis often involves whether to offer revascularization in addition to optimal medical therapy.

Indications for renal artery revascularization proposed by the American College of Cardiology and American Heart Association in 2005 are summarized in Table 32.3. There are both surgical and endovascular revascularization options. Surgical methods include aorto-renal bypass, extra-anatomic bypass (e.g., splenorenal, hepatorenal), and endarterectomy [2]. The only randomized trial of surgical compared to percutaneous revascularization was conducted in the 1980s and was underpowered ($n = 58$) and not applicable to contemporary practice (renal artery angioplasty performed without stenting) [61]. In a large surgical series of 323 patients undergoing surgical revascularization for renal artery stenosis, the perioperative mortality rate was 5.6 % [62]. In another similar report from a different institution, the 30-day mortality for surgical renal artery revascularization was 7.4 % [63]. Due to the higher morbidity and mortality associated with surgical revascularization for renal artery stenosis, endovascular treatment is usually preferred. Accordingly, several randomized trials have compared percutaneous renal artery revascularization with medical therapy [64–68].

Randomized Trials Comparing Percutaneous Renal Artery Revascularization to Medical Therapy

Five randomized trials have been published in which percutaneous renal artery revascularization was compared to medical therapy, and results from a 6th trial are awaited [64–68] (Table 32.4). The initial three trials were small, published in 1998–2000 prior to the routine use of stenting in the renal artery, and included study populations with hypertension. The other two trials were published in 2009 and included larger study populations that consisted primarily of patients

Table 32.4 Trials of percutaneous renal artery revascularization compared to medical therapy

Study	N	Study population	Intervention	Lesion assessment	Primary outcome	Follow-up
EMMA [64]	49	HTN (DBP >95 or on AHM) Unilateral RAS ≥75% or ≥60% + abnormal functional study Functional contralateral kidney CrCl ≥50 cc/min Recent pulmonary edema excluded	Angioplasty	Angiography Scintigraphy IVP Renal vein renin	Ambulatory blood pressure	6 months
SNRASCB [66]	55	HTN (DBP >95 + 2 AHM) Unilateral and bilateral RAS >50% SCr >5.7 mg/dL excluded	Angioplasty	Angiography	Change in mean BP and SCr	6 months
DRASTIC [67]	106	HTN (DBP >95 × 2 + 2 AHM) or increase SCr >0.2 mg/dL on ACEi RAS ≥50% Solitary kidney excluded SCr > 1.7 mg/dL excluded Heart failure excluded	Angioplasty	Angiography	SBP and DBP at 3 and 12 months	12 months
STAR [65]	140	Renal dysfunction (CrCl <80 mL/min) RAS ≥50% CrCl <15 mL/min excluded Malignant HTN excluded	Stenting	CT, MR, or angiography for inclusion Angiography for treatment	≥20% decrease in CrCl	2 years
ASTRAL [69]	806	Unexplained renal dysfunction or uncontrollable HTN thought due to RAS "Substantial" anatomic RAS	Stenting	CT, MR, US, or angiography for inclusion Angiography for treatment	Slope of 1/SCr	34 months
CORAL [70]	1,080 (goal)	SBP≥155 + 2 AHM ≥80% RAS by angiography 60–80 % stenosis by angiography and 20 mmHg systolic gradient Recent HF excluded	Stenting	Angiography Pressure gradient (obtained by catheter, not flow wire)	Composite of CV/renal death, MI, HF hospitalization, stroke, doubling SCr, and dialysis	Ongoing

Abbreviations: *EMMA* Essai Multicentrique Medicaments vs Angioplastie, *SNRASCB* Scottish and Newcastle Renal Artery Stenosis Collaborative Group, *DRASTIC* Dutch Renal Artery Stenosis Intervention Cooperative Study, *STAR* Stent placement in patients with Atherosclerotic Renal artery stenosis and impaired renal function, *ASTRAL* Angioplasty and Stenting for Renal Artery Lesions, *HTN* hypertension, *DBP* diastolic blood pressure, *AHM* antihypertensive medications, *RAS* renal artery stenosis, *CrCl* creatinine clearance, *IVP* intravenous pyelogram, *SCr* serum creatinine, *CV* cardiovascular, *MI* myocardial infarction, *HF* heart failure

with renal insufficiency. The methodology and results of these trials are summarized below.

The 1st randomized trial of percutaneous renal artery revascularization (*Essai Multicentrique Medicaments vs Angioplastie, or EMMA*) compared to medical therapy included 49 patients with unilateral renal artery stenosis and uncontrolled hypertension [64]. No statistically significant change in the primary outcome of 24-h ambulatory blood pressure was found between the two groups. The study was limited by lack of adequate power, lack of adjunctive stenting in the intervention group, and a high crossover rate (7 of 26 in medical therapy group). Furthermore, the trial was not applicable to those with severe disease as only 8 of 23 in angioplasty group had >75 % stenosis, and those with malignant hypertension, pulmonary edema, and creatinine clearance <50 mL/min were excluded.

The second early randomized trial (*Scottish and Newcastle Renal Artery Stenosis Collaborative Group*) of percutaneous renal artery revascularization compared to medical therapy included two parallel arms – patients with bilateral renal artery stenosis and unilateral renal artery stenosis – each compared to medical therapy [66]. This trial was also limited by a small study population and lack of stenting in the interventional group. Despite these limitations which bias against a beneficial effect of angioplasty, those in the angioplasty group with bilateral renal artery stenosis exhibited an impressive benefit in the primary outcome of blood pressure improvement at 6 months compared to baseline (mean 166/90 vs. 185/94, SD not provided, p value not provided). In comparison, the medical therapy arm of the bilateral renal artery stenosis group had minimal change in blood pressure over the prespecified follow-up period of 6 months (177/93 vs. 179/91). The comparison of the change in blood pressure between the two groups (17 mmHg systolic/3 mmHg diastolic) in favor of angioplasty did not reach statistical significance. In those with unilateral renal artery stenosis, the blood pressure improved to a similar degree over 6 months in the angioplasty (−9/−5 mmHg) and medical (−8/−6 mmHg) groups.

Renal angioplasty was also compared with medical therapy in the *DRASTIC* (Dutch Renal Artery Stenosis Intervention Cooperative study) trial [67]. Eligible patients had refractory hypertension or an increase in serum creatinine by 0.2 mg/dL as well as a>=50 % renal artery stenosis due to atherosclerosis by qualitative angiographic assessment by the treating interventionalist. Exclusion criteria included a history of unstable angina or decompensated heart failure, serum creatinine >2.3 mg/dL or >1.7 in presence of solitary kidney, and post-stenotic kidney <8 cm. Though a power analysis was not provided, 106 patients were randomized and followed for 1 year. The primary outcome included the systolic and diastolic blood pressure at 3 and 12 months. Twenty-two of the 50 (44 %) patients in the medical group crossed over to the angioplasty group for either worsening hypertension or renal function. Only two patients who underwent angioplasty received adjunctive stenting. There was no statistical difference in the primary outcome at 3 or 12 months. Regarding secondary outcomes, patients in the angioplasty group were taking fewer antihypertensives than the medical therapy group (1.9 vs. 2.4, $p=0.002$) at 12 months. In eight patients in the medical therapy group who did not cross over, the renal artery stenosis progressed to complete occlusion and was associated with an increase of serum creatinine by>=50 %. Restenosis (>=50 %) within the treated renal artery segment occurred in 23 of the 48 patients who underwent repeat angiography. Blood pressure improved in 38 of 56 patients in the angioplasty group but only 18 of 48 in the medical therapy group.

The DRASTIC trial has been criticized for the high crossover rate of the medical arm to the angioplasty arm as well as lack of adjunctive stenting, which likely explains the high restenosis rate [71]. Several other features of the trial suggest that the study population had moderate, rather than severe disease, and would be less likely to benefit from revascularization over medical therapy: Those with unstable angina or heart failure were excluded, limiting applicability to patients with cardiopulmonary syndromes from renal artery stenosis. Twenty-one percent of the angioplasty group and 30 % of the medical therapy group had stenoses <70 %. Nine percent of the study population had stenoses <50 % as adjudicated by an independent committee.

The *STAR* trial (Stent placement in patients with Atherosclerotic Renal artery stenosis and impaired renal function) was a multicenter European randomized trial of renal artery stenting compared to medical therapy for treatment of patients with renal dysfunction ascribed to atherosclerotic renal artery stenosis [65]. It was the 1st trial of a study population with renal artery stenosis and primarily renal dysfunction, rather than hypertension. It was also the 1st trial in which renal artery stenting, rather than renal angioplasty, was the primary modality of revascularization.

Inclusion criteria were estimated creatinine clearance <80 mL/min and renal artery stenosis >=50 % by noninvasive imaging. The primary outcome was a >=20 % decrease in creatinine clearance during the 2 year follow-up period. The study was powered for a 50 % event rate in the stenting group and a 20 % event rate in the medical therapy group. However, the event rates were much lower: 16 % in the stenting group and 22 % in the medical therapy group, a difference that did not reach statistical significance. One reason for the low event rate was, again, the inclusion of patients with moderate, rather than severe, disease. Surprisingly, only 46 of the 62 patients randomized to the stenting arm actually underwent renal artery stenting, largely because 12 patients had angiographic stenoses <50 %. The fact that only 74 % of patients (46 of 62) in the stenting arm were actually revascularized compounds the limitation of inadequate power in this trial.

Other disturbing data from the STAR trial involved complication rates. Though the mortality rate was the same for the medical and interventional groups (8 % over 2 years), three deaths in the stenting group followed procedural complications (two renal artery perforations and one infected hematoma). Such procedural complications rightfully influenced the general conclusions from this study. However, the mortality rate of 6.5 % in patients receiving stents is markedly higher than that reported in other trials and observational studies of renal artery stenting (~0.8 %) [5].

Like STAR, the *ASTRAL* (Angioplasty and Stenting for Renal Artery Lesions) trial compared renal artery stenting to medical therapy alone in a study population with renal dysfunction and renal artery stenosis [68]. Eight hundred and six patients were randomized and followed for a median of 34 months. The primary outcome was the rate of decline in renal function measured by the reciprocal of the serum creatinine. There was a non-statistical trend in favor of the stenting group (-0.13×10^{-3} vs. -0.07×10^{-3}, $p=0.06$), though the study has been interpreted as a negative one.

Several concerns about the internal validity and generalizability of the ASTRAL trial have been raised [72–77]. First, the results are generalizable to those with moderate disease, rather than severe disease. Approximately 40 % of patients had stenoses <70, and 9 % of patients randomized to the intervention group were thought not to have sufficiently severe lesion to warrant stenting by angiography. Second, there is concern for the lack of assessment of viability and small vessel renal disease. Patients with renal sizes as low as 6 cm were included in the trial as well as patients with polycystic kidney disease. Also, renal resistive indices were not assessed. Third, though not commonly recognized, ASTRAL trial was underpowered. The observed decline in renal function, as assessed by the reciprocal of creatinine, was less severe by a factor of 10 than that expected and used for the power calculation. Thus, though the study was powered to detect a 20 % difference in the primary outcome, the p value was 0.06 despite a 50 % difference in the primary outcome.

Summary of Randomized Trials

In summary, results from the five trials summarized above have dampened enthusiasm for renal artery revascularization. More importantly, lessons from these trials indicate that careful patient selection is paramount to optimal patient outcomes and that benefits are limited in patients with moderate renal artery stenosis associated with excretory dysfunction. It is more difficult to draw conclusions regarding renal artery stenting in patients with renal artery stenosis and hypertension, as relevant trials suffered from small sample sizes and high crossover rates. Finally, this evidence base is not generalizable to patients with cardiopulmonary disturbance syndromes, as such patients were excluded from these trials. Some of these unresolved issues will be addressed by the ongoing CORAL trial, in which patients with refractory hypertension and hemodynamically significant renal artery stenoses (incorporating translesional gradient assessment) will be randomized after catheter-based angiography to optimal medical therapy or renal artery stenting with distal embolic protection. The primary outcome will be a composite of cardiovascular and renal events. The results are expected in 2012 [70].

Patient Selection for Renal Artery Revascularization for Atherosclerotic Renal Artery Stenosis

In the absence of the "perfect" clinical prediction model, the following guidelines may facilitate optimal patient selection for renal artery stenting:

- When considering revascularization of renal artery stenoses associated with hypertension and/or excretory dysfunction, demonstration of a hemodynamically significant stenosis is paramount. A hyperemic mean or systolic gradient of >20 mmHg and a renal fractional flow reserve of <0.8 has been shown to be predictive of improvement in hypertension following renal artery stenting [36–38].
- When considering revascularization for renal artery stenosis associated with excretory dysfunction, viability is important. Proteinuria, renal size, a recent decline in renal function, and the renal resistive index may assist with decisions of viability.
- For patients with suspected hypertension due to renal artery stenosis, blood pressure control may not improve following revascularization in the presence of small vessel disease within the renal parenchyma. A renal resistive index <0.80 and a translesional gradient response to a renal vasodilator may be surrogates for the absence of irreversible small vessel disease.
- In the presence of a renal artery stenosis, causes for nephropathy or hypertension other than the stenosis should be strongly considered prior to revascularization.

Fibromuscular Dysplasia

Fibromuscular dysplasia is an idiopathic, noninflammatory arteriopathy [29, 78]. It accounts for ~10 % of renal artery stenosis [2, 78]. Sixty to seventy percent of cases of fibromuscular dysplasia involve the renal arteries, and 35 % of these cases are bilateral [6, 29].

Fibromuscular dysplasia most commonly affects females aged 15–50 years and is more common in 1st-degree relatives of those with fibromuscular dysplasia than in the general population [29, 78]. It can be an incidental finding or present as hypertension [29]. Rarely, patients with fibromuscular dysplasia develop renal dysfunction [24].

In contrast to atherosclerotic disease of the renal arteries, fibromuscular dysplasia affects the mid and distal renal artery [78]. The angiographic appearance depends on the type of FMD. Medial fibroplasia (>80 % of FMD cases) appears as "beads-on-a-string" [78] (Fig. 32.4a). Intimal fibroplasia (10 % of FMD cases) can appear as a "napkin-ring" stenosis, a long, smooth stenosis resembling a vasculitis (Figs. 32.4, and 32.5), or as redundancy in the affected vessel [78]. Perimedial fibroplasia, medial hyperplasia, and adventitial hyperplasia are much less common.

In a meta-analysis in which catheter-based angiography was the gold standard, CT angiography and MR angiography had excellent specificity but limited sensitivity [79] for renal fibromuscular dysplasia. The specificity of CT angiography was 99 % (95 % CI 98–100 %) and of MR angiography was 96 % (95 % CI 94–97 %), while the sensitivity was only 28 % for CT (95 % CI 15–52 %) and 22 % for MR (12–32 %). Duplex ultrasonography remains an excellent test for renal FMD, however [78].

In 11 observational studies of 456 patients who underwent angioplasty to treat hypertension from renal FMD, 70–98 % of patients enjoyed improvement or cure from hypertension over 9–39 months of follow-up [78, 80]. Thus, the threshold to revascularize patients with renal FMD is lower than for atherosclerotic renal artery stenosis. However,

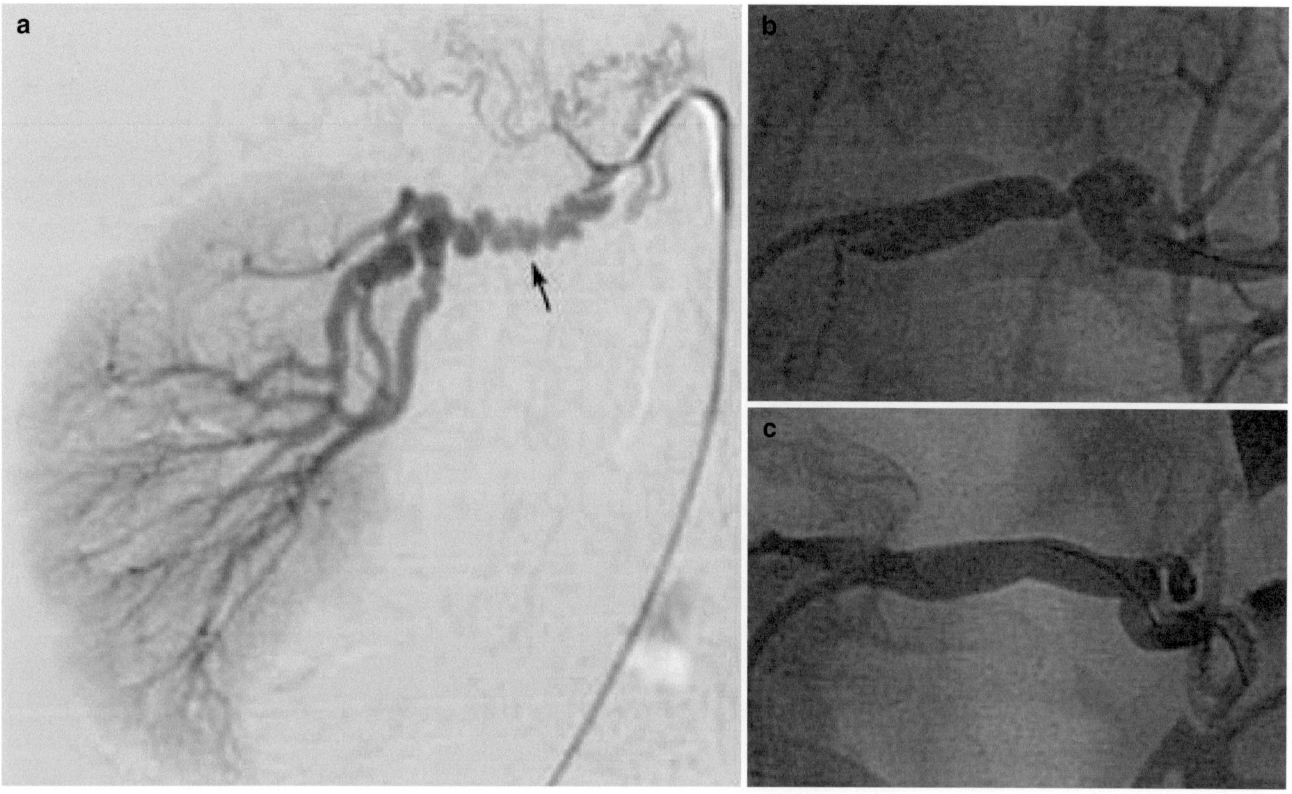

Fig. 32.4 (**a**) Nonselective renal angiogram demonstrating typical "beads-on-a-string" (*arrow*) appearance of medial fibroplasia. (**b**) Selective renal angiogram demonstrating a "napkin-ring" stenosis typical of intimal fibroplasia. (**c**) Final angiogram in the same patient after angioplasty alone

randomized trials of renal revascularization have included patients with atherosclerotic renal artery stenosis, rather than renal FMD. In addition, patients with hypertension due to renal FMD should receive medical therapy for blood pressure control.

It is generally accepted that angiographic assessment of the medial fibroplasia variant of FMD is challenging. Thus, operators should measure translesional gradients and strongly consider using intravascular ultrasound to assess lesion severity [4, 24]. Angioplasty, with bailout stenting, is the recommended revascularization strategy [4, 29, 78]. Distal embolic protection is not thought to be necessary for renal FMD interventions.

Transplant Renal Artery Stenosis

Transplant renal artery stenosis is a rare cause of renal artery stenosis and an infrequent, though not insignificant, occurrence following renal transplant. In a retrospective cohort study of 831 renal transplant patients at a single institution, the incidence of transplant renal artery stenosis was 3.1 % and was diagnosed by catheter-based angiography done to evaluate worsening allograft function [81]. In another large retrospective cohort study of 1,843 patients with renal transplants, the incidence of transplant renal artery stenosis was 0.75 % [82]. Thus, the incidence of clinically significant transplant renal artery stenosis in contemporary practice is likely <3 %.

Transplant renal artery stenosis typically occurs within 12 months following transplant [82, 83]. Causes are usually due to a mechanical problem during surgery or intimal hyperplasia [81, 83]. Other potential contributors to posttransplant renal failure are cytomegalovirus and allograft rejection. The stenosis is often at the anastomosis. However, an upstream aorto-iliac stenosis compromising the inflow into the transplanted renal artery can also cause this syndrome.

The presentation can be quite dramatic, due to rapidly progressive allograft dysfunction, uncontrolled hypertension, or volume overload [83]. Duplex ultrasonography is a reasonable diagnostic test in these patients in whom administration of iodinated contrast is typically contraindicated. However, the transplanted renal artery can be difficult to image with this modality. Catheter-based angiography offers a diagnostic modality in which less contrast is needed than CT angiography, albeit at the higher risk of vascular complications.

Percutaneous angioplasty and stenting is the preferred treatment of clinically significant transplant renal artery stenosis, in the absence of clinical trials, to salvage the allograft [81–83]. From small case series, the technical success

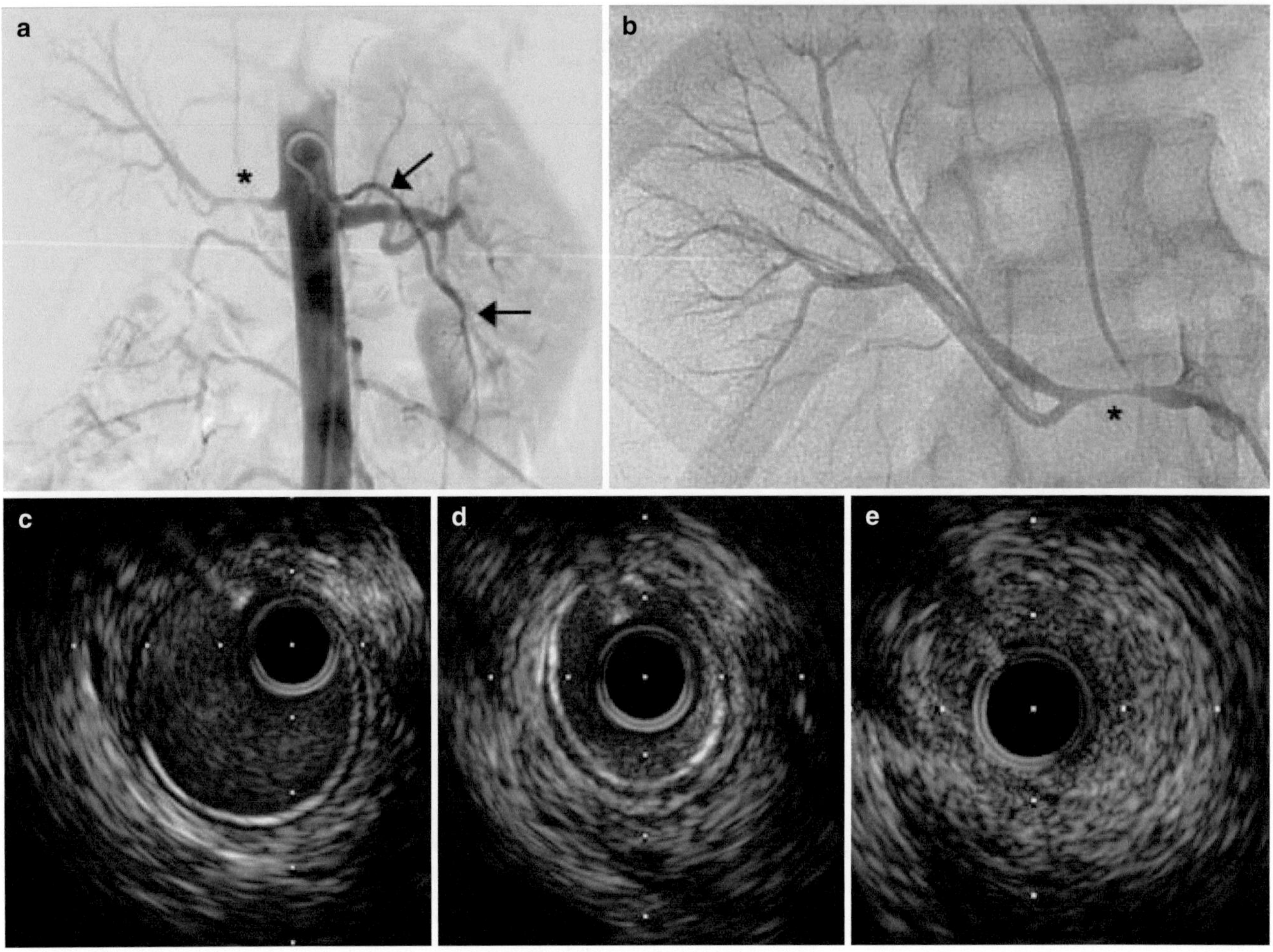

Fig. 32.5 20-year-old female thought to have intimal fibroplasia. (**a**) Severe, long smooth stenosis of the right renal artery (*asterisk*). There is delayed filling of the right nephrogram of the post-stenotic kidney relative to the contralateral normal kidney. Note the right accessory renal artery (*arrows*). (**b**) Selective left renal angiogram in the same patient. (**c**) IVUS image distal to the stenosis in relatively normal vessel. (**d**) IVUS image within the distal lesion. Note intimal thickening from 3 to 8 o'clock. (**e**) IVUS image within the stenosis. There is diffuse intimal thickening such that the IVUS catheter is occlusive

approaches 95–100 % [81, 82, 84], though it is difficult to draw conclusions regarding durability in the "stenting era" due to the rarity of this condition and limited duration of reported follow-up. The angiographic approach depends on the site of the anastomosis. That is, for end-to-end anastomoses of the donor renal artery to the internal iliac artery, contralateral common femoral access is preferred [84]. In contrast, for end-to-side anastomoses of the donor renal artery to the external or common iliac arteries, ipsilateral common femoral artery access is favored (Fig. 32.6). The aorto-iliac inflow to the donor renal artery should be assessed in some fashion – if not angiographically, then noninvasively.

Acute Renovascular Disorders

Acute renovascular disorders can involve occlusions of either the renal arteries or the renal veins. Acute renal arterial occlusion can be caused by thromboembolism, atheroembolism, in situ thrombosis, and spontaneous dissections [26]. Other causes – such as trauma, abdominal aortic dissection, iatrogenic occlusion during abdominal aneurysm endografting, and renal artery aneurysmal rupture – are beyond the scope of this chapter.

Acute renovascular disorders are rare [85]. Similar to acute mesenteric ischemia, the heart is the source of most thromboembolic events [85, 86]. It is more common for emboli to occlude small branches, a situation less amenable to endovascular treatment than occlusion of a main renal artery [26]. Similarly, atheroemboli – either spontaneous or iatrogenic – tend to occlude small vessels [26]. In situ thrombosis can complicate a previously existing atherosclerotic plaque or may occur due to a hypercoagulable state, such as antiphospholipid antibody syndrome. Patients with preexisting renal artery stenosis are more likely to have prolonged viability in the setting of a renal infarct due to

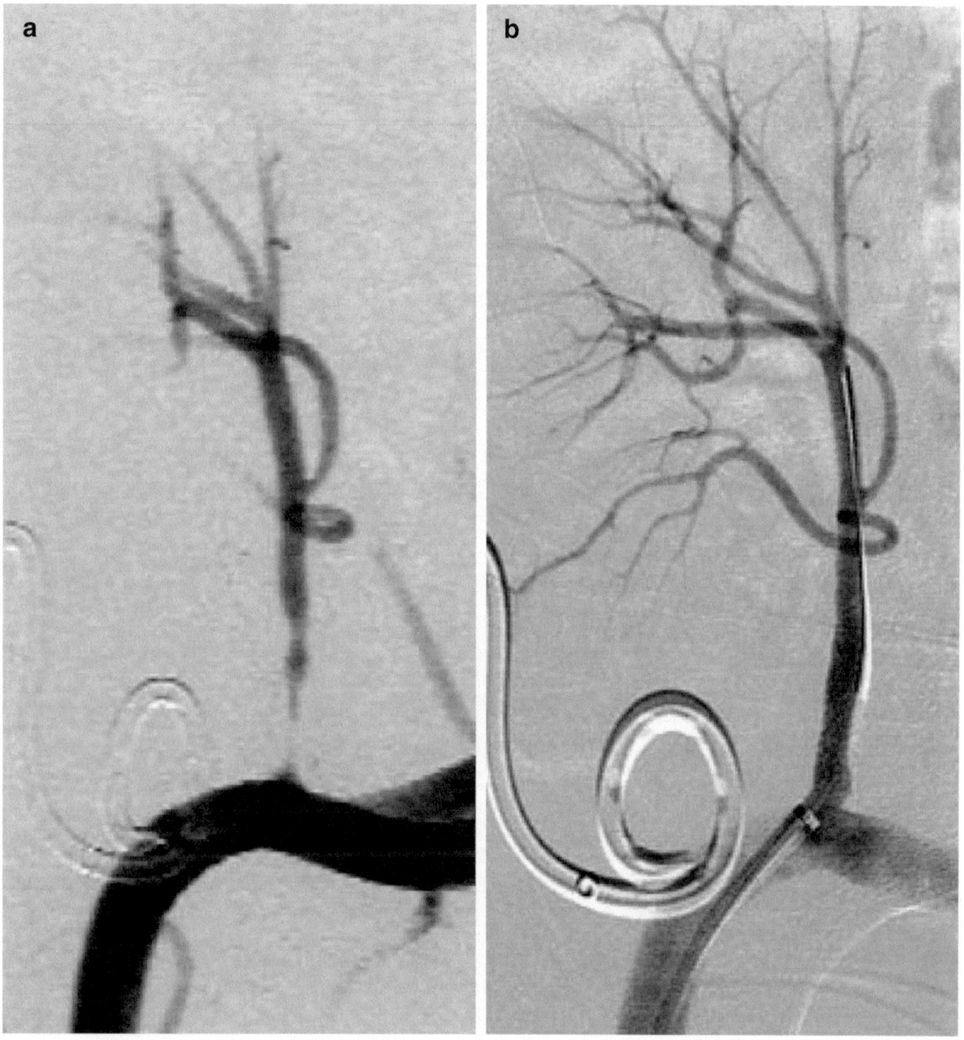

Fig. 32.6 Case of transplant renal artery stenosis. (**a**) The transplanted renal artery has a critical stenosis just distal to the anastomosis with the right external iliac artery. (**b**) Post-intervention (5 × 20 mm balloon-expandable stent), there is improved filling of the nephrogram

preexisting collaterals [26]. An association between Behcet's disease and acute thrombotic occlusion of the renal artery has been described [87]. Spontaneous dissection may occur in a patient with renal artery atherosclerosis, fibromuscular dysplasia, or Vascular Ehlers-Danlos (Ehlers-Danlos Syndrome Type IV). If a dissection propagates into the segmental branches, endovascular therapy is unfavorable (Fig. 32.7).

The result of acute renal artery occlusion is renal infarction. It is believed that the kidney can remain viable for up to 1.5–3 h, in the absence of developed preexisting collaterals [26, 85, 86, 88]. The patient often presents with flank pain, nausea and vomiting, hematuria, and hypertension. An elevated lactate dehydrogenase is nearly always present and has a sensitivity well over 90 % [85, 86, 88]. The serum creatinine will not be elevated if the contralateral kidney is normal. Thus, the trend of serum creatinine is not a good indicator of ongoing infarction; scintigraphy or serum LDH is more accurate in this regard. The renal infarct is usually evident by computed tomography, ultrasonography, or magnetic resonance imaging. The actual arterial occlusion may not be visualized by these imaging modalities if it is located in distal renal artery branches.

There is scant data on the outcome of acute renal infarction due to arterial occlusion. In a series of 44 patients with acute renal infarction due to thromboembolism from atrial fibrillation, 23 of 44 patients had normal renal function as assessed by serum creatinine at follow-up [86]. Only three patients progressed to need dialysis. This cohort was treated predominantly with a noninvasive approach. In another series of 11 patients with acute renal infarction, three patients had deterioration in renal function while eight had stable renal function [85]. There was unsuccessful restoration of renal function in one patient treated invasively.

There are case reports and small series of catheter-directed thrombolysis for acute renal artery occlusion. In a series of 14 patients treated with catheter-directed thrombolysis for acute renal infarction due to thromboembolism, procedural success was achieved in 13 of the 14 patients, but no

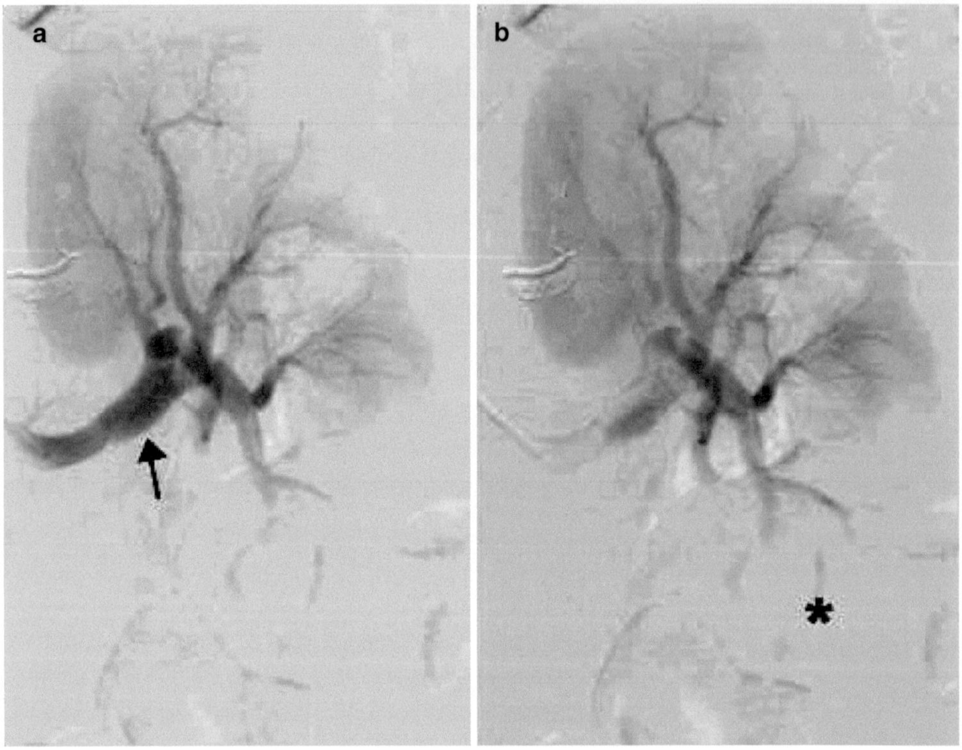

Fig. 32.7 Acute renal artery dissection in 33-year-old female with Ehlers-Danlos IV. (**a**) Dissection flap (*arrow*) involves the main renal artery and extends into multiple segmental branches. (**b**) Nephrogram in the same patient demonstrates no filling of inferior pole of the kidney (*asterisk*)

significant improvement was found in the affected kidney's function by scintigraphy. These patients were diagnosed 12 h to 8 days after symptoms [88]. There are also case reports of successful restoration of renal function following catheter-directed thrombolysis [89, 90].

It is unknown in which situations catheter-directed revascularization is warranted. The decision should be based on the viability of the affected kidney (time to presentation, degree of impairment of perfusion, potential presence of preexisting collaterals), overall renal function (health of contralateral kidney), patient-specific risks and preferences regarding thrombolysis, and local expertise. Regardless, anticoagulation appropriate to the underlying cause of the event is indicated.

Renal vein thrombosis is associated with hypercoagulable states, nephrotic syndrome, inferior vena caval thrombosis, inferior vena caval filter thrombosis, and malignancy [26, 91]. The presentation can vary depending on the acuity of the occlusion. Regardless, endovascular therapy is rarely necessary due to the generous venous collaterals present in most individuals, and anticoagulation alone is typically sufficient. Case reports of catheter-directed thrombolysis with or without adjunctive thrombectomy do exist, however [91]. Occasionally, lack of venous outflow from the kidney results in parenchymal engorgement, renal capsular swelling, and rupture. In the case of an enlarging kidney following renal vein thrombosis, surgical consultation is recommended.

Endovascular Technique for Renovascular Disease

Pre-procedural Management

There is little to no evidence regarding the best pre-procedural medical therapy prior to renal artery intervention. However, most if not all patients referred with atherosclerotic disease should already be taking aspirin. Aggressive measures should be taken to prevent contrast-induced nephropathy and to treat contrast allergies prior to the planned procedure.

Procedure

Access

Renal angiography and intervention can be performed via femoral, brachial, and radial arterial access. The advantages of performing the procedure from access in the arm include coaxial alignment of diagnostic and guiding catheters with the often, slight downward takeoff of the renal arteries and lower rates of bleeding. The disadvantages of radial access, however, include the inability of catheters to reach the renal vessels in tall patients and the inability to use 7F sheaths if necessary.

In general, 5F sheaths are sufficient for diagnostic angiography, while 6–7F sheaths are needed for renal stenting.

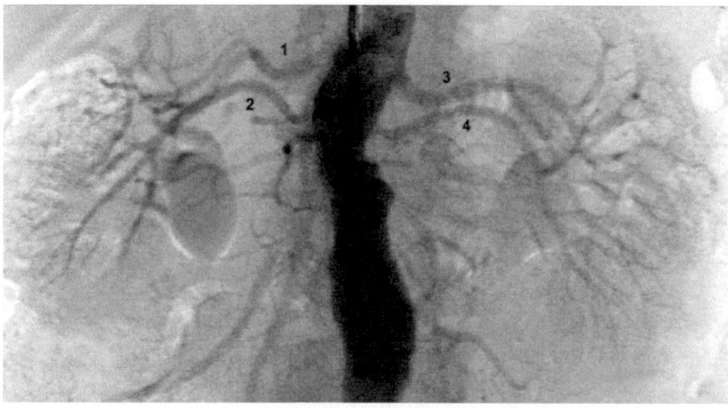

Fig. 32.8 Abdominal aortogram demonstrating dual renal arteries bilaterally (*1* – superior right renal artery; *2* – inferior right renal artery; *3* – superior left renal artery; *4* – inferior left renal artery)

Antithrombotics

For diagnostic angiography alone via a femoral approach, pre-procedural aspirin is sufficient, although some operators may favor addition of an antithrombin agent. For renal intervention, pre-procedural aspirin in addition to an antithrombin (e.g., unfractionated heparin, bivalirudin, low molecular weight heparin, argatroban) is appropriate. The particular antithrombin can be operator-dependent. If unfractionated heparin is used, we recommend a goal activated clotting time (ACT) of 200–250. When the decision to perform renal artery stenting is made, clopidogrel can be administered (300–600 mg load). A small randomized trial showed no benefit of abciximab (bolus and 12-h infusion) in addition to an antithrombin with a goal ACT of 275 s when compared to placebo; however, in a separate arm of this trial, abciximab in addition to an embolic protection device did provide benefit in renal function at 1 month following stenting compared to placebo. There was no statistically significant increase in bleeding associated with the use of abciximab [92]. Thus, if an embolic protection device is used, adjunctive use of a glycoprotein 2b/3a inhibitor should be considered.

Angiography

In general, a nonselective abdominal aortogram is performed initially followed by selective renal angiography (Fig. 32.8). Though abdominal aortography is useful for identifying accessory renal arteries and ostial stenoses, it can be omitted in certain situations to avoid additional contrast administration, depending on pre-procedural imaging (e.g., prior angiography or the presence of previously placed renal artery stents which can serve as fluoroscopic "landmarks").

A variety of 5F side hole catheters are available for abdominal aortography (pigtail, OmniFlush, AngioDynamics, Latham, NY). The catheter should be 100–125 cm if coming from radial access. Abdominal aortography should be performed in a slight left anterior oblique or an anterior-posterior (AP) projection. A power injection of 20–25 cc at a rate of 15–20 cc/s is generally adequate to obtain a complete angiogram.

The abdominal aortogram can refine the choice of diagnostic catheter and angiographic views for selective renal angiography. When performing selective renal angiography from access in the arm, a 5F multipurpose catheter is typically effective. A number of diagnostic catheters – including reverse curve catheters, catheters designed for renal angiography, and catheters used for coronary angiography – are appropriate depending on the angle of the proximal renal artery of interest. Approximately 6–8 cc of contrast at 3–4 cc/s is typically sufficient to obtain a good selective angiogram. The decision to perform bilateral selective renal angiography should be individualized case by case.

Attention should be paid to the nephrogram during angiography. Certain cineangiographic findings, such as renal frame count and renal blush grade, have been quantified and studied; however, lower frame rates for digital subtraction angiography may limit the clinical utility of these parameters.

Translesional Hemodynamic Assessment

Traditionally, translesional pressure gradients were measured with a small caliber (4F) catheter placed distal to the stenosis and a guiding catheter (>=6F) proximal to the stenosis. Recently, there has been increasing interest in using a flow wire to assess translesional hemodynamics. As has been described for the coronary arteries, a flow wire is advanced through a guiding catheter distal to the lesion of interest. Resting fractional flow reserve and translesional gradients are measured. Subsequently, hyperemia is induced with the administration of an intra-arterial vasodilator. Multiple vasodilators have been studied for this purpose including papaverine, dopamine, fenoldopam, and isosorbide dinitrate [40]. Dopamine was shown to be the most powerful inducer of hyperemia and may be preferred. An intrarenal dose of 50 ug/kg is adequate. Alternatively, 30–40 mg of intrarenal papaverine is commonly used. After administration of the vasodilator, it is important to disengage the tip of the guiding catheter from the renal artery ostium when assessing an ostial stenosis. If stenting is performed subsequent to the hemodynamic assessment, it can be done over the flow wire. Translesional hemodynamic assessment is reasonable for any atherosclerotic renal artery lesion in which the severity is in doubt. There should be an even lower threshold to employ hemodynamic assessment of lesions due to fibromuscular dysplasia due to the difficulty in angiographic assessment of these stenoses.

Therapy

The mainstay of percutaneous treatment of atherosclerotic renal artery stenosis is stenting with or without distal embolic protection. For renal artery stenosis due to fibromuscular dysplasia, angioplasty with bailout stenting is the usual strategy. There are rare case reports of catheter-directed thrombolysis for acute renovascular syndromes. Catheter-based renal sympathetic denervation is a promising novel treatment of essential hypertension.

Angioplasty and Stenting

There is evidence from a randomized trial that procedural success and long-term patency are superior for stenting compared to angioplasty alone in the treatment of atherosclerotic renal artery stenosis [21]. This finding has been consistent with observational studies [4, 24]. In contrast, angioplasty alone – guided by hemodynamic lesion assessment and intravascular ultrasound – is usually sufficient for procedural success and a durable result for the treatment of renal artery stenosis due to fibromuscular dysplasia. If angioplasty alone is the desired strategy, a 5F guiding system or sheath is appropriate. In the more common scenario in which stenting is performed adjunctively, a 6F guiding catheter or 5F guiding sheath is necessary for most stent platforms. A 7–8F guiding catheter (6–7F guiding sheath) will be required for most appropriately sized covered stents.

Multiple potential guiding catheters and sheaths are available for renal intervention. The principal advantage of a guiding catheter over a guiding sheath is better torquability and control of the former. The main advantage of a guiding sheath is a smaller arteriotomy necessary to perform the procedure. Thus, a guiding sheath may be preferable when using radial or brachial access, in which manipulation of the guiding system is less of an issue and the size of the guiding system needs to be minimized.

There are two basic techniques to engage a renal artery with a guiding system: *no-touch* and *direct engagement* (Fig. 32.9). In the *no-touch* technique, a guidewire (0.014, 0.018, or 0.035) is advanced into the descending thoracic aorta, assuming access is via the common femoral artery. The guiding catheter or sheath is oriented toward the ostium of the vessel of interest. A 2nd wire – usually a 0.014-in. wire – is then advanced past the lesion into a distal renal artery branch. The original wire is then withdrawn, "seating" the guiding catheter or sheath at the ostium of the vessel. This technique is particularly suited for a guiding catheter from femoral access, in which more challenging catheter manipulation is required to obtain a coaxial position with the frequently downward-going renal vessels as compared to

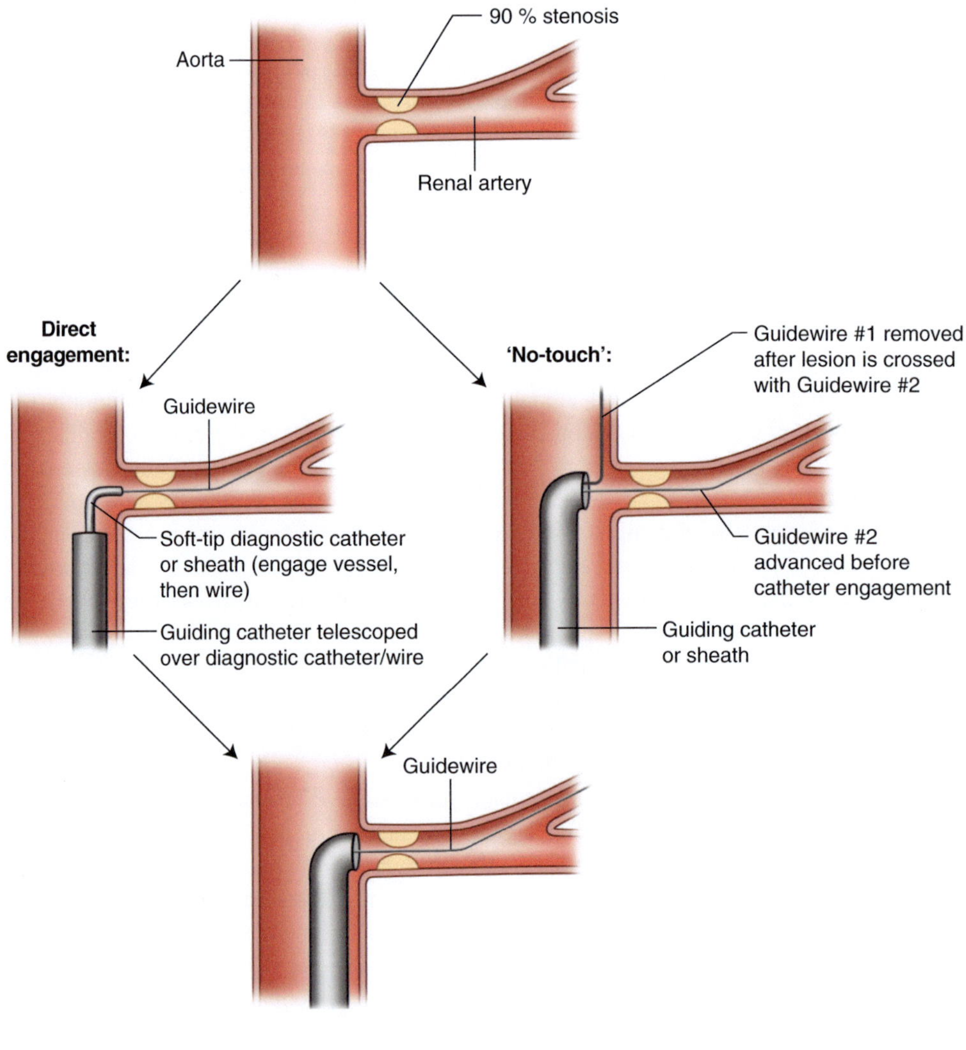

Fig. 32.9 Schematic of "no-touch" and "direct engagement" techniques for engagement of a renal artery

arm access. This technique is more challenging with a guiding sheath, which is more difficult to maneuver towards the renal artery ostium so that it can be wired. To obviate this problem and position a guiding sheath in the ostium of interest, a diagnostic catheter can be telescoped through a guiding sheath. After engaging the mesenteric artery with the diagnostic catheter and wiring the vessel, the guiding sheath can be advanced over the diagnostic catheter/wire combination.

In the *direct engagement* technique, a 4–5F diagnostic catheter is telescoped through a guiding catheter or sheath. The diagnostic catheter is manipulated to engage the ostium of the mesenteric artery. A guidewire (0.014, 0.018, or 0.035) is advanced past the lesion. The guiding catheter or sheath is then advanced over the diagnostic catheter/wire combination. Directly engaging the ostium of a renal artery is not recommended for a guiding catheter; that is, the tip of a guiding catheter is often considered too traumatic to safely engage a vessel with an ostial lesion directly.

Numerous 0.014, 0.018, and 0.035 wires are available for renal artery intervention. 0.014 wires have the advantage of being particularly atraumatic and allow for low-profile balloons and stents, thus ultimately minimizing the caliber of arteriotomy and lowering the risk of bleeding.

Multiple angioplasty balloon catheters are available for treatment of a renal artery stenosis. The diameter of the angioplasty balloon can be sized based on an individual patient's anatomy in combination with the typical renal artery diameter. When treating an ostial lesion, the length of the angioplasty balloon should be ~2 mm longer than the length of the culprit lesion so that the balloon protrudes 2 mm into the aorta to ensure complete treatment of the ostium (Fig. 32.10).

When treating atherosclerotic renal arterial stenoses, balloon-expandable stents are preferred to self-expanding stents for two reasons: increased radial strength, which is desirable to treat the typically heavily calcified stenoses seen with this disorder and increased accuracy in placement of the stent for the typical ostial location of the target lesions. Patency rates between drug-eluting and bare metal stents were compared in the nonrandomized GREAT (sirolimus-eluting vs. bare metal low-profile stent for renal artery treatment) trial [93]. In this study, the target lesion revascularization rate was an impressive 1.9 % at 1 year in the sirolimus-eluting stent group and 11.5 % in the bare metal stent group (p=NS). The drug-eluting stents used in this trial were 5–6 mm in diameter, which are not commercially available currently. Much poorer patency rates have been reported for smaller sirolimus-eluting stents designed for coronary intervention (3.5 mm in diameter, post-dilated to 4–4.5 mm) in the treatment of in-stent restenosis [94]. Thus, it is our practice to match the stent to the diameter of the renal artery, which typically results in a bare metal stent being used for this 5–7 mm vessel. Similar to the technique for angioplasty, ~2 mm of stent should protrude into the aorta, to ensure adequate coverage of ostial lesions. This technique thus requires the guiding catheter or sheath to be retracted >2 mm from the ostium, so that the stent is not inadvertently deployed within the guiding catheter/sheath.

Following stent deployment, the tip of the guiding catheter or sheath can be advanced over the deflating stent balloon, so that the tip of the guide is seated within the lumen of the recently placed stent. Failure to perform this maneuver can complicate delivery of additional equipment (e.g., post-dilatation balloon catheters), as the tip of the post-dilatation balloon catheter will "catch" on the edge of the stent protruding into the aorta. Likewise, the guide often cannot be advanced within the lumen of the stent for the same reason, precluding a completion angiogram. A related issue exists when treating in-stent restenosis within an ostial renal arterial stent. In such a situation, extreme care must be taken to advance the guidewire through the lumen of the stent rather than through a side strut. In our experience, a reverse curve catheter such as an SOS may facilitate access to the "true lumen" of the stent; the catheter is advanced from caudal to the stent, such that the tip "catches" on the inferior border of the protruding stent. With additional forward pressure on the catheter, the tip will "jump" into the lumen of the stent, after which a guidewire can be advanced into the vessel.

Clearly, the ostial nature of atherosclerotic renal artery stenoses increases the complexity of percutaneous renal artery revascularization. Accordingly, several novel devices are in the early stages of translational and clinical development [95–97]. The fundamental concept behind these devices involves a dual balloon delivery system, of which the distal balloon is a traditional stent-mounted system, and the proximal balloon acts as a tactile and visual "locator" balloon that identifies the ostium but can also flare the stent into the aorta.

Distal Embolic Protection. Atheroemboli during intervention are suspected to be a major cause of periprocedural renal injury and failure to preserve renal function following revascularization [4]. In multiple cohort studies in which embolic protection was commonly used, the retrieval of debris occurred in 65–100 % of cases [69, 98–100]. A randomized trial comparing stenting with abciximab and distal embolic protection, stenting with abciximab, stenting with distal embolic protection, and stenting alone showed favorable results with the use of distal embolic protection in conjunction with abciximab [92]. Favorable results were also found in a prospective cohort study of 63 patients with declining renal function and renal artery stenosis, in whom stenting with distal embolic protection resulted in improvement or stabilization of renal function in 94 % of cases at a mean of 16 months [100]. Thus, it is reasonable to consider embolic protection for renal artery interventions.

Unfortunately, it can be technically difficult to achieve complete embolic protection ubiquitously due to the variable

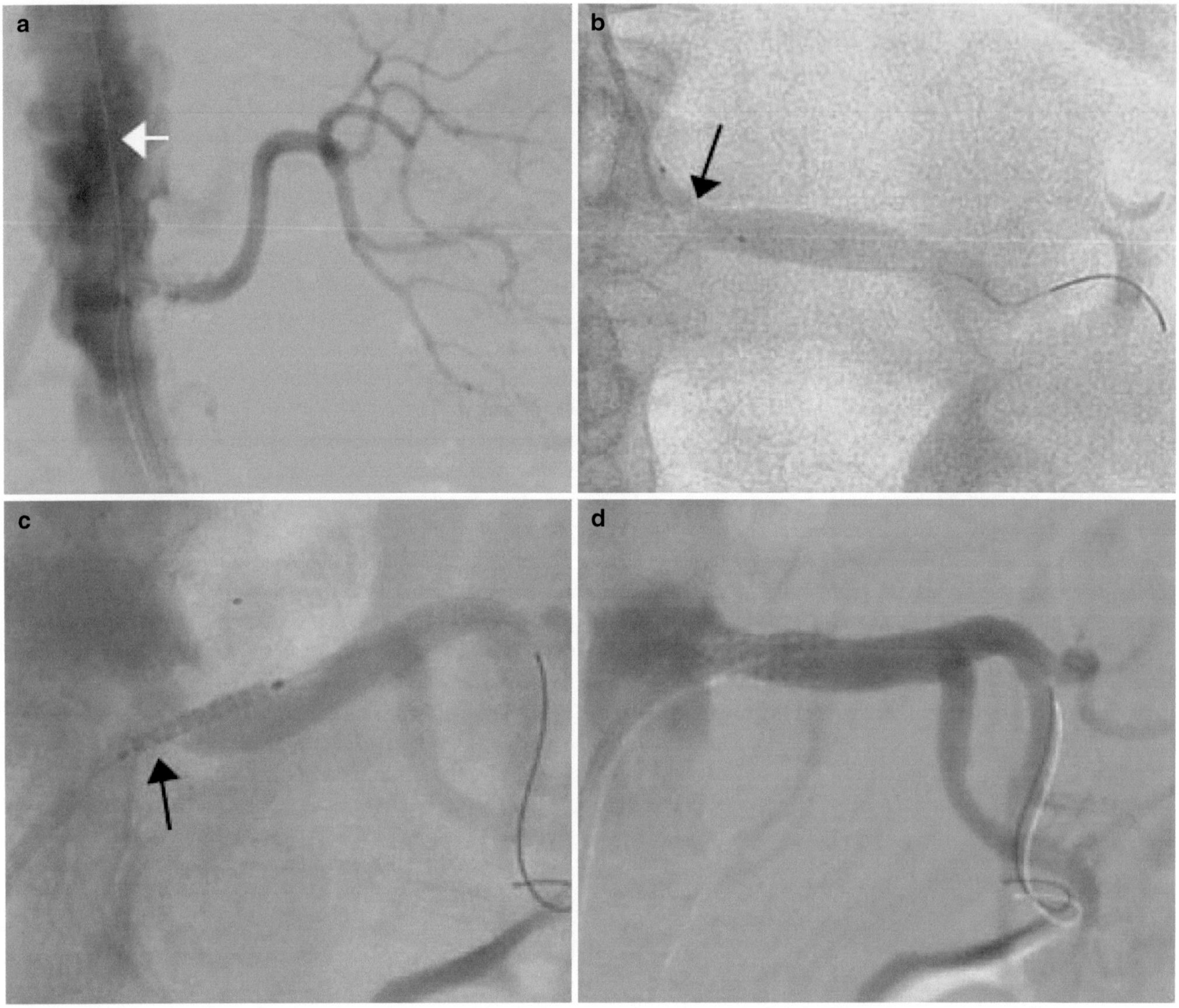

Fig. 32.10 (**a**) Left renal angiogram using the "no-touch" technique, with a guidewire (*arrow*) placed cephalad in the diseased abdominal aorta. (**b**) Positioning of the pre-dilatation balloon to cover the ostial disease (*arrow*) with the proximal balloon marker placed in the aorta. (**c**) Positioning of the stent to cover the ostial disease (*arrow*) with the proximal stent extending into the aorta. The guiding catheter has been retracted into the aorta. (**d**) Post-stent deployment. The guiding catheter was transitioned over the deflating balloon into the lumen of the stent to enable a selective angiogram

branching of the segmental arteries from the main renal artery. Additionally, at least 2 cm between the distal landing zone of the stent and a distal embolic protection device is required. Thus, particularly for the renal artery, a short filtration element is preferable. Another desirable feature of a distal embolic protection device is a wire independent filter, which allows wiring the lesion prior to advancing the filtration element (Table 32.5). This feature is particularly helpful for very tight lesions or tortuous segments in which the additional "purchase" of a wire positioned distally can facilitate device delivery. There are no distal embolic protection devices designed specifically for the renal artery. Currently, the FiberNet filter (Invatec, Bethlehem, PA) has the shortest basket but is wire dependent. Hopefully, the CORAL trial, in which the Angioguard filter (Cordis) was used, will provide additional insight into distal embolic protection for renal artery intervention.

Thrombectomy/Thrombolysis for Acute Renovascular Disorders

There is insufficient evidence to propose a refined procedure for catheter-based treatment of acute renovascular disorders. Regarding acute thrombotic occlusions, catheter-directed thrombolysis has been described [88–90]. The technique has involved delivery of the thrombolytic agent through an end-hole catheter selective placed in the ostium of the renal artery.

Table 32.5 Comparison of distal embolic protection devices

Device	Company	Pore size (uM)	Wire independent?
Accunet	Guidant	120	No
Angioguard	Cordis	100	No
Emboshield NAV6	Abbott	140	Yes
Fibernet	Invatec	40	No
Filterwire EZ	Boston Scientific	80	No
Spider	ev3	50–200	Yes

Infusion times have varied from 1 to 48 h. Careful attention, including serial X-ray studies, must be paid to maintain catheter position in the renal artery ostium for prolonged infusions.

Similarly, there is little evidence for the endovascular technique for renal vein thrombosis. In a series of seven patients, the renal vein of interest was engaged with a multipurpose or renal double curve guiding catheter [91]. The occlusion was crossed with a 0.035 glidewire and angled glide catheter. Venography was performed through the glide catheter. Thereafter, rheolytic thrombectomy was performed for several passes within 1 min or less. For residual thrombus, thrombolysis was performed via an infusion catheter. This technique was associated with 100 % procedural success and favorable clinical results [91].

Renal Sympathetic Denervation

This modality is a promising new catheter-based therapy for essential hypertension. In the randomized trial Symplicity HTN-2, 106 patients with refractory essential hypertension were randomized to denervation in addition to medical therapy or medical therapy alone. At 6 months, there was an impressive reduction in blood pressure of the denervation group of 32/12 mmHg (SD 23/11 mmHg), which was statistically superior to the medical therapy alone group in which blood pressure was essentially unchanged. There were no major complications [101].

The procedural technique involves accessing the common femoral artery with a 6F sheath. Anticoagulation is administered. The renal artery is engaged with a 6F guiding catheter. A steerable radiofrequency catheter, connected to a generator, is then advanced into the renal artery. The tip of the catheter is oriented to contact the wall of the artery, and pulses of radiofrequency energy are delivered which deactivate the sympathetic nerves in the adventitia of the vessel. Multiple areas along the wall of each renal artery are treated. Back pain during the administration of the radiofrequency energy is common.

Post-procedure

There is little evidence to drive decisions regarding antiplatelet therapy and surveillance imaging following renal artery stenting. In general, many operators prescribe aspirin for life and clopidogrel for 4 weeks. Duplex ultrasonography is often performed at 1 month and then 6–12 months thereafter.

Complications of Renal Artery Stenting

Adverse outcomes following renal artery stenting in 2,176 patients in 15 observational studies published in 1994–2007 have been summarized [5]. Indications for these studies included both hypertension and renal dysfunction. Relevant reported outcomes included in-stent restenosis and procedure-related complications [5, 15–22, 47]. Procedural death occurred in 17 of 2,089 patients (0.8 %), which is nearly identical to the pooled mortality rate in randomized trials of renal artery stenting compared to medical therapy (5/593). In-stent restenosis occurred in 5.5–26 % of cases over a mean of 10 months. The rate of restenosis has been found to have an inverse relationship to vessel size [102]. Other major complications included access site complications requiring surgery, bleeding requiring transfusion, renal artery perforation from guidewire misplacement, stroke, and myocardial infarction. The major complication rates varied from 0 to 8 % across studies. Notably, progression to renal replacement therapy was relatively infrequent for this population, occurring in 0–5 % of cases.

References

1. Gruntzig A, Kuhlmann U, Vetter W, Lutolf U, Meier B, Siegenthaler W. Treatment of renovascular hypertension with percutaneous transluminal dilatation of a renal-artery stenosis. Lancet. 1978;1(8068):801–2.
2. Hirsch AT, Haskal ZJ, Hertzer NR, Bakal CW, Creager MA, Halperin JL, et al. ACC/AHA 2005 guidelines for the management of patients with peripheral arterial disease (lower extremity, renal, mesenteric, and abdominal aortic): executive summary a collaborative report from the American Association for Vascular Surgery/ Society for Vascular Surgery, Society for Cardiovascular Angiography and Interventions, Society for Vascular Medicine and Biology, Society of Interventional Radiology, and the ACC/AHA task force on practice guidelines (writing committee to develop guidelines for the management of patients with peripheral arterial disease) endorsed by the American Association of Cardiovascular and Pulmonary Rehabilitation; National Heart, Lung, and Blood Institute; Society for Vascular Nursing; TransAtlantic Inter-society Consensus; and Vascular Disease Foundation. J Am Coll Cardiol. 2006;47(6):1239–312.
3. Safian RD, Textor SC. Renal-artery stenosis. N Engl J Med. 2001;344(6):431–42.
4. White CJ. Catheter-based therapy for atherosclerotic renal artery stenosis. Circulation. 2006;113(11):1464–73.

5. Rosenfield K, Jaff MR. An 82-year-old woman with worsening hypertension: review of renal artery stenosis. JAMA. 2008;300(17):2036–44.
6. Olin JW, Melia M, Young JR, Graor RA, Risius B. Prevalence of atherosclerotic renal artery stenosis in patients with atherosclerosis elsewhere. Am J Med. 1990;88(1N):46N–51.
7. Wollenweber J, Sheps SG, Davis GD. Clinical course of atherosclerotic renovascular disease. Am J Cardiol. 1968;21(1):60–71.
8. Meaney TF, Dustan HP, McCormack LJ. Natural history of renal arterial disease. Radiology. 1968;91(5):881–7.
9. Schreiber MJ, Pohl MA, Novick AC. The natural history of atherosclerotic and fibrous renal artery disease. Urol Clin North Am. 1984;11(3):383–92.
10. Tollefson DF, Ernst CB. Natural history of atherosclerotic renal artery stenosis associated with aortic disease. J Vasc Surg. 1991;14(3):327–31.
11. Dean RH, Kieffer RW, Smith BM, Oates JA, Nadeau JH, Hollifield JW, et al. Renovascular hypertension: anatomic and renal function changes during drug therapy. Arch Surg. 1981;116(11):1408–15.
12. Zierler RE, Bergelin RO, Davidson RC, Cantwell-Gab K, Polissar NL, Strandness Jr DE. A prospective study of disease progression in patients with atherosclerotic renal artery stenosis. Am J Hypertens. 1996;9(11):1055–61.
13. Caps MT, Perissinotto C, Zierler RE, Polissar NL, Bergelin RO, Tullis MJ, et al. Prospective study of atherosclerotic disease progression in the renal artery. Circulation. 1998;98(25):2866–72.
14. Conlon PJ, Little MA, Pieper K, Mark DB. Severity of renal vascular disease predicts mortality in patients undergoing coronary angiography. Kidney Int. 2001;60(4):1490–7.
15. Bates MC, Campbell JE, Stone PA, Jaff MR, Broce M, Lavigne PS. Factors affecting long-term survival following renal artery stenting. Catheter Cardiovasc Interv. 2007;69(7):1037–43.
16. Blum U, Krumme B, Flugel P, Gabelmann A, Lehnert T, Buitrago-Tellez C, et al. Treatment of ostial renal-artery stenoses with vascular endoprostheses after unsuccessful balloon angioplasty. N Engl J Med. 1997;336(7):459–65.
17. Ivanovic V, McKusick MA, Johnson 3rd CM, Sabater EA, Andrews JC, Breen JF, et al. Renal artery stent placement: complications at a single tertiary care center. J Vasc Interv Radiol. 2003;14(2 Pt 1):217–25.
18. Rocha-Singh KJ, Mishkel GJ, Katholi RE, Ligon RA, Armbruster JA, McShane KJ, et al. Clinical predictors of improved long-term blood pressure control after successful stenting of hypertensive patients with obstructive renal artery atherosclerosis. Catheter Cardiovasc Interv. 1999;47(2):167–72.
19. Rodriguez-Lopez JA, Werner A, Ray LI, Verikokos C, Torruella LJ, Martinez E, et al. Renal artery stenosis treated with stent deployment: Indications, technique, and outcome for 108 patients. J Vasc Surg. 1999;29(4):617–24.
20. Tuttle KR, Chouinard RF, Webber JT, Dahlstrom LR, Short RA, Henneberry KJ, et al. Treatment of atherosclerotic ostial renal artery stenosis with the intravascular stent. Am J Kidney Dis. 1998;32(4):611–22.
21. van de Ven PJ, Kaatee R, Beutler JJ, Beek FJ, Woittiez AJ, Buskens E, et al. Arterial stenting and balloon angioplasty in ostial atherosclerotic renovascular disease: a randomised trial. Lancet. 1999;353(9149):282–6.
22. Rocha-Singh K, Jaff MR, Rosenfield K, ASPIRE-2 Trial Investigators. Evaluation of the safety and effectiveness of renal artery stenting after unsuccessful balloon angioplasty: the ASPIRE-2 study. J Am Coll Cardiol. 2005;46(5):776–83.
23. Textor SC, Lerman L, McKusick M. The uncertain value of renal artery interventions: where are we now? JACC Cardiovasc Interv. 2009;2(3):175–82.
24. Safian RD, Madder RD. Refining the approach to renal artery revascularization. JACC Cardiovasc Interv. 2009;2(3):161–74.
25. Casserly I, Ravish S, Yadav JS, editors. Manual of peripheral vascular intervention. 1st ed. Philadelphia: Lippincott Williams & Wilkins; 2005.
26. Cronenwett JL, Johnston KW, editors. Rutherford's vascular surgery. 7th ed. Philadelphia: Elsevier; 2010.
27. Lohse JR, Shore RM, Belzer FO. Acute renal artery occlusion: the role of collateral circulation. Arch Surg. 1982;117(6):801–4.
28. Witz M, Kantarovsky A, Morag B, Shifrin EG. Renal vein occlusion: a review. J Urol. 1996;155(4):1173–9.
29. Fernando D, Garasic J. Percutaneous intervention for renovascular disease: rationale and patient selection. Curr Opin Cardiol. 2004;19(6):582–8.
30. Cooper CJ, Murphy TP. Is renal artery stenting the correct treatment of renal artery stenosis? The case for renal artery stenting for treatment of renal artery stenosis. Circulation. 2007;115(2):263–9. discussion 270.
31. Brewster UC, Setaro JF, Perazella MA. The renin-angiotensin-aldosterone system: cardiorenal effects and implications for renal and cardiovascular disease states. Am J Med Sci. 2003;326(1):15–24.
32. Chade AR, Rodriguez-Porcel M, Grande JP, Krier JD, Lerman A, Romero JC, et al. Distinct renal injury in early atherosclerosis and renovascular disease. Circulation. 2002;106(9):1165–71.
33. Kobayashi S, Ishida A, Moriya H, Mori N, Fukuda T, Takamura T. Angiotensin II receptor blockade limits kidney injury in two-kidney, one-clip goldblatt hypertensive rats with special reference to phenotypic changes. J Lab Clin Med. 1999;133(2):134–43.
34. Eddy AA. Molecular insights into renal interstitial fibrosis. J Am Soc Nephrol. 1996;7(12):2495–508.
35. Scoble JE. Atherosclerotic nephropathy. Kidney Int Suppl. 1999;71:S106–9.
36. Mitchell JA, Subramanian R, White CJ, Soukas PA, Almagor Y, Stewart RE, et al. Predicting blood pressure improvement in hypertensive patients after renal artery stent placement: renal fractional flow reserve. Catheter Cardiovasc Interv. 2007;69(5):685–9.
37. Mangiacapra F, Trana C, Sarno G, Davidavicius G, Protasiewicz M, Muller O, et al. Translesional pressure gradients to predict blood pressure response after renal artery stenting in patients with renovascular hypertension. Circ Cardiovasc Interv. 2010;3(6):537–42.
38. Leesar MA, Varma J, Shapira A, Fahsah I, Raza ST, Elghoul Z, et al. Prediction of hypertension improvement after stenting of renal artery stenosis: comparative accuracy of translesional pressure gradients, intravascular ultrasound, and angiography. J Am Coll Cardiol. 2009;53(25):2363–71.
39. Mounier-Vehier C, Cocheteux B, Haulon S, Devos P, Lions C, Gautier C, et al. Changes in renal blood flow reserve after angioplasty of renal artery stenosis in hypertensive patients. Kidney Int. 2004;65(1):245–50.
40. Manoharan G, Pijls NH, Lameire N, Verhamme K, Heyndrickx GR, Barbato E, et al. Assessment of renal flow and flow reserve in humans. J Am Coll Cardiol. 2006;47(3):620–5.
41. Subramanian R, White CJ, Rosenfield K, Bashir R, Almagor Y, Meerkin D, et al. Renal fractional flow reserve: a hemodynamic evaluation of moderate renal artery stenoses. Catheter Cardiovasc Interv. 2005;64(4):480–6.
42. Siddiqui TS, Elghoul Z, Reza ST, Leesar MA. Renal hemodynamics: theory and practical tips. Catheter Cardiovasc Interv. 2007;69(6):894–901.
43. Makanjuola AD, Suresh M, Laboi P, Kalra PA, Scoble JE. Proteinuria in atherosclerotic renovascular disease. QJM. 1999;92(9):515–18.
44. Beck AW, Nolan BW, De Martino R, Yuo TH, Tanski WJ, Walsh DB, et al. Predicting blood pressure response after renal artery stenting. J Vasc Surg. 2010;51(2):380,5. discussion 385.
45. Cognet F, Garcier JM, Dranssart M, Defraissinette B, Cercueil JP, Ravel A, et al. Percutaneous transluminal renal angioplasty in

atheroma with renal failure: long-term outcomes in 99 patients. Eur Radiol. 2001;11(12):2524–30.
46. Marshall FI, Hagen S, Mahaffy RG, Petrie JC, Roy-Chaudhury P, Russell IT, et al. Percutaneous transluminal angioplasty for atheromatous renal artery stenosis–blood pressure response and discriminant analysis of outcome predictors. Q J Med. 1990;75(277):483–9.
47. Burket MW, Cooper CJ, Kennedy DJ, Brewster PS, Ansel GM, Moore JA, et al. Renal artery angioplasty and stent placement: predictors of a favorable outcome. Am Heart J. 2000;139(1 Pt 1):64–71.
48. Zeller T, Frank U, Muller C, Burgelin K, Sinn L, Bestehorn HP, et al. Predictors of improved renal function after percutaneous stent-supported angioplasty of severe atherosclerotic ostial renal artery stenosis. Circulation. 2003;108(18):2244–9.
49. Muray S, Martin M, Amoedo ML, Garcia C, Jornet AR, Vera M, et al. Rapid decline in renal function reflects reversibility and predicts the outcome after angioplasty in renal artery stenosis. Am J Kidney Dis. 2002;39(1):60–6.
50. Silva JA, Chan AW, White CJ, Collins TJ, Jenkins JS, Reilly JP, et al. Elevated brain natriuretic peptide predicts blood pressure response after stent revascularization in patients with renal artery stenosis. Circulation. 2005;111(3):328–33.
51. Chrysochou C, Cheung CM, Durow M, Middleton RJ, Solomon LR, Craig A, et al. Proteinuria as a predictor of renal functional outcome after revascularization in atherosclerotic renovascular disease (ARVD). QJM. 2009;102(4):283–8.
52. Radermacher J, Chavan A, Bleck J, Vitzthum A, Stoess B, Gebel MJ, et al. Use of doppler ultrasonography to predict the outcome of therapy for renal-artery stenosis. N Engl J Med. 2001;344(6):410–17.
53. Leiner T, de Haan MW, Nelemans PJ, van Engelshoven JM, Vasbinder GB. Contemporary imaging techniques for the diagnosis of renal artery stenosis. Eur Radiol. 2005;15(11):2219–29.
54. Tan KT, van Beek EJ, Brown PW, van Delden OM, Tijssen J, Ramsay LE. Magnetic resonance angiography for the diagnosis of renal artery stenosis: a meta-analysis. Clin Radiol. 2002;57(7):617–24.
55. Gill-Leertouwer TC, Gussenhoven EJ, Bosch JL, Deinum J, van Overhagen H, Derkx FH, et al. Predictors for clinical success at one year following renal artery stent placement. J Endovasc Ther. 2002;9(4):495–502.
56. HERCULES: renal stenting lowers BP, but BNP is not a marker of benefit. http://www.theheart.org/article/1222027.do. Accessed 1 July 2011.
57. Colyer Jr WR, Cooper CJ, Burket MW, Thomas WJ. Utility of a 0.014″ pressure-sensing guidewire to assess renal artery translesional systolic pressure gradients. Catheter Cardiovasc Interv. 2003;59(3):372–7.
58. Voiculescu A, Schmitz M, Plum J, Hollenbeck M, Vupora S, Jung G, et al. Duplex ultrasound and renin ratio predict treatment failure after revascularization for renal artery stenosis. Am J Hypertens. 2006;19(7):756–63.
59. Mahmud E, Smith TW, Palakodeti V, Zaidi O, Ang L, Mitchell CR, et al. Renal frame count and renal blush grade: quantitative measures that predict the success of renal stenting in hypertensive patients with renal artery stenosis. JACC Cardiovasc Interv. 2008;1(3):286–92.
60. Dangas G, Laird Jr JR, Mehran R, Lansky AJ, Mintz GS, Leon MB. Intravascular ultrasound-guided renal artery stenting. J Endovasc Ther. 2001;8(3):238–47.
61. Weibull H, Bergqvist D, Bergentz SE, Jonsson K, Hulthen L, Manhem P. Percutaneous transluminal renal angioplasty versus surgical reconstruction of atherosclerotic renal artery stenosis: a prospective randomized study. J Vasc Surg. 1993;18(5):841,50. discussion 850–2.
62. Cambria RP, Brewster DC, L'Italien GJ, Moncure A, Darling Jr RC, Gertler JP, et al. The durability of different reconstructive techniques for atherosclerotic renal artery disease. J Vasc Surg. 1994;20(1):76,85. discussion 86–7.
63. Hansen KJ, Cherr GS, Craven TE, Motew SJ, Travis JA, Wong JM, et al. Management of ischemic nephropathy: dialysis-free survival after surgical repair. J Vasc Surg. 2000;32(3):472,81. discussion 481–2.
64. Plouin PF, Chatellier G, Darne B, Raynaud A. Blood pressure outcome of angioplasty in atherosclerotic renal artery stenosis: a randomized trial. Essai multicentrique medicaments vs angioplastie (EMMA) study group. Hypertension. 1998;31(3):823–9.
65. Bax L, Woittiez AJ, Kouwenberg HJ, Mali WP, Buskens E, Beek FJ, et al. Stent placement in patients with atherosclerotic renal artery stenosis and impaired renal function: a randomized trial. Ann Intern Med. 2009;150(12):840–8. W150-1.
66. Webster J, Marshall F, Abdalla M, Dominiczak A, Edwards R, Isles CG. Randomised comparison of percutaneous angioplasty vs continued medical therapy for hypertensive patients with atheromatous renal artery stenosis. scottish and newcastle renal artery stenosis collaborative group. J Hum Hypertens. 1998;12(5):329–35.
67. van Jaarsveld BC, Krijnen P, Pieterman H, Derkx FH, Deinum J, Postma CT. The effect of balloon angioplasty on hypertension in atherosclerotic renal-artery stenosis. dutch renal artery stenosis intervention cooperative study group. N Engl J Med. 2000;342(14):1007–14.
68. ASTRAL Investigators, Wheatley K, Ives N, Gray R, Kalra PA, Moss JG, et al. Revascularization versus medical therapy for renal-artery stenosis. N Engl J Med. 2009;361(20):1953–62.
69. Henry M, Henry I, Polydorou A, Hugel M. Embolic protection for renal artery stenting. J Cardiovasc Surg (Torino). 2008;49(5):571–89.
70. Cooper CJ, Murphy TP, Matsumoto A, Steffes M, Cohen DJ, Jaff M, et al. Stent revascularization for the prevention of cardiovascular and renal events among patients with renal artery stenosis and systolic hypertension: rationale and design of the CORAL trial. Am Heart J. 2006;152(1):59–66.
71. Dworkin LD, Jamerson KA. Is renal artery stenting the correct treatment of renal artery stenosis? Case against angioplasty and stenting of atherosclerotic renal artery stenosis. Circulation. 2007;115(2):271,6. discussion 276.
72. Mills NL, Dhaun N, Uren NG. Revascularization for renal-artery stenosis. N Engl J Med. 2010;362(8):763. author reply 763–4.
73. Mann SJ, Sos TA. Misleading results of randomized trials: the example of renal artery stenting. J Clin Hypertens (Greenwich). 2010;12(1):1–2.
74. White CJ. Kiss my astral: one seriously flawed study of renal stenting after another. Catheter Cardiovasc Interv. 2010;75(2):305–7.
75. George JC, White CJ. Renal artery stenting: lessons from ASTRAL (angioplasty and stenting for renal artery lesions). JACC Cardiovasc Interv. 2010;3(7):786–7.
76. Esposito P, Piotti G, Dal Canton A. Revascularization for renal-artery stenosis. N Engl J Med. 2010;362(8):762–3. author reply 763–4.
77. Staub D, Uthoff H, Jaeger KA. Revascularization for renal-artery stenosis. N Engl J Med. 2010;362(8):762. author reply 763–4.
78. Slovut DP, Olin JW. Fibromuscular dysplasia. N Engl J Med. 2004;350(18):1862–71.
79. Vasbinder GB, Nelemans PJ, Kessels AG, Kroon AA, Maki JH, Leiner T, et al. Accuracy of computed tomographic angiography and magnetic resonance angiography for diagnosing renal artery stenosis. Ann Intern Med. 2004;141(9):674,82. discussion 682.
80. Davies MG, Saad WE, Peden EK, Mohiuddin IT, Naoum JJ, Lumsden AB. The long-term outcomes of percutaneous therapy for renal artery fibromuscular dysplasia. J Vasc Surg. 2008;48(4):865–71.
81. Patel NH, Jindal RM, Wilkin T, Rose S, Johnson MS, Shah H, et al. Renal arterial stenosis in renal allografts: retrospective study of predisposing factors and outcome after percutaneous transluminal angioplasty. Radiology. 2001;219(3):663–7.

82. Aktas S, Boyvat F, Sevmis S, Moray G, Karakayali H, Haberal M. Analysis of vascular complications after renal transplantation. Transplant Proc. 2011;43(2):557–61.
83. Safian RD. Transplant renal artery stenosis: what lessons should we learn? Catheter Cardiovasc Interv. 2011;77(2):294–5.
84. Sharma S, Potdar A, Kulkarni A. Percutaneous transluminal renal stenting for transplant renal artery stenosis. Catheter Cardiovasc Interv. 2011;77(2):287–93.
85. Korzets Z, Plotkin E, Bernheim J, Zissin R. The clinical spectrum of acute renal infarction. Isr Med Assoc J. 2002;4(10):781–4.
86. Hazanov N, Somin M, Attali M, Beilinson N, Thaler M, Mouallem M, et al. Acute renal embolism. forty-four cases of renal infarction in patients with atrial fibrillation. Medicine (Baltimore). 2004;83(5):292–9.
87. Fukuda T, Hayashi K, Sakamoto I, Mori M. Acute renal infarction caused by behcet's disease. Abdom Imaging. 1995;20(3):264–6.
88. Blum U, Billmann P, Krause T, Gabelmann A, Keller E, Moser E, et al. Effect of local low-dose thrombolysis on clinical outcome in acute embolic renal artery occlusion. Radiology. 1993;189(2):549–54.
89. Contractor FM, Leicht JP. Intraarterial infusion of low-dose streptokinase after acute thromboembolization of the right renal artery. Cardiovasc Intervent Radiol. 1984;7(1):21–3.
90. Cheng BC, Ko SF, Chuang FR, Lee CH, Chen JB, Hsu KT. Successful management of acute renal artery thromboembolism by intra-arterial thrombolytic therapy with recombinant tissue plasminogen activator. Ren Fail. 2003;25(4):665–70.
91. Kim HS, Fine DM, Atta MG. Catheter-directed thrombectomy and thrombolysis for acute renal vein thrombosis. J Vasc Interv Radiol. 2006;17(5):815–22.
92. Cooper CJ, Haller ST, Colyer W, Steffes M, Burket MW, Thomas WJ, et al. Embolic protection and platelet inhibition during renal artery stenting. Circulation. 2008;117(21):2752–60.
93. Zahringer M, Sapoval M, Pattynama PM, Rabbia C, Vignali C, Maleux G, et al. Sirolimus-eluting versus bare-metal low-profile stent for renal artery treatment (GREAT trial): angiographic follow-up after 6 months and clinical outcome up to 2 years. J Endovasc Ther. 2007;14(4):460–8.
94. Kiernan TJ, Yan BP, Eisenberg JD, Ruggiero NJ, Gupta V, Drachman D, et al. Treatment of renal artery in-stent restenosis with sirolimus-eluting stents. Vasc Med. 2010;15(1):3–7.
95. Suzuki Y, Ikeno F, Lyons JK, Koizumi T, Yeung AC. Novel stent system for accurate placement in aorto-ostial renal artery disease: preclinical study in porcine renal artery model. Cardiovasc Revasc Med. 2007;8(2):99–102.
96. Improved Stents. Balloons and Embolic Protection Devices (EPDs) for renal stenting. http://www.aimsymposium.org/pdf/vei/3634.pdf. Accessed 5 July 2011.
97. BullsEye Ostial Stent Study-I (BOSS-I): a novel flared stent tailored for treatment of aorto-ostial lesions. http://www.google.com/url?q=http://www.leipzig-interventionalcourse.com/index.php%3Foption%3Dcom_docman%26task%3Ddoc_download%26gid%3D37&sa=U&ei=aaALTrCbJY5tgeiu4BV&ved=0CBsQFjAGOBQ&usg=AFQjCNE-ux00eJ9alsRkjih68uqZ2xm05w . Accessed 5 July 2011.
98. Henry M, Henry I, Klonaris C, Polydorou A, Rath P, Lakshmi G, et al. Renal angioplasty and stenting under protection: the way for the future? Catheter Cardiovasc Interv. 2003;60(3):299–312.
99. Holden A, Hill A. Renal angioplasty and stenting with distal protection of the main renal artery in ischemic nephropathy: early experience. J Vasc Surg. 2003;38(5):962–8.
100. Holden A, Hill A, Jaff MR, Pilmore H. Renal artery stent revascularization with embolic protection in patients with ischemic nephropathy. Kidney Int. 2006;70(5):948–55.
101. Symplicity HTN-2 Investigators, Esler MD, Krum H, Sobotka PA, Schlaich MP, Schmieder RE, et al. Renal sympathetic denervation in patients with treatment-resistant hypertension (the symplicity HTN-2 trial): a randomised controlled trial. Lancet. 2010;376(9756):1903–9.
102. Zeller T, Muller C, Frank U, Burgelin K, Sinn L, Horn B, et al. Gold coating and restenosis after primary stenting of ostial renal artery stenosis. Catheter Cardiovasc Interv. 2003;60(1):1,6. discussion 7–8.

Endovascular Therapy for Mesenteric Disease

33

R. Kevin Rogers and Joseph M. Garasic

In 1966, Dr. Trygve Aakhus touted the role of angiography in the evaluation of mesenteric ischemia [1]. Eleven years later in 1977, Boley described the intra-arterial administration of papaverine to treat mesenteric ischemia [2]. The 1st report of mesenteric angioplasty was published in 1980 by Gruntzig et al. [3]. During the past 31 years, percutaneous management of mesenteric vascular disease has expanded considerably. Though endovascular therapy in mesenteric disease is performed for aneurysmal, oncologic, traumatic, and hemorrhagic indications, the most common indication is the treatment of ischemic diseases [4].

It has been estimated that 1 of 1,000 hospital admissions is due to intestinal ischemic disorders [5], which can be classified as chronic and acute mesenteric ischemia [4]. In the general population, the incidence of chronic mesenteric ischemia is 1/100,000; however, in populations with known atherosclerotic disease, the prevalence is much higher [6]. Chronic mesenteric ischemia is most frequently due to multivessel atherosclerotic arterial disease in the abdomen [4, 7, 8]. In contrast, acute mesenteric ischemia can result from arterial embolism, arterial or venous thrombosis, or low cardiac output states complicated by profound mesenteric vasoconstriction [8–10]. Despite advances in imaging and interventional therapies, the mortality rate from acute mesenteric ischemia remains disappointing, ranging from 30 to 80 % depending on the etiology [5, 10]. Endovascular therapy has emerged as the primary revascularization strategy for chronic mesenteric ischemia and offers multiple therapeutic options adjunctive to surgery for acute mesenteric ischemia (Table 33.1) [4, 6–8, 10].

This chapter focuses on the percutaneous treatment of acute and chronic mesenteric ischemia, in the context of a complementary, multidisciplinary approach to these diagnostically and therapeutically challenging disorders. Comprehensive endovascular therapy is reviewed, including patient selection, technical aspects of intervention, catheter-directed delivery of vasodilators and fibrinolytics, percutaneous revascularization, concomitant medical therapy, and follow-up considerations. Relevant anatomic, pathophysiologic, and clinical information is also summarized.

Mesenteric Arterial Anatomy for the Interventionalist

The intestinal blood supply arises from three major branches of the abdominal aorta: the celiac, superior mesenteric, and inferior mesenteric arteries (Fig. 33.1). Each vessel arises anteriorly from the aorta. Typically, the celiac artery has a horizontal takeoff, while the SMA takes a downward course [11, 12]. Appreciation of the level, trajectory, of the origin of these vessels, as well as their caliber and branches, influences the selection of guiding catheters, positioning of guide wires, and choice of angioplasty balloons and stents (Table 33.2).

The celiac trunk is typically a 5–7 mm vessel and arises at the level of the 12th thoracic vertebra [11–13]. It gives rise to the common hepatic and splenic arteries and often the left gastric artery. Any of these branches may arise directly from the aorta, however. The celiac axis supplies the stomach, duodenum, spleen, liver, and pancreas (Table 33.2).

The SMA is 4–6 mm in caliber and arises at the level of the 1st lumbar vertebra, 1.5 cm below the origin of the celiac trunk [11, 13]. Its branches include the inferior pancreaticoduodenal, middle colic, right colic, ileocolic, jejunal, and ileal arteries. Variations of this anatomy include the SMA or its colic branches arising from the celiac trunk. The SMA system supplies the pancreas, jejunum, ileum, ascending colon, and proximal half of the transverse colon (Table 33.2).

The IMA is 3–5 mm in diameter [11, 13] and arises at the level of the 3rd lumbar vertebra, approximately 4 cm above the aortoiliac bifurcation. Its branches include the left colic, sigmoid, marginal, and superior rectal arteries, which have important anastamoses with the inferior rectal arteries of the

R.K. Rogers, MD, MSc (✉) • J.M. Garasic, MD
Division of Cardiology, Massachusetts General Hospital, GRB-8-821, Boston, MA 02114, USA
e-mail: r.kevin.rogers@gmail.com; jgarasic@partners.org

C.A. Thompson (ed.), *Textbook of Cardiovascular Intervention*,
DOI 10.1007/978-1-4471-4528-8_33, © Springer-Verlag London 2014

Table 33.1 Ischemic intestinal disorders

Disorder	Endovascular therapy available?		
	Catheter-directed medical treatment		
	Vasodilator	Fibrinolysis	Revascularization
Chronic intestinal ischemia			
Atherosclerotic			X
Arcuate ligament syndrome			+/–
Rare vascular causes			X
Mesenteric venous thrombosis		X	
Acute intestinal ischemia			
Thromboembolism	X	X	X
Arterial thrombosis	X	X	X
Nonocclusive	X		
Venous thrombosis		X	

internal iliac arteries. The IMA system supplies the distal half of the transverse colon, descending colon, and rectum (Table 33.2).

The development of chronic mesenteric ischemia is usually the result of multivessel disease [4, 7, 8, 12]. This phenomenon is due to the typical ostial location of atherosclerotic lesions and to the presence of multiple, more distal anastomotic connections between the mesenteric vessels (Table 33.3) [11–13]. In contrast, acute mesenteric ischemia most often involves a single vessel, the SMA. Embolization has a predilection for this vessel likely due to its acute, downward-going takeoff from the aorta [12]. A common location of SMA embolization is just distal to the takeoff of the middle colic artery, which compromises multiple pathways of anastomotic supply to the SMA territory – the marginal artery of Drummond, arc of Riolan, and pancreaticoduodenal arcade [12] (Table 33.3).

Clinical Syndromes

Chronic Mesenteric Ischemia

Chronic intestinal ischemia results from inadequate oxygen supply to the gut during digestion. 10 % of cardiac output perfuses the intestines at rest, while up to 35 % is required following a meal [14]. This hyperemic response is directed primarily to the small intestine and pancreas, which are supplied by the SMA and its branches; hence, the SMA is the most frequently diseased mesenteric artery in patients manifesting symptoms of chronic mesenteric ischemia [14, 15].

The incidence of chronic mesenteric ischemia is estimated at 1/100,000 per year in the general population [6]. The most common cause of chronic mesenteric ischemia is atherosclerosis, which affects an older patient population with a slight female preponderance [15]. Over 30 % of patients with chronic intestinal ischemia due to atherosclerosis have concomitant atherosclerotic disease of other vascular beds, and 75 % are smokers [15]. More rare etiologies of chronic mesenteric ischemia include fibromuscular dysplasia and several vasculitides.

The classic presenting symptom of chronic mesenteric ischemia has been described as "abdominal angina," which is a cramping discomfort occurring anywhere from 15 min to 3 h after a meal [16]. Patients develop an aversion to food (sitophobia) resulting in weight loss over the months prior to presentation. In fact, the diagnosis should be questioned in the absence of weight loss. Other symptoms may include nausea, vomiting, and changes in bowel habits [4, 16]. On exam, a systolic bruit may be heard as well as signs of atherosclerosis in other arterial distributions.

Chronic Mesenteric Ischemia due to Atherosclerotic Disease

It is for this entity that percutaneous treatment of mesenteric vascular disease is most frequently employed. As mentioned, due to the various anastomotic pathways (Table 33.3) that allow single-vessel disease to be well tolerated, chronic intestinal ischemia most commonly results from multivessel disease of the mesenteric vessels. In nine reports of 244 cases of chronic mesenteric ischemia published in the 1980s and 1990s, 91 % of cases involved 2-vessel disease, 55 % involved 3-vessel disease, and 9 % had single-vessel disease (7 % SMA, 2 % celiac) by catheter-based angiography [15]. Though uncommon, single-vessel mesenteric disease can result in symptomatic chronic intestinal ischemia in the presence of insufficient collateral reserve. Individuals with prior abdominal surgery are particularly susceptible to disrupted collateral supply. Culprit atherosclerotic lesions most commonly affect the ostium of the mesenteric vessels and are frequently heavily calcified.

Several imaging modalities facilitate the diagnosis of chronic mesenteric ischemia due to atherosclerosis and have largely replaced the need for diagnostic invasive angiography for this disease. Doppler ultrasonography is an excellent

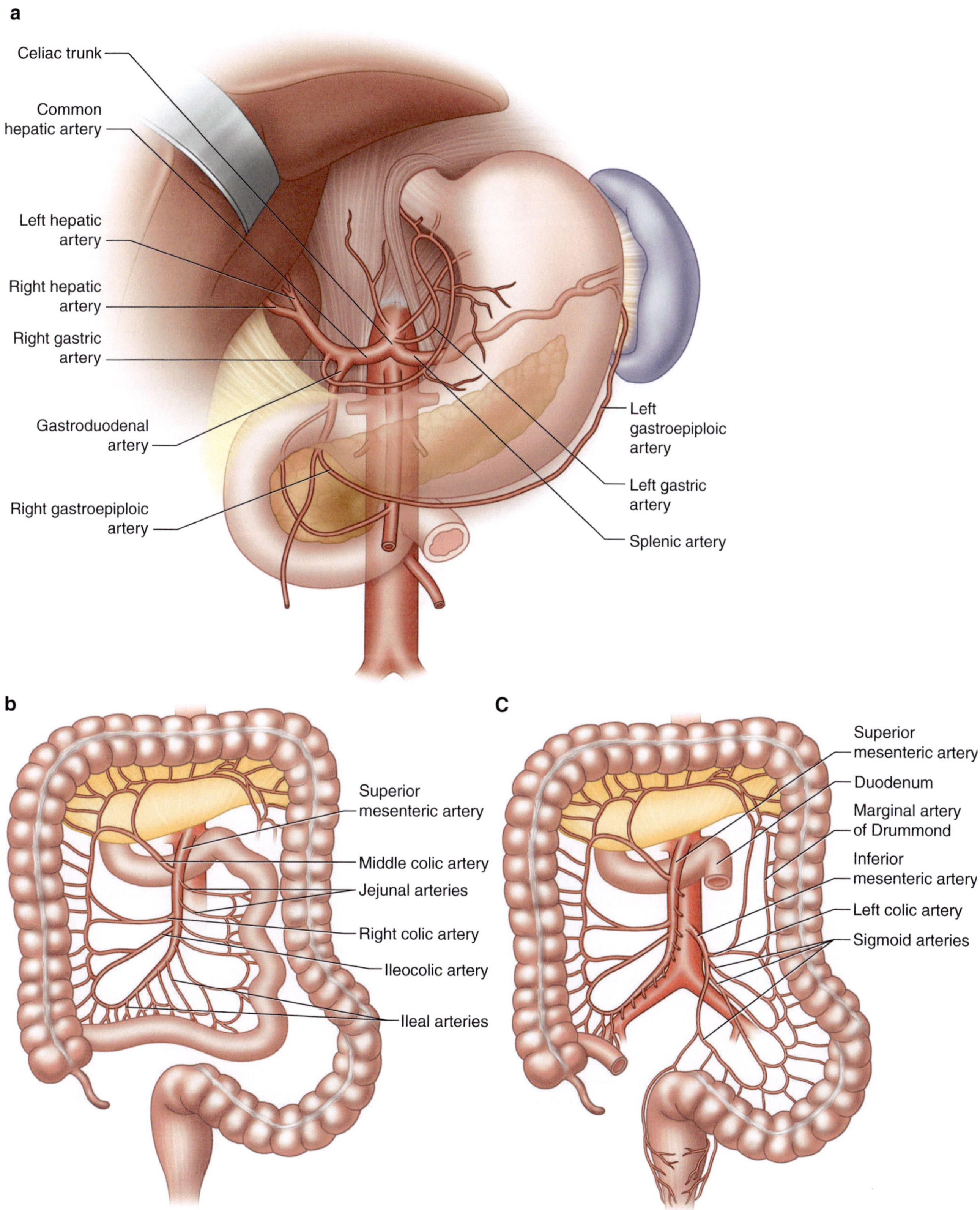

Fig. 33.1 Anatomy of (**a**) celiac, (**b**) superior mesenteric, and (**c**) inferior mesenteric arteries and branches

Table 33.2 First-order mesenteric branches

	Level of takeoff	Diameter	Major branches	Organs supplied
Celiac trunk	T12	5–7 mm	Common hepatic artery Splenic artery Left gastric artery	Stomach Duodenum Spleen Liver Pancreas
SMA	L1 1.5 cm below celiac artery	4–6 mm	Inferior pancreaticoduodenal Middle colic artery Right colic artery Ileocolic artery Jejunal arteries Ileal arteries	Pancreas Jejunum Ileum Ascending colon Proximal half of transverse colon
IMA	L3 4 cm above aortoiliac bifurcation	3–5 mm	Left colic Sigmoid Marginal Superior rectal	Distal half of transverse colon Descending colon Rectum

Abbreviations: *SMA* superior mesenteric artery, *IMA* inferior mesenteric artery

Table 33.3 Major anastamoses in mesenteric arterial circulation

Anastomosis	Anatomy	Major branches connected	Clinical relevance
Inferior phrenic arteries	Inferior phrenic arteries–hepatic arteries	Aorta and celiac axis	Celiac occlusion
Arc of Barkow	Hepatic/gastroduodenal/right gastroepiploic arteries–left gastroepiploic/splenic arteries	Celiac–celiac axis	
Pancreaticoduodenal arcade	Common hepatic/gastroduodenal/superior PD arteries–inferior PD artery	Celiac and SMA	Celiac or proximal SMA occlusion
Arc of Buhler	Persistent embryonic connection	Celiac and SMA	4 % occurrence
Marginal artery of Drummond	Confluence of right and middle colic arteries (SMA) with left colic artery (IMA)	SMA and IMA	Proximal SMA occlusion
Arc of Riolan	Middle colic (SMA)–left colic artery (IMA)	SMA and IMA	Proximal SMA occlusion
Rectal arteries	Superior rectal artery (IMA)–middle and inferior rectal arteries (IIA)	IMA and IIA	Celiac/SMA/IMA occlusions

Abbreviations: *SMA* superior mesenteric artery, *IMA* inferior mesenteric artery, *PD* pancreaticoduodenal, *IIA* internal iliac artery

modality in the diagnosis of obstructive atherosclerotic disease of the celiac and superior mesenteric arteries provided the study is performed by a skilled technician and the patient's body habitus is not prohibitive [15, 17]. Due to the proximal nature of typical atherosclerotic stenoses, computed tomographic angiography and magnetic resonance angiography are also accurate imaging tools. Though superior in its imaging resolution, catheter-based angiography is not a first-line diagnostic test for chronic intestinal ischemia due to a relatively higher rate of vascular complications than other imaging tests and due to the exposure to iodinated contrast and radiation as compared to duplex ultrasonography or magnetic resonance angiography. It should be emphasized that the presence of obstructive lesions on any of these modalities is not sufficient to make the diagnosis of chronic intestinal ischemia; rather, the presence of suggestive clinical symptoms is also necessary. Thus, catheter-based angiography – with an inclination for endovascular treatment – is typically reserved for the patient with suggestive symptoms of chronic mesenteric ischemia in addition to evidence of severe obstructive disease on a less-invasive imaging modality.

Asymptomatic mesenteric atherosclerosis is thought to have a relatively high prevalence but a benign natural history. In a population-based study of 553 elderly individuals, the prevalence of single-vessel mesenteric obstructive disease was 17 % by duplex ultrasonography [18]. The favorable prognosis of asymptomatic mesenteric atherosclerotic disease is largely based on a report from the Cardiovascular Health Study; however, this report suffered from incomplete follow-up [18]. Nonetheless, it is generally accepted that medical therapy, in the absence of revascularization, is warranted for asymptomatic patients [6].

For patients with symptoms and weight loss thought to be due to obstructive, atherosclerotic mesenteric disease, revascularization is warranted. No randomized trials have been conducted comparing the various treatment options of chronic intestinal ischemia due to atherosclerotic disease. Surgical revascularization was 1st done in 1958 [19]. Options include bypass, endarterectomy, and reimplantation. Bypass choices include single-vessel versus multivessel revascularization, prosthetic versus venous conduits, and antegrade (from the supraceliac aorta) versus retrograde (from the internal iliac arteries) approaches [15]. Depending on the study, perioperative mortality has ranged from 0 to 16 %, and reported recurrence rates have varied widely from 0 to 26 % over 3–12 years [8].

Feasible, percutaneous revascularization is generally preferred over surgical revascularization due to the morbidity associated with surgery in the typically elderly population with this disease. However, certain patient subsets are more appropriate for surgery, including those with concomitant aneurysmal disease in need of repair and those with flush occlusions of the culprit mesenteric vessel(s) [6]. The technical aspects of endovascular therapy and its evidence base are discussed later in this chapter.

Nonatherosclerotic Causes of Chronic Mesenteric Ischemia

Less than 10 % of cases of chronic intestinal ischemia are due to nonatherosclerotic diseases, which are summarized in Table 33.4 [16]. In general, catheter-based angiography is employed more frequently for the diagnosis of *fibromuscular dysplasia* and *vasculitis* than for atherosclerotic disease due to involvement of mid and distal mesenteric vessels by these nonatherosclerotic diseases and consequently the need for an imaging modality with higher resolution. There is minimal literature to assist with decision-making regarding revascularization for chronic intestinal ischemia in fibromuscular dysplasia and vasculitis. In the absence of such evidence, extrapolation of data from intervention in other arterial beds seems appropriate. Thus, for chronic intestinal ischemia due to fibromuscular dysplasia, measurement of pressure gradients to assess severity of stenoses and angioplasty alone without stenting should be considered as is done for renal artery interventions for this disorder [20]. Also, endovascular therapy for chronic mesenteric ischemia due to vasculitis should be performed in the chronic fibrotic stage, rather than the active inflammatory stage, to improve durability of the intervention.

Median arcuate ligament syndrome is a controversial entity that refers to compression of the celiac trunk by the arcuate ligament of the diaphragm in the presence of symptoms of chronic mesenteric ischemia and in the absence of alternative etiologies. The stenosis is dynamic, becoming more severe in expiration when the diaphragm moves upward. Duplex ultrasonography shows elevated peak systolic velocities during expiration. CT angiography shows a focal, ostial narrowing with an acutely downward-going proximal segment forming a classic "hooked" appearance [21, 22].

Celiac artery compression by the arcuate ligament occurs not infrequently in the absence of symptoms [23]. Thus, establishing a cause-and-effect relationship between this finding and symptoms is challenging and likely only possible if symptoms improve after revascularization. However, given the uncertain benefit, the indication for revascularization is often suspect. If revascularization is pursued, surgical release of compression with or without celiac trunk revascularization is recommended [6]. Laparoscopic release with or without endovascular revascularization has been described as a minimally invasive option ([24]. It is important for the interventionalist not to mistake this syndrome with atherosclerotic disease of the celiac artery.

Table 33.4 Nonatherosclerotic, nontraumatic causes of chronic intestinal ischemia

	Demographic	Noninvasive imaging	Catheter-based angiographic findings	Endovascular therapy
Fibromuscular dysplasia	Most commonly 20–40-year-old women	Mid-distal lesions may be difficult to visualize. "String of beads" for medial fibroplasias. Long smooth stenoses if intimal fibroplasia. No vessel wall edema as seen in vasculitis	"String of beads" for medial fibroplasia. Long smooth stenoses if intimal fibroplasia. Cause of spontaneous dissection	PTA after assessment with IVUS/pressure gradient with "bailout" stenting
Segmental arterial mediolysis	>40 years	Aneurysmal disease	Aneurysmal disease	No reported cases
Vasculitis	Depends on type	Mid-distal lesions difficult to visualize. MRI and US may show wall edema. Proximal stenoses may be seen in large-vessel vasculitis	Large-vessel vasculitis (e.g., Takayasu's): Smooth stenoses of proximal mesenteric vessels Medium vessel vasculitis (PAN): multiple aneurysms <1 cm +/– stenoses in distal medium-sized branches of mesenteric vessels	For large-vessel vasculitis, PTA/stenting rarely, in chronic fibrotic stage of disease. Not recommended in acute inflammatory stage
Radiation induced	History of >4,500 cGy abdominal radiation	Mid-distal lesions difficult to visualize	Multiple stenoses of small vessels	No reported cases
Median arcuate ligament syndrome	Typically, young thin females	US: elevated velocities in proximal celiac trunk during expiration CT: "hooked" appearance of proximal celiac trunk	Rarely necessary for diagnosis Respirophasic proximal celiac trunk stenosis (worse in expiration)	Stenting – controversial

Abbreviations: *CT* computed tomography, *MRI* magnetic resonance imaging, *US* ultrasound, *PAN* polyarteritis nodosa, *PTA* angioplasty, *IVUS* intravascular ultrasound

Acute Mesenteric Ischemia

Patients with acute intestinal ischemia have a 60–80 % mortality rate [10]. Outcomes can be improved if prompt diagnosis leads to efficient mesenteric reperfusion such that viable bowel can be preserved, the extent of necrotic bowel can be limited, and necrotic intestine can be resected [10, 25].

Surgery – explorative laparotomy, bowel resection, and revascularization – is a mainstay of the management of acute intestinal ischemia [4, 8, 10]. In contemporary medicine, however, multiple endovascular treatments are also available [26–29]. When used in conjunction with surgery, endovascular techniques can optimize prompt and efficient diagnosis and treatment of patients with acute intestinal ischemia.

Given the high mortality rate, challenging diagnosis, and varied treatment options spanning multiple specialties, efficient multidisciplinary collaboration is essential in achieving optimal patient outcomes.

Etiology

Acute mesenteric ischemia can result from arterial occlusion, nonocclusive mesenteric ischemia, or venous thrombosis. *Arterial occlusion* most commonly results from thromboembolism, which accounts for 30–50 % of cases of acute mesenteric ischemia. In situ thrombosis is another common cause of arterial occlusion, contributing to 25–30 % of cases of acute mesenteric ischemia. Less common causes of acute mesenteric arterial occlusion are atheroembolism and dissection [5, 10, 14]. *Nonocclusive mesenteric ischemia (NOMI)* refers to a state of low cardiac output accompanied by profound mesenteric vasoconstriction in the absence of focal mesenteric arterial obstruction. This entity is responsible for 20–30 % of acute mesenteric ischemia cases [10]. It can also be due to intense mesenteric vasospasm from ergotamines, digoxin, cocaine, amphetamine, or vasopressor agents without reduced cardiac output [4]. *Venous thrombosis* of the celiac and/or superior mesenteric veins is typically seen in conditions predisposing to deep venous thrombosis – such as protein C deficiency, protein S deficiency, factor V Leiden, and prothrombin gene mutation – and is reported to account for 15–20 % of acute intestinal ischemia [10, 30]. Other risk factors for mesenteric venous thrombosis include pancreatitis, recent intra-abdominal surgery, and cirrhosis [30].

Presentation

Regardless of etiology, patients with acute mesenteric ischemia present with severe abdominal pain that is classically out of proportion to physical findings. Other symptoms include nausea, vomiting, diarrhea, and gastrointestinal bleeding. On physical exam, a rigid abdomen indicates peritonitis from perforation of necrotic bowel. Such a finding is critical in the early evaluation of this disease as it indicates the need for emergent surgery, the absence of which carries a high mortality rate [4]. Melena may also be present, though the absence of heme-positive stools cannot rule out acute intestinal ischemia [4]. Lactic acidosis is common, but an elevated lactate is nonspecific.

In all comers with acute intestinal ischemia, the median age is 70 years and 2/3 are women [4]. There may be clinical features that suggest a precise etiology in patients presenting with acute mesenteric ischemia, and recognition of these clues can facilitate appropriate initial workup and management. For example, potential sources of thrombotic or atherosclerotic embolism should be sought (e.g., atrial fibrillation, severe left ventricular dysfunction, aortic atheroma, and a recent arterial catheterization procedure), particularly in the nonanticoagulated patient. These patients may also have evidence of embolization elsewhere, causing acute stroke or acute limb ischemia. A history of chronic intestinal ischemic symptoms suggests in situ atherothrombosis as the etiology of acute intestinal ischemia. Critical illness, hypotension from any cause, and certain offending medications (vasopressors, digoxin, ergotamines) are risk factors for NOMI. Finally, a known hypercoagulable state and pancreatitis may be present in patients with mesenteric venous thrombosis.

Diagnosis

Unlike for chronic mesenteric ischemia, duplex ultrasonography is not an appropriate first-line diagnostic study for acute mesenteric ischemia due to the acuity of the disease, time required to complete an adequate study, and typical nonfasting state of the patient. Similarly, magnetic resonance angiography cannot be accomplished in a sufficiently expedient fashion for this acute illness. Computed tomographic (CT) angiography is an accurate and practical diagnostic test, if the patient's clinical status allows. This modality can promptly identify arterial and venous obstruction, evaluate changes in the bowel wall indicative of intestinal ischemia, and search for alternative diagnoses of acute abdominal pain. Though there is evidence that early catheter-based angiography improves outcomes, these studies predate contemporary CT scanning [2, 31, 32]. With the current technology, CT angiography is an appropriate first-line diagnostic study in patients suspected to have acute mesenteric ischemia due to embolization or arterial or venous thrombosis [14].

Catheter-based angiography has traditionally been considered the gold standard diagnostic test for acute intestinal ischemia. Certainly, it remains the diagnostic test of choice for NOMI, and patients suspected to have acute mesenteric ischemia due to NOMI should go immediately to catheter-based angiography if no peritoneal signs are present. However, the greater role of angiography in contemporary practice may be in presurgical planning or for delivery of catheter-based therapies. Nonetheless, not only can catheter-based angiography diagnose mesenteric arterial and venous

Table 33.5 Features of acute intestinal ischemia by pathogenetic mechanism

	Clinical setting/risk factors	Initial diagnostic test of choice	Pattern of bowel involvement	Typical angiographic findings
Thromboembolism	Cardioembolic source (atrial fibrillation, LV thrombus) Concomitant thromboembolic events	CT angiogram	Sparing of jejunum, ascending colon	SMA occlusion distal to middle colic artery
Atheroembolism	Recent arterial catheterization	Clinical	More focal, localized areas of ischemia	Distal mesenteric arterial occlusions
Arterial thrombosis	History of chronic intestinal ischemia	CT angiogram	Small intestine, ascending colon involved	Ostial SMA or celiac arterial occlusion
NOMI	Critical illness, hypotension, low cardiac output, offending medications (vasopressors, digoxin, ergotamines), cocaine/amphetamine use	Catheter-based angiography	Small intestine	Diffuse severe tapering of distal SMA branches "String of sausages" sign
Venous thrombosis	History of DVT/PE, hypercoagulable state, pancreatitis	CT angiogram	Variable	Slow filling and delayed emptying of contrast from mesenteric arteries

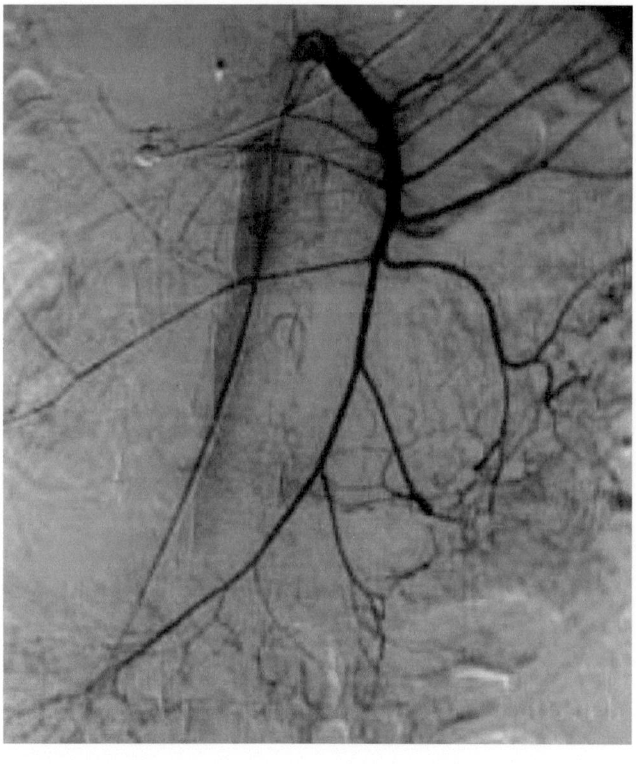

Fig. 33.2 Angiogram from patient with nonocclusive mesenteric ischemia (From Trompeter et al. [33], with permission)

obstruction, but it can also differentiate among the different causes of acute intestinal ischemia (Table 33.5).

The typical angiographic finding of acute mesenteric ischemia due to thromboembolism to the superior mesenteric artery is occlusion just distal to the middle colic artery, where over 50 % of thromboemboli lodge [10, 14]. In contrast, arterial in situ thrombosis usually occurs at the ostium, superimposed on a preexisting atherosclerotic lesion. In NOMI, there is diffuse vasospasm of small mesenteric arteries that may respond to the administration of vasodilators (Fig. 33.2). Angiography in mesenteric venous thrombosis reveals slow filling and delayed emptying of mesenteric arteries.

Management

The key initial step to determine management in patients with acute mesenteric ischemia is to identify signs of necrotic bowel and/or peritonitis based on exam, serology, and initial imaging. If signs of peritonitis are present, the patient should have emergent laparotomy. If no such clinical findings are present, then management can be tailored to the etiology and individual patient. Regardless of cause, intravenous volume resuscitation, anticoagulation (unfractionated heparin infusion being the drug of choice due to its relatively short half-life), and empiric antibiotics are almost always appropriate. If vasopressors are required for hypotension after volume resuscitation, dopamine and epinephrine, rather than pure alpha agonists or vasopressin, may cause less mesenteric vasoconstriction [10].

Surgical revascularization is usually preferred over endovascular therapy for acute intestinal ischemia due to arterial obstruction, largely due to the need to concomitantly assess for and/or resect necrotic bowel. Endovascular treatment options for thromboembolism or in situ thrombosis include catheter-based thrombectomy, catheter-directed fibrinolysis, angioplasty, stenting, and administration of vasodilators (Table 33.5). One or more of these treatment modalities are usually reserved for patients without peritoneal signs on physical examination in whom it is felt safe to defer surgical exploration for necrotic bowel (Table 33.6). Additionally, percutaneous revascularization may be pursued for patients felt to be at prohibitive risk for surgery. Occasionally, vasodilator therapy delivered via a catheter placed selectively in the mesenteric artery of interest can be used as a bridge to surgery in attempts to facilitate preservation of viable bowel.

Table 33.6 Endovascular treatment of acute intestinal ischemia in patients without peritoneal signs[a]

Mechanism	Vasodilator	Catheter-directed fibrinolysis	Catheter thrombectomy	Angioplasty/stenting
Thromboembolism	+ (as bridge to surgery)	+ (if surgical risk prohibitive)	+ (if surgical risk prohibitive or to reduce extent of surgery)	+ (if surgical risk prohibitive or to reduce extent of surgery)
In situ thrombosis	+ (as bridge to surgery)	+ (if surgical risk prohibitive)	+ (if surgical risk prohibitive or to reduce extent of surgery)	+ (if surgical risk prohibitive or to reduce extent of surgery)
NOMI	++	–	–	–
Mesenteric venous thrombosis	–	Rarely	Rarely	–

NOMI nonocclusive mesenteric ischemia
[a]Patients with peritoneal signs should emergently go to surgery

In contrast, such vasodilator therapy is the cornerstone of treatment for NOMI, along with reversal of precipitating causes, if possible. For mesenteric venous thrombosis, there is limited data that catheter-directed fibrinolysis is effective, though this modality would be 2nd line to surgical intervention. The technique of endovascular therapy for acute mesenteric ischemia is discussed in the next section.

Endovascular Therapy

Preprocedural Management

It cannot be overstressed that meticulous clinical evaluation is paramount for appropriate patient selection for endovascular treatment of chronic intestinal ischemia. Similarly, for acute mesenteric ischemia, prompt multidisciplinary collaboration is necessary for optimal patient outcomes.

There is little to no evidence regarding the best preprocedural medical therapy prior to mesenteric intervention. However, most if not all patients referred with chronic mesenteric ischemia should already be taking aspirin. Likewise, patients with acute mesenteric ischemia should be anticoagulated on arrival to the angiographic suite, often with unfractionated heparin. Like catheter-based treatments in other arterial beds, appropriate measures should be taken to prevent contrast-induced nephropathy and to treat contrast allergies prior to the planned procedure.

Extrapolating from the literature for percutaneous coronary intervention, when consenting patients with chronic intestinal ischemia, it is reasonable to quote a minor complication rate of <10 % and a major complication rate <5 %. Complications primarily involve minor vascular complications, such as access site pseudoaneurysm and arteriovenous fistula; however, less common major vascular complications – such as atheroembolism, aortic dissection, distal embolization, and acute mesenteric ischemia – can occur (Fig. 33.3).

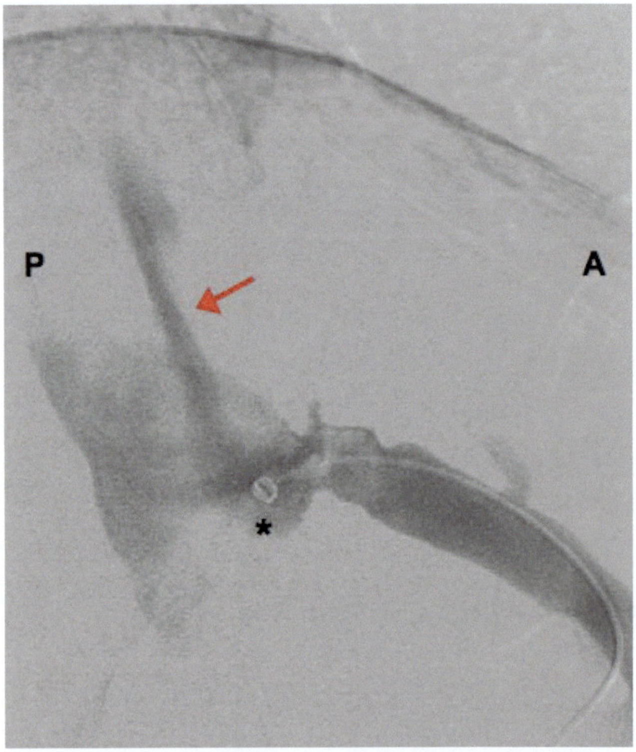

Fig. 33.3 Right lateral view of retrograde aortic dissection following post-dilatation of a celiac artery stent. The patient recovered after covered stenting and conservative management (*A* Anterior, *P* posterior, * – catheter tip; *arrow* – dissection)

Procedure

Access

Mesenteric angiography and intervention can be performed via femoral, brachial, and radial arterial access. The advantages of performing the procedure from access in the arm include coaxial alignment of diagnostic and guiding catheters with the downward takeoff of the mesenteric vessels and lower rates of access site bleeding. The disadvantages of radial access, however, include the inability of catheters to reach the mesenteric vessels in tall patients and the relative inability to use 7F sheaths if necessary.

In general, 5F sheaths are sufficient for diagnostic angiography, while 6–7F sheaths are needed for mesenteric stenting and administering fibrinolytics or vasodilators.

Antithrombotics

There are no randomized trials to guide the most effective antithrombotic therapy during mesenteric intervention. For diagnostic angiography alone, preprocedural aspirin is sufficient. For mesenteric intervention, preprocedural aspirin in addition to an antithrombin (e.g., unfractionated heparin, bivalirudin, low molecular weight heparin, argatroban) is appropriate. The particular antithrombin can be operator dependent. If unfractionated heparin is used, we recommend a goal activated clotting time of 200–250 s for the treatment of chronic mesenteric ischemia and 250–300 s for treatment of acute intestinal ischemia. When the decision to perform mesenteric stenting is made, clopidogrel can be administered (300–600 mg load). Glycoprotein 2b/3a inhibitors are not typically used due to the lack of evidence for benefit and expected increased risk of bleeding. However, in the rare circumstance when catheter-based treatment of acute mesenteric ischemia due to thrombotic arterial occlusion is planned in the absence of surgery or thrombolysis, one could consider adjunctive glycoprotein 2b/3a inhibition.

Angiography

In general, a nonselective abdominal aortogram is performed initially followed by selective mesenteric angiography.

A variety of 5F sidehole catheters are available for abdominal aortography (pigtail, Omni Flush, AngioDynamics, Latham, NY). The catheter should be 110–125 cm if coming from radial access. Abdominal aortography should be performed in anterior–posterior (AP) and lateral projections (Fig. 33.4). In the AP view, the ostia of the mesenteric vessels are not well visualized due to vessel overlap with the aorta. However, careful attention should be paid to mesenteric branch vessels, collateral pathways, and anatomic variants. Understanding collateral flow will provide insight into the best revascularization strategy. The internal iliac arteries should also be visualized, as these vessels may be involved in supplying the mesentery in the event of disease of the superior mesenteric and inferior mesenteric arteries (Fig. 33.5). A power injection of 20–25 cc at a rate of 15–20 cc/s is generally adequate to obtain a complete angiogram.

The abdominal aortogram can refine the choice of diagnostic catheter and angiographic views for selective mesenteric angiography. When performing selective mesenteric angiography from access in the arm, a 5F multipurpose catheter is typically effective. A number of reverse-curve catheters can be used from femoral access. Alternatively, internal mammary, Judkins right, or hockey stick catheters can be

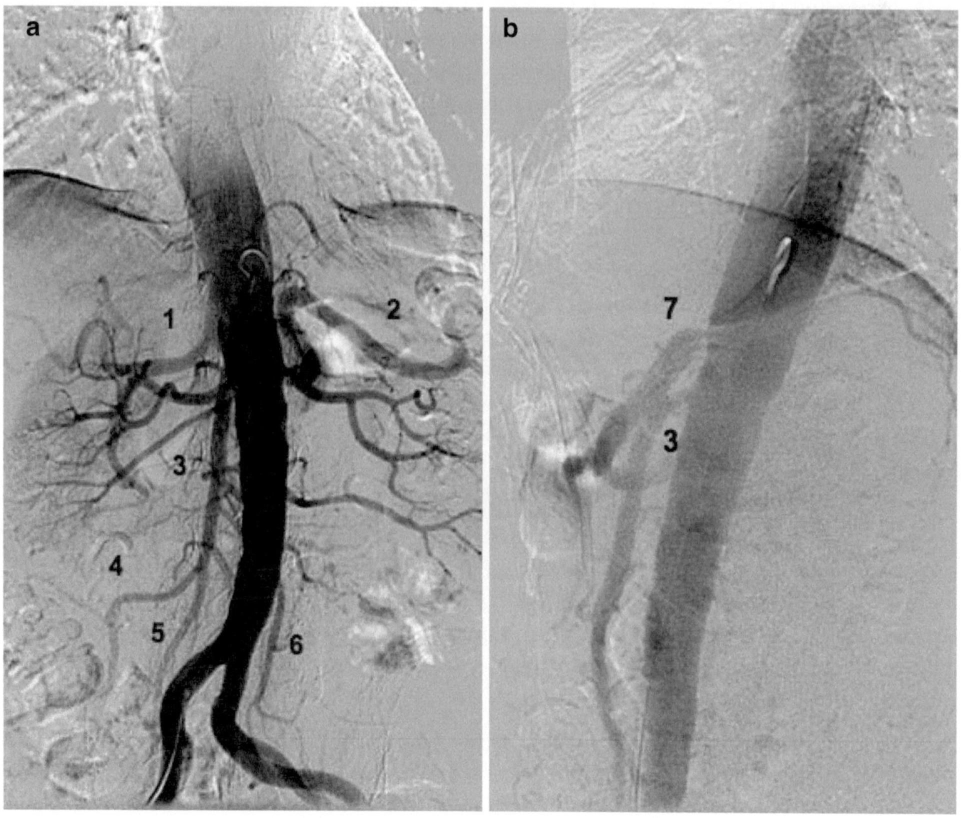

Fig. 33.4 (a) Abdominal aortogram, anteroposterior view. The origin of the mesenteric vessels is not well seen due to overlap, but branch vessels are displayed. (b) Abdominal aortogram, lateral view. The origins of the mesenteric vessels are better visualized. There is a severe ostial celiac artery stenosis and a mild ostial superior mesenteric artery stenosis. *1* – Common hepatic artery; *2* – splenic artery; *3* – superior mesenteric artery; *4* – right colic artery; *5* – ileocolic artery; *6* – inferior mesenteric artery; *7* – celiac artery

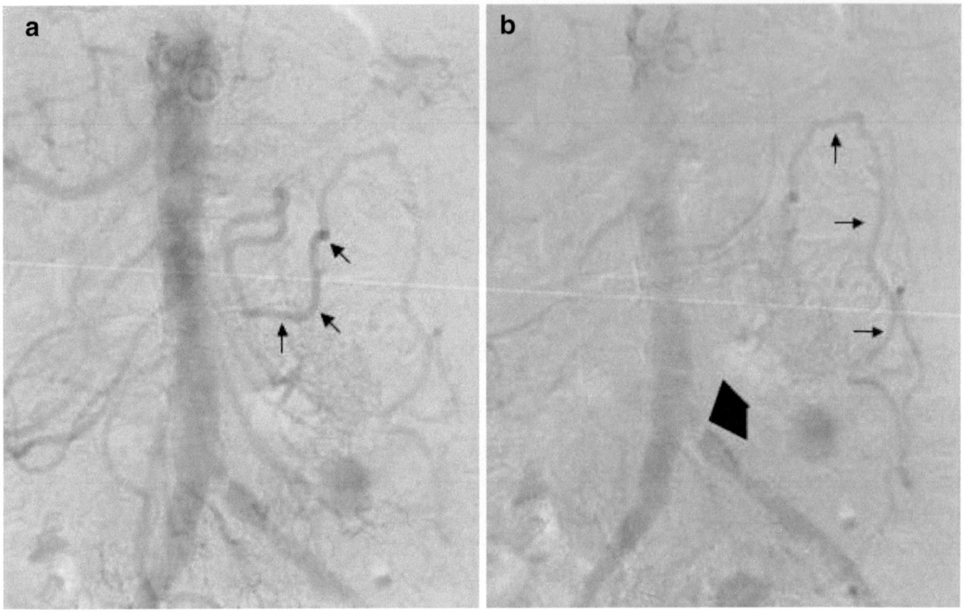

Fig. 33.5 Abdominal aortogram with prominent marginal artery of Drummond (*arrows*) in (**a**) early and (**b**) delayed phases of contrast injection. Typically, a prominent marginal artery of Drummond signifies collateral filling of the SMA territory by the IMA, due to severe SMA disease. In this patient, however, the SMA collateralizes the IMA via the marginal artery of Drummond due to an IMA occlusion. The ipsilateral internal iliac artery fails to collateralize the IMA due to the severe CIA stenosis (*arrowhead*)

used depending on the angle of the proximal mesenteric vessel of interest. Anterior–posterior, lateral, and right anterior oblique caudal views are often helpful but should be tailored for the individual patient's anatomy (Figs. 33.6, and 33.7). Approximately 6–8 cc of contrast at 3–4 cc/s is typically sufficient to obtain a good selective angiogram.

The decision to perform selective mesenteric angiography of all or only a single mesenteric vessel should be case specific, depending on the adequacy of prior imaging, findings on the abdominal aortogram, baseline renal function, and the clinical situation. Selective angiography of the inferior mesenteric artery can be challenging due to its small caliber. A technique for imaging this vessel is to orient the diagnostic catheter anteriorly at the level of L3 and perform a vigorous injection of contrast in the lateral view to nonselectively image the proximal IMA (Fig. 33.8). Selective angiography of the nontarget vessel may be necessary to adequately visualize collateral flow to the reconstituted segment of the occluded target artery, particularly for patients with chronic mesenteric ischemia in which collaterals may be well developed. Knowledge of the reconstituted segment reveals the length of occlusion, facilitating the decision of whether and how to intervene.

Therapy

Several therapeutic options are available for the endovascular treatment of chronic and acute intestinal ischemia: angioplasty, stenting, catheter-directed thrombolysis, catheter-based delivery of vasodilators, and catheter thrombectomy.

Angioplasty and Stenting

The most common indication for angioplasty and stenting of the mesenteric arteries is chronic intestinal ischemia. Angioplasty is rarely performed alone for atherosclerotic disease in this setting, as the culprit lesions are typically heavily calcified and do not respond adequately to balloon dilatation alone. Nonetheless, if angioplasty alone is the desired strategy, a 5F guiding system or sheath is appropriate. In the more common scenario in which stenting is performed adjunctively, a 6–7F guiding catheter or 5–6F guiding sheath is necessary for most stent platforms. A 7–8F guiding catheter (6–7F guiding sheath) will be required for most appropriately sized covered stents.

Multiple potential guiding catheters and sheaths are available for mesenteric intervention. The principal advantage of a guiding catheter over a guiding sheath is better torquability and control of the former. The main advantage of a guiding sheath is a smaller arteriotomy and lower bleeding risk. Thus, a guiding sheath may be preferable when using radial or brachial access, in which manipulation of the guiding system is less of an issue and the size of the guiding system needs to be minimized.

There are two basic techniques to engage the mesenteric artery of choice with a guiding system: *no-touch* and *direct engagement*. In the *no-touch* technique, a guide wire (0.014, 0.018, or 0.035) is advanced into the descending thoracic aorta, assuming access is via the common femoral artery. The guiding catheter or sheath is oriented toward the ostium of the vessel of interest. A 2nd wire – usually a 0.014 in. wire – is then advanced past the lesion into the distal mesenteric artery. The original wire is then withdrawn, "seating" the tip of the guiding catheter or sheath at the ostium of the vessel. This technique is particularly suited for a guiding catheter from femoral access, in which more challenging catheter manipulation is required to obtain a coaxial position with the downward-going mesenteric vessels as compared to arm

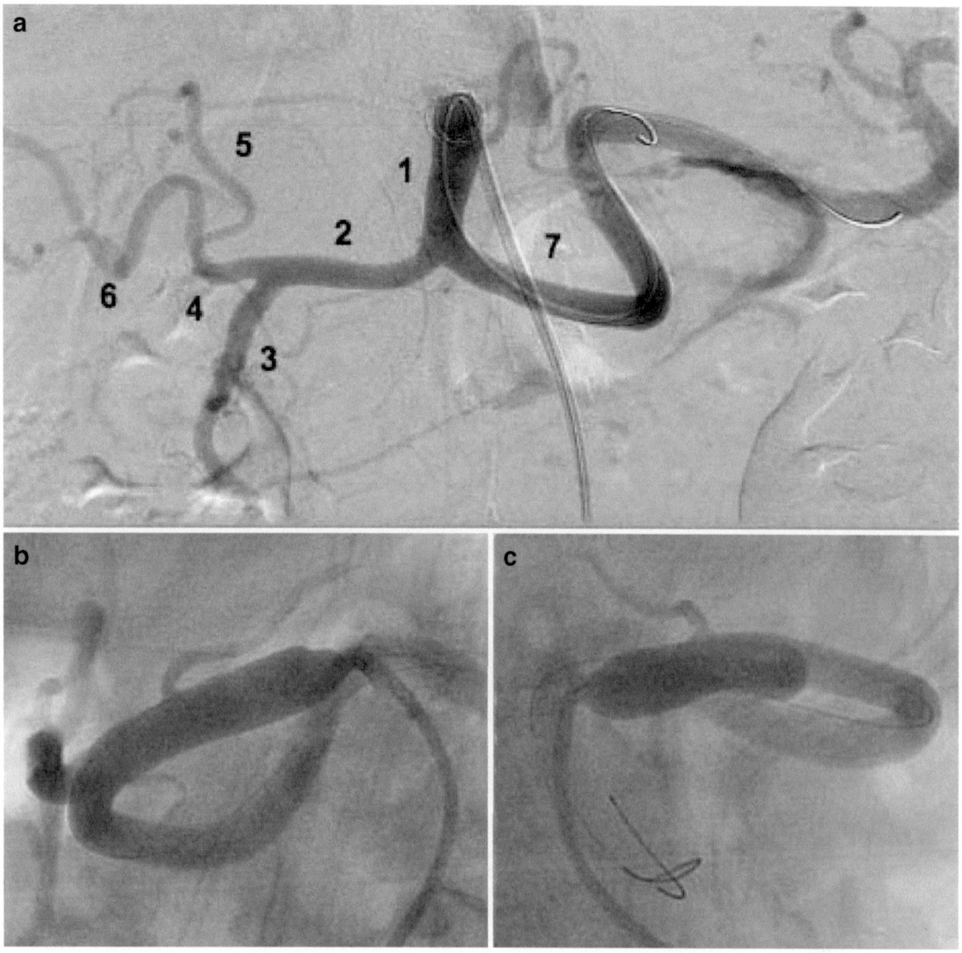

Fig. 33.6 Selective celiac angiography. (**a**) Anteroposterior view. (**b**) Left lateral view. (**c**) Right anterior oblique view. *1* – Celiac trunk; *2* – common hepatic artery; *3* – gastroduodenal artery; *4* – proper hepatic artery; *5* – left hepatic artery; *6* – right hepatic artery; *7* – splenic artery

access. In contrast, this technique is more challenging with a guiding sheath, which is more difficult to maneuver towards the mesenteric artery ostium so that it can be wired. To obviate this problem and position a guiding sheath in the ostium of interest, a diagnostic catheter can be telescoped through a guiding sheath. After engaging the mesenteric artery with the diagnostic catheter and wiring the vessel, the guiding sheath can be advanced over the diagnostic catheter/wire combination.

In the *direct engagement* technique, a 4–5F diagnostic catheter is telescoped through a guiding catheter or sheath. The diagnostic catheter is manipulated to engage the ostium of the mesenteric artery. A guide wire (0.014, 0.018, or 0.035) is advanced past the lesion. The guiding catheter or sheath is then advanced over the diagnostic catheter/wire combination. Directly engaging the ostium of a mesenteric artery is not recommended for a guiding catheter; that is, the tip of a guiding catheter is too traumatic to safely engage a vessel with an ostial lesion directly and could result in occlusion of the target vessel.

When engaging a mesenteric artery, an oblique view is usually best when wiring the proximal vessel, whereas an AP view may facilitate wiring the more distal vessel and its branches. Numerous 0.014, 0.018, and 0.035 wires, borrowed from interventional equipment designed for other arterial beds, are available. 0.014 wires have the advantage of being particularly atraumatic and allow for low-profile balloons and stents, thus ultimately minimizing the caliber of arteriotomy and lowering the risk of bleeding. 0.014 wires have the disadvantage, however, of less support which can result in the guiding system "kicking out" when attempting to delivery balloon and stent catheters. In such a situation, a 2nd 0.014 wire can be advanced into a different branch of the target mesenteric artery to increase support of the guiding system. After crossing an occlusion, the distal vessel should be imaged via an angiogram through a diagnostic catheter. This technique is particularly useful for treating acute mesenteric ischemia, when filling of the distal vessels via collaterals is more likely to be absent.

Multiple angioplasty balloon catheters are available for the treatment of mesenteric stenoses. The diameter of the angioplasty balloon can be sized based on an individual patient's anatomy in combination with the typical mesenteric vessel diameter (Table 33.2). When treating an ostial lesion, the length of the angioplasty balloon should be ~2 mm longer than the length of the culprit lesion so that the balloon

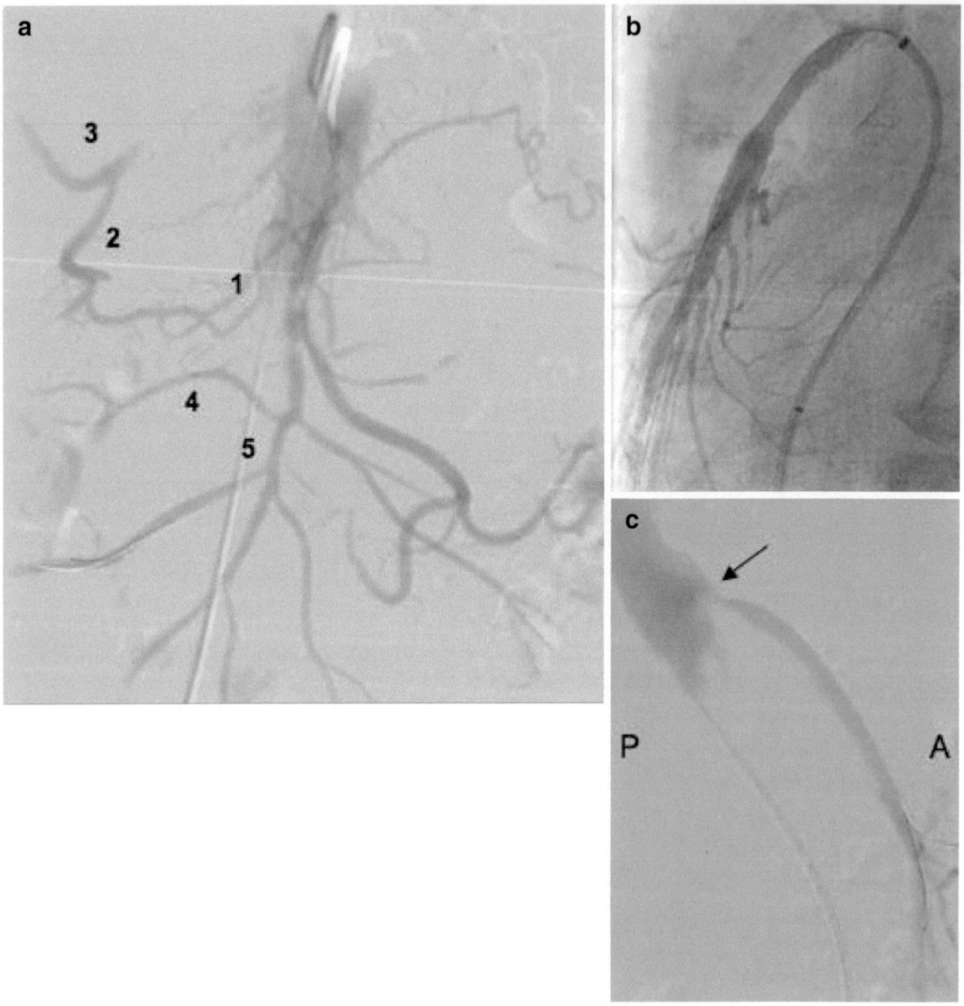

Fig. 33.7 Selective superior mesenteric angiography. (**a**) Anteroposterior view. The proper hepatic artery fills via a pancreaticoduodenal arcade from the superior mesenteric artery. *1* – Inferior pancreaticoduodenal artery; *2* – Gastroduodenal artery; *3* – Proper hepatic artery; *4* – Right colic artery; *5* – Middle colic artery. (**b**) Lateral view. (**c**) Right anterior oblique view. There is a moderate-severe ostial SMA stenosis (*arrow*) (*A* Anterior, *P* posterior)

protrudes 2 mm into the aorta to ensure complete treatment of the ostium (Fig. 33.9).

When treating mesenteric arterial stenoses, balloon-expandable stents are preferred to self-expanding stents for two reasons: increased radial strength, which is desirable to treat the typically heavily calcified stenoses seen with this disorder, and increased accuracy in placement of the stent for the typical ostial location of the target lesions. Only nondrug-eluting stents are currently available in the sizes appropriate for the mesenteric bed. Similar to the technique for angioplasty, ~2 mm of stent should protrude into the aorta, to ensure adequate coverage of ostial lesions. This technique thus requires the guiding catheter or sheath to be retracted >2 mm from the ostium, so that the stent is not inadvertently deployed within the guiding catheter/sheath (Fig. 33.10).

Following stent deployment, the tip of the guiding catheter or sheath can be advanced over the deflating stent balloon, so that the tip of the guide is seated within the lumen of the recently placed stent. Failure to perform this maneuver can complicate delivery of additional equipment (e.g., post-dilatation balloon catheters), as the tip of the post-dilatation balloon catheter will "catch" on the edge of the stent protruding into the aorta. Likewise, the guide often cannot be advanced within the lumen of the stent for the same reason, precluding a completion angiogram. A related issue exists when treating in-stent restenosis within an ostial mesenteric stent. In such a situation, extreme care must be taken to advance the guide wire through the lumen of the stent rather than through a side strut. In our experience, a reverse-curve catheter, such as a SOS (AngioDynamics, Latham, NY), may facilitate access to the "true lumen" of the stent; the catheter is advanced from caudal to the stent, such that the tip "catches" on the inferior border of the protruding stent. With additional forward pressure on the catheter, the tip will "jump" into the lumen of the stent, after which a guide wire can be advanced into the vessel.

Catheter-Directed Fibrinolysis

There is sparse evidence to guide the optimal technique of administering fibrinolytics for acute mesenteric ischemia. A 2005 systematic review of publications of superior

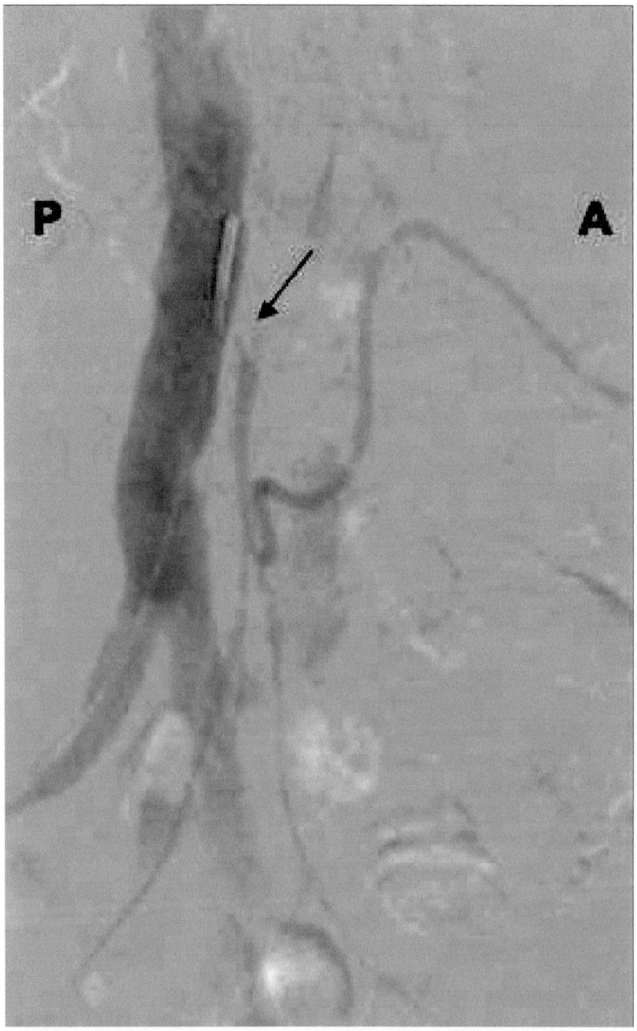

Fig. 33.8 Non-selective angiogram of the inferior mesenteric artery showing a critical ostial stenosis (*arrow*) (*A* Anterior, *P* posterior)

mesenteric arterial fibrinolysis found 27 reports (20 case reports and 7 case series) encompassing 48 patients with acute mesenteric ischemia due to thromboembolism [34]. The dominant fibrinolytic agent used was urokinase (38/48 cases), likely due to its short half-life (~15 min). The dose varied from boluses of 200,000–300,000 units and infusions of 100,000–600,000 units/h. The duration of treatment ranged from a few minutes for a bolus to 48 h. Angiographic success in this review was achieved in 43 of 48 patients, and four of the five patients in whom angiographic success was not achieved survived. Clinical success (angiographic success, symptom resolution, avoidance of need for surgery, and survival to discharge), however, was achieved in 30 of 48 patients. Survival occurred in 43 of 48 patients. These good outcomes are encouraging but may reflect publication bias.

The manner of administering the thrombolytic agent is even less well described. Some authors have reported "lacing" the thrombus through an end-hole catheter and then infusing the agent proximal to the thrombus through an end-hole catheter [34]. Other authors have used an infusion catheter or wire to infuse directly within the clot, similar to the technique of fibrinolysis in the extremities for acute limb ischemia [34, 35]. Regardless, a 5F guiding sheath or 6F guiding catheter is usually needed, through which a 4–5F diagnostic catheter, infusion catheter, or infusion wire is telescoped.

"Re-look" angiography is typically performed sooner (4–6 h) than for fibrinolysis in the extremities, due to the need to urgently assess for reperfusion and possible need for surgery.

There are a few case reports and case series of fibrinolysis for mesenteric venous thrombosis [36–39]. This modality can be performed via access to the portal vein or via arterial access. The portal vein may be entered from a transhepatic approach or from the internal jugular or femoral veins. These techniques are beyond the scope of this chapter. Some authors have reported infusing fibrinolysis through a catheter selectively placed in the SMA, performed in a manner similar to that described above [38, 39].

Catheter Thrombectomy

Catheter thrombectomy, as an adjunct to catheter-directed fibrinolysis, has been described in the treatment of acute mesenteric ischemia due to superior mesenteric arterial thromboembolism. The largest described series to date is a retrospective description of 15 patients with atrial fibrillation and thromboembolism of the SMA causing acute mesenteric ischemia [35]. The technique developed by these authors involved placing a 7–9F sheath in the SMA, crossing the thrombotic occlusion with a 0.035 guide wire, placing a 7–9F guiding catheter over the wire into the thrombus, removing the wire, and manually aspiring from the guiding catheter as it is retracted through the thrombus. A similar technique was used in SMA side branches with a 5F catheter. From their experience, the authors recommend administering a bolus of a fibrinolytic agent prior to and during manual thrombectomy; they also found that 6–7F guiding catheters reduced complications compared to larger guides. The rate of complete procedural success (<30 % residual stenosis) was 73 %, and partial procedural success (improved perfusion but residual stenosis >30 %) was achieved in the other 27 % of patients. Three patients subsequently underwent bowel resection. The 30-day mortality rate was 33 %.

Other reported techniques include the use of rheolytic thrombectomy and rapid exchange thrombectomy catheters designed for the coronary arteries [26, 29, 40].

Catheter Delivery of Vasodilators

Administration of vasodilators via a catheter selectively placed in the superior mesenteric artery is a treatment modality

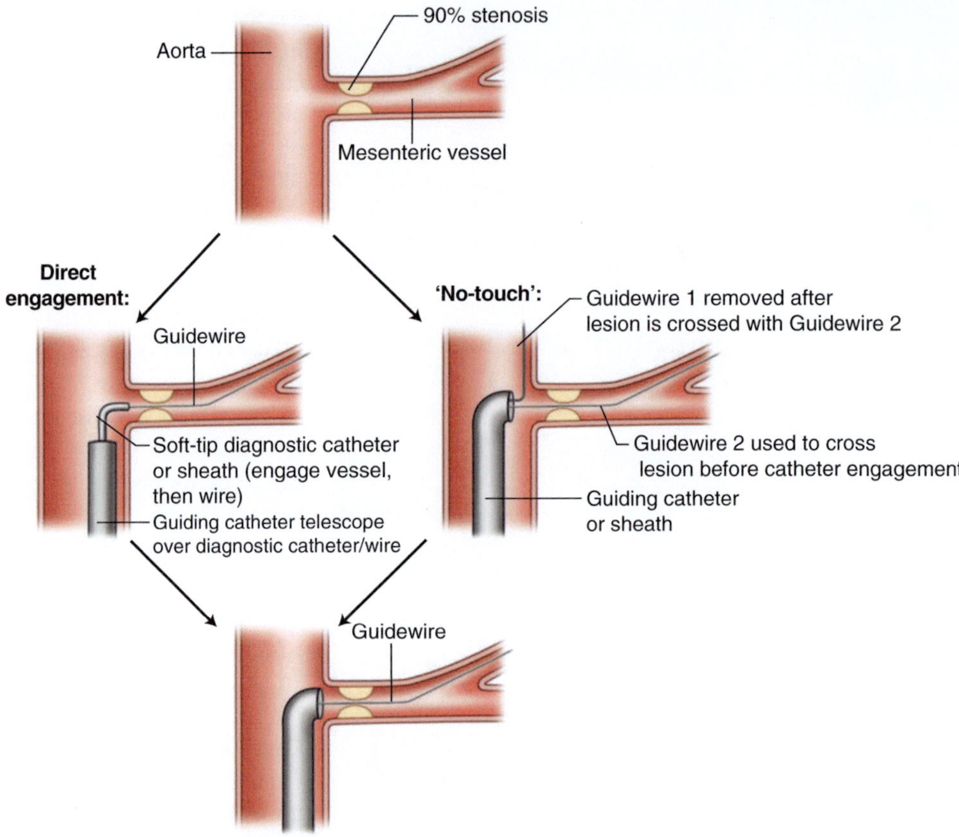

Fig. 33.9 Schematic of "no-touch" and "direct engagement" techniques for engagement of a mesenteric artery

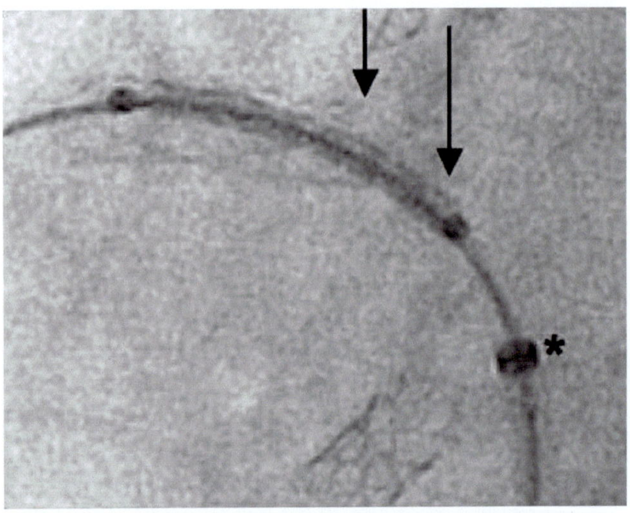

Fig. 33.10 Proximal edge of previously placed stent is at the ostium (*short arrow*). Stent to be placed overhangs ~2 mm into the aorta to adequately cover the ostium (* – catheter tip). This technique thus requires the guiding catheter or sheath to be retracted >2 mm from the ostium, so that the stent is not inadvertently deployed within the guiding catheter/sheath

described for NOMI and occasionally as adjunctive treatment to revascularization for mesenteric arterial or venous occlusive disease causing acute mesenteric ischemia. The primary vasodilator used for this indication is papaverine, though there is some experience with prostaglandin E2 [14, 33, 41, 42].

Papaverine is a phosphodiesterase inhibitor that is rapidly metabolized by the liver and has a half-life of ~1 h [43]. Reported protocols for the administration of papaverine for NOMI involve infusion through a catheter selectively placed in the superior mesenteric artery at a dose of 0.7 mg/kg/h (30–60 mg/h). An abdominal x-ray to confirm the position of the catheter should be performed daily or if hypotension develops. The infusion can be stopped if there is clear clinical improvement, after a repeat angiogram is performed. The duration of papaverine administration has been reported up to 5 days [2, 14, 41, 42]. During the infusion, if peritoneal signs develop, the patient should undergo emergent laparotomy.

Post-procedure

There is little evidence to guide decisions regarding antiplatelet therapy and surveillance imaging following endovascular treatment of mesenteric vessels. In general, many operators prescribe aspirin indefinitely and clopidogrel for 4 weeks. Duplex ultrasonography is often performed at 1 month and 6–12 months thereafter. Unfortunately, no validated duplex criteria are available for in-stent restenosis.

Outcomes

Chronic Mesenteric Ischemia

Though technical success rates reported in contemporary series well exceed 90 %, restenosis rates are higher in the mesentery than other arterial beds [6, 44, 45]. Restenosis rates of 29–40 % have been reported over 1–7 years following stenting of mesenteric arteries. This restenosis rate is marginally inferior to that reported for surgical revascularization; however, stenting is often preferred given the lower morbidity (length of hospital stay and recovery time) and lower reported perioperative mortality (3.7 vs. 15.4 %, $p<0.001$) [6, 46]. These data should be interpreted with caution due to lack of randomization, different definitions of restenosis, lack of duplex criteria for in-stent restenosis, publication bias, and selection bias.

Acute Mesenteric Ischemia

Evidence regarding outcomes for endovascular treatment of acute mesenteric ischemia is limited by small case series and case reports that are subject to publication bias. The largest, single-center study to date from the Cleveland Clinic reported outcomes on 70 consecutive patients undergoing therapy for AMI from 1999 to 2008 [26]. Fifty-six patients underwent primary endovascular treatment, while 24 patients were treated in a traditional manner, receiving laparotomy primarily. Endovascular treatment consisted of rheolytic thrombectomy that was typically followed by fibrinolysis +/− stenting and +/− vasodilator therapy. Thus, the host of endovascular treatment options was tailored to the given clinical situation. Sixty-nine percent of the endovascular group eventually underwent laparotomy. Compared to the traditional therapy group, the patients treated with endovascular therapy had on average shorter length of resected bowel and a lower incidence of acute renal failure and acute pulmonary failure. Mortality was 36 % in the endovascular group and 50 % in the traditional group ($p<0.05$) [26]. This study is encouraging that in contemporary practice, combining endovascular and surgical modalities in a complementary fashion can improve outcomes for patients with acute mesenteric ischemia.

References

1. Aakhus T. The value of angiography in superior mesenteric artery embolism. Br J Radiol. 1966;39(468):928–32.
2. Boley SJ, Sprayregan S, Siegelman SS, Veith FJ. Initial results from an aggressive roentgenological and surgical approach to acute mesenteric ischemia. Surgery. 1977;82(6):848–55.
3. Furrer J, Gruntzig A, Kugelmeier J, Goebel N. Treatment of abdominal angina with percutaneous dilatation of an arteria mesenterica superior stenosis. preliminary communication. Cardiovasc Intervent Radiol. 1980;3(1):43–4.
4. Hirsch AT, Haskal ZJ, Hertzer NR, Bakal CW, Creager MA, Halperin JL, et al. ACC/AHA 2005 guidelines for the management of patients with peripheral arterial disease (lower extremity, renal, mesenteric, and abdominal aortic): Executive summary a collaborative report from the American Association for Vascular Surgery/Society for Vascular Surgery, Society for Cardiovascular Angiography and Interventions, Society for Vascular Medicine and Biology, Society of Interventional Radiology, and the ACC/AHA task force on practice guidelines (writing committee to develop guidelines for the management of patients with peripheral arterial disease) endorsed by the American Association of Cardiovascular and Pulmonary Rehabilitation; National Heart, Lung, and Blood Institute; Society for Vascular Nursing; TransAtlantic Inter-Society Consensus; and Vascular Disease Foundation. J Am Coll Cardiol. 2006;47(6):1239–312.
5. Herbert GS, Steele SR. Acute and chronic mesenteric ischemia. Surg Clin North Am. 2007;87(5):1115–34. ix.
6. Zeller T, Rastan A, Sixt S. Chronic atherosclerotic mesenteric ischemia (CMI). Vasc Med. 2010;15(4):333–8.
7. Sreenarasimhaiah J. Diagnosis and management of intestinal ischaemic disorders. BMJ. 2003;326(7403):1372–6.
8. Brandt LJ, Boley SJ. AGA technical review on intestinal ischemia. american gastrointestinal association. Gastroenterology. 2000;118(5):954–68.
9. Smith JH, Jacobs NL, Ficalora RD. 52-year-old woman with intractable nausea and vomiting. Mayo Clin Proc. 2010;85(3):280–3.
10. Oldenburg WA, Lau LL, Rodenberg TJ, Edmonds HJ, Burger CD. Acute mesenteric ischemia: a clinical review. Arch Intern Med. 2004;164(10):1054–62.
11. Uflacker R, editor. Atlas of vascular anatomy. 2nd ed. Philadelphia: Lippincott Williams & Wilkins; 2007.
12. Paterno F, Longo WE. The etiology and pathogenesis of vascular disorders of the intestine. Radiol Clin North Am. 2008;46(5): 877–85. v.
13. Casserly I, Ravish S, Yadav JS, editors. Manual of peripheral vascular intervention. 1st ed. Philadelphia: Lippincott Williams & Wilkins; 2005.
14. Cronenwett JL, Johnston KW, editors. Rutherford's vascular surgery. 7th ed. Philadelphia: Elsevier; 2010.
15. Moawad J, McKinsey JF, Wyble CW, Bassiouny HS, Schwartz LB, Gewertz BL. Current results of surgical therapy for chronic mesenteric ischemia. Arch Surg. 1997;132(6):613–8. discussion 618–9.
16. Biolato M, Miele L, Gasbarrini G, Grieco A. Abdominal angina. Am J Med Sci. 2009;338(5):389–95.
17. Mohler ER, Gerhard-Herman M, Jaff MR, editors. Essentials of vascular laboratory diagnosis. 1st ed. Malden: Wiley-Blackwell; 2005.
18. Wilson DB, Mostafavi K, Craven TE, Ayerdi J, Edwards MS, Hansen KJ. Clinical course of mesenteric artery stenosis in elderly americans. Arch Intern Med. 2006;166(19):2095–100.
19. Cunningham CG, Reilly LM, Rapp JH, Schneider PA, Stoney RJ. Chronic visceral ischemia. three decades of progress. Ann Surg. 1991;214(3):276–87.
20. Slovut DP, Olin JW. Fibromuscular dysplasia. N Engl J Med. 2004;350(18):1862–71.
21. A-Cienfuegos J, Rotellar F, Valenti V, Arredondo J, Pedano N, Bueno A, et al. The celiac axis compression syndrome (CACS): critical review in the laparoscopic era. Rev Esp Enferm Dig. 2010;102(3):193–201.
22. Ozbulbul NI. CT angiography of the celiac trunk: anatomy, variants and pathologic findings. Diagn Interv Radiol. 2011;17(2):150–7.

23. Soman S, Sudhakar SV, Keshava SN. Celiac axis compression by median arcuate ligament on computed tomography among asymptomatic persons. Indian J Gastroenterol. 2010;29(3):121–3.
24. Roseborough GS. Laparoscopic management of celiac artery compression syndrome. J Vasc Surg. 2009;50(1):124–33.
25. Grace PA, Da Costa M, Qureshi A, Sheehan S, Burke P, Bouchier-Hayes D. An aggressive approach to acute superior mesenteric arterial ischemia. Eur J Vasc Surg. 1993;7(6):731–2.
26. Arthurs ZM, Titus J, Bannazadeh M, Eagleton MJ, Srivastava S, Sarac TP, et al. A comparison of endovascular revascularization with traditional therapy for the treatment of acute mesenteric ischemia. J Vasc Surg. 2011;53(3):698–704. discussion 704–5.
27. Hackworth CA, Leef JA. Percutaneous transluminal mesenteric angioplasty. Surg Clin North Am. 1997;77(2):371–80.
28. Schoots IG, Koffeman GI, Legemate DA, Levi M, van Gulik TM. Systematic review of survival after acute mesenteric ischaemia according to disease aetiology. Br J Surg. 2004;91(1):17–27.
29. Russo MJ, Chaer RA, Lin SC, Kent KC, McKinsey JF. Percutaneous endovascular treatment of acute sequential systemic emboli. J Vasc Surg. 2006;43(2):388–92.
30. Kumar S, Sarr MG, Kamath PS. Mesenteric venous thrombosis. N Engl J Med. 2001;345(23):1683–8.
31. Clark RA, Gallant TE. Acute mesenteric ischemia: angiographic spectrum. AJR Am J Roentgenol. 1984;142(3):555–62.
32. Clark RA, Colley DP, Jacobson ED, Herman R, Tyler G, Stahl D. Superior mesenteric angiography and blood flow measurement following intra-arterial injection of prostaglandin E1. Radiology. 1980;134(2):327–33.
33. Trompeter M, Brazda T, Remy CT, Vestring T, Reimer P. Non-occlusive mesenteric ischemia: etiology, diagnosis, and interventional therapy. Eur Radiol. 2002;12(5):1179–87.
34. Schoots IG, Levi MM, Reekers JA, Lameris JS, van Gulik TM. Thrombolytic therapy for acute superior mesenteric artery occlusion. J Vasc Interv Radiol. 2005;16(3):317–29.
35. Heiss P, Loewenhardt B, Manke C, Hellinger A, Dietl KH, Schlitt HJ, et al. Primary percutaneous aspiration and thrombolysis for the treatment of acute embolic superior mesenteric artery occlusion. Eur Radiol. 2010;20(12):2948–58.
36. Harnik IG, Brandt LJ. Mesenteric venous thrombosis. Vasc Med. 2010;15(5):407–18.
37. Hollingshead M, Burke CT, Mauro MA, Weeks SM, Dixon RG, Jaques PF. Transcatheter thrombolytic therapy for acute mesenteric and portal vein thrombosis. J Vasc Interv Radiol. 2005;16(5):651–61.
38. Rosen MP, Sheiman R. Transhepatic mechanical thrombectomy followed by infusion of TPA into the superior mesenteric artery to treat acute mesenteric vein thrombosis. J Vasc Interv Radiol. 2000;11(2 Pt 1):195–8.
39. Poplausky MR, Kaufman JA, Geller SC, Waltman AC. Mesenteric venous thrombosis treated with urokinase via the superior mesenteric artery. Gastroenterology. 1996;110(5):1633–5.
40. Kawarada O, Sonomura T, Yokoi Y. Direct aspiration using rapid-exchange and low-profile device for acute thrombo-embolic occlusion of the superior mesenteric artery. Catheter Cardiovasc Interv. 2006;68(6):862–6.
41. Klotz S, Vestring T, Rotker J, Schmidt C, Scheld HH, Schmid C. Diagnosis and treatment of nonocclusive mesenteric ischemia after open heart surgery. Ann Thorac Surg. 2001;72(5):1583–6.
42. Niederhauser U, Genoni M, von Segesser LK, Bruhlmann W, Turina MI. Mesenteric ischemia after a cardiac operation: conservative treatment with local vasodilation. Ann Thorac Surg. 1996;61(6):1817–9.
43. Boswell-Smith V, Spina D, Page CP. Phosphodiesterase inhibitors. Br J Pharmacol. 2006;147 Suppl 1:S252–7.
44. Silva JA, White CJ, Collins TJ, Jenkins JS, Andry ME, Reilly JP, et al. Endovascular therapy for chronic mesenteric ischemia. J Am Coll Cardiol. 2006;47(5):944–50.
45. Kasirajan K, O'Hara PJ, Gray BH, Hertzer NR, Clair DG, Greenberg RK, et al. Chronic mesenteric ischemia: open surgery versus percutaneous angioplasty and stenting. J Vasc Surg. 2001;33(1):63–71.
46. Schermerhorn ML, Giles KA, Hamdan AD, Wyers MC, Pomposelli FB. Mesenteric revascularization: management and outcomes in the united states, 1988–2006. J Vasc Surg. 2009;50(2):341.e1–8.e1.

34 Endovascular Management of Aortic Aneurysmal and Stenotic Disease

Giovanni Teruzzi and Antonio L. Bartorelli

From the beginning, the basic idea underlying the development of arterial aneurysm treatment with endoluminal approach was to replace the surgical suture by a different element of fixation of the fabric graft to the arterial wall. Since the introduction of this approach in the early 1990s, the technology has progressed rapidly. The endovascular treatment era started with "home-made" devices, as they were named, and has now improved to third-generation devices that are being manufactured by several medical companies.

The evolution of catheter-based methods stemming from percutaneous transluminal balloon angioplasty (PTA) has made these techniques a viable first-choice option also in the treatment of stenotic disease of the thoracic and abdominal aorta. Based on new devices, improved techniques, and operator skills, a sizable percentage of patients are candidate for treatment with minimally invasive procedures. Improvements in the safety and effectiveness of the endovascular treatment of aneurysmal and stenotic disease of the aorta represent an achievement of which also physicians are responsible and may be justifiably proud.

In the present chapter, we will describe the endovascular treatment of aneurysms located in the abdominal and thoracic aorta. Moreover, endovascular treatment of coarctation of the aorta and abdominal aorta stenosis will also be discussed.

Abdominal Aortic Aneurysm

Indications for Intervention

The main reason to treat asymptomatic patients is to prevent the risk of abdominal aortic aneurysm (AAA) rupture, which brings a high mortality rate. Because mortality in elective AAA repair is dramatically lower than that associated with rupture, the emphasis must be on early detection and elective repair. The risk of rupture is strongly related to AAA size: aneurysms between 5.5 and 5.9 cm in diameter have an annual risk of rupture of 9.4 %, and those between 6 and 6.9 cm have an annual risk of rupture of 10.2 %. The speed of aneurysm growth and the eccentric or saccular shape (which have considerably increased wall stress) are other factors that can influence the rupture risk. ACC/AHA Guidelines for peripheral arterial disease suggest intervention for infrarenal aortic aneurysms larger than 5.5 cm and rapidly expanding aneurysms with lower diameter.

Endovascular Abdominal Aortic Aneurysm Repair

The History

On September 7, 1990, Dr. Juan C. Parodi and his team at the Instituto Cardiovascular de Buenos Aires in Argentina performed the first endovascular AAA repair (EVAR) [1]. The aneurysm was excluded endoluminally with a Dacron graft that was anchored at the proximal infrarenal neck with a stainless steel balloon-expandable stent. The system was assembled by affixing with sutures the fabric tube to an undeployed stent mounted on a large-diameter angioplasty balloon. The system was then sheathed inside a large-bore catheter that served as the delivery system. The access to the aorta for delivery and deployment was obtained through the surgically exposed common femoral artery. This system was the first generation of endografts, the home-made ones, and obtained exclusion and depressurization of the large aneurysm in a patient who had been deemed an unsuitable candidate for standard surgical repair. Two years later, Parodi and Claudio Schonolz performed the first endovascular AAA repair in the United States that ushered in a new era for the interventional vascular practice [2]. Not surprisingly, but unbeknownst to them at the time, they were not alone in these endeavors. The Ukrainian surgeon Nicholas Volodos performed the first endovascular repair of a traumatic

G. Teruzzi, MD • A.L. Bartorelli, MD (✉)
Cardiovascular Section, Department of Clinical Sciences and Community Health, Centro Cardiologico Monzino, University of Milan, Via Carlo Parea 4, Milan 20138, Italy
e-mail: albartorelli@ccfm.it

C.A. Thompson (ed.), *Textbook of Cardiovascular Intervention*, DOI 10.1007/978-1-4471-4528-8_34, © Springer-Verlag London 2014

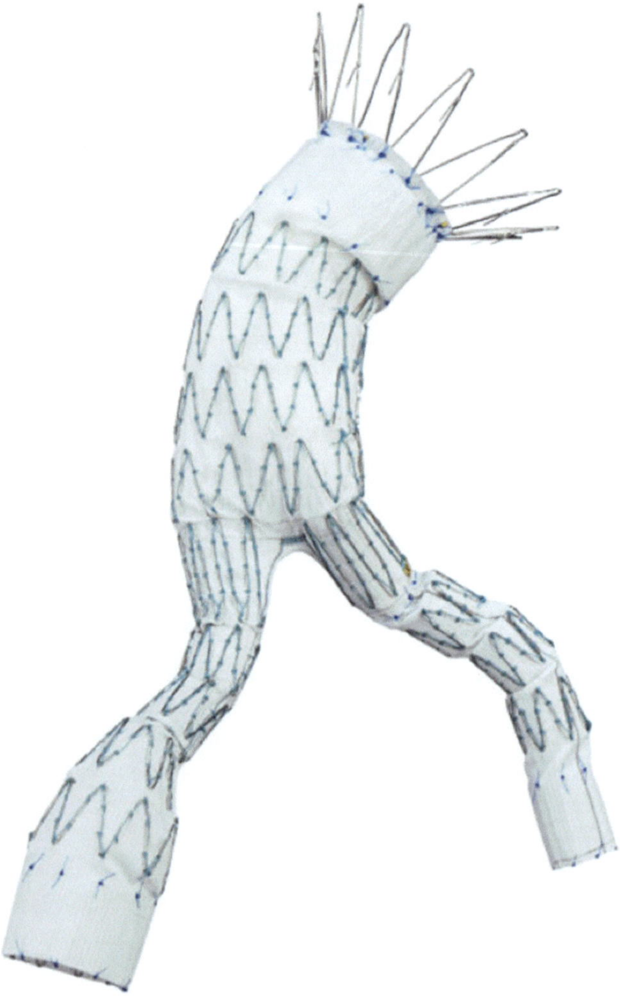

Fig. 34.1 Zenith endovascular stent system (Permission for use granted by William Cook Europe, Bjaeverskov, Denmark)

thoracic aortic aneurysm (TAA) as early as 1986 [3]. These initial experiences were the driving force and stimulus for the truly explosive growth in interest, creativity, and investment that followed. Indeed, subsequent years have seen a tremendous surge in both the number of endovascular AAA repairs performed worldwide, technological improvements in endograft design, and application of the technique to other vascular beds.

EVAR Devices

Zenith Flex Endovascular Graft (Cook Inc., Bloomington, IN)

The Zenith Flex endograft for AAA with the introduction system H&L-B One-Shot is a modular bifurcated stent composed of Z-shaped self-expandable stainless steel exoskeleton, covered with woven polyester (Fig. 34.1). The main body of the endograft includes the aortic portion and is

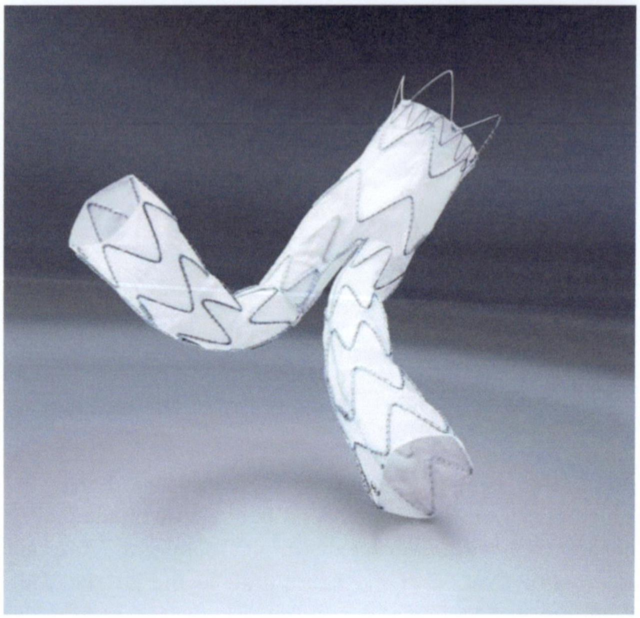

Fig. 34.2 Talent abdominal stent graft (Courtesy of Medtronic Italy Spa, Brescia, Italy)

introduced through the H&L-B One-Shot system. It is provided with a long iliac extremity (ipsilateral) and another short iliac extremity (contralateral), both of which work as a link for the branch extensions. A bare-metal stent is attached to the top of the main body, cephalad to the fabric graft. Multiple steel barbs are welded in a staggered configuration to the bare-metal stent to provide additional aortic fixation.

Talent Abdominal Stent Graft (MedtronicVascular, Santa Rosa, CA)

The device is a self-expanding modular system composed of serpentine-shaped nitinol stents integrated into a woven polyester matrix (Fig. 34.2). The stents are discontinuous and are spaced along a full-length nitinol spine. The latter wire provides columnar strength to a graft that is otherwise flexible enough to accommodate aortoiliac angulations. The spine also prevents twisting and longitudinal infolding of the endograft during deployment. The proximal aortic fixation end has a 1.5-cm uncovered nitinol frame that allows for transrenal fixation of the device. These characteristics may allow increased potential for treating patients with challenging aortic neck configurations [4, 5]. Since its original introduction, the endograft has been modified to include the use of a thinner, low-profile graft fabric to create the Talent Low-Porosity System (LPS). Later, the Talent endograft nitinol springs were chemically treated to enhance durability, and the position of the iliac longitudinal connecting bar was moved from lateral to medial to improve conformability and decrease risk of kinking and thrombosis, resulting in the latest-generation Talent eLPS device. The Talent Abdominal

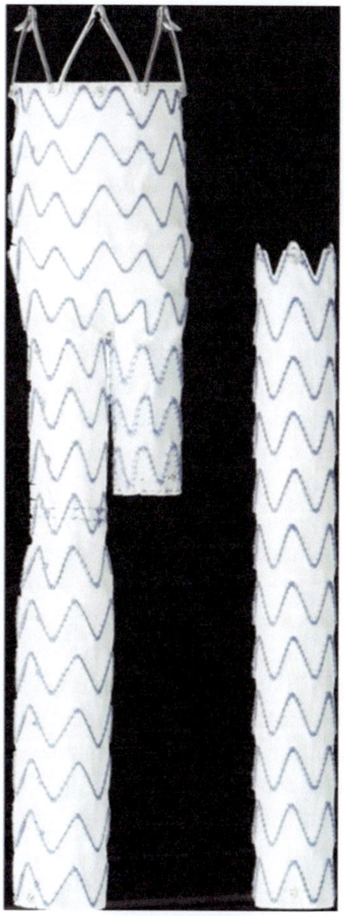

Fig. 34.3 Endurant stent graft (Courtesy of Medtronic Italy Spa, Brescia, Italy)

Stent endograft has a 22F delivery system with a hydrophilic coating which does not require a delivery sheath. A 24F delivery system is required for 30 to 36-mm devices and allows treatment of up to 32-mm neck diameters with a neck length of 10 mm and <60° of angulation.

Endurant Stent Graft (MedtronicVascular, Santa Rosa, CA)

This device features a polyester graft material externally supported by an electropolished nitinol stent structure attached to the graft by sutures (Fig. 34.3). An M-shaped proximal stent with anchoring hooks is designed to fix the endograft above the renal arteries. The hydrophilic, low-profile delivery system for the main body measures between 18F and 20F, while for the iliac extensions, the sizes are 14F and 16F. A tip-capture mechanism allows separate control-release deployment of the suprarenal stent. The Endurant endograft is loaded into a low-profile delivery system, with an outer diameter ranging from 18F to 20F for the main body and from 14F to 16F for the extenders. The delivery system features a tip-capture release mechanism to ensure accurate control of suprarenal stent deployment.

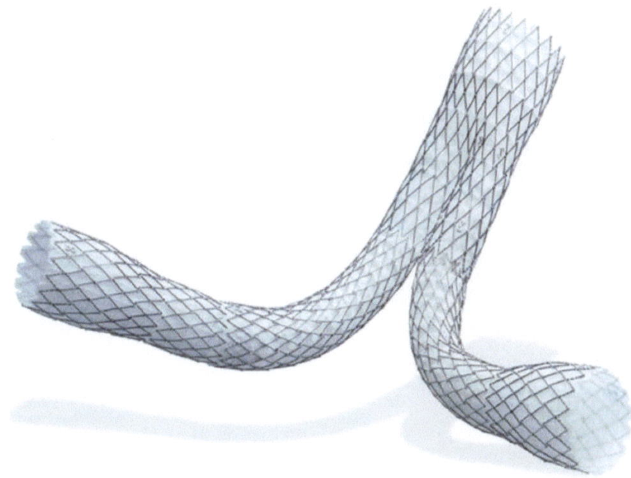

Fig. 34.4 AneuRx abdominal stent graft (Courtesy of Medtronic Italy Spa, Brescia, Italy)

AneuRx Abdominal Stent Graft (MedtronicVascular, Santa Rosa, CA)

This is a modular endograft system that utilizes an exoskeleton of 1-cm self-expanding elements (Fig. 34.4). The self-expanding, thin-wall polyester graft material, supported by diamond-shaped elements, supplies high radial force for reliable and secure sealing without barbs, hooks, or balloons. To date, the AneuRx Abdominal Stent Graft has undergone eight modifications since the original clinical trial. The first-generation device consisted of a stiff-body design with a pre-reduced porosity graft material and a bullet delivery system. In 1998, the endograft flexibility was increased by changing the body of the endograft from a single 5-cm nitinol stent to a series of 1-cm diamond-shaped rings. Furthermore, the graft material was changed to a reduced porosity material. In 2002, the delivery system was changed to the Xpedient Delivery System with a tapered nose cone, allowing the device to be placed without a sheath. In 2004, the graft material was again changed to the Resilient graft material, which was associated with the greatest amount of sac shrinkage as compared to other contemporary graft materials [6]. In 2005, the Xcelerant Delivery System was added, allowing for easier deployment of the endograft. In 2006, the AneuRx AAAdvantage Stent Graft was offered, which added an extended aortic body of 4 cm, contoured stent rings, longer, larger, and flared iliac limbs to decrease the number of components required for repair and enhanced radiopaque markers. Finally, in 2008 a hydrophilic coating was added to the delivery system. Currently, the AneuRx AAAdvantage Stent Graft has a 21F delivery system and may be used to treat up to 26-mm aortic neck diameters that are 15 mm in length with <45° of angulation.

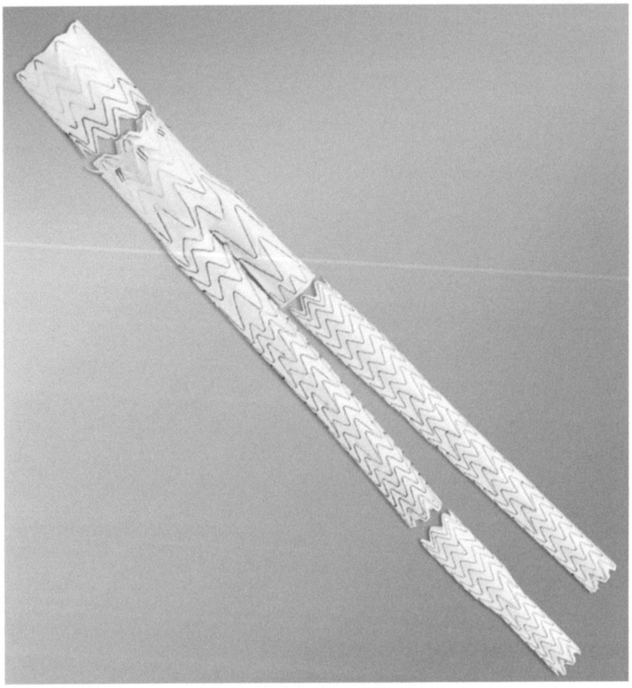

Fig. 34.5 Excluder aortic endograft (Courtesy of W.L. Gore & Associates, Inc., Flagstaff, AZ)

Excluder Aortic Endograft (W.L. Gore & Associates, Flagstaff, AZ)

This device is a modular system covered with expanded polytetrafluoroethylene (ePTFE) and supported by a nitinol stent frame (Fig. 34.5). The endograft material is bonded to the nitinol frame and thus has no suture holes in the material. The microstructure in the original device permitted selective permeability of serous fluid in a subset of patients that could be associated with endotension [7, 8], but with the addition of a non-permeable, very thin, and highly durable fluoropolymer layer, this drawback was overcome [9, 10]. The endograft consists of a bifurcated main body with a single docking limb and assorted iliac limbs. Iliac and proximal extenders are also available. The main proximal portion of the main body has a scalloped end that is entirely covered with paired nitinol anchors for fixation set at 45°. There is no mechanism for suprarenal fixation. The proximal edge is identifiable by three gold markers designed to be placed immediately below the most inferior renal artery. The main body of the device is contained in an ePTFE jacket that is stitched with a single strand of ePTFE string. This is the mechanism for deployment: the string is pulled and the stitches are released, causing endograft deployment (proximal to distal). Rotational orientation is facilitated by different length markers on the ipsilateral and contralateral endograft sides. In the new C3 Delivery System, deployment is now a three-step maneuver, including the option of re-constraining and repositioning the device. If the position is believed to be too high or too low with regard to the renal arteries, the device can be easily adjusted to reach the ideal final location. Similarly, reorientation of the contralateral gate is possible, which makes cannulation easier and less time consuming. Currently, introducer sheaths are available in 30-cm length as 12F, 18F, and 20F sheaths. Main trunks with ipsilateral leg are available in 23-mm, 26-mm, and 28.5-mm diameters with 12-mm and 14.5-mm iliac diameters. The endoprosthetic length ranges from 12 to 18 cm in 2-cm increments. The recommended aortic neck diameter ranges from 19 to 28 mm. The ipsilateral iliac treatment diameter ranges from 10 to 13.5 mm. All these devices can be delivered via the 18F sheath except for the 31-mm endograft, which requires the 20F sheath. The contralateral endograft ranges from 12 to 20 mm in 2-mm increments and is available in 9.5-cm, 10-cm, 11.5-cm, 12-cm, 13.5-cm, and 14-cm length increments. The larger diameter contralateral leg endograft (16, 18, and 20 mm) can also be used as iliac extenders. The Excluder device contains flared iliac extenders to attach to aneurysmal iliac vessels. Dedicated iliac extenders range from 10 to 14.5 mm and are available in 7-cm length increments. The recommended iliac treatment diameters range from 8 to 18.5 mm. All may be delivered via the 12F sheath except for the 16-mm to 20-mm endograft, which requires an 18F sheath. Aortic extenders range 23, 26, and 28.5 mm and are available in 3.3-cm length increments. Their recommended aortic neck diameter is 19 to 26 mm in the United States, and a range of 19 to 29 mm has been used outside the United States.

Anaconda AAA Stent Graft System (Vascutek, Scotland, UK)

The system is tri-modulare and is composed of a bifurcated body to which the ipsilateral and contralateral branch may engage (Fig. 34.6). A wide range of bodies and bifurcated iliac branches allows to treat patients with an aortic neck from 17.5 to 31 mm and iliac arteries from 8.5 to 21 mm. The tri-modulare system allows adapting the stent to the size and characteristic anatomy of each patient. The flexibility of the body is allowed by the fact that distally to the two rings of nitinol for the proximal anchorage, the prosthesis is supported by two other very flexible rings, which, while supporting the bifurcated body, will not impair flexibility. The end of the contralateral side has a thin support of nitinol and radiopaque markers to ensure an open and visible lumen during the procedure of cannulation. The iliac branches, straight and/or flared, are equipped with support rings and radiopaque markers for the correct positioning inside the main body. The rings of support are varied but independent of one another so as to ensure an excellent flexibility to the iliac branches and prevent kinking. The iliac branches can be used to treat isolated aneurysmal iliac arteries. The flexibility characterizes also the introduction and release system that

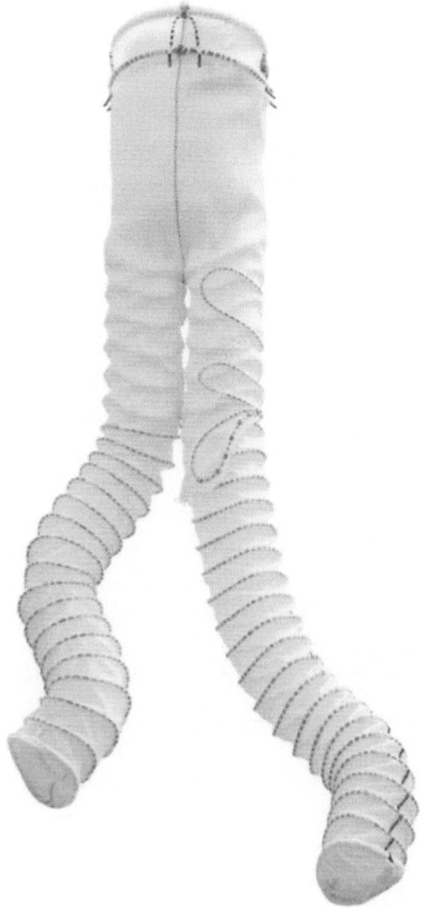

Fig. 34.6 Anaconda AAA stent graft system (Courtesy of Vascutek Ltd., Renfrewshire, Scotland)

allows placing the stent in vessels anatomically very tortuous. The proximal part of the aortic bifurcated body has two rings of nitinol supported by four pairs of hooks that ensure safe anchorage of the device.

AFX Endovascular AAA System (Endologix, Irvine, CA)

This Endovascular AAA System integrates anatomical fixation with an advanced delivery system and graft material technology (Fig. 34.7).

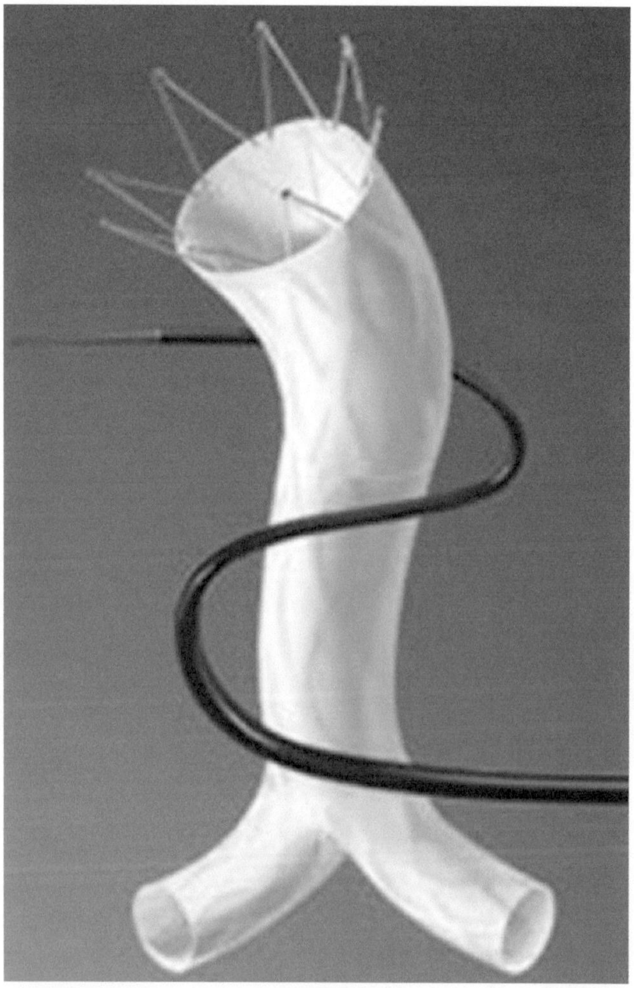

Fig. 34.7 AFX endovascular AAA system (Courtesy of Endologix, Inc., Irvine, CA)

Incraft Stent Graft System (Cordis Corporation, Florida, USA)

This new system was designed so that a few sizes will fit most vessels with respect to both diameters and length (Fig. 34.8). The modular components can be tailored during the implant procedure, with "in situ length adjustment" of the limb prostheses. This permits up to 2–3 cm of variability that can be achieved by varying the modular overlap length on each side reducing the risk of inadvertent coverage of the hypogastric orifice and, at the same time, allowing the maximum length of iliac fixation for migration prevention. The endograft design provides appropriate radial force over a relatively large range of diameters, so that four sizes can be used for aortic diameters ranging from 17 to 31 mm. Similarly, five different iliac limb diameters will accommodate iliac arteries ranging from 7 to 22 mm in size. Each iliac limb is supplied in four distinct lengths ranging from 8 to 14 cm, allowing a total aortoiliac coverage length between 13 and 21 cm. Therefore, a combination of 23 different modular components allows the operator to customize the device to the wide variety of AAA anatomy, with a significant reduction in the complexity of device selection, which is so critical in emergency settings. The Incraft device has a flared bare transrenal stent with 8–10 laser-cut barbs (size depending) located on the most cranial part of the stent for suprarenal fixation. The transrenal stent, the short segmented sealing infrarenal endoskeleton stent and the non-tilting deployment mechanism maximize the proximal seal, especially in the presence of a challenging aortic neck. The endograft is constructed of a seamless, woven polyester material supported

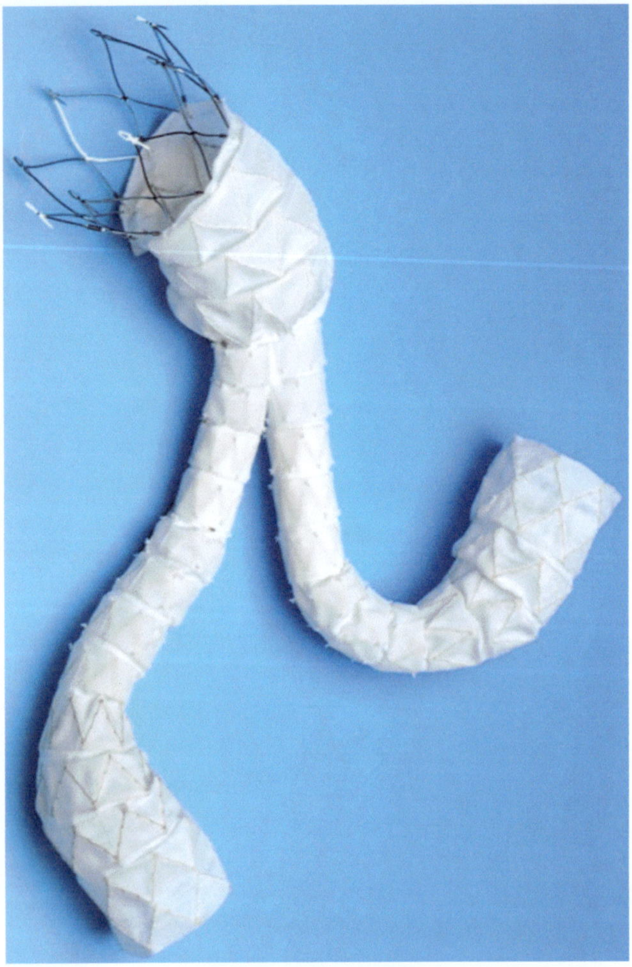

Fig. 34.8 Incraft stent graft system (Courtesy of Cordis Corp., Hialeah, FL)

by a series of laser-cut nitinol stents throughout its entire length. Such a design was chosen for kinking prevention, which has been associated with limb thrombosis. The Incraft stents are attached to the graft with a unique suture scheme to minimize micromotion between the stent and graft component, a mechanism believed to have a negative impact on endograft integrity with prior devices. Finally, one of the most innovative features of the device is the ultra-low profile: the integrated delivery system is 13F with a 14F (4.7 mm) outer diameter. The "catheter-like" flexibility and the elimination of sheath exchange minimize delivery problems, particularly in patients with small, diseased, and otherwise challenging access anatomy.

Selection Criteria for EVAR

General accepted guidelines for EVAR include at least 10–15 mm of non-aneurysmal proximal neck, proximal neck diameter less than 30 mm, adequate access vessels (femoral/iliac arteries) at least 7 mm in diameter, minimal vessel calcification and thrombus, and a neck–body aneurysm angle ≤60°. The 2005 Excluder instructions for use recommend the following selection criteria: adequate iliac/femoral access, infrarenal aortic neck diameter ranging from 19 to 26 mm, minimum aortic neck length of 15 mm, proximal aortic neck angulation ≤60°, iliac artery treatment diameter ranging from 8 to 18.5 mm, and iliac distal vessel seal zone of at least 10 mm. Device delivery may be hindered by excessive tortuosity, calcification, or occlusive disease of femoral or iliac arteries. Additional considerations relate to the adequacy of collateral flow for occluded branches, such as an indispensable inferior mesenteric artery or accessory renal artery. The most common obstacle for EVAR is inadequate proximal anatomy. Self-expanding stents may be used more frequently to treat AAA with neck dilatation compared with balloon-expandable stents. An analysis comparing Excluder and the balloon-expandable Lifepath found this factor to be correlated with a higher rate of device migration seen in the Excluder device in this series [11]. A review from the EUROSTAR database analyzed 1,152 patients treated with EVAR having severe neck angulation (>60°) with Excluder, Talent, or Zenith endografts [12]. All three had acceptable outcomes in patients with severe neck angulation, with the Excluder and Zenith having increased risk for short-term type I endoleak and device migration and the Talent device having increased long-term risk of type I endoleak and secondary intervention. Favorable anatomic criteria allow use of any of the current commercially available endografts for EVAR. However, it has become apparent that certain features of proximal neck diameter, length, and angulation, or iliac anatomy characteristics favor some devices over another. The low-profile delivery is one such example. Also, the scalloped proximal edge makes precision delivery possible for tight proximal anatomy. A unique characteristic of the Excluder is its rapid deployment mechanism. This rapid deployment of a self-expanding device with proximal fixation in the setting of tortuosity and path rotation may lead to unexpected shortening and a more distal position than expected in inexperienced hands. Potential consequences of unexpected distal migration could include inadvertent hypogastric artery occlusion. Whittaker et al. found that this event occurred in 11 % of limbs studied with a shortening of graft path 1 cm or more [13]. Moreover, they noted that graft path shortening was affected more by anatomic factors than by Excluder device factors. Graft rotation was the most difficult pattern to predict preoperatively. Most patients will be assessed with three-dimensional reconstruction of multi-detector CT angiography (MDCTA). This has replaced previous modalities such as "road-map" angiogram or marker catheter as the best method for preintervention planning. Features such as tortuosity and rotation require special consideration in preoperative planning. Whittaker et al. reported that three-dimensional computer-aided measurement, planning, and simulation software was very accurate for preoperative planning with the Excluder device and more accurate than using marker catheter angiography [14]. Availability of several commercial devices with different properties with regard to proximal fixation, deployment accuracy, endograft flexibility, and size of introduction system enables to tailor the device selection according to each patient's AAA anatomy. Zenith endografts were mainly used for short proximal necks in view of the suprarenal fixation of the bare stent with hooks and barbs. In addition, in view of the versatility of the Zenith Tri-Fab system in which the length of both limbs can be chosen after insertion of the main body, the endograft may be appropriate also in aneurysms where accurate length measurement proves difficult (e.g., angulation or short common iliac arteries). This feature is shared also by the Incraft Stent Graft System. The Talent endografts were initially used for proximal necks with a large diameter, but this advantage was lost when the Zenith equally featured larger proximal diameter sizes. Excluder endografts were preferred in patients with narrow and angulated iliac arteries because of flexible and thinner wall limbs. In July 2004, the Excluder underwent an important modification with the introduction of a lower porosity graft material. The Talent prosthesis was recently replaced by Medtronic with the Endurant. This new prosthesis, always with suprarenal attachment, has greater flexibility and conformability in the aortic vessel and requires thinner, dedicated introducers.

EVAR Procedure

The deployment technique for a two-piece modular device involves passage through one femoral artery of a sheath containing a body and the ipsilateral iliac limb. The superior end of the body is positioned just below the lowermost renal artery. The contralateral iliac limb is inserted through the opposite femoral artery and is overlapped with a short stump in the body of the device. The end result is a percutaneous Y-graft, with some important differences as compared to surgical grafts: the attachment sites in the infrarenal aortic neck, iliac arteries, and within the endograft are not sutured, and the aortic side branches are not ligated. Since the attachment sites are not hand sutured, they rely on the radial force of the stents to provide a hemostatic seal. Fixation at the attachment sites is also important to prevent endograft migration. Some manufacturers achieve this by adding hooks or barbs on the infrarenal stent. Some devices incorporate a bare suprarenal stent with or without hooks. This suprarenal stent may extend as high as the superior mesenteric artery.

Access-Related Issues

EVAR requires adequate vessel size in order to place the device and to exclude the aneurysm. Indeed, small external iliac arteries, vessel tortuosity, and heavily calcified vessels with aortoiliac occlusive disease make EVAR more difficult. For each of the currently available devices, the external iliac and common iliac arteries need a minimum diameter of 7 mm for the main device. Certain anatomical conditions will make access more difficult, but certain technical maneuvers can overcome these conditions.

Femoral Artery Access

Standard femoral artery access is achieved via a transverse or longitudinal incision. Use of small transverse incisions just below the inguinal ligament may be beneficial during EVAR. With this exposure, dissection just below the inguinal ligament gains access to the common femoral artery, typically in a relatively soft area of the artery. Furthermore, the femoral bifurcation is avoided, making control of the femoral artery easier and avoiding dissection of the profunda and superficial femoral arteries. When using this approach even in patients with heavily calcified vessels, it is usually possible to find a soft spot on the anterior wall of the femoral artery just distal to the inguinal ligament that can be used to puncture the artery. If the vessel is still heavily calcified, the inguinal ligament can be divided to allow access to the very distal external iliac artery. Once the femoral artery is dissected out, proximal and distal control of the vessel is obtained with vessel loops. Wire access is then obtained using the standard Seldinger technique. There is growing experience with a truly percutaneous approach using a technique, often referred to as the *"pre-close technique."* With this technique, sutures are percutaneously placed before the insertion of the sheath and are used to close the femoral entry site at the end of the procedure. Using ultrasound guidance to confirm access to the common femoral artery, the artery is accessed and a 7F sheath is placed. A femoral arteriography is performed to confirm the sheath is within the common femoral artery. The 7F sheath is removed, and either a single 10F Prostar (Abbott Vascular, Santa Clara, CA) or two 6F ProGlides (Abbott Vascular, Santa Clara, CA), the second 45°–90° to the first, can be advanced over the guidewire with the sutures deployed within the vessel wall. Once the sutures are deployed, guidewire access is regained through the rapid-exchange port of the device. The suture device is then removed, and either an 11F or 16F sheath can be placed for hemostasis. This technique can be used with any of the currently available devices. When first learning this technique, it is best to avoid small, calcified vessels, as well as extremely tortuous vessels. A fully percutaneous procedure presents some advantages: less bleeding, reduced risk of femoral nerve injury, faster recovery, and, in most cases, earlier ambulation.

Aortic Angiogram

After femoral access is achieved, a marker pigtail angiography catheter is inserted into the sheath and advanced over a J-tipped guidewire up to the suprarenal aorta under fluoroscopic control. The guidewire is removed, and an aortogram is obtained with a pressure injector and recorded on the fluoroscopy screen with road-mapping technology. Aortic angiography with the marker catheter, which has radiopaque markers at 1-cm intervals, allows accurate measurement of the distance between the point of proposed placement of the proximal attachment system (below the lowest renal artery) and that of the distal attachment system (above the ipsilateral hypogastric artery). This serves to confirm preoperative MDCTA measurements and to assure that the appropriate endograft length had been selected.

Endograft Positioning and Deployment

Once guidewire access is obtained, before placing any large sheath or device, it is best to have a stiffer guidewire in place for the sheath and device to track. Stiff guidewire that are available to straighten out the vessels include the Amplatz Super Stiff (Cook Medical, Bloomington, IN), the Meier Wire (Boston Scientific Corporation, Natick, MA), and the Lunderquist (Cook Medical, Bloomington, IN). In vessels with extreme tortuosity and calcification, even advancing a stiff guidewire through a catheter can be difficult, with the stiff guidewire not advancing and the catheter coming back. This can sometimes be overcome with the use of a "buddy guidewire." Initially, if a stiff guidewire does not pass through a catheter, a stiff Glidewire (Terumo Interventional Systems, Somerset, NJ) can be passed though the catheter, which will usually track easily. Leaving the stiff Glidewire within the catheter, a second guidewire – typically a Glidewire – can be placed within the sheath and into the descending thoracic aorta. A catheter is then advanced over the Glidewire. With the stiff Glidewire and catheter already in place, a stiffer guidewire, such as an Amplatz Super Stiff or a Lunderquist guidewire, can be advanced through the second catheter to straighten out the external iliac artery for placement of the device. Gradually increasing the size of small vessels bypassing dilators can be an adjunctive maneuver besides using a stiff guidewire for device placement. In some patients with severely diseased external iliac arteries or iliofemoral vessels of inadequate size, a conduit end-to-end sutured to the common iliac artery can be used to obtain adequate access for placement of the endograft. A 10-mm Dacron graft allows for passage of all devices. This can be extremely beneficial in preventing damage and/or rupture of the external iliac artery. Once the endograft sheath is introduced over the stiff guidewire and advanced under fluoroscopic control up the iliac segment and well into the aneurysm, the patients receive 5,000 IU intravenous heparin. With the guidewire left in place, the angiography catheter is removed, and the endovascular deployment assembly (trunk-ipsilateral component) is prepared for insertion into the sheath. The assembly is loaded over the guidewire and advanced under fluoroscopic control up the introducer sheath to the aortic position. The introducer sheath, initially advanced into the aorta, is backed into the external iliac artery, which permits the endovascular prosthesis portion of the assembly to be positioned within the aneurysm. The proximal attachment system is positioned just below the renal arteries, the distal attachment system is positioned in the common iliac artery, and the trunk-ipsilateral component of the endograft is deployed. In order to maximize and improve proximal fixation, there are some maneuvers that can be used. The first of these is magnification views and appropriate angulation of the fluoroscopy unit. Typically, adjustment of the image intensifier in the caudal direction will open up the infrarenal neck and show its true length. Typically, the infrarenal aortic neck begins to angle anteriorly following the course of the lumbar spine. Adjusting the image intensifier 10° to 20° is usually sufficient to open up the proximal neck. After guidewire cannulation of the contralateral "gate," the contralateral leg of the endograft is then inserted in the opposite common femoral artery and advanced until overlap is obtained on the short contralateral leg of the aortic endograft placed in the abdominal aorta. An elastomeric balloon is then used to secure the endograft to the proximal aortic neck. This step is usually performed during cardiac pacing at high frequency to reduce blood pressure and to avoid that the displacing forces of the high aortic flow may push the inflated balloon causing downward migration of the endograft from its position. New balloons, such as the Tri-Lobe (Fig. 34.9), allow blood flow through the device itself and do not require temporary pacing. A pigtail angiography catheter is then reinserted over the guidewire into the suprarenal aorta, and a completion angiogram is obtained. Technical success is achieved when there has been successful access to the arterial system using a remote site, successful deployment of the endograft with secure proximal and distal fixation, absence of either a type I or type III endoleak (see complications), and a patent endograft without significant twist, kinks, or obstruction by intraoperative measurements [13–15]. The sheath and guidewire are removed, and the access site is sutured or hemostasis is obtained with the pre-close technique.

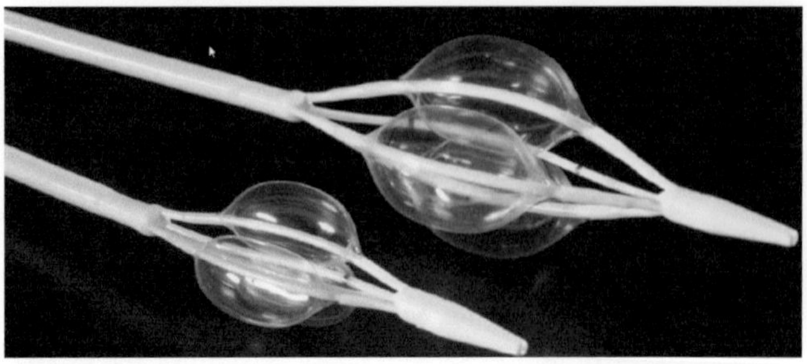

Fig. 34.9 GORE tri-lobe balloon catheter (Courtesy of W.L. Gore & Associates, Inc., Flagstaff, AZ)

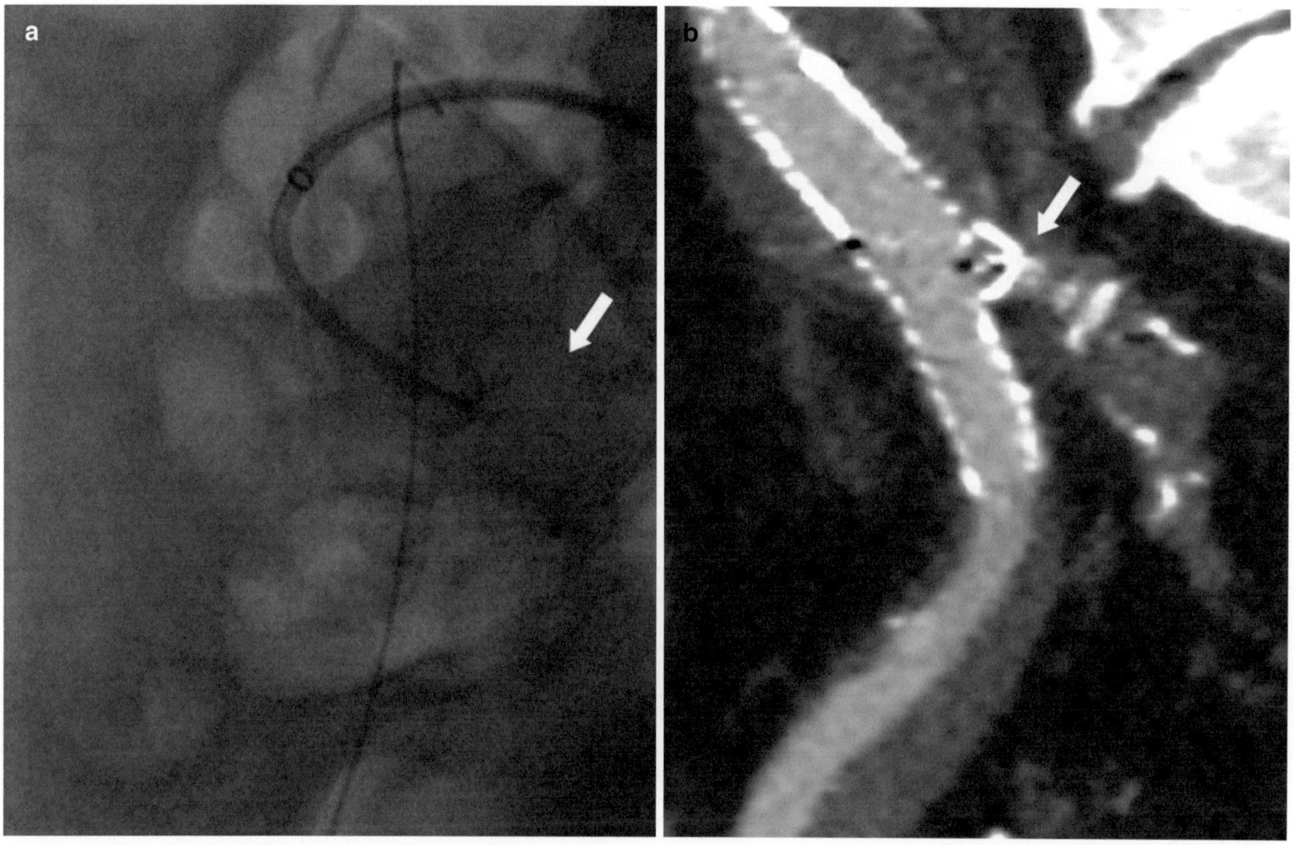

Fig. 34.10 Embolization of the hypogastric artery before EVAR. (**a**) Deployment of an Amplatzer vascular plug (*arrow*) in the right hypogastric artery. (**b**) MDCTA (multiplanar reconstruction) showing final result after EVAR. Note the deployed Amplatzer vascular plug (*arrow*) with complete occlusion of the right hypogastric artery and the endograft leg that was brought into the external iliac artery

Vascular Anatomy Issues

Proximal Aortic Neck

It has been demonstrated that placing the endograft as close to the renal arteries as possible at the original implantation significantly decreases the risk of migration. There are certainly some conditions that are going to increase the risk of migration or proximal type I endoleaks. These risks include a short angled neck as well as a reverse funnel neck. Currently, all devices are approved for use with a proximal neck length of 15 mm except the Talent abdominal endograft, which is approved for use with a 10-mm neck. The technique and precision of device implantation, along with patient selection are significant factors in predisposing patients to subsequent adverse events in the future, especially migration. Migration has been reported with all devices with an incidence between 2.3 and 9.5 % in clinical trials with a follow-up of 1–4 years [16–19]. When evaluating device-specific outcomes, Ouriel et al. found no significant difference among various devices regarding the risk of migration, which ranged from 0 % with the Talent and Ancure to 8.2 % with the Zenith [18]. In a more recent study, Abbruzzese et al. evaluated 177 Zenith, 111 Excluder, and 277 AneuRx endografts [19]. In the study, 39.3 % of devices were placed outside of at least one of the instruction for use parameters. Mean follow-up was 30 ± 21 months and was significantly shorter for the Zenith (20 months) compared to the Excluder (35 months) and AneuRx (31 months), respectively. Overall actuarial 5-year freedom from aneurysm-related death, reintervention, and graft-related event rates were similar among the three devices.

Iliac Artery Aneurysms

In patients with aortoiliac aneurysms, there are three options available to the implanting physician. For ectatic iliac vessels, use of flared limbs has simplified the repair of aneurysms with large common iliac arteries. Flared limbs as large as 24 mm allow vessels up to 20–22 mm to be safely treated without the need of coil embolization of the internal iliac artery. This is possible with both the AneuRx AAAdvantage and Talent abdominal endografts. However, when using these flared limbs, it is still important to try to achieve between 20 and 25 mm of seal to prevent a retrograde type I endoleak. With aneurysmal common iliac arteries, it is usually safer to occlude the hypogastric artery by coil embolization or vascular plug deployment and bring the endograft into the external iliac artery (Fig. 34.10).

Complications Following EVAR

Migration

As the attachment sites are not sutured, there may be movements at the aortic or iliac attachments or at points of connection within modular endografts. Device migration is defined as any report of postprocedure device movement. These migrations include reports of migrations of the trunk-ipsilateral, contralateral leg, and extender components. It is well known that preprocedure planning, which includes appropriate patient anatomical measurements and device selection, will minimize migration events. Even when placing the device as close to the renal arteries as possible during initial deployment, there is continued risk of migration, especially if there is a short aortic neck, significant neck disease, including thrombus and calcification, neck angulation, and adverse neck contour, such as a reverse funnel neck [18–21]. However, it is important to remember that endograft relies on three points of fixation, including the proximal aortic neck and the right and left common iliac arteries. In vivo animal studies have shown that by maximizing the distal iliac fixation, the amount of force required to displace the endograft is increased by 67 %. This has been demonstrated with both infrarenal and suprarenal devices with no significant improvement when hooks were present [22–25].

Endoleaks

The term endoleak was first used in 1996 and defines the persistent perfusion of the aneurysm sac after EVAR due to incomplete sealing. The presence of an endoleak implies failure to exclude the aneurysm or a vessel segment. A leak can appear during the first 30 days after implantation. This type of leak is called "primary endoleak." "Secondary endoleak" is one that occurs after 30 days. Persistent blood flow within the aneurysm sac eventually may result in aneurysm rupture despite endovascular repair. Review of EUROSTAR data suggested that the presence of an endoleak can predict rupture, since 69 % of patients whose aneurysm ruptured following EVAR had a preexisting endoleak [26]. The incidence of endoleak varies from 10 to 50 %, and its treatment depends on the type, site, and size of the endoleak.

Endoleak Classification

The anatomic classification of endoleaks is based upon the source of the inflow into the aneurysm sac, regardless of the number and type of other vessels involved in the outflow. The initial definition differentiated between four types of endoleak, but it was expanded in 1999 to include endotension (type V) (Table 34.1).

Table 34.1 Endoleak classification

Types	Mechanism
I	Flow originates from ineffective endograft seal at fixation zones
A	Proximal
B	Distal
C	Iliac occluded
II	Branch vessel retrograde flow
A	Single vessel (simple)
B	Two or more vessels creating a circuit (complex)
III	Flow results from structural endograft failure
A	Junctional separation (modular devices)
B	Endograft fracture or holes – Minor (<2 mm) – Major (≥2 mm)
IV	Endograft fabric porosity (<30 days after endograft implantation)
V	Endotension

Type I

These endoleaks are caused by failure of the circumferential seal at the fixation points of either the proximal (type IA) or distal (type IB) end of the endograft. Type IC endoleak is due to non-occluded iliac artery in patients with aorto-mono-iliac grafts and fem–fem bypass. With type I endoleaks, the aneurysm is perfused directly from the aorta or iliac arteries (inflows). These leaks usually communicate through a channel (sometimes multiple channels) with the aneurysm sac. There are several outflow vessels, mainly lumbar arteries and inferior mesenteric artery that communicate with the channel and or the sac. The pressure within a type I leak is systemic. The tension on the aortic wall remains high. Causes of primary type I endoleaks include inappropriate anatomy, such as a significantly angulated neck, severe calcification/plaque at the proximal or distal landing zones, a noncircular landing zone, endograft malpositioning and under-dilation, and endograft type. Secondary type I endoleaks can be due to aneurysm remodeling, resulting in endograft migration, progressive dilatation of the proximal neck, design and dimensions of endograft, or unfavorable infrarenal necks, including the conically shaped neck and neck shorter than 15 mm. Treatment is mandatory because the aneurysm sac is at systemic pressure. Untreated type I endoleaks are at high risk of aneurysm rupture. Indeed, a rupture rate of 3.37 % has been reported [27]. Treatment requires satisfactory circumferential apposition between the endoluminal surface of the vessel and the external aspect of the endograft. Gentle expansion of the device with a compliant "molding" balloon will seal the majority of primary type I leaks. Occasionally, despite prolonged molding, the leak will persist. A giant Palmaz stent may then be used to prevent recoil and improve stent apposition to the proximal neck. If this procedure fails and the leak is significant, a limited laparotomy will enable an external band to be placed around the proximal neck, without opening

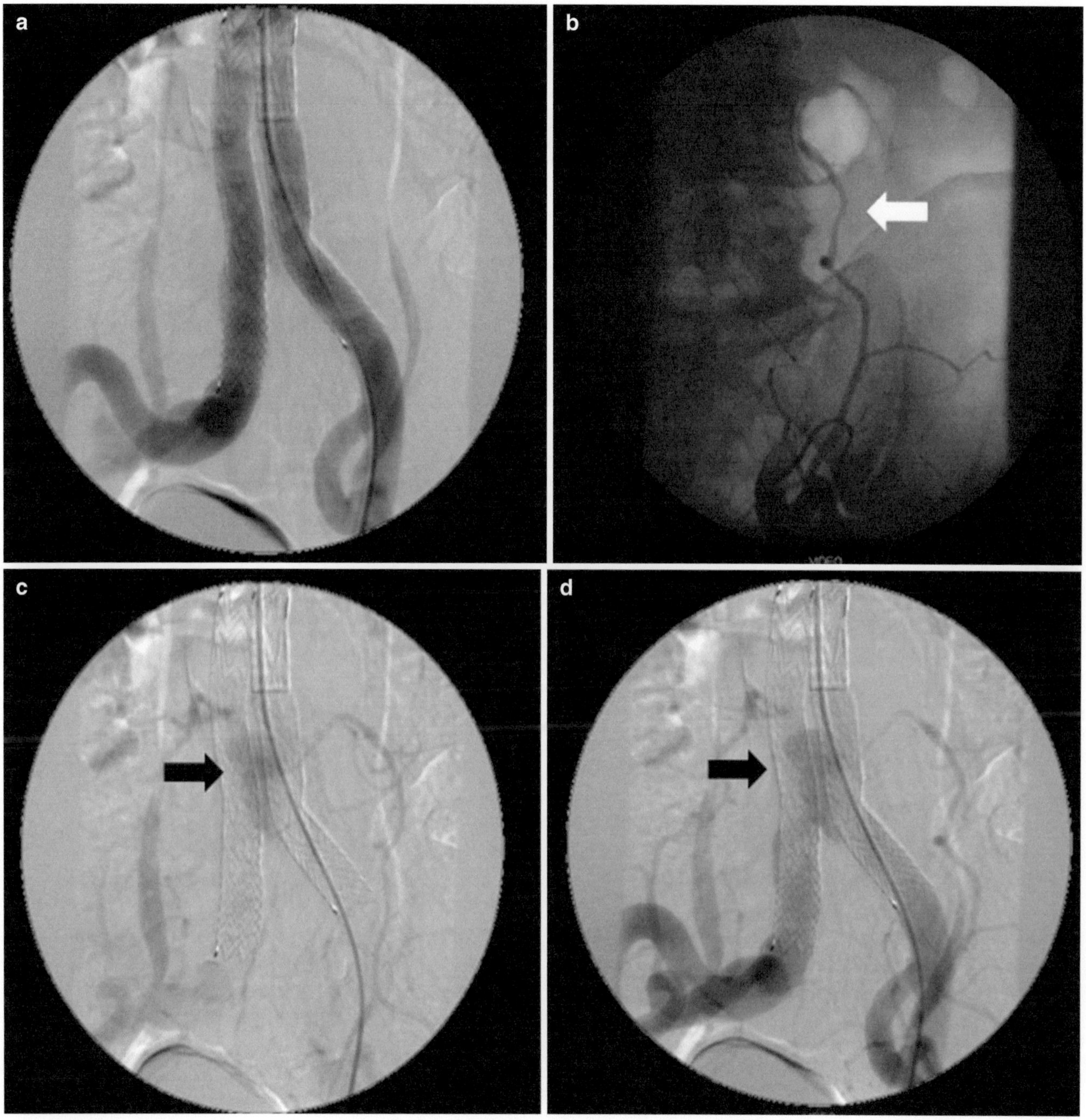

Fig. 34.11 Follow-up angiography after EVAR in a patient with type II endoleak. (**a**) Early-phase subtraction angiography showing patency and correct position of the endograft. (**b**) Selective angiography of the feeding collateral vessel (*arrow*) originating from the external left iliac artery. (**c–d**) Late-phase subtraction angiography showing the endoleak (*arrows*)

the aneurysm sac. Open conversion is occasionally required and was more frequent in the past for very large endoleaks due to the migration of home-made devices. If the endoleak is due to endograft malposition or moderate distal migration, the endograft is extended to increase the length of neck contact or the distal seal in the case of a leaking limb. Hence, a proximal aortic cuff or a graft extension limb may be required, and these are generally oversized by 10–20 % to prevent further endoleaks.

Type II

This type of endoleaks corresponds to the retrograde filling of the aneurysm, mainly from lumbar arteries and/or inferior mesenteric artery but also, in rare situations, from sacral, gonadal, accessory renal artery arteries, or iliac artery branches (Fig. 34.11). The leak always communicates with another "outflow" vessel. These are the commonest endoleaks, affecting up to 43 % of cases, and may be associated with aneurysm expansion and rupture. However, this risk is much less than with the

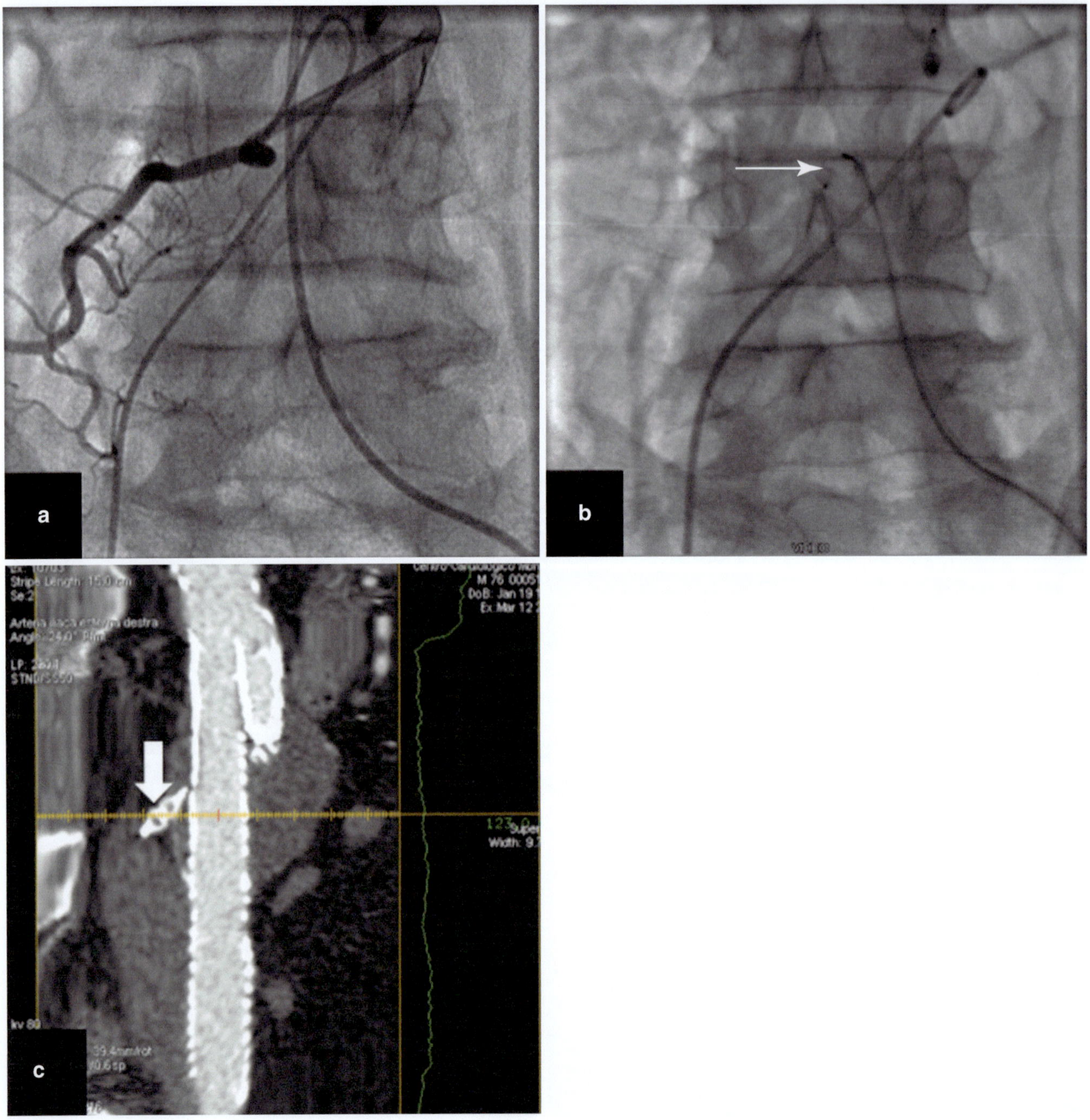

Fig. 34.12 Embolization of a large lumbar artery (**a**) selective angiography before EVAR. (**b**) Amplatzer vascular plug deployment (*arrow*). (**c**) MDCTA (multiplanar reconstruction) showing final result after EVAR. Note the deployed Amplatzer vascular plug (*arrow*) with complete occlusion of the lumbar artery

type I and III endoleaks (0.5 % vs. 3.4 %) [26, 28]. Of note, they are associated with a significant rate (up to 40 %) of spontaneous closure. The current consensus is that a type II endoleak in the setting of a shrinking aneurysm can generally be followed without the need of immediate intervention. Treatment is required only for endoleaks that persist for more than a year in an aneurysm of increasing size. Intervention is usually by percutaneous embolization, either by a transarterial or a translumbar route. Percutaneous CT-guided or ultrasound-guided thrombin injection in appropriate patients can be a useful treatment option and should be considered when the more conventional methods are difficult [29, 30]. In some instances, coil or plug embolization of feeding vessels before endograft deployment is a viable option for type II endoleak prevention [31] (Fig. 34.12).

Type III

These endoleaks are caused by structural failure of the endograft due to separation of its modular components (type IIIA)

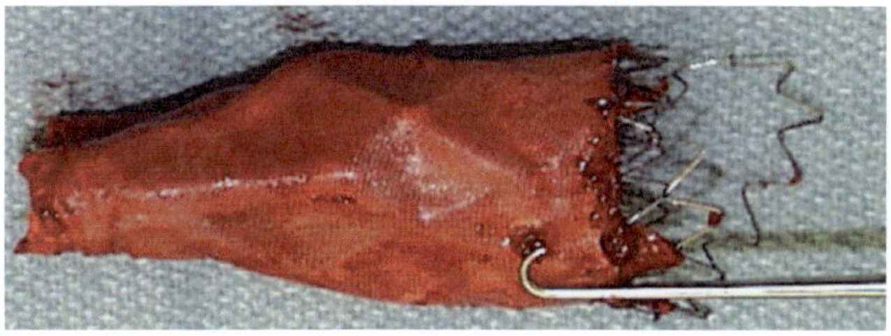

Fig. 34.13 Explanted endograft from a patient with type IIIB endoleak. Note the structural defect and a hole in the graft fabric

or a tear in the graft material (type IIIB) (Fig. 34.13). As in the case of type I endoleaks, type III endoleaks represent direct perfusion of the aneurysm sac at systemic pressure and have a relatively high rupture rate. Primary type IIIA endoleaks are readily apparent during the initial procedure, but it can be difficult to differentiate them from type I endoleaks. They are usually caused by inadequate overlapping of the junctional sections of a modular endograft. Rarely, the cause may be defects in the graft material. Primary type IIIA leaks almost always resolve after balloon molding of the junction(s). If there is insufficient overlap of the components, an additional component may be required. If the endoleak is from the main body of the endograft or at the flow divider, a second endograft should be deployed within the first. Use of an aorto-mono-iliac device and a surgical fem–fem crossover helps to reduce the total amount of graft material. If no suitable graft is available, open surgical conversion must be considered. Delayed type IIIA endoleaks were seen commonly in the first-generation devices due to a short overlap between the main body and the limb [32]. They are generally due to sac remodeling, causing the graft components to separate, or to mechanical stress causing stent and fabric failure. They are very dangerous, since there is acute repressurization of the sac, and should be treated aggressively as primary type I leaks, accepting that there is a significant open conversion rate [26].

Type IV

Type IV endoleaks are caused by porosity of the endograft fabric during the primary procedure and are seen at the time of device implantation, as a faint blush on the postimplantation angiogram, when patients are fully anticoagulated. They were reported almost exclusively with the first-generation devices and seal spontaneously. Rupture has not been reported.

Type V

This type of endoleak is caused by continued expansion of the aneurysm sac in the absence of an endoleak visible on conventional imaging. The term "endotension" has also been coined for this phenomenon, which is thought to reflect the continued pressurization of the aneurysm sac. It is important to exclude the presence of a subtle endoleak by further investigation such as contrast-enhanced ultrasound. If found, this needs to be treated as described previously. In some cases, the expansion may be due to ultrafiltration through first-generation ePTFE endografts, resulting in the formation of a hygroma (Fig. 34.14), or to tiny endoleaks through suture holes in the endograft material. Sac expansion due to ultrafiltration of serous material can be left untreated even if rupture occurs. However, the inside of the endograft can be relined with a second device [33], and open surgical conversion remains a viable option (Fig. 34.15).

Endoleak Diagnosis

Contrast MDCTA is considered the imaging technique of choice for endoleak detection. Indeed, MDCTA is reported to be superior to aortography for the demonstration of small leaks. However, selective angiography is superior to MDCTA for the detection of inflow and outflow vessels (Fig. 34.11b). Deceitful MDCTA images, including calcifications, contrast within the folds of unsupported portions of the endograft, and residual contrast inside the aneurysm sac from the initial procedure may erroneously suggest the presence of endoleaks when noninvasive angiographic follow-up is obtained within 1–3 days after implantation. Of note, "pseudo-endoleaks" are seen in up to 57 % of patients.

Color Doppler ultrasound (CDUS) is a noninvasive and cost-effective imaging modality that can be used for endoleak assessment. It is highly dependent on the operator and has limitations in obese patients and in those with excessive bowel gas. Patients should be evaluated after 5–6 h fasting, in the supine and lateral position. The aorta is evaluated both transversally and longitudinally. A leak is suspected when a reproducible color and Doppler signal inside the aneurysm is visualized. Variable success is reported for the detection and localization of the source of endoleaks with ultrasound, depending on technical factors, imaging protocol, and image quality. Overall, the reported sensitivity for endoleak detection ranges between 12 and 100 %, with specificities ranging between 74 and 99 % [34]. Although these noninvasive techniques are reliable in detecting an endoleak, the characterization and type of endoleak, as well as endovascular treatment planning can still be difficult.

Structural Failure and Graft Distortion

Metals subjected to aortic pulsation pressures may fracture. The iliac limbs of the device may also become distorted and angulated within the residual space of the aneurysm.

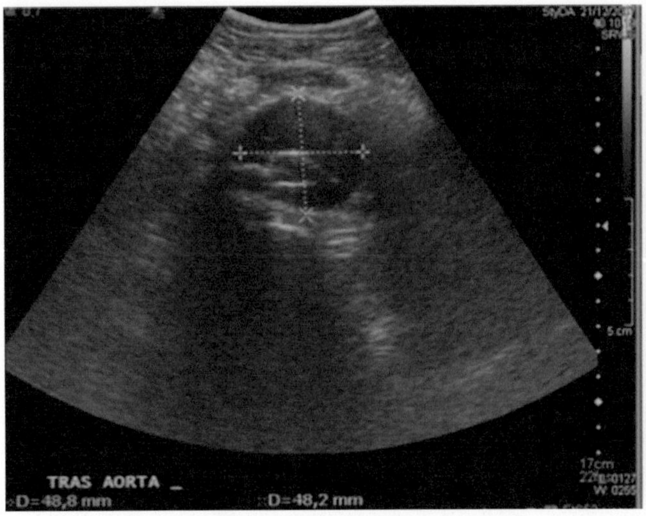

Ultrasound-December 2007
Aneurysm sac diameter= 48.8x48.2 mm

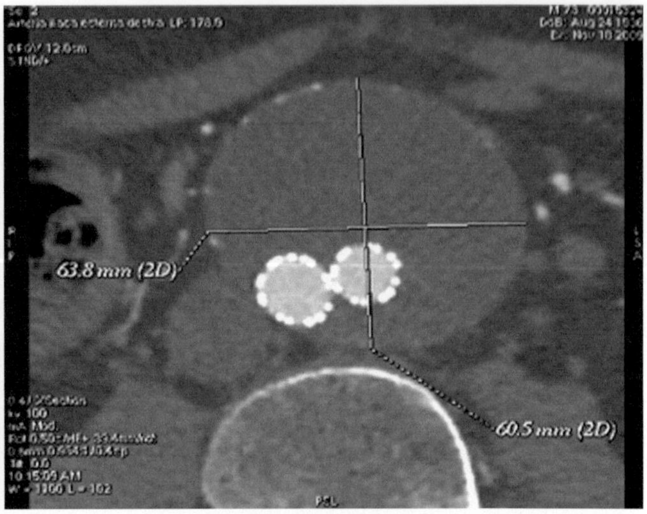

MDCTA-November 2009
Aneurysm sac diameter= 60.5x63.8 mm

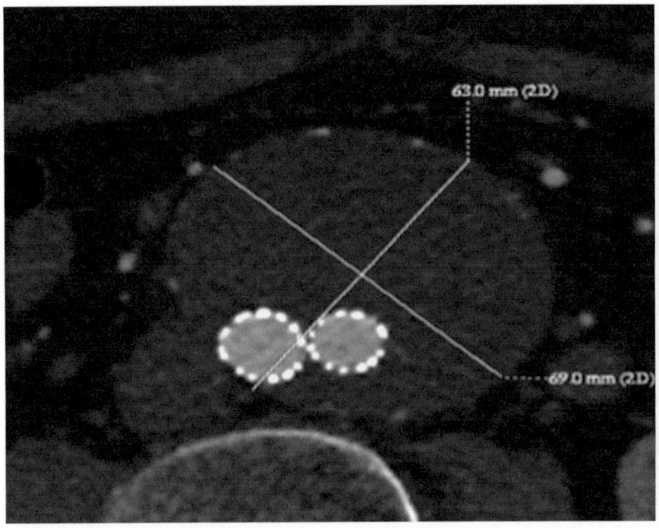

MDCTA-September 2010
Aneurysm sac diameter= 63x69 mm

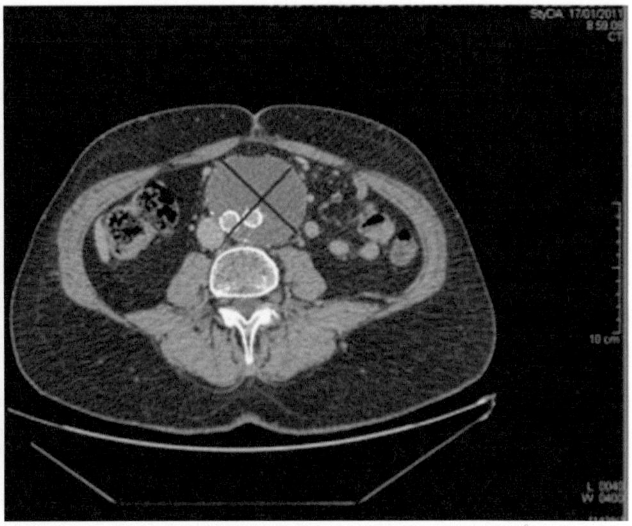

MDCTA-January 2011
Aneurysm sac diameter= 72.6x79.8 mm

Fig. 34.14 Progressive expansion over time of the aneurysm sac in a patient treated with a first-generation Excluder endograft

Non-endoleak-Related Complications

These adverse events during or after EVAR can be categorized as complications owing to surgical exposure of the access arteries or the percutaneous approach, ischemic complications owing to intentional or inadvertent clot embolization or covering of an aortic side branch, stenosis or occlusion of an endograft limb, infection of the endograft or aneurysm sac, and contrast-induced nephropathy.

Local Wound Complications in the Groin

Local wound complications following surgical exposure of the access arteries include groin hematoma, infection, or lymphocele. Their reported incidence is 1–10 % [35]. In some cases, CDUS or MDCTA evaluation may be needed to evaluate the extent of the lesion. Clinical surveillance with or without medical treatment or surgical repair are mostly enough for definitive treatment.

Access Artery Injury

Arterial thrombosis, dissection, or pseudoaneurysm formation can occur in up to 3 % of EVAR procedures. Besides correct surgical and interventional skill, a thorough preoperative CDUS or MDCTA evaluation of the common femoral and iliac arteries with special attention to access vessel diameter, tortuosity, and degree of calcification is mandatory. The introduction of a stiff and large catheter system in the presence of small and heavily calcified iliofemoral arteries can induce vessel wall dissection or even perforation. In case of a postprocedural groin pseudoaneurysm, CDUS-guided

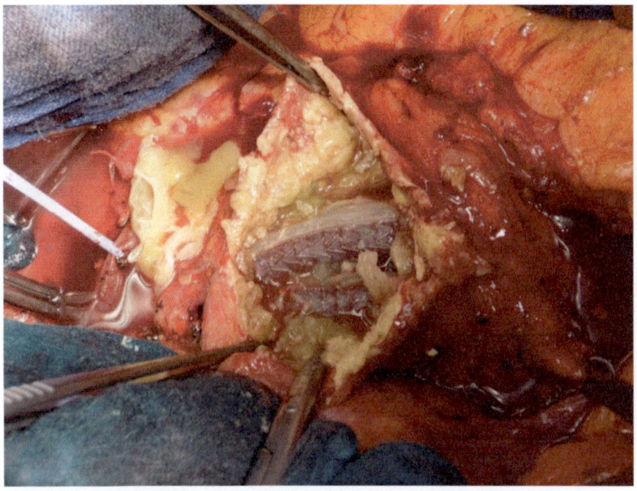

Fig. 34.15 Operating room picture during open surgical conversion (Same patient of Fig. 34.14). Note the proteinaceous material deposited inside the aneurysm sac indicative of hygroma formation

thrombin injection is not always successful as the pseudoaneurysm neck can be too large, making surgical repair the only definitive treatment option.

Ischemic Complications

Ischemic complications may occur immediately after EVAR. They can be due to thrombus formation and embolization into aortic side branches and include colonic, renal, and pelvic ischemia. Another cause of ischemia is endograft misplacement and partial or complete covering of an aortic or iliac side branch, resulting in renal or pelvic ischemia.

Colonic Ischemia

Bowel ischemia occurs in 1–3 % of cases after open aortic aneurysm repair, and the incidence seems to be in the same range for EVAR [36, 37]. Postoperative bowel ischemia after aortic aneurysm repair still remains a serious complication with a mortality rate of 50 % within 1 month. However, the pathophysiological mechanisms of colonic ischemia most probably differ in open versus endovascular repair. Whereas interruption of the inferior mesenteric or iliac arteries has been suggested to be the cause of bowel ischemia in open procedures, the same mechanism does not seem to be important for EVAR. Zhang et al. suggested that thrombotic deposits and atheroma in the suprarenal aorta may play a role in major bowel ischemia in EVAR [38]. Thrombus and atheromatous material may be dislodged while the proximal part of the endograft is being positioned, deployed, and balloon dilated just below the renal arteries. These maneuvers can induce upstream flushing of mural clot or atherosclerotic debris into the superior mesenteric artery. They may also migrate into the renal, inferior mesenteric, and internal iliac and lower-limb circulation resulting in segmental, skipped, or patchy ischemia of the embolized areas. This embolization mechanism may also explain why bowel ischemia after EVAR mostly presents as multifocal patchy ischemia. This type of bowel ischemia is not seen after open repair, most probably because suprarenal aortic and ostial inferior mesenteric arterial clamping during surgery makes distal embolization unlikely. These observations underline the importance of a careful preprocedural evaluation of the proximal aneurysmal neck and the need to identify thrombus and atheroma that may make patients poor candidates for EVAR.

Spinal Cord Ischemia

Spinal cord ischemia after EVAR is very rare. Indeed, in the EUROSTAR database, an incidence of 0.21 % in 2,862 patients has been reported [39]. The mechanism is not completely understood, but atheromatous embolization and interruption of collateral circulation from lumbar and internal iliac arteries together with a variable anatomy of the artery of Adamkiewicz seem to be the most important contributing factors. The treatment is the same as for paraplegia after thoracoabdominal EVAR or open repair and consists in cerebrospinal fluid drainage and, if indicated, recanalization of occluded collateral arteries like the internal iliac artery [40–44].

Renal Artery Occlusion

Inaccurate endograft placement with partial or total coverage of one or both renal arteries occurs in less than 5 % of cases [45] and may be due to lack of high-quality imaging technology for guiding the EVAR procedure and limited experience of the endovascular team. In their early learning curve with EVAR, Kalliafas et al. described renal artery occlusion in 5 of 204 patients, resulting in renal failure with chronic hemodialysis need in two of them [46]. If misplacement is detected during EVAR, a bailout attempt can be made, using a pull-down maneuver with an inflated angioplasty balloon or by tugging caudally on a guidewire placed across the endograft bifurcation and exteriorized from both femoral arteries. Using this technique, Görich et al. could move the stent graft from 5 to 27 mm more distally [47]. It is noteworthy that these authors did not use this bailout technique on endografts with barbs at the proximal part of the suprarenal stent. Finally, in case of partial coverage of one renal artery, stent placement in the renal artery with slight protrusion of the stent over the proximal part of the endograft into the aorta can also be used to manage this complication [48]. Rarely, renal ischemia may also occur when the top of the endograft main body needs to be placed close to the main renal artery in the presence of an accessory renal artery originating from the infrarenal neck (Fig. 34.16).

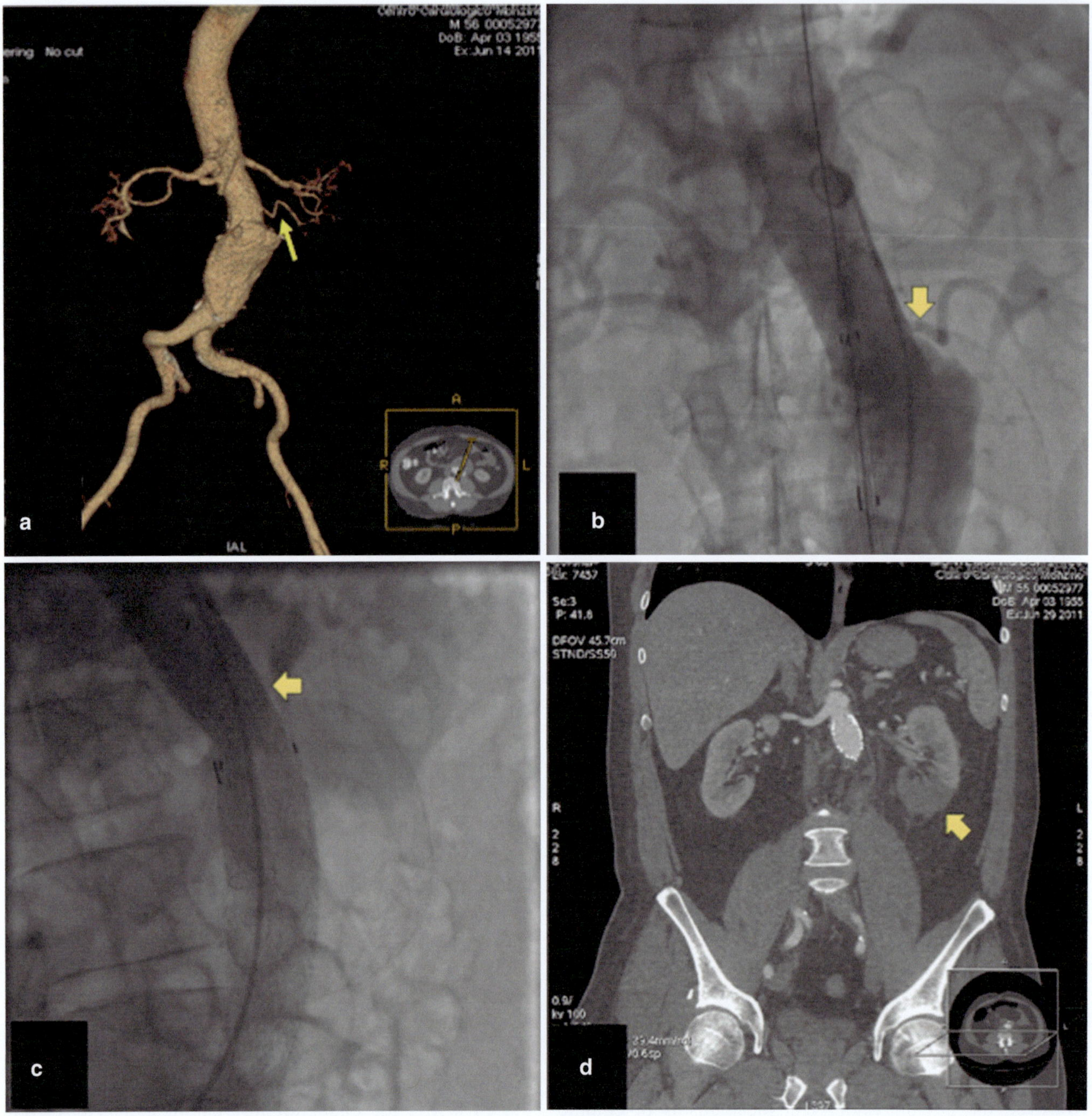

Fig. 34.16 Volume-rendering MDCTA (**a**) and invasive angiography (**b**) showing a left accessory renal artery (*arrows*). (**c**) The endograft main body was deployed close to the main renal artery occluding the accessory renal artery (*arrow*), and (**d**) multiplanar reconstruction MDCTA performed 3 days after EVAR showed infarct of the lower renal pole (*arrow*)

Early and Late Limb Occlusion After EVAR

Endograft limb thrombosis is a known complication of EVAR, especially in unsupported endografts. Indeed, it can occur in as many as 40 % of cases treated with this type of devices [49, 50]. The underlying mechanism is most frequently kinking of the unsupported endograft limb. Second-generation supported endografts perform significantly better with regard to limb thrombosis and have shown a significantly lower rate of limb occlusion, ranging between 0 and 5 % [51]. Most of the limb thrombotic events occur within the first 2 months after EVAR, and the underlying causes are endograft kinking and extension of the small-diameter endograft into the external iliac artery [52, 53]. Recently, it has been demonstrated that limb occlusion may also occur 4–5 years after EVAR [54]. The mechanism of late limb occlusion can be migration and dislocation of an endograft

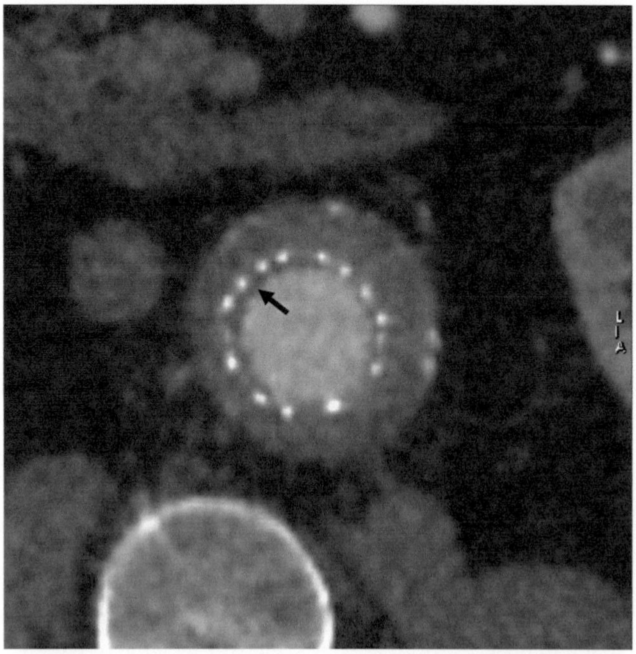

Fig. 34.17 MDCTA (short-axis multiplanar reconstruction) at 6-month follow-up showing a thin circumferential layer of thrombotic material (*arrow*) at the proximal end of an Excluder endograft main body

component causing major hemodynamic turbulence and, eventually, limb or entire endograft thrombosis. Treatment of limb occlusion includes various surgical and endovascular revascularization techniques. The best treatment option depends on the patient's general status as well as on specific endograft and excluded aneurysm changes.

In contrast to limb thrombosis, incidentally found mural thrombotic deposits are much more frequent in both first-generation endografts (20 %) and second-generation supported endografts (17–33 %) [55]. A circumferential layer of thrombotic material has been observed more in the Zenith endografts than in the Excluder endografts, but they are clinically silent and are not associated with potential endograft thrombosis or distal embolization (Fig. 34.17). Additionally, there is no difference in survival among patients presenting with mural deposits in their endograft compared with patients without this thrombotic layer. Based on these observations, additional treatment in the form of relining the endograft with another endograft or administering any type of anticoagulant therapy cannot be recommended.

Infection

The incidence of endograft infection is 0.5–1 %. If untreated, infection can result in generalized sepsis and death [56]. There are multiple causes of this complication. Endograft contamination during EVAR seems to be the source of early infection. Secondary infection from a remote source is another pathophysiological mechanism. van den Berg et al. reported an endograft infection following septic complication of a kidney stone 1 year after EVAR [57]. Another case of endograft infection after EVAR has been reported in a patient who underwent an appendectomy for appendicitis and peri-appendicular abscess formation 1 month prior to EVAR. Another cause of infection is an aortoenteric fistula. Multiple mechanisms of aortoenteric fistula creation have been described and include endograft migration, erosion of the aorta and duodenum by embolization coils, fabric rupture, inflammatory nature of the aneurysm, and bacterial aortitis with chronic duodenal erosion [58–61]. Diagnosis of endograft infection is based on clinical and radiological findings. Leukocytosis, fever, and back pain are typical clinical signs, while MDCTA may show fluid collection around the rim of the aneurysmal sac. Air bubbles may also be seen within the aneurysm sac [62, 63]. Puncture of the collection or sac for microbiological analysis often gives the definitive diagnosis. After intravenous administration of antibiotics, treatment is always resection of the endograft and aneurysm sac, followed by extra-anatomic bypass or in situ venous bypass.

Contrast-Induced Nephropathy and Acute Kidney Injury

Although patients receiving EVAR are spared the ischemic insult of aortic cross-clamping and have less perioperative hemorrhage [64, 65], the potential nephrotoxicity of large contrast volume must be considered. Correct positioning and deployment of the endograft strictly needs high-quality fluoroscopy and digital subtraction angiography imaging using injection of a contrast agent. In addition, repeated administration of contrast during periprocedural evaluation and follow-up surveillance with MDCTA represents an additional risk for progressive renal dysfunction [66, 67]. Although an average contrast volume of 50–100 mL is commonly needed for an EVAR procedure, higher amounts are not infrequently used as a result of multiple angiographies that may be needed, particularly in complex anatomy for correct endograft positioning and for assessment and treatment of type I endoleak at the proximal or distal fixation sites after endograft implantation. Contrast-induced nephropathy, resulting in acute renal failure, occurs in 6.7 % of cases according to a nationwide survey by Wald et al. [68]. To avoid contrast-induced renal complications, carbon dioxide (CO_2) can be used as an alternative contrast agent [69, 70].

In addition to contrast agents, other factors may be responsible for acute kidney injury after EVAR. Manipulation and positioning of the endograft within the aneurysm together with balloon inflation at the proximal fixation site may result in thromboembolism of the renal arteries and renal infarction. Moreover, the type of endograft used for proximal fixation in AAA may have an influence on renal function. Indeed, suprarenal fixation of the endograft is still creating concerns in regards to long-term effects. Interference with renal artery flow, narrowing of the renal ostium, renal infarction, and biological response of the aorta may be the result of continued injury from the suprarenal fixation stent and may play a role in renal function deterioration over time [71, 72].

Post-EVAR Follow-Up

The most common method of evaluating changes in aneurysm sac size is serial MDCTA and measuring the widest diameter for comparison (Fig. 34.14). Ultrasound screening is useful to evaluate sac diameter and to look for evidence of endoleaks, but it may not be sensitive enough to adequately assess early changes. Also, lateral plain X-ray has been used to evaluate graft migration by correlating graft markers with bony landmarks. The most sensitive method for detecting sac changes appears to be three-dimensional volumetric analysis by MDCTA [8]. Serial MDCTA has the benefit of enhanced information compared with ultrasound or plain radiograph. However, the financial burden, cumulative radiation exposure, and potential renal impairment from repeated contrast agent loads are a concern. It has been suggested that if an aneurysm is stable or reduced in size at 12-month MDCTA, it could safely be followed with clinical and ultrasound evaluation. This recommendation is based, in part, on the improved performance of the low-permeability endograft that markedly reduced the rates of endotension and sac expansion at 1-year follow-up. Although this improved short-term performance is encouraging, late expansion is still a concern and the importance of long-term serial evaluation should be emphasized. Another screening approach is to obtain a non-contrast CT image at follow-up. This would provide good information about device migration or deformation, aneurysm sac size, and stent fracture without exposing the patients to contrast agent administration. Screening with magnetic resonance angiography (MRA) is another option and is suitable for the Talent, Excluder, and Quantum low-permeability endografts but not for Zenith or Lifepath endografts due to artifact susceptibility [73].

Thoracic Aortic Aneurysm

Although, in general, cardiac surgeons manage thoracic segments of the aorta and vascular surgeons take care of abdominal aneurysms, the diagnosis and medical care of most aortic pathologies is frequently the responsibility of cardiologists. In light of this fact and considering the emergence of endovascular interventions for this disorder, it is important for cardiologists to gain confidence in managing at least the most frequent presentations of thoracic aortic aneurysms (TAA). Accordingly, it is also important for cardiologists to know the clinical and endovascular management of patients with TAA.

Indications for Intervention

Asymptomatic TAA are initially managed medically. Symptomatic and expanding aneurysms, or those more than 55 mm in diameter in the ascending aorta or more than 60 mm regardless of site or symptoms, are managed surgically. A novel predictor of TAA rupture, the aortic size index, could help predict rupture, dissection, or death. This index uses body surface area information (i.e., mm aortic diameter per m^2 body surface area), enabling improved selection for surgical repair on a case-by-case basis and stratification of patients according to risk. A value of 2.75 cm/m^2 or less represents low risk of rupture (approximately 4 % per year), 2.75–4.24 cm/m^2 represents moderate risk (approximately 8 % per year), and more than 4.25 cm/m^2 represents high risk (approximately 20 % per year), further underlining the importance of relative aortic size for predicting complications [74].

Endovascular Repair of Thoracic Aortic Aneurysm

For aneurysmal disease that encompasses the descending thoracic aorta and, in selected cases, the distal aortic arch, the use of endografts for repair of suitable anatomic conditions is emerging as a promising, nonsurgical alternative. Currently, catheter-based endovascular TAA repair (TEVAR) is undergoing clinical investigation [75–81]. As expected, outcomes have improved with growing technical expertise, use of commercially manufactured endografts, and the availability of appropriate patient selection criteria. Overall, technically successful device deployment is currently achieved in 85–100 % of cases. Data from 457 patients treated with endografts (113 emergency and 344 elective cases) and enrolled in the Talent Thoracic Retrospective Registry showed that among the 422 patients who survived the interventional procedure, mortality during follow-up was 8.5 % [80]. Of the 36 patients who died, 11 died from the aortic disease. Persistent endoleaks were reported in 64 cases, of which 44 cases were primary (9.6 %) and 21 occurred during follow-up (4.9 %). Kaplan-Meier overall survival estimates were 90.9 % at 1 year, 85.4 % at 3 years, and 77.5 % at 5 years [80]. At the same time intervals, the rates of freedom from a second procedure (either open conversion or endovascular) were 92.5 %, 81.3 %, and 70.0 %, respectively. Endovascular treatment for isolated TAA is considered a procedure with low early morbidity and mortality, even in patients treated on an emergency basis or with an arch aneurysm requiring hybrid intervention with surgical de-branching and subsequent endograft placement [80]. Follow-up data suggest substantial durability of such a hybrid procedure with high freedom from procedure-related death and secondary interventions [80]. Notably, patients included in registries had a high burden of comorbidities, and many would, therefore, not have been candidates for open surgery [81]. With only mid-term follow-up data after TEVAR available, any direct comparison with long-term outcome after successful surgical repair is not yet justified. However, the low rate of adverse events and neurological complications could eventually favor endovascular repair.

Hybrid Procedures for Aortic Arch Pathology

The aortic arch morphology is challenging due to angulation and proximity of supra-aortic branches that need to be preserved. Traditionally, the safest open arch reconstruction technique includes hypothermic cardiac arrest, extracorporal circulation, and selective cerebral perfusion. However, open procedures for any arch pathology carry a high risk for in-hospital mortality (2–9 %) and neurological complications (4–13 %) [82–84]. Therefore, surgery is often reserved for low-risk patients. As an alternative strategy, hybrid arch procedures may provide a viable solution in higher-risk patients combining first-stage de-branching bypasses with second-stage endovascular exclusion of the affected arch. Hybrid arch procedures are generally performed without hypothermic circulatory arrest or extracorporal circulation and may expand the treatment option to older patients with severe comorbidities or those who need redo surgery and are currently ineligible for open surgical intervention. To treat distal arch aneurysms involving both the left subclavian and the left common carotid artery, these vessels can be translocated upstream to the right common carotid artery approached via a cervical access [85, 86]. For arch aneurysms extending to the innominate artery, the ascending aorta can be used, via sternotomy, as a donor site for de-branching bypasses and serve as a proximal landing zone for the endograft [87, 88].

TEVAR Devices

The Zenith TX2 Thoracic TAA Endovascular Graft (Cook Inc., Bloomington, IN)

This device is a two-piece modular system allowing the physician to customize a graft system to fit each patient's individual anatomy (Fig. 34.18). Independent, stainless steel z-stent configuration provides graft flexibility. Varied z-stent lengths and diameters promote secure graft/vessel apposition, columnar strength, and graft flexibility. The endograft is covered with a lightweight, strong, and shrink-/stretch-resistant woven polyester (historically used for open surgical TAA and AAA repairs). Four gold markers placed 1 mm from all proximal and distal aspects of the endograft denote its edges to assist in deployment accuracy. Varied proximal component diameters and lengths allow for optimal coverage to fit each patient's specific anatomical requirements. The proximal end of the proximal component has barbs that protrude through the fabric to inhibit downward migration. Varied distal component diameters and lengths allow for optimal coverage to fit each patient's specific anatomical requirements and provide maximum overlap with proximal component. The bare stent at the distal end of the distal component contains fixation barbs to reduce the risk of upward migration. Long, tapered hydrophilic dilator tips minimize vessel trauma and provide increased trackability over the wire guide.

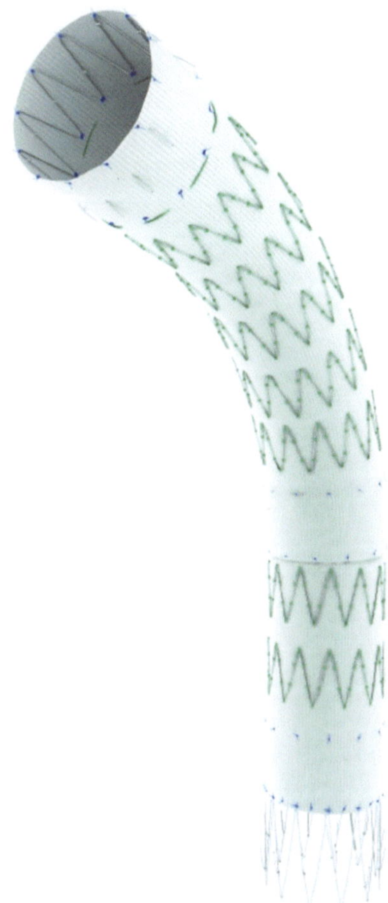

Fig. 34.18 Zenith TX2 thoracic endovascular graft (Permission for use granted by William Cook Europe, Bjaeverskov, Denmark)

Fig. 34.19 Talent (**a**) and Valiant (**b**)thoracic endograft (Courtesy of Medtronic Italy Spa, Brescia, Italy)

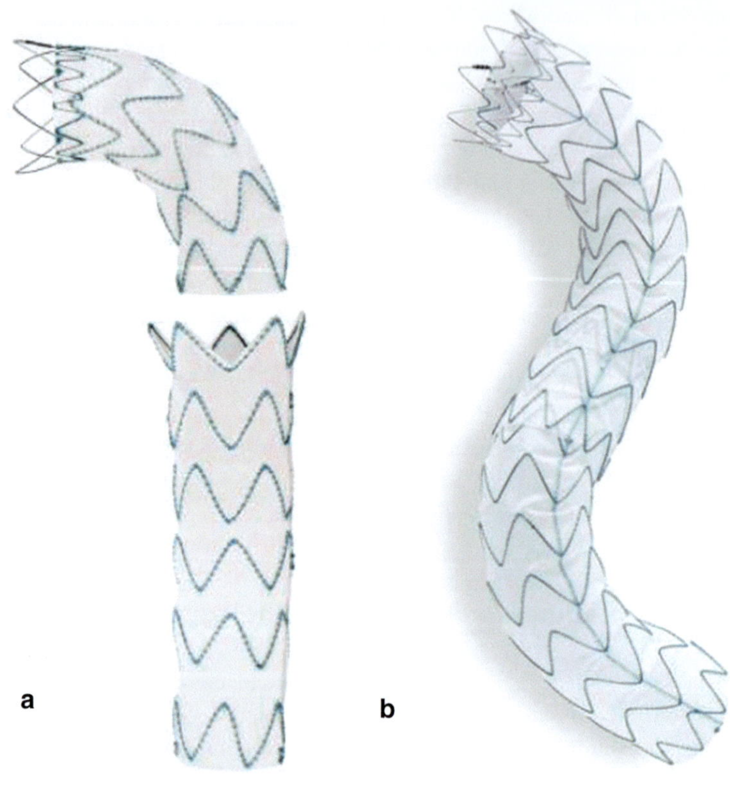

The Talent Thoracic Endograft (MedtronicVascular, Santa Rosa, CA)

The Talent thoracic endograft is composed of a Dacron graft material supported by self-expanding nitinol springs. The springs are sewn to the graft material with polyester sutures (Fig. 34.19a). The graft material is a sheet of monofilament polyester with a seam joining the edges to create a cylindrical tube. Opposite the seam is the connecting bar, which attaches the most proximal and distal springs. The connecting bar provides columnar strength to the device and facilitates deployment. During implantation, the connecting bar should be oriented to the outer radius for endograft conformability and kink resistance. All nitinol components are surface treated to enhance long-term fatigue performance. The Talent endograft has many modular sections that can be used to treat a wide variety of thoracic lesions. The endograft has three proximal and distal configurations. The proximal configurations are FreeFlo, Bare Spring (22 mm only), and Open Web, which all have a flared geometry. The FreeFlo design (different from the Bare Spring configuration) has a bare spring and a mini-support spring, which improves sealing for sizes of 24–46 mm. The distal configurations are Bare Spring, Closed Web, and Open Web. The Open Web configuration was designed for use as distal extensions for the Talent endograft system.

The Valiant Endograft (MedtronicVascular, Santa Rosa, CA)

The Valiant thoracic endograft is an evolution of the previously described Talent thoracic endograft (Fig. 34.19b). The Valiant is composed of a woven, monofilament polyester graft sewn to a self-expanding nickel–titanium (nitinol) wire stent. The nitinol scaffolding is composed of a series of 5 peaked springs stacked in a tubular configuration and sewn with braided polyester non-absorbable sutures onto the outside of the polyester graft material. The proximal and distal stents differ from the "body" springs in that they have 8 peaks and range in height from 15 to 17 mm. The endograft does not have a connecting bar between springs in an attempt to increase conformability of the device. The spring spacing is designed to allow adjacent peaks to contact each other when loaded into the Xcelerant delivery system providing the necessary column strength for deployment. The proximal and distal ends of the endograft come in both open (FreeFlo) and closed (Closed Web) configurations. Seven radiopaque platinum–iridium markers are sewn to the endograft fabric. Four proximal 8-shaped markers and two distal 0-shaped markers indicate the proximal and distal extremities of the stent material. A single 8-shaped "mid-marker" indicates the minimum amount of overlap required when deploying multiple segments. The Closed Web configuration is not designed for use as a primary section or proximal extension. A segment with a FreeFlo configuration should not be deployed within another segment because of the risk of material rupture. The Valiant is currently available in diameters from 24 to 46 mm. Junctions between sections require oversizing to achieve a seal. Multiple sections may be required to achieve disease coverage and fixation. These should be sized to give appropriate oversizing, using tapered segments if necessary, and sufficient length, taking the requirement for adequate overlap into account. The Xcelerant delivery

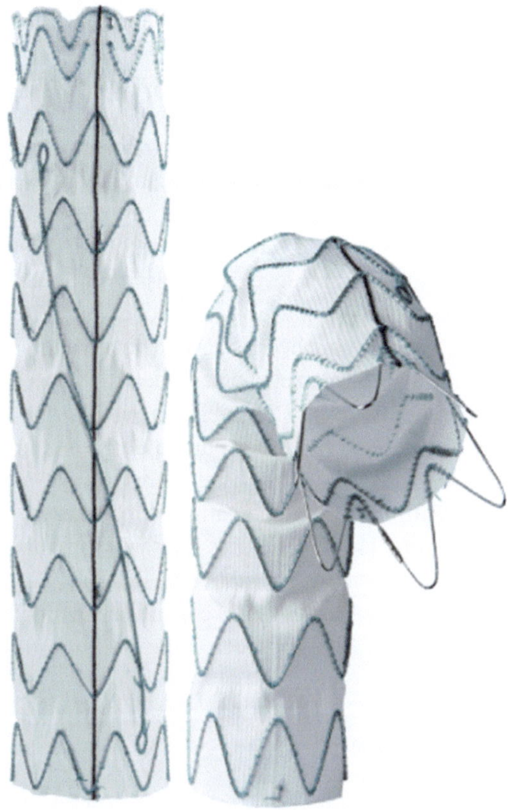

Fig. 34.20 Bolton Medical Relay thoracic endograft (Courtesy of Bolton Medical, Milan, Italy)

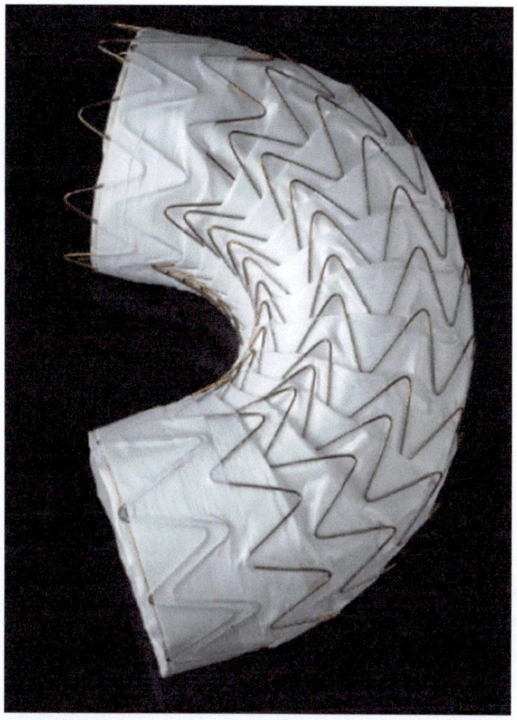

Fig. 34.21 Gore Conformable TAG (Courtesy of W.L. Gore & Associates, Inc., Flagstaff, AZ)

system consists of a single-use, disposable catheter with an integrated handle to provide the user with controlled deployment of the Valiant endograft. The delivery system has a 22–25F outer diameter and is designed to track over a 0.035″ guidewire. The delivery part of the system is composed of an inner member with a flexible tapered tip, a middle member incorporating the stent-stop, and an outer cover. A stainless steel braid stiffens the outer cover. The outer cover restrains the endograft during tracking and releases the endograft upon retraction. The middle member helps tracking through tortuous anatomy and has a flexible stent-stop to maintain the endograft position during deployment. Rotating or releasing and retracting the integrated handle deploy the endograft by retraction of the outer sheath cover. Should the handle jam, it can be disassembled to allow direct retraction of the outer sheath while the inner and middle members are held firmly.

Bolton Medical Relay Thoracic Endograft (Bolton Medical Inc, International Parkway Sunrise, FL)

This device, together with its "Transport" delivery system, has been specifically designed for the thoracic aorta and has an indication to treat every region, particularly the aortic arch (Fig. 34.20). The Relay endograft is made of a Dacron-woven graft and of a proprietary electropolished ultrasmooth nitinol. The device is available in two configurations featuring a proximal bare stent (Relay Plus) or a proximal crown stent (Relay NBS Plus). The device is characterized by a dedicated radial force distribution: the radial force expressed by each stent is different, according to its role (high for proximal and distal sealing stents, intermediate for middle stents, and low for the proximal bare stent). A "spiral support strut," "double S" shaped in three dimensions, is also available with the aim of absorbing the forces expressed by the heartbeat and the blood flow forces onto the aorta, giving columnar strength and support. The "Transport" delivery system is a unique two-stage introducer system: while the primary sheath gives support in the navigation of the iliacs, the flexible secondary inner sheath allows to take the device through every tortuous anatomy. A proximal capture system allows a precise positioning and repositioning of the endograft prior to deployment. Diameters of the Relay endograft vary from 22 to 46 mm, and lengths from 100 to 250 mm, for straight and tapered configurations. A custom-made program is also available.

The TAG (W.L. Gore & Associates, Flagstaff, AZ)

The TAG is a flexible nitinol-supported PTFE device available in diameters of 26–40 mm and in 10-cm, 15-cm, and 20-cm lengths (Fig. 34.21). The exoskeleton is bonded to the graft material without sutures and is constrained by an ePTFE sleeve. The device profile depends on the size of endograft and requires a 20–24F sheath. Deployment is very rapid and occurs with the release of the constraining sleeve. The TAG expansion is designed to start from the middle of the endograft and progress toward its end. This is designed to avoid the displacing forces of the high arterial flow when aortic endografts are partially deployed in a standard deployment mode. The device is then additionally expanded with a specially designed trilobed balloon that allows flow to continue during inflation, thus avoiding the need for rapid pacing (Fig. 34.9). If more than one device is used, the most proximal device should be deployed first, and then the second must follow distal to this with at least 2 cm of overlap. The original device contained two longitudinal spines for columnar support. The device has been redesigned recently: the longitudinal spine was removed, and the ePTFE material was reinforced.

TEVAR Indications

Thoracic Aortic Aneurysm

In approximately 60 % of cases, TAA involves the ascending aorta, in 40 % the descending aorta, and in 10 % the arch, while 10 % of patients show a thoracoabdominal extension. Etiology, natural history, and treatment of TAA differ for each of these segments [89]. The suitability of a given patient for endovascular repair is based on both clinical and anatomical considerations. To date, endograft placement is a first-choice option when TAA is distal to the aortic arch and when an abdominal aorta location is present. As with AAA, the endograft bridges the aneurysm sac to exclude it from high-pressure aortic blood flow, thereby promoting sac thrombosis and aorta remodeling. Successful TAA exclusion similarly requires normal segments of native aorta at both lesion ends of at least 12–25 mm to ensure adequate deployment and contact between the endograft and the aortic wall with a tight circumferential seal. Devices are oversized by 10–20 % in diameter to provide sufficient radial force for fixation. The preferred and most common site of vascular access is the common femoral artery (41–58 %). Less frequently, access to the iliac artery (9–44 %) via an extraperitoneal approach is required [90, 91]. Proximal attachment of the endograft may require intentional coverage of the left subclavian artery ostium [92]. With this technique, it is important to identify patients with anomalous arch vessels in order to allow the requisite revascularization surgery before endograft deployment [93]. Since the first human case of TEVAR was performed in 1986 [94], a primary technical success rate of 80–90 % has been reported [95–101]. Major procedure-related neurological complications, including stroke and spinal cord ischemia, were seen in up to 8 % of patients. However, compared with open surgical repair, endovascular treatment does appear to halve perioperative mortality with similar late survival and almost identical rates of reinterventions and ischemic spinal cord complications [102, 103].

Penetrating Atherosclerotic Ulcer

The term penetrating atherosclerotic ulcer (PAU) describes a condition in which ulceration of an atherosclerotic plaque penetrates the internal elastic lamina and allows hematoma formation within the media of the aortic wall [104]. PAUs are most frequently located in the descending thoracic aorta, and affected patients tend to be elderly with a history of hypertension, smoking, and other atherosclerotic disease, including preexisting TAA. In a quarter of cases, a PAU may penetrate through the media to form a saccular aortic pseudoaneurysm (Fig. 34.22a) or, less often, it may perforate the adventitia to cause transmural aortic rupture [104, 105]. The entity is associated with a variable extent of localized intramural hematoma but may develop to classic aortic dissection in rare cases [104–106]. Currently, no definite treatment strategy has been established for PAU management. Indeed, patients with a PAU diameter and/or depth of 2 cm, those who are hemodynamically unstable, as well as those with evidence of contained rupture should undergo urgent repair. Continued or recurrent pain, distal embolization, and progressive dilatation are also indications for surgery or endovascular therapy [107]. There is growing optimism that TEVAR may become an alternative to open surgery, since limited aortic disease such as PAU constitutes an ideal condition for this less invasive approach (Fig. 34.22b) [108].

TEVAR Procedure

Based on measurements from transesophageal echocardiography, MDCTA, which is the best technique for unstable patients in an emergency situation, or intravascular ultrasound (IVUS), individually selected endografts should be used. The procedure is best performed in the catheterization laboratory or hybrid operating room using digital angiography. Cerebrospinal fluid drainage is recommended for patients with previous AAA repair and in those in whom coverage of the subclavian artery is planned or requires extensive endograft coverage of the aorta. The femoral artery is the preferred access site. In most cases, it can accommodate a 20–24F endograft system. Using the Seldinger technique to place a sheath, a 260-cm stiff guidewire is placed over a pigtail catheter navigated with a soft guidewire in the true lumen under fluoroscopic guidance. In some centers, transesophageal ultrasound guidance is also used. A 6F sheath is placed in the contralateral femoral artery and a second guidewire is positioned in the ascending aorta. If the endograft will be deployed distal to the subclavian artery, a 6F pigtail catheter will be positioned in the ascending aorta. If the left subclavian artery is going to be excluded with the endograft, this guidewire will serve as a “bailout” access guidewire. In case the endograft is deployed inadvertently over the left carotid artery, a balloon catheter of appropriate size will quickly be advanced over the guidewire and inflated across the proximal end of the device, to allow perfusion to the carotid artery. A 4F sheath and subsequent pigtail catheter are placed in the right brachial artery when the left subclavian artery is to be excluded. The pigtail catheter is positioned in the ascending

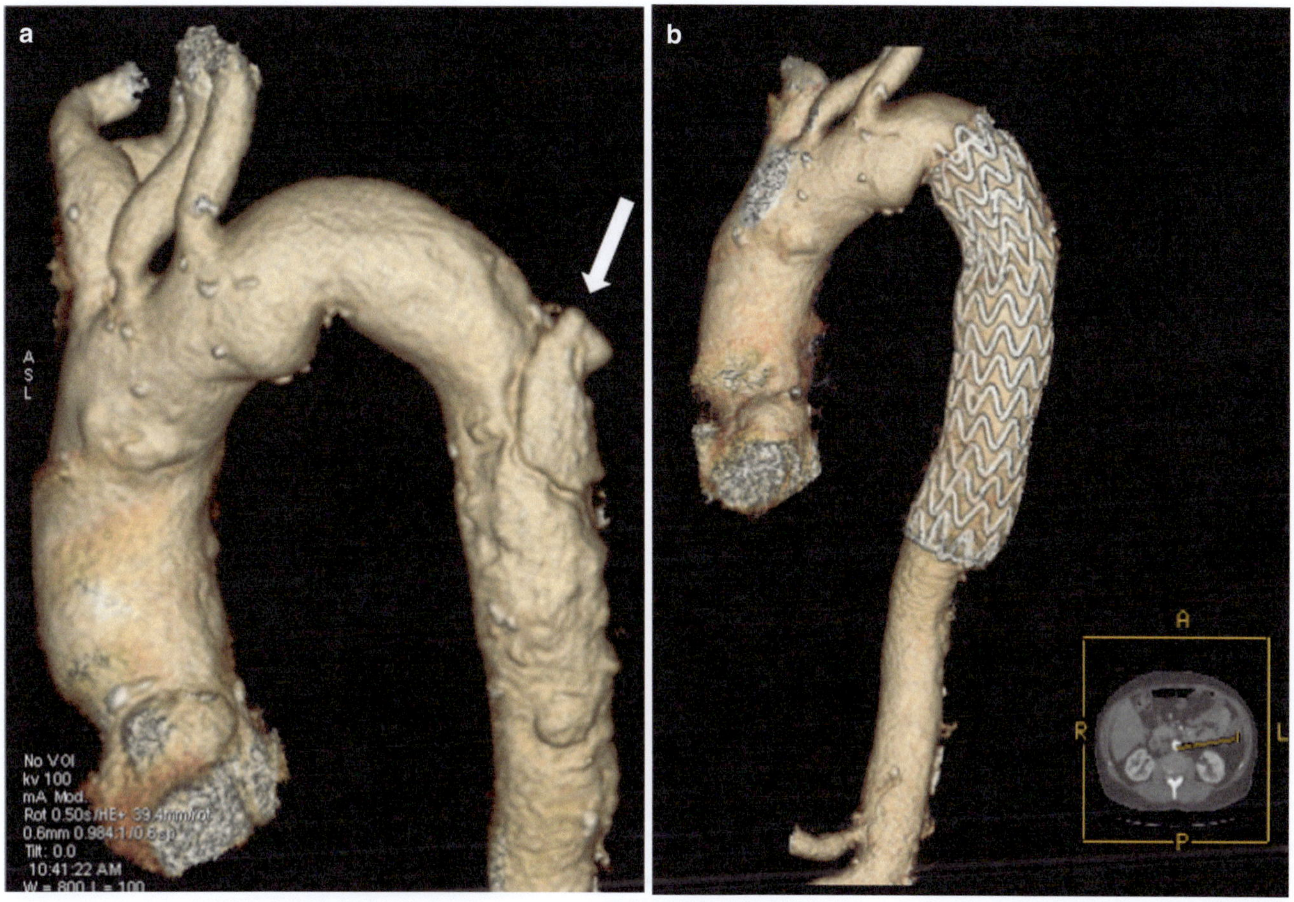

Fig. 34.22 (a) Volume-rendering MDCTA showing a penetrating atherosclerotic ulcer of the descending aorta. (b) MDCTA at 1-year follow-up after implantation of a Gore Conformable TAG showing complete exclusion of the ulcer

aorta. When dealing with a very tortuous aorta or an arch with a small radius, the "body floss" maneuver may be helpful in advancing the endograft through the arch. This is accomplished by advancing a 0.035″×450-cm hydrophilic guidewire from the right brachial artery to the femoral artery. The device may then be advanced over this guidewire. The pigtail catheter (transfemoral or through right brachial/radial access) is used to perform an aortogram of the area of interest. After the angiogram is performed, the proximal neck is evaluated. The length and the diameter of the proximal and distal neck are therefore measured using the preoperative MDCTA, intraoperative IVUS, as well as angiogram. Based on these measurements, the endograft is chosen, flushed with heparinized solution, and carefully advanced, over the stiff guidewire, into the proximal neck. A repeat angiogram is commonly performed to confirm the device position within aorta. Prior to device deployment, the systolic blood pressure is brought down to 100 mmHg. If the patient has a landing zone proximal to the left subclavian artery, adenosine (35 mg for the first dose, 20 mg for subsequent doses) may be administrated to gain a 4–5 s cardiac arrest. The ventilator is stopped for the deployment in patients under general anesthesia. These two measures improve deployment accuracy. Alternatively, endograft deployment is performed with systolic blood pressure briefly lowered by rapid right ventricular pacing [109]. After deployment, short inflation of a latex balloon is performed to improve endograft apposition to the aortic wall but only if proximal sealing is incomplete. Both Doppler ultrasound and contrast fluoroscopy are instrumental for documenting any circumferential stent malapposition to the proximal or distal landing zone that may lead to endoleak. However, a single aortogram may miss endoleak due to projection overlap. A biplane aortogram is more reliable in excluding any significant intraprocedural endoleak. After the completion angiogram, the introducer sheath is removed leaving the guidewire in the aorta. If there is any concern about iliac artery injury, an iliac artery angiogram is performed. If no iliac lesion is detected and the patient remains hemodynamically stable, the guidewire is removed and the femoral artery is repaired in standard fashion.

Post-TEVAR Complications

Postoperative complications in patients undergoing TEVAR are about the same of those described for EVAR in the previous paragraph. We will limit ourselves here to recall briefly the more specific complications of TEVAR. The most severe complications in the W.L. Gore TAG pivotal clinical trial included stroke (4 %), paraplegia/paraparesis (3 %), peripheral vascular injury (14 %), and death (2 %) [110]. Stroke can occur because the guidewires placed in the aortic arch to direct the endograft into position can dislodge a thrombus or atheromatous debris that can embolize via the cerebral vasculature to the brain. Similarly, thromboembolic material can also lead to limb and mesenteric ischemia. Spinal ischemia may occur when the intercostal blood vessels supplying the spinal cord are covered by the endografts. Paraplegia can be occasionally reversed by elevating blood pressure and draining spinal fluid. Due to their large size, thoracic endograft may damage femoral and iliac arteries as they are advanced into position. The most worrisome concern is complete femoral or iliac avulsion, which can be controlled with balloon occlusion. This is the main reason why guidewires must be left in position until the very end of the case. Endoleaks occur when the aneurysm is not completely isolated from the bloodstream. In the W.L. Gore TAG trial, this complication was found in 6 % and 9 % of patients at 1 and 2 years, respectively [111].

Post-TEVAR Therapy and Follow-Up

The long-term follow-up of patients who underwent successful TEVAR begins with the appreciation of a systemic illness. All patients merit aggressive medical therapy, follow-up visits, and serial imaging. Treatment with effective β-blockade is the cornerstone of medical therapy. By lowering both blood pressure and dp/dt, β-blockers have been shown to retard aortic expansion in Marfan's syndrome and that associated with chronic AAA. Blood pressure should be titrated to less than 130/80 mmHg in usual patients and to no more than 120/80 mmHg in those with Marfan's syndrome [112, 113]. Additionally, heart rate should be controlled. Indeed, heart rate <60 bpm significantly decreases secondary adverse events (aortic expansion, recurrent aortic dissection, aortic rupture, and/or need for aortic surgery) compared to conventional control at >60 bpm [114]. Serial imaging of the aorta is an essential component of long-term management after endograft placement (Fig. 34.22b). The choice of imaging modality depends on institutional availability and expertise [112, 113].

Aortic Coarctation and Atherosclerotic Stenosis of the Infrarenal Abdominal Aorta

Coarctation of the aorta (CoA) and atherosclerotic stenosis of the infrarenal abdominal aorta (IAA) will be discussed together because the general and technical principles are similar as well as the devices used for their endovascular treatment.

Aortic Coarctation

CoA is a congenital abnormality that accounts for 5–8 % of the 8/1,000 (4–6/10,000) children born with congenital heart disease. In most cases, CoA is diagnosed in childhood, while in less than 25 % of patients is recognized beyond 10 years. In the adult form, CoA is generally characterized by a narrowing localized in the post-ductal or ligament region, just distal the left subclavian artery origin (Fig. 34.23a). Unlike the infantile CoA, the adult form is typically not associated with a patent arterial duct. Moreover, degenerative aortic wall changes and formation of arterial collateral vessels are usually present (Fig. 34.23b). Coarctation may be an isolated malformation or may occur in association with bicuspid aortic valve and other cardiovascular diseases such as subaortic stenosis, mitral valve abnormalities, ventricular septal defect, and, less frequently, cerebral aneurysms of the Willis circle. In adults, CoA may be recognized because of systemic arterial hypertension and pulse discrepancy between the upper and lower extremities. Patients may complain of exertional headache, leg fatigue, or claudication. Occasionally, the patient may come to medical attention because of a murmur due to a bicuspid aortic valve or ventricular septal defect. Survival in non-operated patients averages 35 years of age, with 75 % mortality by 45 years of age. Systemic arterial hypertension, accelerated coronary artery disease, stroke, aortic dissection, and congestive heart failure are common complications in patients who did not have surgery or underwent surgical correction in later childhood or adult life. Death may be due to congestive heart failure, aortic rupture/dissection, endocarditis/endarteritis, intracerebral hemorrhage, or myocardial infarction [115]. When operated in neonates and small infants, re-coarctation occurs in up to 10 % of cases in most published series. The time of this re-narrowing may vary largely from weeks to years after the first intervention. Patients may also present with aortic wall injury (aneurysm) related to prior CoA repair. Treatment of these aneurysms is surgically challenging.

Atherosclerotic Stenosis of the Infrarenal Abdominal Aorta

Severe, concentric, and diffuse calcific stenosis of the IAA occurs relatively infrequently but presents a challenging management problem [116, 117]. Indeed, focal stenosis of the IAA not extending to the bifurcation or iliac arteries is infrequent and is one of less frequent causes of lower extremity claudication. However, diffuse stenosis of a heavily calcified IAA is an even more uncommon clinical entity and is considered an advanced stage of a severe chronic obliterative atherosclerotic process in the aorta. Patients

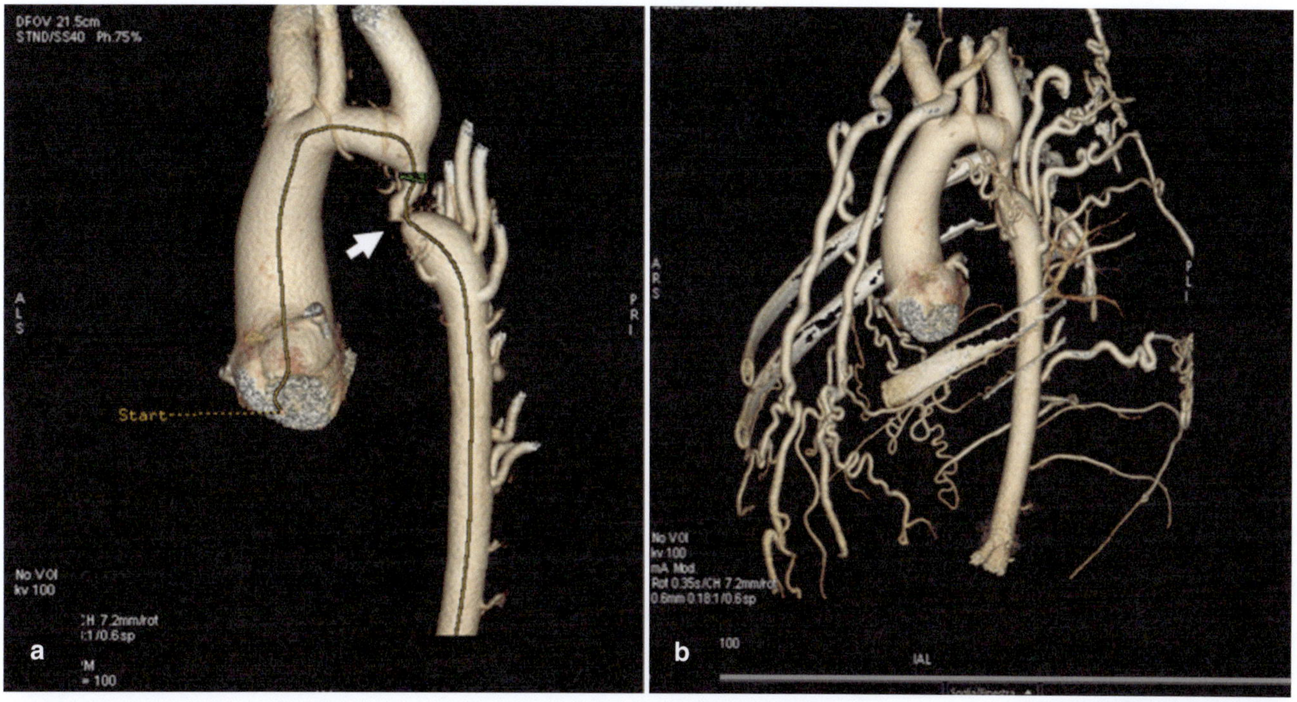

Fig. 34.23 MDCTA (volume rendering) showing aortic coarctation (*arrow*) in an adult patient (**a**) and extensive arterial collateral vessels (**b**)

with IAA stenosis are usually younger and have less extensive atherosclerotic disease than patients who present with iliofemoral or more peripheral disease. These patients have a longer life expectancy than the average patient with claudication. In adult patients, about 90 % of stenosing or occlusive disease of the IAA is caused by atherosclerosis [118]. Open surgery, with either endarterectomy or bypass graft replacement when more extensive disease is present, is an effective treatment modality and traditionally has been the treatment of choice [119, 120]. Both of these treatments have durable results in a high proportion of patients but are highly invasive and carry a significant risk of morbidity and mortality ranging from 9 to 27 % and 1 to 7 %, respectively [121, 122].

Non-invasive Assessment

MRA or MDCTA with three-dimensional reconstruction identifies the precise location and anatomy of CoA and IAA stenosis, as well as collateral vessels (Figs. 34.23 and 34.24). MDCTA is also extremely useful in intervention planning: (1) it helps the physician determine the true diameter of the native aorta that can be underestimated with angiography, and (2) it defines the extent of calcification and (3) the extent of disease (focal or diffuse). Alternatively, IVUS could be used in patients where renal function is suboptimal, but preprocedural MDCTA has the benefit of being able to plan the procedure beforehand. In CoA patients, MRA to search for aneurysms of the intracranial arteries is appropriate and may also be useful to quantify collateral flow.

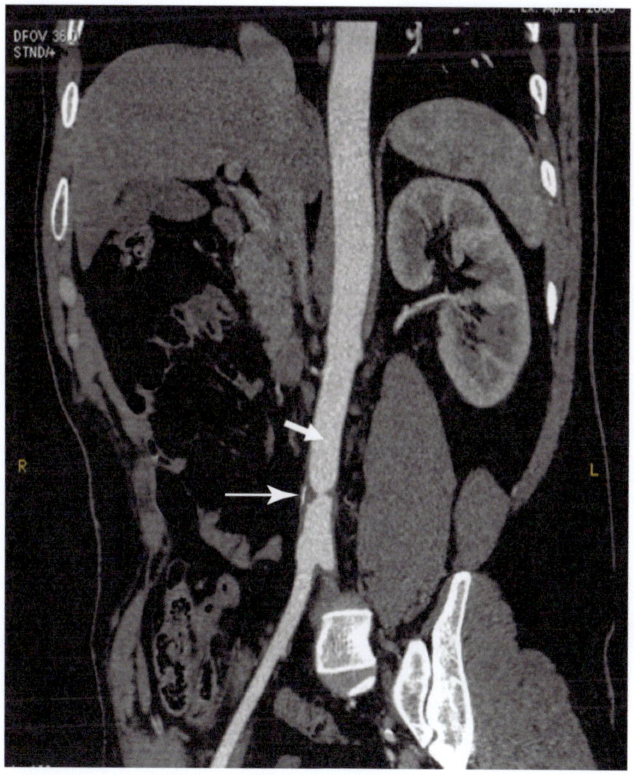

Fig. 34.24 MDCTA (multiplanar reconstruction) showing severe stenosis (*arrow*) of the distal abdominal aorta

Endovascular Treatment

Coarctation of the Aorta

Accepted criteria for CoA treatment in adults (native and post-operative) include an anatomically discrete lesion, upper extremity hypertension, and a resting gradient of at least 20 mmHg or 30 mmHg after exercise. However, the best treatment in adults remains the subject of continuous debate [123, 124]. Surgical repair, first performed by Crafoord and Nylin in 1944 [125], was initially the only available option, but in some cases, it was complicated by restenosis, aneurysm formation [126, 127], late hypertension, and premature death, particularly when the repair was performed after the first year of life [128, 129]. Currently, surgical mortality is very low, but surgery is still associated with a small risk of spinal cord damage and consequent irreversible paraplegia [130]. To deal with postoperative complications such as restenosis after surgical repair, balloon dilation of re-CoA was introduced in 1982 [131–133] and demonstrated to be successful in reducing the gradient to <20 mmHg in 85 % of patients, with a restenosis rate of 8 %. Although widely used since then, balloon dilation has excited controversy. Histology and IVUS studies have established that angioplasty increases the internal aortic diameter by tearing the intima and media of the aorta. Although intimal and medial tears may heal, some may progress to aneurysm formation. The incidence of early and late aneurysm formation after balloon angioplasty has been reported to be between 5 and 11.5 % [128, 132, 134–138], a higher rate as compared to their occurrence after surgical repair (3–4 %). The known major complications of angioplasty are sudden death due to ventricular fibrillation, aortic rupture, and aneurysm formation due to intimal tears and the consequent weakening of the aortic wall. Other problems associated with balloon dilation are residual CoA and re-CoA. Similar complications have been encountered in patients with native CoA treated with balloon dilation [134–136, 139]. In the early 1990s, balloon-expandable stents were introduced for CoA treatment in children, and since then, their use increased dramatically [140–145] due to many advantages over balloon angioplasty. In particular, balloon-expandable stents provide support to the vessel wall and apposition of the torn vessel intima to the media and thereby are associated with a lower rate of residual stenosis, restenosis, and late aneurysm formation. Moreover, they may be redilated to accommodate the patient's somatic growth. Although stenting addresses the concern about angioplasty complications, aortic dissection and aneurysm formation have also been reported after stent implantation in up to 5 % of patients [128, 145, 146]. A meta-analysis of 22 studies performed in adult and adolescent patients with CoA compared interventional to surgical treatment with regard to morbidity, restenosis, requirement for reintervention, and hypertension and found that stenting had the lowest risk of complications, with surgery having a slightly higher risk and angioplasty a significantly higher risk [147]. However, restenosis and reintervention

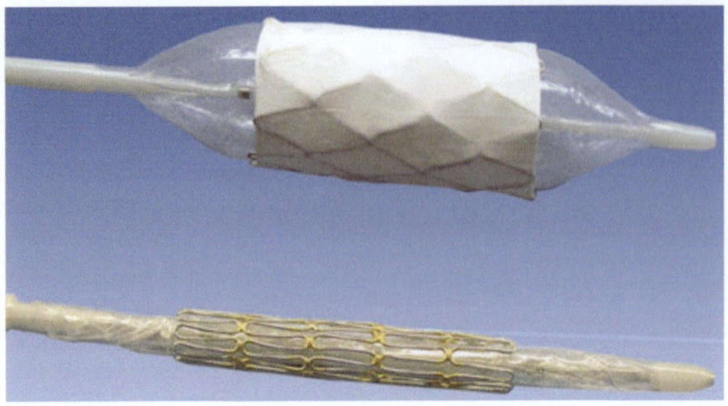

Fig. 34.25 Cheatham-Platinum stent. The covered type (*top*) and bare type (*bottom*) are shown. (Courtesy of NuMED, Inc., Hopkiton, NY)

rates were significantly higher following stenting and angioplasty when compared to surgery, and surgical complications were minor (e.g., vasculitis, bleeding), while endovascular complications tended to be more serious. In 1999, a covered stent was used for the first time to treat coexistent CoA and aneurysm of the aorta in a young man [148]. Since then, covered stent demonstrated to significantly improve endovascular treatment of CoA, reducing the risk associated to angioplasty and bare stent implantation [149–154]. Up to now, several different covered stents have been used: (1) the AneuRx (Medtronic, Watford, England) self-expanding stent covered with a stretchable polytetrafluoroethylene membrane [148], (2) the graft Jomed stent (Jomed, Rangendingen, Germany) [149], (3) the self-expanding stent graft (Braile stent, Braile Biomedica, Sao José do Rio Preto, Brazil) [154], and (4) the balloon-expandable Cheatham-Platinum stent covered with ePTFE (NuMed Inc., Hopkinton, NY) (Fig. 34.25) [150, 151, 153, 154]. Covered stents provide increased safety, reducing the risk associated with aorta rupture by "sealing" the dilated area [155, 156], particularly in patients with extreme narrowing, tortuous lesions, genetic aortic wall weakness, and advanced age. Covered stents have been successfully used even in case of stent fracture and for the treatment of late aortic aneurysm after surgical or endovascular CoA repair and for subatretic native CoA [77, 155, 157]. Although the ability to redilate covered stents has been recently demonstrated [155, 156], their use is limited to patients that are nearly fully grown, because currently they can be redilated up to 25 mm only. Moreover, at diameters of up to 22 mm, they can shorten by one-eighth of their initial length. One of the main initial concerns with the use of covered stents was the occlusion of a significant aortic side branch. It is obviously important to avoid covering the main arteries such as the innominate or the left common carotid arteries, but the left subclavian artery can be covered, if needed, because it has been shown that endograft-induced occlusion of the ostial left subclavian artery is tolerated without chronic functional ischemia in the absence of stenotic vertebral and/or carotid arteries and with a documented intact vertebrobasilar system [92]. Furthermore, occlusion of a spinal artery, which would result in the most severe complication, is unlikely after implantation of a covered stent in the thoracic aorta, because the spinal artery originates below the level of the ninth thoracic vertebra in over 90 % of the patients [158, 159]. The risk of subacute stent thrombosis is low due the brisk aortic flow and the large size of the stent. In conclusion, covered stents have become the therapy of choice in Europe and recently in the USA through the FDA Compassionate Use process in patients with complications after CoA repair. Moreover, they provide a safe alternative to surgery for the treatment of the large part of adult patients with native CoA [160, 161].

Atherosclerotic Stenosis of the Infrarenal Abdominal Aorta

Grollmann et al., Tegtmeyer et al. and Velasques et al. performed the first PTAs of IAA stenoses in 1980 [162–164]. Since then, several authors [162, 163] have shown that PTA is an effective treatment modality of aortic atherosclerotic occlusive disease associated with a high technical and clinical success rate, few major complications, and encouraging mid- and long-term results.[165–174]. The vast majority of lesions treated were relatively short (<2 cm) with a technical success rate ranging from 95 to 100 % and a patency rate approaching 89 % [169, 174]. By comparison, primary patency rates of 75–90 % and 90–95 % have been reported for bypass grafting and endarterectomy, respectively [121, 122]. During the 1990s, some reports were published indicating that stent placement may be an option in cases where PTA of aortic lesions fails, or is inadequate [171, 175, 176]. Growing clinical experience with aortic stenting has demonstrated that this is a safe and effective treatment [171, 177–179]. Indeed, endovascular treatment with stents achieved immediate technical success rates of 100 % and low complication rates in the majority of published series [164, 175, 180–182]. At present, the durability of primary stenting can be considered acceptable in all the studies and appear to be broadly similar or superior to the results obtained by an open surgical approach. Therefore, primary stenting is recommended as a safe and effective treatment strategy and should be offered to patients as "the treatment of choice" in focal atherosclerotic IAA stenoses.

Implantation Technique

Stent Choice

Only a few stents are available that can be dilated to a diameter ≥20 mm. The Palmaz XL (Cordis, Miami, FL) and the Cheatham-Platinum (CP) stent (NuMed Inc., Hopkinton, NY) are designed for treatment of large vessel lesions. The CP stent is composed of 0.013″ platinum/iridium struts arranged in a "zig" pattern. It allows expansion from 8 to 24 mm, and its variability in length is from 11 to 50 mm. The covered-CP stent is the same bare-metal stent covered with an expandable sleeve of ePTFE. A bare and a covered CP stent pre-mounted on a BIB (balloon in balloon) catheter (NuMed Inc., Hopkinton, NY) became recently available in Europe (Fig. 34.25). The BIB catheter is 110 cm in length, utilizes a 0.035″ guidewire, and has an inner balloon half the diameter of the outer balloon and 1 cm shorter in length. The BIB is designed to prevent stent displacement from the balloon during inflation and to allow adjustment of the balloon/stent position after partial dilation of the stent.

Coarctation of the Aorta

The general and technical principles are the same as those used for performing balloon angioplasty or stenting in other vessels. In pediatric patients, the procedure is usually performed under general anesthesia, while sedation with midazolam and propofol and local anesthesia are preferred in adults. Intravenous heparin (100 UI/kg, maximum of 5,000 UI) is given immediately after femoral access is gained percutaneously with an 8 Fr introducer.

Hemodynamic and Angiographic Assessment

The stenotic segment is crossed with a 6F multipurpose catheter over a floppy hydrophilic guidewire (0.035″ Terumo guidewire). Then, the multipurpose catheter is exchanged for a pigtail catheter over a standard 0.035″ exchange 260-cm guidewire. The pressure gradient is measured between the femoral sheath and the pigtail catheter positioned in the ascending aorta. Anteroposterior, 40° left anterior oblique and lateral angiograms are performed and the following measurements are obtained: (1) diameter and length of the stenotic area, (2) diameter of the descending aorta at the level of the diaphragm, (3) diameter of the aorta at the level of the left subclavian artery, and (4) diameter of the transverse arch (Fig. 34.26a). The maximum balloon diameter is usually chosen based on either the transverse or the distal arch diameter, whichever is greater using catheter magnification or the calibration markers on the catheters. The angioplasty balloon diameter is usually 2.5–3.0 times that of the narrowed segment but should be less than 1.5 times the diameter of the aorta proximal to the CoA. It is clear that for some partially elastic stenoses, it is necessary to employ 1–2-mm larger balloons. This strategy may likely play a role in aneurysm formation, but it is not yet clear whether the use of a smaller balloon and elastic recoil prevention by stent implantation [140] may reduce this risk. Some groups suggest a graduated approach, using repeated procedures to gradually enlarge the stenosis, but evidence that graduated ballooning or stenting carries less risk is still lacking.

Stent Delivery

The pigtail catheter is exchanged for a long sheath, usually a Mullins sheath (Cook, Bloomington, IN), ranging from 11F

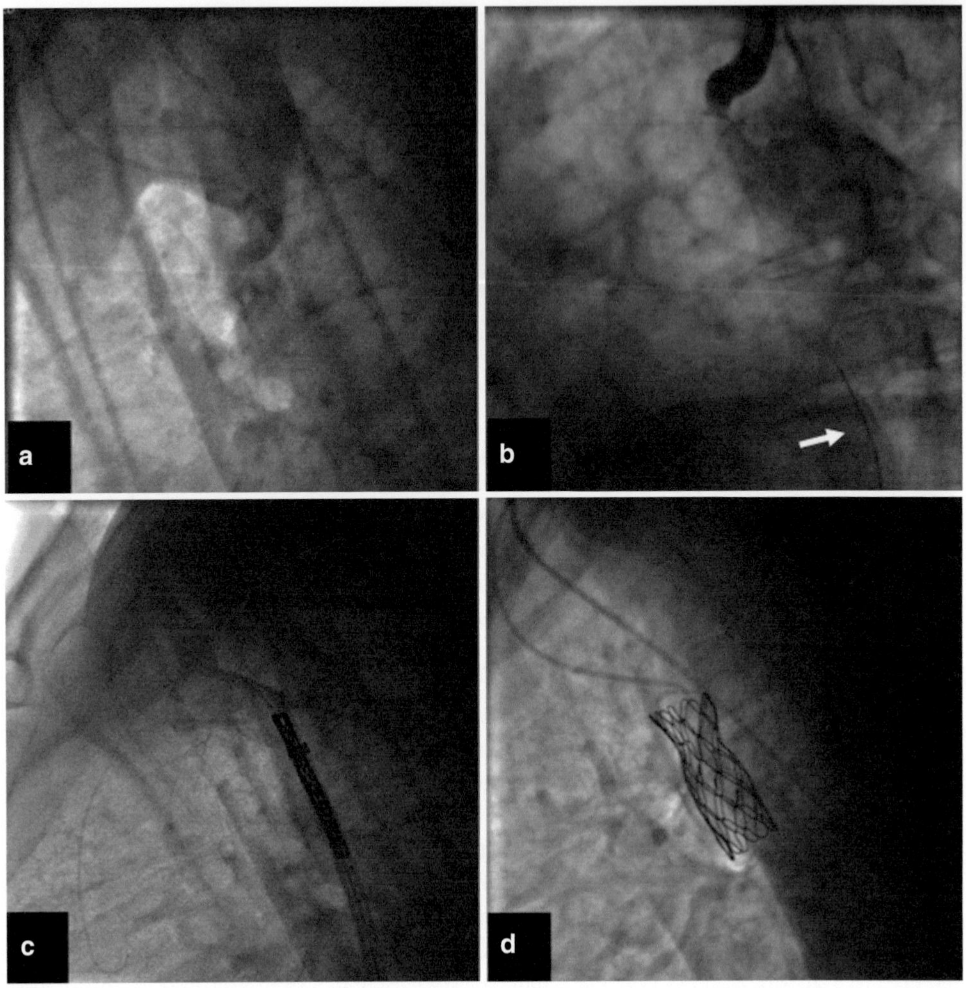

Fig. 34.26 Procedural phases of CoA endovascular treatment. (**a**) Angiography performed with a pigtail cateter advanced in the proximity of the CoA with a transradial approach showing a near-atretic aortic coarctation. (**b**) A 0.014″ coronary guidewire (*arrow*) and a 4.0-mm coronary balloon catheter were needed to predilate the lesion. (**c**) Covered Cheatham-Platinum stent placed across the lesion. (**d**) Stent deployed with BIB balloon inflation

to 14F, over a 0.035″ stiff exchange 260-cm guidewire positioned in the ascending aorta or in the right subclavian artery. The CoA is then predilated with standard peripheral balloons. When a near-atretic CoA is found, predilation with coronary guidewires and balloons may be needed (Fig. 34.26b). The length of the stent is determined by the distance from just beyond the left subclavian artery to about 10–15 mm beyond the CoA site and is always shorter than the balloon length. The stent may be mounted on a BIB catheter. After advancement of the mounted stent to the stenotic site through the long sheath, serial injections of dye through the sheath or a separate catheter confirm the desired position of the stent immediately before implantation. A catheter with radiopaque markers may also be used for this purpose. The fluoroscopic image of the catheter will project over the aortic isthmus and will allow an accurate localization of the narrowing plane, thus confirming that the stent straddles the CoA during balloon inflation (Fig. 34.26c). The balloon is manually inflated up to the pressure recommended by the manufacturer (usually 4–6 atm), and the stent is deployed in the correct position (Fig. 34.26d). Pressure gradient is recorded and angiography is performed after stent placement injecting contrast through the side arm of the long sheath or a pigtail in order to assess the results and to rule out dissection or rupture of the aorta. At the end of the procedure, hemostasis is achieved by manual compression, surgical repair, or percutaneous pre-closure. All patients receive cephalosporin for 24 h and aspirin (≥100 mg) once a day for 6 months after implantation.

Atherosclerotic Stenosis of the Infrarenal Abdominal Aorta

The procedure is usually undertaken under local anesthesia. Initially, bilateral common femoral access is established with a 6F short sheath, followed by systemic anticoagulation with heparin (100 U/kg). Occasionally, transradial access may be used for accurate reference imaging and to pass the initial guidewire in the antegrade direction. This approach may lower the risk of creating a cephalad-extending dissection of the aorta. The IAA-diseased segment is traversed with a 0.035″ hydrophilic guidewire under fluoroscopic guidance, and a pigtail marker angiographic catheter is placed in the aorta for preliminary imaging and to assist in selection of stent length (Fig. 34.27). The hydrophilic guidewire is then

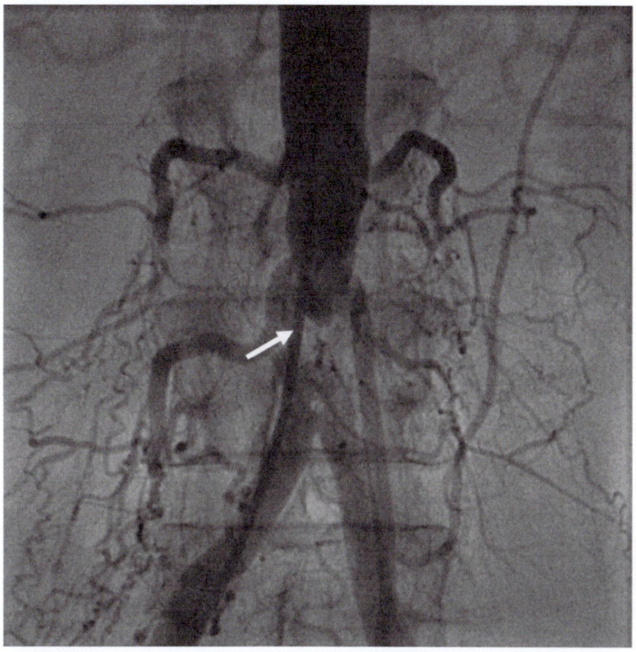

Fig. 34.27 Angiography of the distal abdominal aorta showing nearly complete occlusion of the vessel (*arrow*) and extensive arterial collateral circulation

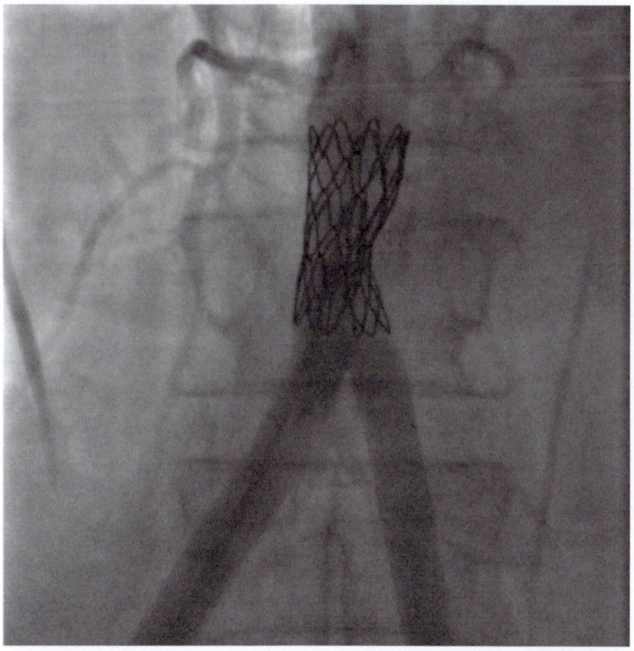

Fig. 34.28 Angiography of the distal abdominal aorta showing final result after covered Cheatham-Platinum stent deployment and post-dilation (Same patient seen in Fig. 34.24)

exchanged for a 0.035″ stiffer guidewire, and a larger (9–12F) long sheath is advanced retrogradely across the stenosis until its tip is proximal to the lesion. The stenotic segment is dilated with balloon angioplasty with standard

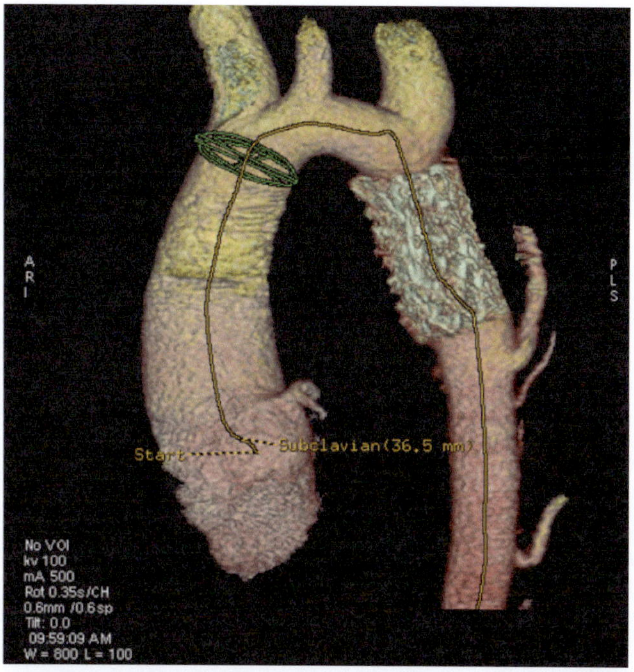

Fig. 34.29 Volume-rendering MDCTA showing correct position and expansion of a covered Cheatham-Platinum stent after endovascular treatment of aortic coarctation

technique. The selection for the balloon catheter size is usually 60–80 % of the diameter of the healthy aorta. A stent of an appropriate diameter for the IAA and length for the lesion (as a rule, the selected stent should be longer then diseased segment by 3 mm) is then positioned, sheath is withdrawn, and the stent is deployed after angiographic control via the contralateral approach for exact placement. After stent deployment, a further angiogram is obtained in two planes to determine whether the stented segment requires any additional dilatation (Fig. 34.28). "Kissing-balloon" technique may be used when dealing with a large IAA. Technical success is determined if residual stenosis is less than 30 % at angiography or there is no hemodynamic pressure gradient across the lesion.

Follow-Up

It is incumbent on all interventionists carrying out endovascular procedures or aortic stenosis treatment to document objective outcomes (e.g., treadmill testing), symptomatic improvement, quality of life, and proof of patency (i.e., duplex ultrasound, MDCTA, MRA, or angiography). Usually, patients undergo MRA or MDCTA (Figs. 34.29 and 34.30) at 3 and 12 months after the procedure. Invasive angiography is usually performed in cases where problems are identified.

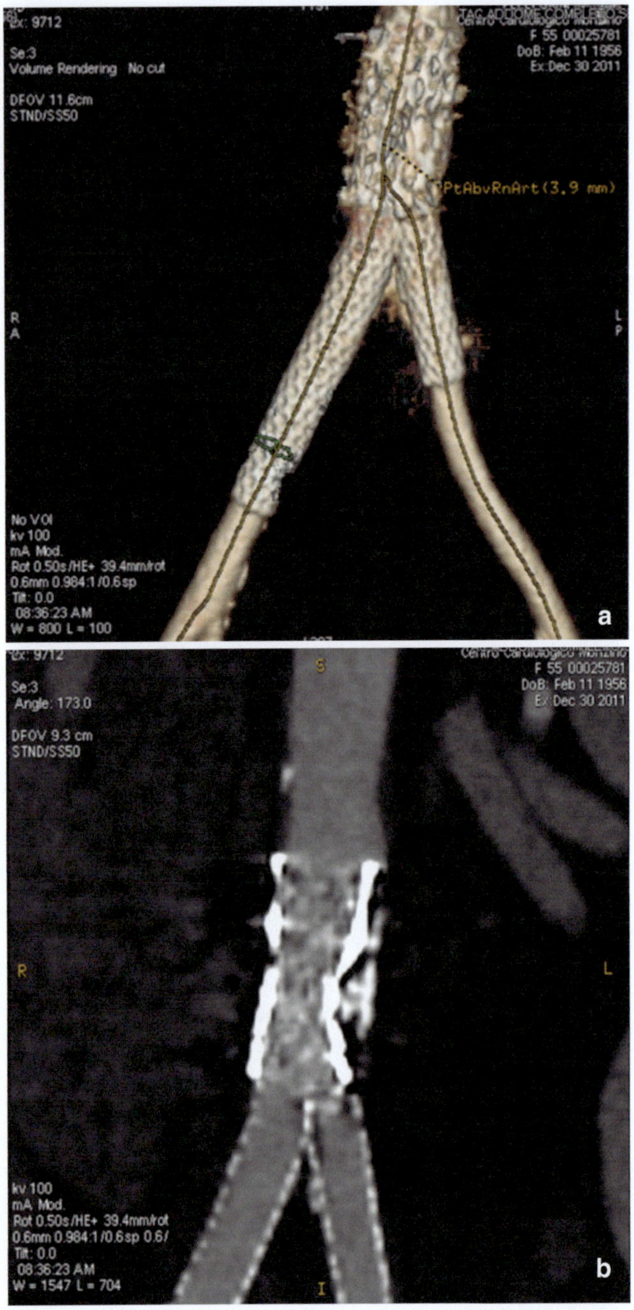

Fig. 34.30 Volume-rendering (**a**) and multiplanar reconstruction (**b**) MDCTA at 1-year follow-up showing correct position and patency of a covered Cheatham-Platinum stent deployed for distal abdominal aorta stenosis. Patency of bilateral stents deployed for treatment of common iliac artery stenoses is also shown

References

1. Parodi JC, Palmaz JC, Barone HD. Transfemoral intraluminal graft implantation for abdominal aortic aneurysms. Ann Vasc Surg. 1991;5:491–9.
2. Parodi JC, Marin ML, Veith FJ. Transfemoral, endovascular stented graft repair of an abdominal aortic aneurysm. Arch Surg. 1995; 130:549–52.
3. Volodos' NL, Goloborod'ko NK, Mikhailenko VV. Surgical treatment of traumatic rupture of the thoracic aorta. Grudn Khir. 1981;6:76–8.
4. Criado FJ, Wilson EP, Wellons E, Abul-Khoudoud O, Gnanasekeram H. Early experience with the talent stent-graft system for endoluminal repair of abdominal aortic aneurysms. Tex Heart Inst J. 2000; 27:128–35.
5. Criado FJ, Fairman RM, Becker GJ. Talent LPS AAA stent graft: results of a pivotal clinical trial. J Vasc Surg. 2003;37:709–15.
6. Broker HS, Foteh KI, Murphy EH, Davis CM, Clagett GP, Modrall JG, Buckley CJ, Arko FR. Device-specific aneurysm sac morphology after endovascular aneurysm repair: evaluation of contemporary graft materials. J Vasc Surg. 2008;47:702–7.
7. Risberg B, Delle M, Eriksson E, Klingenstierna H, Lonn L. Aneurysm sac hygroma: a cause of endotension. J Endovasc Ther. 2001;8:447–53.
8. Fillinger M, Excluder Bifurcated Endoprosthesis Clinical Investigators. Three-dimensional analysis of enlarging aneurysms after endovascular abdominal aortic aneurysm repair in the Gore Excluder Pivotal clinical trial. J Vasc Surg. 2006;43:888–95.
9. Haider SE, Najjar SF, Cho JS, Rhee RY, Eskandari MK, Matsumura JS, Makaroun MS, Morasch MD. Sac behavior after aneurysm treatment with the Gore Excluder low-permeability aortic endoprosthesis: 12-month comparison to the original Excluder device. J Vasc Surg. 2006;44:694–700.
10. Tanski 3rd W, Fillinger M. Outcomes of original and low-permeability Gore Excluder endoprosthesis for endovascular abdominal aortic aneurysm repair. J Vasc Surg. 2007; 45:243–9.
11. Dalainas I, Nano G, Bianchi P, Ramponi F, Casana R, Malacrida G, Tealdi DG. Aortic neck dilatation and endograft migration are correlated with self-expanding endografts. J Endovasc Ther. 2007; 14:318–23.
12. Hobo R, Kievit J, Leurs LJ, Buth J, EUROSTAR Collaborators. Influence of severe infrarenal aortic neck angulation on complications at the proximal neck following endovascular AAA repair: a EUROSTAR study. J Endovasc Ther. 2007;14:1–11.
13. Whittaker DR, Dwyer J, Fillinger MF. Prediction of altered endograft path during endovascular abdominal aortic aneurysm repair with the Gore excluder. J Vasc Surg. 2005;41:575–83.
14. Chaikof EL, Blankensteijn JD, Harris PL, White GH, Zarins CK, Bernhard VM, Matsumura JS, May J, Veith FJ, Fillinger MF, Rutherford RB, Kent KC, Ad Hoc Committee for Standardized Reporting Practices in Vascular Surgery of the Society for Vascular Surgery, American Association for Vascular Surgery. Reporting standards for endovascular aortic aneurysm repair. J Vasc Surg. 2002;35:1048–60.
15. Carpenter JP. Midterm results of the multicenter trial of the Powerlink bifurcated system for endovascular aortic aneurysm repair. J Vasc Surg. 2004;40:849–59.
16. Zarins CK, Bloch DA, Crabtree T, Matsumoto AH, White RA, Fogarty TJ. Stent graft migration after endovascular aneurysm repair: importance of proximal fixation. J Vasc Surg. 2003; 38:1264–72.
17. Ouriel K, Greenberg RK, Clair DG, O'hara PJ, Srivastava SD, Lyden SP, Sarac TP, Sampram E, Butler B. Endovascular repair of abdominal aortic aneurysms: device-specific outcome. J Vasc Surg. 2003;37:991–8.
18. Abbruzzese TA, Kwolek CJ, Brewster DC, Chung TK, Kang J, Conrad MF, LaMuraglia GM, Cambria RP. Outcomes following endovascular abdominal aortic aneurysm repair (EVAR): an anatomic and device-specific analysis. J Vasc Surg. 2008;48:19–28.
19. Albertini J, Kalliafas S, Travis S, Yusuf SW, Macierewicz JA, Whitaker SC, Elmarasy NM, Hopkinson BR. Anatomical risk factors for proximal perigraft endoleak and graft migration following

endovascular repair of abdominal aortic aneurysms. Eur J Vasc Endovasc Surg. 2000;19:308–12.
20. Mohan IV, Harris PL, Van Marrewijk CJ, Laheij RJ, How TV. Factors and forces influencing stent-graft migration after endovascular aortic aneurysm repair. J Endovasc Ther. 2002;9:748–55.
21. Arko FR, Heikkinen M, Lee ES, Bass A, Alsac JM, Zarins CK. Iliac fixation length and resistance to in-vivo stent-graft displacement. J Vasc Surg. 2005;41:664–71.
22. Murphy EH, Johnson ED, Arko FR. Device-specific resistance to in vivo displacement of stent-grafts implanted with maximum iliac fixation. J Endovasc Ther. 2007;14:585–92.
23. Heikkinen MA, Alsac JM, Arko FR, Metsänoja R, Zvaigzne A, Zarins CK. The importance of iliac fixation in prevention of stent graft migration. J Vasc Surg. 2006;43:1130–7.
24. Benharash P, Lee JT, Abilez OJ, Crabtree T, Bloch DA, Zarins CK. Iliac fixation inhibits migration of both suprarenal and infrarenal aortic endografts. J Vasc Surg. 2007;2:250–7.
25. Enzler MA, van Marrewijk CJ, Buth J, Harris PL. Endovascular therapy of aneurysms of the abdominal aorta: report of 4,291 patients of the Eurostar Register. Vasa. 2002;31:167–72.
26. van Marrewijk C, Buth J, Harris PL, Norgren L, Nevelsteen A, Wyatt MG. Significance of endoleaks after endovascular repair of abdominal aortic aneurysms: The EUROSTAR experience. J Vasc Surg. 2002;35:461–73.
27. Zarins CK, White RA, Hodgson KJ, Schwarten D, Fogarty TJ. Endoleak as a predictor of outcome after endovascular aneurysm repair: AneuRx multicenter clinical trial. J Vasc Surg. 2000;32: 90–107.
28. Buth J, Harris PL, van Marrewijk C, Fransen G. The significance and management of different types of endoleaks. Semin Vasc Surg. 2003;16:95–102.
29. Van den Berg JC, Tutein Nolthenius RP, Casparie JWBM, Moll FL. CT-guided thrombin injection into aneurysm sac in a patient with endoleak after endovascular abdominal aortic aneurysm repair. AJR Am J Roentgenol. 2000;175:1649–51.
30. Kasthuri RS, Stivaros SM, Gavan D. Percutaneous ultrasound-guided thrombin injection for endoleaks: an alternative. Cardiovasc Intervent Radiol. 2005;28:110–2.
31. Muthu C, Maani J, Plank LD, Holden A, Hill A. Strategies to reduce the rate of Type II Endoleaks: routine intraoperative embolization of the inferior mesenteric artery and thrombin injection into the aneurysm sac. J Endovasc Ther. 2007;14:661–8.
32. Fransen GA, Vallabhaneni Sr SR, van Marrewijk CJ, Laheij RJ, Harris PL, Buth J, EUROSTAR. Rupture of infra-renal aortic aneurysm after endovascular repair: a series from EUROSTAR registry. Eur J Vasc Endovasc Surg. 2003;26:487–93.
33. Goodney PP, Fillinger MF. The effect of endograft relining on sac expansion after endovascular aneurysm repair with the original-permeability Gore Excluder abdominal aortic aneurysm endoprosthesis. J Vasc Surg. 2007;45:686–93.
34. Bakken AM, Karl A, Illig KA. Long-term follow-up after endovascular aneurysm repair: is ultrasound alone enough? Perspect Vasc Surg Endovasc Ther. 2010;22:145–51.
35. Liaw JV, Clark M, Gibbs R, Jenkins M, Cheshire N, Hamady M. Update: complications and management of infrarenal EVAR. Eur J Radiol. 2009;71:541–51.
36. Becquemin JP, Majewski M, Fermani N, Marzelle J, Desgrandes P, Allaire E, Roudot-Thoraval F. Colon ischemia following abdominal aortic aneurysm repair in the era of endovascular abdominal aortic repair. J Vasc Surg. 2008;47:258–63.
37. Perry RJ, Martin MJ, Eckert MJ, Sohn VY, Steele SR. Colonic ischemia complicating open versus endovascular abdominal aortic aneurysm repair. J Vasc Surg. 2008;48:272–7.
38. Zhang WW, Kulaylat MN, Anain PM, Dosluoglu HH, Harris LM, Cherr GS, Dayton MT, Dryjski ML. Embolization as a cause of bowel ischemia after endovascular abdominal aortic aneurysm repair. J Vasc Surg. 2004;40:867–72.
39. Berg P, Kaufmann D, van Marrewijk CJ, Buth J. Spinal cord ischemia after stent-graft treatment for infra-renal abdominal aortic aneurysm. Analysis of the Eurostar database. Eur J Endovasc Surg. 2001;22:342–7.
40. Fortes DL, Atkins BZ, Chiou AC. Delayed paraplegia following intrarenal abdominal aortic endograft placement: case report and literature review. Vascular. 2004;12:130–5.
41. Reid JA, Mole DJ, Johnston LC, LEE B. Delayed paraplegia after endovascular repair of abdominal aortic aneurysm. J Vasc Surg. 2003;37:1322–3.
42. Garcia ND, Tehrani H, Morasch M, Pearce W, Matsumura J. Spinal cord ischemia following endovascular repair of an infrarenal aortic aneurysm. Ann Vasc Surg. 2002;16:509–12.
43. Rockman CB, Riles TS, Landis R. Lower extremity paraparesis or paraplegia subsequent to endovascular management of abdominal aortic aneurysm. J Vasc Surg. 2001;33:178–80.
44. Bajwa A, Davis M, Moawad M, Taylor PR. Paraplegia following elective endovascular repair of abdominal aortic aneurysm: reversal with cerebrospinal fluid drainage. Eur J Vasc Endovasc Surg. 2008;35:46–8.
45. Kalliafas S, Albertini JN, Macierewicz J, Yusuf SW, Whitaker SC, Macsweeney ST, Wenham PW, Hopkinson BR. Incidence and treatment of intraoperative technical problems during endovascular repair of complex abdominal aortic aneurysm. J Endovasc Ther. 2000;7:123–31.
46. Kalliafas S, Whitaker SC, Hopkinson BR. Use of a bifurcated graft for endovascular repair of a common iliac aneurysm after previous open aortic aneurysm surgery. Eur J Vasc Endovasc Surg. 2000;19:428–9.
47. Görich J, Krämer S, Rilinger N, Sokiranski R, Sunder-Plassmann L, Pamler R, Kapfer X. Malpositioned or dislocated aortic endoprostheses: repositioning using percutaneous pull-down maneuvers. J Endovasc Ther. 2000;7:123–31.
48. van Dijk LV, van Sambeek MR, Cademartiri F, Pattynama PM. Partial blockage of the renal artery ostium after stent-graft placement: detection and treatment. J Endovasc Ther. 2003;10:684.
49. Fairman RM, Baum RA, Carpenter JP, Deaton DH, Makaroun MS, Velazquez OC, Phase II EVT Investigators. Limb interventions in patients undergoing treatment with an unsupported bifurcated aortic endograft system: a review of the Phase II EVT trial. J Vasc Surg. 2002;36:118–26.
50. Amesur NB, Zajko AB, Orons PD, Makaroun MS. Endovascular treatment of iliac limb stenoses or occlusions in 31 patients treated with the Ancure graft. J Vasc Interv Radiol. 2000;11:421–8.
51. Maleux G, Koolen M, Heye S, Nevelsteen A. Limb occlusion after endovascular repair of abdominal aortic aneurysm with supported endografts. J Vasc Interv Radiol. 2008;19:1409–12.
52. Maldonado TS, Rockman CB, Riles E, Douglas D, Adelman MA, Jacobowitz GR, Gagne PJ, Nalbandian MN, Cayne NS, Lamparello PJ, Salzberg SS, Riles TS. Ischemic complications after endovascular abdominal aortic aneurysm repair. J Vasc Surg. 2004;40:703–10.
53. Carroccio A, Faries PL, Morrissey NJ, Teodorescu V, Burks JA, Gravereaux EC, Hollier LH, Marin ML. Predicting iliac limb occlusions after bifurcated aortic stent grafting: anatomic and device-related causes. J Vasc Surg. 2002;36:679–84.
54. Blom AS, Troutman D, Beeman B, Yarchoan M, Dougherty MJ, Calligaro KD. Duplex ultrasound imaging to detect limb stenosis or kinking of endovascular device after midterm follow-up. J Vasc Surg. 2012;55(6):1577–80.
55. Maleux G, Koolen M, Heye S, Heremans B, Nevelsteen A. Mural thrombotic deposits in abdominal aortic endografts are common and do not require additional treatment at short-term and midterm follow-up. J Vasc Interv Radiol. 2008;19:1558–62.
56. Sharif MA, Lee B, Lau LL, Ellis PK, Collins AJ, Blair PH, Soong CV. Prosthetic stent graft infection after endovascular abdominal aortic aneurysm repair. J Vasc Surg. 2007;46:442–8.

57. van der Berg HR, Leijdekkers VJ, Vahl A. Aortic stent-graft infection following septic complications of a kidney stone. Cardiovasc Intervent Radiol. 2006;29:443–5.
58. Saratzis N, Saratzis A, Melas N, Ktenidis K, Kiskinis D. Aortoduodenal fistulas after endovascular stent-graft repair of abdominal aortic aneurysm: single-center experience and review of the literature. J Endovasc Ther. 2008;15:441–8.
59. Bergqvist D, Bjorck M, Nyman R. Secondary aortoenteric fistula after endovascular aortic interventions: a systematic literature review. J Vasc Interv Radiol. 2008;19:163–5.
60. Parra JR, Lee C, Hodgson KJ, Perler B. Endograft infection leading to rupture of aortic aneurysm. J Vasc Surg. 2004;39:676–9.
61. Baker M, Uflacker R, Robinson JG. Stent graft infection after abdominal aneurysm repair: a case report. J Vasc Surg. 2002;36:180–3.
62. Mita T, Arita T, Matsunaga N, Furukawa M, Zempo N, Esato K, Matsuzaki M. Complications of endovascular repair for thoracic and abdominal aortic aneurysm: an imaging spectrum. Radiographics. 2000;20:1263–78.
63. Orton DF, LeVeen RF, Saigh JA, Culp WC, Fidler JL, Lynch TJ, Goertzen TC, McCowan TC. Aortic prosthetic graft infections: radiologic manifestations and implications for management. Radiographics. 2000;20:977–93.
64. Adriansen ME, Bosch JL, Halpern EF, Hunink MGM, Gazelle GS. Elective endovascular versus open surgical repair of abdominal aortic aneurysms: systemic review of short-term results. Radiology. 2002;224:739–47.
65. Zeebregts CJ, Geelkerken RH, van der Palen J, Huisman AB, De Smit P, Van Det RJ. Outcome of abdominal aneurysm repair in the era of endovascular treatment. Br J Surg. 2004;91:563–8.
66. Eggebrecht H, Breuckmann F, Martini S, Baumgart D, Herold U, Kienbaum P, Peters J, Jakob H, Erbel R, Mehta RH. Frequency and outcomes of acute renal failure following thoracic aortic stent-graft placement. Am J Cardiol. 2006;98:458–63.
67. Parmer SS, Fairman RM, Karmacharya J, Carpenter JP, Velazquez OC, Woo EY. A comparison of renal function between open and endovascular aneurysm repair in patients with baseline chronic renal insufficiency. J Vasc Surg. 2006;44:706–11.
68. Wald R, Waikar SS, Liangos O, Pereira BJ, Chertow GM, Jaber BL. Acute renal failure after endovascular vs open repair of abdominal aortic aneurysm. J Vasc Surg. 2006;43:460–6.
69. Gahlen J, Hansmann J, Schumacher H, Seelos R, Richter GM, Allenberg JR. Carbon dioxide digital subtraction angiography for endovascular grafting in high-risk patients with infrarenal abdominal aortic aneurysm. J Vasc Surg. 2001;33:646–9.
70. Chao A, Major K, Kumar SR, Patel K, Trujillo I, Hood DB, Rowe VL, Weaver FA. Carbon dioxide subtraction angiography-assisted endovascular aortic aneurysm repair in azotemic patient. J Vasc Surg. 2007;45:451–8.
71. Blocker D, Krauss M, Mansmann U, Halawa M, Lange R, Probst T, Raither D. Incidence of renal infarction after endovascular AAA repair: relationship to infrarenal versus suprarenal fixation. J Endovasc Ther. 2003;10:1054–60.
72. Sun Z, Stevenson G. Transrenal fixation of aortic stent-grafts: short- to midterm effects on renal function. A systematic review. Radiology. 2006;240:65–72.
73. van der Laan MJ, Bartels LW, Bakker CJ, Viergever MA, Blankensteijn JD. Suitability of 7 aortic stent-graft models for MRI-based surveillance. J Endovasc Ther. 2004;11:366–71.
74. Davies RR, Gallo A, Coady MA, Tellides G, Botta DM, Burke B, Coe MP, Kopf GS, Elefteriades JA. Novel measurement of relative aortic size predicts rupture of thoracic aortic aneurysms. Ann Thorac Surg. 2006;81:169–77.
75. Dake MD, Miller DC, Semba CP, Mitchell RS, Walker PJ, Liddell RP. Transluminal placement of endovascular stent-grafts for the treatment of descending thoracic aortic aneurysms. N Engl J Med. 1994;331:1729–34.
76. Nienaber CA, Fattori R, Lund G, Dieckmann C, Wolf W, von Kodolitsch Y, Nicolas V, Pierangeli A. Nonsurgical reconstruction of thoracic aortic dissection by stent-graft placement. N Engl J Med. 1999;340:1539–45.
77. Ince H, Petzsch M, Rehders T, Kische S, Körber T, Weber F, Nienaber CA. Percutaneous endovascular repair of aneurysm after previous coarctation surgery. Circulation. 2003;108:2967–70.
78. Makaroun MS, Dillavou ED, Kee ST, Sicard G, Chaikof E, Bavaria J, Williams D, Cambria RP, Mitchell RS. Endovascular treatment of thoracic aortic aneurysms: results of the phase II multicenter trial of the GORE TAG thoracic endoprosthesis. J Vasc Surg. 2005;41:1–9.
79. Wheatley 3rd GH, Gurbuz AT, Rodriguez-Lopez JA, Ramaiah VG, Olsen D, Williams J, Diethrich EB. Midterm outcome in 158 consecutive Gore TAG thoracic endoprostheses: single center experience. Ann Thorac Surg. 2006;81:1570–7.
80. Fattori R, Nienaber CA, Rousseau H, Beregi JP, Heijmen R, Grabenwöger M, Piquet P, Lovato L, Dabbech C, Kische S, Gaxotte V, Schepens M, Ehrlich M, Bartoli JM, Talent Thoracic Retrospective Registry. Results of endovascular repair of the thoracic aorta with the Talent Thoracic stent graft: the Talent Thoracic Retrospective Registry. J Thorac Cardiovasc Surg. 2006;132:332–9.
81. Demers P, Miller DC, Mitchell RS, Kee ST, Sze D, Razavi MK, Dake MD. Midterm results of endovascular repair of descending thoracic aortic aneurysms with first-generation stent grafts. J Thorac Cardiovasc Surg. 2004;127:664–7.
82. Kazui T, Washiyama N, Muhammad BA, Terada H, Yamashita K, Takinami M. Improved results of atherosclerotic arch aneurysm operation with a refined technique. J Thorac Cardiovasc Surg. 2001;121:491–9.
83. Spielvogel D, Halstead JC, Meier M, Kadir I, Lansman SL, Shahani R, Griepp RB. Aortic arch replacement using a trifurcated graft: simple versatile, and safe. Ann Thorac Surg. 2005;80:90–5.
84. Nakai M, Shimamoto M, Yamazaki F, Fujita S, Aoyama A, Chin T, Nakata T, Yamada T. Long-term results after surgery for aortic arch non-dissection aneurysm. Kyobu Geka. 2002;55:280–4.
85. Czerny M, Zimpfer D, Fleck T, Hofmann W, Schoder M, Cejna M, Stampfl P, Lammer J, Wolner E, Grabenwoger M. Initial results after combined repair of aortic arch aneurysms by sequential transposition of the supra-aortic branches and consecutive endovascular stent-graft placement. Ann Thorac Surg. 2004;78:1256–60.
86. Schumacher H, Von Tengg-Kobligk H, Ostovic M, Henninger V, Ockert S, Böckler D, Allenberg JR. Hybrid arch procedures for endoluminal arch replacement in thoracic aneurysms and type B dissection. J Cardiovasc Surg (Torino). 2006;47:509–17.
87. Saleh HM, Inglese L. Combined surgical and endovascular treatment of aortic arch aneurysms. J Vasc Surg. 2006;44:460–6.
88. Czerny M, Gottardi R, Zimpfer D, Schoder M, Grabenwoger M, Lammer J, Wolner E, Grimm M. Transposition of the supraaortic branches for extended endovascular arch repair. Eur J Cardiothorac Surg. 2006;29:709–13.
89. Isselbacher EM. Thoracic and abdominal aortic aneurysms. Circulation. 2005;111:816–28.
90. Fann JI, Miller DC. Endovascular treatment of descending thoracic aortic aneurysms and dissections. Surg Clin North Am. 1999;79:551–74.
91. Dake MD, Miller DC, Mitchell RS, Semba CP, Moore KA, Sakai T. The "first generation" of endovascular stent grafts for patients with aneurysms of the descending thoracic aorta. J Thorac Cardiovasc Surg. 1998;116:689–703.

92. Rehders TC, Petzsch M, Ince H, Kische S, Korber T, Koschyk DH, Chatterjee T, Weber F, Nienaber CA. Intentional occlusion of the left subclavian artery during stent-graft implantation in the thoracic aorta: risks and relevance. J Endovasc Ther. 2004; 11:659–66.
93. Peterson BG, Eskandari MK, Gleason TG, Morasch MD. Utility of left subclavian artery revascularization in association with endoluminal repair of acute and chronic thoracic aortic pathology. J Vasc Surg. 2006;43:433–9.
94. Volodos' NL, Shekhanin VE, Karpovich IP, Troian VI, Gur'ev IA. A self-fixing synthetic blood vessel endoprosthesis. Vestn Khir Im I I Grek. 1986;137:123–5.
95. Eggebrecht H, Nienaber CA, Neuhäuser M, Baumgart D, Kische S, Schmermund A, Herold U, Rehders TC, Jakob HG, Erbel R. Endovascular stent-graft placement in aortic dissection: a meta-analysis. Eur Heart J. 2006;27:489–98.
96. Leurs LJ, Bell R, Degrieck Y, Thomas S, Hobo R, Lundbom J, EUROSTAR; UK Thoracic Endograft Registry Collaborators. Endovascular treatment of thoracic aortic diseases: combined experience from the EUROSTAR and United Kingdom Thoracic Endografting registries. J Vasc Surg. 2004;40: 670–9.
97. Cartes-Zumelzu F, Lammer J, Kretschmer G, Hoelzenbein T, Grabenwöger M, Thurnher S. Endovascular repair of thoracic aortic aneurysms. Semin Interv Cardiol. 2000;5:53–7.
98. Heijmen RH, Deblier IG, Moll FL, Dossche KM, van den Berg JC, Overtoom TT, Ernst SM, Schepens MA. Endovascular stent-grafting for descending thoracic aortic aneurysms. Eur J Cardiothorac Surg. 2002;21:5–9.
99. Qu L, Raithel D. Two-year single-center experience with thoracic endovascular repair using the EndoFit thoracic stent-graft. J Endovasc Ther. 2008;15:530–8.
100. Hughes GC, Lee SM, Daneshmand MA, Bhattacharya SD, Williams JB, Tucker Jr SW, McCann RL. Endovascular repair of descending thoracic aneurysms: results with "on-label" application in the post Food and Drug Administration approval era. Ann Thorac Surg. 2010;90:83–9.
101. Stone DH, Brewster DC, Kwolek CJ, Lamuraglia GM, Conrad MF, Chung TK, Cambria RP. Stent-graft versus open-surgical repair of the thoracic aorta: mid-term results. J Vasc Surg. 2006;44:1188–97.
102. Bavaria JE, Appoo JJ, Makaroun MS, Verter J, Yu ZF, Mitchell RS, Gore TAG Investigators. Endovascular stent-grafting versus open surgical repair of descending thoracic aortic aneurysms in low-risk patients: a multicenter comparative trial. J Thorac Cardiovasc Surg. 2007;133:369–77.
103. Coady MA, Rizzo JA, Hammond GL, Pierce JG, Kopf GS, Elefteriades JA. Penetrating ulcers of the thoracic aorta: what is it? How do we recognize it? How do we manage it? J Vasc Surg. 1998;27:1006–15.
104. Vilacosta I, San Román JA, Aragoncillo P, Ferreirós J, Mendez R, Graupner C, Batlle E, Serrano J, Pinto A, Oyonarte JM. Penetrating atherosclerotic aortic ulcer: documentation by transesophageal echocardiography. J Am Coll Cardiol. 1998;32:83–9.
105. Hayashi H, Matsuoka Y, Sakamoto I, Sueyoshi E, Okimoto T, Hayashi K, Matsunaga N. Penetrating atherosclerotic ulcer of the aorta: imaging features and disease concept. Radiographics. 2000;20:995–1005.
106. Tittle SL, Lynch RJ, Cole PE, Singh HS, Rizzo JA, Kopf GS, Elefteriades JA. Midterm follow-up of penetrating ulcer and intramural hematoma of the aorta. J Thorac Cardiovasc Surg. 2002;123:1051–9.
107. Demers P, Miller DC, Mitchell RS, Kee ST, Chagonjian L, Dake MD. Stent-graft repair of penetrating atherosclerotic ulcers in the descending thoracic aorta: mid-term results. Ann Thorac Surg. 2004;77:81–6.
108. Dillavou ED, Makaroun MS. Predictors of morbidity and mortality with endovascular and open thoracic aneurysm repair. J Vasc Surg. 2008;48:1114–20.
109. Nienaber CA, Kische S, Rehders TC, Schneider H, Chatterjee T, Bünger CM, Höppner R, Ince H. Rapid pacing for better placing: comparison of techniques for precise deployment of endografts in the thoracic aorta. J Endovasc Ther. 2007;14:506–12.
110. Cho JS, Haider S, Makaroun MS. Endovascular therapy of thoracic aneurysms: gore TAG trial results. Semin Vasc Surg. 2006; 19:18–24.
111. Hagan PG, Nienaber CA, Isselbacher EM, Bruckman D, Karavite DJ, Russman PL, Evangelista A, Fattori R, Suzuki T, Oh JK, Moore AG, Malouf JF, Pape LA, Gaca C, Sechtem U, Lenferink S, Deutsch HJ, Diedrichs H, Marcos y Robles J, Llovet A, Gilon D, Das SK, Armstrong WF, Deeb GM, Eagle KA. The International Registry of Acute Aortic Dissection (IRAD): new insights into an old disease. JAMA. 2000;283:897–903.
112. Erbel R, Alfonso F, Boileau C, Dirsch O, Eber B, Haverich A, Rakowski H, Struyven J, Radegran K, Sechtem U, Taylor J, Zollikofer C, Klein WW, Mulder B, Providencia LA, Task Force on Aortic Dissection, European Society of Cardiology. Diagnosis and management of aortic dissection. Eur Heart J. 2001;22: 1642–81.
113. Svensson LG, Kouchoukos NT, Miller DC, Bavaria JE, Coselli JS, Curi MA, Eggebrecht H, Elefteriades JA, Erbel R, Gleason TG, Lytle BW, Mitchell RS, Nienaber CA, Roselli EE, Safi HJ, Shemin RJ, Sicard GA, Sundt 3rd TM, Szeto WY, Wheatley 3rd GH, Society of Thoracic Surgeons Endovascular Surgery Task Force. Expert consensus document on the treatment of descending thoracic aortic disease using endovascular stent-grafts. Ann Thorac Surg. 2008;85:S1–41.
114. Kodama K, Nishigami K, Sakamoto T, Sawamura T, Hirayama T, Misumi H, Nakao K. Tight heart rate control reduces secondary adverse events in patients with type B acute aortic dissection. Circulation. 2008;118 Suppl 1:S167–70.
115. Warnes CA, Williams RG, Bashore TM, et al. American College of Cardiology; American Heart Association Task Force on Practice Guidelines (Writing Committee to Develop Guidelines on the Management of Adults with Congenital Heart Disease); American Society of Echocardiography; Heart Rhythm Society; International Society for Adult Congenital Heart Disease; Society for Cardiovascular Angiography and Interventions; Society of Thoracic Surgeons. ACC/AHA 2008 guidelines for the management of adults with congenital heart disease: a report of the American College of Cardiology/American Heart Association Task Force on Practice Guidelines (Writing Committee to Develop Guidelines on the Management of Adults With Congenital Heart Disease). Developed in Collaboration with the American Society of Echocardiography, Heart Rhythm Society, International Society for Adult Congenital Heart Disease, Society for Cardiovascular Angiography and Interventions, and Society of Thoracic Surgeons. J Am Coll Cardiol. 2008;52:e143–263.
116. Ali AT, Modrall JG, Lopez J, Brawley JG, Welborn MB, Clagett GP, Valentine RJ, Jackson MR. Emerging role of endovascular grafts in complex aortoiliac occlusive disease. J Vasc Surg. 2003;38:486–91.
117. Poncyljusz W, Falkowski A, Garncarek J, Karasek M, England S, Zawierucha D. Primary stenting in the treatment of focal atherosclerotic abdominal aortic stenoses. Clin Radiol. 2006;61:691–5.
118. Ramzi Cotran S, Robbins SL, Kumar V. Robbins pathologic basis of disease. 4th ed. Philadelphia: Saunders; 1989.
119. DeLaurentis DA, Friedman P, Wolferth Jr CC. Atherosclerosis and the hypoplastic aortoiliac system. Surgery. 1978;83:27–37.
120. Constantino MJ, Smith RB, Perdue GD. Segmental aortic occlusion. An unusual lesion found in menopausal women. Arch Surg. 1979;114:317–8.

121. Nevelsteen A, Wouters I, Suy R. Aorto-femoral Dacron reconstruction for aortoiliac occlusive disease: a 25 years survey. Eur J Surg. 1991;5:179–86.
122. Ar N, Ah-See AK, Engeset J. Aortoiliac endarterectomy: an 11 year review. Br J Surg. 1990;77:190–3.
123. Rao PS. Should balloon angioplasty be used instead of surgery for native aortic coarctation? Br Heart J. 1995;74:578–9.
124. Fawzy ME, Sivanandam V, Galal O, Dunn B, Patel A, Rifai A, von Sinner W, Al Halees Z, Khan B. One- to ten-year follow-up results of balloon angioplasty of native coarctation of the aorta in adolescents and adults. J Am Coll Cardiol. 1997;30:1542–6.
125. Crafoord C, Nylin G. Congenital coarctation of the aorta and its surgical treatment. J Thorac Surg. 1945;14:347–61.
126. Bromberg BI, Beekman RH, Rocchini AP, et al. Aortic aneurysm after patch aortoplasty repair of coarctation: a prospective analysis of prevalence, screening tests and risks. J Am Coll Cardiol. 1989;14:734–41.
127. Parks WJ, Ngo TD, Plauth WH, et al. Incidence of aneurysm formation after Dacron patch aortoplasty repair for coarctation of the aorta: long term results and assessment utilizing magnetic resonance angiography with three dimensional surface rendering. J Am Coll Cardiol. 1995;26:266–71.
128. Ovaert C, Benson LN, Nykanen D, Freedom RM. Transcatheter treatment of coarctation of the aorta: a review. Pediatr Cardiol. 1998;19:27–44.
129. Cohen M, Fuster V, Steele PM, Driscoll D, McGoon DC. Coarctation of the aorta. Long term follow-up and prediction of outcome after surgical correction. Circulation. 1989;80:840–5.
130. Gibbs JL. Interventional catheterisation. Opening up I: the ventricular outflow tracts and great arteries. Heart. 2000;83:111–5.
131. Singer MI, Rowen M, Dorsey TJ. Transluminal aortic balloon angioplasty for coarctation of the aorta in the newborn. Am Heart J. 1982;103:131–2.
132. Hijazi ZM, Fahey JT, Kleinman CS, Hellenbrand WE. Balloon angioplasty for recurrent coarctation of the aorta: immediate and long term results. Circulation. 1991;84:1150–6.
133. Maheshwari S, Bruckheimer E, Fahey JT, Hellenbrand WE. Balloon angioplasty of postsurgical recoarctation in infants: the risk of restenosis and long term follow-up. J Am Coll Cardiol. 2000;35:209–13.
134. Fletcher SE, Nihill MR, Grifka RG, O'Laughlin MP, Mullins CE. Balloon angioplasty of native coarctation of the aorta: midterm follow-up and prognostic factors. J Am Coll Cardiol. 1995;25:730–4.
135. Rao PS, Galal O, Smith PA, Wilson AD. Five to nine year follow-up results of balloon angioplasty of native coarctation in infants and children. J Am Coll Cardiol. 1996;27:462–70.
136. Mendelsohn AM, Lloyd TR, Crowley DC, Sandhu SK, Kocis KC, Beekman 3rd RH. Late follow-up of balloon angioplasty in children with a native coarctation of the aorta. Am J Cardiol. 1994;74:696–700.
137. Marshall A, Perry SB, Keane JF, Lock JE. Early results and medium-term follow-up of stent implantation for mild residual or recurrent aortic coarctation. Am Heart J. 2000;139:1054–60.
138. McCrindle BW, Jones TK, Morrow WR, Hagler DJ, Lloyd TR, Nouri S, Latson LA. Acute results of balloon angioplasty of native coarctation versus recurrent aortic obstruction are equivalent. J Am Coll Cardiol. 1996;28:1810–7.
139. Tynan M, Finley JP, Fontes V, Hess J, Kan J. Balloon angioplasty for the treatment of native coarctation: results of the valvuloplasty and angioplasty of congenital anomalies registry. Am J Cardiol. 1990;65:790–2.
140. Ebeid MR, Prieto LR, Latson LA. Use of balloon expandable stents for coarctation of the aorta: initial results and intermediate term follow-up. J Am Coll Cardiol. 1997;30:1847–52.
141. Cheatham JP. Stenting of coarctation of the aorta. Catheter Cardiovasc Interv. 2001;54:112–25.
142. Magee AG, Brzezinska-Rajszys G, Qureshi SA, Rosenthal E, Zubrzycka M, Ksiazyk J, Tynan M. Stent implantation for aortic coarctation and recoarctation. Heart. 1999;82:600–6.
143. Thanopoulos BD, Hadjinikolaou L, Konstadopoulou GN, Tsaousis GS, Triposkiadis F, Spirou P. Stent treatment for coarctation of the aorta: intermediate term follow-up and technical considerations. Heart. 2000;84:65–70.
144. Hamdan MA, Maheshwari S, Fahey JT, Hellenbrand WE. Endovascular stents for coarctation of the aorta: initial results and intermediate term follow-up. J Am Coll Cardiol. 2001;38:1518–23.
145. De Lezo JS, Pan M, Romero M. Immediate and follow-up findings after stent treatment for severe coarctation of aorta. Am J Cardiol. 1999;83:400–6.
146. Varma C, Benson LN, Butany J, McLaughlin PR. Aortic dissection after stent dilatation for coarctation of the aorta: a case report and literature review. Catheter Cardiovasc Interv. 2003;59:528–35.
147. Carr JA. The results of catheter-based therapy compared with surgical repair of adult aortic coarctation. J Am Coll Cardiol. 2006;47:1101–7.
148. Gunn J, Cleveland T, Gaines P. Covered stent to treat coexistent coarctation and aneurysm of the aorta in a young man. Heart. 1999;82:351.
149. DeGiovanni JV. Covered stents in the treatment of aortic coarctation. J Interv Cardiol. 2001;14:187–90.
150. Qureshi SA, Zubrzycka M, Brzezinska-Rajszys G, Kosciesza A, Ksiazyk J. Use of covered Cheatham-platinum stents in aortic coarctation and recoarctation. Cardiol Young. 2004;14:50–4.
151. Ewert P, Abdul-Khalid H, Peters B, Nagdyman N, Schubert S, Lange PE. Transcatheter therapy of long extreme subatretic aortic coarctations with covered stents. Catheter Cardiovasc Interv. 2004;63:236–9.
152. Forbes T, Matisoff D, Dysart J, Aggarwal S. Treatment of coexisting coarctation and aneurysm of the aorta with covered stent in a pediatric patient. Pediatr Cardiol. 2003;24:289–91.
153. Sadiq M, Malick NH, Qureshi SA. Simultaneous treatment of native coarctation of the aorta combined with patent ductus arteriosus using a covered stent. Catheter Cardiovasc Interv. 2003;59:387–90.
154. Pedra CA, Fontes VF, Esteves CA, Arrieta SR, Braga SL, Justino H, Kambara AM, Moreira SM, Sousa JE. Use of covered stents in the management of coarctation of the aorta. Pediatr Cardiol. 2005;26:431–9.
155. Butera G, Gaio G, Carminati M. Redilation of e-PTFE covered CP stents. Catheter Cardiovasc Interv. 2008;72:273–7.
156. Butera G, Dua J, Chessa M, Carminati M. Covered Cheatham-Platinum stents for serial dilatation of severe native aortic coarctation. Catheter Cardiovasc Interv. 2010;75:472. author reply 473.
157. Butera G, Piazza L, Chessa M, Abella R, Bussadori C, Negura D, Carminati M. Covered stents in patients with congenital heart defects. Catheter Cardiovasc Interv. 2006;67:466–72.
158. Wada T, Yao H, Miyamoto T, Mukai S, Yamamura M. Prevention and detection of spinal cord injury during thoracic and thoracoabdominal aortic repairs. Ann Thorac Surg. 2001;72:80–4.
159. Connolly JE. Prevention of spinal cord complications in aortic surgery. Am J Surg. 1998;176:92–101.
160. Forbes TJ, Moore P, Pedra CA, et al. Intermediate follow-up following intravascular stenting for treatment of coarctation of the aorta. Catheter Cardiovasc Interv. 2007;70:569–77.

161. Ewert P, Schubert S, Peters B, Abdul-Khaliq H, Nagdyman N, Lange PE. The CP stent-short, long, covered-for the treatment of aortic coarctation, stenosis of pulmonary arteries and caval veins, and Fontan anastomosis in children and adults: an evaluation of 60 stents in 53 patients. Heart. 2005;91:948–53.
162. Velasquez G, Castaneda-Zuniga W, Formanek A, Zollikofer C, Barreto A, Nicoloff D, Amplatz K, Sullivan A. Nonsurgical aortoplasty in Leriche syndrome. Radiology. 1990;134:359–60.
163. Grollman Jr JH, Del Vicario M, Mittal AK. Percutaneous transluminal abdominal aortic angioplasty. AJR Am J Roentgenol. 1980;134:1053–4.
164. Tegtmeyer CJ, Wellons HA, Thompson RN. Balloon dilation of the abdominal aorta. JAMA. 1980;244:2636–7.
165. Heeney D, Bookstein J, Daniels E, Warmath M, Horn J, Rowley W. Transluminal angioplasty of the abdominal aorta: report of 6 cases in women. Radiology. 1983;148:81–3.
166. Tegtmeyer CJ, Kellum CD, Kron IL, Mentzer Jr RM. Percutaneous transluminal angioplasty in the region of the aortic bifurcation. The two-balloon technique with results and long-term follow-up study. Radiology. 1985;157:661–5.
167. Charlebois N, Saint-Georges G, Hudon G. Percutaneous transluminal angioplasty of the lower abdominal aorta. AJR Am J Roentgenol. 1986;146:369–71.
168. Morag B, Rubinstein Z, Kessler A, Schneiderman J, Levinkopf M, Bass A. Percutaneous transluminal angioplasty of the distal abdominal aorta and its bifurcation. Cardiovasc Intervent Radiol. 1987;10:129–33.
169. Yakes WF, Kumpe DA, Brown SB, Parker SH, Lattes RG, Cook PS, Haas DK, Gibson MD, Hopper KD, Reed MD. Percutaneous transluminal aortic angioplasty: techniques and results. Radiology. 1989;172:965–70.
170. Gross-Fengels W, Steinbrich W, Pichlmaier H, Erasmi H. Percutaneous transluminal angioplasty of the infrarenal abdominal aorta. Radiologe. 1990;30:235–41.
171. el Ashmaoui A, Do DD, Triller J, Stirnemann P, Mahler F. Angioplasty of the terminal aorta: follow-up of 20 patients treated by PTA or PTA with stents. Eur J Radiol. 1991;13:113–7.
172. Hallisey MJ, Meranze SG, Parker BC, Rholl KS, Miller WJ, Katzen BT, van Breda A. Percutaneous transluminal angioplasty of the abdominal aorta. J Vasc Interv Radiol. 1994;5:679–87.
173. Steinmetz OK, McPhail NV, Hajjar GE, Barber GG, Cole CW. Endarterectomy versus angioplasty in the treatment of localized stenosis of the abdominal aorta. Can J Surg. 1994;37:385–90.
174. Hedeman Joosten PP, Ho GH, Breuking Jr FA, Overtoom TT, Moll FL. Percutaneous transluminal angioplasty of the infrarenal aorta: initial outcome and long-term clinical and angiographic results. Eur J Vasc Endovasc Surg. 1996;12:201–6.
175. Westcott MA, Bonn J. Comparison of conventional angioplasty with the Palmaz stent in the treatment of abdominal aortic stenoses from the STAR registry. SCVIR transluminal angioplasty and revascularization. J Vasc Interv Radiol. 1998;9:225–31.
176. Therasse E, Cote G, Soulez G. Infrarenal aortic stenting with the Palmaz stent: midterm results. J Vasc Interv Radiol. 1989;9:169–70.
177. Long AL, Gaux JC, Raynaud AC, Faintuch JM, Pagny JY, Lacombe P, Fiessinger JN, Relland JY, Beyssen BM. Infrarenal aortic stents: initial clinical experience and angiographic follow-up. Cardiovasc Intervent Radiol. 1993;16:203–8.
178. Wolf YG, Schatz RA, Knowles HJ, Saeed M, Bernstein EF, Dilley RB. Initial experience with the Palmaz stent for aortoiliac stenoses. Ann Vasc Surg. 1993;7:254–61.
179. Yilmaz S, Sindel T, Yeğin A, Erdoğan A, Lüleci E. Primary stenting of focal atherosclerotic infrarenal aortic stenoses: long-term results in 13 patients and a literature review. Cardiovasc Intervent Radiol. 2004;27:121–8.
180. Audet P, Therasse E, Oliva VL, Soulez G, Côté G, Wistaff R, Nguyen PV, Blair JF, Bui BT, Cusson JR. Infrarenal aortic stenosis: long-term clinical and hemodynamic results of percutaneous transluminal angioplasty. Radiology. 1998;209:357–63.
181. Ravimandalam K, Rao VR, Kumar S, Gupta AK, Joseph S, Unni M, Rao AS. Obstruction of the infrarenal portion of the abdominal aorta: results of treatment with balloon angioplasty. AJR Am J Roentgenol. 1991;156:1257–60.
182. McPherson SJ, Laing AD, Thomson KR, Mitchell PJ, Milne P, Atkinson N, Cox G. Treatment of infrarenal aortic stenosis by stent placement: a 6-year experience. Australas Radiol. 1999;43(2):185–91.

35 Percutaneous Management of Carotid and Vertebral Artery Disease

Zehra Jaffery and Christopher J. White

On average, someone has a stroke every 45 s and someone dies of a stroke every 3 min [1]. Stroke is the third leading cause of death in the USA, with more than three-quarter of a million strokes/year. Stroke is a leading cause of functional impairment in adults, with approximately 20 % of survivors requiring institutional care and up to one-third having a permanent disability [2]. Approximately 80 % of strokes are ischemic (occlusive, embolic, or hemorrhagic) in origin, of which 75 % occur in the distribution of the carotid artery [3]. Approximately 20–25 % of ischemic strokes are located in the posterior circulation involving the vertebrobasilar system [3, 4]. Vertebrobasilar strokes have a worse prognosis when compared to carotid artery strokes. Basilar artery occlusion results in a very high mortality and is associated with severe disability in survivors, whereas ≤8 % of carotid artery strokes are lethal [5, 6].

Carotid Artery Disease

Etiology and Prevalence

Atherosclerosis is the most common cause of extracranial carotid artery disease. Population-based epidemiological studies using ultrasound in patients over age 65 show that the prevalence of asymptomatic atherosclerotic carotid artery stenosis ≥50 % ranges from 4 to 8 %, and 1 % of this otherwise healthy Medicare population has a stenosis ≥75 % [7, 8]. Other less common causes of carotid artery disease include inflammatory disorders such as Takayasu's arteritis [9], fibromuscular dysplasia [10], arterial dissection [8], aneurysm, and psuedoaneurysms [11]. There is very little published data on non-atherosclerotic carotid disease; therefore, their prevalence and natural history are difficult to discern. The incidence of carotid dissection is reported as 2–3 per 100,000 per year [12]. The incidence of carotid artery aneurysm ranges from 0.4 to 4 % of all peripheral artery aneurysms [13, 14].

Natural History of Atherosclerotic Carotid Disease

The risk of progression of atherosclerotic carotid stenosis (defined as an increase in stenosis ≥50 % when baseline stenosis is ≤50 % or an increase in stenosis to a higher category when baseline stenosis is ≥50 %) is 9.3 % per year [15]; however, the annual risk of stroke in asymptomatic patients with carotid artery stenosis depends on both lesion severity and on plaque morphology [16, 17], collateral circulation, patency of the Circle of Willis [18], and clinical presentation [6, 19]. Lesion characteristics per ultrasonography such as grey-scale distribution in the atherosclerotic plaque can predict risk of ipsilateral stroke. With the help of computerized quantification of the atherosclerotic plaque, a grey-scale median (GSM) may be derived, and this expresses the overall reflectance of the lesion. The risk of stroke was found to be related to the GSM value: a GSM value ≤25 when compared to a value ≥25, increased the odds of ipsilateral stroke by 7.11 ($P=0.002$) [20]. Large ulcers have also been related to a higher risk of stroke. In a study of 153 asymptomatic patients with non-stenotic carotid ulceration, an ulcer product (depth × length of the ulcer in mm) ≤10, 10–40, and ≥40 had an annual risk of stroke of 0.9, 4.5, and 7.5 % respectively [21].

Asymptomatic Patients

Natural history studies of asymptomatic ICA stenosis have reported an annual risk of ipsilateral stroke of approximately

Z. Jaffery, MD
John Ochsner Heart and Vascular Institute,
Department of Cardiovascular Diseases,
Ochsner Clinic Foundation, 1514 Jefferson Hwy,
New Orleans, LA 70121, USA

C.J. White, MD (✉)
Department of Cardiovascular Diseases, Ochsner Clinic Foundation,
1514 Jefferson Highway, New Orleans, LA 70121, USA
e-mail: cwhite@ochsner.org

C.A. Thompson (ed.), *Textbook of Cardiovascular Intervention*,
DOI 10.1007/978-1-4471-4528-8_35, © Springer-Verlag London 2014

1–3 % [22, 23]. In the Asymptomatic Carotid Surgery Trial (ACST) study, there was no relationship between the severity of the carotid stenosis and the risk of ipsilateral stroke. In the medically treated patients of the ACST trial, the 5-year risk of stroke was 9.5 % in those with 60–79 % stenosis and 9.6 % in those with 80–99 % stenosis determined by ultrasound [23].

The investigators in the Asymptomatic Carotid Stenosis and Risk of Stroke (ACSRS) study identified medical comorbidities that worsen the prognosis of asymptomatic carotid stenosis. The highest risk group (82–99 % stenosis by NASCET criteria, history of contralateral transient ischemic attacks, and serum creatinine level >0.085 mmol/l) had a 4.3 % annual ipsilateral stroke rate compared with 0.7 % in the lowest risk group patients [24].

Symptomatic Patients

Patients with carotid artery stenosis are considered symptomatic if they experience (1) a transient or permanent focal neurological deficit including retinal symptoms such as amaurosis fugax or (2) hemispheric symptoms such as contralateral weakness or numbness of an arm, leg, or face, dysarthria, and/or aphasia. The risk of recurrent stroke is highest immediately after the initial ischemic event and declines with time (returns to baseline 2–3 years after the initial qualifying cerebral event). A transient ischemic attack (TIA), defined as a neurologic event lasting <24 h, predicts a 15 % risk of stroke at 1 month and a 30 % risk of TIA, stroke, or death within 3 months [25, 26]. In the medical treatment arm of the North American Symptomatic Carotid Endarterectomy Trial (NASCET) study, the 3-year risk of ipsilateral stroke was 10 % after retinal TIAs and 20.3 % after a hemispheric TIA [27].

For symptomatic patients, the risk of stroke increases with increasing lesion severity. In the medical treatment arm of the NASCET trial of symptomatic carotid lesions, the 5-year risk of ipsilateral stroke was 18.7 % for lesions <50 % in severity, 22.2 % in those with 50–69 % stenosis, while the 2-year risk of stroke was 26 % for lesions 70–99 % [6, 28]. Consistent findings were also demonstrated in ECST [29]. In near occlusions, defined in the ECST trial as a severe stenosis with reduced flow in the distal ICA, there was a lower 1-year ipsilateral stroke risk of 11 % [30]. This low rate of events for near occlusions has generated debate over the risk to benefit ratio for revascularization in this group.

In NASCET, the medically treated symptomatic patients with severe carotid stenosis (70–99 %), with an occluded contralateral artery, were more than twice as likely to have an ipsilateral stroke at 2 years than patients with moderate <70 % (hazard ratio: 2.65; 95 % CI: 1.43–4.90) or severe ≥70–99 % (hazard ratio: 2.36; 95 % confidence interval (CI): 1.00–5.62) contralateral carotid artery stenosis (Fig. 35.1) [31]. In both NASCET and ECST trials, the risk of ipsilateral stroke declined 2–3 years after the initial qualifying cerebral event to an annual level of 1–2 % irrespective of the severity of stenosis [6, 28, 29].

Diagnosis of Carotid Disease

Indications for Screening

In asymptomatic patients, there are no guidelines to support routine screening for atherosclerotic carotid artery disease. In patients with carotid bruits discovered on routine examination, further diagnostic tests for identification of carotid disease are recommended if they are candidates for carotid revascularization [1]. In patients scheduled for coronary artery bypass graft surgery (CABG), screening for carotid stenosis is recommended in patients older than 65 years, those with left main coronary stenosis, known peripheral arterial disease, a history of smoking, a history of TIA or stroke, or in the presence of a carotid bruit [32]. Patients with transient retinal or hemispheric neurological deficits should be screened for extracranial carotid artery disease [1, 32].

Diagnostic Modalities

Current management decisions for atherosclerotic carotid disease depend heavily on the severity of luminal stenosis. Therefore, accurate grading of stenosis severity is essential to good decision-making.

Noninvasive Testing

The three noninvasive modalities used for diagnosis of carotid disease are Doppler ultrasound (DUS), magnetic resonance angiography (MRA), and computerized tomographic angiography (CTA). Among the noninvasive imaging techniques, DUS is the most widely available, least toxic, and least expensive. It has been established as an accurate method of assessing carotid stenosis and provides reliable information on the localization and degree of stenosis, plaque structure, and vessel wall characteristics [33, 34]. Diagnostic accuracy of DUS is limited by operator skill and has susceptibility to artifacts from calcified plaques [35]. In addition, it does not provide an overview of vascular anatomy and surrounding structures [36]. Although consensus criteria for interpreting carotid duplex ultrasound results have been published [37], it is important to note that data obtained by individual vascular laboratories will vary owing to differences in equipment, ability, and consistency of vascular technicians and reader interpretability. Therefore, each vascular laboratory needs to internally validate their criteria for definition of carotid stenosis [38]. A meta-analysis of 64 series comparing DUS with digital subtraction angiography (DSA) found a sensitivity of 86 % and a specificity of 87 % for detecting stenosis of 70–99 % by NASCET criteria [39].

MRA can quantify carotid stenosis noninvasively and does not expose the patient to ionizing radiation or ionizing contrast. There is concern about administering gadolinium to patients with renal insufficiency. MRA offers 3D reconstructions of the carotid artery and the possibility of "one-stop" brain imaging. MRA, however, tends to overestimate the degree of stenosis [39]. A meta-analysis of 17 studies looking

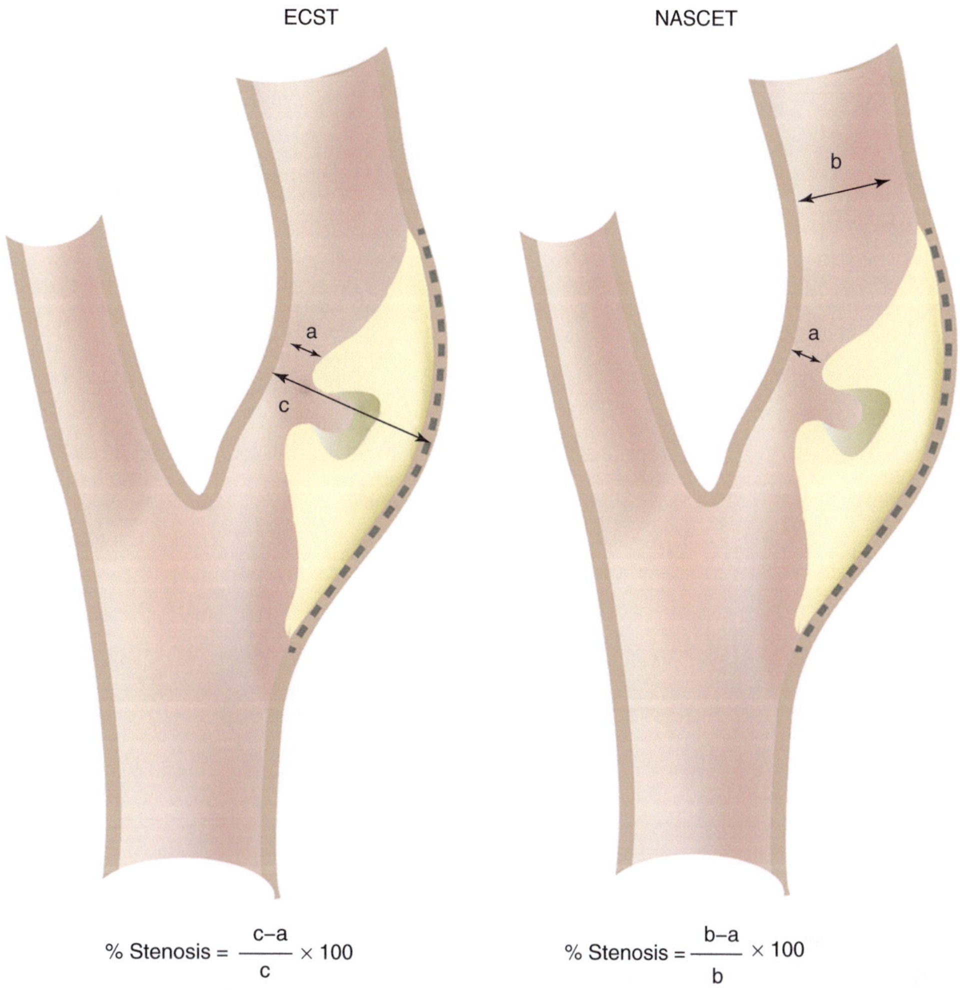

Fig. 35.1 Assessment of severity of carotid stenosis. The NASCET uses the formula b – a/b × 100, where *a* is the residual luminal diameter at the stenosis and *b* is the luminal diameter at a visible, disease-free point above the stenosis. The ECST uses the formula c – a/c × 100, where *c* is the estimated luminal diameter at the level of the lesion based on a visual impression of where the normal arterial wall was before development of the stenosis

at 1,714 carotids in 905 patients comparing contrast-enhanced MRA (CE-MRA) with DSA found a sensitivity of 94 % and a specificity of 92 % for identification of carotid stenosis of 70–99 % by NASCET criteria [40].

CTA exposes the patient to both ionizing radiation and iodinated contrast, but has several advantages over DUS and MRA. CTA has a better spatial resolution than MRA, is less susceptible to artifacts, and details vascular anatomy. A meta-analysis comparing CTA with DSA found sensitivity ranging from 85 to 92 % and specificity ranging from 93 to 97 % for detecting stenosis of 70–99 % by NASCET criteria [41, 42].

Invasive Testing

DSA is considered the gold standard in terms of assessment of luminal stenosis. Cerebral catheter-based angiography carries a risk of cerebral infarction of 0.5–1.2 %; therefore, noninvasive imaging should be the initial strategy for evaluation [19, 43]. Vascular access is most commonly obtained from the femoral artery although brachial or radial access may be used (Fig. 35.2). Prior to selective arch angiography, an arch aortogram is performed with a pigtail catheter placed in the proximal ascending aorta to define the anatomy of the aortic arch. This is done in

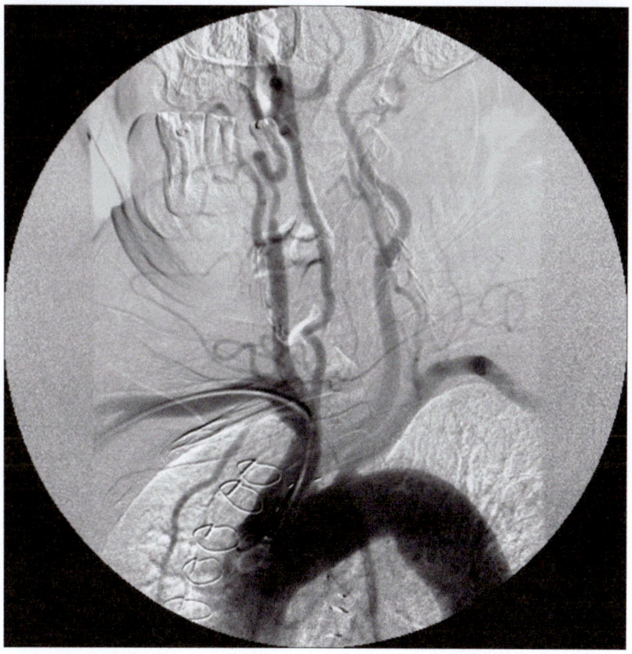

Fig. 35.2 Radial access for aortic arch angiography

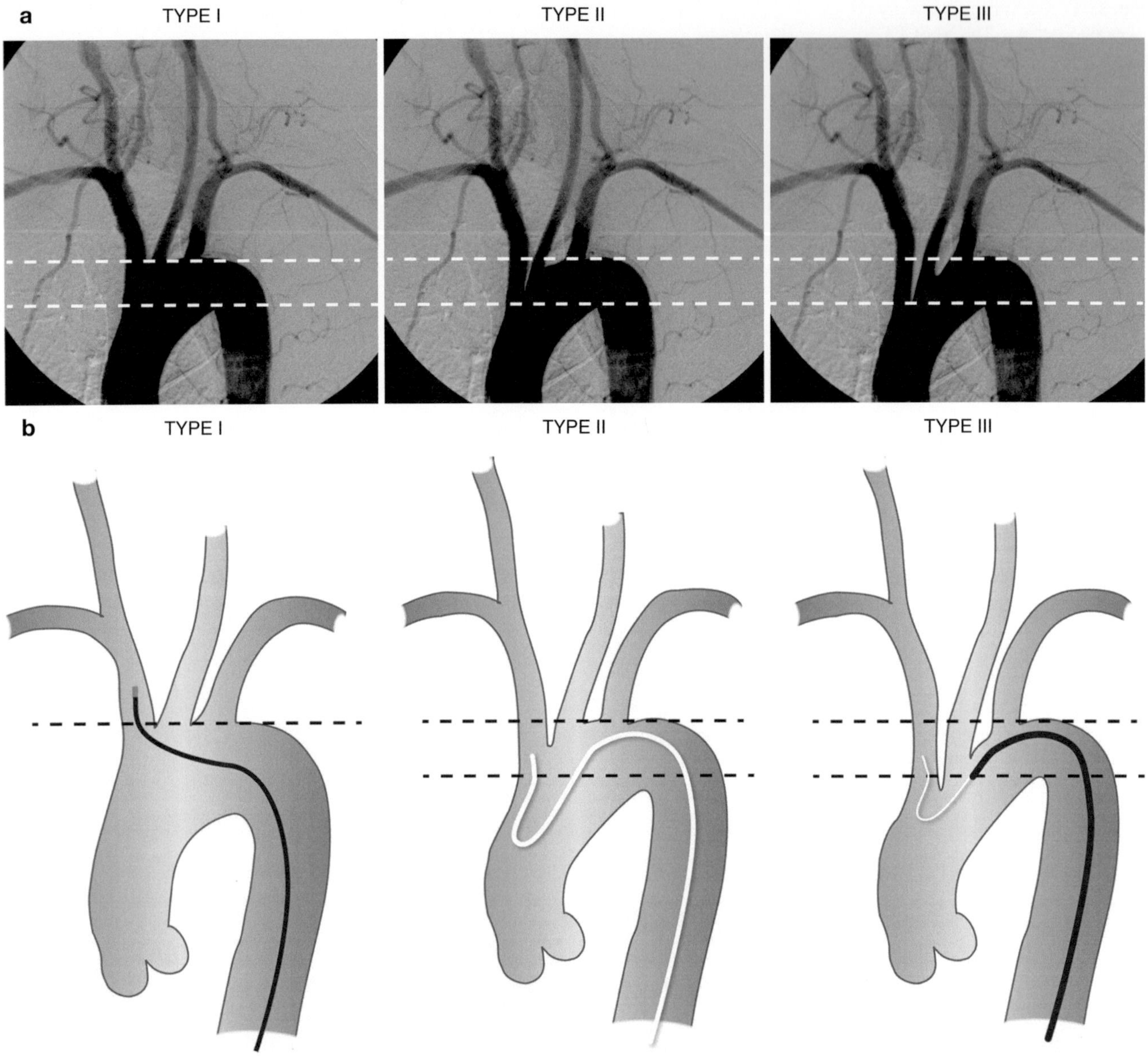

Fig. 35.3 (**a**) Aortic arch morphologies. Type I arch: all vessels originate at the superior margin of the arch. Type II arch: at least 1 vessel originates between the superior and inferior margins of the aortic arch. Type III arch: at least 1 vessel originates below the inferior margin of the aortic arch. (**b**) Aortic arch morphologies with different catheters used to access the right innominate artery. A JR 4 catheter is used in a type 1 arch, Simmons catheter for a type 2 arch, and Vitek catheter for a type 3 arch

the 45° left anterior oblique (LAO) position with a large-format image intensifier (12-in. to 16-in.) using DSA (15 cm^3 per second for 3 s) and a power injector. Once the morphology of the aortic arch is determined (Fig. 35.3a), catheters are chosen for selective angiography of the cervical arteries supplying the brain (right and left carotid and vertebral arteries) and the cerebral vasculature (Fig. 35.3b). In a type I arch, Berenstein or Judkins Right (JR) catheters are often used. In type II or III arch morphologies, shepherd's crook-shaped catheters, i.e., Simmons or Vitek catheters, may be best (Fig. 35.4).

Angiograms are obtained to delineate the anterior and posterior circulation supplying the brain. The intracranial and extracranial portions of each vessel are studied. We routinely obtain three views of carotid bifurcation (anterior, lateral, and a 45° oblique views). Alternatively, some operators use rotational angiography imaging a 90° arc with a single injection. It is important to demonstrate the anatomy of the Circle of Willis to define any baseline abnormalities. DSA may be performed with diluted contrast, using a 1:1 mix of saline and contrast. A reference object is used with carotid angiograms in order to accurately measure the diameter of the artery. The NASCET criteria for measuring carotid stenosis have become the international standard methodology (Fig. 35.1).

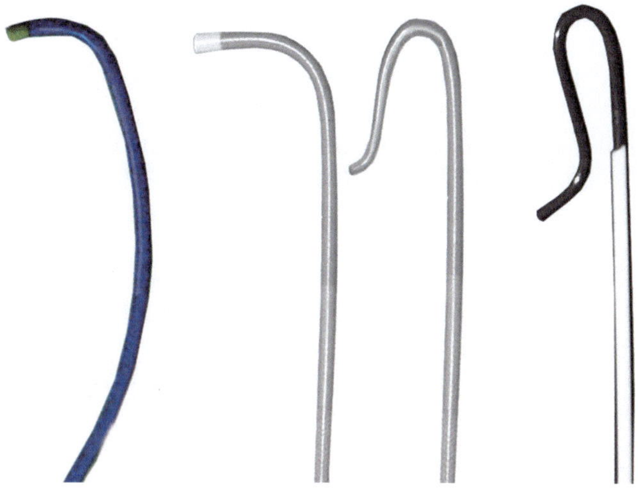

Fig. 35.4 Catheters for accessing the carotid artery. Berenstein or JR 4 catheters are usually best for a type 1 arch. Simmons and Vitek catheter may be best for type 2 or type 3 arches

Medical Therapy

Atherosclerotic risk factor management is recommended for patients with documented atherosclerotic carotid stenosis similar to that for patients with coronary artery disease. This includes blood pressure (BP) control, glycemic control in diabetics, statins for management of dyslipidemia, and cessation of smoking and heavy alcohol consumption [44]. The optimal antihypertensive drug regimen remains uncertain. The recently published extracranial carotid and vertebral artery disease guidelines have recommended a BP goal of less than 140/90 [45]. In patients with symptomatic carotid stenosis, a goal low-density cholesterol (LDL) level of <70 mg/dl or a reduction of at least 50 % in LDL is recommended [44, 46]. In patients with an ischemic stroke or TIA, aspirin monotherapy (50–325 mg/day), aspirin 25 mg and dipyridamole 200 mg twice daily, or aspirin 25 mg and clopidogrel 75 mg daily are all acceptable options for initial therapy. In patients presenting with an ischemic stroke on daily aspirin, there is no benefit for increasing the daily dose of aspirin or adding another antiplatelet agent (clopidogrel or dipyridamole). In patients with underlying symptomatic carotid dissection, antithrombotic treatment (unfractionated heparin, low molecular weight heparin, or Coumadin) for 3–6 months is reasonable [44].

Clinical Trials

Large-scale randomized trials (RTs) have been conducted to compare medical treatment with surgical revascularization in patients with both asymptomatic and symptomatic atherosclerotic carotid artery stenoses. There is current debate whether more aggressive modern anti-atherosclerotic therapy would reduce the magnitude of benefit shown for surgery in the earlier trials.

In the last decade, percutaneous treatment of carotid stenosis with protected carotid artery stenting (CAS) has emerged as an attractive alternative to carotid endarterectomy (CEA). Data on over 24,000 patients undergoing CAS have been published. In addition, more than 12 RTs and several industry-sponsored CAS registries have described outcomes of CAS in patients for patients at average and high risk for CEA [47]. Patients at increased risk for CEA are defined by anatomic characteristics and medical comorbidities as outlined in Table 35.1.

Table 35.1 High-risk criteria for carotid endarterectomy per clinical expert consensus document 2007

Anatomic criteria	Medical comorbidities
Lesion at C-2 or higher	Age ≥ 80
Lesion below clavicle	NYHA class 111/1V congestive heart failure
Prior radical neck surgery or irradiation	CCS class 111/1V angina
Contralateral carotid occlusion	Left main/≥2 vessel coronary artery disease
Prior ipsilateral carotid endarterectomy	Urgent <30 days heart surgery
Contralateral laryngeal nerve palsy	Left ventricular ejection fraction ≤30 %
Tracheostoma	Recent (<30 days) myocardial infarction
	Severe chronic lung disease
	Severe renal disease

Medical Therapy Versus CEA in Asymptomatic Patients

Three randomized trials compared carotid endarterectomy (CEA) plus aspirin with aspirin alone in asymptomatic patients. In the VACS trial, 444 men with asymptomatic stenosis of ≥50 % by angiography (NASCET criteria) were randomized to medical therapy plus CEA or medical therapy alone [48]. There was no difference in ipsilateral stroke (CEA 4.7 % vs. medical 9.4 %, P=NS) or combined end point of stroke and death (CEA 41.2 % vs. medical 44.2 % P=NS) at a mean follow-up of 4 years.

The ACAS trial randomized 1,662 patients with asymptomatic carotid stenosis of ≥60 % by angiography (NASCET criteria) to medical therapy plus CEA or medical therapy alone [19]. The estimated 5-year risk of ipsilateral stroke and any perioperative stroke or death was 11.0 % for the medical group and 5.1 % for the surgical group (relative risk reduction 53 %, 95 % CI, 22–72 %, $P=0.004$). The risk of stroke and death for patients undergoing CEA was the highest during the first month after endarterectomy, whereas the risk for medical patients was evenly distributed throughout 5 years.

Using ACAS eligibility requirements, 19 surgeries would be necessary to prevent one stroke over 5 years. Although not statistically significant, the benefit of CEA was greater in men when compared to women (reduction of 5-year event rate; men 66 %, 95 % CI, 36–82 % vs. women 17 %, 95 % CI, –96–65 %, $P=0.10$). There was no relationship for risk of stroke and increasing percent stenosis in the medical treatment group. A post hoc analysis suggested that CEA in patients with contralateral occlusion provides no long-term benefit and may be harmful [49].

ACST evaluated 3,120 asymptomatic patients with ≥60 % carotid stenosis by ultrasound [23]. The risk of perioperative stroke or death was 3.1 % (95 % CI 2.3–4.1 %). The 5-year risk of perioperative death or total stroke was reduced from 11.8 to 6.4 % with CEA. The benefit of surgery was significant for both men and women and across varying degrees of stenosis (60–99 % stenosis). The 10-year risk of perioperative stroke or death was reduced from 17.9 to 13.4 % with CEA [50]. Half of this reduction was in disabling or fatal strokes.

Medical Therapy Versus CEA in Symptomatic Patients

Three large studies have been performed evaluating the benefit of CEA versus medical therapy in symptomatic patients with carotid artery disease. In these trials, medical therapy included smoking cessation, antiplatelet, antihypertensive, and lipid-lowering agents. However, similar to trials in patients with asymptomatic carotid stenosis, the end points of medical treatment were not specified, and the nature of the medical treatment varied with the time of patient enrollment and randomization [28, 29].

The VA 309 trial screened 5,000 men who presented within 4 months with a small stroke, TIA, or transient monocular blindness and randomized 189 to either CEA with best medical therapy or best medical therapy alone [51]. These patients had angiographically defined internal carotid stenosis >50 %. This trial was ended prematurely when early results from NASCET and ECST confirmed the significant benefit of CEA. At a mean follow-up of 1 year, there was a reduction in ipsilateral stroke or TIA from 19.4 % in the medical treatment arm to 7.7 % in the surgical arm ($P=0.011$).

The NASCET trial investigators randomized 2,885 patients with a TIA or non-disabling stroke within 180 days of enrollment to CEA with medical therapy or medical therapy alone. Patients were originally stratified according to the degree of stenosis: <50, 50–69, and 70–99 %. After randomizing 659 patients with ≥70 % stenosis, that portion of the study was concluded. CEA demonstrated an absolute risk reduction of 17 % (26 % vs. 9 %, $P<0.001$) in the rate of ipsilateral stroke at 2 years [6, 52]. Among patients with a 50–69 % stenosis, there was an absolute risk reduction of 6.5 % in the rate of ipsilateral stroke in those treated with CEA (22.7 % vs. 15.7 %, $P=0.04$) after 5-year follow-up [28]. In patients with <50 % stenosis, there was no benefit for CEA compared to medical therapy. The 5-year rate of ipsilateral stroke was 18.7 % in those treated medically and 14.9 % in those treated with CEA ($P=0.16$) [28]. For patients with stenosis >70 %, the perioperative risk of stroke or death was 5.8 %, whereas for those with stenosis 50–69 %, it was 6.7 %. The number needed to treat to prevent 1 stroke in a 2-year period was 8 for patients with stenosis >70 % and 20 for patients with stenosis 50–69 %.

The ESCT trial investigators randomized 3,024 patients with a TIA or non-disabling stroke within 180 days of enrollment to CEA with medical therapy or medical therapy alone [29]. In patients with ≥80 % stenosis by ESCT criteria (70 % stenosis by NASCET criteria), the rate of major stroke or death at 3 years was 26.5 % in the medical therapy group and 14.9 % in the CEA group, an absolute reduction of 11.6 % favoring surgery ($P<0.001$). There was no benefit for patients who had near occlusion of the carotid artery. The perioperative risk of stroke or death was 7.0 %.

Current Recommendations for Carotid Endarterectomy

Based on the above data, CEA has been established as the preferred treatment to prevent stroke for average surgical risk symptomatic patients with ≥50 % carotid stenosis [28, 29] and average-risk asymptomatic patients with ≥60 % carotid stenosis [19, 23, 48] compared with medical therapy provided the perioperative risk of stroke and death do not exceed 3 % for asymptomatic patients and 6 % for symptomatic patients. Symptomatic patients should undergo CEA within 14 days of presenting event provided there are no contraindications for revascularization. Asymptomatic patients undergoing CEA should have a life expectancy of more than 5 years [44].

CEA Versus CAS in High-Risk Patients

The Stenting and Angioplasty with Protection in Patients at High Risk for Endarterectomy (SAPPHIRE) was a multicenter, prospective RT that compared CAS with an embolic protection device (EPD) to CEA in patients at increased risk for surgery [53]. To be included, patients had to have symptomatic stenosis ≥50 % by angiography or asymptomatic stenosis ≥80 % by ultrasound with one or more high-risk features (Table 35.1) and be eligible for either CEA or CAS. Investigators in this trial had a median experience of 64 CAS procedures (range 20–700). Of 747 patients randomized, 334 were eligible for either CAS or CEA and entered the trial, and 413 patients were entered into a registry. Among 334 patients randomized, 167 underwent CEA and CAS, respectively. The primary end point of the trial was the cumulative incidence of death, stroke, or myocardial infarction within

30 days after the procedure or death or ipsilateral stroke between 31 days and 1 year. The 30-day death or stroke rate was 5.6 % for CEA and 4.8 % for CAS. Rates of 30-day MI were higher, although statistically nonsignificant, for CEA when compared to CAS (6.1 % CEA, 2.4 % CAS, $P=0.10$). At 1 year, the primary composite end point was reached in 20.1 % of patients with CEA as compared to 12.2 % patients with CAS ($P=0.048$ for non-inferiority). In addition, target vessel revascularization at 1 year (CEA 4.3 %, CAS 0.6 %, $P=0.04$) and cranial nerve palsy rates (CEA 4.9 %, CAS 0 %, $P=0.03$) favored stenting. On the basis of this data, in April 2004, an FDA panel advisory recommended approval of the devices used in this trial. Three-year follow-up of the SAPPHIRE trial continues to show no differences for the primary end point between CEA and CAS (CEA 30.3 %, CAS 24.6 %, $P=0.27$) [54].

Following FDA approval of carotid stent systems for symptomatic high surgical risk patients with ≥70 % carotid stenosis, several post-market surveillance registries have been launched. An overview of RTs and registries for patients undergoing CAS is provided in Table 35.2 and Fig. 35.5.

CEA Versus CAS in Average-Risk Patients

The Carotid and Vertebral Artery Transluminal Angioplasty Study (CAVATAS) trial, published in 2001, was the first multicenter clinical trial which randomized 504 symptomatic patients at average risk for CEA in 22 centers to CEA (253 patients) or endovascular revascularization (251 patients) [55]. In patients with technically successful endovascular revascularization, stents were used in only 26 % (55/213). The 30-day outcome of death and stroke was equivalent for both CEA and CAS (10 %). CEA had a higher rate of cranial nerve palsy and hematoma as compared to CAS (cranial nerve palsy 9 % CEA vs. 0 % CAS, $P<0.0001$; hematoma 7 % CEA vs. 1 % CAS, $P<0.0015$). The 1-year death or stroke rate was comparable, 13.4 % CEA versus 14.3 % CAS, P=NS. The 1-year restenosis rate (>70–99 %) was 14 % for CAS as compared to 4 % for CEA ($P<0.001$). At 3-year follow-up, no difference in the rate of death or stroke was noted (14.2 % CEA vs. 14.3 % CAS, P=NS) [56].

Several multicenter randomized trials (RTs) comparing CAS to CEA for average surgical risk patients with both symptomatic and asymptomatic carotid stenoses have been published, while others are ongoing (Table 35.2). The Stent-Supported Percutaneous Angioplasty of the Carotid Artery versus Endarterectomy (SPACE) trial was designed to prove non-inferiority of CAS as compared to CEA in average surgical risk symptomatic patients with ≥50 % carotid stenosis by angiography [57]. It was a multinational, multicenter RT with the primary end point of ipsilateral stroke or death between randomization and 30-day follow-up. Initially, 1,200 patients were randomized between March 2001 and Feb 2006 (595 patients to CEA and 605 patients to CAS). Tutoring of inexperienced interventionalists enrolling study patients was permitted. Surgeons had to provide proof of 25 consecutive carotid endarterectomy procedures. At the time of an interim analysis, the primary end point occurred in 6.4 % of patients randomized to CEA and 6.8 % randomized to CAS (P=NS). The incidence of any stroke was 6.2 % in CEA and 7.5 % in CAS (P=NS). Importantly, EPDs were used in only 27 % of cases. Although no difference was seen between CAS and CEA, this analysis showed that 2,500 patients would be needed to prove non-inferiority of CAS. The SPACE steering committee acknowledged a lack of funds sufficient to enroll the requisite number of patients and suspended the trial.

The Endarterectomy Versus Angioplasty in patients with Symptomatic Severe carotid Stenosis (EVA-3S) trial was similar to the SPACE trial in that it was a RT designed to assess non-inferiority of CAS as compared to CEA in average-risk symptomatic patients with carotid stenosis [58]. The symptomatic carotid stenosis threshold was increased to >60 %. This was a multicenter trial conducted in France from 2000 to 2005. The primary end point was the incidence of 30-day death or any stroke. The trial was stopped after enrolling 527 of the intended 872 patients for reasons of safety and futility. Two hundred and sixty-two patients underwent CEA and 265 received CAS. The primary end point was lower in patients undergoing CEA as compared to CAS (3.8 % CEA vs. 9.4 % CAS, $P=0.01$), and EVA-3S concluded that CAS was inferior to CEA for symptomatic patients with carotid stenosis >60 %. Critics of this study point to the fact that trial operators certified to perform CAS could have little (5 prior cases) or no experience (interventions performed with a tutor), and EPDs were used in a minority of the trial, after 5 out of 20 patients treated without EPD suffered a stroke. This resulted in protocol changes by the EVA-3S safety committee. At 4-year follow-up, excluding periprocedural complications, rates of death or any stroke were comparable between CEA and CAS (HR 1.39, 95% CI 0.96–2.00; $P=0.08$) [58].

The International Carotid Stenting Study (ICSS) was another European RT that enrolled 1,713 (CAS=855 or CEA=858) symptomatic patients at average risk for CEA with carotid stenosis >50 % by angiography (NASCET criteria) [59]. Amazingly for a modern trial, the use of EPDs was optional. To qualify as an experienced center, a surgeon must have performed 50 CEA procedures and an interventionalist (physician or surgeon), 10 CAS procedures. However, if the center had no CAS experience, they could still enroll patients into the trial if they were tutored by a proctor.

The primary outcome of ICSS was the 3-year rate of any fatal or disabling stroke. The 3-month interim analysis demonstrated a similar result between the two groups (4.0 % for CAS and 3.2 % for CEA, $P=0.34$). The 120-day rate of death, stroke, or MI was 8.5 % in the CAS group and 5.2 % in the CEA group ($P=0.006$).

Table 35.2 Randomized trials of Carotid Artery Stenting

Variable	SAPPHIRE¶	CREST	ICSS	EVA-3S	SPACE	Kentucky 2001	Wallstent	BACASS	KENTUCKY 2004	CAVATAS	LEICESTER
	N=334			*N*=527	*N*=1183	*N*=104	*N*=219	*N*=20	*N*=85	*N*=504	*N*=17
Inclusion Criteria	High-risk CEA with symptomatic carotid stenosis ≥50 % or asymptomatic carotid stenosis ≥80 %	Symptomatic carotid stenosis ≥50 % Asymptomatic carotid stenosis ≥60 %	Symptomatic carotid stenosis >50 %	Symptomatic carotid stenosis ≥60 %	Symptomatic carotid stenosis ≥50 %	Symptomatic carotid stenosis >70 %	Symptomatic carotid stenosis >60 %	Symptomatic carotid stenosis ≥70 %	Asymptomatic carotid stenosis >80 %	Symptomatic Carotid stenosis	Symptomatic Carotid stenosis >70 %
Stent system	PRECISE	Acculink Carotid Stent	Wallstent, Precise, Acculink Smart Exponent	Wallstent, Precise, Acculink Zilver	Wallstent, Precise, Acculink	Wallstent	Wallstent	Wallstent	Wallstent	Wallstent, Stricker Palmaz (26 %)	Wallstent
EPD	Angioguard XP	Accunet Embolic Protection Device	Percusurge, Angioguard, Filterwire EZ, Mednova, parody, Emboshield, etc. (operator discretion)	Percusurge Guardwire, Angioguard, Filterwire, EZ, Spider, Emboshield, Accunet	Percusurge, FilterWire EX, Neuroshield, carotid trap (in 27 %)	None	None	FilterWire, Angioguard RX	None	None	None
Termination	Premature (%)	Trial completion (%)	Interim analysis (%)	Premature (%)	Premature (%)	Trial completion (%)	Premature (%)	Premature (%)	Trial completion (%)	Exploratory trial (%)	Premature (%)
30-day death CEA, CAS	2.5, 1.2	0.3, 0.7	0.1, 0.1	1.2, 0.8	0.9, 0.7	2, 0	NA	0, 0	0, 0	2, 3	0, 0
30-day stroke CEA, CAS	3.1, 3.6	2.3, 4.1	3.2, 7.0	2.7, 8.8	6.2, 7.5	0, 0	NA	10, 0	0, 0	8, 8	0, 71
30-day MI CEA, CAS	6.1, 2.4	2.3, 1.1	0.6, 0.3	0.8, 0.4	0, 0	0, 0	NA	0, 0	0, 0	NA	NA
30-day death/stroke CEA, CAS	8.4, 5.5	2.3, 4.4	3.4, 7.1	3.8, 9.4	6.5, 7.7	2, 0	4.5, 12.1	10, 0	0, 0	10, 10	0,71
30-day death/stroke/MI CEA, CAS	9.8, 4.8	6.8, 7.2	4.0, 7.4	6.1, 11.7	6.5, 7.7	2, 0	NA	10, 0	0, 0	NA	NA

SAPPHIRE – Only randomized trial which included high-risk CEA patients
CABERNET, BEACH, and CREATE reported data on age ≥75 years
CABERNET reported data on dialysis-dependent renal failure only
ARCHER, CABERNET, and CREATE resulted in FDA device approval

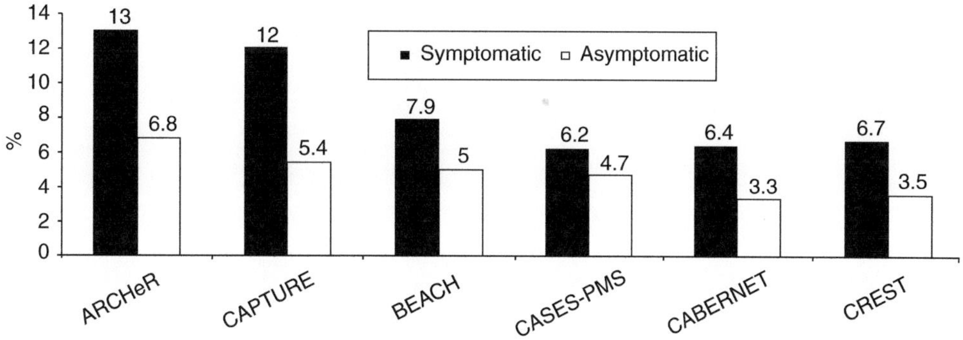

Fig. 35.5 30-day rates of death, stroke, and myocardial infarction for carotid artery stenting

The Carotid Revascularization Endarterectomy versus Stenting Trial (CREST) is the largest randomized trial published comparing CAS with EPD to CEA [60]. There were 2,502 average surgical risk patients with symptomatic (1,321) and asymptomatic (1,181) carotid stenosis randomized to either CEA or CAS. The primary outcome of periprocedural stroke, death, or MI or follow-up ipsilateral stroke was not different between the two groups at 4 years (7.2 % for CAS and 6.8 % for CEA). The 30-day risk of all stroke was higher for CAS (4.1 % vs. 2.3 %, $P=0.01$), whereas CEA was associated with a higher 30-day risk of MI (2.3 % vs. 1.1 %, $P=0.03$). The rate of ipsilateral stroke over a mean follow-up of 2.5 years was similar between the two groups. CAS trended safer than CEA for patients ≤69 years of age, while CEA yielded better outcomes in those >70 years of age.

The Asymptomatic Carotid Stenosis Stenting versus Endarterectomy (ACT I) trial will further help evaluate risk of CAS versus CEA in asymptomatic patients at average risk for CEA. This trial is enrolling 1,540 patients with asymptomatic stenosis greater than 70 % at average risk for CEA and randomizing them, on a 3:1 basis, to CAS or CEA [35]. The aim is to demonstrate the non-inferiority of CAS using the Emboshield Embolic Protection System and Emboshield Pro Embolic Protection System with the Xact Carotid Stent System (Abbott Vascular Corporation, Abbott Park, Illinois) to CEA for the treatment of asymptomatic extracranial carotid atherosclerotic disease. The primary end point is death, stroke, or MI at 30 days and ipsilateral stroke between 31 and 365 days. Secondary end points include target lesion revascularization, device and procedural success, ipsilateral stroke at 5 years, and economic and quality of life indicators.

Guidelines for Carotid Artery Stenting

The American College of Cardiology Foundation/Society for Cardiovascular Angiography and Interventions/Society for Vascular Medicine and Biology/Society of Interventional Radiology/American Society of Interventional and Therapeutic Neuroradiology (ACCF/SCAI/SVMB/SIR/ASITN) published a clinical expert consensus document on carotid stenting in 2007 [1]. Per this consensus statement, CAS is recommended in patients with symptomatic stenosis greater than 50 % and asymptomatic stenosis greater than 80 % (NASCET criteria) who are at high risk for CEA.

For average surgical risk patients, the recently published American Heart Association stroke guidelines make CAS a level 1 indication for symptomatic patients with carotid stenosis >50 % by angiography at average risk for CEA. In patients at high-risk for CEA, CAS is indicated among patients with symptomatic stenosis >70 % provided perioperative risk morbidity and mortality rates are 4–6 %, respectively [44]. This document did not comment on revascularization for patients with asymptomatic carotid stenosis. The recently published guidelines on extracranial carotid and vertebral artery disease make CAS a class 1 indication for symptomatic patients with carotid stenosis >50 % by angiography (NASCET method) provided the anticipated rate of stroke or death is less than 6 %. For asymptomatic patients with carotid stenosis >60 % by angiography (NASCET method), CAS can be considered in highly selected patients [45]. A summary of recommendations for CAS by various professional societies is provided in Table 35.3.

In patients with carotid dissection, endovascular intervention is recommended when a patient experiences recurrent symptoms on antithrombotic therapy [44]. No guideline has addressed endovascular management of carotid aneurysm. Based on few case reports, endovascular treatment appears feasible and safe for selected patients [11, 61].

Carotid Artery Stenting

Choosing the Right Patient: Who Should Not Undergo CAS?

Appropriate patient selection and technical considerations are required to achieve optimal results with CAS. The risks of periprocedural complications after CAS appear to be independent of severity of stenosis (unless the lesion contains a large thrombus load) [62, 63].

CAS is contraindicated in the presence of a bleeding diathesis or renal dysfunction [1]. Advanced age >80 years has

Table 35.3 Recommendation for carotid artery stenting by professional societies

Professional society	Asymptomatic CAS	Symptomatic CAS
ASITN/ASNR/SIR guideline 2003	≥90 % with high-risk features £	≥70 % with high-risk features £
SVS guideline 2008	Not recommended	≥50 % with high-risk features £
ESVS guideline 2009	In high-volume centers with documented low periprocedural death or stroke rates (≤3 %) or within well-conducted clinical trials	In high-volume centers with documented low periprocedural death or stroke rates (≤6 %) or within well-conducted clinical trials or when anatomy is not amenable for CEA
	Stenosis threshold are not validated	Stenosis threshold are not validated
SPREAD Italian guideline 2009	In patients with difficult to access anatomy for CEA or medical comorbidities	In patients with difficult to access anatomy for CEA or medical comorbidities
	Stenosis threshold are not mentioned	Stenosis threshold are not mentioned
ACCF/SCAI/SVMB/SIR/ASITN Consensus statement 2007	>70 % with high-risk features £	>50 % with high-risk features £
AHA stroke guidelines 2010	>70 % with high-risk £ features/>50 % at average risk for CEA	NA
ASA/ACCF/AHA/AANN/AANS/ACR/ ASNR/CNS/SAIP/SCAI/SIR/SNIS/SVM/ SVS extracranial carotid and vertebral artery disease guidelines 2011	>60 % by angiography	>50 % by angiography

CAS carotid artery stenting, *CEA* carotid endarterectomy, *ASA* American Stroke Association, *AANN* American Association of Neurosciences Nurses, *AANS* American Association of Neurological Surgeons, *ACR* American College of Radiology, *CNS* Congress of neurological surgeons, *SAIP* Society of Atherosclerosis Imaging and Prevention, *SNIS* Society of Neurointerventional Surgery, *SVS* Society of Vascular Surgery, *ASITN* American Society of Therapeutic and Interventional Neuroradiology, *ASNR* American Society of Neuroradiology, *SIR* Society of Interventional Radiology, *SVS* Society of Vascular Surgery, *ACCF* American College of Cardiology Foundation, *SCAI* Society for Cardiovascular Angiography and Interventions, *SVMB* Society for Vascular Medicine and Biology, *AHA* American Heart Association, *SPREAD* Stroke Prevention and Education Awareness Diffusion

£ – for details on high risk, please see text

Table 35.4 High-risk features for carotid stenting

Angiographic criteria	Clinical features
Poor vascular access	Age ≥ 75/80
≥2 acute (90°) bends	Dementia
Circumferential calcification	Bleeding disorder
Intracranial microangiopathy	Multiple lacunar strokes
Evidence of thrombus	Renal failure

Adapted from Roubin et al. [67], with permission

been shown to increase the risk of periprocedural complications in patients undergoing CAS [64, 65]. In the CREST trial, age did interact with treatment efficacy ($P = 0.002$). CAS tended to show greater efficacy at younger ages (<70 years) and CEA at older ages (>70 years) [65]. Other reports, however, have suggested favorable outcomes in octogenarians undergoing CAS when performed in high-volume centers with experienced operators [66].

Angiographic characteristics which make CAS a high-risk procedure include patients with difficult vascular access, a tortuous aorta with ≥2 acute (90°) bends within 5 cm of the lesion and a circumferential heavily calcified lesion (Table 35.4). These features increase the potential for prolonged catheter/guidewire manipulation in the aortic arch and render lesion crossing more difficult, increasing procedural hazard [1, 67]. An angiographic string sign (tapering of the vessel lumen with a post-stenotic region of significantly reduced caliber) has been considered a contraindication to CAS; however, recent small case series have shown safety and feasibility in string-sign patients with CAS [68, 69].

Procedural Details

On the day of the procedure, oral antihypertensive therapy is withheld, and adequate volume status is ensured. This will help in managing hemodynamic instability that might occur during carotid stenting. Aspirin (81–325 mg daily) is begun at least 24 h prior to the procedure and is continued indefinitely. A second antiplatelet agent (clopidogrel 75 mg daily or alternatively ticlopidine 250 mg twice daily) is given for 5 consecutive days preceding stent placement and continued for at least 1 month after stent deployment. Minimal, if any, sedation is used during the procedure to facilitate neurological assessments during the procedure. Unfractionated heparin should be given to prolong the activated clotting time (ACT) which is ≥250 s. Additional boluses of heparin may be required during the procedure. Glycoprotein IIb/IIIa antagonists are not routinely used [70]. Although small case series report the use of bivalirudin for percutaneous carotid interventions [71], there is no data to suggest a benefit over unfractionated heparin.

Key anatomic information needed before CAS includes evaluation of the aortic arch, patency of the Circle of Willis, anatomy of the CCA and carotid bifurcation, and ipsilateral intracranial anatomy. A 4/5 Fr diagnostic catheter is used to engage the common carotid artery (CCA), and a road-map angiogram is made of the carotid bifurcation. A 0.035″ stiff angled hydrophilic glidewire is advanced into the external carotid artery (ECA), and the diagnostic catheter is advanced into the ECA over the wire. The glidewire is exchanged for a 0.035″ exchange length stiff Amplatz wire over which an 8 Fr guiding catheter or a 6 Fr sheath may be advanced to the common carotid artery. Care must be taken to avoid plaque disruption with wires and catheters, and at this point in the procedure, the plaque in the internal carotid artery should remain untouched. For procedures performed with a distal EPD, the target lesion is crossed with the EPD. If the distal EPD will not cross the lesion, the stenosis may be crossed with a conventional 0.014-in. guidewire and pre-dilated with a small (2.5 mm) balloon. Then the EPD should be placed. After distal EPD deployment, the lesion is often pre-dilated with an undersized coronary balloon, typically 4 mm in diameter. A self-expanding carotid stent (open or closed cell) is then placed across the lesion. The stent is typically oversized for the ICA in order to fit the common carotid artery. There is no advantage for using tapered stents. It is routine practice, when treating a carotid bifurcation lesion, to place the stent across the ostium of the external carotid artery.

For aorto-ostial or common carotid lesions, the lesion is pre-dilated with a slightly undersized balloon. As the predilation balloon is deflated, the guide is gently advanced or "telescoped" over the balloon and across the lesion. This will protect the balloon-expandable stent as it is delivered to the lesion. The pre-dilation balloon is removed, and a balloon-expandable stent is placed (in arteries protected by the axial skeleton, balloon-expandable stents are more often used). After positioning the stent at the target lesion, the guide catheter is withdrawn, uncovering the stent. The proximal stent should protrude very slightly into the aorta to ensure adequate lesion coverage. After verifying adequate placement with contrast injections through the guide catheter, the stent is deployed at nominal pressure. As the stent deployment balloon deflates, the guide is again gently telescoped over the balloon across the lesion to facilitate additional stents to be delivered distally if needed. A post-stent carotid diameter stenosis of ≤50 % is an acceptable result.

With completion angiography, it is important to confirm that the carotid artery is free of dissection and that the intracranial cerebral vasculature is intact. Prior to removal of equipment, a neurologic exam assessing speech, movement, and mental status is performed. If a neurologic deficit is found, the culprit lesion is sought and neurovascular rescue attempted. Sheath removal is performed when the ACT is ≤170 s if a closure device is not used.

Embolic Protection Devices

Periprocedural neurological complications, the major determinant of the risk-benefit ratio of CAS, are due primarily to embolization of friable atheromatous material from the aortic arch or the carotid lesion that has undergone intervention [72, 73]. EPDs include (1) a distal occlusion balloon, (2) distal filter devices, and (3) proximal protection devices with and without flow reversal (Table 35.5). Although, there have been no randomized trials to demonstrate the safety and efficacy of any carotid EPD, one early meta-analysis concluded that EPDs did reduce the risk of stroke with CAS [74]. Currently, Medicare reimbursement for patients undergoing CAS requires the use of an EPD.

Table 35.5 Carotid embolic protection devices

Embolic protection device	Manufacturer
Distal occlusion balloon	
Percusurge Guardwire	Medtronic, Minneapolis, Minnesota
Distal filter devices	
AccuNet	Abbott Vascular, Abbott Park, Illinois
AngioGuard	Cordis Corporation, Miami Lakes, Florida
FilterWire	Boston Scientific, Natick, Massachusetts
Emboshield	Abbott Vascular, Abbott Park, Illinois
Spider	Ev3 Inc, Plymouth, Minnesota
Interceptor	Medtronic, Minneapolis, Minnesota
Rubicon	Rubicon Medical, Salt Lake City, Utah
FiberNet	Lumen Biomedical Inc, Plymouth, Minnesota
Proximal endovascular occlusion	
Mo.Ma	Medtronic, Minneapolis, Minnesota
Gore Flow Reversal System	Gore & Associates, Flagstaff, Arizona

The ideal EPD should be easy to deliver, use, and remove. It should provide protection during all phases of the intervention, with easy lesion visualization and few mishaps related to the device. No EPDs protect against embolization due to catheter manipulation of the aortic arch. With distal EPD, embolization may occur during lesion crossing, and even after deployment of the device, embolization can occur to the intracranial circulation via external to internal carotid artery collaterals. Distal occlusion balloons are characterized by occasional patient intolerance to interruption of cerebral blood flow and an inability to angiographically visualize the lesion during stent deployment. Distal filter-type EPDs although easier to use can be difficult to retrieve, and a filter can become so full that the overflowing debris must be removed or aspirated separately to avoid spilling the contents of the filter during retrieval. Moreover, small emboli can pass through filters. Proximal EPDs theoretically should be more effective at preventing embolization than filters. This EPD is placed and functioning before the lesion is crossed with the operator's choice of guidewire. They are limited by their more complicated, bulky design. Approximately 5–10 % of patients will develop some level of intolerance during the procedure, making it more difficult for the operator, and the operator cannot angiographically visualize the target lesion during stent deployment.

There has been no head-to-head comparison between different types of EPDs. A study using transcranial Doppler as a surrogate marker for atheroembolism has shown less embolic signals with a proximal EPD versus a distal filter-type EPD [75]. However, the clinical significance of these embolic signals remains uncertain. A recent single-center registry of 1,300 patients after CAS using proximal EPD reported a 30-day stroke and death rate of 1.4 % with independent neurological assessment [73]. These results if reproducible will dramatically improve the safety of CAS.

Complications

Complication of CAS can be divided into two categories: cervical and intracranial [69]. Cervical complications can be proximal to the stent (arterial dissection), within the stent (plaque prolapse, acute stent thrombosis, or incorrect stent deployment), and distal to the stent (arterial dissection, difficult retrieval of EPD, or distal filter occlusion). Intracranial complications include embolic events, hyperperfusion syndrome, and contrast encephalopathy. Other complications of CAS include hemodynamic instability (bradycardia and hypotension) and access site (hemorrhage or occlusive) complications. Mental status changes *after* CAS warrants CT evaluation to rule out intracranial bleeding.

Hypotension during CAS might be a result of stimulation of the carotid sinus baroreceptor or a manifestation of blood loss due to access site hemorrhage. Carotid sinus stimulation presents as acute hypotension with bradycardia during the procedure. Acute hypotension can lead to brain hypoperfusion and neurological symptoms due to impaired cerebral autoregulation. Aggressive fluid administration is important in treating hypotension, but vasopressor medications are often needed to maintain a systolic blood pressure of ≥120 mm Hg. Repeated boluses, as needed, of 25–50 mcg of phenylephrine can be administered. A continuous infusion may be required if hypotension persists. In most patients, however, phenylephrine can be weaned within several hours of the procedure, and the patient can ambulate in preparation for discharge the next day. Midodrine 2.5–10 mg three times daily can be useful to support blood pressure in the setting of prolonged hypotension. Adjusting the patient's antihypertensive regimen will be necessary over the short term. Atropine (0.5–1 mg) may be used to treat bradycardia. A prophylactic dose can be considered before stent deployment if the patient was sensitive to pre-dilation.

Procedural risk of arterial dissection increases with increasing vessel tortuosity, unfavorable aortic arch anatomy (bovine or type 2/3 arch), increasing number of maneuvers to cannulate the common carotid artery and passage of bulky oversized rigid EPDs. Flow-limiting dissections of the common carotid or internal carotid artery must be treated by stent implantation.

No reflow after stent deployment may be due to spasm, dissection, or a large quantity of material obstructing the filter. Aspiration must be performed before filter retrieval, minimizing the risk of debris dislodgment as the filter is captured.

Entrapment/difficult retrieval of a distal EPD, usually a filter, usually occurs in cases of tortuous anatomy. Maneuvers such as rotating the patient's neck or using of a diagnostic catheter have been suggested for cases with difficult filter retrieval. Aggressively pulling the filter downward should never be attempted since it may result in dumping the filter or stent damage [76].

Emboli during CAS procedures usually consist of solid plaque material. Performing intracranial cerebral angiography before CAS in two orthogonal views (including the capillary phase of blood–brain perfusion) allows comparison of these images with those after CAS and is the best way to detect subtle signs of cerebral embolization. Once symptomatic intracranial embolization is detected, catheters can be advanced for embolectomy or stent deployment.

Cerebral hyperperfusion syndrome has been defined as a neurological deficit (or seizure) ipsilateral to the carotid artery treated, not related to cerebral embolism [77]. Sudden reperfusion of chronically ischemic brain with reduced preoperative cerebrovascular reactivity predisposes a patient to hyperperfusion injury. Risk factors associated with reperfusion injury include severe and/or bilateral carotid artery stenosis, contralateral occlusion, poor collateral blood supply, preexisting cerebral infarctions, periprocedural hypertension, and advanced age [77, 78]. The presenting symptoms are usually nonspecific, such as mental confusion or atypical migraine. They may appear as early as 30 min or as late as 2 weeks after the procedure. Sometimes specific neurological deficits ("stroke-like" symptoms) or even epileptic seizures may be present. In the early phase, the stroke-like symptoms are associated with diffuse cerebral edema on the CT scan and effacement of the cortical sulci [78, 79]. There are no evidence-based data regarding the optimal management of patients at risk of or with evident hyperperfusion syndrome. Symptomatic treatment of the cerebral edema associated with the hyperperfusion syndrome includes intravenous administration of corticosteroids and mannitol. In the periprocedural period, aggressive monitoring and control of systemic blood pressure (goal systolic pressure of 120–140 mm Hg) is desirable.

Contrast encephalopathy is a rare complication associated with local contrast administration particularly with older hyperosmolar contrast agents [80, 81]. This syndrome presents with transient neurological deficits [81]. The radiological findings are compatible with disruption of the blood–brain barrier caused by direct neurotoxic effect of contrast, which allows contrast to enter the brain where staining of the cortical and the basal ganglia may be seen on the brain CT. Acute blood–brain barrier breakdown may allow fluid extravasation, leading to cerebral edema. Generally, both the symptoms and the radiological findings resolve within 24 and 48 h. Patient outcome is considered excellent.

Follow-Up

In-stent restenosis (ISR) after CAS has been documented at 3–6 % over 12–17 month follow-up [82, 83]. CEA restenosis is associated with an increased risk of carotid ISR [84]. Doppler ultrasonography is not as reliable for post-stent restenosis when compared to native artery stenosis due to lack of well-established criteria and falsely increased velocities associated with increased stiffness of the stented carotid artery. The optimal treatment of asymptomatic ISR following CAS is unclear. However, limited data suggests that a conservative strategy is appropriate until a severe obstruction is apparent when repeat endovascular intervention is an effective strategy [82, 83].

Vertebral Artery Disease

Etiology and Prevalence

In marked contrast with prevalence of revascularization for carotid artery disease, vertebral artery disease has received limited attention. This has been due to the lack of surgical options for treating posterior circulation lesions. The vertebral artery is affected by several pathological processes, the most common being atherosclerosis which will be the main focus of this chapter [85]. Other pathologies include dissection, aneurysm, vasculitis, and arteriovenous fistulas.

There are no population-based prevalence data for vertebral artery stenosis. Patients with atherosclerotic peripheral arterial disease have a 40 % incidence of atherosclerotic VAS [86]. In patients presenting with symptoms of posterior circulation, stroke, TIA, or both, reported prevalence of atherosclerotic vertebral artery stenosis ≥50 % ranges from 20 to 40 % [87–89]. The most frequent site of atherosclerotic involvement is the origin of the vertebral artery from the subclavian artery.

Natural History of Atherosclerotic Vertebral Artery Disease

The prognosis of *asymptomatic vertebral artery stenosis* is unclear. A prospective single-center series of 96 patients with asymptomatic vertebral artery stenosis ≥50 % by angiography reported a stroke rate of 5.3 % per year and a 5-year survival rate of 60 %. More than 50 % of the deaths were related to cardiac disease, reflecting the widespread underlying atherosclerotic burden in this patient population [90].

Posterior-circulation ischemia rarely causes only one symptom but rather produces a collection of symptoms and signs depending on which area of the brain is ischemic [91]. Stenosis at or near the origin of a vertebral artery often manifests as brief attacks of dizziness and altered vision with loss of balance [88]. Bilateral vertebral artery stenosis will present with brief episodes of dizziness, ataxia, and diplopia with perioral paresthesias [91]. Stenosis or occlusion of the intracranial portion of the vertebral artery may cause the Wallenberg, or lateral medullary, syndrome, characterized by dizziness, limb ataxia, facial pain, hoarseness, and dysphagia with decreased pain and temperature sensation on ipsilateral face and contralateral trunk, limbs, or both [4]. Distal vertebrobasilar occlusions can present acutely as coma, "locked-in" syndrome, oculomotor disturbances, and bilateral motor deficits [92].

In a population-based study of 91,000 patients, 37 patients with symptomatic vertebral artery stenosis ≥50 % were identified by MRA. Within 90 days, 46 % had a recurrent TIA or a minor stroke [87]. In this study, the annual incidence of TIA or minor stroke in patients with symptomatic vertebral artery stenosis (13.5 patients per 100,000) was higher than the incidence in patients with symptomatic carotid stenosis (9.0 per 100,000). Other studies have shown that medically refractory, symptomatic vertebral artery stenosis carries a 5–11 % incidence of stroke or death at 1 year [93, 94]. Acute basilar artery occlusion is often fatal, with death occurring in the majority from 2 days to 5 weeks after the event [95].

Diagnosis of Vertebral Disease

There are no recommendations for routine screening of an asymptomatic patient for vertebral artery stenosis [44]. In patients presenting with symptoms suggestive of posterior (vertebrobasilar) ischemia, they should first be imaged noninvasively. The role of DUS in vertebral artery dissection is limited to documenting vessel patency and antegrade or retrograde flow.

Invasive arterial angiography (IAA), however, remains the gold standard for diagnosis of vertebral disease.

Noninvasive Testing

The limited available data suggests that contrast-enhanced MRA and CTA have a higher sensitivity than DUS (93.9 %, 100 % vs. 70.2 %, respectively) for vertebrobasilar stenosis [96]. CTA in addition to offering comparable sensitivity and specificity to contrast-enhanced MRA for diagnosis of vertebral artery stenosis is more widely available. Further studies are required to directly compare CTA with MRA.

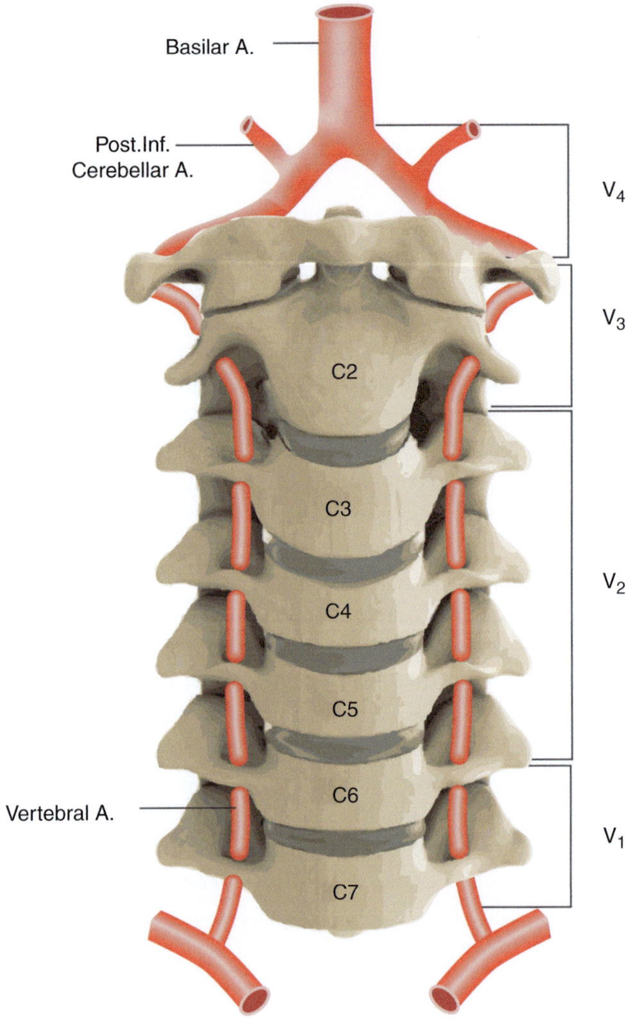

Fig. 35.6 Anatomy of the vertebral artery (From Jenkins et al. [113], with permission)

Invasive Testing

The gold standard for diagnosis of vertebral artery stenosis is DSA. The technique for diagnostic angiography is similar to that described earlier for diagnosis of carotid stenosis. Anatomically, the vertebral artery can be divided into four parts: three extracranial and one intracranial (Fig. 35.6) [85]. Stenosis at the vertebral arch origin can be missed with standard arch views, because of superimposition of the subclavian artery; therefore, additional oblique views are required.

Important anatomic variants of the vertebral artery include termination of the vertebral artery in posterior inferior communicating artery instead of the basilar artery in 1 % of the population, atretic vertebral artery (<2 mm in diameter) in 15 % of the population, and an anomalous origin of left vertebral artery in 1–5 % (most common as a branch of the aortic arch, arising between the left common carotid and left subclavian artery) [97]. The left vertebral artery is dominant in 50 %, right vertebral artery is dominant in 25 %, and both vertebral arteries are of similar caliber in 25 % of patients [85].

Medical Therapy

There is limited data regarding medical therapy in patients with symptomatic vertebral artery stenosis. Atherosclerotic risk factor modification is recommended [44]. In the prospective Warfarin and Aspirin for Symptomatic Intracranial Arterial Stenosis (WASID) trial, 19 % of the patients (107/569) had symptomatic vertebral artery stenosis. Patients were randomized to 650 mg twice daily aspirin or 5 mg warfarin (target range, 2.0–3.0). This trial reported no difference in annual rates of stroke in the territory of the symptomatic artery in patients randomized to aspirin or warfarin (15 % vs. 13 %, $P=0.31$). Warfarin when compared to aspirin had a higher rate of hemorrhagic complications (8.3 % vs. 3.2 %, $P=0.01$) [98].

Similar to the strategy for treatment of acute anterior circulation stroke, intracranial hemorrhage must first be excluded by CT, and then patients presenting within 3–4.5 h after an acute posterior circulation stroke should be administered with intravenous tissue plasminogen (t-PA) [5, 99]. However, unlike middle cerebral artery acute occlusions, the stroke guidelines do not discuss the role of intra-arterial thrombolysis for an acute vertebral occlusions [5].

Revascularization

Indications for surgical revascularization remain unattractive. Three *surgical revascularization* techniques for symptomatic VAS have been described including (1) transection of the vertebral artery above the stenosis with reimplantation into the ipsilateral subclavian or carotid artery, (2) vertebral artery endarterectomy, and (3) vein patch angioplasty [100]. None have been successfully adopted in clinical medicine. Perioperative mortality rates remain low (0–0.6 %); however, postoperative morbidity is high (10–20 %) [101–103]. One series reported recurrent laryngeal nerve palsy in 2 %, Horner's syndrome in 15 %, lymphocele in 4 %, chylothorax in 0.5 %, and immediate thrombosis in 1 % of patients undergoing vertebral artery reconstruction [102].

Currently for patients with recurrent symptoms on medical therapy (medical therapy failures), endovascular revascularization is recommended [44]. The severity of stenosis at which an intervention should be performed is not specified, but in most studies, VAS is performed for stenosis ≥70–99 %. Endovascular treatment (stenting and coil embolization) is also increasingly replacing surgical treatment for VA dissections and aneurysms [104]. Since the first reported vertebral artery intraoperative transluminal angioplasty in 1980

[105], multiple case reports and clinical series have described the use of balloon angioplasty and stenting to treat vertebrobasilar atherosclerotic disease [100, 106, 107].

The only randomized trial comparing VAS stent placement with medical therapy was Carotid and Vertebral Artery Transluminal Angioplasty Study (CAVATAS) which only randomized 16 patients [108]. A Cochrane Review identified 313 cases of vertebral artery intervention and found a 30-day major stroke and death rate of 3.2 % and a 30-day TIA and non-disabling stroke rate of 3.2 % [109]. We have reported the largest single-center series of 105 patients (112 arteries) undergoing VAS stenting with a procedural stroke and death rate of 0 %. At 1-year follow-up, the mortality and posterior circulation stroke rate was 5.7 and 4.8 %, respectively [100]. VAS in experienced hands is a technically safe procedure; however, due to a lack of reimbursement, there remains limited published data on vertebral interventions.

Vertebral Artery Stenting

Procedural Details

All patients are empirically placed on dual-antiplatelet therapy. Aspirin (81–325 mg daily) is begun at least 24 h prior to the procedure and is continued indefinitely. A second antiplatelet agent (clopidogrel 75 mg daily) (or alternatively ticlopidine 250 mg twice daily) should be given for 5 consecutive days preceding stent placement and continued for at least 1 month after bare metal and 1 year after drug-eluting stent deployment. Minimal, if any, sedation is used during the procedure since the patient requires neurological assessments during the procedure. Intravenous unfractionated heparin should be given such that the activated clotting time (ACT) is ≥250 s. Additional boluses of heparin may be required during the procedure.

Vascular access is most commonly obtained from the femoral artery, although brachial or radial access may be used. Selective engagement of the vertebral artery is performed via a 4 F Judkins right-4, internal mammary artery, or multipurpose diagnostic coronary catheter. A 0.014 in steerable guidewire is advanced across the stenosis. EPDs are not routinely used due to the small size of the vessel. The diagnostic catheter is removed and an appropriately shaped 6 F coronary guiding catheter is advanced over the wire to the stenosis. Pre-dilation with a balloon sized to match the reference vessel diameter is performed. Stent placement is performed with a coronary balloon-expandable stent. A post-stent stenosis ≤30 % is considered a technically successful result. After stent deployment, completion angiography should be performed to demonstrate the posterior circulation. Sheath removal is performed when the ACT is ≤170 s if a closure device is not used.

Follow-Up

In the prospective, multicenter feasibility study of the NEUROLINK System (Guidant Corporation, Menlo Park, CA) Stenting of Symptomatic Atherosclerotic Lesions in the Vertebral or Intracranial Arteries (SSYLVIA) study, presence of diabetes mellitus, vertebral ostial lesions, increasing age, low pretreatment vessel diameter, and posttreatment stenosis ≥30 % predicted ISR [110]. Rates of ISR are higher in patients treated with a bare metal stents when compared to a drug-eluting stent (38–43 % vs. 11–17 %, respectively, in a median follow-up of 15–21 months) [111, 112]. Interestingly, ISR does not correlate with symptom recurrence [106, 112]. Asymptomatic ISR should be followed noninvasively. Re-intervention with either angioplasty or a stent-in-stent technique should be performed in patients with progressive or symptomatic ISR [111].

Conclusion

CAS in suitable patients with the use of an EPD is a well-validated alternative to surgical revascularization for stroke prevention in patients with carotid artery stenosis. For optimal outcomes, all patients undergoing CAS need to be carefully selected, based on readily available clinical and angiographic features. Proximal embolic protection offers a strategy that will likely dramatically improve the safety of CAS. Patients who have symptomatic vertebral artery stenosis and have failed medical therapy should be considered candidates for percutaneous intervention in experienced hands. Larger trials of patients with vertebral artery stenosis are needed, both to further understand the natural history of the disease and to validate currently available treatment options.

References

1. Bates ER, Babb JD, Casey Jr DE, et al. ACCF/SCAI/SVMB/SIR/ASITN 2007 clinical expert consensus document on carotid stenting: a report of the American College of Cardiology Foundation Task Force on Clinical Expert Consensus Documents (ACCF/SCAI/SVMB/SIR/ASITN Clinical Expert Consensus Document Committee on Carotid Stenting). J Am Coll Cardiol. 2007;49(1):126–70.
2. Lloyd-Jones D, Adams RJ, Brown TM, et al. Heart disease and stroke statistics–2010 update: a report from the American Heart Association. Circulation. 2010;121(7):e46–215.
3. Bamford J, Sandercock P, Dennis M, et al. Classification and natural history of clinically identifiable subtypes of cerebral infarction. Lancet. 1991;337(8756):1521–6.
4. Savitz SI, Caplan LR. Vertebrobasilar disease. N Engl J Med. 2005;352(25):2618–26.
5. Adams Jr HP, del Zoppo G, Alberts MJ, et al. Guidelines for the early management of adults with ischemic stroke: a guideline from the American Heart Association/American Stroke Association Stroke Council, Clinical Cardiology Council, Cardiovascular Radiology and Intervention Council, and the Atherosclerotic Peripheral Vascular Disease and Quality of Care

Outcomes in Research Interdisciplinary Working Groups: The American Academy of Neurology affirms the value of this guideline as an educational tool for neurologists. Circulation. 2007;115(20):e478–534.
6. Barnett HJM, Taylor DW, Sackett DL, et al. Beneficial effect of carotid endarterectomy in symptomatic patients with high-grade carotid stenosis. North American Symptomatic Carotid Endarterectomy Trial Collaborators. N Engl J Med. 1991;325(7):445–53.
7. O'Leary DH, Polak JF, Kronmal RA, et al. Distribution and correlates of sonographically detected carotid artery disease in the Cardiovascular Health Study. The CHS Collaborative Research Group. Stroke. 1992;23(12):1752–60.
8. Longstreth Jr WT, Shemanski L, Lefkowitz D, et al. Asymptomatic internal carotid artery stenosis defined by ultrasound and the risk of subsequent stroke in the elderly. The Cardiovascular Health Study. Stroke. 1998;29(11):2371–6.
9. Sharma BK, Jain S, Bali HK, et al. A follow-up study of balloon angioplasty and de-novo stenting in Takayasu arteritis. Int J Cardiol. 2000;75 Suppl 1:S147–52.
10. Finsterer J, Strassegger J, Haymerle A, et al. Bilateral stenting of symptomatic and asymptomatic internal carotid artery stenosis due to fibromuscular dysplasia. J Neurol Neurosurg Psychiatry. 2000;69(5):683–6.
11. Longo GM, Kibbe MR. Aneurysms of the carotid artery. Semin Vasc Surg. 2005;18(4):178–83.
12. Lucas C, Moulin T, Deplanque D, et al. Stroke patterns of internal carotid artery dissection in 40 patients. Stroke. 1998;29(12):2646–8.
13. El-Sabrout R, Cooley DA. Extracranial carotid artery aneurysms: Texas Heart Institute experience. J Vasc Surg. 2000;31(4):702–12.
14. McCollum CH, Wheeler WG, Noon GP, et al. Aneurysms of the extracranial carotid artery. Twenty-one years' experience. Am J Surg. 1979;137(2):196–200.
15. Muluk SC, Muluk VS, Sugimoto H, et al. Progression of asymptomatic carotid stenosis: a natural history study in 1004 patients. J Vasc Surg. 1999;29(2):208–14. discussion 214–206.
16. Mathiesen EB, Joakimsen O, Bonaa KH. Prevalence of and risk factors associated with carotid artery stenosis: the Tromso Study. Cerebrovasc Dis. 2001;12(1):44–51.
17. Polak JF, Shemanski L, O'Leary DH, et al. Hypoechoic plaque at US of the carotid artery: an independent risk factor for incident stroke in adults aged 65 years or older. Cardiovascular Health Study. Radiology. 1998;208(3):649–54.
18. Yonas H, Smith HA, Durham SR, et al. Increased stroke risk predicted by compromised cerebral blood flow reactivity. J Neurosurg. 1993;79(4):483–9.
19. Toole JF, Baker WH, Castaldo JE, et al. Endarterectomy for asymptomatic carotid artery stenosis. Executive Committee for the Asymptomatic Carotid Atherosclerosis Study. JAMA. 1995;273(18):1421–8.
20. Biasi GM, Froio A, Diethrich EB, et al. Carotid plaque echolucency increases the risk of stroke in carotid stenting: the Imaging in Carotid Angioplasty and Risk of Stroke (ICAROS) study. Circulation. 2004;110(6):756–62.
21. Dixon S, Pais SO, Raviola C, et al. Natural history of nonstenotic, asymptomatic ulcerative lesions of the carotid artery. A further analysis. Arch Surg. 1982;117(11):1493–8.
22. Rockman CB, Riles TS, Lamparello PJ, et al. Natural history and management of the asymptomatic, moderately stenotic internal carotid artery. J Vasc Surg. 1997;25(3):423–31.
23. Halliday A, Mansfield A, Marro J, et al. Prevention of disabling and fatal strokes by successful carotid endarterectomy in patients without recent neurological symptoms: randomised controlled trial. Lancet. 2004;363(9420):1491–502.
24. Nicolaides AN, Kakkos S, Griffin M, et al. Severity of asymptomatic carotid stenosis and risk of ipsilateral hemispheric ischaemic events: results from the ACSRS study. Eur J Vasc Endovasc Surg. 2005;30:275–84. Nicolaides et al. 2006;31(3):336.
25. Kleindorfer D, Panagos P, Pancioli A, et al. Incidence and short-term prognosis of transient ischemic attack in a population-based study. Stroke. 2005;36(4):720–3.
26. Thacker EL, Wiggins KL, Rice KM, et al. Short-term and long-term risk of incident ischemic stroke after transient ischemic attack. Stroke. 2010;41(2):239–43.
27. Streifler JY, Eliasziw M, Benavente OR, et al. The risk of stroke in patients with first-ever retinal vs hemispheric transient ischemic attacks and high-grade carotid stenosis. North American Symptomatic Carotid Endarterectomy Trial. Arch Neurol. 1995;52(3):246–9.
28. Barnett HJ, Taylor DW, Eliasziw M, et al. Benefit of carotid endarterectomy in patients with symptomatic moderate or severe stenosis. North American Symptomatic Carotid Endarterectomy Trial Collaborators. N Engl J Med. 1998;339(20):1415–25.
29. Farrell B, Fraser A, Sandercock J, et al. Randomised trial of endarterectomy for recently symptomatic carotid stenosis: final results of the MRC European Carotid Surgery Trial (ECST). Lancet. 1998;351(9113):1379–87.
30. Rothwell PM, Gutnikov SA, Warlow CP. Reanalysis of the final results of the European Carotid Surgery Trial. Stroke. 2003;34(2):514–23.
31. Henderson RD, Eliasziw M, Fox AJ, et al. Angiographically defined collateral circulation and risk of stroke in patients with severe carotid artery stenosis. North American Symptomatic Carotid Endarterectomy Trial (NASCET) Group. Stroke. 2000;31(1):128–32.
32. Eagle KA, Guyton RA, Davidoff R, et al. ACC/AHA 2004 guideline update for coronary artery bypass graft surgery: a report of the American College of Cardiology/American Heart Association Task Force on Practice Guidelines (Committee to Update the 1999 Guidelines for Coronary Artery Bypass Graft Surgery). Circulation. 2004;110(14):e340–437.
33. Eliasziw M, Rankin RN, Fox AJ, et al. Accuracy and prognostic consequences of ultrasonography in identifying severe carotid artery stenosis. North American Symptomatic Carotid Endarterectomy Trial (NASCET) Group. Stroke. 1995;26(10):1747–52.
34. Chen JC, Salvian AJ, Taylor DC, et al. Predictive ability of duplex ultrasonography for internal carotid artery stenosis of 70%-99%: a comparative study. Ann Vasc Surg. 1998;12(3):244–7.
35. Mikkonen RH, Kreula JM, Virkkunen PJ. Reproducibility of Doppler ultrasound measurements. Acta Radiol. 1996;37(4):545–50.
36. Tang TY, JM U-K-I, Walsh SR, et al. Invasive and non-invasive modalities of imaging carotid stenosis. J Cardiovasc Surg (Torino). 2009;50(6):715–25.
37. Grant EG, Benson CB, Moneta GL, et al. Carotid artery stenosis: grayscale and Doppler ultrasound diagnosis–Society of Radiologists in Ultrasound consensus conference. Ultrasound Q. 2003;19(4):190–8.
38. AbuRahma AF, Srivastava M, Stone PA, et al. Critical appraisal of the Carotid Duplex Consensus criteria in the diagnosis of carotid artery stenosis. J Vasc Surg. 2011;53(1):53–9. discussion 59–60.
39. Nederkoorn PJ, van der Graaf Y, Hunink MG. Duplex ultrasound and magnetic resonance angiography compared with digital subtraction angiography in carotid artery stenosis: a systematic review. Stroke. 2003;34(5):1324–32.
40. Menke J. Diagnostic accuracy of contrast-enhanced MR angiography in severe carotid stenosis: meta-analysis with metaregression of different techniques. Eur Radiol. 2009;19(9):2204–16.
41. Hollingworth W, Nathens AB, Kanne JP, et al. The diagnostic accuracy of computed tomography angiography for traumatic or atherosclerotic lesions of the carotid and vertebral arteries: a systematic review. Eur J Radiol. 2003;48(1):88–102.
42. Koelemay MJ, Nederkoorn PJ, Reitsma JB, et al. Systematic review of computed tomographic angiography for assessment of carotid artery disease. Stroke. 2004;35(10):2306–12.

43. Fayed AM, White CJ, Ramee SR, et al. Carotid and cerebral angiography performed by cardiologists: cerebrovascular complications. Catheter Cardiovasc Interv. 2002;55(3):277–80.
44. Furie KL, Kasner SE, Adams RJ, et al. Guidelines for the prevention of stroke in patients with stroke or transient ischemic attack: a guideline for healthcare professionals from the American Heart Association/American Stroke Association. Stroke. 2011;42(1): 227–76.
45. Brott TG, Halperin JL, Abbara S, et al. 2011 ASA/ACCF/AHA/AANN/AANS/ACR/ASNR/CNS/SAIP/SCAI/SIR/SNIS/SVM/SVS guideline on the management of patients with extracranial carotid and vertebral artery disease. A report of the American College of Cardiology Foundation/American Heart Association Task Force on Practice Guidelines, and the American Stroke Association, American Association of Neuroscience Nurses, American Association of Neurological Surgeons, American College of Radiology, American Society of Neuroradiology, Congress of Neurological Surgeons, Society of Atherosclerosis Imaging and Prevention, Society for Cardiovascular Angiography and Interventions, Society of Interventional Radiology, Society of NeuroInterventional Surgery, Society for Vascular Medicine, and Society for Vascular Surgery developed in collaboration with the American Academy of Neurology and Society of Cardiovascular Computed Tomography. J Am Coll Cardiol. 2011;57(8):1002–44.
46. Amarenco P, Labreuche J, Lavallee P, et al. Statins in stroke prevention and carotid atherosclerosis: systematic review and up-to-date meta-analysis. Stroke. 2004;35(12):2902–9.
47. Goodney PP, Powell RJ. Carotid artery stenting: what have we learned from the clinical trials and registries and where do we go from here? Ann Vasc Surg. 2008;22(1):148–58.
48. Hobson 2nd RW, Weiss DG, Fields WS, et al. Efficacy of carotid endarterectomy for asymptomatic carotid stenosis. The Veterans Affairs Cooperative Study Group. N Engl J Med. 1993;328(4):221–7.
49. Baker WH, Howard VJ, Howard G, et al. Effect of contralateral occlusion on long-term efficacy of endarterectomy in the asymptomatic carotid atherosclerosis study (ACAS). ACAS Investigators. Stroke. 2000;31(10):2330–4.
50. Halliday A, Harrison M, Hayter E, et al. 10-year stroke prevention after successful carotid endarterectomy for asymptomatic stenosis (ACST-1): a multicentre randomised trial. Lancet. 2010;376(9746):1074–84.
51. Mayberg MR, Wilson SE, Yatsu F, et al. Carotid endarterectomy and prevention of cerebral ischemia in symptomatic carotid stenosis. Veterans Affairs Cooperative Studies Program 309 Trialist Group. JAMA. 1991;266(23):3289–94.
52. Barnett HJM, Taylor DW, Sackett DL, et al. Clinical alert: benefit of carotid endarterectomy for patients with high-grade stenosis of the internal carotid artery. National Institute of Neurological Disorders and Stroke Stroke and Trauma Division. North American Symptomatic Carotid Endarterectomy Trial (NASCET) investigators. Stroke. 1991;22(6):816–7.
53. Yadav JS, Wholey MH, Kuntz RE, et al. Protected carotid-artery stenting versus endarterectomy in high-risk patients. N Engl J Med. 2004;351(15):1493–501.
54. Gurm HS, Yadav JS, Fayad P, et al. Long-term results of carotid stenting versus endarterectomy in high-risk patients. N Engl J Med. 2008;358(15):1572–9.
55. Brown MM, Rogers L, Bland JM, et al. Endovascular versus surgical treatment in patients with carotid stenosis in the Carotid and Vertebral Artery Transluminal Angioplasty Study (CAVATAS): a randomised trial. Lancet. 2001;357(9270):1729–37.
56. Ederle J, Bonati LH, Dobson J, et al. Endovascular treatment with angioplasty or stenting versus endarterectomy in patients with carotid artery stenosis in the Carotid and Vertebral Artery Transluminal Angioplasty Study (CAVATAS): long-term follow-up of a randomised trial. Lancet Neurol. 2009;8(10):898–907.
57. Ringleb PA, Allenberg J, Bruckmann H, et al. 30 day results from the SPACE trial of stent-protected angioplasty versus carotid endarterectomy in symptomatic patients: a randomised non-inferiority trial. Lancet. 2006;368(9543):1239–47.
58. Mas JL, Trinquart L, Leys D, et al. Endarterectomy versus angioplasty in patients with symptomatic severe carotid stenosis (EVA-3S) trial: results up to 4 years from a randomised, multicentre trial. Lancet Neurol. 2008;7(10):885–92.
59. International Carotid Stenting Study Investigators, Ederle J, Dobson J, Featherstone RL, et al. Carotid artery stenting compared with endarterectomy in patients with symptomatic carotid stenosis (International Carotid Stenting Study): an interim analysis of a randomised controlled trial. Lancet. 2010;375(9719):985–97.
60. Clark WM, for the Crest Investigators. Carotid revascularization and endarterectomy versus stenting trial. Paper presented at: American Stroke Association, San Antonio, TX; 2010.
61. McCready RA, Divelbiss JL, Bryant MA, et al. Endoluminal repair of carotid artery pseudoaneurysms: a word of caution. J Vasc Surg. 2004;40(5):1020–3.
62. Mathur A, Roubin GS, Iyer SS, et al. Predictors of stroke complicating carotid artery stenting. Circulation. 1998;97(13): 1239–45.
63. Roubin GS, New G, Iyer SS, et al. Immediate and late clinical outcomes of carotid artery stenting in patients with symptomatic and asymptomatic carotid artery stenosis: a 5-year prospective analysis. Circulation. 2001;103(4):532–7.
64. Hobson 2nd RW, Howard VJ, Roubin GS, et al. Carotid artery stenting is associated with increased complications in octogenarians: 30-day stroke and death rates in the CREST lead-in phase. J Vasc Surg. 2004;40(6):1106–11.
65. Brott TG, Hobson 2nd RW, Howard G, et al. Stenting versus endarterectomy for treatment of carotid-artery stenosis. N Engl J Med. 2010;363(1):11–23.
66. Grant A, White C, Ansel G, et al. Safety and efficacy of carotid stenting in the very elderly. Catheter Cardiovasc Interv. 2010; 75(5):651–5.
67. Roubin GS, Iyer S, Halkin A, et al. Realizing the potential of carotid artery stenting: proposed paradigms for patient selection and procedural technique. Circulation. 2006;113(16):2021–30.
68. Barker CM, Gomez J, Grotta JC, et al. Feasibility of carotid artery stenting in patients with angiographic string sign. Catheter Cardiovasc Interv. 2010;75(7):1104–9.
69. Nikas DN, Ghany MA, Stabile E, et al. Carotid artery stenting with proximal cerebral protection for patients with angiographic appearance of string sign. JACC Cardiovasc Interv. 2010;3(3): 298–304.
70. Chan AW, Yadav JS, Bhatt DL, et al. Comparison of the safety and efficacy of emboli prevention devices versus platelet glycoprotein IIb/IIIa inhibition during carotid stenting. Am J Cardiol. 2005; 95(6):791–5.
71. Bush RL, Lin PH, Mureebe L, et al. Routine bivalirudin use in percutaneous carotid interventions. J Endovasc Ther. 2005;12(4):521–2.
72. Cremonesi A, Manetti R, Setacci F, et al. Protected carotid stenting: clinical advantages and complications of embolic protection devices in 442 consecutive patients. Stroke. 2003;34(8):1936–41.
73. Stabile E, Salemme L, Sorropago G, et al. Proximal endovascular occlusion for carotid artery stenting: results from a prospective registry of 1,300 patients. J Am Coll Cardiol. 2010;55(16): 1661–7.
74. Kastrup A, Groschel K, Krapf H, et al. Early outcome of carotid angioplasty and stenting with and without cerebral protection devices: a systematic review of the literature. Stroke. 2003;34(3):813–9.
75. Garami ZF, Bismuth J, Charlton-Ouw KM, et al. Feasibility of simultaneous pre- and postfilter transcranial Doppler monitoring during carotid artery stenting. J Vasc Surg. 2009;49(2):340–344, 345 e341–2; discussion 345.

76. Ganim RP, Muench A, Giesler GM, et al. Difficult retrieval of the EPI Filterwire with a 5 French FR4 coronary catheter following carotid stenting. Catheter Cardiovasc Interv. 2006;67(2):309–11.
77. Coutts SB, Hill MD, Hu WY. Hyperperfusion syndrome: toward a stricter definition. Neurosurgery. 2003;53(5):1053–8. discussion 1058–1060.
78. Abou-Chebl A, Yadav JS, Reginelli JP, et al. Intracranial hemorrhage and hyperperfusion syndrome following carotid artery stenting: risk factors, prevention, and treatment. J Am Coll Cardiol. 2004;43(9):1596–601.
79. Terada T, Tsuura M, Matsumoto H, et al. Hemorrhagic complications after endovascular therapy for atherosclerotic intracranial arterial stenoses. Neurosurgery. 2006;59(2):310–8. discussion 310–318.
80. Studdard WE, Davis DO, Young SW. Cortical blindness after cerebral angiography. Case report. J Neurosurg. 1981;54(2):240–4.
81. Dangas G, Monsein LH, Laureno R, et al. Transient contrast encephalopathy after carotid artery stenting. J Endovasc Ther. 2001;8(2):111–3.
82. Zhou W, Lin PH, Bush RL, et al. Management of in-sent restenosis after carotid artery stenting in high-risk patients. J Vasc Surg. 2006;43(2):305–12.
83. Willfort-Ehringer A, Ahmadi R, Gschwandtner ME, et al. Single-center experience with carotid stent restenosis. J Endovasc Ther. 2002;9(3):299–307.
84. Setacci C, Pula G, Baldi I, et al. Determinants of in-stent restenosis after carotid angioplasty: a case–control study. J Endovasc Ther. 2003;10(6):1031–8.
85. Cloud GC, Markus HS. Diagnosis and management of vertebral artery stenosis. QJM. 2003;96(1):27–54.
86. Phatouros CC, Higashida RT, Malek AM, et al. Endovascular treatment of noncarotid extracranial cerebrovascular disease. Neurosurg Clin N Am. 2000;11(2):331–50.
87. Marquardt L, Kuker W, Chandratheva A, et al. Incidence and prognosis of > or = 50% symptomatic vertebral or basilar artery stenosis: prospective population-based study. Brain. 2009;132(Pt 4):982–8.
88. Wityk RJ, Chang HM, Rosengart A, et al. Proximal extracranial vertebral artery disease in the New England Medical Center Posterior Circulation Registry. Arch Neurol. 1998;55(4):470–8.
89. Fields WS, North RR, Hass WK, et al. Joint study of extracranial arterial occlusion as a cause of stroke. I. Organization of study and survey of patient population. JAMA. 1968;203(11):955–60.
90. Moufarrij NA, Little JR, Furlan AJ, et al. Vertebral artery stenosis: long-term follow-up. Stroke. 1984;15(2):260–3.
91. Caplan LR, Wityk RJ, Glass TA, et al. New England Medical Center Posterior Circulation registry. Ann Neurol. 2004;56(3):389–98.
92. Hacke W, Zeumer H, Ferbert A, et al. Intra-arterial thrombolytic therapy improves outcome in patients with acute vertebrobasilar occlusive disease. Stroke. 1988;19(10):1216–22.
93. Ausman JI, Diaz FG, Sadasivan B, et al. Intracranial vertebral endarterectomy. Neurosurgery. 1990;26(3):465–71.
94. Hopkins LN, Budny JL. Complications of intracranial bypass for vertebrobasilar insufficiency. J Neurosurg. 1989;70(2):207–11.
95. Kubik CS, Adams RD. Occlusion of the basilar artery; a clinical and pathological study. Brain. 1946;69(2):73–121.
96. Khan S, Cloud GC, Kerry S, et al. Imaging of vertebral artery stenosis: a systematic review. J Neurol Neurosurg Psychiatry. 2007;78(11):1218–25.
97. Tay KY, U-King-Im JM, Trivedi RA, et al. Imaging the vertebral artery. Eur Radiol. 2005;15(7):1329–43.
98. Chimowitz MI, Lynn MJ, Howlett-Smith H, et al. Comparison of warfarin and aspirin for symptomatic intracranial arterial stenosis. N Engl J Med. 2005;352(13):1305–16.
99. Del Zoppo GJ, Saver JL, Jauch EC, et al. Expansion of the time window for treatment of acute ischemic stroke with intravenous tissue plasminogen activator: a science advisory from the American Heart Association/American Stroke Association. Stroke. 2009;40(8):2945–8.
100. Jenkins JS, Patel SN, White CJ, et al. Endovascular stenting for vertebral artery stenosis. J Am Coll Cardiol. 2010;55(6): 538–42.
101. Imparato AM. Vertebral arterial reconstruction: a nineteen-year experience. J Vasc Surg. 1985;2(4):626–34.
102. Berguer R, Flynn LM, Kline RA, et al. Surgical reconstruction of the extracranial vertebral artery: management and outcome. J Vasc Surg. 2000;31(1 Pt 1):9–18.
103. Thevenet A, Ruotolo C. Surgical repair of vertebral artery stenoses. J Cardiovasc Surg (Torino). 1984;25(2):101–10.
104. Rabinov JD, Hellinger FR, Morris PP, et al. Endovascular management of vertebrobasilar dissecting aneurysms. AJNR Am J Neuroradiol. 2003;24(7):1421–8.
105. Sundt Jr TM, Smith HC, Campbell JK, et al. Transluminal angioplasty for basilar artery stenosis. Mayo Clin Proc. 1980;55(11): 673–80.
106. Albuquerque FC, Fiorella D, Han P, et al. A reappraisal of angioplasty and stenting for the treatment of vertebral origin stenosis. Neurosurgery. 2003;53(3):607–14. discussion 614–606.
107. Mukherjee D, Roffi M, Kapadia SR, et al. Percutaneous intervention for symptomatic vertebral artery stenosis using coronary stents. J Invasive Cardiol. 2001;13(5):363–6.
108. Coward LJ, McCabe DJ, Ederle J, et al. Long-term outcome after angioplasty and stenting for symptomatic vertebral artery stenosis compared with medical treatment in the Carotid And Vertebral Artery Transluminal Angioplasty Study (CAVATAS): a randomized trial. Stroke. 2007;38(5):1526–30.
109. Coward LJ, Featherstone RL, Brown MM. Percutaneous transluminal angioplasty and stenting for vertebral artery stenosis. Cochrane Database Syst Rev. 2005;(2):CD000516.
110. Lutsep HL, Barnwell S, Mawad M, et al. Stenting of Symptomatic Atherosclerotic Lesions in the Vertebral or Intracranial Arteries (SSYLVIA): study results. Stroke. 2004;35(6):1388–92.
111. Eberhardt O, Naegele T, Raygrotzki S, et al. Stenting of vertebrobasilar arteries in symptomatic atherosclerotic disease and acute occlusion: case series and review of the literature. J Vasc Surg. 2006;43(6):1145–54.
112. Ogilvy CS, Yang X, Natarajan SK, et al. Restenosis rates following vertebral artery origin stenting: does stent type make a difference? J Invasive Cardiol. 2010;22(3):119–24.
113. Jenkins JS, White CJ, Ramee SR, et al. Vertebral insufficiency: when to intervene and how? Curr Interv Cardiol Rep. 2000;2(2):91–4.

Acute Stroke Intervention

36

James T. DeVries

Stroke currently affects 750,000 patients yearly in the United States and is projected to increase in frequency to one million per year by 2025 [1]. As such, stroke represents the third leading cause of death in the United States and is the most common cause of adult disability, with healthcare expenditures of approximately 73 billion dollars in hospitalization and lost productivity in 2010 [2]. The vast majority of all strokes (>80 %) are ischemic in nature [3]. Treatment for stroke has undergone rapid advances in the past two decades, beginning with the first FDA-approved therapy for acute ischemic stroke, intravenous thrombolysis, in 1995 [4]. New understanding of the pathophysiology of stroke in conjunction with advances in endovascular equipment have created the field of stroke intervention, which has fostered a host of new devices and technologies to treat acute stroke in patients not eligible for thrombolysis [5–11]. Many of these new techniques and devices have shown promise for offering improved outcomes following ischemic stroke in small case series, yet the field remains very much in its infancy with little in the way of large randomized trials to guide policy-level decision making or guideline generation.

Moreover, acute stroke cannot be treated in isolation or by a single specialty provider. Instead, it requires complex coordination between multiple providers from different specialties, organized towards a single goal [12]. Whereas the patient with an acute ST-elevation myocardial infarction can be treated by a single interventional cardiologist throughout his or her hospital stay, stroke patients are unique in their requirements for coordinated, multidisciplinary care. The fields of emergency medicine, neurology, neurosurgery, radiology, interventional neuroradiology, vascular surgery, and interventional cardiology all have important contributions to the care of the individual patient and advancement of the field. As a result, it is difficult to develop a stroke program without cooperation between colleagues across disciplines. In fact, the American Stroke Association's Task Force on the Development of Stroke Systems identifies fragmentation of care as a major contributor to suboptimal treatment of stroke and inefficient use of healthcare resources [13]. As such, coordinated systems of care which integrate prevention and treatment and provide patient and community education should be a primary focus in the development of stroke programs. This chapter will focus on the current treatment modalities that exist for acute ischemic stroke management, with a primary focus on new devices targeted for the endovascular specialist.

Intravenous Thrombolysis

For the appropriately selected patients, intravenous (IV) thrombolysis represents the current standard of care for treating acute stroke [14]. Whereas the initial window for administration of IV thrombolytics extended to 3 h from symptom onset in early trials [4], more recent European data has suggested that with the proper patient selection, the window can be extended to four and a half hours from symptom onset [15]. The concern with later administration of thrombolytics involves higher rates of hemorrhagic transformation of the infracted brain tissue, particularly in large territory strokes which are more susceptible to hemorrhagic conversion. Because of this, there has been much interest in finding novel mechanisms for identifying patients at high risk for hemorrhage. Evidence suggests that advanced MRI-based perfusion techniques may be able to select late-presenting patients least likely to have hemorrhagic transformation following administration of IV thrombolytics [16, 17]. Nevertheless, the benefit of intravenous thrombolysis is clearly time related, with a decreasing benefit the later the administration of drug occurs from the onset of symptoms [18].

J.T. DeVries, MD
Division of Cardiology,
Dartmouth-Hitchcock Medical Center,
1 Medical Center Dr, Lebanon, NH 03756, USA

Department of Medicine,
Dartmouth Medical School, Lebanon, NH, USA
e-mail: james.t.devries@hitchcock.org

C.A. Thompson (ed.), *Textbook of Cardiovascular Intervention*,
DOI 10.1007/978-1-4471-4528-8_36, © Springer-Verlag London 2014

The National Institute of Neurological Disorders and Stroke (NINDS) published the landmark trial of intravenous recombinant tissue plasminogen activator (t-PA) in 1995 [4]. In the trial, 624 patients who presented with an acute ischemic stroke within 3 h of symptom onset and had no evidence of brain hemorrhage by CT scanning were randomized to t-PA or placebo infusions. All patients received baseline National Institutes of Health Stroke Score (NIHSS), a 42-point scale which quantifies the degree of neurologic deficit in 11 categories [19]. Outcomes including neurologic recovery and overall survival were assessed at 24 h and 90 days. In this trial, patients who received t-PA were 30 % more likely than those who received placebo to have minimal or no neurologic deficits at 90 days and had no increase in mortality [4]. Moreover, this benefit was maintained out to 1 year, with continued neurologic benefit for treatment with t-PA and no adverse effect on overall mortality [20]. Nevertheless, t-PA treatment was not risk-free and was associated with higher rates of intracranial hemorrhage within the first 36 h, and some have suggested that the stroke severity was lower in the t-PA group, which may have skewed the results [21]. In spite of the controversy, the FDA-approved intravenous thrombolytic therapy for appropriate patients and it remains the standard of care.

More recently, the strict 3-h time window cutoff was tested in a European setting of acute ischemic stroke [15] in which the time window was extended to 4.5 h after symptom onset in appropriate patients. In this trial, 821 patients who were between 3 and 4.5 h from stroke symptoms onset were randomly assigned to intravenous t-PA or placebo, and neurologic outcomes were assessed at 90 days using the modified Rankin score, which scores functional capacity on a 6-point scale (lower numbers are higher functional capacity, with 0 indicating no deficit and 6 indicating death) [22]. In patients who received thrombolytic therapy, 52 % had a favorable outcome versus only 45 % in the placebo group. Of note, intracranial hemorrhage was higher in those treated with t-PA (27 % vs. 18 %), but there was no difference in overall survival [15].

Despite the results of the above trials, time restrictions continue to exclude a significant number of patients from candidacy for IV thrombolysis. In addition to patients presenting more than 4.5 h beyond symptom onset, many patients present with "wake-up" strokes where the time on onset cannot be calculated and therefore are excluded from receiving thrombolytic therapy. As a result of the time limitations in conjunction with fear of litigation and lack of appropriate treatment algorithms, less than five percent of all stroke patients who present for medical care receive intravenous thrombolysis [23]. Additionally, intravenous thrombolysis is less effective for large vessel occlusive disease (particularly distal carotid), and in these cases, which typically have high stroke scores and larger clot burden, catheter-based devices may hold an advantage in terms of more effective reperfusion and lower risk for hemorrhagic transformation [24].

Endovascular Therapies for Stroke: An Overview

Because of the limitations of intravenous thrombolysis, multiple catheter-based thrombectomy approaches have been developed to allow for reperfusion of ischemic brain tissue. Advantages to this approach include a longer time window (6–8 h after symptom onset) [25] for treatment than intravenous thrombolysis, where guidelines dictate administration within 3 h of symptom onset [14]. Recent data suggests that there may be benefit to intravenous thrombolysis up to 4.5 h from symptom onset in select patients, although the benefits are small and there is increased risk of intracranial hemorrhage [15]. Moreover, only a small fraction (~2 %) of patients with ischemic stroke receive intravenous thrombolysis, largely due to the narrow time window in which it can be administered [26]. Efforts to predict which patients outside the 3-h window for thrombolysis will benefit from catheter-based intervention have relied on several imaging modalities to identify jeopardized brain tissue, or ischemic penumbra, including CT perfusion and MRI perfusion/diffusion mismatch [27, 28]. The penumbra represents the brain tissue which is at risk for permanent injury, but has not yet been irreversibly damaged. A large penumbra signifies more brain tissue at jeopardy and therefore higher potential benefit for reperfusion therapy. Current data suggests that more than three-fourths of ischemic strokes will have a penumbra size which would favor reperfusion within the first 6–8 h following symptom onset [29]. Mechanical reperfusion strategies which facilitate recanalization of the culprit vessel may therefore be helpful during this time to salvage brain tissue.

There is no one "ideal" endovascular treatment for stroke. The goal of all technologies currently available is to reperfuse the culprit artery while avoiding the most feared complication of intracranial intervention: brain hemorrhage. Symptomatic intracranial hemorrhage is associated with high morbidity and mortality [20] and occurs in roughly 5–12 % of patients undergoing endovascular stroke therapy [9, 25, 30]. Initial efforts at reperfusion outside the intravenous thrombolytic time window focused on intra-arterial (IA) delivery of thrombolytics adjacent to the obstructing thrombus in selected patients with middle cerebral artery occlusions [25, 31]. In this population of patients, IA thrombolysis compared with placebo improved both recanalization rates (66 % with IA thrombolysis and 18 % with placebo) and 90-day neurologic outcomes as measured by the modified Rankin score [25]. Nevertheless, IA thrombolysis remains non-FDA approved for stroke treatment [14]. Mechanical reperfusion with the Merci Retrieval System (Concentric Medical, Mountain View, CA) in selected patients ineligible for intravenous thrombolysis up to 8 h after symptom onset resulted in recanalization rates approaching 70 %, and those patients who were successfully revascularized had improved functional status at 90 days [9, 10] (Fig. 36.1). Another extraction device (Fig. 36.2), the Penumbra System (Penumbra, San Leandro, CA), has demonstrated excellent results at restoring artery patency up to 8 h after symptom onset in a cohort of patients with severe stroke (mean NIHSS of 21) [7].

Mechanical strategies can broadly be divided into several groupings: clot retrievers, aspiration- or suction-type devices, balloons and stents, and ultrasonography-based devices [32]. Ultimately, each of these techniques requires detailed understanding of not only the operational

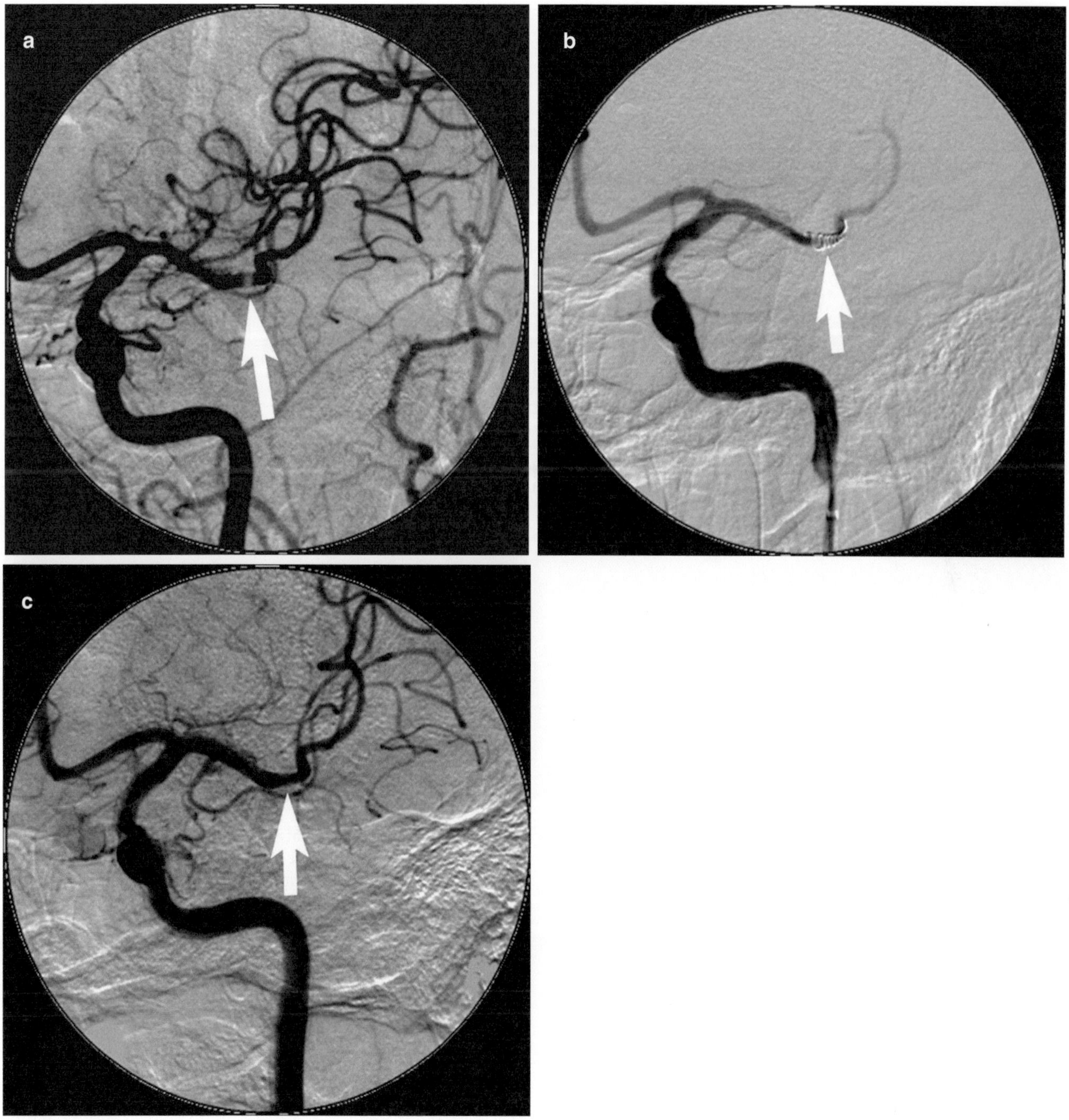

Fig. 36.1 MERCI device. The MERCI device: (**a**) Left middle cerebral artery thrombus in a patient with acute right-sided weakness (*arrow* shows thrombus). (**b**) MERCI device engaged in the thrombus. (**c**) Angiogram of the left middle cerebral artery post embolectomy with the MERCI device (*arrow* shows resolution of thrombus)

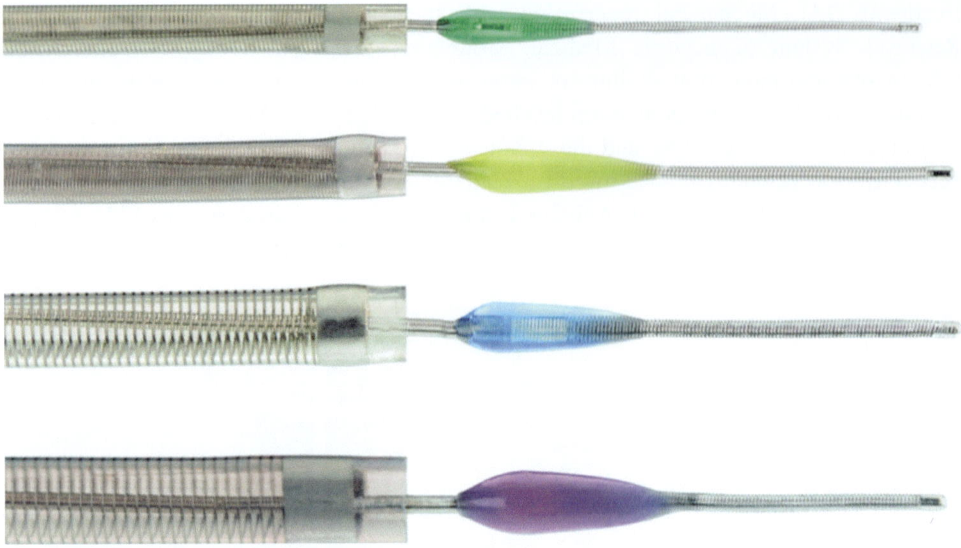

Fig. 36.2 The Penumbra device: Stators with aspiration catheters used for thrombus removal

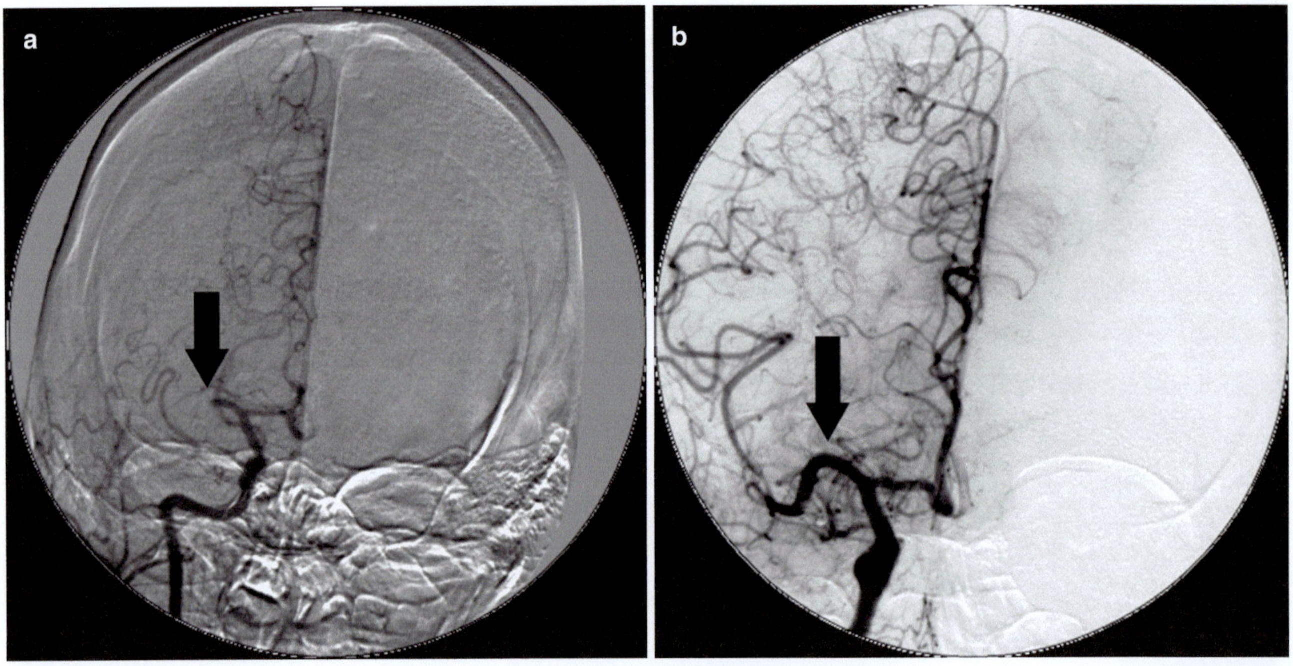

Fig. 36.3 Microcatheter for primary reperfusion. The patient presented with an acute stroke but was lytic ineligible and received catheter-based therapy with local delivery of t-PA via a microcatheter. (**a**) Occlusion of the right middle cerebral artery (*arrow*). (**b**) Reestablished patency of the right middle cerebral artery post-local delivery of t-PA via microcatheter

characteristics of the device but also the methods for delivering these potentially bulky tools to the intracranial circulation. As such, injury to the neurovasculature, distal embolization of clot, and conversion of ischemic injury to hemorrhagic injury are all possible complications. Specialized training is required not only to learn the individualized techniques for operation of these devices but also for approaches to selecting the optimal patient population who may benefit from their use.

Intra-arterial Thrombolysis

The concept of intra-arterial (IA) thrombolysis for acute stroke was a logical progression from IV thrombolysis in that it allowed local delivery of the thrombolytic drug directly to the thrombus rather than systemic administration (Fig. 36.3). In theory, this technique offers fewer systemic side effects and more effective thrombolysis. As a result, the therapeutic window for delivery was broader in time scope, as well as patient inclusion [33]. Downsides of this approach include the need for highly skilled interventionalists who can identify the culprit thrombus and successfully navigate the tortuous brain arteries to deliver drug locally as well as appropriate facilities and support staff to allow for successful patient treatment during and after the procedure.

The PROACT-II trial [25] was a randomized and placebo-controlled trial of patients with middle cerebral artery occlusions and moderately high NIH Stroke Scores (mean 17) who presented within 6 h of symptom onset. The 180 patients enrolled were randomly assigned to treatment with intra-arterial catheter-delivered recombinant prourokinase or low-dose heparin, and standard neurologic outcomes were examined at 90 days, including the modified Rankin Scale score (mRS) which measures functional status. The protocol allowed for placement of a microcatheter up to the thrombotic occlusion, but no mechanical disruption of the clot with wires or catheters. Patients enrolled were highly selected, with over 12,000 patients screened to identify the 180 patients who were enrolled. In this trial, patients who received the thrombolytic therapy had higher rates of artery reperfusion (66 % vs. 18 %) and had better neurologic outcomes as measured by the mRS (40 % had mRS 2 or less in lytic arm versus only 25 % in the control arm). The overall mortality was about 25 % and not different between the two groups, despite a higher rate of intracranial hemorrhage in the patients who received thrombolysis during the first 24 h (35 % vs. 13 %) [25].

Despite the improvements in neurologic outcomes seen in PROACT-II, intra-arterial thrombolytic therapy has not been approved in the United States. Nevertheless, enthusiasm remains for off-label use of commercially available thrombolytics including urokinase and recombinant t-PA, both as stand-alone therapy and when used in combination with intravenous thrombolytics [6]. The concept of a dual thrombolytic approach is appealing in that it allows for rapid treatment of patients in the emergency room setting with IV thrombolytics, followed by local, intra-arterial delivery of additional thrombolytic directly at the site of occlusion (Fig. 36.4). Intra-arterial thrombolysis allows for a higher recanalization rate than systemic intravenous administration, which is less effective in large clots. The Emergency Management of Stroke Bridging Trial (EMS) [34] examined the feasibility and safety of combining intravenous with intra-arterial thrombolytics in patients with acute stroke. In this small study, which enrolled 35 patients with stroke, patients randomized to intravenous and intra-arterial thrombolytics had improved rates of recanalization of infarct arteries compared with those randomized to placebo followed by intra-arterial thrombolysis. Despite no difference in intracerebral bleeding rates, there was no improvement which was noted in overall neurologic outcomes [34]. Since then, other trials have examined the safety endpoints of combined therapy in a nonrandomized fashion, but there has not been overwhelming adoption of this approach [35].

The Interventional Management of Stroke II Study (IMS II) [6] used a combined approach of intravenous thrombolysis followed by immediate cerebral angiography with additional intra-arterial delivery of thrombolytics for patients with persistent cerebral artery occlusion. IMS II also employed the EKOS ultrasound catheter for enhanced thrombolysis in a portion of the patients. Overall, this trial found that, when compared with IV thrombolysis alone as in the NINDS trial, the combined approach had no higher rates of intracranial hemorrhage and numerically improved survival when compared to the treatment or placebo arms of the NINDS trial [6]. This encouraging result leads to the organization of the IMS III trial, which is currently enrolling and is randomizing acute stroke patients to intravenous thrombolytic versus combination therapy [36].

Mechanical Thrombectomy

In addition to thrombolytic therapies, there has been an explosion of devices in the past few years which are designed to mechanically remove thrombus from the infarct-related artery. The Mechanical Embolus Removal in Cerebral Ischemia (MERCI) device is FDA approved for the treatment of intracranial clot removal in acute stroke [10]. It has a corkscrew shape and is designed to engage a clot and allow for physical removal of the clot from the cerebral circulation (see Fig. 36.1). It is deployed via a specialized delivery system which is equipped with an occlusion balloon. In theory, this allows for cessation of forward blood flow while the thrombus is being removed and also allows for aspiration of the affected artery so as to prevent further embolization of clot fragments to distal vessels. The pivotal MERCI trial enrolled patients with acute stroke within the first 8 h of symptom onset who were ineligible for intravenous thrombolytic therapy. Successful recanalization was achieved in 48 % of the patients in whom the device was used, with a symptomatic intracranial hemorrhage rate of about 8 % [10]. In patients in whom successful recanalization was achieved, univariate analysis of neurologic outcomes at 90 days showed improvement in mRS, which leads to much excitement about the device and its possible role in thrombolytic-ineligible patients. Interestingly, with multivariate analysis, successful recanalization was no longer a predictor of a good neurologic outcome [37], and there remains much debate about the benefits of the MERCI device and the role that this device should have in the treatment of acute stroke. Newer versions of the MERCI device which incorporate Prolene microfilaments were used in the nonrandomized

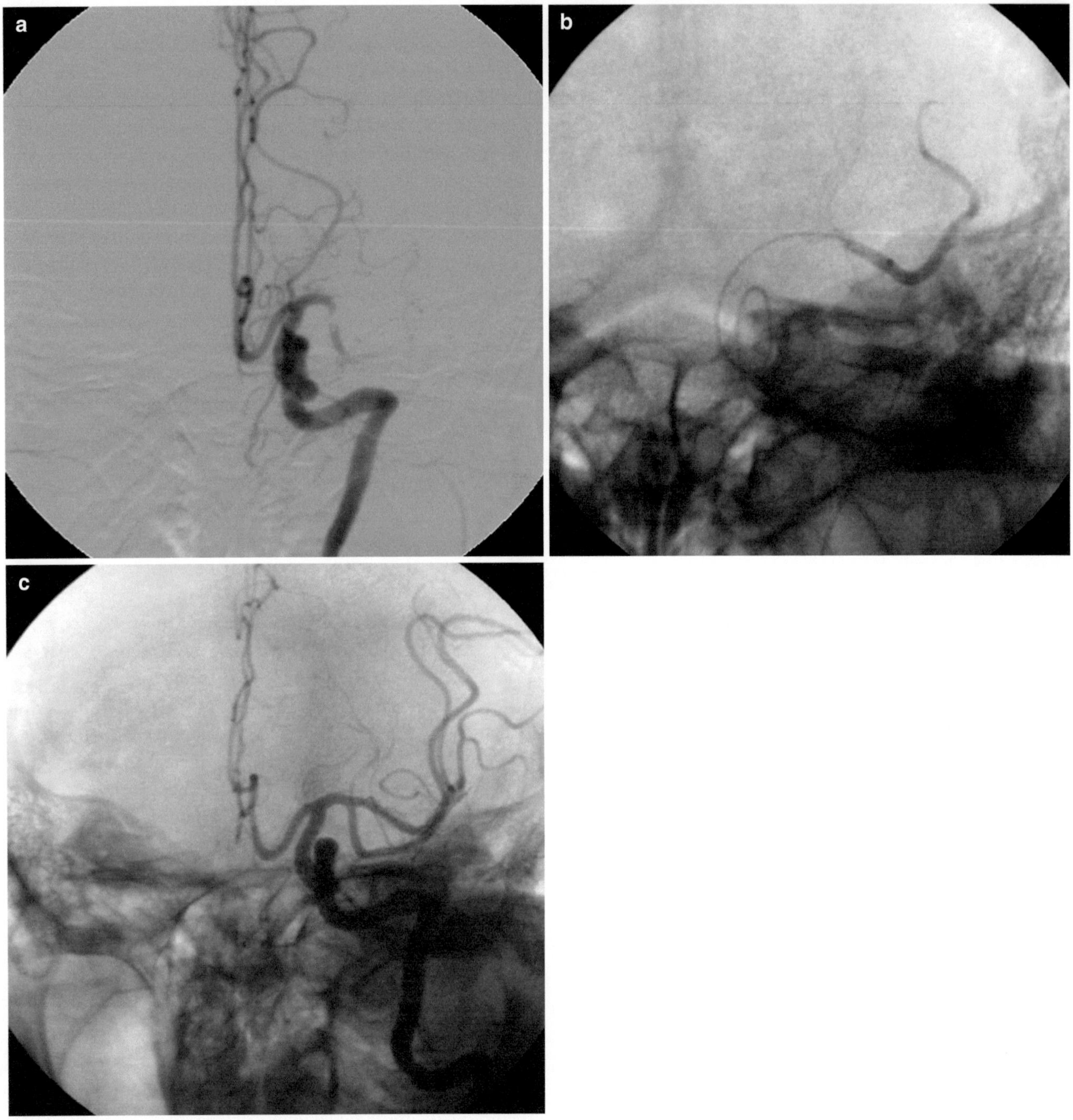

Fig. 36.4 Microcatheter for assisted reperfusion after failed systemic thrombolytics. The patient presented with an acute stroke to an outside hospital and received full-dose systemic thrombolysis. Her symptoms did not improve and she was transferred for rescue intervention. Local delivery of t-PA via a microcatheter allowed for successful reperfusion. (**a**) Thrombotic occlusion of the left MCA with visible thrombus despite intravenous thrombolytic administration. (**b**) A microcatheter is delivered distal to the obstruction in the left middle cerebral artery and contrast injection is performed to confirm intraluminal placement. Thrombolytics (t-PA) are then delivered locally to the thrombus via the microcatheter. (**c**) Final cerebral angiogram demonstrating patency of the left middle cerebral artery after local delivery of thrombolytics. Clinically, this patient had a nearly complete neurologic recovery

phase I Multi-MERCI trial, where high rates of successful recanalization were seen when the device was used alone (54 %) or in conjunction with intra-arterial thrombolytics (69 %) [30].

The Penumbra System is another mechanical thrombectomy device which is designed to allow removal of thrombus in the setting of acute stroke. The system consists of an aspiration catheter and a stator which fits through the lumen of the catheter and helps facilitate thrombus maceration and removal (see Fig. 36.2). It was utilized in a single-arm, multicenter registry in 125 patients who presented within 8 h of acute stroke and allowed for successful recanalization in 81 % on the arteries in which it was attempted [38]. Intracranial hemorrhage occurred in 28 % of patients in whom the device was used, with just less than half of hemorrhages classified as symptomatic. Yet despite the high rate of successful recanalization, the rate of favorable clinical outcomes as determined by the mRS was only 25 %, and mortality at 90 days remained high at 33 % [38]. Results such as this have called into question the continued focus on recanalization as a surrogate for success in treating acute stroke, but trials continue to try to define the role for mechanical thrombectomy devices in acute stroke.

Intracranial Stenting

Taking a lesson from the world of coronary intervention, the use of intracranial stents has emerged in the past few years as a means of providing immediate restoration of flow in an acute stroke. Whereas thrombolytics may fail because of the fibrous nature of a more mature embolus, and other mechanical approaches may fail because of embolic adherence to the vessel wall, intracranial stenting is very effective at reestablishing artery patency [39]. Initial attempts at intracranial stenting utilized balloon-expandable stents, which resulted in reasonably high recanalization rates (79 %) but continued high mortality of over 30 % [40]. Part of the difficulty with balloon-expandable stents is the bulky nature of the devices, which have to be delivered to the intracranial circulation via highly tortuous vessels. Moreover, cerebral vessels lack a robust external elastic membrane and have little mobility to stretch and move as a stiff stent travels through because of extensive fixation from branching and perforating arteries [41]. As a result, the chances of vessel damage via dissection or perforation are higher than would be expected when working in the coronary realm. In addition, the consequences of plaque shifting with subsequent compromise of a small perforator artery can be disastrous in the cerebral circulation, making intracranial stenting with balloon-expandable stents a potentially risky proposition.

Because of these unique challenges discussed above, self-expanding stents have gained popularity in the intracranial circulation. They have more flexible delivery systems and are able to track more easily to the target vessel with less risk of vessel injury [42]. There are currently five commercially available stents for use in the intracranial circulation: Wingspan (Stryker, former Boston Scientific, Fremont, CA), Solitaire (ev3, Plymouth, MN), Enterprise (Cordis, Miami Lakes, FL), Leo (Balt, Montmorency, France), and Neuroform (Boston Scientific, Natick, MA). These devices can all be used for the treatment of acute stroke, although they are actually indicated for use in coiling wide-neck aneurysms in the cerebral circulation. Several small single-center experiences with these devices have been reported, including one which included nine patients who were treated just over 5 h after symptom onset and found an 89 % recanalization rate with one intracranial hemorrhage and one acute stent thrombosis [43].

The Stent-Assisted Recanalization in Acute Ischemic Stroke (SARIS) trial is a prospective trial examining the role for stenting in acute stroke [44]. In the trial, 20 patients who either failed intravenous thrombolysis or were not eligible to receive thrombolysis underwent stent-assisted recanalization of the infarct-related artery. Successful recanalization (TIMI 3 or TIMI 2 flow) was achieved in 100 % of the patients, and at 1 month, roughly 60 % of patients had mRS of 3 or less. Many other smaller studies and case series have validated these findings, suggesting that a stent-based approach has real merit in the management of patients with acute stroke [45–47]. An interesting approach which has been utilized in the intracranial circulation is the use of "temporary" stent placement to allow for rapid reestablishment of flow at which point the stent is then retrieved, essentially leaving nothing behind in the intracranial circulation. This approach has several advantages. First, there is no need for dual antiplatelet therapy which can increase the risk of bleeding, particularly intracranial bleeding. Second, stents in the intracranial circulation have been noted to have very high rates of restenosis in small angiographic follow-up studies, although the Wingspan stent used in the SARIS trial had low rates of restenosis at follow-up angiography 6 months after placement [48]. The first case report of temporary endovascular bypass was published in 2008 and detailed a case involving a patient with an unsuccessful mechanical thrombectomy of a large M1 clot where an Enterprise stent was used to successfully reestablish flow to the occluded segment [49]. The stent was left in place for only 20 min and then retrieved from the circulation once flow was restored. The patient did well clinically with a significant fall in NIH Stroke Scale following the procedure. Since then, there have been additional reports which detail similar successes in using stents in a retrievable manner [50]. Based on the high success rates with recanalization and good clinical outcomes, it seems that stent-based therapies for acute stroke hold much promise in the future of stroke therapy.

Neuroprotection

The concept of neuroprotection for acute stroke involves the administration of a drug or other therapy to help minimize ischemic brain injury. While enticing to imagine a drug treatment which blocks the effects of ischemia or protects from cellular damage, the field of neuroprotection has been littered with many "wonder drugs" which held great promise in early animal models yet demonstrated no benefit when studied in man [51]. Many of these drugs are targeted at modulating mediators of neuronal damage, including free radicals, excitatory neurotransmitters, inflammatory markers, and even temperature. There has also been enthusiasm for therapeutic hypothermia in the setting of acute stroke, as it seems to provide benefit following cardiac arrest [52]. However, concerns exist about complications from the required intubation and paralysis which accompanies hypothermia, and the beneficial cerebral effects seen during cooling may be lessened by the requisite rewarming phase [53]. Because of the lack of evidence, there are no current recommendations for administration of neuroprotective agents in the setting of acute stroke, although research continues in this area.

Manpower Issues

Widespread adoption of reperfusion strategies outside intravenous thrombolysis will require a sizable pool of appropriately trained "stroke interventionalists" who are capable of delivering therapy to the brain 24 h a day and 365 days a year. Recent surveys have indicated that fewer than 400 interventional neuroradiologists are currently working in the United States, an inadequate supply to treat even a fraction of the 700,000 strokes which occur in this country every year [54]. Proposals for increasing neuroendovascular manpower have focused on utilizing the pool of carotid-stent-trained interventionalists, a diverse group of providers including neurologists, surgeons, and cardiologists [12]. Specific universal guidelines and training qualifications for acute stroke intervention do not currently exist, but the Society for Coronary Angiography and Interventions (SCAI) is now offering small, multidisciplinary meetings specifically designed to build competence in stroke intervention, including the use of simulators to teach intracranial intervention [55]. More widespread effort to grow the cadre of stroke interventionalists at the community level is the best strategy for impacting stroke outcomes at the national and health policy level.

Despite the multitude of options for the endovascular treatment of stroke, it is clear that not all patients will benefit from this therapy. The role of the "team approach" is to help select the patients who are best suited to catheter-based therapies, determined through assessing the degree of neurologic deficit, duration of symptoms, and size of penumbra as well as incorporating anatomic variables such as degree of collateral circulation. A stroke neurologist is a crucial component of the stroke team and can help guide decision making for the endovascular specialist.

Stroke Centers

Stroke centers are a key component of building a successful stroke program. The concept of stroke centers is relatively new, outlined by the Brain Attack Coalition (BAC) in the year 2000 [56] in response to earlier publications detailing the potential benefits of such centers [57, 58]. The model which has evolved through these efforts is similar to the model for trauma centers or for ST-elevation myocardial infarction (MI). Both trauma care and acute myocardial infarction care share similarities to acute stroke treatment in that they require rapid identification and triage of patients in order to provide timely access to care. This systems-based approach requires community-wide coordination and planning in order to execute in an efficient manner, beginning with empowering ambulances to bypass hospitals in order to bring stroke patients to facilities with appropriate treatment capabilities. To improve stroke care, the BAC has delineated specific components for both Primary Stroke Centers (PSC) [56] and Comprehensive Stroke Centers (CSC) [59]. PSCs are organized to provide a basic infrastructure for acute stroke care, including thrombolytic therapy administration by stroke teams, stroke units, and 24-h access to computed tomography scanning, while CSCs build upon this framework to allow for more comprehensive care.

The components of CSC have been outlined in the BAC consensus document [59] and broadly include (1) adequately trained personnel, (2) specific neuroimaging capability, (3) surgical and endovascular interventional capabilities, and (4) the infrastructure to support the above activities. Each of these components plays a key role in the rapid and effective diagnosis and treatment of stroke. Adequately trained personnel form the backbone of comprehensive stroke centers. Providers are needed to rapidly assess a stroke patient, determine time of symptom onset, and perform a neurologic exam which includes a National Institutes of Health Stroke Score (NIHSS) [19]. Timely assessment is important because of the narrow window (3 h from symptom onset) in which to administer intravenous thrombolytic therapy in eligible patients [14]. Imaging capability includes a CT scanner which is available around the clock, preferably with CT perfusion imaging capability, along with magnetic resonance imaging and angiography (MRI/MRA), angiography suites with digital subtraction angiography (DSA) to allow for percutaneous catheter-based therapy when appropriate, carotid duplex and transcranial Doppler scanning, and transesophageal echo. An endovascular specialist and a neurosurgeon need to be available for consultation and immediate procedural support, including aneurysm clipping, ventriculostomy placement, intracranial pressure transducer placement, and percutaneous, catheter-based therapy. Dedicated stroke units or neuroscience ICUs with appropriate staffing allow for close monitoring of stroke patients by providers accustomed to treating stroke patients and familiar with their unique needs. Part of the infrastructure of CSCs includes rigorous data collection and outcomes assessment for stroke patients, with the goal of national presentations and peer-reviewed publication in order to advance the field of stroke care. Additionally, community education about recognition of stroke risk factors in conjunction with ambulance bypass systems are crucial components to building successful stroke systems.

Beyond the manpower necessary, organizational components include written protocols that detail the treatment for stroke in a concise and easy-to-follow algorithm. Ideally, these algorithms should be posted in conspicuous locations in the emergency rooms, where any provider who may have contact with stroke patients can have easy access to them. Additionally, the algorithms should spell out the steps to activate the stroke alert teams and what testing (imaging, lab panels, etc.) needs to be performed immediately in stroke patients. Stroke team activation should involve a single call to a standard number, to minimize confusion and response time. Members of the stroke alert teams, including an endovascular specialist, need to be ready to respond to stroke alerts rapidly, including the technicians and nurses which are necessary to operate the angiography suite. Thrombolytic eligibility criteria and contraindications should be included in the algorithms, along with dosing guidelines for intravenous thrombolysis. Pharmacies should have thrombolytics prepackaged and ready to administer within emergency rooms. Again, there is a heavy emphasis on rapid assessment and triage because of the narrow time window in which therapy can be effective in stroke patients. Many of these practices have already been successfully utilized in reducing door-to-balloon times in acute myocardial infarction [60] and are logical to apply to reducing door-to-treatment times for acute stroke. The "time is muscle" paradigm used for treating heart attacks is an excellent model from which to construct a "time is brain" paradigm for treating acute stroke.

Starting a Stroke Program

The development of a new stroke program should incorporate the various components discussed above in an integrated package to provide complete care for stroke patients. A systematic approach to building a stroke program can help the process proceed in manageable steps. The first step is to analyze the available resources in the community, assess what care systems are currently in place for acute stroke, and determine who is providing this care. Next, stroke providers need to come together to form a multidisciplinary consortium to discuss the resources which exist in the community and the benefits of multidisciplinary cooperation, as well as establish a written plan outlining how the available resources can be utilized in unified and systematic way to treat stroke. Part of this process includes setting goals and expectations for how stroke care can be improved in the community, preferably with an understanding of the local stroke outcomes at baseline. A method for tracking outcomes must be established, ideally in the form of a database which can collect key patient and procedural variables and measure both functional outcomes and survival at prespecified time intervals (ideally at discharge, 1 month, and 3 months). Finally, the multidisciplinary consortium must arrange to meet on a regular basis to assess progress, discuss outcomes, and review new developments in the field.

The first step in building a stroke program is to assess what resources are currently available in the community. This includes both physical resources (CT scanners, MRI, etc.) and manpower resources. Remember that these providers can be from multiple disciplines, including neurology, cardiology, vascular surgery, and neurosurgery. Importantly, rehabilitation services following an acute hospital stay are a crucial component of comprehensive stroke care and should not be overlooked. Additionally, emergency services including ambulance crews and emergency physicians should be included in the survey of community resources, as they play an important role in controlling the flow of stroke patients and are the first responders for the majority of stroke patients. Once assessed, the resources should be recorded in a systematic way so that any deficiencies can be recognized. Unique solutions to a lack of community resources may exist in the form of telemedicine, a technology which has been used successfully to help improve outcomes in the treatment of stroke [61].

Following a thorough assessment of resources, the next step in beginning a stroke program is to bring together the key community providers in a forum to discuss the benefits and goals of a stroke program. Ideally, this discussion will be led by the person wishing to form the stroke program, acting as a "cheerleader" to raise awareness of the potential benefits of a stroke program. This meeting is a time to outline the information collected about community resources which are available, discuss acute stroke treatment (including thrombolytic and catheter-based therapy), and identify the barriers which may exist to implementation of these resources. Discussion points include rational for program development, assessment of availability for round-the-clock care, and a plan for how to arrange subsequent meetings. Part of the process is setting expectations for what can be achieved in stroke care. It should be emphasized that the mortality for acute stroke patients is high (approximately 20 % at 3 months for both arms of the NINDS thrombolytic trial [4]) no matter what treatment is rendered and that the benefits of thrombolytic therapy and catheter-based therapy are realized not immediately but at 30–90-day timepoints [4, 5]. Because much of the benefit comes late, it is important to establish a system to follow patients after they receive stroke care. A database which collects pertinent baseline and follow-up clinical variables allows for tracking outcomes and providing feedback to providers. At a minimum, this database should include demographic data, time from symptom onset to presentation, treatments delivered, baseline and follow-up NIHSS and modified Rankin scores [22], and mortality. The rational for cost saving with increased utilization of intravenous thrombolysis for acute stroke should also be discussed [62].

Finally, regularly scheduled meetings need to occur to discuss progress and outcomes. This will allow a forum for the various providers to discuss successes as well as difficulties which they may face in implementing stroke care. A review of the written protocols should be conducted regularly, along with a periodic comprehensive review of new publications and guidelines in the field. As the program takes form, marketing to the community can help educate the public and local providers, which can then fuel further program growth.

Conclusions

Acute stroke is common, has high morbidity and mortality, and is grossly undertreated in the United States. The goals for ischemic stroke therapy should be rapid and safe reperfusion of the culprit artery, either through the use of thrombolytic drugs or mechanical therapies in appropriate patients. Many options currently exist for mechanical embolectomy of stroke and each has unique advantages and disadvantages. The field of stroke intervention is constantly evolving as new devices and new insights are employed. Nevertheless, the "optimal" therapy for acute stroke remains elusive, as the field searches for large-scale multicenter randomized trials which can help build consensus and shape guideline recommendations.

The stroke center concept, which has been outlined by the BAC, provides guidance as to the important components which should be present in order to safely and effectively treat stroke. Current treatment options for ischemic stroke include intravenous thrombolysis as well as catheter-based therapy. Because of the narrow time window and broad exclusion criteria for intravenous thrombolytic therapy, a very small number of patients receive this therapy. Catheter-based therapy offers hope to patients who are ineligible for intravenous thrombolysis by extending the time window for treatment, but is limited by both the small number of providers who are currently performing this therapy and the lack of guidelines for which devices are "best" to use for an individual patient. Efforts are being undertaken by the SCAI and other organizations to increase the number of "stroke interventionalists" who are capable of providing round-the-clock catheter-based therapy. Carotid-stent operators, a broad group of providers from multiple disciplines, are the natural fit to expand the pool of stroke interventionalists, as they are familiar with cannulation of arch vessels and intracerebral anatomy. To realize the full benefits of stroke therapy, organization needs to exist at the community level to treat stroke with the same urgency and systemized approach that has been used for acute MI. This can be accomplished by conducting a thorough assessment of community resources, cooperating across disciplines, and developing written protocols for the standardization of stroke care. Importantly, we need more data in the form of randomized trials as we move forward into the twenty-first century in order to determine the safest and most efficacious ways to treat acute ischemic stroke.

References

1. Rosamond W, Flegal K, Furie K, et al. Heart disease and stroke statistics–2008 update: a report from the American Heart Association Statistics Committee and Stroke Statistics Subcommittee. Circulation. 2008;117(4):e25–146.
2. Lloyd-Jones D, Adams RJ, Brown TM, et al. Heart disease and stroke statistics–2010 update: a report from the American Heart Association. Circulation. 2010;121(7):e46–215.
3. Bozzao L, Fantozzi LM, Bastianello S, et al. Ischaemic supratentorial stroke: angiographic findings in patients examined in the very early phase. J Neurol. 1989;236(6):340–2.
4. Tissue plasminogen activator for acute ischemic stroke. The National Institute of Neurological Disorders and Stroke rt-PA Stroke Study Group. N Engl J Med. 1995;333(24):1581–87.
5. Combined intravenous and intra-arterial recanalization for acute ischemic stroke: the Interventional Management of Stroke Study. Stroke. 2004;35(4):904–11.
6. The Interventional Management of Stroke (IMS) II Study. IMS II Trial Investigators. Stroke; a journal of cerebral circulation. 2007; 38(7):2127–35.
7. Bose A, Henkes H, Alfke K, et al. The penumbra system: a mechanical device for the treatment of acute stroke due to thromboembolism. AJNR Am J Neuroradiol. 2008;29(7):1409–13.
8. Ramee SR, Subramanian R, Felberg RA, et al. Catheter-based treatment for patients with acute ischemic stroke ineligible for intravenous thrombolysis. Stroke. May 2004;35(5):e109–11.
9. Smith WS, Sung G, Saver J, et al. Mechanical thrombectomy for acute ischemic stroke. Final results of the multi MERCI trial. Stroke. 2008;39:1205–12.
10. Smith WS, Sung G, Starkman S, et al. Safety and efficacy of mechanical embolectomy in acute ischemic stroke: results of the MERCI trial. Stroke. Jul 2005;36(7):1432–8.
11. DeVries JT, White CJ, Collins TJ, et al. Acute stroke intervention by interventional cardiologists. Catheter Cardiovasc Interv. 2009; 73(5):692–8.
12. White CJ, Cates CU, Cowley MJ, et al. Interventional stroke therapy: current state of the art and needs assessment. Catheter Cardiovasc Interv. 2007;70(3):471–6.
13. Schwamm LH, Pancioli A, Acker III JE, et al. Recommendations for the establishment of stroke systems of care: recommendations from the American Stroke Association's Task Force on the Development of Stroke Systems. Circulation. 2005;111(8):1078–91.
14. Adams Jr HP, del Zoppo G, Alberts MJ, et al. Guidelines for the early management of adults with ischemic stroke: a guideline from the American Heart Association/American Stroke Association Stroke Council, Clinical Cardiology Council, Cardiovascular Radiology

and Intervention Council, and the Atherosclerotic Peripheral Vascular Disease and Quality of Care Outcomes in Research Interdisciplinary Working Groups: The American Academy of Neurology affirms the value of this guideline as an educational tool for neurologists. Circulation. 2007;115(20):e478–534.

15. Hacke W, Kaste M, Bluhmki E, et al. Thrombolysis with alteplase 3 to 4.5 hours after acute ischemic stroke. N Engl J Med. 2008;359(13):1317–29.
16. Albers GW, Thijs VN, Wechsler L, et al. Magnetic resonance imaging profiles predict clinical response to early reperfusion: the diffusion and perfusion imaging evaluation for understanding stroke evolution (DEFUSE) study. Ann Neurol. Nov 2006;60(5):508–17.
17. Schaefer PW, Barak ER, Kamalian S, et al. Quantitative assessment of core/penumbra mismatch in acute stroke. CT and MR perfusion imaging are strongly correlated when sufficient brain volume is imaged. Stroke. 2008 Nov;39(11):2986–92.
18. Hacke W, Donnan G, Fieschi C, et al. Association of outcome with early stroke treatment: pooled analysis of ATLANTIS, ECASS, and NINDS rt-PA stroke trials. Lancet. 2004;363(9411):768–74.
19. NIHSS Web Page. www.strokecenter.org/trials/scales/nihss.html. Accessed 28 Feb 2008.
20. Kwiatkowski TG, Libman RB, Frankel M, et al. Effects of tissue plasminogen activator for acute ischemic stroke at one year. National Institute of Neurological Disorders and Stroke Recombinant Tissue Plasminogen Activator Stroke Study Group. N Engl J Med. 1999;340(23):1781–7.
21. Magid D, Naviaux N, Wears RL. Stroking the data: re-analysis of the NINDS trial. Ann Emerg Med. Apr 2005;45(4):385–7.
22. Modified Rankin Scores. www.strokecenter.org/trials/scales/rankin.html. Accessed 28 Feb 2008.
23. Demaerschalk BM, Yip TR. Economic benefit of increasing utilization of intravenous tissue plasminogen activator for acute ischemic stroke in the United States. Stroke. Nov 2005;36(11):2500–3.
24. Thomassen L, Bakke SJ. Endovascular reperfusion therapy in acute ischaemic stroke. Acta Neurol Scand Suppl. 2007;187:22–9.
25. Furlan A, Higashida R, Wechsler L, et al. Intra-arterial prourokinase for acute ischemic stroke. The PROACT II study: a randomized controlled trial. Prolyse in Acute Cerebral Thromboembolism. JAMA. 1999;282(21):2003–11.
26. Kleindorfer DO, Khatri P, Katzan I. Reasons for exclusion from thrombolytic therapy following acute ischemic stroke. Neurology. 2005;65(11):1844; author reply 1844.
27. Davalos A, Blanco M, Pedraza S, et al. The clinical-DWI mismatch: a new diagnostic approach to the brain tissue at risk of infarction. Neurology. 2004;62(12):2187–92.
28. Kidwell CS, Warach S. Mismatch and defuse: harvesting the riches of multicenter neuroimaging-based stroke studies. Stroke. Jun 2007;38(6):1718–19.
29. 2005 American Heart Association Guidelines for Cardiopulmonary Resuscitation and Emergency Cardiovascular Care. Circulation. 2005;112(24 Suppl):IV1-203.
30. Smith WS. Safety of mechanical thrombectomy and intravenous tissue plasminogen activator in acute ischemic stroke. Results of the multi Mechanical Embolus Removal in Cerebral Ischemia (MERCI) trial, part I. AJNR Am J Neuroradiol. 2006;27(6):1177–82.
31. del Zoppo GJ, Higashida RT, Furlan AJ, Pessin MS, Rowley HA, Gent M. PROACT: a phase II randomized trial of recombinant prourokinase by direct arterial delivery in acute middle cerebral artery stroke. PROACT Investigators. Prolyse in Acute Cerebral Thromboembolism. Stroke. 1998;29(1):4–11.
32. Baker WL, Colby JA, Tongbram V, et al. Neurothrombectomy devices for the treatment of acute ischemic stroke: state of the evidence. Ann Intern Med. 2011;154(4):243–52.
33. Meyers PM, Schumacher HC, Higashida RT, et al. Indications for the performance of intracranial endovascular neurointerventional procedures: a scientific statement from the American Heart Association Council on Cardiovascular Radiology and Intervention, Stroke Council, Council on Cardiovascular Surgery and Anesthesia, Interdisciplinary Council on Peripheral Vascular Disease, and Interdisciplinary Council on Quality of Care and Outcomes Research. Circulation. 2009;119(16):2235–49.
34. Lewandowski CA, Frankel M, Tomsick TA, et al. Combined intravenous and intra-arterial r-TPA versus intra-arterial therapy of acute ischemic stroke: Emergency Management of Stroke (EMS) Bridging Trial. Stroke. Dec 1999;30(12):2598–605.
35. Flaherty ML, Woo D, Kissela B, et al. Combined IV and intra-arterial thrombolysis for acute ischemic stroke. Neurology. 2005;64(2):386–8.
36. Mackey J, Khatri P, Broderick JP, Investigators II. Increasing use of CT angiography in interventional study sites: the IMS III experience. AJNR Am J Neuroradiol. 2010;31(3):E34.
37. Becker KJ, Brott TG. Approval of the MERCI clot retriever: a critical view. Stroke. Feb 2005;36(2):400–3.
38. Penumbra Pivotal Stroke Trial I, Clark W, Lutsep H, et al. The penumbra pivotal stroke trial: safety and effectiveness of a new generation of mechanical devices for clot removal in intracranial large vessel occlusive disease. Stroke J Cereb Circ. 2009;40(8):2761–8.
39. Velat GJ, Hoh BL, Levy EI, Mocco J. Primary intracranial stenting in acute ischemic stroke. Curr Cardiol Rep. 2010;12(1):14–9.
40. Levy EI, Ecker RD, Horowitz MB, et al. Stent-assisted intracranial recanalization for acute stroke: early results. Neurosurgery. 2006;58(3):458–63. discussion 458-463.
41. Lee VH, Samuels S, Herbst TJ, et al. Histopathologic description of Wingspan stent in acute ischemic stroke. Neurocrit Care. 2009;11(3):377–80.
42. Levy EI, Sauvageau E, Hanel RA, Parikh R, Hopkins LN. Self-expanding versus balloon-mounted stents for vessel recanalization following embolic occlusion in the canine model: technical feasibility study. AJNR Am J Neuroradiol. 2006;27(10):2069–72.
43. Zaidat OO, Wolfe T, Hussain SI, et al. Interventional acute ischemic stroke therapy with intracranial self-expanding stent. Stroke J Cereb Circ. 2008;39(8):2392–5.
44. Levy EI, Siddiqui AH, Crumlish A, et al. First Food and Drug Administration-approved prospective trial of primary intracranial stenting for acute stroke: SARIS (stent-assisted recanalization in acute ischemic stroke). Stroke J Cereb Circ. 2009;40(11):3552–6.
45. Weber W, Kis B, Siekmann R, Kuehne D. Endovascular treatment of intracranial arteriovenous malformations with onyx: technical aspects. AJNR Am J Neuroradiol. 2007;28(2):371–7.
46. Castano C, Dorado L, Guerrero C, et al. Mechanical thrombectomy with the Solitaire AB device in large artery occlusions of the anterior circulation: a pilot study. Stroke J Cereb Circ. 2010;41(8):1836–40.
47. Roth C, Papanagiotou P, Behnke S, et al. Stent-assisted mechanical recanalization for treatment of acute intracerebral artery occlusions. Stroke J Cereb Circ. 2010;41(11):2559–67.
48. Levy EI, Rahman M, Khalessi AA, et al. Midterm clinical and angiographic follow-up for the first Food and Drug Administration-approved prospective, Single-Arm Trial of Primary Stenting for Stroke: SARIS (Stent-Assisted Recanalization for Acute Ischemic Stroke). Neurosurgery. 2011;69(4):915–20. discussion 920.
49. Kelly ME, Furlan AJ, Fiorella D. Recanalization of an acute middle cerebral artery occlusion using a self-expanding, reconstrainable, intracranial microstent as a temporary endovascular bypass. Stroke J Cereb Circ. 2008;39(6):1770–3.
50. Hauck EF, Mocco J, Snyder KV, Levy EI. Temporary endovascular bypass: a novel treatment for acute stroke. AJNR Am J Neuroradiol. 2009;30(8):1532–3.
51. O'Collins VE, Macleod MR, Donnan GA, Horky LL, van der Worp BH, Howells DW. 1,026 experimental treatments in acute stroke. Ann Neurol. 2006;59(3):467–77.
52. Hypothermia after Cardiac Arrest Study G. Mild therapeutic hypothermia to improve the neurologic outcome after cardiac arrest. N Engl J Med. 2002;346(8):549–56.

53. Ueda Y, Suehiro E, Wei EP, Kontos HA, Povlishock JT. Uncomplicated rapid posthypothermic rewarming alters cerebrovascular responsiveness. Stroke J Cereb Circ. 2004;35(2):601–6.
54. Suzuki S, Saver JL, Scott P, et al. Access to intra-arterial therapies for acute ischemic stroke: an analysis of the US population. AJNR Am J Neuroradiol. 2004;25(10):1802–6.
55. SCAI first to offer multidisciplinary course in acute stroke intervention. Cathet Cardiovas Interv. 2008;71:445–6.
56. Alberts MJ, Hademenos G, Latchaw RE, et al. Recommendations for the establishment of primary stroke centers. Brain Attack Coalition. JAMA. 2000;283(23):3102–9.
57. Skolnick BE. Guidelines for acute stroke treatment centers. Phys Med Rehabil Clin N Am. 1999;10(4):801–13. viii.
58. Furlan AJ, Murdock MM, Spilker JA. NSA stroke center network stroke center recommendations. J Stroke Cerebrovas Dis. 1997;6(4):299–302.
59. Alberts MJ, Latchaw RE, Selman WR, et al. Recommendations for comprehensive stroke centers: a consensus statement from the Brain Attack Coalition. Stroke. Jul 2005;36(7):1597–616.
60. Antman EM. Time is muscle: translation into practice. J Am Coll Cardiol. 2008;52(15):1216–21.
61. Meyer BC, Raman R, Hemmen T, et al. Efficacy of site-independent telemedicine in the STRokE DOC trial: a randomised, blinded, prospective study. Lancet Neurol. 2008;7(9):787–95.
62. Demaerschalk BM, Yip TR. Economic benefit of increasing utilization of intravenous tissue plasminogen activator for acute ischemic stroke in the United States. Stroke. 2005;36(11):2500–3.

Venous Thromboembolic Disease

37

Ido Weinberg and Michael R. Jaff

Venous thromboembolic disease (VTE) is common. The incidence is estimated to be 108 per 100,000 population with an annual incidence of 250,000 in the United States alone. The incidence of DVT in early studies was 30 % following surgery [1]. The combined 30-day survival rate is 74.8 % following VTE, higher for deep vein thrombosis (DVT) than for pulmonary embolism (PE) [2].

Deep Vein Thrombosis

Deep vein thrombosis (DVT) most commonly arises in the deep venous system of the lower extremities. The natural history involves three phases: adherence of loose thrombus to the vein wall, organization of thrombus coupled with inflammation, and recanalization that occurs within 1 year of the event, depending on thrombus location and extent [3]. DVT is divided according to their anatomical location, as the distribution of a thrombus may predict early and late clinical outcomes. Proximal DVT in the lower extremity is located in the vena cava, iliac, femoral, profunda femoris (rarely), and popliteal veins. Distal deep vein thrombi of the lower extremity are those located in the veins of the calf (both muscular and crural veins) [4]. Iliofemoral DVT is considered more prone to systemic and long-term local complications, as blood has no anatomical route by which to bypass the obstruction [5]. In the upper extremity, DVT occurs in the jugular, subclavian, axillary, and brachial veins.

DVT may also be divided into provoked (i.e., DVTs that are secondary to a specific, etiology such as trauma, surgery, comorbid illness (i.e., congestive heart failure or immobility)) [6] or unprovoked (otherwise known as idiopathic) [7]. Risk factors for DVT are shown in Table 37.1 [6–8].

Symptoms of DVT include pain and swelling of the affected extremity (or extremities). While not all DVTs are symptomatic and not all DVTs result in complications, they may result in long-term morbidity. This may include pulmonary emboli, venous insufficiency, post-thrombotic syndrome (PTS), and lymphedema. Venous insufficiency after DVT may be as prevalent as 56 %, depending on the exact location, extent, and initial treatment [3]. PTS develops in as many as 40 % of patients within 5 years of a DVT [9]. Clinical manifestations of PTS include pain in the affected limb, cramps, heaviness, paresthesia and pruritus, pretibial edema, skin induration or ulceration, hyperpigmentation, pain during calf compression, venous ectasia, and erythema [10].

Furthermore, left untreated, mortality from VTE may be as high as 30 %. Even with treatment, death rates are not negligible [11]. DVT is a recurring disease, even with adequate treatment. Recurrence rates vary and depend on the presence or absence of an underlying cause and on other clinical characteristics and may range from less than 1 %/year to as high as 27 % in 1 year after stopping anticoagulation [12]. In a series of 355 patients, recurrence rates increased with time since the inciting event. At 8 years, the cumulative incidence was 30.3 % [9]. The risk of fatal PE was as high as 0.49 per 100 person-years after a complete course of anticoagulation in a prospective surveillance of 2,052 patients with VTE [13].

Diagnosis of DVT

The diagnosis of DVT mandates a high index of suspicion as derived from a careful history and physical examination, combined with judicious use of imaging. Classic symptoms of DVT include pain and swelling of the involved extremity. A DVT in the inferior vena cava may present as bilateral lower extremity swelling. Catheter-associated DVT may present with malfunction of the catheter. The clinical likelihood that a DVT is present is assessed by using the Wells criteria.

I. Weinberg, MD, MSc
Department of Cardiology, Massachusetts General Hospital, 55 Fruit St., Boston, MA, USA

M.R. Jaff, DO (✉)
Section of Vascular Medicine, Department of Medicine, Massachusetts General Hospital, 55 Fruit St., Boston, MA, USA
e-mail: mjaff@partners.org

C.A. Thompson (ed.), *Textbook of Cardiovascular Intervention*,
DOI 10.1007/978-1-4471-4528-8_37, © Springer-Verlag London 2014

Table 37.1 Risk factors for the development of DVT

Cause	Example
Obstruction to venous outflow	May-Thurner syndrome
Immobility	Postsurgical or acute illness
Inflammation	Postsurgical or acute illness
Genetic predisposition	Factor V Leiden
Estrogen supplementation	Oral contraceptives, hormone replacement therapy, and prostate cancer hormonal treatment
Smoking	
Obesity	
Malignancy	Adenocarcinoma (e.g., pancreatic cancer)
Congestive heart failure	
Advanced age	
Trauma	Spinal cord injury and limb fracture
Central venous catheter	
Previous DVT	
Venous varicosities	
Pregnancy and the postpartum period	
Diet rich in red meat and low in fruit and fish	

Once the pretest probability has been formulated, ancillary testing may be added including quantitative D-dimer laboratory assays and duplex ultrasonography (DUS). An elevated quantitative D-dimer does not confirm the diagnosis, while a negative value has a high negative predictive value for DVT [14]. DUS findings that support the presence of DVT include lack of compression of the vein that is being tested, lack of augmentation of blood flow in response to distal compression, and lack of respiratory variation in the venous Doppler blood flow pattern. Color flow ultrasonography may show lack of flow or partial recanalization. When clinical suspicion is high, yet duplex ultrasonography is negative or when DVT is suspected in the pelvis or inferior vena cava, computed tomography (CTV) and magnetic resonance venography (MRV) should be used. A diagnostic algorithm is shown in Fig. 37.1.

Treatment of DVT

Anticoagulation

Anticoagulation is the mainstay of treatment of DVT [15]. Duration of anticoagulant treatment varies according to the underlying etiology, comorbidities, and the location of

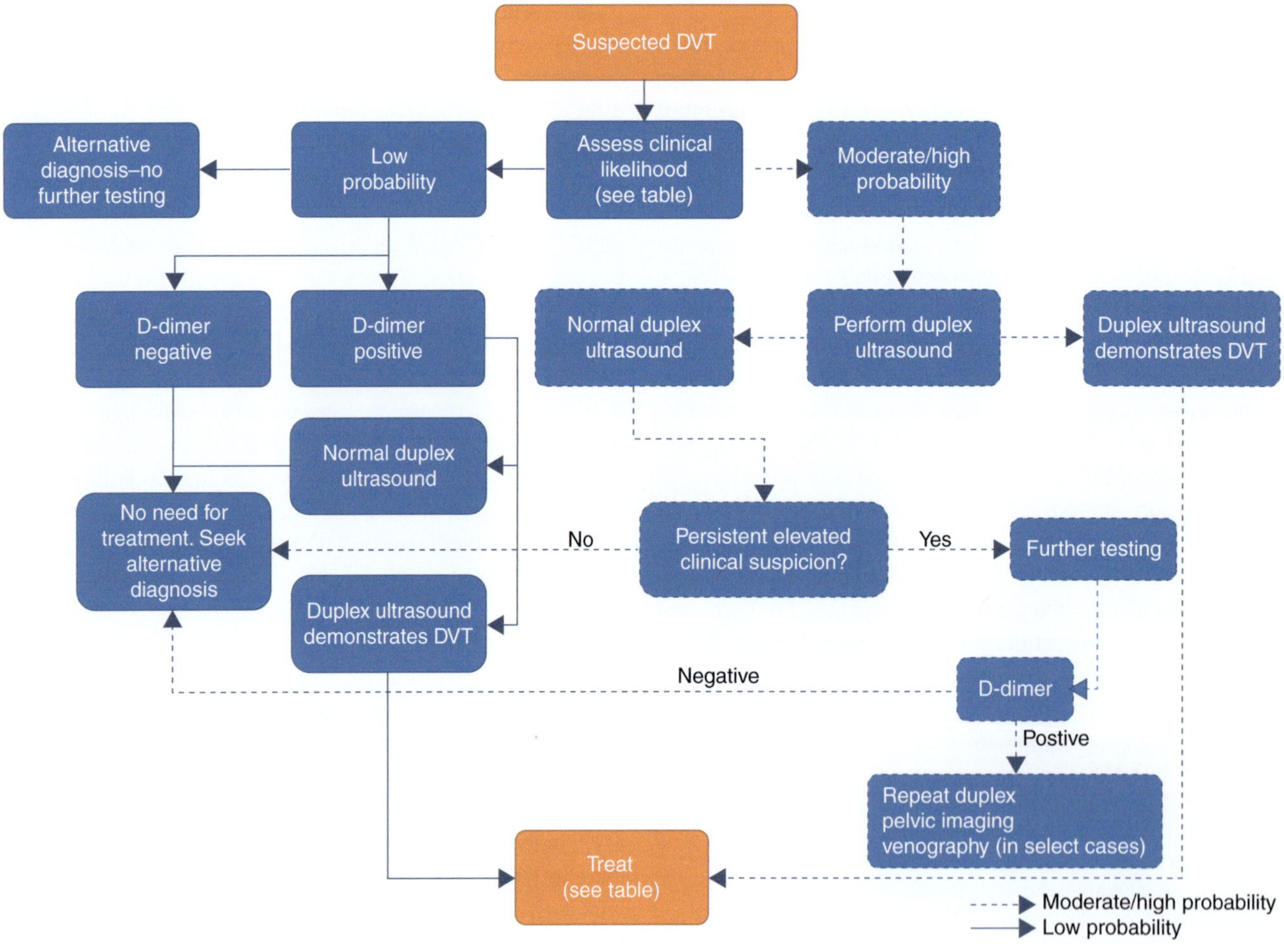

Fig. 37.1 Diagnostic algorithm for deep vein thrombosis

Table 37.2 Duration of treatment of DVT according to location and provocation[a]

Thrombus location	Type of treatment	Duration of treatment	Comments
Proximal, provoked	Full-dose anticoagulation	3–6 months	
Proximal, unprovoked	Full-dose anticoagulation. After 6 months, consider reduced target INR of 1.5–2.0 [20]	At least 6 months. Consider indefinite according to assessed risk of bleeding	In patients with malignancy, low molecular weight heparin is preferred; utilize adjunctive testing to determine duration of treatment; if second event, consider long-term treatment (see text)
Calf (distal), unprovoked	Nonsteroidal anti-inflammatory drugs (if no anticoagulation and serial DUS) or full-dose anticoagulation	≤3 months	Treatment type and duration should be driven by location and extent of the clot as well as progression over repeat testing. Attention should be paid to patient symptoms and preferences
Superficial venous thrombus	Topical heat with optional nonsteroidal anti-inflammatory drugs or preventive-dose heparin or low molecular weight heparin or fondaparinux [120]	4 weeks	When the superficial vein thrombus in the greater saphenous vein extends to within 8 cm of the saphenofemoral junction, treat as DVT
Catheter associated	Full-dose anticoagulation	No more than 3 months after catheter removal	

Data from [15, 16]
[a]Treatment duration should weigh the benefits of anticoagulation with the risk of bleeding and the inconvenience of treatment

Table 37.3 Pharmacological options for systemic anticoagulation

Method	Mode of administration	Main characteristics	Monitoring	Comments
Unfractionated heparin	Administered intravenously and subcutaneously	Short acting; has antidote (protamine sulfate)	aPTT	Mandates frequent testing and dose adjustments
Low molecular weight heparin	Administered subcutaneously; dose adjustment by body weight and renal function	Intermediate half-life	Anti-Xa	Protamine sulfate results in partial reversal of action
Oral vitamin K antagonist	Dose adjusted by total weekly dose	Many drug and food interactions; narrow therapeutic range	INR	Classically must be preceded by heparin in order to prevent transient hypercoagulable state (see text)
Factor Xa inhibitor	Either subcutaneously (fondaparinux) or orally (rivaroxaban and apixaban) [86, 121]	Intermediate half-life; no antidote	None available; perhaps drug levels in plasma	No intermediate dose available
Direct thrombin inhibitor	Oral (ximelagatran[a], dabigatran), subcutaneous (hirudins, melagatran[a]), or intravenous (hirudins, bivalirudin, argatroban, melagatran[a])	Short half-life (bivalirudin, argatroban, and intravenous hirudin), intermediate (subcutaneous hirudin, melagatran[a], ximelagatran[a], dabigatran); no antidote	None available	Various options with varying metabolic pathways

[a]Not available in the United States

the thrombus. Duration of systemic anticoagulation ranges from several weeks to indefinite treatment [16]. Table 37.2 summarizes the main factors that need to be considered when planning the duration of treatment for a VTE episode. Full-dose anticoagulation may be achieved by several methods (Table 37.3). Special consideration needs to be given to the initiation of warfarin treatment, if it is the chosen method of anticoagulation. Though warfarin dose varies among different patients, the usual method for initiating treatment is to administer a loading dose of 5 or 10 mg for 2 days and then make adjustments according to INR measurements. In at-risk patient populations such as people who are elderly, are malnourished, or have liver disease, a lower loading dose should be given [17]. Starting warfarin with 10 mg as compared to 5 mg has not resulted in excess bleeding [18, 19] and may achieve a more rapid effect [18]. Target INR is 2.0–3.0. After 6 months, consideration may be given to reducing to a target INR of 1.5–2.0 [20]. The first days after the administration of warfarin represent a *pro*-thrombotic state as vitamin K antagonists affect both *pro*coagulant factors (II, VII, IX, and X) and *anti*coagulant cofactors (protein S and protein C). Upon first administration, levels of protein S and protein C are reduced, while factor II levels remain relatively high, because it has a relatively long half-life. This allows for unopposed pro-thrombotic activity of factor II. Therefore, for most patients, warfarin must be administered in conjunction with another method of anticoagulation such as heparin, low molecular heparin, or fondaparinux until the INR has been therapeutic for 24 h (typically INR ≥2). Treatment duration with anticoagulation may be extended in several situations including recurrent unprovoked DVT, persistent elevation of the serum D-dimer levels 1 month after completion of an adequate initial course of anticoagulation [21, 22], and, potentially, residual thrombus detected by serial duplex studies [23]. This latter indication has been disputed [24]. A prospective study examined the value of combining both D-dimer and residual thrombus and showed that DVT recurrence correlated only with D-dimer [25]. Patients with antiphospholipid antibody syndrome (APLS) anticoagulation who had a thrombotic event should usually be treated indefinitely with anticoagulation as recurrence rate is often high. However, patients with APLS are a heterogeneous group, carrying varying degrees of risk for recurrent thrombosis. Therefore, for some, treatment can be shorter. Current recommendations favor warfarin with a target INR of 2.0–3.0 [26]. Nevertheless, in the general population of patients with thrombosis, DVT may recur during treatment in up to 27 % of cases, particularly among patients with underlying malignancy. One study compared DVT recurrence rates in 842 patients with and without malignancy who suffered their first episode of DVT. The incidence was 30 per 100 patient-years in patients with cancer as compared with 12.8 per 100 years in patients without malignancy [27].

Compression Stockings

Graduated compression stockings (GCS) are important adjuncts to the treatment of DVT as they have been proven to be effective in the prevention of post-thrombotic syndrome. A comparison of compression stockings in 194 consecutive patients with proximal DVT showed a reduction in post-thrombotic syndrome from 47 to 20 % after a mean follow-up of 76 months [28]. Another, prospective, non-blinded, randomized comparison of GCS versus no stockings was conducted in 180 patients after a first symptomatic proximal leg deep vein thrombosis for 3–5 years. Stockings were knee-high and 30–40 mmHg compression at the ankle and were worn for 2 years. PTS developed in 44/90 patients in the control group and only 23/90 in the treatment group. The number needed to treat to prevent one episode of PTS was four patients for 1 year [29]. Severity of PTS was also reduced in these trials.

Thrombolytic Therapy for DVT

Catheter-directed thrombolysis (CDT) is a treatment option for proximal iliofemoral DVT. Indications for thrombolysis for DVT stem from several limitations of anticoagulation. First, thrombolysis has the theoretical advantage of reducing thrombus burden. Second, anticoagulation has not been shown to reduce the incidence of PTS, a cause of significant morbidity and reduced quality of life. A prospective trial compared anticoagulation with a target INR <1.7 with anticoagulation targeted at an INR >2.5 in 145 patients with proximal DVT. This trial did not find a reduction of PTS in the higher intensity group. The combined incidence of PTS in both groups was 37 %, similar to other series. Time in therapeutic range also did not correlate with PTS [30].

Thrombolytic therapy aims at achieving greater thrombus lysis than anticoagulation and theoretically less PTS. In a 50-month follow-up of 101 patients undergoing CDT for iliofemoral DVT in 103 extremities, 10 patients were reported to have mild chronic venous insufficiency symptoms. Compression stockings and anticoagulation were prescribed for 12 months as well. Vein patency was 82 % at 6 years [31]. Mewissen et al. reported CDT for treatment of lower extremity DVT in 303 limbs in 287 patients. Proximal DVT was detected in 74 % of limbs and 65 % of these were acute (less than 10 days). Primary patency at 1 year was 59.7 %, more in iliofemoral DVT than in femoral-popliteal (64 % vs. 47 %, respectively) and more in acute rather than chronic DVT. Of note, 45 % of patients also received a stent [32]. A nonrandomized comparison of thrombolysis with anticoagulation to anticoagulation alone for iliofemoral DVT in 51 patients reported 5-year results. Patency was 69 % in the combined treatment group and 18 % in the anticoagulation group, and symptom resolution was more common in the CDT group (78 % vs. 30 %) [33]. Another trial, the largest trial to date comparing CDT with anticoagulation to anticoagulation alone for treatment of DVT, is the catheter-directed venous thrombolysis in acute iliofemoral vein thrombosis trial (CaVenT). This is a multicenter, prospective, non-blinded, randomized controlled trial [34]. The first set of results was published regarding outcome at 6 months after initiating treatment. Bleeding was greater in the CDT group (10/49 vs. 2/53; 4 major bleeding). Patency was greater in the CDT group (64 % vs. 35.8 %). There was no difference in femoral vein reflux between the two groups (66 % vs. 60 %). The CaVenT trial lacked information regarding the use of compression stockings, so the results must be viewed with limited applicability. It is anticipated that 2-year follow-up will be reported.

The ATTRACT trial is an ongoing trial sponsored by the National Institutes of Health. ATTRACT is randomizing patients with iliofemoral DVT to optimal anticoagulation versus pharmacomechanical thrombolysis (PMT) followed by optimal anticoagulation. ATTRACT will systematically determine the incidence of PTS over 24-month follow-up [35]. Patients undergoing thrombolysis need to be treated with anticoagulation following intervention. Unfractionated heparin is appropriate for use during CDT, albeit in a reduced dose [34]. Dose should increase if aggressive manipulation of the clot is performed [36].

The American College of Chest Physicians Evidence-Based Clinical Practice Guidelines (8th edition) recommend that for patients with a low risk of bleeding who have a proximal acute DVT, good functional status, and reasonable life expectancy, thrombolysis may be used. In patients with extensive proximal DVT with symptoms ≤14 days, who have a reasonable life expectancy and who have a low bleeding risk, CDT is reasonable, potentially with PMT [15]. An American Heart Association position statement suggested indications for CDT to include phlegmasia cerulea dolens, thrombus progression, and symptoms worsening despite treatment with anticoagulation [5]. As mentioned above, PTS prevention is still being studied as an indication. Contraindications to CDT are viewed as absolute and relative and are shown in Table 37.4.

Table 37.4 Contraindications to pharmacological thrombolysis

Absolute contraindications
Active internal bleeding or severe coagulopathy such as disseminated intravascular coagulation
Cerebrovascular event, neurosurgical procedure (including spinal and paraspinal), and cerebral trauma in the past 3 months
Contraindication to anticoagulation
Aortic dissection
Relative contraindications
Recent cardiopulmonary resuscitation
Recent surgery including major surgery, organ biopsy, and trauma in the past 10 days or eye surgery in the past 3 months
Obstetrical delivery
Intracranial tumor
Seizures
Uncontrolled hypertension (systolic >180 mmHg and diastolic >110 mmHg)
Gastrointestinal bleed in the past 3 months
Allergy to one of the agents needed for the procedure
Hemodynamic instability
Severe thrombocytopenia
Left ventricular thrombus or right to left heart shunt or bacterial endocarditis
Suspected infected thrombus
Severe renal failure or severe hepatic dysfunction
Pregnancy or lactation
Diabetic hemorrhagic retinopathy

Data from [5, 122]

Percutaneous Mechanical Thrombectomy

Percutaneous mechanical thrombectomy (PMT) utilizes fragmentation, maceration, and aspiration of thrombus. Devices include rotational, rheolytic, and ultrasound-enhanced catheters. Mechanical methods utilize various types of devices to macerate the thrombus. Rheolytic devices spray the thrombus with thrombolytic agents while aspirating the debris. Ultrasound-enhanced devices have multiple high-frequency ultrasound transducers. The ultrasound waves cause disruption of the venous thrombus matrix, thus exposing plasminogen receptors and allowing for better targeting of the thrombus to the lytic agent. PMT is usually combined with pharmacological thrombolysis as it is not sufficiently effective as standalone treatment. PMT has only been studied in retrospective cohorts and not in a prospective manner, although several trials are underway [37]. Nonetheless, one study of 27 patients who underwent aspiration thrombectomy for iliofemoral DVT reported 88.9 % immediate success without thrombolysis. Two patients had recurrent DVT during follow-up. No other complications were reported; however, all patients received an IVC filter prior to PMT [38]. A trial comparing 26 limbs in which DVT was treated with CDT alone with 19 limbs in which PMT was added showed that addition of PMT to CDT reduced the thrombolytic drug dose and infusion time and thus reduced hospitalization time and resource utilization [39]. Others have reported complications with PMT including bleeding, local vessel damage, and PE [40]. The Society of Interventional Radiology guidelines suggest that there is still need for further research regarding pharmacomechanical techniques as compared to CDT alone for treatment of proximal DVT [41]. The American Heart Association consensus statement suggests that PMT may be combined with CDT [36].

Surgical Venous Thrombectomy

In light of the advent of less invasive procedures, surgical venous thrombectomy is suitable for a minority of patients with iliofemoral DVT. A single center reported both 6-month and 5-year results of surgical venous thrombectomy compared to anticoagulation for iliofemoral DVT. In the short term, more patients in the surgical group were free of PTS (42 % vs. 7 %, $P<0.005$) [42]. In the long term, there were also fewer symptoms in this group, though not statistically significant (18 % vs. 37 %) [43]. Ten-year results of the same patient cohort demonstrated that the surgical group again had non-statistically significant better clinical outcomes. Vein patency was higher in this group as well, demonstrating statistical significance [44].

Vena Cava Filters

The practice of interrupting the passage of thrombi from the lower extremity veins to the pulmonary vasculature has been entertained for decades. Early procedures included physical ligation of the inferior vena cava. These have been replaced by peripherally inserted vena cava filters.

Inferior vena cava (IVC) filters are permanent and retrievable (Table 37.5). All retrievable filters can theoretically remain in the body and function permanently, though long-term durability data is lacking [5].

Indications for IVC filters include secondary prevention of PE in a patient with DVT and a contraindication to anticoagulation or failure of anticoagulation treatment such as recurrent VTE despite adequate anticoagulation [15].

Table 37.5 Inferior vena cava filters

Filter	Company
Non-retrievable	
Stainless steel Greenfield filter	Boston Scientific, Natick, MA
Titanium Greenfield filter	Boston Scientific, Natick, MA
Vena Tech LGM filter	B. Braun, Boulogne, France
Vena Tech LP filter	B. Braun, Boulogne, France
Simon Nitinol filter	Bard, Nordic, Sweden
Bird's Nest filter	Cook Medical, Bloomington, IN
TrapEase filter	Cordis Corporation, Bridgewater, NJ
G2 Recovery filter	Bard, Nordic, Sweden
SafeFlo permanent filter	Rafael Medical, Dover, DE
Retrievable	
Recovery filter	Bard, Nordic, Sweden
Gunther Tulip filter	Cook Medical, Bloomington, IN
Celect filter	Cook Medical, Bloomington, IN
OptEase filter	Cordis Corporation, Bridgewater, NJ
Antheor filter	Boston Scientific, Natick, MA
Tempofilter[a]	B. Braun, Boulogne, France
Prolyser filter[a]	B. Braun, Boulogne, France
ALN filter[a]	ALN, Bormes-les-Mimosas, France

[a]Not FDA approved

The latest American Heart Association scientific statement also addressed IVC filter insertion in patients with iliofemoral DVT. This committee assigned a lower rate of evidence to IVC filter insertion when there is recurrent DVT despite anticoagulation (level of evidence IIb) than to recurrent PE (level of evidence IIa). This document also suggests that trying a different type of anticoagulation ("second-line" anticoagulation) for recurrent DVT may be suitable [5]. Contraindications for IVC filter insertion are few and include lack of access site and severe coagulopathy.

Despite widespread use of IVC filters [45], most data regarding their efficacy is retrospective in nature [46, 47]. Use of IVC filters was examined in a retrospective community-based observational study. Medical charts of patients who had a diagnosis of VTE were reviewed and the indications for IVC filters were examined along with patient outcomes. Mean follow-up was 926 days. Overall, a panel of reviewers found that in 51 % of patients, the filters had been inserted without proper indications, while in 26 % of cases, the panel found that the filters were inserted for sufficiently evidence-supported reasons. When the reviewers disagreed, it was most commonly due to perceived risk of bleeding. Patients with filters had fewer PE (1.7 % vs. 5.3 %, $P=0.18$), but more DVT (21 % vs. 14.9 %, $P=0.009$) at 3 years of follow-up. Mortality was higher in this group as compared to patients who did not receive a filter. Importantly, patients enrolled in this study were treated until 2003 and most received permanent filters [48]. Furthermore, a population-based study examining discharge data for over 67,000 patients with DVT in California examined the effect of IVC filters on rehospitalization. While IVC filters reduced the readmissions for PE, patients were admitted more for DVT and overall admission rate was not lower [49]. A possible explanation for lack of a mortality benefit in "real-life" series is that the need for a filter may be a marker of sicker patients, in whom survival benefit is difficult to attain [47].

Only two prospective high-quality studies have examined the efficacy of IVC filters. Both studies evaluated permanent filters. In these studies, mortality was not reduced despite reduction in the incidence of PE. The pivotal Prévention du Risque d'Embolie Pulmonaire par Interruption Cave (PREPIC) study was a two-by-two factorial trial comparing filter to no filter and low molecular weight heparin to unfractionated heparin for the treatment of acute VTE in 400 patients. Filters were non-retrievable. At 2 years, there was no difference in mortality or in PE, but patients with filters had a higher incidence of DVT (20.8 % vs. 11.6 %, $P=0.02$). Some of the recurrent DVTs were directly attributable to filter thrombosis [50].

Complications of IVC filters are also not uncommon. Complications during insertion have been reported in 4–15 % and include puncture site-related problems, misplacement, migration, filters failing to deploy properly, and vena cava perforation [51]. A rare complication is access site DVT [52]. Complications of retained IVC filters include strut fracture and erosion into the IVC wall and adjacent structures, need for long-term anticoagulation, and thus continued bleeding risk, recurrent PE, and IVC filter thrombosis leading to advanced PTS. In the aforementioned PREPIC trial, 20.8 % of patients with indwelling filters had thrombotic complications, versus 11.6 % in patients without filters ($P=0.02$) [50]. Many of the thrombotic complications of IVC filters can be avoided by prompt removal of retrievable IVC filters. Only 20 % of filters are retrieved in clinical practice, although there are appropriate reasons for not extracting a retrievable filter, including retained filter thrombus and persistent contraindication to anticoagulation. However, the majority of filters are not retrieved due to lack of follow-up. A dedicated IVC filter clinic with planned follow-up with patients and referring physicians may increase retrieval rate [5, 53]. This has been studied in a single-center comparison of retrospective retrieval data to prospectively collected data after establishing a dedicated clinic. Retrieval rates were 29 % in 369 patients before the clinic was established and 60 % in 100 patients afterward [54].

Axillosubclavian Deep Venous Thrombosis

Upper extremity DVTs probably comprise less than 10 % of all DVT and are often related to indwelling venous catheters, pacemaker/defibrillator leads, and thoracic outlet syndrome [55]. As more central catheters are used in patient care, more of their complications are being seen. The risk for catheter-associated upper extremity DVT has been reported to be 2–5 % [56]. Risk factors for catheter-associated DVT include active cancer and larger lines [56, 57].

Compared with lower extremity DVT, there is a relative lack of data regarding upper extremity DVT. A recent review of the literature found PE to complicate upper extremity DVT in 5.6 % of the time, some of which were fatal [55]. Though effort-related upper extremity DVT (see below) is a non-life-threatening cause of upper extremity DVT, in other cases patients are typically systemically ill and the 1-year survival of all patients with upper extremity DVT is as low as 50 % [58]. As in lower extremity DVT, PTS is a potential complication of upper extremity DVT, albeit at a lower frequency. Recurrence is also less frequent [55].

Symptoms of upper extremity DVT include pain, swelling, paresthesias, and weakness of the limb. The diagnosis of upper extremity DVT relies first of all on compression duplex ultrasonography. Sometimes, when proximal subclavian or brachiocephalic DVT is suspected, formal venography, CT, or MRI is needed to confirm the diagnosis. D-dimer to rule out DVT is often not practical as many patients have multiple reasons for it to be elevated.

Anticoagulation forms the basis for the treatment of upper extremity DVT. There is no high-quality data regarding the intensity and duration of treatment. Practically, extrapolation from lower extremity DVT data is used. Treatment of catheter-associated DVT may include catheter removal, especially when there is catheter malfunction, though recurrence rate is not affected by this and catheter removal is not routinely indicated [55, 59]. An anticoagulation course of at least 3 months should be completed, even if the catheter has been removed. Data regarding CDT is poor and decided upon on a case-by-case basis according to symptom severity. Other catheter-based intervention such as aspiration, fragmentation, angioplasty, and stent placement should be performed only if thrombolysis and anticoagulation have failed. Stent placement in the subclavian vein in the costoclavicular junction results in high rates of stent deformity and fracture and should be avoided [55]. The treatment of "Paget-Schroetter" syndrome is discussed below.

Superior vena cava (SVC) filters are the upper extremity equivalent of IVC filters. Limited data suggests a higher complication rate with SVC filters in comparison with IVC filters. As for IVC filters, indications for superior vena cava filter insertion include inability to administer anticoagulation and failure of anticoagulation. Complications are also similar to IVC filters; however, risk of perforation into adjacent structures seems to be higher as a result of SVC characteristics and of anatomical proximity of the superior vena cava to the heart and lungs [60].

Paget-Schroetter Syndrome

Paget-Schroetter syndrome (PSS) is also known as effort-related thrombosis of the subclavian vein. It is caused by compression of the subclavian vein in the thoracic outlet and is a form of venous thoracic outlet syndrome (TOS). While most cases of TOS are neurogenic, the incidence of PSS has never been assessed directly. One center reported it to be 1 patient per 100,000 population a year [61]. PSS tends to occur in younger, muscular, active adults, and there have been many notable episodes among professional athletes [62].

The pathophysiology of PSS cannot be understood without first appreciating the anatomy of the thoracic outlet. The subclavian vein traverses in a potential space bordered by the clavicle, scalene muscle, and the first rib. In some people, the costoclavicular ligament courses laterally and thus may compress the subclavian vein during activity, especially if it is brought forward by a hypertrophied scalene muscle [63].

The clinical symptoms of PSS are directly related to thrombus formation in the subclavian vein. The onset of symptoms is usually acute, although preceding intermittent symptoms may be described. In a series of 626 limbs with PSS over 50 years, the most common symptoms were upper extremity venous dilatation, subcutaneous venous collaterals around the shoulder (Urschel's sign), arm swelling, bluish discoloration, and aching pain with exercise [63].

Left untreated, patients with PSS develop long-term morbidity that includes post-thrombotic venous insufficiency [64], potentially resulting in limited recreational and employment abilities [63]. Treatment with anticoagulation without invasive intervention was customary until the mid-1970s [65], but this may result in an incidence of long-term morbidity and recurrence in patients with PSS as high as 50 % [63, 66]. Furthermore, after thrombolysis alone, the recurrence rate of PSS is also high [63]. Two therapeutic approaches may be deduced from the above. The first approach advocates prompt thrombolysis followed by surgical resection of the compressive structure. The second approach is to follow patients after thrombolysis and intervene surgically only in those patients in whom thrombosis recurs or symptoms persist despite treatment. A retrospective analysis of a prospectively organized cohort reported a comparison of the two approaches. Of 64 patients, 29 were operated upon after thrombolysis with a long-term success rate of 93 %. Of 35 patients who were followed after thrombolysis, 8 eventually required surgical intervention [67]. These results are different than those reported by Urschel et al., who described persistent symptoms in 25 of 42 (60 %) patients treated by initial thrombolysis and further expectant management. These patients had good to excellent long-term results after surgical intervention [63].

Surgery for PSS involves mechanical alleviation of compression. The most common surgical approach is transaxillary first rib resection. This is not a benign procedure. Complications include hemopneumothorax, long thoracic nerve injury, and inadvertent removal of the second rib instead of the first. Other methods for thoracic outlet decompression include supra-, para-, and infraclavicular first rib resection, sternal disarticulation of the first rib, and medial claviculectomy [61].

Superior Vena Cava Syndrome

Obstruction of the superior vena cava, either by external compression by causes such as malignant tumor compression, fibrosing mediastinitis, infectious masses, or thoracic aortic aneurysms or internally because of tumor invasion or thrombosis, may lead to the superior vena cava syndrome (SVCS) [68, 69]. The annual incidence of SVCS in the United States is estimated to be 15,000 [68]. SVCS is present at diagnosis in 10 % of patients with small cell lung carcinoma and 1.7 % of patients with non-small cell lung carcinoma [70]. Malignant causes are responsible for most SVCS, while iatrogenic obstruction secondary to indwelling catheters and mediastinal fibrosis are the most common nonmalignant causes [71].

Clinical manifestations of SVCS are a direct result of increased upper body venous pressure. Symptoms characteristically develop gradually, over several weeks, and should usually be investigated for the causative process rather than regarded as a true medical emergency [72, 73]. When obstruction to venous flow is mild, symptoms may include dilatation of arm, neck, and chest-wall veins and edema of the upper body. Mild symptoms may include cough, dysphagia, chest pain, and dyspnea. More severe cases may present with conjunctival injection, respiratory distress, and cyanosis. The final, albeit rare, endpoint of SVCS is brain edema, coma, convulsions, and death [74].

The diagnosis of SVCS is based on the clinical presentation and imaging studies. CT with intravenous contrast is probably the best method to diagnose the cause of SVCS, while MR angiography and positron emission tomography CT (PET-CT) may be useful in selected cases [69]. Venography, still considered to be the "gold standard," is needed for demonstrating degree of obstruction within the SVC prior to interventional treatment [75]. Ancillary tests such as pleural tap, bronchoscopy, mediastinoscopy, or open biopsy are often needed to diagnose the cause of SVCS.

Treatment of SVCS aims at treating both the obstruction and the causative disorder. Treatment modalities may include chemotherapy, radiotherapy, superior vena cava stenting, and surgery (debulking and vascular reconstruction). Medical treatment may include glucocorticoids [70] and diuretics [69], despite lack of evidence. Palliative measures include elevation of the patient's upper body to assist in venous return.

Treating SVCS with SVC stents may be performed as secondary, rescue, treatment after failure of chemotherapy and/or radiotherapy or as first-line therapy. SVC stenting for malignant causes of SVCS is usually durable at least as patient prognosis demands. Recurrence of SVCS after stent deployment has been reported to depend on operator experience and range 0–41 % [76]. While stents have been reported more commonly as being used after the failure of other forms of treatment, arguments for using it as a primary choice include advances in endovascular technique, proven durability, low rate of complications, rapidity of clinical relief of symptoms, and the ability to treat the underlying disease more appropriately since the SVCS has subsided. Stent timing is still a matter of controversy [70]. There are several stents that are commonly used for SVC stenting, both balloon-expandable and self-expanding [75, 76]. The most common complications after stent placement for superior vena cava syndrome include stent occlusion by thrombosis or tumor invasion. Other complications that are directly related to the procedure include stent misplacement, stent migration, rupture of the vena cava during insertion [74], pericardial tamponade, groin hematoma, recurrent laryngeal nerve palsy, epistaxis, and hematemesis [75]. Other complications include anticoagulation-related bleeding [77], cardiac arrhythmia, infection, and pulmonary emboli. Another type of complication after stent placement stems from the rapid relief of obstruction and therefore the sudden increase in venous return. This may cause cardiac ischemia and pulmonary edema in the first 48 h after the procedure [76]. Most complications are minor and their reported incidence is under 10 % [75, 76]. Anticoagulation after SVC stent placement is still an area of uncertainty. Most authors report using anticoagulation for relatively prolonged periods.

Relative contraindications for stent placement in patients with SVCS include no symptoms, inability of the patient to lie flat, and when there is potential for rapid response of tumor to chemotherapy or radiotherapy (such as lymphoma) [74, 77].

Thrombolysis, most commonly catheter directed, may serve as an adjunct for treatment of SVCS or as a treatment on its own [78]. Surgical reconstruction or bypass to treat SVCS is usually performed for nonmalignant causes, as patients with nonmalignant obstruction of the SVC are typically younger than patients with malignant SVCS and usually have a good long-term prognosis. Furthermore, there is lack of information regarding stent durability in this population.

Pulmonary Embolism

Pulmonary embolism is the most serious and feared acute complication of venous thromboemboli. PE occur in 0.07–0.2 % of hospitalized patients [2, 79, 80]. In a single

Table 37.6 Wells model of the clinical pretest probability of PE

Clinical feature	Score
Clinical signs and symptoms of DVT (minimum of leg swelling and pain with palpation of the deep veins)	3
An alternative diagnosis is less likely than PE	3
Heart rate greater than 100	1.5
Immobilization or surgery in the previous 4 weeks	1.5
Previous DVT/PE	1.5
Hemoptysis	1
Malignancy (on treatment, treated in the last 6 months, or palliative)	1

From Wells et al. [123], with permission
Interpretation: High probability >6; moderate probability ≥2 and ≤6; low probability <2. If the D-dimer is negative, a cutoff point of 4 points or less makes a PE unlikely

center, PE was revealed by autopsy in 14.6 % of patients and was thought to have contributed to the patients' death in most cases [80]. This translates to over 140,000 cases a year in the United States. More than one quarter of patients with PE present as sudden death and the overall 30-day survival is 59.1 % [2]. PE-related death was estimated at 1–4.8 % in several cohorts [81, 82], while mortality in patients with massive PE has been reported to exceed 50 % [36]. It is now estimated that PE represents the most common preventable cause of death among hospitalized patients.

Diagnosis of PE is made by combining clinical symptoms and signs with proper imaging. The Wells criteria for PE, shown in Table 37.6, are a series of bedside-derived clinical characteristics that can accurately divide patients into low and high probability for PE.

Accuracy can be augmented by D-dimer for patients with low clinical probability [83]. For patients with moderate and high-probability scores, the diagnosis can be validated with further imaging. This may include computed tomography, ventilation perfusion scan, and lower extremity venous duplex ultrasonography. When clinical suspicion is high, diagnostic imaging should be used to its full extent when ruling out PE.

Hemodynamic instability is a marker of massive PE and is associated with increased mortality. Predicting mortality in patients with PE who are hemodynamically stable is achieved by combining patient characteristics, clinical measures, and data derived from laboratory and imaging studies. Patient characteristics can be organized into clinical scores that assign points to comorbidities and clinical features such as cancer, heart failure, previous DVT, and hypoxemia [84]. According to the RIETE Registry that examined predictors of mortality in 15,520 consecutive patients with VTE, 3-month mortality correlated with PE (as opposed to DVT), advanced age, cancer, and prolonged immobilization [36]. Laboratory tests that predict poor outcome include elevated troponin and brain natriuretic peptide (BNP) levels as markers of myocardial necrosis and right ventricular dysfunction. Many electrocardiographic changes may occur in patients with PE. Some, including sinus tachycardia, atrial arrhythmias, and new bundle branch block, correlate with adverse outcomes. Right ventricular (RV) dysfunction or RV dilatation has been found to correlate with PE mortality. Echocardiographic measures that have been found to correlate with mortality in the presence of PE include RV hypokinesis, RV end-diastolic area to left ventricular end-diastolic area ratio >0.6, RV end-diastolic diameter to left ventricular end-diastolic diameter >0.9 or >1, and ventricular septal bowing. Dilatation can also be seen on CT [5]. Embolic burden found on CT does not correlate with mortality [85].

Anticoagulation for PE

Anticoagulation is the foundation of treatment of PE. The various agents used for anticoagulation are listed in Table 37.3. Rivaroxaban, an oral Xa inhibitor, has been found to be effective for DVT [86], but is still being evaluated for PE. The initial treatment for PE should include low molecular weight heparin, unfractionated heparin, or fondaparinux. Patients with intermediate or high clinical suspicion for PE should receive treatment pending definitive diagnosis [85] unless there is an absolute contraindication to anticoagulation. The duration of treatment with anticoagulation depends on the inciting event. Provoked PE should be treated for a minimum of 3 months [15]. Prolonged treatment should be considered in patients with low bleeding risk [87]. Patients who suffer a first unprovoked PE should be treated for at least 3 months and long-term anticoagulation should be given, unless bleeding risk is high. A second unprovoked PE necessitates indefinite anticoagulation [15]. Patients with cancer should receive low molecular weight heparin for the first 3–6 months and then treatment should be continued with either low molecular weight heparin or warfarin for life or until the malignancy is considered cured. When choosing vitamin K antagonists, the goal INR should be 2–3.

Thrombolysis for PE

Thrombolytic treatment for PE may affect resolution of symptoms, hemodynamic stabilization, improved exercise tolerance, and prolonged survival. It is indicated in massive PE and in some cases of submassive PE. The International Cooperative Pulmonary Embolism Registry (ICOPER) followed 2,454 patients from 52 centers in seven countries.

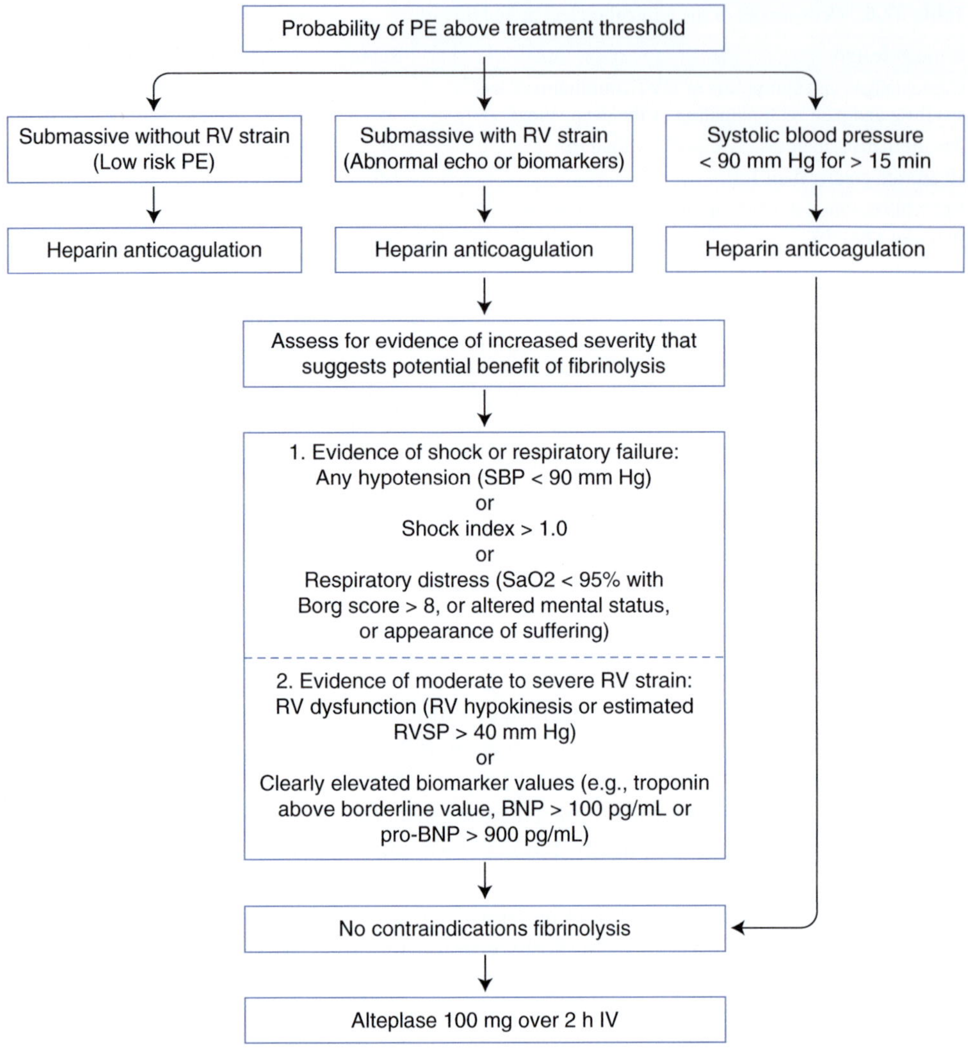

Fig. 37.2 Diagnostic algorithm for PE

Of these, 108 patients had massive PE and 33 of these patients received thrombolysis. Thrombolysis did not reduce 90-day mortality [88]. A pooled analysis of 13 trials examining the effect of thrombolysis on overall mortality showed a trend in favor of treatment [36]. A Cochrane database review included 8 trials with 679 patients and did not show benefit of thrombolysis over anticoagulation. Some trials in this review actually excluded patients who were hemodynamically unstable [89]. Thrombolysis is indicated if there is presence of respiratory or hemodynamic instability or if there is evidence of moderate or severe right ventricular dysfunction attributable to the PE (Fig. 37.2). It is commonly administered via a peripheral vein. Contraindications for thrombolysis for PE are the same as for thrombolysis for DVT as described above [5].

Catheter-Directed Treatment for PE

Catheter-based treatments for PE are most often adjuncts to thrombolysis [90]. They include aspiration thrombectomy, thrombus fragmentation, and rheolytic thrombectomy. Aspiration thrombectomy involves securing and removing clots with suction with a device such as the Greenfield suction embolectomy catheter (Meditech/Boston Scientific, Natick, MA). Thrombus fragmentation can be performed with a balloon catheter, with a rotating pigtail catheter, or with the Amplatz catheter (ev3 Endovascular, Plymouth, MN). Rheolytic catheters use a high-velocity saline jet to fragment thrombi. Debris is removed to an evacuation lumen. While there are no randomized controlled trials of catheter-based treatments for PE, a pooled analysis of data from 348 patients showed an overall success rate of 81 % [90]. Catheter-directed embolectomy has been described after failure of systemic thrombolysis, as repeat thrombolysis may increase the chances of intracranial bleeding. A retrospective analysis of 12 patients with shock secondary to PE reported success rate of 83 % for catheter-directed interventions. Of these patients, seven failed thrombolysis and five had a contraindication to thrombolysis. No major complications were reported [91].

The AngioVac suction (Vortex Medical, Norwell, MA, USA) cannula and circuit is a novel minimally invasive endovenous suction cannula aimed at removing "undesirable intravascular material" (UIM) from the venous, right atrial, or pulmonary arterial system. Initial clinical experience with 40 patients suggested that the AngioVac device is a possible alternative for removal of UIM. Atrial or ventricular perforation represents a rare but serious complication. In early cases, the AngioVac appeared more effective for catheter-associated or nonadherent right atrial or iliocaval UIM, than for pulmonary emboli, especially in the distal main pulmonary arteries and tricuspid valve vegetations [92]. There is minimal experience with this device, and further study is required.

Surgical Embolectomy for PE

Surgical embolectomy involves manually extracting thrombus from the pulmonary arteries. Though old series reported high mortality rates, newer series are more promising. A retrospective analysis of 190 patients with PE revealed that among those who had right ventricular dilatation, patients who underwent surgical embolectomy had a mortality of 11 %, much lower than among patients treated with thrombolytic therapy (33 %) [93]. One single-center analysis of 47 patients that underwent surgical embolectomy for various indications including contraindications or failure of thrombolysis reported 94 % survival. An IVC filter was inserted in most (81 %) patients [94]. A single-center prospective comparison of repeat thrombolysis versus surgical embolectomy in 30 patients that failed initial thrombolysis and were still in shock secondary to PE was performed. In 14 patients, embolectomy was performed, while in 26 repeat thrombolysis. Repeat thrombolysis resulted in less favorable outcome (79 % vs. 31 %, $p=0.004$), most commonly due to more recurrent PE (35 % vs. 0 %, $p=0.015$). A trend toward mortality reduction was also seen (38 % vs. 7 %, $p=0.07$). Of note is that all patients in the surgical group received an IVC filter compared to only 31 % in the thrombolysis group. Long-term follow-up of survivors failed to show a difference in outcome [95]. Current guidelines recommend that the decision of whether to choose surgical or catheter-directed embolectomy should depend on local expertise [5].

IVC Filter in Patients with PE

The data and recommendations regarding IVC filters for DVT have been described above and are relevant also when considering these devices for patients with PE. In the ICOPER Registry, 11 patients with massive PE received an IVC filter [88]. Their 90-day survival was 90.9 %, higher than patients who did not receive a filter (56.7 %, $p=0.002$). As with DVT, IVC filters are not routinely indicated for patients with PE. IVC filters should be inserted when anticoagulation cannot be given. Once the contraindications pass, anticoagulation should be given. Other indications include recurrent PE despite anticoagulation. Filters may also be considered in patients with acute PE and very poor cardiopulmonary reserve [5].

May-Thurner Syndrome

Compression of the left iliac vein by the overlying right iliac artery may cause extensive left lower extremity thrombosis. This is termed "May-Thurner syndrome" (MTS). MTS is typically a disease of young women [96]. Patients often present with left lower extremity swelling that is disproportionate to the extent of the thrombus and poor response to initial medical management. Once suspected, the diagnosis of MTS is confirmed by imaging studies. Choice of imaging technique depends on local expertise and patient factors. CT venography, while offering anatomical information, exposes patients to ionizing radiation. MR venography, on the other hand, also offers anatomical information, but is not available in all centers and may not be practical for acutely ill patients because of the prolonged scan times. Ascending contrast venography, while considered the gold standard, is invasive and should be reserved for patients in which invasive therapy has been determined to be optimal. The final diagnosis becomes certain during venography, after the thrombus has been removed and the compression becomes evident.

The treatment for iliofemoral venous thrombosis secondary to MTS combines anticoagulation followed by CDT and placement of a stent in the compressed iliac vein. At 10 years of follow-up, 71 % of patients with MTS treated with anticoagulation alone had persistent leg swelling [44], while a retrospective series demonstrated that 64 % of patients who received a stent had little to no edema [97]. The long-term patency of this procedure has been reported to be excellent. In a retrospective analysis of 35 patients treated with CDT and stent placement for MTS, the patency rate at 1 year was 93.6 % [96]. Anticoagulation should be administered following similar considerations as for patients with iliofemoral DVT [5]. Though antiplatelet agents are commonly used in conjunction to anticoagulation after venous stent placement, their efficacy in prevention of re-obstruction and the duration of treatment have never been assessed.

Chronic Venous Insufficiency

Chronic venous insufficiency (CVI) is a term describing venous valve insufficiency, venous obstruction, and venous hypertension [98, 99]. The anatomy of the lower extremity

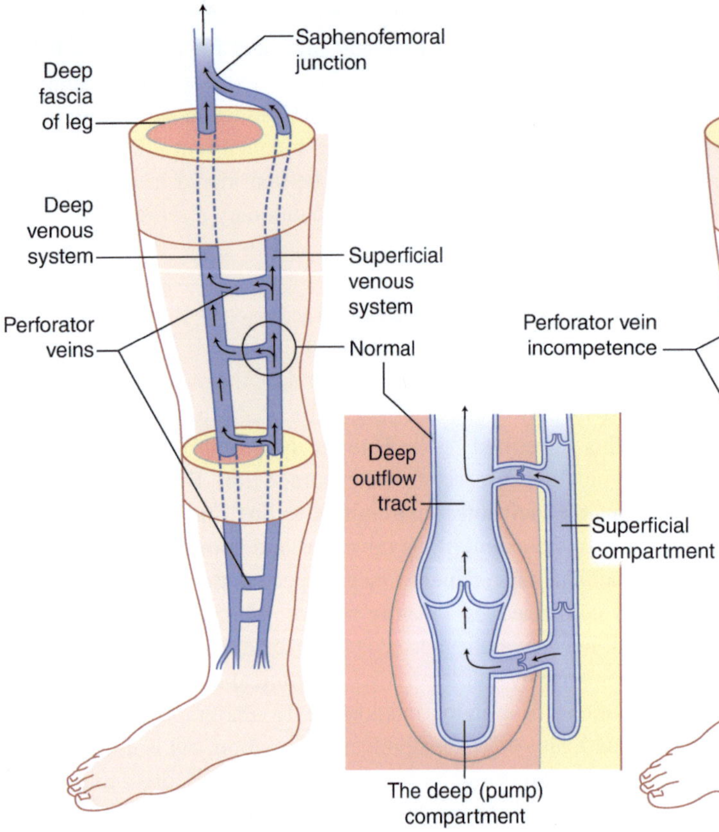

Fig. 37.3 Sites of valvular incompetence

venous system is divided into deep veins, superficial veins, and perforator veins that connect the other two systems. The veins of the superficial system have tributaries that drain the skin and subcutaneous tissues. Varicose veins represent dilatation of these tributaries (Fig. 37.3). The pathophysiology of CVI, including the relative roles of obstruction and reflux, is not well understood [100]. Venous valve dysfunction may be primary because of weakness of the vein wall or valve leaflets or secondary to damage, most commonly DVT or superficial vein thrombophlebitis. Definitions of CVI vary in different publications. Thus, while CVI is prevalent, the true prevalence is not known and varies by clinical feature [98, 101]. Varicose veins, for example, are as prevalent as 40 %, while the prevalence of venous ulcers is estimated between 0.3 and 1 % of the adult population. Incidence of CVI increases with age and in women, also worsening during pregnancy. Other risk factors include obesity, DVT, and leg injury.

Clinical Manifestations of Chronic Venous Insufficiency

The clinical presentation of CVI includes lower extremity swelling, venous varicosities, skin changes, skin ulceration, and rarely, venous claudication. In some instances, a venous etiology may be hard to identify; however, most often leg pain from venous causes is different from arterial causes. Pain from venous insufficiency is often described as heaviness and aching. It is usually relieved by leg elevation. Pulses are classically preserved when the etiology is venous. Typical skin changes include hyperpigmentation, eczema, stasis dermatitis, lipodermatosclerosis (subcutaneous tissue fibrosis), atrophie blanche, and ulcers. Ulcer location is typically perimalleolar on the medial aspect, and delayed healing is typical. The ulcerations have a classic appearance with healthy granulation tissue, significant overlying exudate, and minimal discomfort. Combinations of these signs and symptoms can cluster into several clinical patterns [100].

A clinical scoring system has been devised to aid in the management of patients with CVI and includes the following measures: pain or discomfort; varicose veins ≥3 mm in the standing position; venous edema; skin pigmentation that is not focal over a varicose vein or secondary to another presumed condition; inflammation (more than pigmentation); induration (skin and subcutaneous changes, white atrophy, and lipodermatosclerosis); active ulcers, their number and duration; the size of the longest active ulcer; and the use of compression therapy. Each characteristic is assigned points between 1 and 3 if it is mild, moderate, or severe and a score of 0–30 is calculated for each leg [102].

Diagnostic Procedures for Chronic Venous Insufficiency

Duplex ultrasound has a central role in the evaluation of venous insufficiency. Venous reflux is assessed by applying tourniquets or valsalva while measuring direction of blood flow across valves. Reverse flow for longer than 1 s denotes reflux. Interestingly, duplex-measured reflux time and volume have shown a weak correlation to plethysmographic quantification of reflux. Duplex also offers anatomical information about the distribution of varicose veins. If there is variation from the expected distribution of venous insufficiency, complex disease and congenital anomalies should be suspected [103]. Continuous wave Doppler can supplement duplex as an office-based alternative for screening for saphenofemoral and sapheno-popliteal junction venous incompetence. Other diagnostic methods, less commonly used in everyday clinical practice, include air or photo-plethysmography [98, 104]. Imaging of the iliocaval venous system may be achieved with CT, MRI, venography, and intravascular ultrasound (IVUS). There is no standard for quantification of hemodynamic significance of venous obstruction [105]. Ambulatory venous pressure measurement, obtained by a cannula inserted to a superficial vein on the dorsum of the foot, remains standard for assessing venous hypertension, but is rarely used in clinical practice due to its invasive nature [104]. Imaging studies should be used according to the clinical stage of CVI and suspected findings as shown in Fig. 37.4.

Treatment of Chronic Venous Insufficiency

The goal in treating CVI is to alleviate symptoms and prevent limb ulcerations and refractory limb edema. Treatment is divided into conservative measures and invasive procedures. The mainstay of conservative treatment for CVI is compression therapy in order to oppose the elevated venous pressure. Graduated compression, compressing more at the ankles, rather than using uniform compression, is preferred. Daily compression of 30–40 mmHg has been shown to significantly reduce symptoms. Stockings were found to be effective in ulcer healing according to the latest Cochrane database review [106]. Compression has not been shown to prevent CVI progression in primary CVI [106], while post DVT it has [28].

Another important aspect of conservative treatment of CVI is skin and wound care. Skin emollients should be routinely used to prevent dryness, fissures, cellulitis, and ulceration. Pharmacotherapy has a limited role in treating CVI. A group of compounds, phlebotonics or venoactive drugs (VAD), has been suggested to address venous hypertension

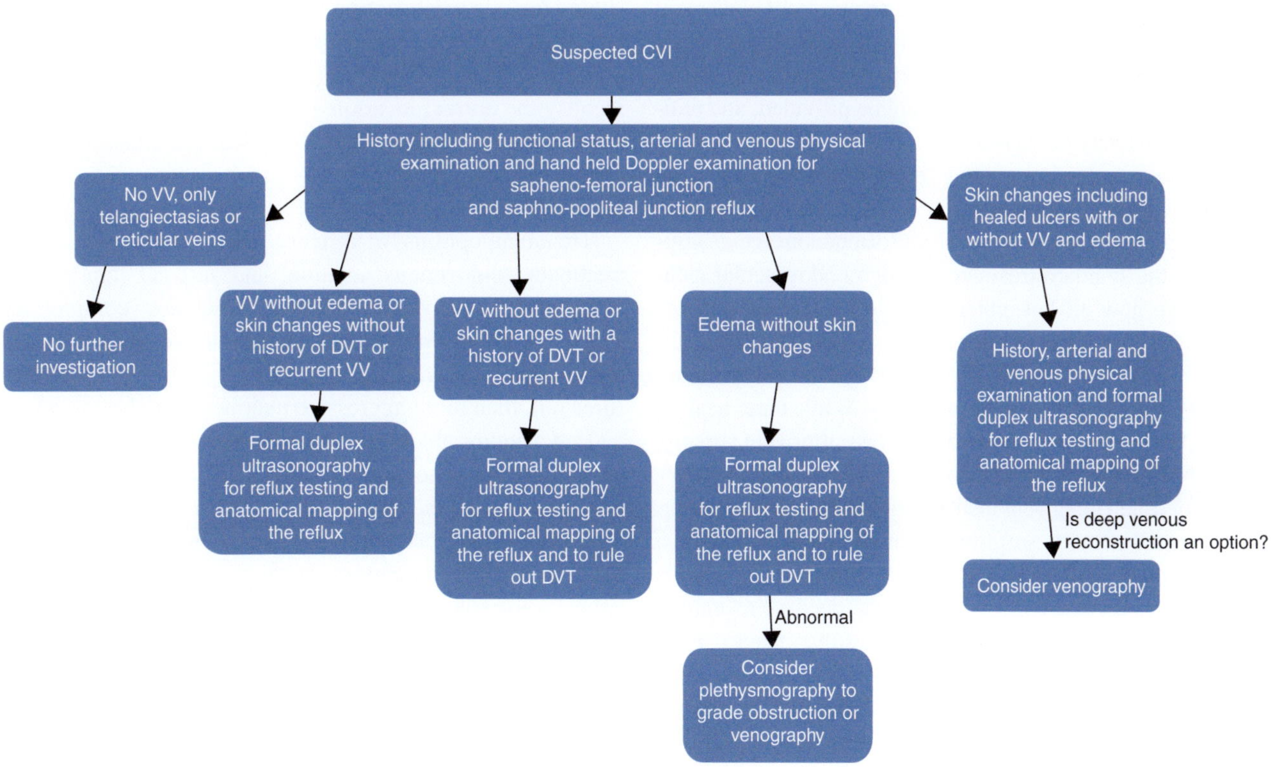

Fig. 37.4 Investigation of patients with suspected chronic venous insufficiency

and capillary leak [99]. A Cochrane review questioned the quality of present data [107]. Horse chestnut (*Aesculus hippocastanum*) has been reviewed in a separate Cochrane review and found to reduce leg pain and swelling [108]. Pentoxifylline in high dose was also found to be safe as an adjunct to compression in promoting ulcer healing [109].

Failure of conservative measures or advanced disease must prompt consideration of invasive procedures. There are several modalities for interventional treatment of CVI. Injection venous sclerotherapy is suitable for treatment of spider veins, venous lakes, and varicose veins that are smaller than 4 mm. It may be used as a single treatment or in conjunction with other treatments aimed at larger varicose veins. There are multiple sclerosing agents in clinical use, including hypertonic sodium chloride, sodium tetradecyl sulfate, and sodium morrhuate, among others. Foam sclerotherapy, utilizing foam detergents, has gained recent popularity. Ultrasound guidance may help avoid complications. Side effects of sclerotherapy include hyperpigmentation, hypopigmentation, persistent pain, damage to overlying tissue resulting in limb ulceration, thrombophlebitis, and deep vein thrombosis [110].

Chronic obstruction of the iliac vein is being recognized as a prevalent cause for symptomatic CVI. A large single-center study examined long-term results of iliac vein balloon angioplasty and stenting for CVI. Primary assisted and secondary patency rates were 100 % at 72 months. Pain, swelling, and ulcer healing were significantly improved [105]. The benefit of percutaneous intervention and stent placement has also been cited as potentially beneficial, a recent American Heart Association scientific statement [5]. After this procedure, anticoagulation should be provided, and antiplatelet agents may be considered.

Preventing saphenous venous reflux has been cited as an important factor in ulcer healing and recurrence prevention. Saphenofemoral venous ligation and saphenous vein stripping were the standard treatment, though endovascular techniques have now all but replaced surgery for most patients (see below). The effect of surgery and compression on healing and recurrence (ESCHAR) trial compared compression with and without saphenous vein surgery. While ulcer healing was similar, long-term recurrence was less after vein surgery, especially in patients with isolated superficial venous insufficiency or when deep vein insufficiency was limited [111].

In selected patients suffering from recurrent ulcerations, in which valve malfunction is felt to contribute to venous insufficiency, valve reconstruction of the deep veins can be offered in specialized centers. Results have been conflicting.

Most would agree that when superficial and deep venous insufficiencies coincide, the superficial system should be addressed first. Outflow obstruction is also treated earlier, rather than later [105].

Venous Varicosities

It is estimated that the annual incidence of varicose veins is 2 % while the lifetime prevalence is as high as 40 % in modern series. Venous varicosities occur more often in women than men [101, 112]. It is thought that the mechanism underlying the formation of varicose veins is venous hypertension. Normally, the pressure in the veins does not exceed 15 mmHg. Incompetence of venous valves is a cause for varicose vein formation. This is further exacerbated when the perforating and tributary veins are not functioning normally, thus allowing a further rise in venous pressure. Various risk factors for varicose vein formation have been identified including prolonged standing, obesity, pregnancy, prior deep vein thrombosis, and even tight garments. Other factors include family history, female sex, and age. Despite the strong tendency for familial distribution of varicose veins, the genetic component is most likely multifactorial. There are however some rare disorders in which varicose veins are common, and specific genetic components have been postulated including Klippel-Trenaunay-Weber syndrome and Chuvash polycythemia [113].

Typical complaints of patients with varicose veins include itching, burning, pain, limb heaviness, and limb fatigue. Aesthetic considerations are common. Varicose veins also pose an increased risk for venous thromboembolic events [114].

Physical examination of patients with varicose veins should include a description of the veins and associated findings such as edema, hyperpigmentation, and venous ulcers, as well as their distribution (Fig. 37.5). Failure to properly identify the correct location and cause of the varicose veins may result in treatment failure. Physical examination is often complemented by duplex ultrasonography with venous reflux testing.

Treatment options for varicose veins include conservative treatment, endovenous ablation, and surgical ligation and stripping. Conservative treatment includes compression stockings, elevating the lower extremities as much as possible, weight loss, and physical activity. If conservative measures fail, then more aggressive treatment may be sought.

Endovenous ablation is usually performed by laser or radiofrequency. The target for ablation should be the superficial vein that is the source of venous insufficiency. Many times this is the great saphenous vein. The actual technique for venous ablation includes inserting a catheter that delivers either radiofrequency energy (radiofrequency ablation, RFA) or laser energy (endovascular laser ablation, EVLA) to the vein. This, in turn, causes thermal injury, destroying the endothelium and disrupting the collagen in the vein wall. This promotes thrombosis and fibrosis of the vein, thus eliminating the source of venous insufficiency and venous hypertension [115]. Before starting the procedure, tumescent

Fig. 37.5 Vein anatomy

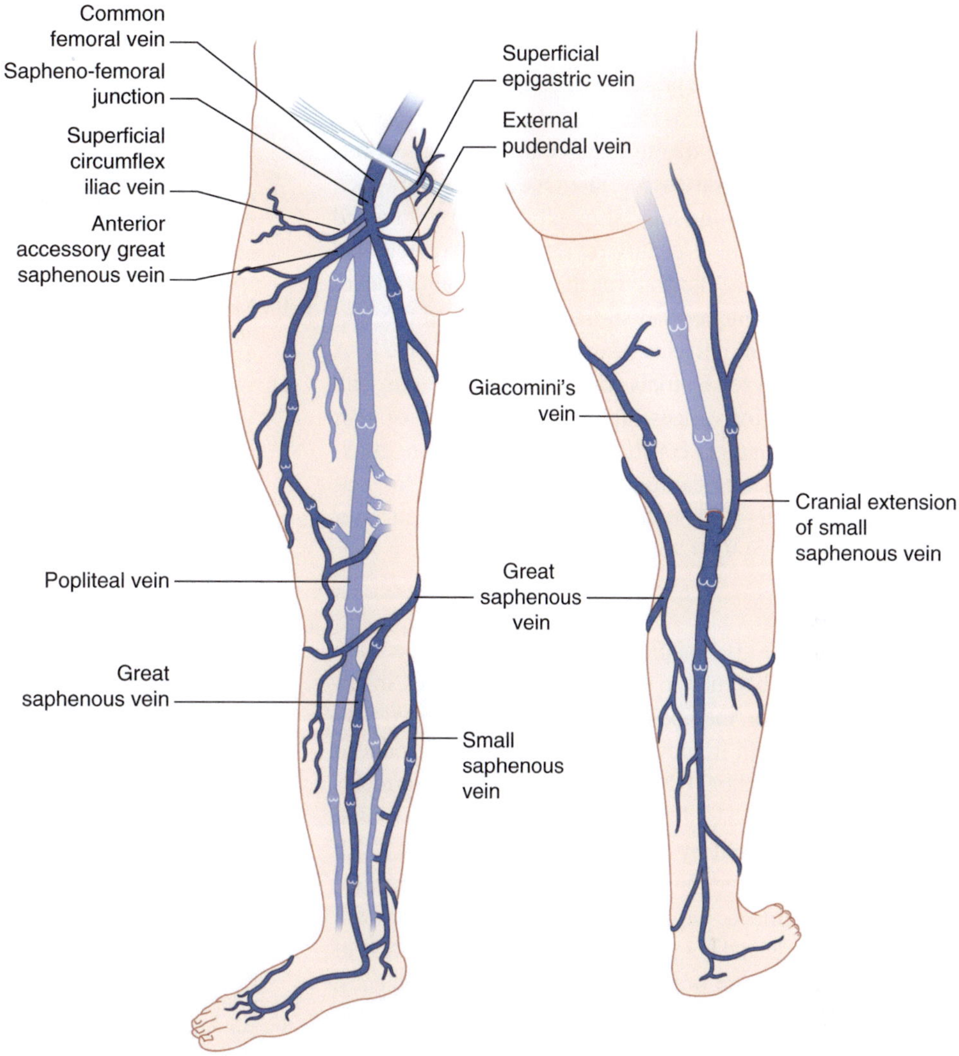

anesthesia is injected into a potential space around the vein of interest. Injection is performed under ultrasound guidance. Anesthesia is also injected into the subcutaneous tissue. This is usually performed with a mechanical injector and serves two purposes: prevention of discomfort during the ablation procedure and creating a fluid barrier between the vein and the overlying skin, thus preventing thermal injury. Subsequently, the ablation catheter is inserted under ultrasound guidance into the vein. As the catheter emits energy from the area close to the tip, it is gradually retracted, thus delivering energy to the venous segment of interest. Common complications of endovenous ablation include soreness and bruising. Less common but more severe complications include DVT, paresthesia, and burns [116].

After the ablation, the venous tributaries that constitute the varicose veins need to be treated. If the varicose veins are larger than 4 mm, the preferred method is excision by phlebectomy. If they are smaller than 4 mm, injection venous sclerotherapy can be employed. Bleeding is infrequent as the trauma of the phlebectomy serves to promote thrombus formation. Once the varicose veins have been treated, a compression stocking is put over the region for up to 1 week while the patient ambulates. Superficial vein thrombosis may develop over the phlebectomies and should be treated conservatively. Contraindications for vein ablation include DVT, pregnancy, severe peripheral artery disease, or inability to ambulate.

Surgical treatment of varicose veins includes vein ligation and stripping. Ligation involves tying the saphenofemoral or sapheno-popliteal junction. Then, a metal rod called a "stripper" is inserted into the vein, along its course. The end of the vein is tied to the stripper. Extraction of the stripper removes the vein as well. Perforator veins can be treated with subfascial endoscopic perforator surgery (SEPS). Although there is debate regarding the role of perforator vein treatment, a meta-analysis reviewing 1,140 lower extremities showed 88 % of ulcer healing and only 13 % recurrence at an average of 21-month follow-up. In most cases, saphenous vein ablation was also performed. Complications included wound infection, hematoma, and deep vein thrombosis [117]. SEPS does not have a role in the presence of correctable main stem disease [103].

There is lack of high-quality data comparing the various treatment options for varicose veins. One review, however, attempted to compare the highest quality data (randomized controlled trials and high-quality reviews). This review had two main conclusions. The first was that surgery and endovenous treatment techniques had similar efficacy and the second was that major adverse events were rare [112]. A meta-analysis analyzed 64 trials comparing endovenous with surgical treatment for varicose veins. In an analysis of over 12,300 limbs, the authors concluded that laser is more effective than RFA and surgical ligation and stripping. This was true even after long-term follow-up at 5 years, when laser had a success rate of 92.9 % [118].

Conclusions

Venous disease is unique, encompassing a spectrum between thromboembolic phenomena and venous insufficiency. Correct therapeutic choices for patients with VTE can result in improved mortality rates and reduced long-term morbidity. While anticoagulation, thrombolysis, and catheter-based treatments are extensively used and often supported by high-quality data, there are still many areas of uncertainty such as patient selection for invasive treatment, improving patient compliance with anticoagulation and compression stockings, prevention of PTS, and prediction of recurrence. Venous insufficiency, on the other hand, is seldom fatal, but often detrimental to patients' quality of life. Conservative, catheter-based, and surgical treatments are available; however, there is still much to be known, including mechanism of disease and patient selection for catheter-based interventions.

References

1. Kakkar VV, Howe CT, Flanc C, Clarke MB. Natural history of postoperative deep-vein thrombosis. Lancet. 1969;2(7614):230–2.
2. Roger VL, Go AS, Lloyd-Jones DM, Adams RJ, Berry JD, Brown TM, et al. Heart disease and stroke statistics – 2011 update: a report from the American Heart Association. Circulation. 2011;123(4):e18–209.
3. Yamaki T, Nozaki M. Patterns of venous insufficiency after an acute deep vein thrombosis. J Am Coll Surg. 2005;201(2):231–8.
4. Galanaud JP, Sevestre MA, Genty C, Laroche JP, Zizka V, Quere I, et al. Comparison of the clinical history of symptomatic isolated muscular calf vein thrombosis versus deep calf vein thrombosis. J Vasc Surg. 2010;52(4):932, 8, 938.e1–2.
5. Jaff MR, McMurtry MS, Archer SL, Cushman M, Goldenberg N, Goldhaber SZ, et al. Management of massive and submassive pulmonary embolism, iliofemoral deep vein thrombosis, and chronic thromboembolic pulmonary hypertension: a scientific statement from the American Heart Association. Circulation. 2011;123(16):1788–830.
6. Eichinger S, Heinze G, Jandeck LM, Kyrle PA. Risk assessment of recurrence in patients with unprovoked deep vein thrombosis or pulmonary embolism: the Vienna prediction model. Circulation. 2010;121(14):1630–6.
7. Anderson Jr FA, Spencer FA. Risk factors for venous thromboembolism. Circulation. 2003;107(23 Suppl 1):I9–16.
8. Goldhaber SZ. Risk factors for venous thromboembolism. J Am Coll Cardiol. 2010;56(1):1–7.
9. Prandoni P, Lensing AW, Cogo A, Cuppini S, Villalta S, Carta M, et al. The long-term clinical course of acute deep venous thrombosis. Ann Intern Med. 1996;125(1):1–7.
10. Kahn SR. Measurement properties of the Villalta scale to define and classify the severity of the post-thrombotic syndrome. J Thromb Haemost. 2009;7(5):884–8.
11. White RH. The epidemiology of venous thromboembolism. Circulation. 2003;107(23 Suppl 1):I4–8.
12. Rodger MA, Kahn SR, Wells PS, Anderson DA, Chagnon I, Le Gal G, et al. Identifying unprovoked thromboembolism patients at low risk for recurrence who can discontinue anticoagulant therapy. CMAJ. 2008;179(5):417–26.
13. Douketis JD, Gu CS, Schulman S, Ghirarduzzi A, Pengo V, Prandoni P. The risk for fatal pulmonary embolism after discontinuing anticoagulant therapy for venous thromboembolism. Ann Intern Med. 2007;147(11):766–74.
14. Bounameaux H, Perrier A, Righini M. Diagnosis of venous thromboembolism: an update. Vasc Med. 2010;15(5):399–406.
15. Kearon C, Kahn SR, Agnelli G, Goldhaber S, Raskob GE, Comerota AJ, et al. Antithrombotic therapy for venous thromboembolic disease: American College of Chest Physicians evidence-based clinical practice guidelines (8th edition). Chest. 2008;133(6 Suppl):454S–545.
16. Goldhaber SZ, Piazza G. Optimal duration of anticoagulation after venous thromboembolism. Circulation. 2011;123(6):664–7.
17. Ansell J, Hirsh J, Hylek E, Jacobson A, Crowther M, Palareti G, et al. Pharmacology and management of the vitamin K antagonists: American College of Chest Physicians evidence-based clinical practice guidelines (8th edition). Chest. 2008;133(6 Suppl):160S–98.
18. Kovacs MJ, Rodger M, Anderson DR, Morrow B, Kells G, Kovacs J, et al. Comparison of 10-mg and 5-mg warfarin initiation nomograms together with low-molecular-weight heparin for outpatient treatment of acute venous thromboembolism. A randomized, double-blind, controlled trial. Ann Intern Med. 2003;138(9):714–19.
19. Quiroz R, Gerhard-Herman M, Kosowsky JM, DeSantis SM, Kucher N, McKean SC, et al. Comparison of a single end point to determine optimal initial warfarin dosing (5 mg versus 10 mg) for venous thromboembolism. Am J Cardiol. 2006;98(4):535–7.
20. Ridker PM, Goldhaber SZ, Danielson E, Rosenberg Y, Eby CS, Deitcher SR, et al. Long-term, low-intensity warfarin therapy for the prevention of recurrent venous thromboembolism. N Engl J Med. 2003;348(15):1425–34.
21. Cosmi B, Palareti G. Update on the predictive value of D-dimer in patients with idiopathic venous thromboembolism. Thromb Res. 2010;125 Suppl 2:S62–5.
22. Witt DM. Review: positive D-dimer results predict recurrence after first unprovoked VTE regardless of test timing or cutpoint, or patient age. Ann Intern Med. 2011;154(2):JC1,4, JC1-5.
23. Prandoni P, Prins MH, Lensing AW, Ghirarduzzi A, Ageno W, Imberti D, et al. Residual thrombosis on ultrasonography to guide the duration of anticoagulation in patients with deep venous thrombosis: a randomized trial. Ann Intern Med. 2009;150(9):577–85.
24. Cosmi B, Legnani C, Iorio A, Pengo V, Ghirarduzzi A, Testa S, et al. Residual venous obstruction, alone and in combination with D-dimer, as a risk factor for recurrence after anticoagulation withdrawal following a first idiopathic deep vein thrombosis in the prolong study. Eur J Vasc Endovasc Surg. 2010;39(3):356–65.

25. Cosmi B, Legnani C, Cini M, Guazzaloca G, Palareti G. D-dimer and residual vein obstruction as risk factors for recurrence during and after anticoagulation withdrawal in patients with a first episode of provoked deep-vein thrombosis. Thromb Haemost. 2011;105(5):837–45.
26. Ruiz-Irastorza G, Cuadrado MJ, Ruiz-Arruza I, Brey R, Crowther M, Derksen R, et al. Evidence-based recommendations for the prevention and long-term management of thrombosis in antiphospholipid antibody-positive patients: report of a task force at the 13th International Congress on Antiphospholipid Antibodies. Lupus. 2011;20(2):206–18.
27. Prandoni P, Lensing AW, Piccioli A, Bernardi E, Simioni P, Girolami B, et al. Recurrent venous thromboembolism and bleeding complications during anticoagulant treatment in patients with cancer and venous thrombosis. Blood. 2002;100(10):3484–8.
28. Brandjes DP, Buller HR, Heijboer H, Huisman MV, de Rijk M, Jagt H, et al. Randomised trial of effect of compression stockings in patients with symptomatic proximal-vein thrombosis. Lancet. 1997;349(9054):759–62.
29. Prandoni P, Lensing AW, Prins MH, Frulla M, Marchiori A, Bernardi E, et al. Below-knee elastic compression stockings to prevent the post-thrombotic syndrome: a randomized, controlled trial. Ann Intern Med. 2004;141(4):249–56.
30. Kahn SR, Kearon C, Julian JA, Mackinnon B, Kovacs MJ, Wells P, et al. Predictors of the post-thrombotic syndrome during long-term treatment of proximal deep vein thrombosis. J Thromb Haemost. 2005;3(4):718–23.
31. Baekgaard N, Broholm R, Just S, Jorgensen M, Jensen LP. Long-term results using catheter-directed thrombolysis in 103 lower limbs with acute iliofemoral venous thrombosis. Eur J Vasc Endovasc Surg. 2010;39(1):112–17.
32. Mewissen MW, Seabrook GR, Meissner MH, Cynamon J, Labropoulos N, Haughton SH. Catheter-directed thrombolysis for lower extremity deep venous thrombosis: report of a National Multicenter Registry. Radiology. 1999;211(1):39–49.
33. AbuRahma AF, Perkins SE, Wulu JT, Ng HK. Iliofemoral deep vein thrombosis: conventional therapy versus lysis and percutaneous transluminal angioplasty and stenting. Ann Surg. 2001;233(6):752–60.
34. Enden T, Klow NE, Sandvik L, Slagsvold CE, Ghanima W, Hafsahl G, et al. Catheter-directed thrombolysis vs. anticoagulant therapy alone in deep vein thrombosis: results of an open randomized, controlled trial reporting on short-term patency. J Thromb Haemost. 2009;7(8):1268–75.
35. Comerota AJ. The ATTRACT trial: rationale for early intervention for iliofemoral DVT. Perspect Vasc Surg Endovasc Ther. 2009;21(4):221,4; quiz 224–5.
36. Laporte S, Mismetti P, Decousus H, Uresandi F, Otero R, Lobo JL, et al. Clinical predictors for fatal pulmonary embolism in 15,520 patients with venous thromboembolism: findings from the Registro Informatizado de la Enfermedad TromboEmbolica Venosa (RIETE) Registry. Circulation. 2008;117(13):1711–16.
37. Karthikesalingam A, Young EL, Hinchliffe RJ, Loftus IM, Thompson MM, Holt PJ. A systematic review of percutaneous mechanical thrombectomy in the treatment of deep venous thrombosis. Eur J Vasc Endovasc Surg. 2011;41(4):554–65.
38. Kwon SH, Oh JH, Seo TS, Ahn HJ, Park HC. Percutaneous aspiration thrombectomy for the treatment of acute lower extremity deep vein thrombosis: is thrombolysis needed? Clin Radiol. 2009;64(5):484–90.
39. Kim HS, Patra A, Paxton BE, Khan J, Streiff MB. Adjunctive percutaneous mechanical thrombectomy for lower-extremity deep vein thrombosis: clinical and economic outcomes. J Vasc Interv Radiol. 2006;17(7):1099–104.
40. Nazir SA, Ganeshan A, Nazir S, Uberoi R. Endovascular treatment options in the management of lower limb deep venous thrombosis. Cardiovasc Intervent Radiol. 2009;32(5):861–76.
41. Gogalniceanu P, Johnston CJ, Khalid U, Holt PJ, Hincliffe R, Loftus IM, et al. Indications for thrombolysis in deep venous thrombosis. Eur J Vasc Endovasc Surg. 2009;38(2):192–8.
42. Plate G, Einarsson E, Ohlin P, et al. Thrombectomy with temporary arteriovenous fistula: the treatment of choice in acute iliofemoral venous thrombosis. J Vasc Surg. 1984;1(6):867–76.
43. Plate G, Akesson H, Einarsson E, Ohlin P, Eklof B. Long-term results of venous thrombectomy combined with a temporary arterio-venous fistula. Eur J Vasc Surg. 1990;4(5):483–9.
44. Plate G, Eklof B, Norgren L, Ohlin P, Dahlstrom JA. Venous thrombectomy for iliofemoral vein thrombosis – 10-year results of a prospective randomised study. Eur J Vasc Endovasc Surg. 1997;14(5):367–74.
45. Stein PD, Kayali F, Olson RE. Twenty-one-year trends in the use of inferior vena cava filters. Arch Intern Med. 2004;164(14):1541–5.
46. Crowther MA. Inferior vena cava filters in the management of venous thromboembolism. Am J Med. 2007;120(10 Suppl 2):S13–17.
47. Young T, Tang H, Hughes R. Vena caval filters for the prevention of pulmonary embolism. Cochrane Database Syst Rev. 2010;2:CD006212.
48. Spencer FA, Bates SM, Goldberg RJ, Lessard D, Emery C, Glushchenko A, et al. A population-based study of inferior vena cava filters in patients with acute venous thromboembolism. Arch Intern Med. 2010;170(16):1456–62.
49. White RH, Zhou H, Kim J, Romano PS. A population-based study of the effectiveness of inferior vena cava filter use among patients with venous thromboembolism. Arch Intern Med. 2000;160(13):2033–41.
50. Decousus H, Leizorovicz A, Parent F, Page Y, Tardy B, Girard P, et al. A clinical trial of vena caval filters in the prevention of pulmonary embolism in patients with proximal deep-vein thrombosis. prevention du risque d'embolie pulmonaire par interruption cave study group. N Engl J Med. 1998;338(7):409–15.
51. Stein PD, Alnas M, Skaf E, Kayali F, Siddiqui T, Olson RE, et al. Outcome and complications of retrievable inferior vena cava filters. Am J Cardiol. 2004;94(8):1090–3.
52. Vaziri K, Bhanot P, Hungness ES, Morasch MD, Prystowsky JB, Nagle AP. Retrievable inferior vena cava filters in high-risk patients undergoing bariatric surgery. Surg Endosc. 2009;23(10):2203–7.
53. Dabbagh O, Nagam N, Chitima-Matsiga R, Bearelly S, Bearelly D. Retrievable inferior vena cava filters are not getting retrieved: where is the gap? Thromb Res. 2010;126(6):493–7.
54. Minocha J, Idakoji I, Riaz A, Karp J, Gupta R, Chrisman HB, et al. Improving inferior vena cava filter retrieval rates: impact of a dedicated inferior vena cava filter clinic. J Vasc Interv Radiol. 2010;21(12):1847–51.
55. Kucher N. Clinical practice. Deep-vein thrombosis of the upper extremities. N Engl J Med. 2011;364(9):861–9.
56. Evans RS, Sharp JH, Linford LH, Lloyd JF, Tripp JS, Jones JP, et al. Risk of symptomatic DVT associated with peripherally inserted central catheters. Chest. 2010;138(4):803–10.
57. King MM, Rasnake MS, Rodriguez RG, Riley NJ, Stamm JA. Peripherally inserted central venous catheter-associated thrombosis: retrospective analysis of clinical risk factors in adult patients. South Med J. 2006;99(10):1073–7.
58. Owens CA, Bui JT, Knuttinen MG, Gaba RC, Carrillo TC. Pulmonary embolism from upper extremity deep vein thrombosis and the role of superior vena cava filters: a review of the literature. J Vasc Interv Radiol. 2010;21(6):779–87.
59. Jones MA, Lee DY, Segall JA, Landry GJ, Liem TK, Mitchell EL, et al. Characterizing resolution of catheter-associated upper extremity deep venous thrombosis. J Vasc Surg. 2010;51(1):108–13.
60. Usoh F, Hingorani A, Ascher E, Shiferson A, Tran V, Marks N, et al. Long-term follow-up for superior vena cava filter placement. Ann Vasc Surg. 2009;23(3):350–4.

61. Illig KA, Doyle AJ. A comprehensive review of Paget-Schroetter syndrome. J Vasc Surg. 2010;51(6):1538–47.
62. Melby SJ, Vedantham S, Narra VR, Paletta Jr GA, Khoo-Summers L, Driskill M, et al. Comprehensive surgical management of the competitive athlete with effort thrombosis of the subclavian vein (Paget-Schroetter syndrome). J Vasc Surg. 2008;47(4):809, 820. discussion 821.
63. Urschel Jr HC, Patel AN. Surgery remains the most effective treatment for Paget-Schroetter syndrome: 50 years' experience. Ann Thorac Surg. 2008;86(1):254, 60. discussion 260.
64. Elman EE, Kahn SR. The post-thrombotic syndrome after upper extremity deep venous thrombosis in adults: a systematic review. Thromb Res. 2006;117(6):609–14.
65. Prescott SM, Tikoff G. Deep venous thrombosis of the upper extremity: a reappraisal. Circulation. 1979;59(2):350–5.
66. Tilney ML, Griffiths HJ, Edwards EA. Natural history of major venous thrombosis of the upper extremity. Arch Surg. 1970;101(6): 792–6.
67. Lee JT, Karwowski JK, Harris EJ, Haukoos JS, Olcott IV C. Long-term thrombotic recurrence after nonoperative management of Paget-Schroetter syndrome. J Vasc Surg. 2006;43(6): 1236–43.
68. Lanciego C, Pangua C, Chacon JI, Velasco J, Boy RC, Viana A, et al. Endovascular stenting as the first step in the overall management of malignant superior vena cava syndrome. AJR Am J Roentgenol. 2009;193(2):549–58.
69. Wilson LD, Detterbeck FC, Yahalom J. Clinical practice. superior vena cava syndrome with malignant causes. N Engl J Med. 2007;356(18):1862–9.
70. Rowell NP, Gleeson FV. Steroids, radiotherapy, chemotherapy and stents for superior vena caval obstruction in carcinoma of the bronchus. Cochrane Database Syst Rev. 2001;4:CD001316.
71. Kalra M, Gloviczki P, Andrews JC, Cherry Jr KJ, Bower TC, Panneton JM, et al. Open surgical and endovascular treatment of superior vena cava syndrome caused by nonmalignant disease. J Vasc Surg. 2003;38(2):215–23.
72. Bagheri R, Rahim M, Rezaeetalab F, Akbari H, Shojaian R. Malignant superior vena cava syndrome: is this a medical emergency? Ann Thorac Cardiovasc Surg. 2009;15(2):89–92.
73. Schraufnagel DE, Hill R, Leech JA, Pare JA. Superior vena caval obstruction. Is it a medical emergency? Am J Med. 1981;70(6): 1169–74.
74. Watkinson AF, Yeow TN, Fraser C. Endovascular stenting to treat obstruction of the superior vena cava. BMJ. 2008;336(7658): 1434–7.
75. Ganeshan A, Hon LQ, Warakaulle DR, Morgan R, Uberoi R. Superior vena caval stenting for SVC obstruction: current status. Eur J Radiol. 2009;71(2):343–9.
76. Nguyen NP, Borok TL, Welsh J, Vinh-Hung V. Safety and effectiveness of vascular endoprosthesis for malignant superior vena cava syndrome. Thorax. 2009;64(2):174–8.
77. Sheikh MA, Fernandez Jr BB, Gray BH, Graham LM, Carman TL. Endovascular stenting of nonmalignant superior vena cava syndrome. Catheter Cardiovasc Interv. 2005;65(3):405–11.
78. Kee ST, Kinoshita L, Razavi MK, Nyman UR, Semba CP, Dake MD. Superior vena cava syndrome: treatment with catheter-directed thrombolysis and endovascular stent placement. Radiology. 1998;206(1):187–93.
79. Silverstein MD, Heit JA, Mohr DN, Petterson TM, O'Fallon WM, Melton III LJ. Trends in the incidence of deep vein thrombosis and pulmonary embolism: a 25-year population-based study. Arch Intern Med. 1998;158(6):585–93.
80. Stein PD, Henry JW. Prevalence of acute pulmonary embolism among patients in a general hospital and at autopsy. Chest. 1995;108(4):978–81.
81. Heit JA, Silverstein MD, Mohr DN, Petterson TM, O'Fallon WM, Melton III LJ. Predictors of survival after deep vein thrombosis and pulmonary embolism: a population-based, cohort study. Arch Intern Med. 1999;159(5):445–53.
82. Pollack CV, Schreiber D, Goldhaber SZ, Slattery D, Fanikos J, O'Neil BJ, et al. Clinical characteristics, management, and outcomes of patients diagnosed with acute pulmonary embolism in the emergency department: Initial report of EMPEROR (Multicenter Emergency Medicine Pulmonary Embolism in the Real World Registry). J Am Coll Cardiol. 2011;57(6):700–6.
83. Wells PS, Anderson DR, Rodger M, Stiell I, Dreyer JF, Barnes D, et al. Excluding pulmonary embolism at the bedside without diagnostic imaging: management of patients with suspected pulmonary embolism presenting to the emergency department by using a simple clinical model and D-dimer. Ann Intern Med. 2001;135(2):98–107.
84. Bova C, Pesavento R, Marchiori A, Palla A, Enea I, Pengo V, et al. Risk stratification and outcomes in hemodynamically stable patients with acute pulmonary embolism: a prospective, multicentre, cohort study with three months of follow-up. J Thromb Haemost. 2009;7(6):938–44.
85. Subramaniam RM, Mandrekar J, Chang C, Blair D, Gilbert K, Peller PJ, et al. Pulmonary embolism outcome: a prospective evaluation of CT pulmonary angiographic clot burden score and ECG score. AJR Am J Roentgenol. 2008;190(6):1599–604.
86. EINSTEIN Investigators, Bauersachs R, Berkowitz SD, Brenner B, Buller HR, Decousus H, et al. Oral rivaroxaban for symptomatic venous thromboembolism. N Engl J Med. 2010;363(26):2499–510.
87. Spurzem JR, Geraci SA. Outpatient management of patients following pulmonary embolism. Am J Med. 2010;123(11): 987–90.
88. Kucher N, Rossi E, De Rosa M, Goldhaber SZ. Massive pulmonary embolism. Circulation. 2006;113(4):577–82.
89. Dong BR, Hao Q, Yue J, Wu T, Liu GJ. Thrombolytic therapy for pulmonary embolism. Cochrane Database Syst Rev. 2009; 3:CD004437.
90. Skaf E, Beemath A, Siddiqui T, Janjua M, Patel NR, Stein PD. Catheter-tip embolectomy in the management of acute massive pulmonary embolism. Am J Cardiol. 2007;99(3):415–20.
91. Kuo WT, van den Bosch MA, Hofmann LV, Louie JD, Kothary N, Sze DY. Catheter-directed embolectomy, fragmentation, and thrombolysis for the treatment of massive pulmonary embolism after failure of systemic thrombolysis. Chest. 2008;134(2):250–4.
92. Sakhuja R, Gandhi S, Rogers RK, Margey RJP, Weinberg I, Jaff M, Schainfeld R, Rosenfield K. Initial case series treated with the AngioVac suction cannula and circuit: A possible novel endovenous approach for treatment of central venous or pulmonary arterial pathology. Poster Presentation at American College of Cardiology, 60th Annual Scientific Session, New Orleans, LA, 2011. (Abstract #12530).
93. Sukhija R, Aronow WS, Lee J, Kakar P, McClung JA, Levy JA, et al. Association of right ventricular dysfunction with in-hospital mortality in patients with acute pulmonary embolism and reduction in mortality in patients with right ventricular dysfunction by pulmonary embolectomy. Am J Cardiol. 2005;95(5):695–6.
94. Leacche M, Unic D, Goldhaber SZ, Rawn JD, Aranki SF, Couper GS, et al. Modern surgical treatment of massive pulmonary embolism: results in 47 consecutive patients after rapid diagnosis and aggressive surgical approach. J Thorac Cardiovasc Surg. 2005;129(5):1018–23.
95. Meneveau N, Seronde MF, Blonde MC, Legalery P, Didier-Petit K, Briand F, et al. Management of unsuccessful thrombolysis in acute massive pulmonary embolism. Chest. 2006;129(4):1043–50.
96. O'Sullivan GJ, Semba CP, Bittner CA, Kee ST, Razavi MK, Sze DY, et al. Endovascular management of iliac vein compression (May-Thurner) syndrome. J Vasc Interv Radiol. 2000;11(7):823–36.
97. Titus JM, Moise MA, Bena J, Lyden SP, Clair DG. Iliofemoral stenting for venous occlusive disease. J Vasc Surg. 2011;53(3): 706–12.
98. Eberhardt RT, Raffetto JD. Chronic venous insufficiency. Circulation. 2005;111(18):2398–409.

99. Perrin M, Ramelet AA. Pharmacological treatment of primary chronic venous disease: rationale, results and unanswered questions. Eur J Vasc Endovasc Surg. 2011;41(1):117–25.
100. Raju S, Neglen P. Clinical practice. Chronic venous insufficiency and varicose veins. N Engl J Med. 2009;360(22):2319–27.
101. Beebe-Dimmer JL, Pfeifer JR, Engle JS, Schottenfeld D. The epidemiology of chronic venous insufficiency and varicose veins. Ann Epidemiol. 2005;15(3):175–84.
102. Vasquez MA, Rabe E, McLafferty RB, Shortell CK, Marston WA, Gillespie D, et al. Revision of the venous clinical severity score: venous outcomes consensus statement: special communication of the American Venous Forum Ad Hoc Outcomes Working Group. J Vasc Surg. 2010;52(5):1387–96.
103. Parnaby CN, Welch GH, Stuart WP. An overview of the surgical aspects of lower limb venous disease. Scott Med J. 2009;54(3):30–5.
104. Nicolaides AN, Cardiovascular Disease Educational and Research Trust, European Society of Vascular Surgery, The International Angiology Scientific Activity Congress Organization, International Union of Angiology, Union Internationale de Phlebologie at the Abbaye des Vaux de Cernay. Investigation of chronic venous insufficiency: a consensus statement (France, March 5-9, 1997). Circulation. 2000;102(20):E126–63.
105. Neglen P, Writing Group II of the Pacific Vascular Symposium 6, Eklof B, Kulwicki A, Davies A, Deschamps T, et al. Prevention and treatment of venous ulcers in primary chronic venous insufficiency. J Vasc Surg. 2010;52(5 Suppl):15S–20S.
106. O'Meara S, Cullum NA, Nelson EA. Compression for venous leg ulcers. Cochrane Database Syst Rev. 2009;1:CD000265.
107. Martinez MJ, Bonfill X, Moreno RM, Vargas E, Capella D. Phlebotonics for venous insufficiency. Cochrane Database Syst Rev. 2005;3:CD003229.
108. Pittler MH, Ernst E. Horse chestnut seed extract for chronic venous insufficiency. Cochrane Database Syst Rev. 2006; 1:CD003230.
109. Jull A, Arroll B, Parag V, Waters J. Pentoxifylline for treating venous leg ulcers. Cochrane Database Syst Rev. 2007;3: CD001733.
110. Stucker M, Kobus S, Altmeyer P, Reich-Schupke S. Review of published information on foam sclerotherapy. Dermatol Surg. 2010;36 Suppl 2:983–92.
111. Gohel MS, Barwell JR, Taylor M, Chant T, Foy C, Earnshaw JJ, et al. Long term results of compression therapy alone versus compression plus surgery in chronic venous ulceration (ESCHAR): randomised controlled trial. BMJ. 2007;335(7610):83.
112. Leopardi D, Hoggan BL, Fitridge RA, Woodruff PW, Maddern GJ. Systematic review of treatments for varicose veins. Ann Vasc Surg. 2009;23(2):264–76.
113. Lim CS, Davies AH. Pathogenesis of primary varicose veins. Br J Surg. 2009;96(11):1231–42.
114. Huerta C, Johansson S, Wallander MA, Garcia Rodriguez LA. Risk factors and short-term mortality of venous thromboembolism diagnosed in the primary care setting in the United Kingdom. Arch Intern Med. 2007;167(9):935–43.
115. Desmyttere J, Grard C, Stalnikiewicz G, Wassmer B, Mordon S. Endovenous laser ablation (980 nm) of the small saphenous vein in a series of 147 limbs with a 3-year follow-up. Eur J Vasc Endovasc Surg. 2010;39(1):99–103.
116. Kouri B. Current evaluation and treatment of lower extremity varicose veins. Am J Med. 2009;122(6):513–15.
117. Tenbrook Jr JA, Iafrati MD, O'donnell Jr TF, Wolf MP, Hoffman SN, Pauker SG, et al. Systematic review of outcomes after surgical management of venous disease incorporating subfascial endoscopic perforator surgery. J Vasc Surg. 2004;39(3):583–9.
118. van den Bos R, Arends L, Kockaert M, Neumann M, Nijsten T. Endovenous therapies of lower extremity varicosities: a meta-analysis. J Vasc Surg. 2009;49(1):230–9.
119. Wells PS, Anderson DR, Bormanis J, Guy F, Mitchell M, Gray L, et al. Value of assessment of pretest probability of deep-vein thrombosis in clinical management. Lancet. 1997;350(9094): 1795–8.
120. Decousus H, Prandoni P, Mismetti P, Bauersachs RM, Boda Z, Brenner B, et al. Fondaparinux for the treatment of superficial-vein thrombosis in the legs. N Engl J Med. 2010;363(13): 1222–32.
121. Lassen MR, Gallus A, Raskob GE, Pineo G, Chen D, Ramirez LM, et al. Apixaban versus enoxaparin for thromboprophylaxis after hip replacement. N Engl J Med. 2010;363(26): 2487–98.
122. Vedantham S, Thorpe PE, Cardella JF, Grassi CJ, Patel NH, Ferral H, et al. Quality improvement guidelines for the treatment of lower extremity deep vein thrombosis with use of endovascular thrombus removal. J Vasc Interv Radiol. 2009;20(7 Suppl): S227–39.
123. Wells PS, Anderson DR, Rodger M, Ginsberg JS, Kearon C, Gent M, et al. Derivation of a simple clinical model to categorize patients probability of pulmonary embolism: Increasing the models utility with the SimpliRED D-dimer. Thromb Haemost. 2000;83(3):416–20.

Index

A
Abdominal aortic aneurysm
  endovascular management (*see* Endovascular abdominal aortic aneurysm repair (EVAR))
  indications for intervention, 445
Academic Research Consortium (ARC), 125
ACC/AHA. *See* American College of Cardiology and American Heart Association (ACC/AHA)
Access artery injury, 458–459
Acute coronary syndrome (ACS)
  fractional flow reserve, 199–200
  GRACE risk score, 44
  pathogenesis, 44
  PCI in elderly, 247
  timing of intervention, 45
  TIMI risk score, 44–45
  in women, 232
Acute kidney injury, 461–462
Acute mesenteric ischemia
  clinical presentation, 434
  diagnosis, 434–435
  etiology, 434
  management, 435–436
  mortality, 443
  restenosis rate, 443
Acute myocardial infarction. *See also* Primary percutaneous coronary intervention
  percutaneous cell therapy
    intracoronary delivery, 182–184
    intramyocardial injection, 184–185
  in women, 232–233
Acute renovascular disorders
  antiphospholipid antibody syndrome, 418
  catheter-directed thrombolysis, 419
  causes, 418
  renal artery dissection, 419–420
  renal infarction, 419
  renal vein thrombosis, 420
  thrombectomy/thrombolysis, 424–425
Acute stroke intervention
  endovascular therapies, 500–502
  intra-arterial thrombolysis, 502–503
  intracranial stenting, 505
  intravenous thrombolysis, 499–500
  manpower issues, 506
  mechanical thrombectomy, 503–505
  neuroprotection, 505–506
  new stroke program, 507–508
  stroke centers, 506–507
Adenosine
  coronary flow reserve, 81
  ischemic heart disease, 195
  myocardial perfusion imaging, 42
  PCI, 215
Adenosine diphosphate P2Y12 receptor antagonist, 249–250
Adipose-derived stem cells (ADSCs), 174–175
Adjunctive pharmacology, for coronary intervention
  factor Xa inhibitors
    apixaban, 152
    otamixaban, 153
    rivaroxaban, 152–153
  fondaparinux, 148
  glycoprotein IIb/IIIa inhibitors
    clinical evidence, 148–149
    pharmacokinetics, 148
  heparin
    low-molecular-weight heparins (LMWH), 147–148
    unfractionated heparin (UFH), 146–147
  intravenous direct thrombin inhibitors
    argatroban, 149–150
    bivalirudin, 150–151
    hirudin, 149
  oral antiplatelet agents
    aspirin, 143–144
    thienopyridines and ticagrelor, 144–146
  oral direct thrombin inhibitors, 151–152
Adjunctive pharmacotherapy, for PCI in elderly
  periprocedural, 248–249
  post-procedural, 249–250
AFX endovascular, 449
Allen's/Barbeau tests, 69, 70
American College of Cardiology and American Heart Association (ACC/AHA)
  intra-aortic balloon pump, 217
  for oral antiplatelet therapy, 144, 145
  UFH usage, 147
Amplatz left catheter, 82
Anaconda AAA stent graft system, 448–449
Anchor technique, 86
AneuRx Abdominal Stent Graft, 447
Angiographic aneurysms, 33–34
Angiographic technique
  applications, 20
  complications
    abrupt closure, 19
    aneurysm formation, 19
    coronary dissection and perforation, 19
    distal embolization, 19
    no reflow, 19
    spasm, 19
  endovascular therapy, 437–438
  image acquisition
    biologic variability, 10
    coronary anatomy, 10–13

C.A. Thompson (ed.), *Textbook of Cardiovascular Intervention*,
DOI 10.1007/978-1-4471-4528-8, © Springer-Verlag London 2014

Angiographic technique (*cont.*)
data compression variability, 10, 12
error sources, 10, 13
factors, 10
vessel orientation, 10–13
morphologic characteristics
ACC/AHA lesion, 16
angulation, 17
bifurcation lesions, 17–18
collateral assessment, 18
lesion calcification and length, 17
ostial lesions, 17
saphenous vein graft degeneration, 17
SCAI lesion classification system, 16, 17
thrombus, 17
total occlusions, 18
myocardial perfusion measurements
TFC, 19
TIMI flow grade system, 18
TMPG, 19
procedural results
binary angiographic restenosis, 20
late lumen loss, 20
QCA analysis
coronary atherosclerosis, 14–15
2-dimensional system, 13, 14
3-dimensional system, 13–14
generation systems, 12–13
limitations of, 12
measurement factors, 15–16
Angiojet, 111
Angioplasty and stenting, 438–440
Angioplasty and Stenting for Renal Artery Lesions (ASTRAL) trial, 415–416
Angioplasty balloons
characteristics of, 96–97
evolution of, 96
general construction, 96
Gruentzig's catheter, 91, 92
over-the-wire design, 97
Angio-Seal device, 72–73
Antegrade double balloon technique, 319, 320
Anterograde aortic valvuloplasty, 334–335
Anticoagulants, 235
Anticoagulation, 512–514
Antiplatelet agents, 233
Antiproliferative drugs
paclitaxel, 119–120
restenosis, 116
sirolimus and limus analogues, 118–119
Antithrombotics, 437
Anti-Xa agents
apixaban, 152
otamixaban, 153
rivaroxaban, 152–153
Aortic aneurysm
abdominal (*see* Abdominal aortic aneurysm)
thoracic (*see* Thoracic aortic aneurysm)
Aortic coarctation, of infrarenal abdominal aorta
diagnosis and incidence, 468
endovascular treatment, 471
implantation technique, 471
Aortic stenosis, 332, 333
Aortic valve therapy. *See* Transcatheter aortic valve therapy
Aortic valvuloplasty. *See* Balloon aortic valvuloplasty (BAV)
Apixaban, 152
Appropriate use criterion (AUC). *See* Chronic total occlusions (CTO) angioplasty
Argatroban, 149–150
Arterial disease in lower extremity. *See* Peripheral arterial disease (PAD)
ARTS II trail, 268–269
Aspirin
clinical evidence, 143–144
PCI
in elderly, 249
in women, 233
pharmacokinetics, 143
Asymptomatic vertebral artery stenosis, 493
Atherectomy device
excisional, 401
laser, 400–401
PAD, 400
rotational (*see* Rotational atherectomy)
TurboHawk and SilverHawk plaque excision system, 401
AtheroCath, 106
Atherosclerosis renal artery stenosis
anatomy, 406, 407
association with adverse outcomes, 405–406
catheter-based evaluation
angiography, 411–412
intravascular ultrasound, 412–413
renal vein renin sampling, 412
translesional pressure gradients, 411–412
diagnostic evaluation, 409
vs. fibromuscular dysplasia, 405
management, 413
noninvasive imaging, 410–411
pathophysiology, 406–407
patient selection for renal artery revascularization, 416
percutaneous revascularization *vs.* medical therapy
ASTRAL trial, 415–416
CORAL trial, 416
DRASTIC trial, 415
EMMA, 414
randomized trials of, 413–414
Scottish and Newcastle Renal Artery Stenosis Collaborative Group, 414–415
STAR trial, 415
presentation, 408–409
prevalence of, 405
progression, 405
renal translesional hemodynamics, 407–408
serologic studies, 409–410
urine studies, 410
Atherosclerotic stenosis, of infrarenal abdominal aorta
diagnosis and incidence, 468–469
endovascular treatment, 470–471
implantation technique, 472–473
Atrial fibrillation, 327
Attenuated plaques, 28, 29
Automated contrast injectors, 58, 59
Avinger device, 398–399
Axillary artery, upper extremity interventions, 372

B

Balloon angioplasty, 99
Balloon aortic valvuloplasty (BAV)
complications
brady-and tachyarrhythmia, 335
cardiac tamponade, 336

death, 336
embolic events, 336
massive aortic regurgitation, 336
vascular injury, 336
ventricular perforation, 336
decription, 330
long-term results, 335
patient selection and indications
children and young adults, 331
rheumatic aortic valve stenosis, 331
symptoms, 331
transcatheter aortic valve implant, 331
procedure
anterograde aortic valvuloplasty, 334–335
aortic stenosis severity assessment, 332, 333
coronary arteries assessment, 332, 333
evaluation of, 331
post-catheterization orders, 335
retrograde balloon valvuloplasty, 332–334
vascular access and preclosure, 332
Benephit catheter system, 59
BioCardia's HelixT catheter, 181–182
BioHeart injection catheter, 180–181
Biolimus, 118, 119
Biolimus-eluting stent (BES), 134, 136
Bioresorbable stents (BRS), 134–136
BioTronix, 133–134
Bivalirudin
PCI, 213–214
PCI and NSTEMI, 150–151
PCI in women, 235
ST segment elevation MI, 151
Bolton medical Relay thoracic endograft, 465
Bone marrow-derived mononuclear/stem cells (BMSCs), 175–176
Boomerang device, 71, 72
Boston Scientific catheter, 181
Brachial artery
closure methods, 73–74
upper extremity interventions, 372–373
vascular access
anatomy, 65, 67
cut-down and percutaneous approach, 69
risks, 75
Brachiocephalic atery. *See* Upper extremity interventions
Bradyarrhythmia, 335
Brockenbrough-Braunwald-Morrow sign, 5

C

CABG. *See* Coronary artery bypass surgery (CABG)
Calcification and tortuosity, 244, 247
Carabello sign, 4, 5
Cardiac Dimensions Carillon Device, 359–360
Cardiac power output (CPO), 222
CARDia trail, 269
Cardiogenic shock
hemodynamic support in PCI, 221–222
intra-aortic balloon pump, 217, 222
Cardiosolutions Percu-Pro™ system, 358–359
Cardiovascular disease (CVD)
barriers to, 229
risk factors, 229
women with, 228
Carillon Mitral Contour System, 359–360
Carotid artery disease
asymptomatic patients, 481–482
carotid endarterectomy, 486
CEA *vs.* CAS, 486–487, 489
clinical trials, 485
diagnosis
indications for screening, 482
invasive testing, 483–484
noninvasive testing, 482–483
etiology and prevalence, 481
medical therapy
vs. CEA, 485–486
risk factor management, 485
natural history, 481
stenting
complication, 492–493
embolic protection devices, 491–492
guidelines for, 489
patient selection, 489–490
procedure, 490–491
randomized trials of, 488
symptomatic patients, 482
Carpentier Type I, 351, 353
Carpentier Type II dysfunction, 351–352
Catheter-directed fibrinolysis, 440–441
Catheter-directed thrombolysis (CDT), 514–515
Cell delivery methods
cell mobilization, 177
coronary sinus infusion, 177–178
intracoronary infusion, 178
intramyocardial injection
open surgical transepicardial injection, 178
percutaneous transendocardial injection, 178–182
TVIM injection, 182
peripheral intravenous infusion, 177
Cell mobilization, 177
Cell therapy, 173. *See also* Percutaneous cell therapy
Cerclage annuloplasty, 361
Chronic heart failure
clinical trials, 185–186
intracoronary delivery, 187
transendocardial delivery, 186–187
Chronic mesenteric ischemia
atherosclerotic causes, 430, 432–433
incidence of, 430
nonatherosclerotic causes, 433
restenosis rate, 443
Chronic stable angina (CSA)
agents, 41
diagnostic coronary angiography, 42
National Institute for Health and Clinical Excellence guideline, 41
tolerance test, exercise, 42
Chronic total occlusion (CTO). *See* Retrograde approach, chronic total occlusion PCI
Chronic total occlusion percutaneous intervention (CTO PCI)
IVUS (*see* Intravascular ultrasound (IVUS))
Chronic total occlusions (CTO) angioplasty
appropriate use criterion
aim of, 290
asymptomatic patients, 291–292
clinical scenarios, 290
definition, 290
rational for, 290
symptomatic patients, 290–291
technical panel, 290

Chronic total occlusions (CTO) angioplasty (*cont.*)
dogmatic approach, 293
hybrid technique
antegrade and retrograde tools, 295
clinical utility, 293
goal of, 293, 294
initial strategies, 294
reasons for, 293
secondary strategies, 294
variables, 294
wires, 295
methodical wire technique, 293
in north America
attempt rate, 289
Canadian registry, 289
NHLBI and NCDR registry, 289
survival hypothesis
acute myocardial infarction, 292
baseline ischemic burden, 292
EXPLORE trial, 292, 293
ischemia, 292
mortality, 292
retrospective analysis, 292
VACTO study, 292
symptoms, 289
Chronic venous insufficiency (CVI)
clinical presentation, 522
diagnosis, 523
pathophysiology, 522
treatments, 523–524
venous varicosities, 524–526
Classic T-stenting technique, 257
Clinical Outcomes Utilizing Revascularization and Aggressive Drug Evaluation (COURAGE) study, 43
Clinical syntax score (CSS), 271
Clopidogrel
with bivalirudin, 151
clinical evidence, 145
PCI, 48
PCI in women, 233–234
vs. prasugrel, 146
for STEMI PCI, 214–215
Closed-and open-cell stent design, 117
Colonic ischemia, 459
Complex two-stents techniques, 257
Comprehensive Stroke Centers (CSC), 506
Computed tomographic (CT) angiography, 434
Congestive heart failure, 200
Contrast-induced acute kidney injury (CI-AKI)
cardiac catheterization and surgery, 60–61
diagnosis
biomarkers, 56
clinical risk prediction, 56–57
creatinine elevation, 56
definition, 55
Kaplan-Meier survival curve, 56
discharge planning and follow-up, 61
pathophysiology
CT image, 54
mechanisms, 53, 54
probability of, 55, 56
prevention of
automated contrast injectors, 58, 59
Benephit catheter system, 59
contrast agents and volume, 58, 60
hydration and N-acetylcysteine, 58
iloprost, 60
iron chelators, 60
meta-analysis, 59
NPO orders, 57, 58
pleiotropic effects, 60
Reitan pump, 59
Renal Guard, 59, 60
sodium bicarbonate, 58
volume depletion, 57
quality improvement monitoring, 61
USRDS reports, 53
Controlled antegrade and retrograde tracking (CART), 305–307
Cordis. *See* FRONTRUNNER device; OUTBACK LTD reentry catheter
Coronary angiography, TRA. *See* Transradial approach (TRA)
Coronary artery bypass surgery (CABG)
LMCA disease
off-pump, 253
patients outcomes, 253
vs. stents theraphy, 260–262
multivessel disease
vs. bare metal stenting, 266–268
vs. drug-eluting stents, 268
meta-analyses, 268
vs. POBA, 266
PCI in women, 235–236
Coronary atherectomy
balloon angioplasty, 99
directional coronary atherectomy, 106–107
laser atherectomy, 106
manual aspiration catheters, 109–110
mechanical disruption and extraction, 111–112
percutaneous transluminal atherectomy, 100–101
rotational atherectomy
in drug-eluting stent era, 105–106
early studies, 104
instrumentation, 99, 101
mechanism, 101–102
perforation, 105
procedure, 102, 104
Rotablator, 99, 101, 105
Rotalink burr catheter, 102, 104
Rota rescue case, 103–104
RotaWire specifications, 103
stent expansion, MicroCT, 102
thrombus extraction
distal protection, 108–109
ischemic time frame, 108
late stent thrombosis, 107
serial manual aspiration, 107
Coronary bifurcation lesions
classification systems
Lefevre, 278
Medina, 278
three number designation system, 278
definition, 277
drug eluting stents
balloon expandable, 285, 286
main branch, 285, 286
self-expanding design, 286
side branch, 286
randomized datas for
BBC-One trial, 284
BBK trial, 284
Cactus trial, 284
DKCrush-II trial, 284, 285

MACE, 284
Nordic trial, 283, 284
treatment for
crush stent, 279, 280
culotte/Y stent, 281, 282
double barrel technique, 281
kissing balloon angioplasty, 279
provisional approach, 278, 279
side branch stent, 279
simultaneous kissing stent technique, 280, 281
T-stent, 279
V-stent, 281
Coronary bypass graft surgery, 248
Coronary catheters, TRA, 171
Coronary flow reserve (CFR), 194, 202
Coronary microcirculation assessment, 201–202
Coronary sinus infusion, 177–178
CorPath robotic system
clinical experience, 164–165
CorPath 200 robotic system, 162–164
Counterpuncture approach, 70
Covidien. *See* CTO crossing system
Critical limb ischemia (CLI)
acute and chronic, 384
anticoagulation with heparin, 385
definition, 384
inflow and outflow disease, 384
targeted therapy, 385
CROSSER catheter, 397
Crush stent, 279, 280
Crush techniques, 257, 259
Cryoplasty
BTK-CHILL trial, 390
endovascular treatment, 388
mid-SFA CTO, 389
PolarCath® balloon dilation system, 389
vs. conventional angioplasty, 389
CTO crossing system, 399–400
Culotte techniques, 259
Culotte/Y stent, 281, 282
Cyclooxygenase-1, 143

D
Dabigatran/pradaxa, 151–152
Deep vein thrombosis (DVT)
diagnosis of, 511–512
treatment of
anticoagulation, 512–514
graduated compression stockings, 514
percutaneous mechanical thrombectomy, 515
surgical venous thrombectomy, 515
thrombolytic therapy, 514–515
vena cava filters, 515–516
Degenerative mitral regurgitation (DMR), 351–352
Delivering cell therapy. *See* Cell delivery methods
Diamondback Stealth Orbital system, 402
2-dimensional QCA system, 13, 14
3-dimensional QCA system, 13–14
Direct engagement technique, 422, 423
Directional coronary atherectomy, 106–107
Direct thrombin inhibitors
intravenous
argatroban, 149–150
bivalirudin, 150–151
hirudin, 149
oral, 151–152
PCI in women, 235
Distal bifurcation
benefits, 256
classic T-stenting technique, 257
clinical data, 256
complex two-stents techniques, 257
crush techniques, 257, 259
culotte techniques, 259
single stent techniques with optional T stenting, 256–257
SKS techniques, 259
Distal embolic protection devices, 424, 425
Double balloon technique, 328
Double barrel technique, 281
Double-lumen pigtail catheter, 4, 5
Drug-eluting stents (DES)
vs. bare-metal stents, 248
characteristics, 118
development, 133–136
everolimus, 126–127
high-resolution radiographs, 117
on-label *vs.* off-label use, 122–124
paclitaxel, 120–121
PCI in women *vs.* BMS, 230
safety, 127–133
coronary aneurysms, 129
in-stent restenosis, 132–133
restenosis, 130–133
stent fracture, 129–130
stent thrombosis, 127–129
sirolimus, 120
sirolimus *vs.* paclitaxel, 121–122
zotarolimus, 124–126
zotarolimus *vs.* bare-metal stents, 124–125
Duke classification, 17–18
Dutch Renal Artery Stenosis Intervention Cooperative study (DRASTIC) trial, 415

E
Echocardiographic scores, 319, 323, 328
Echolucent plaques, 28–29
Edwards Monarc Device, 360–361
Edwards SAPEIN THV, 344–346, 348–349
Elective PCI, 246–247
Electrocardiogram (ECG), 229
Eliquisr, 152
Embolic/distal protection, 216–217
Embryonic stem cells (ESCs), 174
Endoleaks
classification
type I, 454–455
type II, 455–456
type III, 456–457
type IV, 457
type V, 457
diagnosis, 457
primary and secondary, 454
Endovascular abdominal aortic aneurysm repair (EVAR)
access artery injury, 458–459
complications, 454
devices
AFX endovascular, 449
Anaconda AAA stent graft system, 448–449
AneuRx Abdominal Stent Graft, 447
endurant stent graft, 447

Endovascular abdominal aortic aneurysm repair (EVAR) (*cont.*)
excluder aortic endograft, 448
Incraft stent graft system, 449–450
talent abdominal stent graft, 446–447
Zenith Flex endograft, 446
endoleak (*see* Endoleaks)
groin injury, 458
infection, 461
ischemic complications, 459
limb occlusion, 460–461
migration, 454
nephropathy and acute kidney injury, 461–462
non-endoleak-related complications, 457
post-EVAR follow-up, 462
procedure
access, 451
aortic angiogram, 452
endograft positioning and deployment, 452
femoral artery access, 451
selection criteria, 450–451
structural failure and graft distortion, 457
vascular anatomy issues, 453
Endovascular management
abdominal aortic aneurysm
EVAR (*see* Endovascular abdominal aortic aneurysm repair (EVAR))
history, 445–446
indications, 445
acute stroke, 500–502
infrarenal abdominal aorta (*see* Infrarenal abdominal aorta)
mesenteric ischemia
access, 436–437
angiography, 437–438
angioplasty and stenting, 438–440
antithrombotics, 437
catheter delivery of vasodilators, 441–442
catheter-directed fibrinolysis, 440–441
catheter thrombectomy, 441
post-procedure, 442
preprocedural management, 436
stenotic diseases, 468–474
thoracic aortic aneurysm (*see* Thoracic aortic aneurysm)
Endovascular Valve Edge-to-Edge Repair Study (EVEREST) trials, 355–356
Endurant stent graft, 447
Enoxaparin, 147–148
Epicardium-derived progenitor cells (EPDCs), 175
ERAC III trail, 269
Essai Multicentrique Medicaments vs Angioplastie (EMMA), 414
Everolimus, 119
Everolimus-eluting stents (EES), 126–127
Excluder aortic endograft, 448
Expanded polytetrafluoroethylene (ePTFE), 448

F
Factor Xa inhibitors
apixaban, 152
otamixaban, 153
rivaroxaban, 152–153
FAME trial, 273
Femoral artery
access (*see* Vascular access)
closure methods and devices
active closure, 71, 72
Angio-Seal, 72–73
assisted compression, 70–71
Boomerang, 71, 72
FemoStop, 71
manual compression, 70
Perclose ProGlide, 73
Safeguard, 71
safety of, 72
StarClose, 73
FemoStop device, 71
Fibromuscular dysplasia, 416–417
Fibrous plaques, 28
Fondaparinux
clinical evidence, 148
PCI, 213
pharmacokinetics, 148
Fractional flow reserve (FFR)
acute coronary syndromes, 199–200
after stenting, 201
complications, 196
congestive heart failure, 200
and Grey Zone, 197
guided PCI in MVD, 273
inducing hyperemia, 194–195
in intermediate coronary disease, 196–197
left main disease, 200–201
left ventricular hypertrophy, 200
multivessel coronary disease, 197–199
patient selection, 42–43
practical aspects, 194
serial stenoses, 201
unique aspects of, 193–194
7-Fr catheters, 170
FRONTRUNNER device
MicroGuide, 395, 396
post stent angiogram, 396
principle of, 395
XP blunt microdissection, 396
Functional MR (FMR), 351, 353

G
Global Positioning System (GPS), 157
Global Registry of Acute Coronary Events (GRACE) risk score, 44
Global risk score (GRC), 271–272
Glycoprotein IIb/IIIa inhibitors
clinical evidence, 148–149
PCI in women, 234–235
pharmacokinetics, 148
Glycoprotein IIb/IIIa receptor antagonists, 214
Gorlin's formula, 4
Graduated compression stockings (GCS), 514
Granulocyte-stimulating factor (G-CSF), 177
Guided Delivery Systems, 364
Guided measurement catheters (GMC), 158
Guideliner catheter, 86, 87
Guidewires, construction
characteristics, 91
core material, 91–93
features of, 95
hydrophobic and hydrophilic coating, 93–94
polymer jackets/covers, 94–95
stress-strain curve, 93
wire tip, 94, 95

H
Hakki formula, 4
Hazy lesions, 35
HelixT catheter, 181–182
Hemodynamics
  aortic and pulmonic artery pressures, 1–3
  atrial pressure waveform, 1, 2
  cardiac outputs, 2–3
  constriction *vs.* restriction, 6–7
  hypertrophic obstructive cardiomyopathy, 5–6
  in PCI
    cardiogenic shock, 221–222
    intra-aortic balloon pump (IABP), 222–223
    left ventricular dysfunction, 221
    mechanical support, 222
    percutaneous left ventricular assist devices (LVADs), 223–224
  percutaneous mitral valvuloplasty, 325, 328
  pericardial tamponade, 6
  post-PVC, 5–6
  pulmonary artery wedge pressure, 2, 3
  valvular area calculations
    Carabello sign, 4, 5
    double-lumen pigtail catheter, 4, 5
    Gorlin's and Hakki formula, 4
    pressure recovery, 5
  vascular resistance, 4
  ventricular waveform, 1
Heparin
  low-molecular-weight heparins (LMWH), 147–148
  for STEMI PCI, 213
  unfractionated heparin (UFH), 146–147
Hirudin, 149
Hybrid technique, for CTO angioplasty
  antegrade and retrograde tools, 295
  clinical utility, 293
  goal of, 293, 294
  initial strategies, 294
  reasons for, 293
  secondary strategies, 294
  variables, 294
  wires, 295
Hyperechoic plaque, 26, 27
Hyperemic agents, 195
Hypertrophic obstructive cardiomyopathy (HOCM), 5–6

I
iCoapsys system, 364–365
Iliac arteries, lower extremity arterial disease
  ACTIVE trial, 385
  covered balloon-mounted stents, 386
  endovascular treatment through radial artery access, 386
  occluded segment, 387
  self-expanding stents, 386
  TASC guidelines, 385
Iliac artery aneurysms, 453
Iloprost, 60
Impella, 217, 223–224
Implantation technique, of infrarenal abdominal aorta
  hemodynamic and angiographic assessment, 471
  stent choice, 471
  stent delivery, 471–472
Incraft stent graft system, 449–450
Indirect mitral annuloplasty, 359–360
Inducible pluripotent stem cells (iPSCs), 174
Inducing hyperemia, 194–195
Infrainguinal arterial disease, 387–388
Infrarenal abdominal aorta
  aortic coarctation
    diagnosis and incidence, 468
    endovascular treatment, 471
    implantation technique, 471
  atherosclerotic stenosis
    diagnosis and incidence, 468–469
    endovascular treatment, 470–471
    implantation technique, 472–473
  implantation technique
    hemodynamic and angiographic assessment, 471
    stent choice, 471
    stent delivery, 471–472
  non-invasive assessment, 469
  volume-rendering and multiplanar reconstruction, 473–474
Inoue balloon technique, 328
In-stent restenosis (ISR)
  morphology, 132
  treatment, 133
Intermediate coronary disease, 196–197
Intra-aortic balloon pump (IABP)
  hemodynamic support in PCI, 222–223
  primary PCI, 217
Intra-arterial thrombolysis, 502–503
Intracoronary delivery/infusion, 178
  acute myocardial infarction, 182–184
  chronic heart failure, 187
  refractory angina, 188
Intracranial stenting, 505
Intramyocardial injection
  acute myocardial infarction, 184–185
  open surgical transepicardial injection, 178
  percutaneous cell therapy
    in acute myocardial infarction, 184–185
    in refractory angina, 188
  percutaneous transendocardial injection, 178–182
  refractory angina, 188
  TVIM injection, 182
Intravascular ultrasound (IVUS)
  anatomic factors, 311
  guide wire, 312, 313
  histopathologic features, 311, 312
  imaging diagnosis
    angiographic aneurysms, 33–34
    hazy lesions, 35
    myocardial bridges, 34, 35
    spontaneous dissection, 34–35
    stenosis severity, 31–32
    unstable lesion morphology, 32–33
  lesion and reference segment assessment, 29, 30
    vs. coronary angiography, 30
    distal, 30
    lengths and volumes, 31
    plaque burden *vs.* stenosis, 30
    remodeling, 30
    volumetric analysis, 31
  neointimal hyperplasia, 37
  pre-intervention diagnostic uses, 23
  qualitative analyses
    attenuated plaques, 28, 29
    echolucent plaques, 28–29
    fibrous plaques, 28
    hyperechoic plaque, 26, 27
    thrombus, 29

Intravascular ultrasound (IVUS) (*cont.*)
quantitative analyses
external elastic membrane, 25–26
lumen borders, 24, 25
media, 25, 26
non-uniform rotational distortion, 24
plaque, 25, 26
ring-down artifacts, 24
re-entry device options, 313–315
retrograde approach, 313, 315, 316
roles for, 311
saphenous vein grafts, 36
stent malapposition, 36
structure sequences, 23, 24
sweet spot, 311, 312
Intravenous direct thrombin inhibitors
argatroban, 149–150
bivalirudin, 150–151
hirudin, 149
Intravenous thrombolysis, 499–500
Invasive hemodynamics. *See* Hemodynamics
Iodixanol, 375
Iron chelators, 60
Ischemic heart disease
clinical background, 193
coronary microcirculation assessment, 201–202
fractional flow reserve
acute coronary syndromes, 199–200
after stenting, 201
complications, 196
congestive heart failure, 200
and Grey Zone, 197
inducing hyperemia, 194–195
in intermediate coronary disease, 196–197
left main disease, 200–201
left ventricular hypertrophy, 200
multivessel coronary disease, 197–199
practical aspects, 194
serial stenoses, 201
unique aspects of, 193–194

J
Jetstream Navitus device, 401
J-tip wire, 169
Judkins catheter, 81

K
Kissing balloon angioplasty, 279

L
Laser atherectomy, 106
Leaflet repair in mitral regurgitation
European registries, 356–357
EVEREST trials, 355–356
MitraClip therapy, 353–355, 358
Mobius device, 358
Percu-Pro system, 358–359
Lefevre classification system, 278
Left internal mammary (LIMA), 82
Left main coronary artery (LMCA) disease
CABG
off-pump, 253
patients outcomes, 253
vs. stents theraphy, 260–262
distal bifurcation
benefits, 256
classic T-stenting technique, 257
clinical data, 256
complex two-stents techniques, 257
crush techniques, 257, 259
culotte techniques, 259
single stent techniques with optional T stenting, 256–257
SKS techniques, 259
guidelines, 262
ostial stenting
catheter selection, 255
clinical data, 254–255
intravascular ultrasound, 255
technical tips, 255
types, 255
randomized trials, 261
relative indication/contraindication, 260
stenting
clinical experience, 254
fractional flow reserve, 254
intravascular ultrasound guidance, 254
safety and efficacy issues, 254
Left main disease
fractional flow reserve, 200–201
PCI in elderly, 248
Left ventricles
dysfunction of, 221
hypertrophy, 200
Left ventricular ejection fraction (LVEF), 173
Limb occlusion, 460–461
LMWH. *See* Low-molecular-weight heparins (LMWH)
Lower extremity arterial disease. *See also* Peripheral arterial disease (PAD)
atherectomy, 400
Avinger devices, 398–399
CROSSER catheter, 397
CTO crossing system, 399–400
FRONTRUNNER device
MicroGuide, 395, 396
post stent angiogram, 396
principle of, 395
XP blunt microdissection, 396
laser atherectomy, 400–401
reentry devices, 399–400
rotational atherectomy
Diamondback Stealth Orbital system, 402
Jetstream Navitus device, 401
OUTBACK LTD reentry catheter, 402
pioneer, 402–403
true-lumen reentry catheters, 402
subintimal angioplasty, 395
TruePath crossing device, 397–398
TurboHawk and SilverHawk plaque excision system, 401
Low-molecular-weight heparins (LMWH)
clinical evidence, 147–148
PCI, 213
PCI in women, 235
pharmacokinetics, 147

M
Magnetic navigation system (MNS)
clinical experience, 160–161
3D reconstruction angiogram, 161
left coronary artery, 160
magnetic wires, 160–161

Magnetic positioning system
  clinical experience, 158–159
  guided measurement catheters, 158
  instrumentation, 158
Main branch stent
  balloon expandable, 285
  self-expanding design, 286
Manual aspiration catheters, 109–110
May-Thurner syndrome (MTS), 521
Medical Positioning System (MPS), 157–158
Medina bifurcation classification, 17–18
Medina classification system, 17–18, 278
Medtronic CoreValve Revalving System, 344, 345, 347–349
Medtronic device. *See* Pioneer catheter
Mesenteric ischemia
  acute
    clinical presentation, 434
    diagnosis, 434–435
    etiology, 434
    management, 435–436
    mortality, 443
    restenosis rate, 442–443
  chronic
    atherosclerotic causes, 430, 432–433
    incidence of, 430
    nonatherosclerotic causes, 433
    restenosis rate, 442
  endovascular therapy (*See* Endovascular management, mesenteric ischemia)
  intestinal disorders, 430
  mesenteric arterial anatomy, 429–431
Methodical wire technique, 293
Millipede system, 364
MitraClip therapy
  description, 353
  double-orifice valve generation, 355
  future aspects, 358
  mitral paravalvular leaks, percutaneous closure, 365–367
  percutaneous mitral valve replacement, 364–365
  procedure, 353–354
  supraannular rings, 364
  ventricular reshaping technologies, 364–365
Mitralign Percutaneous Annuloplasty System, 363
Mitral regurgitation (MR)
  apparatus, 351–352
  Cardiac Dimensions Carillon Device, 359–360
  Cerclage annuloplasty, 361
  degenerative, 351–352
  direct annuloplasty, 363
  Edwards Monarc Device, 360–361
  functional MR, 351, 353
  indirect mitral annuloplasty, 359–360
  leaflet repair
    European registries, 356–357
    EVEREST trials, 355–356
    MitraClip therapy, 353–355, 358
    Mobius device, 358
    Percu-Pro system, 358–359
  mitralign percutaneous annuloplasty system, 363
  NeoChord device, 358–359
  percutaneous therapies, 353
  QuantumCor System, 364
  septal sinus shortening procedure, 362
  surgical annuloplasty, 359
  Viacor PTMA Device, 361
Mitral valvuloplasty. *See* Percutaneous mitral valvuloplasty (PMV)
Mother-in-child technique, 86
Multivessel disease (MVD)
  ARTS II trail, 268–269
  balloon angioplasty, 265
  CABG
    vs. bare metal stenting, 266–268
    vs. drug-eluting stents, 268
    meta-analyses, 268
    vs. POBA, 266
  CARDia trail, 269
  clinical syntax score, 271
  complete *vs.* incomplete revascularization, 272–273
  considerations, 273–274
  ERAC III trail, 269
  FAME trial, 273
  FFR in, 197–199
  fractional flow reserve, 273
  global risk score, 271–272
  incidence of, 265
  NERS score, 272
  PCI in elderly, 247
  SYNTAX trail, 269–270
    limitations, 270–271
    score, 271
    at 4 years, 270
  treatment of, 265
MyoCathT/BioHeart injection catheter, 180–181
MyoStar™ mapping catheter system, 179–180

N
N-acetylcysteine, 58
Navigation and positioning systems, 157–160. *See also* Robotic-assisted coronary intervention
NeoChord device, 358–359
Neointimal hyperplasia, 37
Nephropathy, 461–462
NERS score, 272
NOGA® system, 179–180
Nonocclusive mesenteric ischemia (NOMI), 434
Non-uniform rotational distortion (NURD), 24
No-touch technique, 422–423

O
Ocelot device, 398–399
Oral antiplatelet therapy
  ACCF/AHA guidelines, 144, 145
  aspirin, 143–144
  PCI, 214–215
  thienopyridines and ticagrelor, 144–146
Oral direct thrombin inhibitors, 151–152
Ostial stenting
  catheter selection, 255
  clinical data, 254–255
  intravascular ultrasound, 255
  technical tips, 255
  types, 255
Otamixaban, 153
OUTBACK LTD reentry catheter, 402

P
Paclitaxel, 119–120
Paclitaxel-eluting stents (PES)
  clinical results of patients, 121
  vs. sirolimus-eluting stenting, 121–122

Paget–Schroetter syndrome (PSS), 517–518
PCI. *See* Percutaneous coronary intervention (PCI)
Perclose ProGlide device, 73
Percu-Pro system, 358–359
PercuSurge GuardWire Plus distal protection, 109
Percutaneous cell therapy
  in acute myocardial infarction
    intracoronary delivery, 182–184
    intramyocardial injection, 184–185
  in chronic heart failure
    clinical trials, 185–186
    intracoronary delivery, 187
    transendocardial delivery, 186–187
  in refractory angina
    clinical trials, 187
    intracoronary infusion, 188
    intramyocardial injection, 188
  stem cell biology (*see* Stem cell biology)
Percutaneous coronary intervention (PCI). *See also* Chronic total occlusions (CTO) angioplasty
  acute coronary syndrome
    GRACE risk score, 44
    pathogenesis, 44
    timing of intervention, 45
    TIMI risk score, 44–45
  aspirin, 48
  backup force
    alignment of, 85, 86
    anchor technique, 86
    with angle, 84, 85
    buddy wire strategy, 86
    catheter size and supporting characteristics, 84
    deep seating and engagement, 86
    friction of, 85
    Guideliner catheter, 86, 87
    mother-in-child technique, 86
    retrospective analysis, 84
    TFI *vs.* TRI, 85
  bivalirudin, 48
  chronic stable angina
    agents, 41
    diagnostic coronary angiography, 42
    National Institute for Health and Clinical Excellence guideline, 41
    tolerance test, exercise, 42
  COURAGE study, 43
  fractional flow reserve, 42–43
  guiding catheter
    advantages, 80
    complications, 87, 88
    construction, 80–81
    designs, 84
    disadvantages, 80
    longer soft tip, 82–83
    passive *vs.* active support, 79–80
    selection and functions, 79, 84
    side holes, 81
    transradial and transfemoral procedures, 83
  patient selection with fibrinolysis, 46–48
  prasugrel, 48
  rescue PCI, 48
  STEMI, 45–46
  and stent development, 116
  SYNTAX, 43–44
  thrombectomy, 48–49
  ticagrelor, 48
  transfemoral (*see* Transfemoral interventions, PCI)
  transradial (*see* Transradial interventions, PCI)
  transradial approach, 170
Percutaneous left ventricular assist devices (LVADs)
  Impella, 223–224
  TandemHeart™, 223
Percutaneous mechanical thrombectomy (PMT), 515
Percutaneous mitral valvuloplasty (PMV)
  antegrade double balloon technique, 319, 320
  cardiac output, 318
  clinical follow-up
    actuarial and event-free survival rates, 325
    atrial fibrillation, 327
    echocardiographic scores, 319, 323, 328
    in elderly, 326
    functional deterioration, 325, 326
    hemodynamic improvement, 325, 328
    mitral valve calcification, 327
    patients characteristics, 328
    previous surgical commissurotomy, 327
    pulmonary artery hypertension, 327
    restenosis, 325, 326
    tricuspid regurgitation, 328
  complications, 324–325
  double balloon *vs.* inoue balloon technique, 328
  guide wires, 319
  inoue technique, 319–321
  mechanism of, 321
  metallic valvulotome, 320
  outcomes, 321–322, 330
  patient selection, 317–318
  in pregnant women, 330
  procedure
    age, 324
    atrial fibrillation, 324
    balloon size and EBDA, 323–324
    echocardiographic score, 319, 323
    mitral valve calcification and regurgitation, 324
    multiple stepwise regression analysis, 323
    surgical commissurotomy, 324
    univariate analysis, 322, 323
  vs. surgical mitral commissurotomy, 328–330
  transseptal left heart catheterization, 318, 319
Percutaneous septal sinus shortening (PS3) procedure, 362
Percutaneous transluminal atherectomy, 100–101
Peripheral arterial disease (PAD)
  biodegradable stents, 390–391
  claudication management
    aortoiliac occlusive disease, 384
    class I indication, 381
    failed iliac PTA, 383
    translesional pressure gradients, 381
  critical limb ischemia (CLI)
    acute and chronic, 384
    anticoagulation with heparin, 385
    definition, 384
    inflow and outflow disease, 384
    targeted therapy, 385
  cryoplasty
    BTK-CHILL trial, 390
    endovascular treatment, 388
    mid-SFA CTO, 389
    PolarCath® balloon dilation system, 389
    vs. conventional angioplasty, 389

drug-eluting stents and balloons, 390
iliac arteries
ACTIVE trial, 385
covered balloon-mounted stents, 386
endovascular treatment through radial artery access, 386
occluded segment, 387
self-expanding stents, 386
TASC guidelines, 385
infrainguinal vessels, 387–388
popliteal and infrapopliteal vessels, 388
TASC documents
aortoiliac disease, 381, 382
femoropopliteal disease, 381, 383
Peripheral intravenous infusion, 177
Periprocedural antithrombotic therapy, 248–249
Pharmaco-invasive PCI, 210–211
Pharmacology for coronary intervention. *See* Adjunctive pharmacology, for coronary intervention
Phosphorylcholine, 116
Pioneer catheter, 402–403
Planned percutaneous coronary intervention (PCI) and NSTEMI, 150–151
Platelets role, in acute coronary syndrome, 144
Poly-D,L-lactic acid (PDLLA), 134
Poly-L-lactic acid (PLLA), 134
Polymer coating stents, 116, 118
Popliteal and infrapopliteal arterial disease, 388
Post-premature ventricular contraction (PVC), 5–6
Post-procedural antithrombotic therapy, 249–250
Prasugrel, 146, 215, 234
Primary percutaneous coronary intervention. *See also* Retrograde approach, chronic total occlusion PCI
access route, 217
adjunctive pharmacology
adenosine, 215
bivalirudin, 213–214
fondaparinux, 213
glycoprotein IIb/IIIa receptor antagonists, 214
LMWH, 213
oral antiplatelet agents, 214–215
effect of timing/door-to-balloon time, 208–209
in elderly
acute coronary syndromes, 247
calcification and tortuosity, 244, 247
drug-eluting *vs.* bare-metal stents, 248
elective PCI, 246–247
left main disease, 248
multivessel disease, 247
pathophysiology, 244–246
periprocedural adjunctive pharmacotherapy, 248–249
post-procedural adjunctive pharmacotherapy, 249–250
prior coronary bypass graft surgery, 248
risk, 243–244
vascular complications, 245–246
embolic/distal protection, 216–217
evolution in STEMI
bare metal *vs.* drug-eluting stents, 208
PTCA *vs.* thrombolysis, 207–208
stents *vs.* PCTA, 208
stents *vs.* thrombolysis, 208
hemodynamic support in
cardiogenic shock, 221–222
intra-aortic balloon pump (IABP), 222–223
left ventricular dysfunction, 221
mechanical suppor, 222
percutaneous left ventricular assist devices (LVADs)
percutaneous left ventricular assist devices (LVADs): Impella, 223–224
percutaneous left ventricular assist devices (LVADs): TandemHeart™, 223
impella, 217
intra-aortic balloon pump, 217
in non-PCI-capable hospitals
facilitated PCI *vs.* thrombolytics, 210
PCI *vs.* thrombolytics, 209–210
pharmaco-invasive PCI, 210–211
primary reperfusion, 211
STEMI care systems, 211
rheolytic thrombectomy, 216
therapeutic hypothermia, 216
thrombolytics
facilitated PCI *vs.* PCI, 211–212
pharmaco-invasive PCI *vs.* PCI, 212
rescue PCI, 212–213
thrombus aspiration, 215–216
in women
acute coronary syndrome, 232
acute myocardial infarction, 232–233
anticoagulants, 235
antiplatelet agents, 233
biological characteristics, 228
bleeding and vascular complications, 231–232
CABG, 235–236
clinical features, 227
comorbidities, 227–228
diagnostic testing, 228–229
direct thrombin inhibitors, 235
drug-eluting (DES) *vs.* bare-metal stents (BMS), 230
glycoprotein IIb/IIIa inhibitors, 234–235
healthcare provider barriers, 229
incidence of, 232
mortality, 229–230
patient presentation, 228
restenosis and revascularization, 230–231
social and educational barriers, 229
statins, 235
thienopyridines, 233–234
Primary reperfusion, 211
Primary Stroke Centers (PSC), 506
Proximal aortic neck, 453
Pulmonary artery hypertension, 327
Pulmonary artery wedge pressure (PAWP), 2, 3
Pulmonary embolism (PE)
anticoagulation, 519
catheter-directed treatment, 520–521
diagnosis, 519
IVC filters, 521
surgical embolectomy, 521
thrombolysis, 519–520
Puncture technique, TRA, 167–169
P2Y12, 145

Q

Quantitative coronary angiography (QCA) analysis
coronary atherosclerosis, 14–15
2-dimensional system, 13, 14
3-dimensional system, 13–14
generation systems, 12–13
limitations of, 12
measurement factors, 15–16
QuantumCor System, 364

R

Radial artery
closure methods, 74
intervention (*see* Transradial approach (TRA))
vascular access
Allen's/Barbeau tests, 69, 70
anatomy, 66, 68
anterior wall approach, 70
benefits, 75–76
counterpuncture approach, 70
risks, 76
transradial approach, 69
Reentry devices, 399–400
Refractory angina, percutaneous cell therapy
clinical trials, 187
intracoronary infusion, 188
intramyocardial injection, 188
Reitan pump, 59
Renal artery occlusion, 459–460
Renal artery stenosis
abdominal aortogram, 421
access, 420
acute renovascular disorders
antiphospholipid antibody syndrome, 418
catheter-directed thrombolysis, 419
causes, 418
renal artery dissection, 419–420
renal infarction, 419
renal vein thrombosis, 420
thrombectomy/thrombolysis, 424–425
angioplasty and stenting
comparison of devices, 424, 425
diameter of angioplasty balloon, 423–424
direct engagement technique, 422, 423
distal embolic protection, 423
5F guiding system, 422
no-touch technique, 422–423
antithrombotics, 421
atherosclerosis (*see* Atherosclerosis renal artery stenosis)
complications of, 425
distal embolic protection, 421
fibromuscular dysplasia, 416–417
post-procedure, 425
pre-procedural management, 420
renal sympathetic denervation, 425
translesional hemodynamic assessment, 421
transplant, 417–419
Renal Guard, 59, 60
Renovascular disease. *See* Renal artery stenosis
Resident cardiac stem cells, 175
RESOLUTE stents, 125–126
Restenosis
in-stent, 132–133
mechanisms, 131–132
PCI in women, 230–231
Retrograde approach, chronic total occlusion PCI
CART, 305–307
catheter selection and setup, 300–301
collateral angiography, 301–302
collateral wiring, 303–304
diagnostic angiogram, 299–300
guidelines, 299
hybrid algorithm, 299–300
lesion crossing, 304–305
operators toolbox
Corsair microcatheter, 302–303
OTW balloon catheter, 302–303
wires, 302
procedural anticoagulation, 301
recanalization techniques
delivery of stents, 308
18-3 Merit EN Sare, 307–308
techniques, 305
ViperWire Advance, 308
vascular access, 300
Retrograde approach, IVUS, 313, 315, 316
Retrograde balloon valvuloplasty, 332–334
Rheolytic thrombectomy, 216
Rheumatic aortic valve stenosis, 331
Right coronary artery (RCA), 82
Ring-down artifacts, 24
Rivaroxaban, 152–153
Robotic-assisted coronary intervention
CorPath robotic system
clinical experience, 164–165
CorPath 200 robotic system, 162–164
magnetic positioning system
clinical experience, 158–159
Guided Measurement Catheters, 158
instrumentation, 158
navigation and positioning systems, 157–158
Stereotaxis magnetic navigation system
clinical experience, 161–162
3D reconstruction angiogram, 161
left coronary artery, 160
magnetic wires, 160
Rotablator, 99, 101, 105
Rotational atherectomy
Diamondback Stealth Orbital system, 402
in drug-eluting stent era, 105–106
early studies, 104
instrumentation, 99, 101
Jetstream Navitus device, 401
mechanism, 101–102
OUTBACK LTD reentry catheter, 402
perforation, 105
pioneer, 402–403
procedure, 102, 104
Rotablator, 99, 101, 105
Rotalink burr catheter, 102, 104
Rota rescue case, 103–104
RotaWire specifications, 103
true-lumen reentry catheters, 402

S

Safeguard device, 71
Saphenous vein graft (SVG)
degenerated, 17
intravascular ultrasound, 36
SCAI lesion classification system, 16, 17
Scottish and Newcastle Renal Artery Stenosis Collaborative Group, 414–415
Serial stenoses, 201
Side branch stent
balloon expandable, 286
self-expanding design, 286
treatment, 279
Simultaneous kissing stent (SKS) technique, 280, 281
Single stent techniques with optional T stenting, 256–257

Sirolimus, 118
Sirolimus-eluting stenting (SES)
  clinical studies, 120
  clinical trial and pooled analysis, 120
  vs. paclitaxel-eluting stenting, 121–122
Skeletal myoblasts, 175
SKS techniques, 259
Sodium bicarbonate, 58
Spinal cord ischemia, 459
StarClose device, 73
STAR trial, 415
Statins, 235
Stem cell biology
  adipose-derived stem cells, 174–175
  BMSCs, 175–176
  cell types, 174
  embryonic stem cells, 174
  epicardium-derived progenitor cells, 175
  iPSCs, 174
  resident cardiac stem cells, 175
  skeletal myoblasts, 175
Stents
  antiproliferative drugs
    paclitaxel, 119–120
    restenosis, 116
    sirolimus and limus analogues, 118–119
  carotid artery disease
    complication, 492–493
    embolic protection devices, 491–492
    guidelines for, 489
    patient selection, 489–490
    procedure, 490–491
    randomized trials of, 488
  drug-eluting
    characteristics, 118
    development, 133–136
    everolimus, 126–127
    high-resolution radiographs, 117
    on-label *vs.* off-label use, 122–124
    paclitaxel, 120–121
    safety, 127–133
    sirolimus, 120
    sirolimus *vs.* paclitaxel, 121–122
    zotarolimus, 124–126
    zotarolimus *vs.* bare-metal stents, 124–125
  historical perspective, 115
  vs. PCTA, 208
  polymer coating, 116, 118
  stent platform
    metallurgy, 115–116
    stent architecture, 116, 117
  vs. thrombolysis, 208
  vertebral artery disease, 495
Stent thrombosis
  ARC definitions, 125
  DES safety, 127–129
Stereotaxis magnetic navigation system (MNS)
  clinical experience, 161–162
  3D reconstruction angiogram, 161
  left coronary artery, 160
  magnetic wires, 160–161
Stiletto™ (Boston Scientific) catheter, 181
Stroke centers, 506–507
Stroke intervention
  endovascular therapies, 500–502
  intra-arterial thrombolysis, 502–503
  intracranial stenting, 505
  intravenous thrombolysis, 499–500
  manpower issues, 506
  mechanical thrombectomy, 503–505
  neuroprotection, 505–506
  new stroke program, 507–508
  stroke centers, 506–507
Subclavian atery. *See* Upper extremity interventions
Subintimal angioplasty, 395
Superior vena cava (SVC) filters, 517
Superior vena cava syndrome (SVCS), 518
Surgical venous thrombectomy, 515
Synergy Between Percutaneous Coronary Intervention with TAXus and Cardiac Surgery (SYNTAX), 43–44
SYNTAX score, 199

T

Tachyarrhythmia, 335
TAG, 465–466
Talent abdominal stent graft, 446–447
Talent thoracic endograft, 464
TandemHeart™, 223
Target lesion failure (TLF), 127
TAXUS, 120–121
Telescoping technique, 376
Therapeutic hypothermia (TH), 216
Therapy of transcatheter aortic valve. *See* Transcatheter aortic valve therapy
Thienopyridines
  clinical evidence, 144–145
  PCI in women, 233–234
  pharmacokinetics, 145–146
Thoracic aortic aneurysm
  aortic arch pathology, 463
  complications, 467–468
  endovascular repair, 462–463 (*see also* Thoracic endovascular aortic repair (TEVAR))
Thoracic endovascular aortic repair (TEVAR)
  indications
    for intervention, 462
    penetrating atherosclerotic ulcer, 466
    TAA, 466
  post-TEVAR therapy and follow-up, 468
  procedure, 466–467
  TEVAR devices
    Bolton medical Relay thoracic endograft, 465
    TAG, 465–466
    talent thoracic endograft, 464
    Valiant endograft, 464–465
    Zenith TX2 Thoracic TAA endovascular graft, 463
Thrombolytics
  vs. facilitated PCI, 210
  facilitated PCI *vs.* PCI, 211–212
  PCI *vs.*, 209–210
  pharmaco-invasive PCI *vs.* PCI, 212
  rescue PCI, 212–213
Thromboxane A2 receptor, 143
Thrombus aspiration, 215–216
Thrombus extraction and coronary atherectomy
  distal protection, 108–109
  ischemic time frame, 108
  late stent thrombosis, 107
  serial manual aspiration, 107

Ticagrelor, 215
  clinical evidence, 144–145
  PCI in women, 234
  pharmacokinetics, 145–146
TIMI flow grade system, 18
TIMI frame count (TFC), 19
TIMI myocardial perfusion grade (TMPG), 19
TRA. *See* Transradial approach (TRA)
TransAtlantic Inter-Society Consensus (TASC) documents
  aortoiliac disease, 381, 382
  femoropopliteal disease, 381, 383
Transcatheter aortic valve therapy
  anatomy of aortic valve
    annulus measurement from sinus to commissure, 342
    aortic root and annulus, 341
    conduction system, 342
    trileaflet, 341
  balloon-expandable prosthesis, 344, 345
  clinical evidence
    Edwards SAPIEN THV, 348–349
    Medtronic CoreValve, 349
  coronary angiography, 343
  echocardiographic evaluation, 342, 343
  multislice computed tomography, 343–344
  patient selection, 342–343
  procedure
    aortic valvuloplasty and valve implantation, 347–348
    Edwards SAPEIN THV, 344, 346, 348
    femoral vascular access, 345–347
    Medtronic CoreValve, 344, 347, 348
    vascular access closure, 348
  self-expanding aortic prosthesis, 344, 345
Transendocardial delivery, 186–187
Transfemoral interventions, PCI
  Amplatz left catheter, 82
  Judkins catheter, 81
  left internal mammary, 82
  right coronary artery, 82
Transplant renal artery stenosis, 417–419
Transradial approach (TRA)
  coronary catheters exchange, 171
  diagnostic catheters, 169–170
  guide catheter selection and support, 170
  inability to cannulate the wire, 170
  percutaneous coronary intervention, 170
  puncture technique, 167–169
  radial artery, 69, 76
  radial artery assessment, 167
  right radial vs left radial, 167
  therapeutic devices, 170
Transradial interventions, PCI
  accessor system, 89
  designs and functions, 84
  drawbacks, 83
  JR catheter, 83
  RCA and AL catheters, 83
  sheath, 87, 88
  slender system, 89
Tricuspid regurgitation, 328
True-lumen reentry catheters, 402
TruePath crossing device, 397–398
T-stent, 279
TurboHawk and SilverHawk plaque excision system, 401

U
UFH. *See* Unfractionated heparin (UFH)
Ulnar artery, upper extremity interventions, 373
Ultrasound (US), 68–69
Unfractionated heparin (UFH)
  clinical evidence, 147
  PCI in women, 235
  pharmacokinetics, 146
Upper extremity interventions
  anatomy
    arch variants, 372
    brachial and hand circulation, 373
    classification of subclavian artery, 372
    normal aortic arch, 371
  angiography, 375–376
  balloon angioplasty, 377
  choice of access site, 376
  coronary-subclavian steal, CABG, and anterior ischemia, 377
  occlusive lesion, brachial access, 378
  patient selection
    distal embolization, 375
    endovascular revascularization, 373
    indications, 374
  pharmacology, 376–377
  post-procedural management, 379
  technical success rate, 379

V
Valiant endograft, 464–465
Vascular access
  brachial
    anatomy, 65, 67
    cut-down and percutaneous approach, 69
    risks, 75
  femoral
    anatomy, 65–67
    closure methods (*see* Femoral artery)
    head fluoroscopy, 67–68
    inguinal crease and ligament, 66, 67
    management, 75
    pulsation, 67
    risks, 75
    ultrasound, 68–69
  patent hemostasis technique, 74
  radial
    Allen's/Barbeau tests, 69, 70
    anatomy, 66, 68
    anterior wall approach, 70
    benefits, 75–76
    counterpuncture approach, 70
    risks, 76
    transradial approach, 69
Vascular injury, 336
Vena cava filters, 515–516
Venous thromboembolic disease (VTE)
  axillosubclavian deep venous thrombosis, 516–517
  chronic venous insufficiency (*see* Chronic venous insufficiency (CVI))
  deep vein thrombosis
    diagnosis of, 511–512
    treatment of, 512–516

May-Thurner syndrome, 521
Paget-Schroetter syndrome, 517–518
pulmonary embolism
anticoagulation, 519
catheter-directed treatment, 520–521
diagnosis, 519
IVC filters, 521
surgical embolectomy, 521
thrombolysis, 519–520
superior vena cava syndrome, 518
Venous thrombosis, 434
Venous varicosities, 524–526
Vertebral artery disease
diagnosis
invasive testing, 494
noninvasive testing, 493
etiology and prevalence, 493
medical therapy, 494
natural history, 493
revascularization, 494–495
stenting, 495
Viacor percutaneous transvenous mitral annuloplasty (PTMA) device, 361
Viance Catheter. *See* CTO crossing system
Visipaque, 375
V-stent, 281

W

Warfarin and Aspirin for Symptomatic Intracranial Arterial Stenosis (WASID), 494
Women, PCI in. *See* Primary percutaneous coronary intervention, in women

X

Xareltor, 152–153

Z

Zenith Flex endograft, 446
Zenith TX2 Thoracic TAA endovascular graft, 463
Zotarolimus, 118, 119
Zotarolimus-eluting stents (ZES)
vs. bare-metal stents, 124–125
composition, 124
new-generation, 125–126
vs. PES, 125

MIX
Papier aus verantwortungsvollen Quellen
Paper from responsible sources
FSC® C105338

If you have any concerns about our products,
you can contact us on
ProductSafety@springernature.com

In case Publisher is established outside the EU,
the EU authorized representative is:
Springer Nature Customer Service Center GmbH
Europaplatz 3, 69115 Heidelberg, Germany

Printed by Libri Plureos GmbH
in Hamburg, Germany